THE
RENIN–ANGIOTENSIN SYSTEM

Volume 2

PATHOPHYSIOLOGY
THERAPEUTICS

THE RENIN–ANGIOTENSIN SYSTEM

Edited by

Professor J Ian S Robertson
BSc MB BS FRCP(London) MD(Brussels) FRCP(Glasgow) FIBiol FRS(Edin)
Scientific Adviser
Janssen International Research Council
Senior Consultant in Cardiovascular Medicine
Janssen Research Foundation
Beerse
Belgium

Professor M Gary Nicholls
MB ChB MD(Otago) FRACP FRCP(Glasgow) FRCP(Edin) FRCP(London) FACC
Head, Department of Medicine
The Christchurch School of Medicine
Christchurch Hospital
Christchurch
New Zealand

Volume 2

PATHOPHYSIOLOGY
THERAPEUTICS

Gower Medical Publishing · London · New York

Distributed in USA and Canada by:

Raven Press Ltd
1185 Avenue of the Americas
New York
New York 10036
USA

Distributed in the rest of the world by:

Gower Medical Publishing
Middlesex House
34–42 Cleveland Street
London W1P 5FB
UK

ISBN   1-56375-550-5

CIP data are available on request from the British
Library and the Library of Congress

Publisher:	Angela Bellamy
Project manager:	Moira Sarsfield
Editor:	Saba Zafar
Cover design:	James Evoy
Production:	Adam Phillips Susan Bishop
Index:	Nina Boyd

Printed in the UK by The Bath Press

Tigerstedt and Bergman would look with amazement at the story that has unfolded since 1898 when they first injected saline extracts of kidney and observed the initial depressor and subsequent long-acting pressor responses. Readers of this book will be equally amazed by the expansion of knowledge based on new ideas and techniques, and particularly by the application of molecular biology, during the last several years.

As with many physiological systems based on enzymes and peptides, we have become accustomed to their initial naming and assessment by their site of predominant presence, and by their most obvious biological effect. This is almost always succeeded by the demonstration of wider distribution and wider activities. Gut peptides and neuropeptides become more safely subsumed under the heading of regulatory peptides. And so it has been with the renin–angiotensin–aldosterone system; from the brain, to the heart and to the vessel wall, both active and inactive renins abound, and interrelationships of angiotensin with the nervous system and with other hormonal systems, have acquired better definition. Immunohistochemistry, *in situ* hybridization of renin mRNA, and, most striking of all, the renin transgenic animal, all add to the complexity, as well as to the rapidity of accretion of new knowledge. The expansion of selective methods of blockade of renin and angiotensin has led to real therapeutic advances in heart failure, in hypertension, and in some forms of renal disease, as well as to a more precise definition of the roles of renin and angiotensin in physiology and pathology.

This book is a great tribute to all involved in its production. It is unique in both its range and its detail, and is an absolute necessity for all interested in physiological advances and the pathological deviations which occur in disease.

Sir Stanley Peart

Before the appearance of the present work, no book of this size, scope and detail had been attempted on the subject of the renin–angiotensin system, so far as we are aware. This is remarkable, indeed surprising, given the approaching centenary of the discovery of renin, its pervasion into so many aspects of physiology and pathology, and the therapeutic importance of agents designed to interrupt the system and its actions.

Indeed, the continuing and increasing interest in the renin–angiotensin system, and the burgeoning research into so many of its ramifications, was advanced as one reason why we should not embark on the production of the present work. To have heeded such arguments would have been to accept that the time is hardly ever opportune to write extensively on any scientific topic exciting current concern, together with the corollary that the only suitable fields for such treatment would be those in which research endeavors and enthusiasm had already waned. These notions we took to be self-evidently fallacious.

The need for a wide-ranging and particular exegesis of the subject of the renin–angiotensin system, including the attempt to put contemporary research into its historical perspective, was not always accepted readily by our invited contributors. On more than one occasion we encountered reluctance on the part of an author to consider any aspect of his or her topic on which publications antedated the last few years. We consistently attempted to persuade such recalcitrants otherwise, and we nearly always, but not quite invariably, succeeded. In justification of such intendedly gentle coercion, we can observe that more than one contributor believed, for example, that the discovery of tissue renin–angiotensin systems, or that knowledge of the direct renal actions of angiotensin II, were no older than the late 1980s. Requiring emphasis, therefore, is that, despite the crudeness of many of the early assays for renin and angiotensin II, it is remarkable how broadly correct were the qualitative conclusions reached in studies which employed such methods. Even 50 years ago, investigations into the renin system, with the unavoidable limitations of the then available methodology, proceeded, with only occasional erroneous digressions, in the true direction. To mention probably the most strikingly perceptive of the investigators of the 1940s, Goormaghtigh's interpretations of histological specimens anticipated correctly many of the conclusions derived from assay of renin and angiotensin II some 20 and 30 years later.

Truly quantitative progress was by comparison much slower and much less certain, in which connection the lack, for many years, of a suitable renin standard must be blamed (see *Appendix II* and *Chapters 1, 5* and *17*). This deprivation hindered ready comparison of results obtained in different laboratories and has delayed the recognition of defective methodology. Assays for plasma angiotensin II have not been so subject to these deficiencies; whilst enthusiasm for angiotensin II assay was initially tardy, quantitative inter-laboratory comparisons were easier. Although this latter field is certainly not free from controversy (see *Chapters 9, 15* and *23*), progress has been quicker and less unsure than was the case with renin assay.

From the foregoing it should be evident that we have not acted as passive editors, but have, at some risk of wounding the *amour propre* of our authors and of losing their goodwill, exhorted them, wherever we felt it necessary, to expand their texts and to enlarge their bibliography. All of those stimulated complied, sometimes reluctantly and also, unsurprisingly, not invariably. Nevertheless, we have also striven to give due exposure to those opinions and findings which are contrary to our own.

It was not intended, possible or desirable to attain agreement between the various authors on every aspect. Also, inevitably, certain subjects appear in more than one chapter. We as editors have regarded these occurrences as advantages rather than blemishes, and have, wherever possible, indicated such disputes and encroachments by cross-referencing. The cross-references are attributable solely to us as editors.

We are privileged and grateful to have attracted such a distinguished and scholarly, if unavoidably disputatious, group of writers. We are proud of our good fortune in working with them on this project. Only five of those originally invited to contribute were unable, for diverse reasons, to take part. Sad as we were to lose those authors, their successors were no less distinguished, and we suffered no palpable diminution in quality.

It is thus our pleasure to thank our contributors, and also the staff of Gower Medical Publishing, for their industry, tolerance and good humor. We are also grateful to Lidi Van Gool, Dorothy Neal and Frances Tsui for their secretarial skills, and to Mignon for assiduous checking of references and scrutiny of proofs. For such defects as remain we as editors accept responsibility.

J.I.S. Robertson
M.G. Nicholls

CONTENTS

VOLUME 2   The Renin–Angiotensin System PATHOPHYSIOLOGY · THERAPEUTICS

CONTRIBUTORS

Phyllis August
Hypertension Center, Cardiovascular Center, The
New York Hospital, Cornell Medical Center, New
York, New York, USA

George L Bakris
The University of Texas, Health Science Center at San
Antonio, San Antonio, Texas, USA

Sarah Barnes
Servier Laboratories, IRIS, Courbevoie, France

Terence Bennett
Department of Physiology & Pharmacology,
University of Nottingham Medical School, Queen's
Medical Centre, Nottingham, England

Giuseppe Bianchi
Department of Nephrology, Dialysis & Hypertension,
Milan University, San Raffaele Hospital, Milan, Italy

Jacob Bouhnik
Service de Médecine 9, Centre de Médecine
Preventive Cardio-Vasculaire, Hôpital Broussais,
Paris, France

Chantal M Boulanger
Center for Experimental Therapeutics, Baylor College
of Medicine, Houston, Texas, USA

Michael W Brands
Department of Physiology & Biophysics, University of
Mississippi Medical Center, Jackson, Mississippi,
USA

Virginia L Brooks
Department of Physiology, School of Medicine,
Oregon Health Sciences University, Portland,
Oregon, USA

Fiona Broughton Pipkin
Department of Obstetrics & Gynaecology, University
of Nottingham Medical School, Nottingham,
England

Hans R Brunner
Division of Hypertension, Department of Medicine,
University Hospital, Lausanne, Switzerland

Bernd Bunnemann
Department of Biochemistry, Glaxo Research
Laboratories,Verona, Italy

Duncan J Campbell
St. Vincent's Institute of Medical Research,
Melbourne, Australia

Kevin J Catt
Endocrinology and Reproduction Research Branch,
NICHD, National Institutes of Health, Bethesda, MD,
USA

Anne Charru
INSERM U36, Laboratoire de Médecine
Expérimentale, College de France, Paris, France

Eric Clauser
Service de Médecine 9, Centre de Médecine
Preventive Cardio-Vasculaire, Hôpital Broussais,
Paris, France

James Conway
John Radcliffe Hospital, Oxford, England

Pierre Corvol
INSERM U36, Laboratoire de Médecine
Expérimentale, College de France, Paris, France

Ian G Crozier
Cardiology Department, The Princess Margaret
Hospital, Christchurch, New Zealand

John M Cruickshank
Wythenshawe Hospital, Manchester, England

Daniele Cusi
Department of Nephrology, Dialysis & Hypertension,
San Raffaele Hospital, Milan, Italy

Björn Dahlöf
Department of Medicine, University of Gothenburg,
Östra Hospital, Gothenburg, Sweden

Carolyn F Deacon
Department of Animal & Plant Sciences, School of
Biological Sciences, University of Sheffield, Sheffield,
England

Frans HM Derkx
Department of Internal Medicine I, Academisch
Ziekenhuis Dijkzigt, Rotterdam, The Netherlands

John Doig
University of Glasgow, Department of Medicine &
Therapeutics, Western Infirmary, Glasgow, Scotland

Sir Colin T Dollery
Royal Postgraduate Medical School, Hammersmith Hospital, London, England

Victor J Dzau
Falk Cardiovascular Research Center, Stanford University School of Medicine, Stanford, California, USA

Christopher RW Edwards
Faculty of Medicine, University Medical School, Edinburgh, Scotland

Ervin G Erdös
Laboratory of Peptide Research, Departments of Pharmacology and Anesthesiology, University of Illinois College of Medicine at Chicago, Illinois, USA

Eric A Espiner
Department of Medicine, Christchurch Hospital, Christchurch, New Zealand

Paolo Ferrari
Division of Hypertension, Medizinische Poliklinik, University of Berne, Inselspital, Switzerland

James T Fitzsimons
Physiological Laboratory, University of Cambridge, Cambridge, England

Astrid E Fletcher
Royal Postgraduate Medical School, Hammersmith Hospital, London, England

Kjell Fuxe
Department of Histology & Neurobiology, Karolinska Institute, Stockholm, Sweden

Detlev Ganten
Department of Pharmacology and German Institute for High Blood Pressure Research, University of Heidelberg, Heidelberg, Germany

Sheila M Gardiner
Department of Physiology and Pharmacolology, University of Nottingham Medical School, Queen's Medical Centre, Nottingham, England

Haralambos Gavras
Hypertension & Atherosclerosis Section, Boston University Medical Center, Boston, Massachusetts, USA

Irene Gavras
Hypertension & Atherosclerosis Section, Boston University Medical Center, Boston, Massachusetts, USA

Theodore L Goodfriend
Department of Veteran's Affairs, University of Wisconsin and Veteran's Hospital, Madison, Wisconsin, USA

Richard D Gordon
Endocrine-Hypertension Research Unit, Department of Medicine, University of Queensland, Greenslopes Hospital, Brisbane, Australia

Edgar Haber
Division of Biological Sciences, Harvard School of Public Health, Boston, Massachusetts, USA

Eberhard Hackenthal
Department of Pharmacology, University of Heidelberg, Heidelberg, Germany

John E Hall
Department of Physiology & Biophysics, University of Mississippi Medical Center, Jackson, Mississippi, USA

Lennart Hansson
Department of Medicine, University of Gothenburg, Östra Hospital, Gothenburg, Sweden

Anthony M Heagerty
Department of Medicine, University Hospital of South Manchester, Manchester, England

Ian W Henderson
Department of Animal & Plant Sciences, School of Biological Sciences, University of Sheffield, Sheffield, England

Anders Himmelmann
Department of Medicine, University of Gothenburg, Östra Hospital, Gothenburg, Sweden

Norman K Hollenberg
Departments of Medicine and Radiology, Harvard Medical School and Brigham & Women's Hospital, Boston, Massachusetts, USA

Kwan Y Hui
Lilly Research Laboratories, Lilly Corporate Center, Indianapolis, Indiana, USA

Hamid Ikram
Cardiology Department, The Princess Margaret Hospital, Christchurch, New Zealand

Tadashi Inagami
Department of Biochemistry, Vanderbilt University School of Medicine, Vanderbilt University Medical Center, Nashville, Tennessee, USA

Bruce Jackson
Department of Medicine, University of Melbourne, Preston & Northcote Community Hospital, Victoria, Australia

Jørgen Jacobsen
Institute for Anatomy and Physiology, The Royal Veterinary & Agricultural University, Copenhagen, Denmark

Xavier Jeunemaître
INSERM U36, Laboratoire de Médecine Expérimentale, College de France, Paris, France

Colin I Johnston
Department of Medicine, The University of Melbourne, Austin Hospital, Heidelberg, Victoria, Australia

Roberto SN Kalil
Division of Nephrology, Department of Medicine, Hennepin County Medical Center, University of Minnesota Medical School, Minneapolis, Minnesota, USA

Stephen A Katz
Division of Nephrology, Department of Medicine, Hennepin County Medical Center, University of Minnesota, Minneapolis, Minnesota, USA

William F Keane
Division of Nephrology, Department of Medicine, Hennepin County Medical Center, University of Minnesota Medical School, Minneapolis, Minnesota, USA

Shelley A Klemm
Endocrine-Hypertension Research Unit, Department of Medicine, University of Queensland, Greenslopes Hospital, Brisbane, Australia

Wilhelm Kriz
Institute for Anatomy & Cell Biology, University of Heidelberg, Heidelberg, Germany

Kar Neng Lai
Department of Medicine, Prince of Wales Hospital, The Chinese University of Hong Kong, Shatin, Hong Kong

Siu Fai Lui
Department of Medicine, Prince of Wales Hospital, The Chinese University of Hong Kong, Shatin, Hong Kong

Brenda J Leckie
MRC Blood Pressure Unit, Western Infirmary, Glasgow, Scotland

Kennedy R Lees
Department of Medicine and Therapeutics, University of Glasgow, Western Infirmary, Glasgow, Scotland

Kevin V Lemley
Institute for Anatomy & Cell Biology, University of Heidelberg, Heidelberg, Germany

Nancy W Y Leung
Department of Medicine, Prince of Wales Hospital, The Chinese University Hong Kong, Shatin, Hong Kong

Anthony F Lever
MRC Blood Pressure Unit, Western Infirmary, Glasgow, Scotland

Bernard I Levy
Inserm U141, Lariboisiere Hospital, Paris, France

George BM Lindop
Department of Pathology, University of Glasgow, Western Infirmary, Glasgow, Scotland

Eugenie R Lumbers
School of Physiology & Pharmacology, University of New South Wales, Kensington, New South Wales, Australia

Richard L Malvin
Department of Physiology, University of Michigan, Ann Arbor, Michigan, USA

Joël Menard
Service de Médecine 9, Centre de Médecine Preventive Cardio-Vasculaire, Hôpital Broussais, Paris, France

Frederick AO Mendelsohn
Department of Medicine, University of Melbourne, Austin Hospital, Heidelberg, Victoria, Australia

Jean-Baptiste Michel
Service de Médecine 9, Centre de Médecine Preventive Cardio-Vasculaire, Hôpital Broussais, Paris, France

James S Milledge
Northwick Park Hospital, Harrow, Middlesex, England

Edward D Miller Jr
Department of Anesthesiology, College of Physicians and Surgeons of Columbia University, New York, New York, USA

Albert Mimran
Polyclinique, Hôpital Lapeyronie, Montpellier, France

James J Morton
Medical Research Council Blood Pressure Unit,
Western Infirmary, Glasgow, Scotland

Jean-Vivien Mombouli
Center for Experimental Therapeutics, Baylor College
of Medicine, Houston, Texas, USA

Patrick J Mulrow
Department of Medicine, Medical College of Ohio,
Toledo, Ohio, USA

Pascal Nicod
Department of Medicine, Service B, University
Hospital, Lausanne, Switzerland

Arne Høj Nielsen
Institute for Anatomy & Physiology, The Royal
Veterinary & Agricultural University, Copenhagen,
Denmark

Rainer Nobiling
Department of Physiology, University of Heidelberg,
Heidelberg, Germany

Jürg Nussberger
Division of Hypertension, Department of Medicine,
University Hospital, Lausanne, Switzerland

Alexander A Oldham
Bioscience Department II, ICI Pharmaceuticals,
Macclesfield, Cheshire, England

Paul L Padfield
Department of Medicine, University of Edinburgh,
Western General Hospital, Edinburgh, Scotland

Rose B Perich
Department of Medicine, The University of
Melbourne, Austin Hospital, Heidelberg, Victoria,
Australia

Pierre-François Plouin
Service de Médecine 9, Centre de Médecine
Preventive Cardio-Vasculaire, Hôpital Broussais,
Paris, France

Stephen Poole
Division of Endocrinology, National Institute for
Biological Standards and Control, Potters Bar,
England

Knud Poulsen
Institute for Anatomy and Physiology, The Royal
Veterinary and Agricultural University, Copenhagen,
Denmark

Richard E Pratt
Falk Cardiovascular Research Center, Stanford
University School of Medicine, Stanford, California,
USA

John L Reid
Department of Medicine & Therapeutics, University
of Glasgow, Western Infirmary, Glasgow, Scotland

A Mark Richards
Cardiology Department, The Princess Margaret
Hospital, Christchurch, New Zealand

AJ Günter Riegger
Department of Internal Medicine, University of
Regensburg, Regensburg, Germany

Juan Carlos Romero
Division of Hypertension, Division of Physiology
and Biophysics, Mayo Clinic, Rochester, Minnesota,
USA

Gerhard H Scholz
Ewen Downie Metabolic Unit, Monash University,
Department of Medicine, Alfred Hospital,
Melbourne, Australia

Michel E Safar
Department of Internal Medicine, Broussais
Hospital, Paris, France

Maarten ADH Schalekamp
Department of Internal Medicine I, Academisch
Ziekenhuis Dijkzigt, Rotterdam, The Netherlands

Sidney G Shaw
Division of Hypertension, Medizinische Poliklinik,
University of Berne, Inselspital, Switzerland

Randal A Skidgel
Laboratory of Peptide Research, Departments of
Pharmacology and Anesthesiology, University of
Illinois College of Medicine, Chicago, Illinois, USA

Sandford L Skinner
Department of Physiology, University of Melbourne,
Parkville, Victoria, Australia

Florent Soubrier
INSERM U36, Laboratoire de Médecine
Expérimentale, College de France, Paris, France

Iain B Squire
Department of Medicine and Therapeutics,
University of Glasgow, Western Infirmary, Glasgow,
Scotland

Andrea Stella
Institute of General Clinical Medicine & Therapeutics, University of Milan, Center of Clinical Physiology and Hypertension, Ospedale Maggiore, Milan, Italy

Jan R Stockigt
Ewen Downie Metabolic Unit, Monash University, Department of Medicine, Alfred Hospital, Melbourne, Australia

Jeffrey S Stoff
Renal Division, University of Massachusetts Medical School, Worcester, Massachusetts, USA

David M Strick
Division of Hypertension, Department of Physiology and Biophysics, Mayo Clinic, Rochester, Minnesota, USA

Steven L Strongwater
University of Massachusetts Medical Center, Worcester, Massachusetts, USA

Anders Svensson
Department of Medicine, University of Gothenburg, Östra Hospital, Gothenburg, Sweden

John D Swales
Department of Medicine, School of Medicine, University of Leicester, Leicester Royal Infirmary, Leicester, England

Roland Taugner
Department of Physiology, University of Heidelberg, Heidelberg, Germany

Terry J Tunny
Endocrine-Hypertension Research Unit, Department of Medicine, University of Queensland, Greenslopes Hospital, Brisbane, Australia

Paul M Vanhoutte
Center for Experimental Therapeutics, Baylor College of Medicine, Houston, Texas, USA

Maria Vidal
Department of Cardiology, Scientific Institute San Raffaele, Milan, Italy

Bernard Waeber
Division of Hypertension, Department of Medicine, University Hospital, Lausanne, Switzerland

Peter Weidmann
Division of Hypertension, Medizinische Poliklinik, University of Berne, Inselspital, Switzerland

Judith A Whitworth
Department of Medicine, St. George Hospital, Kogarah, New South Wales, Australia

Alberto Zanchetti
Institute of General Clinical Medicine & Therapeutics, University of Milan, Center of Clinical Physiology and Hypertension, Ospedale Maggiore, Milan, Italy

Jialong Zhuo
Department of Medicine, University of Melbourne, Austin Hospital, Heidelberg, Victoria, Australia

Sir Stanley Peart
Master, Hunterian Institute, Royal College of Surgeons, London, England

GLOSSARY

We give here a short list of some of the abbreviations used in this book, the alternative names for certain substances where appropriate, and the English synonyms for American words used in the text.

Abbreviations

ACE	angiotensin-converting enzyme
ACTH	adrenocorticotropin; adreno-corticotropic hormone
ANF/ANP	atrial natriuretic factor/atrial natriuretic peptide
Ang I	angiotensin I
Ang II	angiotensin II
Ang III	angiotensin III
DOC/DOCA	deoxycorticosterone/deoxy-corticosterone acetate;
	desoxycorticosterone/desoxy-corticosterone acetate
PRA	plasma renin activity
PRC	plasma renin concentration
RAS	renin–angiotensin system

Alternative terms

angiotensinogen	*also known as*	renin substrate
vasopressin	*also known as*	arginine vasopressin; antidiuretic hormone; ADH

American term / English term

American term	English term
epinephrine	adrenaline
furosemide	frusemide
isoproterenol	isoprenaline
licorice	liquorice
lidocaine	lignocaine
norepinephrine	noradrenaline

COLOR PLATES: VOLUME 2

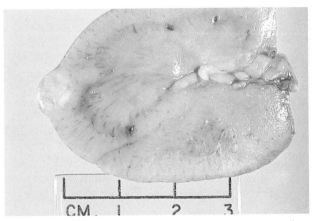

Plate 40 The lower pole of a human kidney, showing a small discrete juxtaglomerular cell tumor in the outer part of the renal cortex (extreme left).

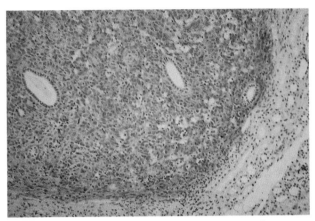

Plate 41 A light micrograph showing the outer part of a juxtaglomerular cell tumor stained with an immunoperoxidase technique using an antiserum to human renin and counterstained with hematoxylin. The encapsulated tumor has a population of tubules among the renin-secreting cells, which are stained brown.

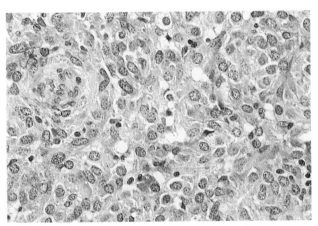

Plate 42 Conventional histological stain showing that juxtaglomerular tumor cells are polygonal and plump spindle cells which contain fine cytoplasmic granules. They are densely packed and are intimately related to fine capillary blood vessels. Hematoxylin and eosin stains have been used.

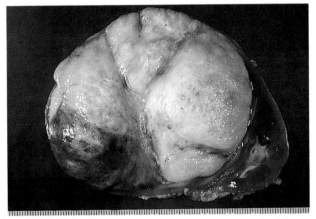

Plate 43 A nephrectomy specimen from a two-year-old child, showing a large nephroblastoma occupying much of the lower pole of the kidney (scale in mm). Reproduced with permission of Dr AAM Gibson.

1

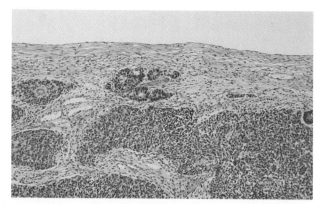

Plate 44 A typical nephroblastoma showing a dark-staining undifferentiated blastema that contains a few primitive tubules intermixed with well-differentiated mesenchyme that contains three blood vessels (top left).

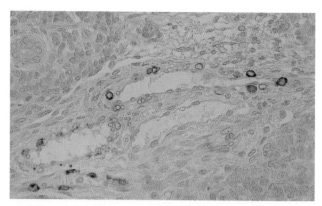

Plate 45 Three blood vessels within the nephroblastoma seen in Plate 44 have been stained with an immunoperoxidase stain using an antiserum to human renin. The renin-containing cells are situated in the mesenchyme intimately associated with the blood vessels external to the endothelium.

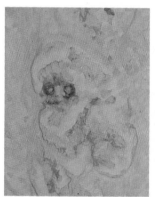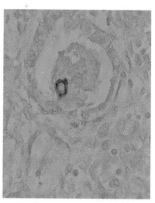

Plate 46 Renin-secreting cells in the mesangium of glomeruloid structures within a well-differentiated nephroblastoma. A renin peroxidase–antiperoxidase stain counterstained with periodic acid/Schiff has been used.

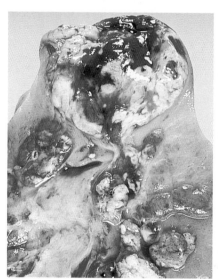

Plate 47 A renal cell carcinoma in the upper pole of a kidney. There is extensive peripelvic infiltration.

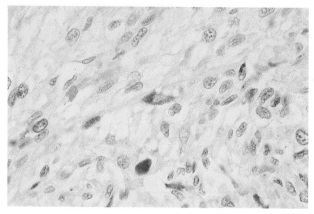

Plate 48 A spindle-cell renal cell carcinoma stained using the renin peroxidase–antiperoxidase technique. The renin-secreting cells are otherwise indistinguishable from adjacent tumor cells.

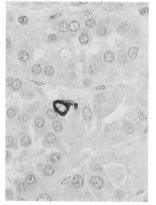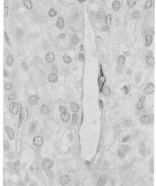

Plate 49 An alveolar renal cell carcinoma where the renin-secreting cells are perivascular, being situated outside the tumor acini. They do not resemble the tumor cells. The renin peroxidase–antiperoxidase technique has been used.

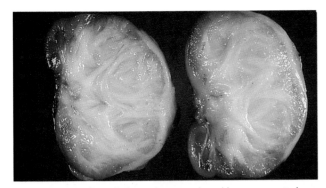

Plate 50 An infant's kidney almost replaced by a congenital mesoblastic nephroma. It has a diffuse edge that merges with the surrounding renal parenchyma. There is a rim of residual renal cortex infiltrated by tumor. Reproduced with permission of Dr AAM Gibson.

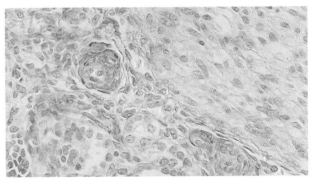

Plate 51 A congenital mesoblastic nephroma stained with the renin peroxidase–antiperoxidase technique. Brown-staining renin-secreting cells are seen in and around the blood vessels which are in an area of developing renal cortex included within the tumor. There is no stainable renin in the spindle-shaped tumor cells (top right).

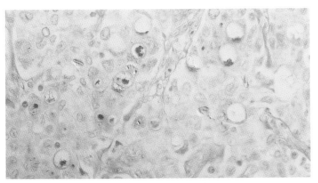

Plate 52 A section of renin-secreting ovarian mucinous adenocarcinoma stained using the renin peroxidase–antiperoxidase technique and counterstained with periodic acid/Schiff. This shows that the renin-secreting cells are tumor cells and that the same cell as contains granular immunoreactive renin also secretes mucin which stains magenta (arrow).

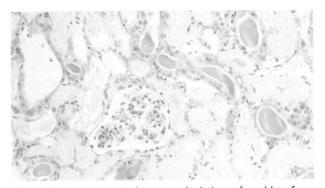

Plate 53 Acute necrotic changes in the kidney of a rabbit after intravenous Ang II infusion at 0.9–1.8μg/kg/min for three days.

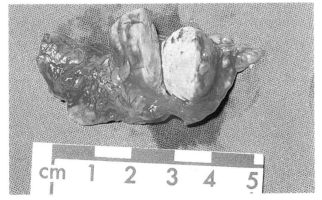

Plate 54 An excised aldosterone-secreting adrenocortical adenoma, showing the characteristic golden yellow of the cut surface.

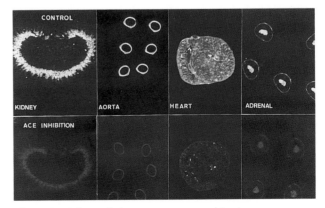

Plate 55 Color-coded computer-generated *in vitro* autoradiographs of ACE in rat tissues before and after administration of an ACE inhibitor.

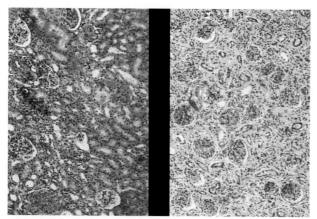

Plate 56 Histological views of kidneys from treated and untreated 2-kidney, 1-clip hypertensive rats (Masson's trichrome). Clipped kidney. No treatment (left): normal aspect of renal cortical tissue. Chronic ACE inhibition treatment (right): diffuse ischemia involving all the structures of the renal parenchyma (tubular and glomerular atrophy, inflammatory cellular infiltration, and diffuse fibrosis).

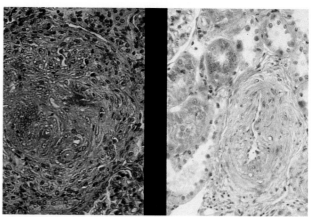

Plate 57 Histological views of kidneys from treated and untreated 2-kidney, 1-clip hypertensive rats (Masson's trichrome). Untouched kidney. No treatment (left): nephroangiosclerosis of an interlobular arteriole. Note the increase in thickness and fibrosis (green) of the arteriolar wall. Chronic ACE inhibition treatment (right): normal aspect of an interlobular arteriole.

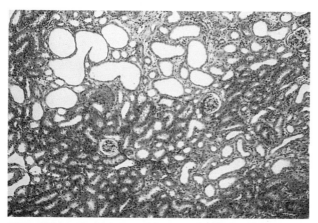

Plate 58 Histological view of the untouched kidney from a 2-kidney, 1-clip hypertensive rat (Masson's trichrome) following ACE inhibition treatment. Nephroangiosclerosis-induced segmental ischemia, corresponding to 'lacunes'. On the left part, note the area of localized tubular dilations associated with fibrosis (green).

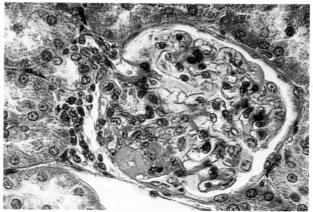

Plate 59 Histological view of the untouched kidney from an untreated 2-kidney, 1-clip hypertensive rat (Masson's Trichrome). Segmental glomerulosclerosis (green), involving part of a glomerulus.

52

THE RENIN–ANGIOTENSIN–ALDOSTERONE SYSTEM IN HYPERTENSION IN HUMAN PREGNANCY

PHYLLIS AUGUST

INTRODUCTION: CLASSIFICATION OF HYPERTENSION IN PREGNANCY

Elevated blood pressure, a common complication of human pregnancy, is separable into several categories on the basis of clinical significance and pathogenesis. An early, convenient, diagnostic framework for the hypertensive disorders of pregnancy was that of the Committee on Terminology of the American College of Obstetricians and Gynecologists of 1972 [1]. In that report, women with hypertension in pregnancy were classified into four groups: chronic hypertension; pre-eclampsia; chronic hypertension with superimposed pre-eclampsia; and transient hypertension. European authors have sometimes employed slightly different terms [2,3]. The US terminology was re-evaluated in 1991 [4].

CHRONIC HYPERTENSION

Chronic hypertension refers to elevated blood pressure existing before the onset of gestation. The preceding hypertension is most often primary (essential) hypertension, and more rarely, a secondary form (see later). Chronic hypertension can give rise to diagnostic problems if no blood pressure readings are available before pregnancy. Nevertheless, the diagnosis of chronic hypertension is very likely if the blood pressure is found to be over 140/90mmHg in the first trimester. Diagnostic confusion can arise if the woman is not seen until later in pregnancy, when differentiation from one of the pregnancy-induced forms of hypertension can be difficult. In these circumstances, absence of proteinuria and a normal serum urate value strongly support a diagnosis of chronic pre-existent hypertension; in most of these women, blood pressure decreases substantially during gestation, and the pregnancies proceed uneventfully and end successfully. A significant minority, however, develops superimposed pre-eclampsia, and this group has a high incidence of hypertension-related complications [5].

PRE-ECLAMPSIA

Pre-eclampsia is diagnosed when hypertension appears for the first time in pregnancy, and is accompanied by proteinuria and hyperuricemia. This occurs usually in a nulliparous woman, in the latter half of pregnancy. When pre-eclampsia develops early in gestation (<30 weeks) there may be an especially high danger of maternal and fetal morbidity and mortality. Pre-eclampsia appearing before 24 weeks of gestation is almost invariably due to the presence of a hydatidiform mole rather than a fetus [3]. Whichever the cause, once the placenta is delivered, the condition always resolves.

ECLAMPSIA

Eclampsia denotes the appearance of tonic or clonic seizures in a woman who has usually, but not invariably, had pre-existing pre-eclampsia.

Since in pre-eclampsia and eclampsia, blood pressure has risen very rapidly from normal values, the vasculature would be expected to be particularly vulnerable to the lesions of the malignant (accelerated) phase of hypertension [6] (see *Chapter 60*). In fact, there is considerable uncertainty and controversy as to what extent the various features of pre-eclampsia and eclampsia represent, in this syndrome, the malignant phase. The issues have been well, and succinctly, reviewed by Redman [2]. Redman points out that in pre-eclampsia and eclampsia, retinal hemorrhages and papilledema are unusual, and malignant nephrosclerosis rare; he therefore prefers to distinguish these features when they appear in pre-eclampsia and eclampsia from malignant hypertension. However, both in eclampsia and in hypertensive encephalopathy from other causes, headache, nausea, vomiting, convulsions, and cortical blindness are features. The medical and obstetric syndromes are thus similar in several important respects and may well involve some of the same mechanisms [2].

The cause of pre-eclampsia or superimposed eclampsia, the most serious of the hypertensive disorders of pregnancy, is not fully understood. Current evidence suggests that impaired utero-placental blood flow, alterations in vascular reactivity, abnormal prostaglandin metabolism, and perhaps changes in vascular endothelial cell function contribute, at least in part, to pathogenesis [7]. The RAS has been a particular focus of investigation into the hypertensive disorders of pregnancy. This latter line of enquiry is indicated by the evident importance of the RAS in the regulation of blood pressure, electrolyte balance, and renal function in normal human pregnancy, as is discussed in detail in Chapter 50.

TRANSIENT HYPERTENSION

Transient hypertension, a diagnosis which has a benign prognosis and which can usually only be established retrospectively, refers to elevation of blood pressure late in gestation, with a return to normal in the immediate postpartum period.

In this chapter, the RAS is considered in various syndromes of human pregnancy hypertension.

HUMAN PRE-ECLAMPSIA AND ECLAMPSIA

For many years, investigators have studied the RAS in preeclampsia with the hope of obtaining insight into the causes of this common, yet still mysterious, affliction. One obstacle to progress has been the lack of uniformity in diagnostic criteria as was hinted at in the introduction to this chapter. This has, in several instances, resulted in apparently contradictory information derived from populations that were in fact not comparable. In the following discussion therefore, it should be appreciated that some of the uncertainty has been due to such problems of classification.

PRE-ECLAMPSIA DE NOVO

Pre-eclampsia, as mentioned above, occurs mostly in primigravidae after the 20th week of gestation, and is characterized by elevated blood pressure, proteinuria, hyperuricemia, generalized edema, and at times, abnormalities of coagulation and/ or liver function. The central pathogenetic feature is severe vasospasm, with reduced perfusion via multiple organs including the uterus, placenta, kidney, brain, and liver. Indeed, although elevated blood pressure and proteinuria are distinctive clinical aspects of pre-eclampsia, they are usually late manifestations of a subclinical process that has been present since early pregnancy. An elevated plasma (or serum) urate value is valuable diagnostically, not only as an early indicator of preeclampsia, but also as a means of differentiation from chronic hypertension [3]. Pre-eclampsia may at times progress rapidly

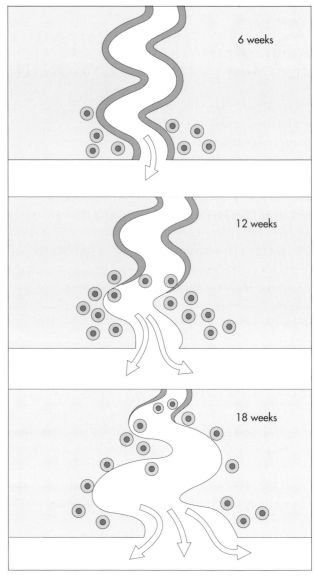

Fig. 52.1 Diagram of fetal trophoblast infiltration of the placental bed and subsequent invasion of wall of maternal spiral arteries supplying the intervillous space of the placenta. Trophoblast cells initially invade the decidua (shaded area), then the myometrium (from 12–18 weeks) and infiltrate the wall of the spiral artery. This destroys the musculo-elastic structure, rendering the artery thin walled, dilated, and capable of transmitting a greater flow of blood. In pre-eclampsia, the process does not proceed beyond the state normally reached at 12 weeks. Modified from Redman C [2].

without warning to the convulsive phase, eclampsia, which is a dramatic and life-threatening complication.

Deviations from many of the normal physiologic adjustments to pregnancy are common in women with pre-eclampsia;

for example, there is increased peripheral vascular resistance, a lower than usual cardiac output, lower plasma volume, reduced glomerular filtration rate (GFR), reduced renal blood flow, abnormalities in sodium excretion, and increased vascular responsiveness to pressor substances.

It has been shown that in pre-eclampsia, there is abnormal placentation due to failure of the trophoblast to invade properly the muscular walls of the maternal spiral arteries, the vessels supplying blood to the placenta [2,8,9]. These arteries retain abnormally their ability to constrict in response to vasoactive substances and to neural stimuli, resulting in inadequate blood flow to the fetoplacental unit (Fig. 52.1). It is hypothesized that several of the clinical features of pre-eclampsia, such as hypertension, are a consequence of this abnormal placentation. Women with pre-existing vascular disease due to chronic hypertension or diabetes are more likely to develop inadequate uteroplacental blood flow and superimposed pre-eclampsia, although it is not yet known whether failure of trophoblast invasion of the spiral arteries is primarily responsible in these circumstances.

THE RENIN–ANGIOTENSIN SYSTEM IN PRE-ECLAMPSIA

Despite the difficulties in evaluating information on pre-eclampsia as against other hypertensive disorders of pregnancy, there is extensive evidence that plasma renin activity (PRA) (Fig. 52.2), plasma renin concentration (PRC) (Fig. 52.3), Ang II (Figs. 52.4 and 52.5), angiotensinogen (Fig. 52.6), and plasma aldosterone levels (Fig. 52.7) are all lower than in normal pregnancy, but usually higher than in nonpregnant women [10–14]. Beilin et al [14] found that in women past the 26th week of gestation, plasma Ang II fell during the day in normotensives and in those with apparent chronic hypertension, whereas pre-eclamptics showed loss of this pattern, as well as having significantly lower Ang II levels (see *Fig. 52.5*). In conformity with these observations of relative suppression of the RAS in pre-eclampsia [10–14] was the finding by others that in kidney biopsies from pre-eclamptic women, the juxtaglomerular cells contained less immunoreactive renin than did specimens obtained from normal pregnant women [15].

The incidence of pre-eclampsia in a population of primigravid women ranges from only 3–8%; therefore, longitudinal studies are difficult and expensive. To date, there are only a few reports of abnormalities in the RAS in early pregnancy in women who later developed pre-eclampsia. Two studies found, perhaps surprisingly, slightly higher PRA values in the second trimester in women who later become hypertensive [16,17].

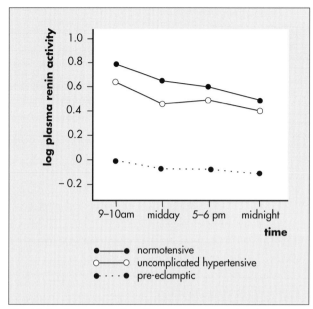

Fig. 52.2 Group mean log plasma renin activity (PRA) at various diurnal sampling times and after 24 weeks of gestation in 10 normotensive women, 13 women with chronic hypertension, and 8 women with pre-eclampsia. Plasma renin activity was significantly lower in the pre-eclamptics than in the other groups (*P*<0.05). All three groups showed a fall in PRA from morning to midnight (*P*<0.005). Modified from Beilin LJ *et al* [14].

Some apparently discordant reports require mention. Gordon *et al* [17] found no difference in the mean plasma Ang II concentration between women with pre-eclampsia and normal pregnant women. Only six measurements were, however, made in pre-eclampsia, and showed a wide scatter, thus limiting statistical analysis. These results [17] are therefore not necessarily in disagreement with reports of relatively low plasma Ang II in pre-eclampsia [12–14]. Symonds and his colleagues reported raised values of Ang II at term in a pre-eclamptic as compared with normotensive pregnant women [18,19]. Symonds and Broughton Pipkin also found a positive correlation between diastolic blood pressure and plasma Ang II levels in 50 primigravid women at term [19]. It should be emphasized that since in these studies [18,19], blood samples were obtained at term with the subjects in the labor suite, the results are not strictly comparable with those obtained earlier in pregnancy [12–14,17]. Symonds and Broughton Pipkin [19] suggested that Ang II may have been secreted from the placental bed and they found evidence that Ang II levels in cord venous blood are higher in infants of mothers with pregnancy-induced hypertension [20] They proposed that excessive Ang II

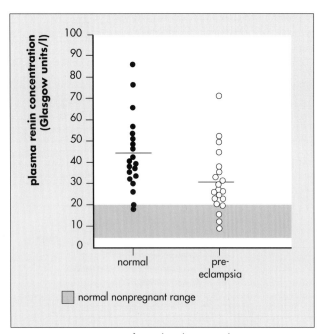

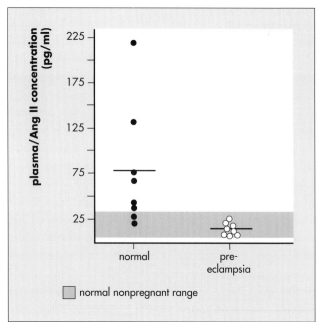

Fig. 52.3 Measurement of peripheral venous plasma renin concentration (in Glasgow units) in a group of 20 women in normal pregnancy and in 20 women with pre-eclampsia, matched for age, parity, and time of gestation. Bars indicate mean. Values are significantly lower in pre-eclampsia (P<0.01). Modified from Weir RJ *et al* [13].

Fig. 52.4 Peripheral venous plasma Ang II concentrations in eight normal pregnant women and in eight women with pre-eclampsia, matched for age, parity, and time of gestation. Bars indicate mean. Values are significantly lower in the pre-eclamptics (P<0.01). Modified from Weir RJ *et al* [13].

originating from the fetoplacental unit may be central to both suppression of maternal renin secretion (due to feedback inhibition) and to the maternal hypertension.

Consistent with the marked elevation of plasma Ang II in normal human pregnancy (see *Chapter 50*) is the long-established decrease in pressor sensitivity to Ang II [21]. Women with pre-eclampsia, have, in comparison with those with normal pregnancy, enhanced pressor responsiveness to Ang II. This presumably reflects in large measure [2] simply their significantly lower plasma Ang II levels [12–14]; the threshold of the pressor response to infused Ang II is in several circumstances established to be in proportion to the basal (preinfusion) plasma Ang II concentration (Fig. 52.8). There are, however, other possible explanations, which are considered later. In a landmark paper by Gant and colleagues, women who subsequently developed pre-eclampsia demonstrated increased sensitivity to the pressor effects of Ang II as early as 18 weeks, and well before the appearance of hypertension and proteinuria [22]. Indeed, the Ang II infusion test is a sensitive method of identifying women likely to develop pre-eclampsia. While these results of Gant *et al* [22] are consistent with the notion that PRA and

Ang II levels are lower in women at risk of pre-eclampsia, measurements of components of the RAS were, unfortunately, not performed in their study.

Platelet Ang II binding in human pregnancy has been examined by several investigators [23–26]. They found that very early in pregnancy, there was a fall in platelet binding from preconceptual levels. Platelet Ang II binding was also significantly lower in both early and late pregnancy in normal women than in the nonpregnant state; these changes paralleled alterations in the vascular responsiveness to Ang II. In pregnancy-induced hypertension, platelet Ang II binding was significantly higher than in normotensive pregnant women [23]. In a prospective trial, Baker *et al* [26] found that a significant relative elevation of platelet Ang II binding successfully predicted pre-eclampsia, and this was more reliable in their view than any variable derived from Ang II infusion studies.

PRE-ECLAMPSIA SUPERIMPOSED ON CHRONIC HYPERTENSION

Studies have been conducted on women with chronic hypertension serially throughout pregnancy [27]. In this high-risk

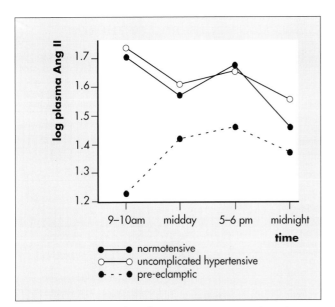

Fig 52.5 Group mean log plasma Ang II at various diurnal sampling times and after 26 weeks of gestation in 10 normotensive women, 13 women with chronic hypertension, and 8 women with pre-eclampsia. Angiotensin II values were significantly lower in pre-eclampsia (*P*<0.025). There was a significant fall in Ang II from morning to midnight in the normotensive and chronic hypertensive women (*P*<0.05). The pre-eclamptics show a significantly different diurnal pattern (*P*<0.05). Modified from Beilin LJ *et al* [14].

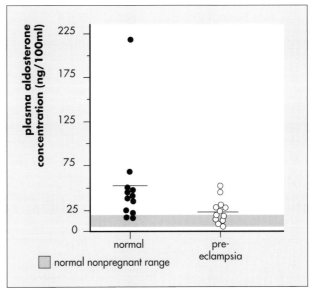

Fig. 52.7 Plasma aldosterone concentrations in 12 normal pregnant women and in 12 women with pre-eclampsia, matched for age, parity, and time of gestation. Bars indicate mean. Values are significantly lower in pre-eclampsia (*P*<0.05). Modified from Weir RJ *et al* [13].

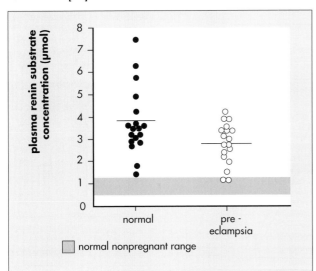

Fig. 52.6 Plasma renin substrate (angiotensinogen) concentrations in 18 normotensive pregnant women and in 18 women with pre-eclampsia, matched for age, parity, and time of gestation. Bars indicate mean. Values are significantly lower in pre-eclampsia (*P*<0.01). Modified from Weir RJ *et al* [13].

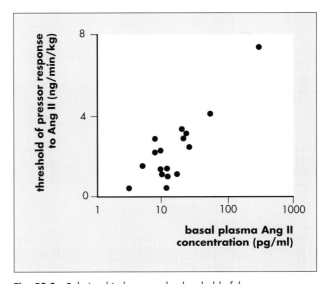

Fig. 52.8 Relationship between the threshold of the pressor response to infused Ang II and the basal (pre-infusion) plasma Ang II concentration in a group of nonpregnant normal and hypertensive subjects. The pressor responsiveness is diminished in proportion to the height of the endogenous plasma Ang II concentration (r = 0.855; *P*<0.001). Modified from Chinn RH and Düsterdieck G [77].

group, 13 of 30 women developed superimposed pre-eclampsia. Plasma renin activity and aldosterone increased in the normal fashion in the first and second trimesters; that is, the values were indistinguishable from those in normotensive pregnant women and in women with uncomplicated chronic hypertension in pregnancy (Fig. 52.9). Shortly before pre-eclampsia was diagnosed, or at the time of diagnosis, PRA and urinary aldosterone excretion fell significantly compared with levels in normal pregnancy (Fig. 52.9). Interestingly, in women who developed pre-eclampsia in the third trimester, blood pressure did not decrease in the second trimester as it did in the other groups (Fig. 52.10).

CONCLUSIONS ON THE ROLE OF THE RENIN–ANGIOTENSIN SYSTEM

It appears therefore that the hypertension associated with human pre-eclampsia is not caused by increased activity of the RAS. Rather, the RAS is suppressed and can perhaps be regarded as responding appropriately to elevated blood pressure and decreased vasodilatation. The possibility remains, nevertheless, that suppression of the RAS is insufficient and that the levels of renin and Ang II are still inappropriately high, and thereby contribute to the development of hypertension.

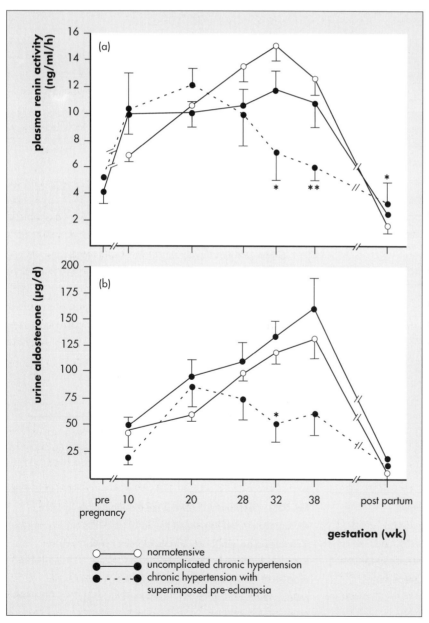

Fig. 52.9 Serial changes in plasma renin activity (PRA) (a) and urine aldosterone excretion (b) before, during, and after pregnancy in normotensive women, women with uncomplicated chronic hypertension, and women with chronic hypertension with superimposed pre-eclampsia (mean ± SEM). (a) In women with superimposed pre-eclampsia, PRA at 32 and 38 weeks was significantly lower (*, $P<0.05$; **, $P<0.01$) than the 20-week value, and at 32 weeks was lower ($P<0.05$) than in normotensive women at the same time. (b) In women with superimposed pre-eclampsia, urine aldosterone was lower ($P<0.05$) at 32 weeks than in normotensive women and women with uncomplicated chronic hypertension. Modified from August P et al [27].

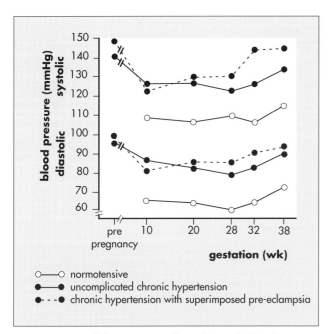

Fig. 52.10 Serial changes in systolic and diastolic blood pressure throughout pregnancy in normotensive women (n=14), women with uncomplicated chronic hypertension (n=17), and women with chronic hypertension with superimposed pre-eclampsia (n=13) (mean ± SEM). Modified from August P *et al* [27].

ANIMAL MODELS OF PRE-ECLAMPSIA

A great hindrance to the study of pre-eclampsia has been the absence of a suitable animal model. There is no animal species that is known to suffer pre-eclampsia naturally, except perhaps the patas monkey, which develops a condition in late pregnancy which has some similarities to the human disease [28].

Over the years, many investigators have attempted to reproduce pre-eclampsia in experimental animals by mechanically reducing uterine perfusion. It has been shown that reduced uterine blood flow in pregnant, but not in nonpregnant, animals of several species causes systemic hypertension, and in some species also other features of pre-eclampsia [29–33].

Several studies have been made of the role of the RAS in hypertension associated with reduced uteroplacental perfusion pressure. Woods and Brooks reported that such hypertension in pregnant dogs was not prevented by pretreatment with captopril [33]. Similar observations have been made in pregnant rabbits [34]. Of some concern, however, with respect to the possible applicability of these experiments to women were the low PRA values in the pregnant dogs and the absence of suppression of either PRA or Ang II when hypertension developed [33].

Nevertheless, the animal work does support the evidence that in women, the hypertension of pre-eclampsia is not due to increased activity of the RAS, but may result from release of some other vasoconstrictor from the ischemic uteroplacental unit, or from failure to secrete a vasodilator.

An Australian group has made considerable progress in developing a model of pre-eclampsia in the pregnant baboon [35]; studies of the RAS in these animals will be of great interest.

OTHER RELEVANT PATHOPHYSIOLOGIC CHANGES IN PRE-ECLAMPSIA

VASCULAR REACTIVITY

As mentioned, whereas normal pregnancy is characterized by refractoriness to the pressor effects of Ang II, pre-eclamptic women demonstrate increased pressor responsiveness to Ang II [22,36]. The most obvious explanation is that, as would be predicted, pressor sensitivity to infused Ang II is inversely related to the endogenous circulating level of Ang II [2], and this is lower in women with pre-eclampsia [12–14]. There are however, possibly, additional contributing factors.

It has been suggested that deficiency of vascular prostacyclin might be a further mechanism underlying this phenomenon. In this regard, it has been shown that normal pregnant women given inhibitors of prostaglandin synthesis become more sensitive to the pressor effects of Ang II [36]. Indeed, considerable evidence has accumulated implicating alterations in prostaglandin metabolism in the pathogenesis of pre-eclampsia [37,38]. Specifically, there appears to be a relative deficiency of vascular prostacyclin synthesis with increased platelet thromboxane generation. Prostacyclin deficiency is thus believed to contribute to vasoconstriction, to increased pressor responsiveness to Ang II, and to the suppression of PRA.

VOLUME REGULATION

Normal pregnancy is associated with a progressive increase in plasma volume. There is still some controversy, however, as to whether the circulating volume is perceived as normal or as underfilled by volume sensors. Using the Evans Blue dye-dilution method, many investigators have documented either a reduced plasma volume in women with pre-eclampsia, or a failure of plasma volume to expand in the normal way [39].

The significance of the relatively reduced plasma volume of pre-eclampsia is not clear. It is uncertain whether this abnormality of plasma volume develops before the other manifestations of the disease, or is secondary to vasoconstriction. If pre-eclamptic women are truly hypovolemic then one would expect circulating renin levels to be high rather than low. In this regard, Brown and colleagues studied sodium excretion in normal and pre-eclamptic women and, in agreement with earlier reports, found that the pre-eclamptics excreted less of an intravenous saline load than did normotensive women [40]. Since the pre-eclamptic subjects had lower plasma volumes (as measured by Evans Blue dye), the sodium retention was believed to be a consequence of volume contraction. It was concluded that the relatively low levels of PRA, PRC, Ang II, and aldosterone in pre-eclampsia represent the consequences of an inadequate response of the juxtaglomerular apparatus to plasma volume contraction, and may be, in part, responsible for inadequate plasma volume expansion. If this were the case, however, one would expect blood pressure to be low rather than high. Alternatively, the reduced plasma volume could be a consequence of an increase in peripheral vascular resistance. Suppression of renin secretion could be due to absence of a vasodilator (for example, prostacyclin), and to hypertension. Inability to excrete sodium normally would be an expected outcome of renal vasoconstriction and the resultant decrease in GFR.

PLASMA ATRIAL NATRIURETIC FACTOR

Studies of atrial natriuretic factor (ANF) are of interest in this connection. As discussed in *Chapter 36*, this peptide has been shown in many circumstances to suppress renin release, and to antagonize the vasoconstrictor action of Ang II [41]. Most investigators have observed that, in normal pregnancy at term, ANF concentrations are either unchanged or slightly higher than in nonpregnant women [42]. There are also several reports of plasma ANF concentrations in pre-eclampsia [42–47]. In the majority of cases, ANF levels are higher than in normal pregnancy, sometimes markedly so. This profile of elevated plasma ANF, depressed PRA and Ang II, and hypertension would not be expected in a state of primary volume contraction and underfilling of the circulation. In an attempt to explain the apparent inconsistency, it has been suggested that in pregnancy, ANF secretion is dependent on stimuli other than volume or atrial stretch, but that ANF still retains its ability to suppress renal renin release. It seems reasonable, however, to consider an alternative explanation — that the plasma volume contraction is secondary to increased vasoconstriction and is not perceived as being a contraction nor is the vasculature perceived as being underfilled. This issue is of more than academic interest, since some authorities recommend volume expansion therapy in pre-eclampsia, to correct the presumed volume contraction, whereas others report this approach to be potentially hazardous [48–50].

UTEROPLACENTAL BLOOD FLOW

As mentioned, several components of the RAS have been identified in uterine and placental tissue, and there is evidence that the RAS regulates uteroplacental blood flow [51–55] (see *Chapters 49* and *50*). Reduced uteroplacental blood flow appears to be central to the pathogenesis of pre-eclampsia. Therefore, it is possible that alterations in either the circulating RAS or a locally functioning prorenin-RAS may be involved. There is evidence that blockade of the RAS in pregnant animals leads to reduced uteroplacental blood flow, possibly through a decrease in production of prostaglandins [52,56,57] (see *Chapter 50*), although it is not clear whether this has relevance to pre-eclampsia. *In vitro* studies of perfused placentae from women with pre-eclampsia have shown impaired prostaglandin PGI_2 generation in both umbilical artery and vein [58,59], but similar experiments have not been performed with either ACE inhibitors or excess Ang II in the system.

If circulating Ang II is a modulator, via prostaglandins, of uteroplacental blood flow, it is possible that suppression of the RAS in pre-eclampsia might further compromise uteroplacental blood flow (that is, decreased Ang II levels could result in there being insufficient vasodilator prostaglandins). Indeed, it has been reported that in women with pregnancy hypertension, there is a correlation between low PRA and intrauterine growth retardation [60].

Further studies of components of the uteroplacental RAS (particularly of prorenin, since it is present in such large quantities in uterine and placental tissue) will, it is hoped, shed light on the role of the uteroplacental RAS in normal and hypertensive pregnancy. At present, however, there is no convincing evidence that this local RAS has physiologic relevance, or that it contributes to levels of circulating renin in the blood of pregnant women (see *Chapters 49, 50,* and *51* for other perspectives on this point).

THE RENIN–ANGIOTENSIN SYSTEM IN PREGNANT WOMEN WITH CHRONIC HYPERTENSION

Chronic hypertension was defined in the introduction to this chapter. Most often, the preceding condition is essential (primary) hypertension. However, secondary forms of hypertension, including that due to intrinsic renal disease, to renovascular lesions, to primary hyperaldosteronism, or to pheochromocytoma for example, must also be considered. Little has been written regarding the RAS in pregnant women with chronic hypertension.

ESSENTIAL HYPERTENSION

Most women with essential hypertension have successful pregnancies and undergo the same physiologic adaptations during gestation as were described earlier in normotensive women, that is, vasodilation, a fall in blood pressure, and increases in GFR and cardiac output (see *Chapter 50*). The behavior of the RAS in pregnant women with essential hypertension is similar to that in normotensive women [14,27,61,62]. There is the usual normal stimulation of the RAS and a rise in aldosterone if the pregnancy is uncomplicated.

If superimposed pre-eclampsia develops, PRA and urine aldosterone excretion decrease, and plasma ANF levels rise [27]. Indeed, a fall in PRA may precede the more obvious clinical signs of superimposed pre-eclampsia, and may therefore be helpful in diagnosis or in identifying women who need closer surveillance.

RENOVASCULAR HYPERTENSION

Fibromuscular dysplasia affecting renal arteries is a not uncommon cause of secondary hypertension in young women, and frequently presents in the second and third decades (see *Chapter 55*). In one series of patients who developed severe pre-eclampsia, postpartum renal angiography showed the prevalence of renal artery stenosis to be 12% [63], suggesting that this diagnosis may frequently be missed. Successful pregnancy has been achieved following previous malignant hypertension in a woman with renovascular disease [64]. Little is known regarding the RAS under these various circumstances.

Plasma renin activity has been measured serially during pregnancy in a woman with hypertension and renovascular disease. Her PRA rose earlier than usual and was at the upper limit of the normal pregnant range throughout most of gestation [65], She then proceeded to develop superimposed pre-eclampsia. Shortly before pre-eclampsia supervened, her PRA dropped precipitously to below her prepregnancy value.

ALDOSTERONE-SECRETING TUMOR

Several cases of primary hyperaldosteronism have been reported in pregnancy [66–68]. Gordon and colleagues [66] were the first to measure PRA in a pregnant woman with primary hyperaldosteronism, and reported that it remained suppressed, as is typical of this disease, in nonpregnant patients (see *Chapter 63*), and in contrast to normal pregnancy, in which both PRA and aldosterone are elevated (see *Chapter 50*). In most of the described cases of aldosterone-secreting tumor in pregnancy, hypertension and hypokalemia have persisted through gestation, although this is not always the case. Biglieri and Slaton reported

a patient with primary hyperaldosteronism in whom metabolic abnormalities and blood pressure were improved in pregnancy, an effect which they attributed to elevated progesterone levels [67]. A similar phenomenon has been observed in a pregnant woman with aldosterone excess and bilateral nodular adrenal hyperplasia [65]. In this latter patient, both the blood pressure and serum potassium became normal during pregnancy. Plasma renin activity was lower than expected in a healthy pregnant woman, but was clearly higher than her nonpregnant levels; urinary aldosterone excretion remained high throughout. After delivery, her blood pressure again rose and serum potassium fell.

Suppression of PRA may therefore be useful in the diagnosis of primary hyperaldosteronism in pregnancy, as it is in nonpregnant individuals.

PHEOCHROMOCYTOMA

The presence of a pheochromocytoma in a pregnant woman presents formidable therapeutic problems [69]. However, little seems to be known of the response of the RAS in these circumstances (see *Chapter 67*).

SECONDARY HYPERTENSION, PREGNANCY, AND RENIN SECRETION

It is of interest that in two patients studied with secondary hypertension during pregnancy, one with renovascular disease and one with bilateral nodular adrenal hyperplasia, the RAS in both appeared to respond appropriately to physiologic signals [65]. This supports the belief that during pregnancy, circulating maternal renin is probably entirely of renal origin.

ANTIHYPERTENSIVE DRUGS, THE RENIN–ANGIOTENSIN SYSTEM, AND HYPERTENSION IN PREGNANCY

ANGIOTENSIN-CONVERTING ENZYME INHIBITORS

The marked activation of the RAS in normal human pregnancy (see *Chapter 50*) strongly suggests that this subserves an important physiologic function. This has been a powerful argument against the use of ACE inhibitors in hypertension in pregnancy. Thus, ACE inhibitors have not been widely or systematically employed in human pregnancy, and an evaluation of their possible dangers and benefits is not easy, in part because of bias in the tendency to report apparent adverse effects and the unexpected. This difficult topic has been the subject of several papers and reviews [70–73].

In rabbits and guineapigs, the earlier in pregnancy that ACE inhibitor treatment is started, the greater the fetal loss. There appear to be no accounts of direct teratogenicity in animals administered ACE inhibitors over the period of conception and pregnancy. There are, however, at least two reports of a rare form of skull ossification defect in the fetus of women who became pregnant while taking ACE inhibitors. Of 31 women who conceived while on either captopril or enalapril, there were three spontaneous first-trimester abortions and two therapeutic terminations of pregnancy. There is suggestive evidence that when ACE inhibitor treatment is stopped in the first trimester, the baby is likely to be born at or near term and to have a birth weight near normal. Continued treatment with an ACE inhibitor, however, appears to carry a risk of early delivery and low birth weight [73]. This same review [73] reports on 15 patients who started ACE inhibitor treatment between 12 and 34 weeks (median 25 weeks) of gestation; 14 of these continued treatment to term. Among these pregnancies, there were two intrauterine fetal deaths, two stillbirths, and two neonatal deaths. Of 17 women who started treatment with either captopril or enalapril between 31 and 37 weeks of pregnancy, however, there was a successful outcome in all instances. Smith [74] reported a patient with severe renal disease and hypertension, who took either enalapril or captopril combined with other antihypertensive drugs before, between, and throughout four pregnancies, three of which were successful.

There are no adequate and well-controlled studies of ACE inhibition in pregnant women. However, data are available that indicate that ACE inhibitors can cause fetal and neonatal morbidity and mortality when administered to pregnant women; therefore, the use of ACE inhibition during pregnancy is not recommended unless needed in a situation where other drugs cannot be used or are ineffective. The association of severe oligohydramnios and/or neonatal anuria with maternal treatment with ACE inhibitors has led to a widespread opinion that these agents are contraindicated in pregnancy [70].

BETA-ADRENOCEPTOR BLOCKERS

Although β-adrenoceptor blocking agents also interfere with renal renin release (see *Chapters 24* and *84*), there are fewer reservations than is the case with ACE inhibitors, concerning their prescription in pregnancy; for example, propranolol, acebutolol, metoprolol, atenolol, oxprenolol, and labetalol have all been extensively, and largely safely, employed to treat hypertensive pregnant women [75]. Nevertheless, a report of a higher incidence of babies with low birth weight in association with β-blocker use early in pregnancy [76] emphasizes the need for caution when using any drug during pregnancy.

OTHER ANTIHYPERTENSIVE DRUGS

A range of other agents, including methyldopa, hydralazine, diazoxide, nitroprusside, and diuretics, several of which can affect the RAS in various ways (see *Chapters 24, 80,* and *83*) has been used in pregnancy [7]. Of these, methyldopa has been most extensively prescribed, from early gestation if necessary; it has a good safety record [2,75].

As mentioned earlier, the employment of diuretics in pregnancy-induced hypertension is controversial [48–50]. Hydralazine, diazoxide, and nitroprusside are reserved for severe hypertension in late pregnancy. There is little experience with calcium-channel blockers [75].

CONCLUSIONS

The RAS plays an integral role in the physiology of normal human pregnancy (see *Chapter 50*). During pregnancy, circulating renin and Ang II levels are raised, probably in response to prostaglandin- and hormonally mediated vasodilation, and to counteract progesterone-induced natriuresis. Elevated levels of Ang II and aldosterone are necessary for the maintenance of blood pressure and sodium balance. It is also likely that the RAS and prostaglandins participate in the regulation of fetal–utero–placental blood flow.

In pre-eclampsia, the RAS is suppressed, probably because of decreased vasodilation. The mediators of the decreased vasodilation in pre-eclampsia are not known. It is possible that a circulating or local vasodilator is absent, or that a vasoconstrictor is produced in excess. Renal involvement, with sodium retention, may also contribute to suppression of the RAS. Pre-eclamptic women are more sensitive to the pressor effects of Ang II; this is predictable from their lower PRA and Ang II levels. It is also possible, however, that increased Ang II sensitivity may, in part, be responsible for the elevated blood pressure in this condition. Changes in plasma levels of renin during pregnancy may aid in the differential diagnosis of hypertensive disorders such as aldosterone-secreting tumor, renovascular disease, and the most common form of hypertension in pregnancy, pre-eclampsia.

REFERENCES

1. Hughes ED. *Obstetric-gynecology terminology*. Philadelphia: FA Davis Co, 1972.

2. Redman C. Hypertension in pregnancy. In: Ginsburg J, ed. *The circulation in the female: From the cradle to the grave*. New Jersey: Parthenon Press, 1989:63–77.

3. Rubin PC. Hypertension in pregnancy: Clinical features. In: Rubin PC, ed. *Handbook of hypertension, Vol 10: Hypertension in pregnancy*. Amsterdam: Elsevier, 1988:10–15.

4. Gifford RW, August PA, Chesley LC, Cunningham G, Ferris TF, Lindheimer MD, Redman CWG, Roberts JM, Zuspan MJ, McNellis D, Rocella EJ. Working Group Report on high blood pressure in pregnancy. *US Dept of Health and Human Services. NIH Publication* 1991;**91–3029**:1–38.

5. Lin C–C, Lindheimer MD, River P, Moawad H. Fetal outcome in hypertensive disorders of pregnancy. *American Journal of Obstetrics and Gynecology* 1985;**142**:255–60.

6. Spence JD, Arnold JMO, Gilbert JJ. Vascular consequences of hypertension and effects of antihypertensive therapy. In: Robertson JIS, ed. *Handbook of hypertension, Volume 15: Clinical aspects of hypertension*. Amsterdam: Elsevier, 1992:chapter 23.

7. August P, Lindheimer MD. Pre-eclampsia revisited. In: Lee RV, Barron WM, Cotton DB, Coustan D, eds. *Current obstetric medicine*. Chicago: Mosby-Year Book, 1991:249–73.

8. Fox H. The placenta in pregnancy hypertension. In: Rubin PC, ed. *Handbook of hypertension, Volume 10: Hypertension in pregnancy*. Amsterdam: Elsevier, 1988:16–37.

9. Zuspan FP, O'Shaughnessy R. The uteroplacental bed: Its anatomic and neuroendocrine alterations. In: Laragh JH, Brenner BM, Kaplan NM, eds. *Endocrine mechanisms in hypertension*. New York: Raven Press, 1989:173–88.

10. Brown JJ, Davies DL, Doak PB, Lever AF, Robertson JIS, Trust P. Plasma renin concentration in hypertensive disease of pregnancy. *Lancet* 1965;**ii**:1219.

11. Tapia HR, Johnson CE, Strong CG. Renin–angiotensin system in normal and in hypertensive disease of pregnancy. *Lancet* 1972;**ii**:847–50.

12. Weir RJ, Doig A, Fraser R, Morton JJ, Parboosingh J, Robertson JIS, Wilson A. Studies of the renin–angiotensin–aldosterone system, cortisone, DOC, and ADH in normal and hypertensive pregnancy. In: Lindheimer M, Katz A, Zuspan F, eds. *Hypertension in pregnancy*. New York: John Wiley & Sons, 1976:251–61.

13. Weir RJ, Brown JJ, Fraser R, Kraszewski A, Lever AF, McInnes GM, Morton JJ, Robertson JIS, Tree M. Plasma renin, renin substrate, angiotensin II, and aldosterone in hypertensive disease of pregnancy. *Lancet* 1973;**i**:291–4.

14. Beilin LJ, Deacon J, Michael CA, Vandongen R, Labor CM, Barden AE, Davidson L, Rouse I. Diurnal rhythms of blood pressure, plasma renin activity, angiotensin II and catecholamines in normotensive and hypertensive pregnancies. *Clinical and Experimental Hypertension* 1983;**B2**:271–93.

15. Nochy D, Bariety J, Camilleri JP, Corvol P, Menard J. Diminished number of renin-containing cells in kidney biopsy samples from hypertensive women immediately postpartum. An immunomorphometric study. *Kidney International* 1984;**26**:85–7.

16. Gordon RD, Parsons S, Symonds EM. A prospective study of plasma renin activity in normal and toxaemic pregnancy. *Lancet* 1969;**i**:347–9.

17. Gordon RD, Symonds EM, Wilmhurst EG, Pawsey K. Plasma renin activity, plasma angiotensin and plasma and urinary electrolytes in normal and toxaemic pregnancy, including a prospective study. *Clinical Science and Molecular Medicine* 1973;**45**:115–27.

18. Symonds EM, Broughton Pipkin F, Craven DJ. Changes in the renin–angiotensin system in primigravidae with hypertensive disease of pregnancy. *British Journal of Obstetrics and Gynaecology* 1975;**82**:643–50.

19. Symonds EM, Broughton Pipkin F. Pregnancy hypertension, parity, and the renin–angiotensin system. *American Journal of Obstetrics and Gynecology* 1978;**132**:473–9.

20. Broughton Pipkin F, Craven DJ, Symonds EM. The uteroplacental renin–angiotensin system in normal and hypertensive pregnancy. *Contributions to Nephrology* 1981;**25**:49–52.

21. Abdul-Karim R, Assali NS. Pressor response to angiotensin in pregnant and nonpregnant women. *American Journal of Obstetrics and Gynecology* 1961;**82**:246–51.

22. Gant NF, Daley GL, Chand S, Whalley PJ, MacDonald PC. A study of angiotensin II pressor response throughout primigravid pregnancy. *Journal of Clinical Investigation* 1973;**52**:2682–9.

23. Baker PN, Broughton Pipkin F, Symonds EM. Platelet angiotensin II binding sites in hypertension in pregnancy. *Lancet* 1989;**ii**:1151.

24. Pawlak MA, MacDonald JG. Possible regulatory disorder of angiotensin II receptors in pregnancy induced hypertension. *Clinical and Experimental Hypertension* 1991;**B10**:153.

25. Baker PN, Broughton Pipkin F, Symonds EM. Platelet angiotensin II binding and plasma renin concentration, plasma renin substrate, and plasma angiotensin II in normal pregnancy. *Clinical Science* 1990;**79**:403–8.

26. Baker PN, Broughton Pipkin F, Symonds EM. Predicting pre-eclampsia: The use of platelet angiotensin II binding. *Clinical Science* 1991;**80** (supp 24):26–7.

27. August P, Lenz T, Ales KL, Druzin ML, Edersheim TG, Hutson JM, Müller FB, Laragh JH, Sealey JE. Longitudinal study of the renin–angiotensin–aldosterone system in hypertensive pregnant women: Deviations related to the development of superimposed pre-eclampsia. *American Journal of Obstetrics and Gynecology* 1990;**163**:1612–21.

28. Palmer AE, London WT, Sly DL, Rice JM. Spontaneous pre-eclamptic toxemia of pregnancy in the patas monkey (Erythrocebus patas). *Laboratory Animal Science* 1979;**29**:102–6.

29. Abitbol MM, Gallo GR, Pirani CL, Ober WB. Production of experimental toxemia in the pregnant rabbit. *American Journal of Obstetrics and Gynecology* 1976;**124**:460–70.

30. Abitbol MM, Ober WB, Gallo GR, Driscoll SG, Pirani CL. Experimental toxemia of pregnancy in the monkey, with a preliminary report on renin and aldosterone. *American Journal of Pathology* 1977;**86**:573–90.

31. Abitbol MM, Pirani CL, Ober WB, Driscoll SG, Cohen MW. Production of experimental toxemia in the pregnant dog. *Obstetrics and Gynecology* 1976;**48**:537–48.

32. Cavanagh D, Rao PS, Tung K, Gaston LW. Toxemia of pregnancy. The development of an experimental model in the primate. *Obstetrics and Gynecology* 1972;**39**:637–8.

33. Woods LL and Brooks VL. Role of the renin–angiotensin system in hypertension during reduced utero-placental perfusion pressure. *American Journal of Physiology* 1989;**257**:R204–9.

34. Losonczy GY, Brown G, Venuto RC. Increased peripheral resistance during reduced uterine perfusion pressure hypertension in pregnant rabbits. *American Journal of the Medical Sciences*;1992;**303**:233–40.

35. Phippard A, Horvath J, Thompson J, Mclean J, Gillin A, Tiller D. Experimental uteroplacental ischemia in the conscious unrestrained pregnant baboon (Papio hamadryas). *Clinical and Experimental Hypertension* 1989;**B8**:181.

36. Gant NF, Worley RJ, Everett RB, MacDonald PC. Control of vascular responsiveness during human pregnancy. *Kidney International* 1980;**18**:253–8.

37. Friedman SA. Pre-eclampsia: A review of the role of prostaglandins. *Obstetrics and Gynecology* 1988;**71**:122–37.

38. Fitzgerald DJ, Fitzgerald GA. Eicosanoids in the pathogenesis of pre-eclampsia. In: Laragh JH, Brenner BM, eds. *Hypertension: Pathophysiology, diagnosis, and management*. New York: Raven Press, 1990:1789–807.

39. Chesley LC. Plasma and red cell volumes during pregnancy. *American Journal of Obstetrics and Gynecology* 1972;**112**:440–9.

40. Brown MA, Gallery EDM, Ross MR, Esber RP. Sodium excretion in normal and hypertensive pregnancy: A prospective study. *American Journal of Obstetrics and Gynecology* 1988;**159**:297–307.

41. Atlas SA, Laragh JH. Atrial natriuretic factor and its involvement in hypertensive disorders. In: Laragh JH, Brenner BM, eds. *Hypertension: Pathophysiology, diagnosis and management*. New York: Raven Press, 1990: 861–84.

42. Bond AL, August P, Druzin MD, Atlas SA, Sealey JE, Laragh JH. Atrial natriuretic factor in normal and hypertensive pregnancy. *American Journal of Obstetrics and Gynecology* 1989;160:1112–6.

43. Thomson JK, Storm TL, Thamsborg G, Nully M, Bodker B, Skouby S. Atrial natriuretic factor concentration in pre-eclampsia. *British Medical Journal* 1987;294:1508.

44. Miyamoto S, Shimokawa H, Sumioki, Nakano H. Circadian rhythm of plasma atrial natriuretic peptide, aldosterone and blood pressure during the third trimester in normal and pre-eclamptic pregnancies. *American Journal of Obstetrics and Gynecology* 1988;158:393.

45. Hirai N, Yanaihara T, Nakayama T, Ishibashi M, Yamaji T. Plasma levels of atrial natriuretic peptide during normal pregnancy and in pregnancy complicated by hypertension. *American Journal of Obstetrics and Gynecology* 1988;159:27.

46. Hatjis CG, Greelish JP, Kofinas AD, Stroud A, Hashimoto K, Rose JC. Atrial natriuretic factor maternal and fetal concentrations in severe pre-eclampsia. *American Journal of Obstetrics and Gynecology* 1989;161:1015–9.

47. Stratta P, Canavese C, Gurioli L, Porcu M, Todros T, Mattone GC, Fianchino O, Gagliardi L, Vercellone A. Ratio between aldosterone and atrial natriuretic peptide in pregnancy. *Kidney International* 1989;36:908–14.

48. Collins R, Yusuf S, Peto R. Overview of randomised trials of diuretics in pregnancy. *British Medical Journal* 1985;290:17–23.

49. De Swiet M, Fayers P. Overview of randomised trials of diuretics in pregnancy. *British Medical Journal* 1985;290:788.

50. Rubin P. Overview of randomised trials of diuretics in pregnancy. *British Medical Journal* 1985;290:788–9.

51. Gorden P, Ferris TF, Mulrow PJ. Rabbit uterus as a possible site of renin synthesis. *American Journal of Physiology* 1967;212:703–6.

52. Ferris TF, Weir EK. Effect of captopril on uterine blood flow and prostaglandin E synthesis in the pregnant rabbit. *Journal of Clinical Investigation* 1983;71: 809–15.

53. Elder MG, Glance DG, Rose M, Myatt L. Arachidonic acid metabolites in human placental tissue: Their role in controlling placental blood flow. *Advances in Prostaglandin, Thromboxane, and Leukotriene Research* 1983;15:627.

54. Parisi VM, Rankin JHG. The effect of prostacyclin on angiotensin II-induced placental vasoconstriction. *American Journal of Obstetrics and Gynecology* 1985;151:444–9.

55. Franklin CO, Dowd AJ, Caldwell BV, Speroff L. The effect of angiotensin II intravenous infusion on plasma renin activity and prostaglandin A, E, and F levels in the uterine vein of the pregnant monkey. *Prostaglandins* 1974;6: 261–80.

56. Broughton Pipkin F, Symonds EM, Turner SR. The effect of captopril (SQ14,225) upon mother and fetus in the cannulated ewe and in the pregnant rabbit. *Journal of Physiology* 1982;323:415–22.

57. Olsson K, Fyhrquist F, Benlamilih K. Effects of captopril on arterial blood pressure, plasma renin activity and vasopressin concentration in sodium-depleted and sodium-deficient goats: A serial study during pregnancy, lactation and anestrus. *Acta Physiologica Scandinavica* 1984;121:73–80.

58. Stuart MJ, Clark DA, Sunderji SG, Allen JB, Yombo T, Elrad H, Slott JH. Decreased prostacyclin production: A characteristic of chronic placental insufficiency syndrome. *Lancet* 1981;i:1126.

59. Walsh SW, Behr MJ, Allen NH. Placental prostacyclin production in normal and toxemic pregnancies. *American Journal of Obstetrics and Gynecology* 1985;151:110–15.

60. Taufield PA, Druzin ML, Edersheim TE, Sealey JE, Laragh JH. Correlation between plasma renin activity and birthweight in hypertensive pregnancy. *Journal of Hypertension* 1986;4 (suppl 5):S96–8.

61. Weinberger MH, Kramer NJ, Petersen LP, Cleary RE, Young PCM. Sequential changes in the renin–angiotensin–aldosterone system and plasma progesterone concentrations in normal and abnormal pregnancy. In: Lindheimer MD, Katz A, Zuspan FP, eds. *Hypertension in pregnancy*. New York: John Wiley & Sons, 1976:263–70.

62. Broughton Pipkin F, Symonds EM, Lamming GD, Jadoul FAC. Renin and aldosterone concentration in pregnant essential hypertensives; a prospective study. *Clinical and Experimental Hypertension* 1983;B2:255–69.

63. Koskela O, Kaski P. Renal angiography in the follow-up examination of toxemia of late pregnancy. *Acta Obstetricia et Gynecologica Scandinavica* 1971;50:41.

64. Weir RJ, Willocks J. A successful pregnancy following malignant phase hypertension. *British Journal of Obstetrics and Gynaecology* 1976;83:584–6.

65. August P, Sealey JE. The renin–angiotensin system in normal and hypertensive pregnancy and in ovarian function. In: Laragh JH, Brenner BM, eds. *Hypertension: Pathophysiology, diagnosis and management*. New York: Raven Press, 1990:1761–78.

66. Gordon RD, Fishman LM, Liddle GW. Plasma renin activity and aldosteronism. *Journal of Clinical Endocrinology* 1967;27:1628.

67. Biglieri EG, Slaton PE. Pregnancy and primary aldosteronism. *Journal of Clinical Endocrinology* 1967;27:1628.

68. Lotgering FK, Derkx FMH, Wallenburg HCS. Primary hyperaldosteronism in pregnancy. *American Journal of Obstetrics and Gynecology* 1986;155:986–8.

69. Ball SG. Treatment of pheochromocytoma: Pregnancy. In: Robertson JIS, ed. *Handbook of hypertension, vol 2: Clinical aspects of secondary hypertension*. Amsterdam: Elsevier, 1983:262–4.

70. Hanssens M, Keirse MJNC, VanKelecom F, Van Assche FA. Fetal and neonatal effects of treatment with angiotensin-converting enzyme inhibitors in pregnancy. *Obstetrics and Gynecology* 1991;78:128–35.

71. Moschizuki M, Maruo T, Motoyame S. Treatment of hypertension in pregnancy by a combined drug regimen including captopril. *Clinical and Experimental Hypertension* 1986;B5:69–78.

72. deLigny BH, Ryckelynck JPH, Mintz PH, Levy G, Muller G. Captopril therapy in pre-eclampsia. *Nephron* 1987;46:329–30.

73. Editorial. Are ACE inhibitors safe in pregnancy? *Lancet* 1989;ii:482–3.

74. Smith AM. Are ACE inhibitors safe in pregnancy? *Lancet* 1989;ii:750–1.

75. Lees KR, Rubin PC. Prescribing in pregnancy: Treatment of cardiovascular diseases. *British Medical Journal* 1987;294:358–60.

76. Butters L, Kennedy S, Rubin PC. Atenolol in essential hypertension during pregnancy. *British Medical Journal* 1990;301:587–9.

77. Chinn RH, Düsterdieck G. The response of blood pressure to infusion of angiotensin II: Relation to plasma concentrations of renin and angiotensin II. *Clinical Science* 1972;42:489–504.

53 ORAL CONTRACEPTIVES AND THE RENIN–ANGIOTENSIN SYSTEM

MAARTEN ADH SCHALEKAMP AND FRANS HM DERKX

INTRODUCTION

Two decades of studies have shown that most women who take oral contraceptives (or the 'pill') for at least six months, in developed and developing countries alike, will experience significant elevations in blood pressure, which generally remit after the oral contraceptive is stopped. The magnitude of these changes has, for the most part, been limited to a few millimeters of mercury [1–6], although one carefully controlled trial documented increases of 9/5mmHg after three years of use and 12/8mmHg after five years of use [7]. The incidence of oral contraceptive-related hypertension has been reported with reasonable consistency to be 4-5%, and the risk variously said to be between 2.5 and 6 times than in nonusers of oral contraceptives [1,7–11]. Hypertension sufficiently severe to enter the malignant phase (see *Chapter 60*) has been infrequently, but regularly, reported with oral contraceptive use [3,43].

The estrogen component has been implicated as the principal determinant of increased blood pressure in pill users. Early studies of blood-pressure changes were conducted in women taking high-dose (50–100μg) estrogen formulations, and the results of later studies of 30-μg estrogen preparations have been more variable, with some demonstrating significant elevations in blood pressure [2,3] and others showing no change [12–14]. Even so, malignant hypertension has been reported as a complication with the 30-μg estrogen pill [43]. It has been claimed that postmenopausal estrogen therapy may also elevate blood pressure [15], although one study has challenged this assumption by reporting a protective effect against age-related changes in diastolic blood pressure [16].

Progestogens alone do not affect blood pressure [17–19]. Nevertheless, for the same estrogen dose, a slight influence of progestogen dose on the magnitude of blood-pressure change has been suggested by two reports, [2,11], one of which [2] was

nonstandardized and must be interpreted cautiously. This dose–response relationship is not a universal finding, however [7].

Oral estrogen markedly increases the synthesis of renin substrate (angiotensinogen) by the liver [20,21] (see *Chapter 8*). Since, under physiological circumstances, renin substrate concentration is as important as renin concentration in determining the generation of Ang I (and II) (see *Chapter 5*), considerable attention has been focused on a possible role of the RAS in the development of oral contraceptive-related blood-pressure changes. This chapter re-examines evidence on the impact of oral contraceptives on components of the RAS and explains why a fresh look at this issue, using more accurate and less ambiguous contemporary assays, may be in order.

EFFECTS OF ORAL CONTRACEPTIVES ON PLASMA LEVELS OF COMPONENTS OF THE RENIN–ANGIOTENSIN SYSTEM AND ALDOSTERONE

RENIN SUBSTRATE

Renin substrate levels in plasma are frequently determined by quantifying the maximum amount of Ang I which can be generated after the addition of an excess of human renin (see *Chapter 14*). An alternative approach is radioimmunoassay, employing antisera raised against purified angiotensinogen [22] (see *Chapter 14*). These different methods can give divergent results during estrogen therapy (see below).

Early work by Helmer and Griffith [20] in rats had already shown that the plasma level of renin substrate is markedly increased by estrogen administration. This effect, which was neutralized by the administration of androgen, did not occur with progesterone and was not altered by removal of the pituitary or adrenal glands. It is now known that the increase in renin substrate in plasma after estrogen administration is caused by stimulation of substrate production from the liver. An increased plasma level of renin substrate is a consistent finding in women who use oral contraceptives containing estrogen, and this is true for both normotensive and hypertensive women. This increase

53.1

is, in fact, the most conspicuous biochemical abnormality in plasma observed in these women. High angiotensinogen levels have been detected as early as one week after oral contraceptive use is started, with peak values after 2–3 months [23,24]. A 3–5-fold increase in plasma renin substrate level has been observed with oral contraceptives containing 50μg or more estrogen [21,23–29], as well as the oral contraceptives containing 30–37.5μg estrogen [30]. With oral contraceptive therapy, consistently higher angiotensinogen values are obtained on incubating with excess of renin than by radioimmunoassay [22,44]. Electrophoresis has shown that with estrogen treatment, three different molecular forms of renin substrate are present, only one of which is recognized by the usual antiserum, although all three are enzymically relevant (see *Chapter 14*).

In normal nonpregnant women who are not taking oral contraceptives, renin substrate concentration in plasma is approximately at the level of K_m for the hydrolysis of substrate by renin at physiological pH (see *Chapter 5*). This means that the increments in substrate that occur with the use of oral contraceptives may be expected to double the plasma renin reactivity (PRA) that is, the velocity of Ang I generation at a given renin concentration. This has indeed been observed when renin reactivity is determined after the addition of renin to the plasma samples in concentrations high enough to overcome the influence of differences in endogenous renin concentration. The results of two studies of renin reactivity have suggested that plasma factors other than changes in the molar concentration of renin substrate influence PRA in oral contraceptive users [22, 31]. This, however, could not be confirmed in a study by Derkx *et al* [30]. In this account, PRA was calculated from the measured plasma concentrations of renin [PRC] and renin substrate (taking into account the values of K_m and V_{max} measured in a purified system), and calculated PRA values were compared with PRA values that were actually measured. There was no difference between calculated and measured levels of PRA either in oral contraceptive users or in control women. Thus, there is no convincing evidence to date that PRA is determined by factors other than the molar concentrations of the active enzyme renin and its substrate.

RENIN ACTIVITY, RENIN CONCENTRATION, AND ANGIOTENSIN II

In contrast with the findings on renin substrate, the results of PRA measurements are not uniform. Elevated PRA with the use of estrogen-containing oral contraceptives has been found in some studies [15,21–23,25,32,33], but not in others [28–30, 34–36]. None of the studies of women using an oral

contraceptive that contained less than 50μg estrogen has documented increased PRA. In an early report on oral contraceptive-induced hypertension, Laragh *et al* [21] stressed that, despite the presence of high levels of substrate and increased renin reactivity, persistent increases in PRA were not observed in all patients. This finding indicates that the 'true' renin concentration (PRC) must have been actually reduced at times as a consequence of oral contraceptive use.

Later studies specifically addressed this issue by simultaneously measuring PRA and PRC. Plasma renin activity is measured as the velocity of Ang I generation *in vitro* from endogenous renin substrate. Plasma renin concentration, in contrast, is measured as the velocity of Ang I generation *in vitro* at a saturating concentration of exogenous renin substrate, so that reaction velocity is maximal and independent of the endogenous substrate concentration (see *Chapter 13*). In two reports, PRA was found to be elevated in oral contraceptive users, whereas PRC was suppressed [25,27]. In these studies, PRC was measured after acidification of the plasma to destroy the endogenous substrate. However, it is now known that acidification causes the conversion of inactive prorenin into active renin (acid activation) (see *Chapter 6*). Thus, PRC determined in this way reflects not only the renin concentration in native plasma, but also includes prorenin converted to renin *in vitro*. In fact, this PRC measurement is grossly overestimating the *in vivo* concentration of renin in plasma, since the concentration of prorenin is much higher than that of renin and because most prorenin is activated by acid treatment.

In a later study by Derkx *et al* [30], such distortions were avoided by measuring PRC in plasma that had not been pretreated with acid and by taking care to prevent inadvertent activation of prorenin during blood sampling and preparation and handling of the plasma samples. A high concentration of exogenous renin substrate was added to the plasma so that differences in endogenous substrate concentration had virtually no influence on the velocity of Ang I generation *in vitro*. With this method, PRC was found to be markedly reduced in oral contraceptive users as compared with control women (Fig. 53.1). In contrast to the two studies cited above [25,27], however, PRA was not elevated in the oral contraceptive users despite a 3–4-fold higher concentration of renin substrate. It was therefore concluded that the effect of increased substrate concentration on the reactivity of renin was fully compensated for by suppression of the active enzyme renin. It is important to note that all three studies that measured PRA and PRC simultaneously were performed in normotensive women. The finding of suppressed PRC in the face of increased renin substrate raised the interesting

Source of plasma	Renin substrate (pmol/ml)	Prorenin (μu/ml)	Active renin (μu/ml)	Plasma renin activity		Fraction of renin that is active (%)
				measured (pmol Ang I/ml/h)	calculated (pmol Ang I/ml/h)	
normal women (n=54)	1,545 (745–2,340)	151 (62–357)	15.4 (4.7–59)	0.88 (0.24–3.25)	1.04 (0.27–3.95)	9.1 (2.9–29.0)
oral contraceptive users (n=44)	4,560* (1,940–7,620)	94* (33–268)	8.9* (2.434)	1.02 (0.26–3.82)	1.02 (0.30–3.66)	8.8 (30.0–25.1)
pregnant women (n=44)	5,130* (3,050–7,210)	645* (263–1,583)	32.8* (10–103)	4.36* (1.25–16.6)	3.90* (1.20–12.7)	4.8* (1.4–18.0)

Fig. 53.1 Concentrations of renin substrate and different forms of renin and plasma renin activity. Mean values and 95% confidence interval (in parentheses) are shown. Statistical analysis was performed after logarithmic transformation of the results to obtain a Gaussian distribution. Results are expressed as the antilog. For calculating plasma renin activity (PRA), the plasma concentration of active renin, which is expressed as microunits of the International human kidney renin standard per milliliters of plasma (μu/ml) (*Appendix II*), was converted into picograms per milliliter. The concentrations of active renin and renin substrate were entered in the Michaelis–Menten equation, and calculations were based on V_{max}=0.08pmol Ang I/h/pg of active renin and K_m=1,200pmol/ml. The measured and calculated values of PRA were not significantly different. *$P<0.001$ versus normal women (by unpaired t test). Modified from Derkx FHM *et al* [30].

possibility that insufficient suppression of renin release by the kidney might be a mechanism underlying the development of hypertension caused by oral contraceptives [21,37]. However, as is discussed later, the finding of an elevated PRA in both normotensive and hypertensive oral contraceptive users might well be a methodological artifact, at least in some cases.

Circulating Ang II levels have been reported to be elevated in oral contraceptive users [32,33]. However, some of these results may be disputed because the plasma Ang II levels in normal controls were 3–4 times higher than those currently measured with more specific assays. No increase in plasma Ang II was found in a prospective study by Weir *et al* [38]. In another report from the latter department [45], however, a comparison was made of women who developed hypertension on oral contraceptive use, with age-matched female patients with essential hypertension. Renin substrate was raised in the women taking oral contraceptives, while plasma concentrations of active renin were similar in both groups; thus, plasma Ang II was significantly elevated in the pill users. Total body sodium was normal with the oral contraceptives. The rise in plasma Ang II in conjunction with the normal body sodium was thought by these investigators probably to contribute to the increase in blood pressure induced by oral contraceptives.

PRORENIN AND THE PROBLEM OF SPONTANEOUS CRYOACTIVATION

As described in *Chapter 6*, plasma prorenin is converted to renin through limited proteolysis by endogenous plasma kallikrein, when plasma is kept at 0–4°C (spontaneous irreversible cryoactivation). In women on oral contraceptives, plasma prorenin concentration is approximately 10 times higher than the renin concentration. Thus, inadvertent activation *in vitro* of even a small fraction of prorenin will lead to a significant percentage increase in the measured levels of PRC and PRA. Cryoactivation is a slow process but is fast enough to have this effect.

Cryoactivation of prorenin can be prevented by collecting the blood in syringes or tubes containing an appropriate serine protease inhibitor [30,39]. As noted above, when this precaution was taken, PRC was found to be suppressed in normotensive oral contraceptive users to the extent that PRA was not elevated despite 3–4-fold increases in renin substrate concentration. Spontaneous cryoactivation of prorenin proceeds faster in plasma from oral contraceptive users [30] and from pregnant women [40,41] than from nonpregnant women not using an oral contraceptive (Fig. 53.2). This enhanced cryoactivation is probably an estrogen-induced effect. Enhanced spontaneous cryoactivation of prorenin could explain, at least in part, earlier reports of increased PRA in oral contraceptive users.

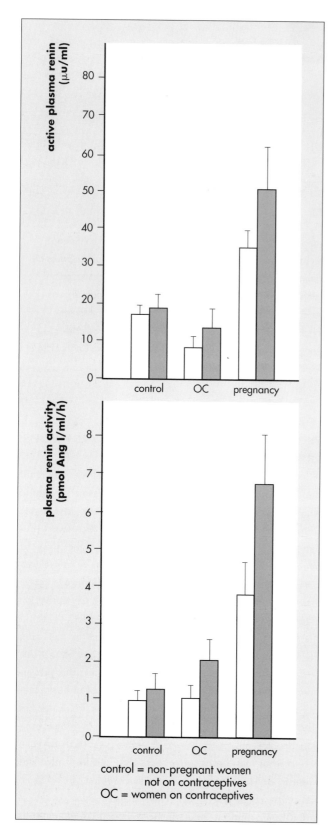

Fig. 53.2 Activation of prorenin during collection and handling of blood samples. Open bars: blood was collected in anticoagulant containing soybean trypsin inhibitor and immediately centrifuged at room temperature; the plasma was snap frozen and stored at −70°C. Tinted bars: blood was collected in anticoagulant without soybean trypsin inhibitor and kept at 0°C for two hours and then centrifuged at 4°C; the plasma was stored at −20°C. Data are mean ± SEM of six plasma samples. Modified from Derkx FHM *et al* [30].

ALDOSTERONE

Although it is now understood that the increase in renin substrate associated with oral contraceptive use does not necessarily lead to increased PRA, early reports of elevated PRA gave rise to the expectation that aldosterone secretion would be stimulated in oral contraceptive users. Modest increases (by a factor of 1.5–2) in urinary aldosterone excretion were reported by Laragh *et al* [21] in three out of eight women who developed hypertension during oral contraceptive use. However, a community survey [29] and a few small-scale studies [35,42] failed to show increases in plasma aldosterone with oral contraceptive use. In a study of 13 women with oral contraceptive-induced hypertension, plasma levels of aldosterone appeared normal, but seven of these women failed to show the suppression of aldosterone normally seen after partial immersion in water [42] (see *Chapter 74*). Theoretically, the lack of aldosterone supressibility, which was also observed one month after the oral contraceptive was discontinued, might contribute to the development of oral contraceptive-induced hypertension.

ROLE OF THE RENIN–ANGIOTENSIN SYSTEM IN HYPERTENSION INDUCED BY ORAL CONTRACEPTIVES

Since oral contraceptives markedly increase renin substrate concentration, the RAS has been implicated as a major culprit in the pathogenesis of oral contraceptive-induced hypertension. It has thus been hypothesized that adaptive suppression of the renal release of renin, in response to the increased level of renin substrate, may be insufficient in some women [21,37,45]. This would then lead to increased production of Ang II and aldosterone. Hyperactivity of the renin–angiotensin–aldosterone system was thought to explain the estrogen-induced hypertension in oral contraceptive users. This hypothesis became muted, but not abandoned [45], when a prospective study [38] showed that, in most women who had developed oral contraceptive-related hypertension, PRA, Ang II, and aldosterone were within the normal range and were not higher than those in oral contraceptive users who remained normotensive. In this particular study, plasma concentrations of renin substrate, cortisol, and deoxycorticosterone were significantly elevated in the oral contraceptive users, but again there was no correlation with blood pressure. In addition, infusion of Ang II antagonist into women with oral contraceptive-induced hypertension did not lower blood pressure [35].

Do these negative results really prove that the RAS does not play a role in the pathogenesis of oral contraceptive-induced hypertension? Both normal and increased levels of PRA and plasma Ang II have been measured in normotensive, as well as hypertensive, oral contraceptive users. However, these results were obtained with assays that did not always measure the levels of renin and Ang II *in vivo*. The levels of PRA, PRC, and Ang II reported in several of these studies are higher than those currently measured. The reasons behind the overestimation of PRA and PRC have been discussed above.

Fortunately, with modern low-estrogen oral contraceptives, the risk of developing hypertension is smaller (although not absent) than that posed by older preparations containing more estrogen. Nonetheless, detailed studies of the more subtle changes in the various components of the RAS may still be in order. Such investigations are now feasible thanks to the availability of more accurate and specific assays. These new methods avoid many of the pitfalls of the older assays. The fallibility of direct radioimmunoassay for renin substrate with oral contraceptive therapy [22,44] has been discussed earlier. Problems stemming from acid treatment of plasma and from handling plasma samples in the cold are now better understood. Inadvertent generation *in vitro* of renin and Ang I can be prevented by the addition of an appropriate serine protease inhibitor and a specific renin inhibitor, respectively. Highly specific and sensitive assays of renin and prorenin, which make use of monoclonal antibodies that react with either renin or prorenin, are now being developed. The new assays of Ang I and II, in which high-performance liquid chromatography separation is carried out prior to radioimmunoassay, are also more specific than the older assays of Ang-like material (see *Chapters 5, 9, 13, and 15*). Finally, the finding that an Ang II antagonist failed to lower the blood pressure in oral contraceptive-induced hypertension [35] does not strongly argue against a role of the RAS, since such agents may not be full antagonists of Ang II (see *Chapter 86*). Perhaps the advent of the orally active Ang II antagonists (see *Chapter 86*) will help to clarify the contribution of the RAS to oral contraceptive-induced hypertension.

REFERENCES

1. Ramcharan S, Pellegrin FA, Hoag EJ. The occurrence and course of hypertensive disease in users and nonusers of oral contraceptive drugs. In: US Department of Health Education and Welfare. *The Walnut Creek Contraceptive Drug Study: A prospective study of the side effects of oral contraceptives, volume 2. Publication no (NIH)* 76–563. Washington DC: Government Printing Office, 1976:1–16.

2. Khaw K, Peart WS. Blood pressure and contraceptive use. *British Medical Journal* 1982;285:402–7.

3. Weinberger MH, Weir RJ. Oral contraceptives and hypertension. In: Robertson JIS, ed. *Handbook of hypertension: Clinical aspects of secondary hypertension, volume 2*. Amsterdam: Elsevier Science Publishers, 1983:196–207.

4. Cook NR, Scherr PA, Evans DA, Laughlin LW, Chapman WG, Rosner B, Kass EH, Taylor JO, Hennekens CH. Regression analysis of changes in blood pressure with oral contraceptive use. *American Journal of Epidemiology* 1985;121:530–40.

5. Woods JW. Oral contraceptives and hypertension. *Hypertension* 1988;11 (suppl II):II-11–15.

6. The WHO Multicentre Trial of the Vasopressor Effects of Combined Oral Contraceptives. Comparisons with IUD. *Contraception* 1989;40:129–45.

7. Weir RJ, Briggs E, Mack A, Naismith L, Taylor L, Wilson E. Blood pressure in women taking oral contraceptives. *British Medical Journal* 1974;1:533–5.

8. Clezy TM, Foy BN, Hodge RL, Lumbers ER. Oral contraceptives and hypertension. An epidemiological survey. *British Heart Journal* 1972;34:1238–43.

9. Fisch IR, Freedman SH, Myatt AV. Oral contraceptives, pregnancy and blood pressure. *Journal of the American Medical Association* 1972;222:1507–10.

10. Report of the Royal College of General Practitioners. Hypertension. In: *Oral contraceptives and health*. London: Pitman, 1974:37–42.

11. Royal College of General Practitioners Oral Contraceptive Study. Effect on hypertension and benign breast disease of progestogen component in combined oral contraceptives. *Lancet* 1977;i:624.

12. Briggs M, Briggs M. Oestrogen content of oral contraceptives. *Lancet* 1977;ii:1233.

13. Liukko P, Erkkola R, Gronroos M, Lammintausta R. Plasma renin activity, blood pressure and body weight during two years oral contraception with two different low-estrogen combinations. *Annales Chirurgiae et Gynaecologiae* 1987; 76 (suppl 202):50–3.

14. The WHO Multicentre Trial of the Vasopressor Effects of Combined Oral Contraceptives. Lack of effect of estrogen. *Contraception* 1989;40:147–56.

15. Crane MG, Harris JJ, Winsor W. Hypertension, oral contraceptive agents and conjugated oestrogens. *Annals of Internal Medicine* 1971;74:13–21.

16. Hassager C, Riis BJ, Strom V, Guene TT, Christiansen C. The long-term effect of oral and percutaneous estradiol on plasma renin substrate and blood pressure. *Circulation* 1987;76:753–8.

17. Mackay EV, Khoo SH, Adam R. Contraception with a six monthly injection of progestagen. Effects on blood pressure, body weight, and uterine bleeding pattern, side effects, efficacy and acceptability. *Australian and New Zealand Journal of Obstetrics and Gynaecology* 1971;11:148–53.

18. Spellacy WN, Birk SA. The effect of intra-uterine devices, oral contraceptives and progestagens on blood pressure. *American Journal of Obstetrics and Gynecology* 1972;112:912–9.

19. Hawkins DF, Benster B. A comparative study of three low dose progestagens, chlormadinone acetate, megestrol acetate and norethisterone, as oral contraceptives. *British Journal of Obstetrics and Gynaecology* 1977;84:708–13.

20. Helmer OM, Griffith. Effect of the administration of estrogens on the renin-substrate (hypertensinogen) content of rat plasma. *Endocrinology* 1952;51:421–6.

21. Laragh JH, Sealey JE, Ledingham JGG, Newton MA. Oral contraceptives. Renin, aldosterone and high blood pressure. *Journal of the American Medical Association* 1967;201:918–22.

22. Eggena P, Hidaka H, Barrett JD, Sambhi MP. Multiple forms of human plasma renin substrate. *Journal of Clinical Investigation* 1978;62:367–72.

23. Beckerhoff R, Luetscher JA, Beckerhoff I, Nokes GW. Effects of oral contraceptives on the renin–angiotensin system and on blood pressure of normal young women. *Johns Hopkins Medical Journal* 1973;132:80–7.

24. Oparil SL. Hypertension and oral contraceptives. *Journal of Cardiovascular Medicine* 1981;6:381–7.

25. Skinner SL, Lumbers ER, Symonds EM. Alteration by oral contraceptives of normal menstrual changes in plasma renin activity, concentration and substrate. *Clinical Science* 1969;36:67–76.

26. Weinberger MH, Collins RD, Dowdy AJ, Nokes GW, Luetscher JA. Hypertension induced by oral contraceptives containing estrogen and gestagen. *Annals of Internal Medicine* 1969;71:891–902.

27. Beckerhoff R, Luetscher JA, Wilkinson R, Gonzalez C, Nokes GW. Plasma renin concentration, activity, and substrate in hypertension induced by oral contraceptives. *Journal of Clinical Endocrinology and Metabolism* 1972;34:1067–73.

28. Krakoff L. Measurement of plasma renin substrate by radio immunoassay of angiotensin I: Concentration in syndromes with steroid excess. *Journal of Clinical Endocrinology and Metabolism* 1973;37:110–7.

29. Goldhaber S, Hennekens CH, Spark PHRF, Evans DA, Rosner B, Taylor JO, Kass EH. Plasma renin substrate, renin activity, and aldosterone levels in a sample of oral contraceptive users from a community survey. *American Heart Journal* 1984;107:119–22.

30. Derkx FHM, Stuenkel C, Schalekamp MPA, Visser W, Huisveld IH, Schalekamp MADH. Immunoreactive renin, prorenin, and enzymatically active renin in plasma during pregnancy and in women taking oral contraceptives. *Journal of Clinical Endocrinology and Metabolism* 1986;63:1008–15.

31. McDonald WJ, Cohen EL, Lucas CP, Conn JW. Renin–renin substrate kinetic constant in the plasma of normal and estrogen-treated humans. *Journal of Clinical Endocrinology and Metabolism* 1977;45:1297–304.

32. Hollenberg NK, Williams GH, Burger B, Chenitz W, Hoosmand I, Adams DF. Renal blood flow and its response to angiotensin II: An interaction between oral contraceptive agents, sodium intake, and the renin–angiotensin system in healthy young women. *Circulation Research* 1976;38:35–40.

33. Cain MD, Walters WA, Catt KJ. Effects of oral contraceptive therapy on the renin–angiotensin system. *Journal of Clinical Endocrinology and Metabolism* 1971;33:671–6.

34. Weinberger MH, Kramer NJ, Grim CE, Petersen LP. The effect of posture and saline loading on plasma renin activity and aldosterone concentration in pregnant, non-pregnant and estrogen-treated women. *Journal of Clinical Endocriniology and Metabolism* 1977;44:69–77.

35. Ogihara T, Hata T, Maruyama A, Nakamaru M, Mikami H, Kumahara Y. Effects of an angiotensin II antagonist, (sarcosine 1, isoleucine 8) angiotensin II, on blood pressure, plasma renin activity and plasma aldosterone in hypertensive and normotensive subjects taking oral contraceptives. *Endocrinologia Japonica* 1979;26:591–7.

36. Leenen FH, Boer P, Dorhout Mees EJ. Oral contraceptives and responsiveness of plasma renin activity and blood pressure in normotensive women. *Clinical and Experimental Hypertension* 1980;2:197–211.

37. Saruta T, Saade GA, Kaplan NM. A possible mechanism for hypertension induced by oral contraceptives: Diminished feedback suppression of renin release. *Archives of Internal Medicine* 1970;126:621–6.

38. Weir RJ, Davies DL, Fraser R, Morton JJ, Tree M, Wilson A. Contraceptive steroids and hypertension. *Journal of Steroid Biochemistry* 1975;6:961–4.

39. Derkx FHM, Bouma BN, Schalekamp MADH. Prorenin–renin conversion by the contact activation system in plasma: Role of plasma protease inhibitors. *Journal of Laboratory and Clinical Medicine* 1984;103:560–73.

40. Rowe J, Gallery EDM, Györy AZ. Cryoactivation of renin in plasma from pregnant and non pregnant subjects, and its control. *Clinical Chemistry* 1979;25:1972–4.

41. Gordon EM, Douglas J, Ratnoff OD. Influence of augmented Hageman factor (factor XII) titers on the cryoactivation of plasma prorenin in women using oral contraceptive agents. *Journal of Clinical Investigation* 1983;72:1833–8.

42. Crane MG, Harris JJ. Estrogens and hypertension: Effect of discontinuing estrogens on blood pressure, exchangeable sodium, and the renin–aldosterone system. *American Journal of the Medical Sciences* 1978;276:33–55.

43. Hodsman GP, Robertson JIS, Semple PF, Mackay A. Malignant hypertension and oral contraceptives: Four cases, with two due to the 30μg oestrogen pill. *European Heart Journal* 1982;3:255–9.

44. Hidaka H, Itoh T, Sato R, Oda T. A new direct radio-immunoassay for human renin substrate and heterogeneity of human renin substrate in pathological states. *Japanese Circulation Journal* 1980;44:375–83.

45. McAreavey D, Cumming AMM, Boddy K, Brown JJ, Fraser R, Leckie BJ, Lever AF, Morton JJ, Robertson JIS, Williams ED. The renin–angiotensin system and total body sodium and potassium in hypertensive women taking oestrogen–progestagen oral contraceptives. *Clinical Endocrinology* (Oxford) 1983;18:111–8.

54 RENIN-SECRETING TUMORS

GEORGE BM LINDOP, BRENDA J LECKIE, AND
ALBERT MIMRAN

INTRODUCTION

Conn [1] proposed the term primary reninism for the clinical syndrome of hypertension with hypokalemia caused by high plasma levels of active renin secreted by a tumor. Tumors can also lead to raised plasma renin levels by inducing the kidney to secrete excess renin but the term 'secondary reninism' is seldom used. This latter may occur when any mass compresses the kidney or compromises its blood supply (see *Chapter 55*). Alternatively, a humoral factor produced by the tumor may increase secretion of renin by the kidney. The purpose of this chapter is to assess the clinical, pathological, and biological significance of these phenomena.

CRITERIA FOR THE DIAGNOSIS OF A RENIN-SECRETING TUMOR

It is essential to show high levels of renin and/or prorenin (inactive renin) in the blood. Plasma renin levels should fall following removal of the tumor, and may rise again if the tumor recurs. To confirm the diagnosis, renin should be demonstrated within the tumor, either by immunohistochemistry or, preferably, by biochemical analysis. In some cases, electron microscopy may show typical renin storage granules within tumor cells, but renin-specific mRNA detected in tumor tissue by Northern blot analysis or by *in situ* hybridization techniques constitutes good evidence of renin synthesis. As an adjunct, it is useful to compare the renin levels in the tumor and in the normal kidney tissue by biochemical measurement or by immunocytochemical studies.

Primary reninism is caused most often by renal tumors — specifically, juxtaglomerular cell tumors (JGCT), by some nephroblastomas, by occasional renal cell carcinomas, and rarely, by nonrenal malignant tumors.

RENAL RENIN-SECRETING TUMORS

JUXTAGLOMERULAR CELL TUMORS

In 1967, Robertson *et al* reported the first case of a benign renin-secreting renal tumor in a 16-year-old male patient who presented with malignant hypertension which was cured by nephrectomy [2]. In the same year, Kihara *et al* described a similar case and coined the term 'juxtaglomerular cell tumor' [3]. Since then, at least 40 additional cases have been reported [4–35].

Histogenesis and nomenclature

The first tumor was diagnosed by Robertson *et al* as a hemangiopericytoma [2]. It is important to distinguish JGCT, which are invariably benign, from true renal hemangiopericytomas which may metastasize [36], and from metastatic hemangiopericytoma which could have spread to the kidney from elsewhere. The term 'hemangiopericytoma' is clearly misleading and should not be used in this context. Other workers have since argued that JGCT are hamartomas or malformations of the juxtaglomerular apparatus [11]. However, although JGCT are seen usually in young people, no congenital cases have been reported, and other tumors are also composed of several tissues including nerves. Therefore, these lesions are best regarded as benign tumors. Renin-secreting cells also occur in the intraglomerular mesangium and in the renal arterial tree distant from the juxtaglomerular apparatus (JGA) (see *Chapters 18* and *19*). Although some tumors may arise in such sites, JGCT seems the best term available.

Pathology

Juxtaglomerular cell tumors are usually approximately 1cm in diameter (Plate 40, see Color Plate Section); some are tiny but the biggest are 5–6cm across. The cut surface is tan or greyish yellow, and scattered hemorrhages are common. Histological examination shows an encapsulated tumor (Plate 41, see Color Plate Section) with polygonal or plump spindle cells which contain cytoplasmic granules (Plate 42, see Color Plate Section). A variable population of tubules, adrenergic nerves [34,35], and mast cells (30% of the cell population of some tumors) are less constant features [35].

The renin-secreting tumor cells have an intimate relationship with capillary and sinusoidal blood vessels in the manner of a hemangiopericytoma. Some tumors contain unusual thick-walled arteries [37,38]. The demonstration of renin granules by immunostaining or by electron microscopy confirms the diagnosis of JGCT. The granular renin-secreting cells show the ultrastructural features of myoepithelioid cells in a state of high secretory activity (Fig. 54.1).

Clinical findings

Juxtaglomerular cell tumors can occur in childhood but are most common in adolescence and young adulthood: of 41 cases reviewed (Fig. 54.2), 76% were less than 30 years old and 44% were aged 8–20 years. Only two cases occurred in older subjects, aged, respectively, 53 and 57 years. The female to male ratio is 1.7:1.

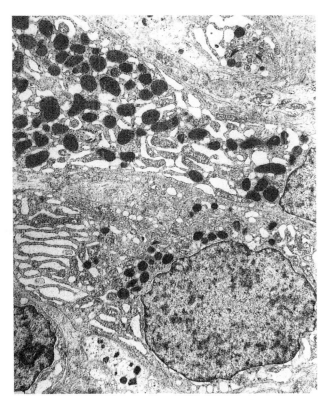

Fig. 54.1 An electron micrograph showing two cells in a juxtaglomerular cell tumor. The lower cell is packed with typical renin storage granules. Prominent dilated cisterns of rough endoplasmic reticulum are also present indicating a cell in a phase of active protein synthesis.

Patients with JGCT usually present with severe hypertension which may be in the malignant (accelerated) phase. In one case, the hypertension was paroxysmal [15]. Significant hypokalemia (<3mmol/l) is present in the majority (61%) but serum potassium levels are occasionally normal [6,10,18,20]. Occasionally [22,23], hyponatremia occurs, possibly due to either pressure natriuresis (see *Chapter 55*) or to Ang II-mediated stimulation of thirst (see *Chapter 32*) and production of vasopressin (see *Chapter 35*).

Proteinuria (>0.4g/24hr — the minimum level for a positive albustix test) is common (55%) and in one patient, this reached a nephrotic level [22]. In patients with high plasma renin levels, both severe hypertension and high circulating levels of Ang II [39,40] could cause proteinuria (see *Chapter 58*). Interestingly, unlike malignant hypertension or renovascular disease, renal function is usually normal in patients with JGCT; this may be the consequence of high renal perfusion and/or Ang II-mediated preferential constriction of the efferent glomerular arterioles. These possibilities are supported by the fall in glomerular filtration rate (GFR) from 142 to 13ml/min/1.73m^2 and a fall in mean arterial pressure from 181 to 123mmHg following infusion of the Ang II antagonist, saralasin, in a personally studied case [14].

Blockade of the RAS consistently lowers the mean arterial blood pressure (from -15 to -60mmHg) [14,22,25,26,28,31,33]. The fall in GFR and blood pressure in response to blockade of the RAS suggests that endogenous Ang II participates in the regulation of renal blood flow and renal function. In the absence of renovascular disease, a dramatic fall in blood pressure in response to inhibition of the RAS should initiate a search for a renin-secreting tumor. Investigations are then directed towards lateralization of renin secretion, assessment of autonomy of renin secretion, and localization of the tumor. A plan is summarized in Fig. 54.3.

Lateralization of renin secretion

Lateralization of renin secretion is defined as a plasma renin ratio between the two renal veins greater than 1.2. It must be emphasized that because renal blood flow is not usually lowered in this condition, the renal vein renin ratio, even with a high rate of renin secretion from the tumor, is usually much less than in unilateral renovascular hypertension [7] (see *Chapter 55*). Lateralization is often found in patients studied in basal conditions (supine and maintained on unrestricted sodium intake). Lateralization may be unmasked by the administration of captopril or furosemide, or by assuming the upright posture (see Fig. 54.2). By contrast, chronic high-dose captopril treatment in one

number of reported cases	41
sex distribution	26 female/15 male
age at diagnosis	8–57 (31/41 below 30)
duration of hypertension	1 month to 16 years
Characteristics of hypertension	
malignant (accelerated)	7/41
average arterial pressure (mmHg)	206/131
serum potassium	
<3mmol/l	26/41
>3.5mmol/l	4/41
hyponatremia	3/41
proteinuria >0.4g/24h	12/22
supine plasma renin (times normal)	3–70
Positive diagnostic indices	
positive lateralization of renin secretion	
in basal condition	19/35 (16/26 patients with positive arteriograms)
unmasked by captopril	2/3
unmasked by furosemide	1/1
unmasked by upright posture	1/1
positive arteriograms	28/40 (size ≥15mm in 27/28)
negative arteriograms	12/40 (size 10–30mm in 4/12 size ≤16mm in 7/12)
positive computerized tomography	11/12 (size ≥10mm in 10/11)
positive renal echography	9/11 (size ≥20mm in all)
Size of tumor (diameter) (mm)	2–50 (14/40 less than 16mm)
Renin response to various maneuvers	
increase in response to upright posture	11/16
increase in response to low sodium intake	4/10
increase in response to renin blockade	4/11
decrease in response to Ang II	0/1
decrease in response to β-blockade	4/4

patient was thought to have obscured the diagnostic usefulness of renal vein renin measurements [41]. Interestingly, of 12 patients with negative arteriograms, all nine who were tested showed positive renin lateralization. In contrast, only 50% of cases with positive arteriograms showed lateralization of renin secretion (see *Fig. 54.2*). Cases with positive lateralization of renin secretion had smaller tumors than those without lateralization (16+9.8 versus 36+8.7mm $P<0.001$) (Fig. 54.4). Patients with bigger tumors were probably hypertensive for longer; therefore, as in hypertensive patients with unilateral renovascular disease, failure of lateralization could be due to increased renin secretion from the contralateral kidney caused by hypertensive vascular damage (see *Chapter 55*).

Autonomy of renin secretion

Renin release from JGCT usually responds to changes in posture and in sodium intake (see *Fig. 54.2*), but perhaps not to the negative feedback mediated by Ang II. In one case, administration of exogenous Ang II failed to decrease circulating renin levels [29]. Conversely, Ang II antagonists and converting-enzyme inhibitors interrupt the negative feedback loop between Ang II and renin and thus lower the systemic blood pressure without altering circulating renin levels [14,28]. This suggests autonomous renin secretion by a tumor. Such apparent autonomy may be absent in patients whose tumors contain adrenergic nerves, since these may respond to change in posture or to the fall in blood pressure. Interestingly, administration of a β-blocker may

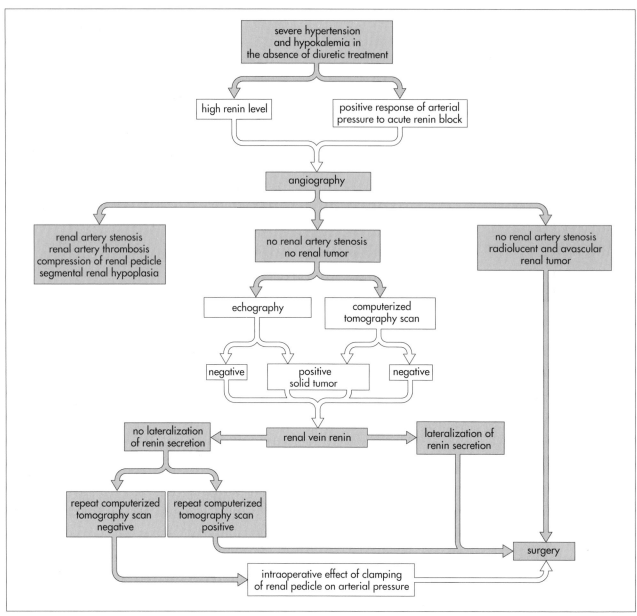

Fig. 54.3 Decision tree for the diagnosis of renin-secreting renal tumors.

lower plasma renin levels without affecting blood pressure [14,22,28].

Tumor localization

Localization is important in planning the surgical management of JGCT. Three techniques have been used: ultrasound, arteriography, and computerized tomography (CT) scanning.

On selective arteriography, the most important finding is the absence of renovascular disease. Juxtaglomerular cell tumors appear as characteristic 'avascular' radiolucent areas on the external contour of the kidney. In patients with positive arteriograms,

the tumor is usually 15mm or greater in diameter. Renal arteriography may be negative in cases with larger tumors (see *Fig. 54.2*); four cases had tumors which were 20–30mm in diameter. Therefore, whatever the result of arteriography, CT scanning should be performed. Computerized tomography confirmed the arteriographic findings of a hypodense tumor in all cases; in addition, tumors 10–16mm in diameter were detected in four patients with negative arteriograms. Unfortunately, CT scanning was not performed in the six cases with tumors less than 10mm in diameter.

In summary, from the available data, the discrimination size

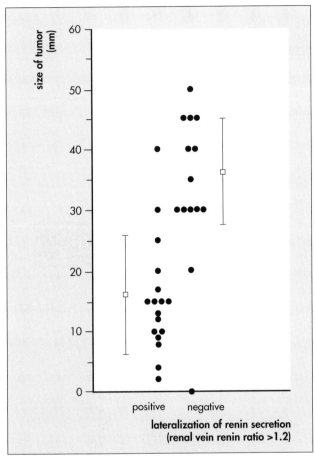

Fig. 54.4 Influence of tumor size on lateralization of renin secretion in patients with juxtaglomerular cell tumors. Data are also presented as mean ± SD.

for CT scanning appears to be 10mm, and possibly less, compared with 15mm for arteriograms and 20mm for echography. Computerized tomography scanning therefore is the most reliable method of tumor localization.

Surgical management

Primary reninism was cured by unilateral nephrectomy (24 cases), partial nephrectomy (3 cases) and removal of the tumor by enucleation (9 cases). Juxtaglomerular cell tumors do not metastasize or recur, and therefore the optimum treatment is simple removal of the tumor. The size range of JGCT, however, overlaps with that of the malignant renal tumors, some of which can also cause primary reninism (see below). Intraoperative scrutiny of a cryostat section will establish the diagnosis and govern the decision between carrying out local excision and

nephrectomy for the larger tumors. Only obvious peripheral tumors are suitable for enucleation; partial nephrectomy should be performed in the others.

If arteriograms and CT scans fail to localize the tumor, the change in renal blood pressure caused by clamping extrarenal renal artery branches can be assessed at operation. This procedure should confirm the segmental renal vein renin measurements and may be a good guide to the type of partial nephrectomy required to conserve the maximum amount of renal tissue. Following removal of the tumor, the high plasma levels of renin and Ang II and the blood pressure usually fall rapidly to normal, even though hypertension may have been present for many years. One follow-up study, however, showed that some cases have persistent mild hypertension [20], possibly due to hypertensive changes in the arterial tree and/or in the contralateral kidney.

Plasma and tumor renin

Plasma renin activity is usually high — more than five-fold the upper limit of normal in 90% of cases. This causes high levels of Ang II and consequently of aldosterone (*Chapter 33*), which result in hypertension. Juxtaglomerular cell tumors always contain high concentrations of renin — often 10,000-fold higher than the surrounding renal cortex, where renin synthesis is suppressed by high circulating levels of Ang II. Immunoreactive renin [17,38,42] and renin mRNA [42] are present in the granular cells, but not in the vascular or tubular elements. In some cases, plasma prorenin is also raised but forms only a small proportion of the total circulating renin [7]. *In vitro* cultured cells initially secrete a high proportion of active renin [1,43], but after some weeks in culture, only prorenin is secreted [43].

NEPHROBLASTOMA (WILMS' TUMOR)

Incidence and clinical findings

Nephroblastoma constitutes 13% of all nonleukemic malignancies in childhood [44,45]. Most cases present with an abdominal mass before the age of five and 95% are diagnosed before the age of 15, but occasional cases occur in adults [46]. In the UK, the incidence is 0.5 cases per 100,000 children per year [44]. As with retinoblastoma, sporadic and familial cases occur. Familial cases are often bilateral and may be associated with aniridia and genitourinary abnormalities. Chromosomal deletions involving the 11p 13 locus have been described and the culprit gene codes for a transcription protein that controls genitourinary development [47]. Other cases are associated with hemihypertrophy of the body and other somatic overgrowth syndromes and at least two other gene loci are involved [48].

Pathology

Nephroblastomas arise from nephrogenic blastema, which may persist in the mature kidney. They are large tumors, usually greater than 5cm and often more than 10cm in diameter (Plate 43, see Color Plate Section), and huge tumors weighing 2–10kg sometimes occur.

Histologically, nephroblastomas may differentiate into a mixture of mesenchymal (stromal) and epithelial components in varying proportion. The mesenchymal areas may remain primitive (blastematous) or differentiate into mature connective tissue (Plate 44, see Color Plate Section). Structures representing all stages in the development of tubules and glomeruli may be identified in the epithelial component.

The reported incidence of hypertension varies widely but probably occurs in approximately 60% of cases [49]. In 1938, Bradley and Pincoffs reported that the hypertension associated with nephroblastoma resolved on treatment of the tumor [50]. Irradiation of the recurrent tumor deposits also lowered blood pressure [51], suggesting that the hypertension was caused by a humoral agent secreted by the tumor. This was first shown to be renin by Mitchell et al in a hypertensive case with primary reninism [52]; other cases with primary reninism followed [53–58].

Tumor and plasma renin

Day and Luetscher [59] studied a case of nephroblastoma where both tumor and plasma contained high molecular-weight inactive renin and suggested that this 'big' renin might be prorenin. A prospective study showed that most cases of nephroblastoma have raised plasma prorenin levels (up to 100 times normal). Following nephrectomy, plasma renin concentrations fall to normal [60].

Plasma prorenin from patients with nephroblastoma elutes from gel filtration columns or affinity columns in a manner identical to normal purified human prorenin. It is also similarly activated by either trypsin or acidification, and the resulting active renin is indistinguishable from normal active renin by the affinities of its binding to antibodies and to peptide inhibitors of renin (Leckie BJ, unpublished data).

Even in cases with high circulating levels of prorenin, tumor tissue usually contains relatively low concentrations of both prorenin and active renin: for example, in one patient with circulating prorenin concentrations of 703µu/ml (upper limit of normal 200µu/ml) the tumor contained only 1.5µu of prorenin per mg of tissue, while the adjacent renal cortex contained 24.0µu/mg of tissue. Active renin concentrations were 180µu/ml in plasma, 0.9µu/mg in tumor, and 126µu/mg in renal cortex

(Leckie BJ unpublished data). This is in agreement with the paucity of renin-containing cells revealed by immunohistochemical study [57,61–63]. Cells containing immunostainable renin are present in primary nephroblastomas [58,61–63] and in metastatic deposits [61]. Perivascular renin-containing cells often occur at the junction between the areas of stromal differentiation and the primitive blastemal areas (Plate 45, see Color Plate Section) and occasionally in the mesangial areas of tumor glomeruli (Page 46, see Color Plate Section). The amount of immunostainable renin in the JGA of the adjacent renal cortex is usually normal [61].

Nephroblastoma tissue contains renin mRNA [63], confirming that renin synthesis occurs in vivo. Cells cultured from nephroblastoma secrete renin in vitro; in one case, the proportions of prorenin and active renin were similar to those in the blood of the patient from whom the tumor was derived [64]. Unlike JGCT cells, the renin-secreting cells in nephroblastoma may be unable to process the newly synthesized enzyme, which is usually secreted as prorenin without being stored.

Since nephroblastomas are large tumors, in some cases they can also cause secretion of excess active renin from the adjacent kidney by compression of renal parenchyma or blood vessels [49]. This could explain why nephrectomy may cure hypertension in some cases with metastatic tumor [49].

In summary, nephroblastoma may secrete both active and inactive renin. Most cases of nephroblastoma secrete predominantly prorenin which, although biologically inert and not accompanied by hypertension, may prove to be a tumor marker. Occasional nephroblastomas secrete active renin which causes primary reninism, and some patients may also become hypertensive due to secondary reninism if a large tumor compresses the kidney or its blood supply.

RENAL CELL CARCINOMA

Renal cell carcinoma (hypernephroma) comprises 1–2% of all malignancies. There is a male/female ratio of 1.5–2:1. It may affect all age groups but is rare in childhood, and the incidence increases with age, rising steeply above 50 years [65].

Pathology

Renal cell carcinoma is an encapsulated tumor (Plate 47, see Color Plate Section) that usually shows pure or partial epithelial differentiation. Some renal cell carcinomas are predominantly sarcomatous and have only a minor epithelial component. Renal cell carcinoma is composed of various cell types in different arrangements. The cells may be clear, granular, basophilic, oncocytic, or spindle shaped and the architecture of the tumor may be alveolar, trabecular, or papillary; in the sarcomatous variety, the cells are arranged in interlacing bundles [66].

Plasma and tumor renin

Mild hypertension is present in 25% of patients with renal cell carcinoma and a similar proportion have a paraneoplastic syndrome [66]. As in nephroblastoma, renal cell carcinoma can occasionally cause primary reninism [67–69]. The renin in tumor tissue from both primary [70–72] and metastatic tumors [70] is mainly inactive. Cells containing immunoreactive renin (Plate 48, see Color Plate Section) are present in renal cell carcinoma [71–73]. In some cases, the renin-containing cells are tumor cells, but in a few cases that have been carefully studied [69,74] these renin-containing cells were perivascular and did not resemble surrounding tumor cells (Plate 49, see Color Plate Section, and Fig. 54.5). Renin-containing cells occur in metastatic renal cell carcinomas that have spread to other tissues, but not in secondary carcinomas originating from other sites and growing in the renal cortex [73]. This suggests that they are tumor cells rather than stromal cells which have colonized the tumor by growing in with the blood vessels from the surrounding renal cortex.

In one personally studied case [70], high levels of plasma prorenin fell to normal following nephrectomy; plasma prorenin levels subsequently rose when a rib metastasis appeared and fell with its excision (Fig. 54.6). In a prospective study, however, only 30% of patients had raised plasma prorenin and, in many of these, the levels were only slightly above normal [75]. Unlike nephroblastoma, prorenin is not significantly raised in the majority of cases of renal cell carcinoma.

In summary, hypertension in renal cell carcinoma is rarely due to primary reninism; in a few other cases, hypertension may be due to compression of the kidney or interference with its blood supply. Most cases of hypertension associated with renal cell carcinoma are probably due to coincidental essential hypertension. Renal cell carcinomas often contain cells that probably secrete prorenin, but, unlike nephroblastoma, plasma prorenin levels are rarely high enough to be useful as a tumor marker.

OTHER RENAL TUMORS

CONGENITAL MESOBLASTIC NEPHROMA

Congenital mesoblastic nephromas (CMN) are large benign tumors of infancy and childhood which most often present as an abdominal mass in the first few months of life [66]. They are composed of fibromyomatous tissue. The edge is diffuse and

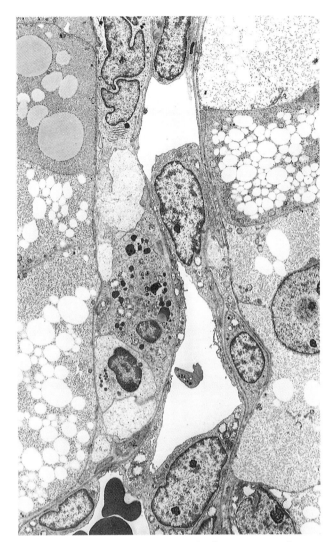

Fig. 54.5 An area in an alveolar renal cell carcinoma similar to that in plate 49 (see Color Plate Section) examined by electron microscopy, showing a capillary within the tumor. External to the endothelium, there is a cell that contains granules morphologically compatible with renin storage granules. It is external to the acini of tumor cells and is morphologically different from the surrounding tumor cells but does not resemble a myoepithelioid cell.

merges with the adjacent kidney, causing inclusions of renal tissue within the tumor. (Plate 50, see Color Plate Section).

Patients with CMN may have high-renin hypertension [76, 77] and renin has been detected biochemically in tumor tissue associated with reduced immunostainable renin in the adjacent renal cortex [76,78]. Renin (Plate 51, see Color Plate Section) and renin mRNA are detectable in perivascular cells within the tumor [78–80]. This suggests secretion of renin by the tumor. The renin-secreting cells have mainly been found in inclusions

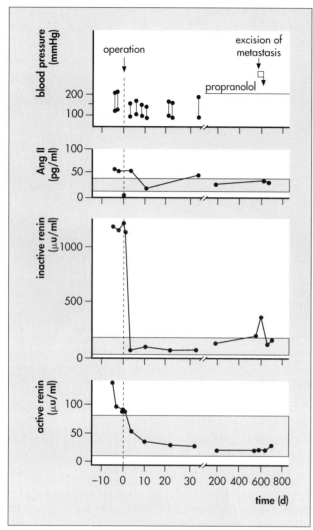

Fig. 54.6 Changes in blood pressure and in the circulating RAS in a case of renal cell carcinoma secreting mainly prorenin. Modified from Leckie B *et al* [70]. Shading indicates the normal range.

of renal tissue which often contain glomeruli and their associated JGA. In areas with no visible renal structures, renin-secreting cells have also been related to tumor blood vessels, the tumor cells being renin negative [80].

In summary, the perivascular renin-secreting cells in mesoblastic nephroma are probably derived from renal tissue included in the tumor. Nephrectomy is curative and the hypertension, whether it is due to true primary or to secondary reninism, nearly always then resolves.

Cells with ultrastructural characteristics of renin-secreting myoepithelioid cells have been described in a renal angiomyolipoma [81], and renin-containing cells have been detected

in two cases of oncocytoma [71]; whether these tumors can cause primary reninism remains to be established.

EXTRARENAL RENIN-SECRETING TUMORS

Extrarenal renin–angiotensin systems are now well recognized in tissues such as the adrenal and pituitary glands, brain, heart, pancreas, and gonads (see *Chapters 41–48* and 78). In 1970, Hauger-Klevene reported the first extrarenal renin-secreting tumor — an oat cell carcinoma of lung [82] that presented with primary reninism. Primary reninism was subsequently reported in other carcinomas variously of lung [83], pancreas [84], small bowel [85], adrenal cortex [86], parovarian region [87], and ovary [88] (Plate 51, see Color Plate Section). Renin production has also been reported in ovarian stromal tumors [89–91], a chemodectoma [92], and a hamartoma of liver [93]. Renin-secreting sarcomas have also been described: hemangiopericytoma of the orbit [94], epithelioid sarcoma of the thigh [95], leiomyosarcomas of the ovary [96], and retroperitoneal tissue [97,98]; these have all caused primary reninism. To date, however, less than 20 cases of extrarenal renin-secreting tumors have been reported.

CLINICAL FEATURES

In the series of 14 cases of extrarenal renin-secreting tumors reviewed by Anderson *et al* [96], all but one were female and the mean age was 32 years. The clinical features of primary reninism were similar to those of patients with renin-secreting renal tumors, but physiological studies of the control of renin release are lacking. As in renin-secreting renal tumors, complete surgical excision usually cures the hypertension. The prognosis is governed by the aggressiveness of the tumor. In a case of primary reninism, failure to find a renal tumor on CT scanning, and the absence of lateralization of renal vein renin levels, should raise the possibility of an extrarenal renin-secreting tumor. This diagnosis should also be considered in any patient with a tumor who has hypertension and hypokalemia.

TUMOR RENIN

As with renal tumors, extrarenal tumors may secrete mainly active renin or a mixture with prorenin in varying proportions. Both renin storage granules [96] and immunoreactive renin (Plate 52, see Color Plate Section) occur in tumor cells. In one ovarian tumor case, typical renin storage granules were scanty and there was morphological evidence that the renin may have been secreted by an alternative pathway [96]. Whether renal and extrarenal tissues and the tumors that arise from them secrete renin via different intracellular pathways is uncertain.

CONCLUSIONS

As yet, there are too few reported cases to suggest that extrarenal renin-secreting tumors predominate in tissues that possess an RAS. Some cases may represent random genetic derepression in a malignant tumor. With increasing awareness of extrarenal renin–angiotensin systems, such terms as 'ectopic' or 'inappropriate' renin secretion are best avoided.

OTHER TUMORS ASSOCIATED WITH HYPERRENINISM

In neuroblastoma, plasma levels of active renin may be raised [99], even in cases with thoracic tumors which do not involve the kidney. Neuroblastoma cell lines contain all components of the RAS, including renin *in vitro* [100]. Whether or not neuroblastoma secretes renin *in vivo* is uncertain, but such tumors could cause hyperreninism via the secretion of catecholamines. In pheochromocytoma, there is often juxtaglomerular hyperplasia in the renal cortex (see *Chapter 67*). This suggests that the raised plasma renin levels could likewise be due to stimulation of the JGA by catecholamines secreted by the tumor.

Functioning parathyroid tumors [101], tumors that cause Cushing's syndrome [102], and angiotensinogen-secreting hepatocellular carcinoma [103] (*Chapter 8*) have all been associated with high plasma renin levels, although the mechanisms are often unclear. This emphasizes the necessity to adhere to the criteria for the diagnosis of primary reninism as outlined above.

RENIN SECRETION IN NORMAL AND NEOPLASTIC TISSUES

THE NATURE OF RENIN-SECRETING CELLS IN TUMORS

In JGCT, and in most extrarenal tumors, the cells that secrete renin are undoubtedly tumor cells. In nephroblastoma and in renal cell carcinoma, some renin-secreting cells are also tumor cells. However, other perivascular renin-secreting cells in some tumors do not resemble the adjacent tumor cells (Plate 49, see Color Plate Section). It is likely, but by no means certain, that they are also tumor cells which have differentiated into renin-secreting cells. Tumors induce blood vessels and stroma to grow into them, and stromal cells such as smooth-muscle cells [104]

and endothelial cells [105] can secrete renin *in vitro*. It therefore remains possible that some perivascular renin-secreting cells could be stromal cells which have been induced to secrete renin by tumor cells. Clinical studies designed to assess autonomy of secretion of these malignant tumors are indicated as are experiments designed to study the phenotypes of renin-secreting cells cultured from these tumors.

THE NATURE OF RENIN SECRETED BY TUMORS

At present, all techniques used have suggested that tumor renin is similar to normal renal renin and prorenin [106] (*Chapters 4 and 6*). It is simply secreted in excess and in an unregulated fashion. Analysis of the upstream controlling sequences show that the excess transcription in JGCT is not due to a structural abnormality of the 5' part of the renin gene [107]. As with normal kidney renin, the biosynthesis of renin in JGCT cells also involves a precursor prorenin [106]. Plasma prorenin levels have shown promise as tumor markers in nephroblastoma and perhaps in other tumors. One preliminary study has suggested a gross error in renin gene transcription in a case of nephroblastoma [63]; more subtle abnormalities are clearly possible. The identification of a specific 'tumor renin' or prorenin is an exciting prospect.

In a case of suspected renin-secreting tumor, it is therefore important to make best use of the excised tissue, some of which must be processed immediately for molecular and cell-culture studies. To subject the tissues to thorough investigation without jeopardizing the priorities of obtaining adequate material for diagnosis requires co-operation between clinician, pathologist, and scientist. Examples of the optimal use of tumor tissue are described by Conn *et al* [1] and Anderson *et al* [96].

CONCLUSIONS

Renin-secreting tumors present the clinician with the opportunity to study pure renin-dependent hypertension in man. Culture of the renin-secreting cells derived from them have provided useful systems to study the biosynthesis and processing of renin in human tissues. The application of modern techniques of cell and molecular biology will establish whether the renin-secreting cells in tumors are tumor cells or stromal cells, or both. The transcription of the renin gene by tumor cells, the processing of the transcripts, and the intracellular pathways traveled by the precursor renin molecule during its processing and secretion, will be elucidated. Molecular studies may also be able to distinguish tumor renin from nontumor renin. Renin-secreting tumors remain a challenging area of research for the scientist, the pathologist, and the clinician.

REFERENCES

1. Conn JW, Cohen EL, Lucas CP, McDonald WJ, Mayor GH, Blough WM, Eveland WC, Bookstein JJ, Lapides J. Primary reninism. Hypertension, hyperreninemia and secondary aldosteronism due to renin-producing juxtaglomerular-cell tumors. *Archives of Internal Medicine* 1972;**130**:682–96.

2. Robertson PW, Klidjian A, Harding LK, Walters G, Lee MR, Robb-Smith AHT. Hypertension due to a renin-secreting renal tumour. *American Journal of Medicine* 1967;**43**:963–76.

3. Kihara I, Kitamura S, Hoshino T, Seida H, Watanabe T. A hitherto unreported vascular tumor of the kidney: A proposal of 'juxtaglomerular cell tumor'. *Acta Pathologica Japonica* 1968;**18**:197–206.

4. Eddy RL, Sanchez SA. Renin-secreting renal neoplasm and hypertension with hypokalemia. *Annals of Internal Medicine* 1971;**75**:725–9.

5. Bonnin JM, Hodge RL, Lumbers ER. A renin-secreting renal tumour associated with hypertension. *Australian and New Zealand Journal of Medicine* 1972;**2**:178–81.

6. Schambelan M, Howes EL, Stockigt JR, Noakes CA, Biglieri EG. Role of renin and aldosterone in hypertension due to a renin-secreting tumor. *American Journal of Medicine* 1973;**55**:86–92.

7. Brown JJ, Fraser R, Lever AF, Morton JJ, Robertson JIS, Tree M, Bell PRF, Davidson JK, Ruthven IS. Hypertension and secondary hyperaldosteronism associated with a renin-secreting renal juxtaglomerular cell tumour. *Lancet* 1973;**ii**:1228–32.

8. Gherardi GJ, Arya S, Hickler RB. Juxtaglomerular body tumor: A rare occult but curable cause of lethal hypertension. *Human Pathology* 1974;**5**:236–40.

9. Orjavik OS, Aas M, Fauchald P, Hovig T, Oystese B, Brodwall EK, Flatmark A. Renin-secreting renal tumor with severe hypertension. *Acta Medica Scandinavica* 1975;**197**:329–35.

10. Connor G, Bennett CM, Lindstrom RR, Brosman SA, Barajas L, Edelbaum D. Juxtaglomerular cell tumor. *Nephron* 1978;**21**:325–33.

11. Hirose M, Arakawa A, Kikuchi M, Kawasaki T, Omoto T, Kato H, Nagayama T. Primary reninism with renal hamartomatous alteration of the kidney. *Journal of the American Medical Association* 1974;**230**:1288–92.

12. Takahashi T, Miura T, Sue A, Saito K, Sakaue M, Yamagata Y, Fukuchi S, Sato Z, Hirai T, Terashima K, Oka K, Imai Y. A case of juxtaglomerular cell tumor diagnosed preoperatively. *Nephron* 1976;**17**:483–95.

13. Bonnin JM, Cain MD, Jose JS, Mukherjee TM, Perrett LV, Scroop GC, Seymour AE. Hypertension due to a renin-secreting tumour localized by segmental renal vein sampling. *Australian and New Zealand Journal of Medicine* 1977;**7**:630–5.

14. Mimran A, Leckie BJ, Fourcade JC, Baldet P, Navratil H, Barjon P. Blood pressure, renin–angiotensin system and urinary kallikrein in a case of juxtaglomerular cell tumor. *American Journal of Medicine* 1978;**65**:527–36.

15. Hanna W, Tepperman B, Logan AG, Robinette MA, Colapinto R, Phillips MJ. Juxtaglomerular cell tumor (reninoma) with paroxysmal hypertension. *Canadian Medical Association Journal* 1979;**120**:957–9.

16. Valdes G, Lopez JM, Martinez P, Rosenberg H, Barriga P, Rodriguez JA, Otipka N. Renin-secreting tumor. *Hypertension* 1980;**2**:714–8.

17. Camilleri J-P, Hinglais N, Bruneval P, Bariety J, Tricottet V, Rouchon M, Mancilla–Jimenez R, Corvol P, Menard J. Renin storage and cell differentiation in juxtaglomerular cell tumors. *Human Pathology* 1984;**15**:1069–79.

18. El-Matri A, Slim R, Hamida CH, Chadli A, Ben Maiz H, Haddad S, Milliez P, Camilleri JP, Zmerli S, Ben Ayed H. Hypertension artérielle secondaire a une 'tumeur a rénine'. *Nouvelle Presse Médicale* 1980;**9**:157–9.

19. Tetu B, Totovic V, Bechtelsheimer H, Smend J. Tumeur rénale a secrétion de rénine. *Annales de Pathologie* 1984;**4**:55–9.

20. Squires JP, Ulbright TM, Deschryver-Kecskemeti K, Engleman W. Juxtaglomerular cell tumor of the kidney. *Cancer* 1984;**53**:516–23.

21. Moss AH, Peterson LJ, Scott CW, Winter K, Olin DB, Garber RL. Delayed diagnosis of juxtaglomerular cell tumor hypertension. *North Carolina Medical Journal* 1982;**43**:705–7.

22. Baruch D, Corvol P, Alhenc-Gelas F, Dufloux MA, Guyenne TT, Gaux JC, Raynaud A, Brisset JM, Duclos JM, Ménard J. Diagnosis and treatment of renin-secreting tumors. *Hypertension* 1984;**6**:760–6.

23. Dennis RL, McDougal WS, Glick AD, MacDonell RC. Juxtaglomerular cell tumor of the kidney. *Journal of Urology* 1985;**134**:334–8.

24. Jordon JM, Gunnells JC. Juxtaglomerular apparatus tumor: A rare but curable cause of secondary hypertension. *Southern Medical Journal* 1985;**78**:1353–7.

25. Hermus ARMM, Pieters GFFM, Lamers APM, Smals AGH, Hanselaar AGJM, Van Haelst UJG, Kloppenborg PWC. Hypertension and hypokalaemia due to a renin-secreting kidney tumour. *Netherlands Journal of Medicine* 1986;**29**:84–91.

26. Handa N, Fukunaga R, Yoneda S, Kimura K, Kamada T, Ichikawa Y, Takaha M, Sonoda T, Tokunaga K, Juroda C, Onishi S. State of systemic hemodynamics in a case of juxtaglomerular cell tumor. *Clinical and Experimental Hypertension. Part A, Theory and Practice* 1986;**A8**:1–19.

27. Martinez-Amenos A, Carreras L, Rama H, Romero M, Sarrias X, Alsina J. Tumor de celulas del aparto juxtaglomerular secretor de renina. *Medicina Clinica* 1987;**88**:157–9.

28. Corvol P, Pinet F, Galen FX, Plouin PF, Chatellier G, Pagny JY, Corvol MT, Ménard J. Seven lessons from seven renin-secreting tumors. *Kidney International* 1988;**34** (suppl 25):S38–44.

29. Gordon RD, Tunny TJ, Klemm SA, Finn WL, Hawkins PJ, Hunyor SJ, Norris JJ. A renin-secreting tumour sensitive to central blood volume but not to circulating angiotensin II. *Clinical and Experimental Pharmacology and Physiology* 1990;**17**:185–9.

30. Lam ASC, Bedard YC, Buckspan MB, Logan AG, Steinhardt MI. Surgically curable hypertension associated with reninoma. *Journal of Urology* 1982;**128**:572–5.

31. Pedrinelli R, Graziadei L, Taddei S, Lenzi M, Magagna A, Bevilacqua G, Salvetti A. A renin-secreting tumor. *Nephron* 1987;**46**:380–5.

32. Duprez D, De Smet H, Roels H, Clement D. Hypertension due to a renal renin-secreting tumour. *Journal of Human Hypertension* 1990;**4**:59–61.

33. Ducret F, Pointet P, Lambert C, Pin J, Baret M, Botta JM, Mutin M, Colon S, Vincent M. Tumeur a rénine et hypertension artérielle sévère. *Nephrologie* 1991;**12**:17–24.

34. Barajas L, Bennett CM, Connor G, Lindstrom RR. Structure of a glomerular cell tumor: The presence of a neural component. *Laboratory Investigation* 1977;**37**:357–68.

35. Phillips G, Mukherjee TM. Juxtaglomerular cell tumour: Light and electron microscopic studies of a renin-secreting kidney tumour containing both juxtaglomerular cells and mast cells. *Pathology* 1972;**4**:193–204.

36. Weiss JP, Pollack HM, McCormick JF, Malloy TM, Hanno PM, Carpiniello VL. Renal hemangiopericytoma: Surgical, radiological and pathological implications. *Journal of Urology* 1984;**132**:337–42.

37. More IAR, Jackson AM, MacSween RNM. Renin-secreting tumor associated with hypertension. *Cancer* 1974;**34**:2093–102.

38. Lindop GBM, Stewart JA, Downie TT. The immunocytochemical demonstration of renin in a juxtaglomerular cell tumour by light and electron microscopy. *Histopathology* 1983;**7**:421–31.

39. Holman ND, Donker AJM, Van Der Meer J. Disappearance of renin-induced proteinuria by an ACE-inhibitor: A case report. *Clinical Nephrology* 1990;**34**:70–1.

40. Eisenbach GM, van Liew JB, Boylan JW. Effects of angiotensin in the filtration of protein in the rat kidney. *Kidney International* 1975;**8**:80–7.

41. Brand G, Beilin LJ, Vandongen R, Matz L. Juxtaglomerular tumour: Diagnostic renal vein renin measurements obscured by chronic captopril therapy. *Australian and New Zealand Journal of Medicine* 1985;**15**:755–7.

42. Bruneval P, Fournier J-G, Soubrier F, Belair M-F, da Silva J-L, Guettier C, Pinet F, Tardivel I, Corvol P, Bariety J, Camilleri J-P. Detection and localization of renin messenger RNA in human pathologic tissues using *in situ* hybridization. *American Journal of Pathology* 1988;**131**:320–30.

43. Galen FX, Devaux C, Houot AM, Menard J, Corvol P, Corvol MT, Gubler MC, Mounier F, Camilleri JP. Renin biosynthesis by tumoral juxtaglomerular cells. *Journal of Clinical Investigation* 1984;73:1144–55.

44. Ledlie EM, Mynors LS, Draper GJ, Gorbach PD. Natural history and treatment of Wilms' tumours: An analysis of 335 cases of Wilms' tumour occurring in England and Wales 1962–6. *British Medical Journal* 1970;4:195–200.

45. Staszewski J. Cancer of the kidney: International mortality patterns and trends. *WHO Statistics Quarterly* 1988;33:42–9.

46. Roth DR, Wright J, Cawood Jr CD, Pranke DW. Nephroblastoma in adults. *Journal of Urology* 1984;132:108–10.

47. Pritchard-Jones K, Fleming S, Davidson D, Bickmore W, Porteous D, Gosden C, Bard J, Buckler A, Pelletier J, Housman D, van Heyningen V, Hastie N. The candidate Wilms' tumour gene is involved in genitourinary development. *Nature* 1991;346:194–7.

48. Weinberg R. Tumour suppressor genes. *Science* 1991;254:1138–46.

49. Sukarochana W, Tolentino W, Kiesewetter WB. Wilms' tumour and hypertension. *Journal of Pediatric Surgery* 1972;7:573–8.

50. Bradley JE, Pincoffs MC. The association of adeno-myosarcoma of the kidney (Wilms' tumour) with arterial hypertension. *Annals of Internal Medicine* 1938;11:1613–28.

51. Bradley JE, Drake ME. The effect of preoperative roentgen-ray therapy on arterial hypertension in embryoma (kidney). *Journal of Pediatrics* 1949;35:710–4.

52. Mitchell JD, Baxter TJ, Blair-West JR, McCredie DA. Renin levels in nephroblastoma (Wilms' tumour). *Archives of Diseases of Childhood* 1970;45:376–84.

53. Masovari I, Kontor E, Kallay K. Renin-secreting Wilms' tumour. *Lancet* 1972;i:1180.

54. Ganguly A, Gribble J, Tune B, Kempson RL, Luetscher JA. Renin secreting Wilms' tumor with severe hypertension. *Annals of Internal Medicine* 1973;79:835–7.

55. Sheth KJ, Tang TT, Blaedel ME, Good TA. Polydipsia, polyuria and hypertension associated with renin-secreting Wilms' tumour. *Journal of Pediatrics* 1978;92:921–4.

56. Luciana J-C, Baldet P, Dumas R, Jean R. Etude du systeme renine–angiotensine dans deux cas de tumeur de Wilms avec hypertension arterielle severe. *Archives Francaises de Pediatrie* 1979;36:240–9.

57. Spahr J, Demers LM, Sochat SJ. Renin producing Wilms' tumor. *Journal of Pediatric Surgery* 1981;16:32–4.

58. Yokomori K, Hori T, Takemura T, Tsuchida Y. Demonstration of both primary and secondary reninism in renal tumours in children. *Journal of Pediatric Surgery* 1988;23:403–9.

59. Day RP, Leutscher JA. Big renin: A possible prohormone in kidney and plasma of a patient with Wilms' tumor. *Journal of Clinical Endocrinology and Metabolism* 1974;38:923–6.

60. Carachi R, Lindop GBM, Leckie BJ. Inactive renin: A tumour marker in nephroblastoma. *Journal of Pediatric Surgery* 1987;22:278–80.

61. Lindop GBM, Fleming S, Gibson AAM. Immunocytochemical localisation of renin in nephroblastoma. *Journal of Clinical Pathology* 1984;37:738–42.

62. Lindop GBM, Millan DWM, Murray D, Gibson AAM, McIntyre GD, Leckie BJ. Immunocytochemistry of renin in renal tumours. *Clinical and Experimental Hypertension. Part A, Theory and Practice* 1987;A9:1305–23.

63. Lindop GBM, Duncan K, Millan DWM, Gibson AAM, Patrick WJA, Leckie BJ, Birnie GD. Renin gene expression in nephroblastoma. *Journal of Pathology* 1990;161:93–7.

64. Inglis GC, Leckie BJ. Renin production by nephroblastoma cells in culture. *American Journal of Hypertension* 1990;3:148–50.

65. Muir CS, Nectoux J. Geographical distribution and aetiology of kidney cancer. In: Suffrin G, Beckley JA, eds. *Renal adenocarcinoma*. Geneva: UICC, 1980:133–46.

66. Millan JC. Tumours of the kidney. In: Hill GS, ed. *Uropathology*. New York: Churchill Livingstone, 1989:23–701.

67. Hollifield JW, Page DL, Smith C, Michelakis AM, Staab E, Rhamy R. Renin-secreting clear cell carcinoma of the kidney. *Archives of Internal Medicine* 1975;135:859–64.

68. Lebel M, Talbot J, Grose J, Morin J. Adenocarcinoma of the kidney and hypertension: Report of 2 cases with special emphasis on renin. *Journal of Urology* 1977;118:923–7.

69. Lindop GBM, Leckie BJ, Winearls CG. Malignant hypertension due to a renin-secreting renal cell carcinoma — an ultrastructural and immunocytochemical study. *Histopathology* 1986;10:1077–88.

70. Leckie B, Brown JJ, Fraser R, Kyle K, Lever AF, Morton JJ, Robertson JIS. A renal carcinoma secreting inactive renin. *Clinical Science* 1978;55 (suppl):159–615.

71. Steffens J, Bock R, Braedel HU, Isenberg E, Bührle CP, Ziegler M. Renin-producing renal cell carcinoma. *European Urology* 1990;18:56–60.

72. Tomita T, Poisner A, Inagami T. Immunohistochemical localisation of renin in renal tumours. *American Journal of Pathology* 1987;126:73–80.

73. Lindop GBM, Fleming S. Renin in renal cell carcinoma — an immunocytochemical study using an antibody to pure human renin. *Journal of Clinical Pathology* 1984;37:27–31.

74. Lindop GBM, More IAR, Leckie BJ. An ultrastructural and immunocytochemical study of a renal carcinoma secreting inactive renin. *Journal of Clinical Pathology* 1983;36:639–45.

75. Leckie BJ, McIntyre GD, Millan WD, Lindop GBM, Carachi R. Renin and inactive renin (prorenin) in the plasma of patients with malignant renal tumours. *Clinical and Experimental Hypertension. Part A Theory and Practice* 1987;A9:1325–32.

76. Bauer JH, Durham J, Miles J. Congenital mesoplastic nephroma presenting with primary reninism. *Journal of Pediatrics* 1984;95:268–72.

77. Malone PS, Duffy PG, Ransley PG, Risdon RA, Cook T, Taylor M. Congenital mesoblastic nephroma, renin production and hypertension. *Journal of Pediatric Surgery* 1989;24:599–603.

78. Yokimori K, Hori T, Takamura T, Tsuchida Y. Demonstration of both primary and secondary reninism in renal tumours in children. *Journal of Pediatric Surgery* 1988;23:403–9.

79. Cook HT, Taylor GM, Malone P, Risdon RA. Renin in mesoblastic nephroma — an immunohistochemical study. *Human Pathology* 1988;19:1347–51.

80. Taylor M, Cook T, Pearson C, Risdon RA, Pearl S. Renin messenger RNA localisation in congenital mesoblastic nephroma using *in situ* hybridisation. *Journal of Hypertension* 1989;7:733–40.

81. Yum M, Ganguly A, Donohue JP. Juxtaglomerular cells in renal angiomyolipoma. *Urology* 1984;24:283–6.

82. Hauger-Klevene JH. High plasma renin activity in an oat cell carcinoma: A renin-secreting carcinoma? *Cancer* 1970;26:1112–4.

83. Genest J, Rojo-Ortega JM, Kuchel O, Boucher R, Nowaczynski W, Lefebvre R, Chretien M, Cantin J, Granger P. Malignant hypertension with hypokalemia in a patient with renin-producing pulmonary carcinoma. *Transactions of the Association of American Physicians* 1975;88:192–201.

84. Ruddy MC, Atlas SA, Salerno FG. Hypertension associated with a renin-secreting adenocarcinoma of the pancreas. *New England Journal of Medicine* 1982;307:993–7.

85. Saito T, Fukamizu A, Okada K, Ishikawa S-E, Iwamoto Y,Kuzuya T, Kawai T, Naruse K, Hirose S, Murakami K. Ectopic production of renin by ileal carcinoma. *Endocrinologica Japonica* 1989;36:117–24.

86. Iimura O, Shimamoto K, Hotta D, Nakata T, Mito T, Kumamoto Y, Dempo K, Ogihara T, Naruse K. A case of adrenal tumor producing renin, aldosterone and sex hormones. *Hypertension* 1986;8:951–6.

87. Aurell M, Rudin A, Rudin A, Kindblom L, Tisell L, Derkx F, Schalekamp M. A case of renin-producing non-renal tumour and the effect of treatment with captopril. In: Blaufox MD, Bianchi C, eds. *Secondary forms of hypertension*. New York: Grune & Stratton, 1981:179–85.

88. Atlas SA, Sherman RL, Parmantier MW, Taufield D, Sealey JA, Laragh JH. Responses of active and inactive renins, aldosterone and blood pressure to chemotherapy in a patient with a possible renin-secreting tumor. *Clinical Research* 1982;**30**:333A.

89. Ehrlich EN, Dominguez OV, Samuels LT, Lynch D, Oberhelman H, Warner NE. Aldosteronism and precocious puberty due to an ovarian androblastoma (Sertoli cell tumor). *Journal of Clinical Endocrinology and Metabolism* 1963;**23**:358–67.

90. Korzets A, Nouriel H, Steiner Z, Griffel B, Kraus L, Freund U, Klajman A. Resistant hypertension associated with a renin-producing ovarian Sertoli cell tumor. *American Journal of Clinical Pathology* 1986;**85**:242–7.

91. Tetu B, Lebel M, Camilleri JP. Renin-producing ovarian tumour. A case with immunohistochemical and electron microscopic study. *American Journal of Surgical Pathology* 1988;**12**:634–40.

92. Morris BJ, Pinet F, Michel J-B, Soubrier F, Corvol P. Renin secretion from malignant pulmonary metastatic tumour cells of vascular origin. *Clinical and Experimental Pharmacology and Physiology* 1987;**14**:227–31.

93. Cox JN, Paunier L, Vallotton MB, Humbert JR, Rohner A. Epithelial liver hamartoma, systemic arterial hypertension and renin hypersecretion. *Virchows Archiv. A, Pathological Anatomy and Histology* 1975;**336**:15–26.

94. Yokoyama H, Yamane Y, Takahara J, Yoshinouchi T, Ofuji T. A case of ectopic renin-secreting orbital hemangiopericytoma associated with juvenile hypertension and hypokalemia. *Acta Medica Okoyama* 1979;**33**:315–22.

95. Chauveau D, Julien J, Pagny J-Y, Jeunemaitre X, Bruneval P, Guyenne TT, Le Chevalier T, Plouin P-F, Corvol P. Epithelioid sarcoma of soft tissues: A case report of extrarenal renin-secreting tumour. *Journal of Human Hypertension* 1988;**2**:261–4.

96. Anderson PW, MacAuley L, Yung SD, Sherrod A, d'Ablaing G, Koss M, Shinagawa T, Tran B, Montz J, Hsueh WA. Extrarenal renin-secreting tumors: Insights into hypertension and ovarian renin production. *Medicine* 1989;**68**:257–68.

97. Fromme M, Streicher E, Kraus B, Kruse–Jarres J. Arterial hypertension associated with a renin-producing retroperitoneal leiomyosarcoma. *Klinische Wochenschrift* 1985;**63**:158–63.

98. Geddy PM, Main J. Renin-secreting retroperitoneal leiomyosarcoma: An unusual cause of hypertension. *Journal of Human Hypertension* 1990;**4**:57–8.

99. Leckie BJ, Carachi R, Wheldon T, Lindop GBM. Plasma renin levels in patients with thoracic neuroblastoma. *Journal of Pediatric Surgery* 1989;**24**:601–3.

100. Okamura T, Clemens DL, Inagami T. Renin, angiotensins, and angiotensin-converting enzyme in neuroblastoma cells: Evidence for intracellular formation of angiotensins. *Proceedings of the National Academy of Sciences of the USA* 1981;**78**:6940–3.

101. Naomi S, Umeda T, Iwaoki T, Sato T, Uemura K. A case of functioning parathyroid carcinoma with hyperreninemic hypertension. *Japanese Journal of Medicine* 1983;**22**:129–33.

102. Jacob C, Menage J-J, Bagros P, Choutet P, Neel J-L. Hypercorticisme paraneoplastique. Hypokaliemie, hypoaldosteronisme au cours d'un cancer du pancreas. *Nouvelle Presse Medicale* 1984;**3**:1805–8.

103. Ueno N, Yoshida K, Hirose S, Yokoyama H, Uchara H, Murakami K. Angiotensinogen-producing hepatocellular carcinoma. *Hypertension* 1984;**16**:931–3.

104. Re RJ, Fallon V, Dzau V, Quay SC, Haber E. Renin synthesis by canine aortic smooth muscle cells in culture. *Life Sciences* 1982;**30**:99–106.

105. Lilly LS, Pratt RE, Alexander RW, Larson DM, Ellison KE, Gumbrone MA, Dzau VJ. Renin expression by vascular endothelial cells in culture. *Circulation Research* 1985;**57**:312–8.

106. Soubrier F, Devaux C, Galen F-X, Skinner SL, Aurell M, Genest J, Menard J, Corvol P. Biochemical and immunological characterisation of ectopic tumoral renin. *Journal of Clinical Endocrinology and Metabolism* 1982;**54**:139–44.

107. Fukamizu A, Nishi K, Mishimatsu SC, Miyazaki H, Hirose S, Murakami K. Human renin gene of renin-secreting tumour. *Gene* 1986;**49**:139–45.

55 RENIN AND THE PATHOPHYSIOLOGY OF RENOVASCULAR HYPERTENSION

J IAN S ROBERTSON

INTRODUCTION

In 1934, [1] Goldblatt and his colleagues published the results of a classical study in which they showed that experimental constriction of a renal artery could lead to sustained systemic hypertension (Fig. 55.1).

Goldblatt *et al* characterized particularly what came to be known as the 1-kidney, 1-clip and the 2-kidney, 2-clip models of experimental hypertension. They also described 2-kidney, 1-clip hypertension, but noted that the blood-pressure increase in this form was less consistent, less severe, and more often only transient.

Their original concept was that such investigations would illuminate pathogenetic aspects of primary ('essential') hypertension; indeed, at that time, human clinical renovascular hypertension was not clearly perceived. Moreover, Goldblatt *et al* did not at first recognize the possible relevance of their work to the

RAS [2], which had been discovered by Tigerstedt and Bergman in 1898 [3] (see *Chapter 1*). Nevertheless, there was a resultant enthusiastic revival of interest in the RAS [4–6], in which Goldblatt joined [2]. Shortly after, the clinical syndrome of renovascular hypertension was defined [7], with the further recognition that the high blood pressure could be lowered in man either by relief of a responsible pathological renal artery constriction, or by excision of the kidney distal to the stenotic renal artery [10]. Consequently, emphasis shifted from essential hypertension to renovascular hypertension, and from this, the present extensive knowledge of the RAS and its ramifications grew.

Even so, the passage of more than 50 years since the historic experiments of Goldblatt and his colleagues, and intense laboratory and clinical studies, have so far failed to define clearly the role of the RAS in the pathogenesis of the various forms of renovascular hypertension. Some writers have expressed scepticism concerning any important participation by the RAS in the pathophysiology of renovascular hypertension [8]. More often, and contrariwise, authors refer to hypertension accompanying a

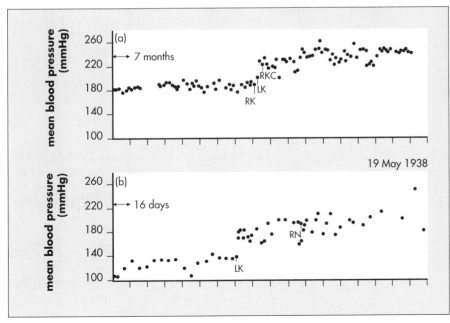

Fig. 55.1 Two illustrative experiments from Goldblatt H *et al* [1]. (a) Effect on blood pressure of bilateral moderate constriction of the renal arteries in the dog. (b) Effect of unilateral renal artery constriction followed by contralateral nephrectomy. RK = moderate constriction of right renal artery; LK = moderate constriction of left renal artery; RKC = occlusion of right renal artery; and RN = right nephrectomy.

renal arterial lesion as 'renin dependent' without evincing any evident comprehension of pathogenesis.

This chapter represents an attempt to expound these often complex, difficult, and still in several respects controversial, issues.

Since, as will be seen, changes in sodium balance can have important influence in various forms of renovascular hypertension, and since hypertension can be produced experimentally in the rat simply by sodium restriction, this latter form of hypertension is also considered in this chapter.

TERMINOLOGY

The terminology of the several forms of experimental Goldblatt hypertension is as follows:

- **2-kidney, 1-clip hypertension**
  One kidney with a main renal artery constriction, the other intact.
- **1-kidney, 1-clip hypertension**
  One kidney removed, the other with renal artery constriction.
- **2-kidney, 2-clip hypertension**
  Both renal arteries constricted.

'Unclipping' and 'unclipped' refer to the removal of a previous experimental renal artery constriction [9]. It is important to avoid the confusion sometimes perpetrated by wrongly using the term 'unclipped' when 'untouched' or 'intact' is intended.

All three of the above forms of Goldblatt experimental hypertension have their clinical counterparts, most often from atherosclerotic (Color Plate 17) or fibromuscular dysplastic renal arterial disease, but also from a wide range of other lesions that can constrict a renal artery or its branches [10] (see *Chapters 60, 67,* and *88–90*). The 2-kidney, 1-clip model is that most often represented clinically. Requiring emphasis is that the conjunction of a clinical renal artery lesion with systemic hypertension does not establish the entity of 'renovascular hypertension'. Confirmation of the diagnosis requires demonstration of relief of the hypertension following correction of the renal arterial narrowing or excision of the afflicted kidney [10,11].

A wide range of unilateral renal diseases, including for example, tumors and cysts, can cause clinical hypertension, often corrected if the kidney bearing the lesion is removed [10]. It is likely that these share a common pathophysiological etiology, via renal ischemia, and thus are akin to 2-kidney, 1-clip hypertension [10].

The special example of adult polycystic renal disease (Color Plate 23), and its uncertain relationship to the RAS, are considered in *Chapter 57*. Hypertension due to renin-secreting tumor is discussed in *Chapter 54*.

Renal hypertension can be produced by cellophane wrapping of the kidney [12]; a clinical counterpart of this experimental model ('Page kidney') has been described following the development of perinephric fibrosis [13]. Hypertension can also be caused experimentally by applying a figure-of-8 ligature around the kidney [14].

INVOLVEMENT OF THE RENIN–ANGIOTENSIN SYSTEM IN THE PATHOGENESIS OF GOLDBLATT HYPERTENSION

The pressor effect of a given dose of Ang II is directly proportional to the body sodium status [15] (see *Chapters 28* and *33*). Thus, consideration and interpretation of the pattern of changes in renin and Ang II during the development of renovascular hypertension are facilitated by information on the concurrent state of body sodium content; this aspect is covered later in this chapter.

Since the evolutionary changes in both the RAS and body sodium, as well as of other participating factors, differ substantially between the different models, these models, together with their clinical counterparts, are considered separately.

TWO-KIDNEY, ONE-CLIP HYPERTENSION

Two-kidney, one-clip hypertension is the form that is most often encountered in man. It has been extensively studied in various experimental animals, especially the dog and the rat. Although some early workers held that 2-kidney, 1-clip hypertension did not readily develop in the rabbit [4], it has been described also in that species [16].

In 1976, a schema was set out [17] in which an attempt was made to describe the evolution of 2-kidney, 1-clip hypertension in relationship to changes in the RAS. This still appears to retain useful validity. In this schema, the course of the disease was divided arbitrarily into three phases (Fig. 55.2). Phase I is seen usually only in the experimental animal. Within minutes of the application of a renal artery constriction, there is a rise of arterial pressure which parallels a rise in circulating renin and Ang II. If the renal artery constriction is relieved, or if the kidney beyond the constriction is removed, there is,

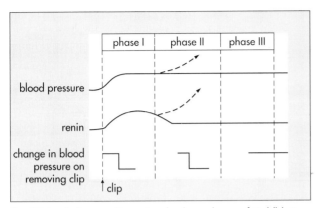

Fig. 55.2 A diagram illustrating the three phases of Goldblatt 2-kidney, 1-clip hypertension. The arrows in phase II indicate the course in the hyponatremic hypertensive syndrome. Modified from Robertson JIS *et al* [18].

equally promptly, a fall in both renin and Ang II in blood, accompanied by a fall in blood pressure to control values.

Within days or weeks, depending on the species, this first phase is succeeded by a second phase, in which, although the blood pressure remains elevated, there is less marked elevation of renin and Ang II. This at least partial dissociation between the hypertension and stimulation of the RAS has led to doubts about the continued relevance of renin to pathogenesis in the second phase. Nevertheless, in phase II, the hypertension can still be relieved either by correction of the renal artery stenosis or by removal of the affected kidney. Occasionally, in phase II, in a minority of patients and in some experimental animals with a very severe unilateral renal artery stenosis, there is progressive and severe elevation of renin and Ang II accompanied by increasing hypertension (Fig. 55.2). This is the hyponatremic hypertensive syndrome which is described in detail later in this chapter (see also *Chapter 88*).

If phase II renovascular hypertension does not progress to the severe hyponatremic syndrome, there will be a very gradual progression over many months or years to phase III. In phase III, although the blood pressure remains high, there is no longer clear elevation of renin or Ang II (although some dispute this). Phase III of experimental renovascular hypertension in the rat has been extensively considered by Floyer [9]. Relief of the renal artery stenosis does not in phase III reduce the arterial pressure, although it can be corrected if the contralateral kidney is subsequently removed. It appears that the sustained hypertension in the late third phase is due to hypertension-induced changes in the contralateral kidney. Some investigators [17,18] consider that these lesions in the contralateral kidney do not mediate hypertension via the circulating RAS; yet others [19] believe that the RAS is involved. Clearly, phase III is important to recognize

clinically, because then ill-judged surgical adventures can be unrewarding.

EVOLUTION OF CHANGES IN BLOOD PRESSURE AND IN THE RENIN–ANGIOTENSIN SYSTEM

Rat

The evolution of renovascular hypertension has been followed in some detail in relationship to the RAS in 2-kidney, 1-clip hypertension in the rat [20] In animals subjected to a sham-clipping operation, no change was observed in blood pressure, or in plasma active renin concentration or Ang II up to 20 weeks after the procedure (Fig. 55.3). In rats in which a constricting clip had been placed on one renal artery, blood pressure was elevated as early as the first and second days after operation, in parallel with a rise in the peripheral plasma concentrations of active renin and Ang II. However, in the second and third weeks after clipping, although the blood pressure remained high, both active renin and Ang II fell back from the early high levels towards or into the upper part of the normal range. From the fourth week onwards, there was on average, another, and often quite marked, rise in arterial pressure which was sustained for the remainder of the 20 weeks of the experiment. This secondary rise in blood pressure was accompanied by a further increase in the average levels of active renin and Ang II. It deserves emphasis, nevertheless, that even in the late stages after clipping, individual rats were seen in which the blood-pressure elevation remained more modest and in which the circulating levels of renin and Ang II lay within or just above the upper limits of the normal range.

When the relationship between Ang II and arterial pressure was examined on the first and second days after the application of the clip, there was seen to be a significant positive correlation between Ang II and arterial pressure (Fig. 55.4). In rats studied between 8 and 20 weeks after clipping, there was similarly a highly significant positive correlation between plasma Ang II and arterial pressure. However, in the rats with established later hypertension, the pressor dose–response curve had been shifted upwards; similar findings have been reported also by Hutchinson *et al* [21]. The lower relationship, that seen on the first and second days after application of the clip, corresponded almost exactly to the acute pressor dose–response curve of Ang II administered to normal rats. If, at these two stages after clipping in the rat, circulating Ang II concentration was altered, either upwards by infusion of the peptide or downwards by the administration of an ACE inhibitor, Ang II and blood pressure moved also the respective regression lines shown in Fig. 55.4.

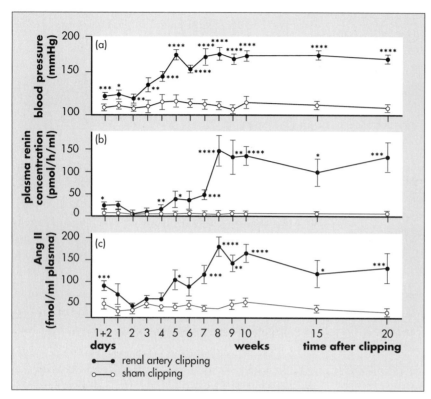

Fig. 55.3 Changes in blood pressure (a), plasma active renin concentration (b), and plasma Ang II concentration (c) in the 2-kidney, 1-clip rat, after renal artery clipping or sham clipping. Significance levels of differences from sham-clip group: *$P<0.05$, **$P<0.02$, ***$P<0.01$, ****$P<0.001$. Modified from Morton JJ and Wallace ECH [20].

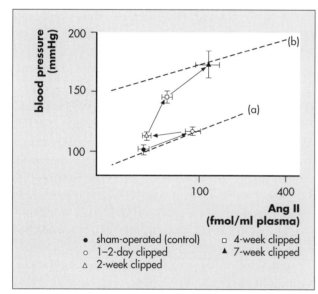

Fig. 55.4 Progressive changes in Ang II and blood pressure during the onset, development, and establishment of hypertension in the 2-kidney, 1-clip hypertensive rat in relation to the upward parallel shift in the Ang II/blood-pressure regression line from that found for acute (a) (1–2 days) hypertensive rats to that found for chronic (b) (8–20 weeks) hypertensive rats. Values are shown as the mean ± SEM for all sham-operated rats, 1–2 day clipped rats, two-week clipped rats, four-week clipped rats, and seven-week clipped rats. Modifed from Morton JJ and Wallace ECH [20].

Dog

Caravaggi *et al* [22] examined the acute effects of unilateral renal artery constriction in trained conscious dogs, the opposite kidney and renal artery remaining untouched. Such renal artery constriction led to an immediate rise in circulating plasma renin concentration (PRC) and Ang II, paralleled by an increase in arterial pressure. Acute infusion of exogenous Ang II into these same dogs when the renal artery was not constricted caused an immediate increase in arterial pressure. The relationships between the arterial blood pressure and plasma Ang II concentration following renal artery constriction and with Ang II infusion were almost identical (Fig. 55.5). Thus, in the dog, as in the rat, the early increase in blood pressure following renal artery constriction in this model (phase I) appears to be fully explained by the immediate direct pressor action of the rise in peripheral arterial concentration of Ang II.

The later course of changes in blood pressure and the RAS in 2-kidney, 1-clip hypertension in the dog have been studied by several groups, most notably by Bianchi *et al* [23] and Anderson *et al* [24,25]. Bianchi *et al* [23] found, within one week of the application of a unilateral renal artery constriction, that, while blood pressure remained high, PRC was less markedly so than initially. Thus, in the dog, as in the rat, evolution into phase II of 2-kidney, 1-clip hypertension is seen to accompany a

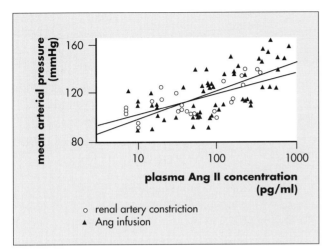

Fig. 55.5 The relationship between arterial pressure and plasma Ang II concentration in conscious dogs before and during infusion of Ang II and before and after renal artery constriction. Modified from Caravaggi AM *et al* [22].

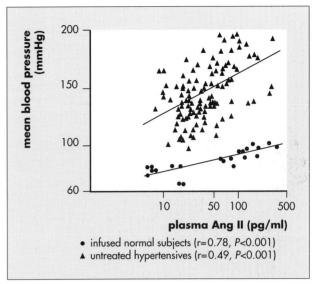

Fig. 55.6 The relationship between peripheral venous plasma Ang II and mean blood pressure (diastolic plus one-third pulse pressure) in a group of patients with untreated hypertension, either in the malignant phase or with an associated renal or renal arterial lesion. A similar relationship is also shown in normal subjects, before and during incremental infusion of Ang II. Throughout the range, arterial pressure is higher for a given plasma Ang II concentration in the hypertensive patients than in the infused normal subjects. Modified from Brown JJ *et al* [26].

disproportionately high arterial pressure in relation to the RAS, in comparison with the relationship in phase I.

Man

For obvious reasons, data in phase I of 2-kidney, 1-clip hypertension in its human counterpart are not available. However, acute Ang II/blood-pressure dose–response curves are established for normal volunteers [15] (Fig. 55.6). These data provide a basis upon which to evaluate the Ang II/blood-pressure relationships in the later, presumed phase II, of human renovascular hypertension.

To this end, a study was made of a large series of patients with untreated hypertension associated with a renal, or renal arterial, lesion [26]. In these subjects, blood samples were taken for the assay of endogenous plasma Ang II, the conditions of blood sampling being closely similar to those in which the normal volunteers had been studied [15]. Although this was a very diverse series of patients, there was a significant positive overall correlation between the level of Ang II and the concurrent blood pressure. However, when a comparison was made of the data in the patients who had established renal hypertension with the acute pressor dose–response curve in the normal volunteers, it could be seen that, for any level of circulating Ang II, in established renal hypertension there was a much higher level of blood pressure than could be achieved by the brief administration of Ang II to normal volunteers (Fig. 55.6). This was, of course, in large part, a clinical study and subject to all of the difficulties of control and other constraints imposed by the necessities of

medical practice. Nevertheless, the findings replicated, in man, almost exactly the relationship between Ang II and arterial pressure seen in phase II of 2-kidney, 1-clip hypertension in strictly controlled experimental circumstances in the rat (Fig. 55.4). It should be emphasized further that the positive correlation between plasma Ang II and arterial pressure in these hypertensive patients with renal or renovascular disease is in contrast to the relationship seen in normal subjects and in patients with essential hypertension, in whom the correlation between blood pressure and the RAS is usually inverse (see *Chapter 74*).

Particularly revealing in this context were observations made before and after removal of a renin-secreting tumor in a patient with severe hypertension [27]. In this subject, it could be assumed that the sole original cause of the hypertension was hypersecretion of renin and hence abnormally high peripheral plasma concentrations of Ang II. Before operation in this patient very high endogenous levels of plasma Ang II were matched in the volunteers only at the highest rates of Ang II infusion (Fig. 55.7). With long-term exposure to these very high plasma Ang II concentrations, blood pressure in the patient was very much higher than in the infused volunteers who were sustaining, acutely, similar Ang II levels. Removal of the renin-secreting tumor returned plasma Ang II and blood pressure to strictly normal values (Fig. 55.7).

Although in clinical renovascular hypertension, renin and Ang II levels may be elevated in peripheral blood, the findings are in no way specific for that disease. Moreover, in a number of patients with unilateral renal artery stenosis, who may eventually show satisfactory reduction in blood pressure after corrective surgery and who therefore can be accepted as having genuine renovascular hypertension, peripheral plasma values of renin and Ang II can lie within the overall normal range [10].

Summary

The foregoing comprises a substantial body of evidence, broadly consistent in rat, dog, and man. The immediate rise of blood pressure in phase I of 2-kidney, 1-clip hypertension can be fully explained by an immediate, direct pressor action of increases in peripheral plasma Ang II. In phase II, arterial pressure is as high as, or higher than, in phase I, but is disproportionately so in relation to concurrent plasma Ang II, as judged from acute

Ang II/pressor dose–response curves established in both rats and normal volunteers (see *Figs. 55.4, 55.6,* and *55.7*). Even so, there remains clamant evidence that actions of the RAS could still be responsible for hypertension in phase II, amongst which data quoted above from the patient with a renin-secreting tumor (Fig. 55.7) are prominent.

SLOW PRESSOR EFFECT OF LOW-DOSE ANGIOTENSIN II

It can be seen from the preceding section that, in both experimental animals and man, established 2-kidney, 1-clip hypertension is associated with an upward shift of the Ang II/pressor dose–response curve. The upward shift could well be due to factors extraneous to the RAS. However, for reasons already given, it is probable that the upward shift might, at least in part, be a result of an action of Ang II itself.

Dickinson and Lawrence [28] showed, in 1963, that the intravenous infusion of Ang II in the rabbit, in doses that were not at first pressor, could lead eventually to marked hypertension. This slow pressor action of Ang II has been much neglected but is of great physiological importance, and is dealt with in detail in *Chapter 28*. One aspect is described briefly here.

A low dose of Ang II was infused intravenously into trained, conscious dogs, combining the study with measurements of circulating Ang II [29]. The aim was, over a two-week period, to raise the circulating level of Ang II to a roughly constant value, but one which was within the physiological range. These animals were given for the first week, an infusion of physiological saline alone, for the succeeding two weeks, a low dose of Ang II, and then for the fourth and final week, physiological saline again. It can be seen from Fig. 55.8 that the infusion of Ang II led to a steady elevation of plasma Ang II, the mean value rising distinctly but modestly from approximately 25pg/ml to some 50pg/ml; the slow pressor effect of this low dose of Ang II is also shown. On the first day after the infusion was started, there was no significant elevation of blood pressure, but from then onwards, there was a clear and progressive rise in the blood-pressure level. When the Ang II infusion was discontinued, blood pressure remained above control values 24 hours after stopping the infusion, but thereafter fell back to levels slightly below the original control. This experiment provided clear evidence that Ang II, administered chronically at low dose, moved its own pressor dose–response curve in an upward direction.

There are several possible ways in which elevated plasma Ang II could reinforce its own pressor action. These have been reviewed previously [18] and are discussed in detail in *Chapter 28*.

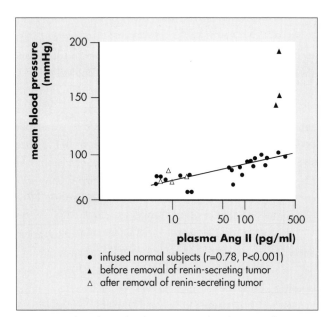

Fig. 55.7 The relationship between peripheral venous plasma Ang II and mean blood pressure (diastolic plus one-third pulse pressure) in a patient with a renin-secreting tumor, before and after excision of the tumor. A similar relationship is also shown in normal subjects, before and during incremental infusion of Ang II. Modified from Brown JJ *et al* [26,27].

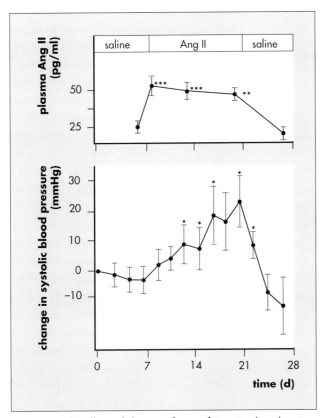

Fig. 55.8 The effects of chronic infusion of Ang II at low dose into conscious dogs. *P<0.05, **P<0.01, ***P<0.001. Modified from Bean BL et al [29].

THE RENIN–ANGIOTENSIN SYSTEM AND DEVELOPMENT OF COLLATERAL CIRCULATION

A variant of 2-kidney, 1-clip hypertension was produced in the rat by Fernandez et al [30] by aortic ligation between the origins of the renal arteries. This procedure caused both left renal ischemia and transient (less than two hours in duration) hindlimb paralysis, the latter due to muscular, not spinal cord, ischemia.

If the ischemic left kidney was removed at the time of aortic ligation, the usual rise in plasma renin activity (PRA) did not occur and hypertension was curtailed, while the paralysis persisted for 24 hours after surgery.

Administration of saralasin or an ACE inhibitor also prevented recuperation from paralysis after aortic ligation. Independent manipulations of renin and systemic blood pressure showed that the presence or absence of paralysis was dependent on PRA rather than arterial pressure. Infusion of Ang II into aortic-ligated, left-renoprival rats restored hindlimb muscle blood flow.

These investigators concluded that after renal ischemia, the RAS, independently of its pressor effect, promotes the development of a collateral arterial circulation.

CHANGES IN ALDOSTERONE

As is discussed in detail in *Chapter 33*, the RAS is one of the principal stimuli to aldosterone secretion. Thus, the elevation of plasma renin and Ang II following renal artery constriction in this model is paralleled by increases in plasma aldosterone, as has been demonstrated, for example, in the dog [31,32] and rabbit [33].

The particular importance of secondary aldosteronism in the hyponatremic hypertensive syndrome in patients [34,35] is discussed in detail later in this chapter.

INTRARENAL AND TRANSRENAL CHANGES IN RENIN AND ANGIOTENSIN II: DIAGNOSTIC APPLICATIONS

As is described in detail in *Chapter 21*, in several mammalian species, normally most of the extractable renal renin is to be found in association with superficial (cortical) glomeruli, with much less in the juxtamedullary glomeruli [36,37]. In 2-kidney, 1-clip hypertension, it has been shown, for example in the rabbit, that the total content of renin is increased in the kidney with the stenosis ('clipped kidney') (see Color Plates 14 and 15). The global increase in intrarenal renin involves the appearance of substantial quantities also in the normally renin-poor juxtamedullary glomeruli [16]. By contrast, the contralateral ('untouched') kidney becomes low in extractable renin, with little to be found even in the superficial glomeruli.

The affected kidney in human unilateral renal artery stenosis shows markedly increased secretion of active renin in comparison with the kidney in essential hypertension; there is also secretion of inactive renin, which is not normally the case [38]. There is with renal artery stenosis, consequent demonstrably increased local formation of both Ang I and Ang II [38,39]. The human contralateral ('untouched') kidney shows, in comparison with the kidney in essential hypertension, suppression of secretion of active renin, no secretion of inactive renin, and 50% net transrenal extraction of Ang II.

Comparison of the renin values in the two renal veins (the 'renal-vein renin ratio') was first described in this condition by Judson and Helmer [40] and is now widely employed as a clinical diagnostic method for unilateral renal artery stenosis. With the Seldinger [41] technique, blood samples (preferably in triplicate) are obtained simultaneously from both main renal veins and from an artery or peripheral vein [42]. Some workers perform the test under conditions of normal controlled sodium intake, supine posture and, so far as possible, freedom from the effects of drugs [10,38]. This approach facilitates an evaluation of the prevailing quantitative function of each kidney, providing data that can be integrated with other measurements, for example of renal plasma flow and glomerular filtration rate (GFR). A detailed evaluation of typical findings in such circumstances, and a comparison with essential hypertension, are given in the paper of Webb *et al* [38]. Others advocate stimulation of renin release (see below) by administering agents such as hydralazine, furosemide, or ACE inhibitors during the test; by tilting the patient upright; or by restricting sodium intake before the study [43–46].

Typically, higher renin values are found in the vein draining the affected kidney, while renin secretion is suppressed from the contralateral side. For theoretical reasons reviewed in detail elsewhere [10,47], increased renin secretion from one side, with contralateral suppression of renin release, can elevate the differential renal vein ratio in the resting state only to approximately 1.5:1. Higher ratios than this can, however, be achieved by mechanisms additional to increased renin secretion on the ischemic side. These include removal of renin from the circulation by the 'untouched kidney', and reduction in blood flow through the ischemic kidney. The ratio can be temporarily enhanced by acutely stimulating renin release [46]. This latter is the reason for administering, as described earlier, hydralazine, furosemide, or captopril during the test, or for tilting the patient. Detection of high renin values in a segmental renal vein may be a useful means of confirming segmental renal artery stenosis [48].

The usual suppression of renin secretion by the 'untouched' kidney is overcome in the hyponatremic hypertensive syndrome, to be discussed below [35]. Enhanced, rather than suppressed, contralateral renin secretion has in other circumstances, been taken as evidence that phase III has been entered [19], although this is controversial (see earlier).

It should be borne in mind that elevation of renal vein renin on one side may also be seen in a variety of unilateral renal diseases other than renal artery stenosis. including notably renin-secreting tumor, although as discussed in *Chapter 54*, the renal vein ratio in this last condition is often much less than in renal artery stenosis [27] because renal blood flow is usually not then diminished.

The changes in the pattern of renin in renal venous plasma in relation to ACE inhibition in man are described later in this chapter.

Meignan *et al* [49] studied renin secretion from both kidneys in Wistar rats for 40 minutes after partial clamping of the left renal artery. ^{14}C inulin and ^{3}H *p*-aminohippuric acid clearance, and the arterial and venous PRC, were measured in each kidney during control and experimental procedures. After clamping, the arterial PRC increased and correlated positively with the PRC in both renal veins. However, the PRC of the right renal vein was lower than the arterial concentration ($P<0.01$). The slope correlating the two variables was significantly lower than unity ($P<0.05$). As the left kidney secreted a large amount of renin, calculated secretion by the right kidney decreased to negative values, implying renin uptake by this kidney.

These data suggest the existence of a balance between the two kidneys. Renin secretion appears to maintain an equilibrium between release by the juxtaglomerular apparatus and removal from the blood into interstitial space. Release seems to predominate in the hypoperfused kidney, and removal in the contralateral kidney. This may result from the increase of circulating Ang II, because there was a direct correlation between renin uptake and the arterial PRC.

ATRIAL NATRIURETIC FACTOR

Rat

Gauquelin *et al* [50] found plasma atrial natriuretic factor (ANF) concentrations (see *Chapter 36*) to be elevated in rats with 2-kidney, 1-clip hypertension as compared with controls, at 3.5 and 7 weeks after operation. Lower ANF levels were found in the right atrium in the hypertensive rats at week three, but not thereafter. The glomerular receptor ANF population was reduced in the clipped left kidney at all stages; in the untouched right kidney, the glomerular receptor population was larger at three weeks, but reduced at five and seven weeks, after surgery. It was concluded that these changes in ANF may play a role in the differential sodium excretion by the two kidneys during various stages of the development of hypertension in this model (see later).

Paul [51] evaluated, in 2-kidney, 1-clip hypertensive rats, the hypothesis that the impaired natriuretic response of the clipped kidney might be due to downregulation of ANF receptors. He found, however, that the blunted natriuretic response in clipped kidneys was not associated with any relative decrease in number or function of glomerular or papillary ANF receptors.

In a further study [52], Garcia *et al* examined rats who sustained a systolic pressure of 150mmHg or more for 2–3 weeks. They found that those rats having an acute reduction in blood pressure with saralasin infusion showed increased density of ANF receptors in the untouched kidney, whereas the density was decreased in the untouched kidney in the saralasin-resistant rats. Receptor numbers were decreased in the clipped kidney in both groups. It was speculated that these differences might result in greater sodium retention and volume expansion, with resulting resistance to saralasin and ANF, in that group [52,53]. Garcia et al [52] did indeed observe expanded blood volume in their saralasin-resistant rats. However, as noted later [54], sodium retention has not been unequivocally demonstrated at any stage in this model.

Man

Larochelle et al [55] determined plasma ANF in eight hypertensive patients with unilateral renal artery stenosis. They found significantly higher values in plasma from aorta and inferior vena cava than in plasma of seven patients with essential hypertension. In the patients with renal artery stenosis, plasma ANF in the renal veins tended to be higher than that drawn from other sites, but not significantly so; the side of the renal artery stenosis did not seem to influence the relative plasma ANF concentrations in the two renal veins.

The absence of the normal inverse relationship between the RAS and ANF in this condition deserves emphasis. These findings are of interest in view of the demonstration [56] that the usual inhibitory effect of ANF on renin release is lost in circumstances in which renal perfusion is diminished (see *Chapter 36*).

VASOPRESSIN

The possibility that vasopressin may participate in the hypertension of the 2-kidney, 1-clip model has attracted repeated attention. As described in *Chapter 35*, circulating Ang II, if sufficiently high, can stimulate the secretion of vasopressin in man. However, chronic exposure of patients to high levels of endogenous vasopressin because of a vasopressin-secreting bronchial neoplasm, while causing gross electrolyte disturbance, does not lead to hypertension [57]. Conversely, rats of the Brattleboro strain, which have vasopressin deficiency, can develop 2-kidney, 1-clip hypertension [58]. Nevertheless, it is possible that vasopressin excess could, in some circumstances, contribute to renovascular hypertension.

Rat

In severely hypertensive 2-kidney, 1-clip rats, manifesting features akin to the hyponatremic hypertensive syndrome in man

(see later), Möhring et al [59] found plasma vasopressin to be raised in approximately 50% of the animals. Moreover, the administration of a specific vasopressin antiserum was found to lower blood pressure.

However, contrary findings were reported by Rabito et al [60] in this same rat model with severe hypertension. They found that a specific vasopressin pressor antagonist failed to alter the blood pressure.

Likewise, Filep et al [61], in careful experiments, showed that neither of two structurally different vasopressin pressor antagonists altered mean arterial pressure or heart rate, when given to rats with severe 2-kidney, 1-clip hypertension. Concurrently, both antagonists completely abolished the pressor effect of exogenous vasopressin.

Dog

Ben et al [62], in the dog, reported rather different findings. Following unilateral renal artery constriction, the opposite kidney remaining intact, the development of hypertension was accompanied by clear increases in PRA and Ang II, and by rather less clear, but significant, increases in plasma vasopressin. Vasopressin concentration rose by at least 50% in all animals. The timing of the greatest increase varied, although it was always seen between days 8 and 16. Over the 30-day period of study, there was only a loose correlation between plasma Ang II and plasma vasopressin. Acute blockade of the RAS with saralasin or captopril, while producing the expected changes in PRA and Ang II, did not lower vasopressin. Thus, the antihypertensive action of captopril in this model and in these circumstances did not seem to involve suppression of vasopressin, nor did the increase in vasopressin appear to be mediated via Ang II.

Man

In the hyponatremic hypertensive syndrome with unilateral renal artery occlusion in man, Atkinson et al [35] found that a gross increase in plasma Ang II concentration could be accompanied by abnormally high vasopressin concentrations. When plasma Ang II was lowered with captopril, vasopressin also returned promptly to the normal range, showing that the enhanced vasopressin secretion was, in these circumstances, dependent on the excessively stimulated RAS (see *Chapters 35 and 88*).

Thus, the results of different studies are not all consistent, and there may well be critical differences between species and between different stages and degrees of severity of the disease. While a contribution from elevated vasopressin cannot be excluded in all circumstances, participation by vasopressin does not seem to be required for the development of 2-kidney, 1-clip hypertension.

BILATERAL CHANGES IN RENAL FUNCTION

Rat

The alterations in bilateral renal function in 2-kidney, 1-clip hypertension in the rat has been reviewed in detail by Ploth and his colleagues [63–66]. Acute constriction of one renal artery causes a decrease in blood flow via the clipped kidney. This blood flow then returns towards normal as systemic arterial pressure rises, with values at or near control within a few days to a few weeks. Blood flow via the untouched kidney increases immediately after clipping and may remain elevated or fall slightly towards values seen for control rats within 1–3 weeks. There is a controversial suggestion that the blood flow in the untouched kidney may be mainly via deep nephrons. The untouched kidney exhibits markedly elevated vascular resistance, since blood flow is at most modestly elevated despite markedly increased systemic arterial pressure. Antagonists of the RAS consistently reduce vascular resistance in the untouched kidney even if given when peripheral plasma renin and Ang II are not much elevated, a circumstance parallel to that noted in the dog [24,25] (see later).

Glomerular filtration rate, urine flow, and sodium excretion are consistently depressed in the clipped kidney and elevated in the untouched kidney as compared with kidneys of normotensive control rats. With acute blockade of the RAS, GFR is raised in the untouched, but decreased in the clipped, kidney.

A consistent, and critically important, observation is that both the clipped and untouched kidneys show shifts in the relationships of pressure natriuresis such that each kidney can excrete a given sodium load only at a higher blood pressure than for a normal kidney.

With acute application of an antagonist of the RAS, urine flow, absolute and fractional sodium excretion, and absolute and fractional potassium excretion, increase several-fold in the untouched kidney, and in contrast decrease in the clipped kidney.

Rabbit

The rabbit deserves especial mention in the present context because of the seminal observations of Thompson and Dickinson [67]. They found that in rabbits with 2-kidney, 1-clip hypertension, isolated perfused kidneys, both clipped and untouched, required a higher perfusion pressure than normal in order to excrete a given quantity of sodium (Fig. 55.9).

Dog

Very similar evolutionary changes to those summarized in the rat and rabbit were reported up to 28 days after unilateral renal artery plication in the dog by DeForrest et al [68]. Sodium and water excretion were markedly reduced in the kidney with the stenosed renal artery, and after the first two days, were increased in the contralateral kidney. These changes in sodium and water excretion were frequently associated with similar directional changes in GFR and renal plasma flow. An exception was noted in that renal sodium and water excretion remained low throughout the 28 days in the kidney with the constricted renal artery, whereas GFR returned to near the control level by the end of two weeks. Altered filtration fraction did not appear to be a determining factor in the control of the rate of sodium excretion.

Man

The differential renal functional characteristics of the untreated clinical counterpart of 2-kidney, 1-clip hypertension have been examined in considerable detail in patients with unilateral renal artery stenosis. Data obtained at bilateral ureteric catheterization provide the most extensive quantitative information on the disordered renal function in this condition [10], especially if inulin

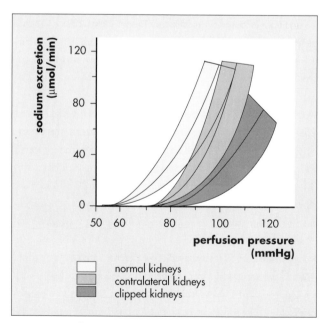

Fig. 55.9 Perfusion pressure of normal donor blood in the renal artery, and rate of urinary sodium excretion in 16 normal rabbit kidneys and in the clipped and contralateral kidneys in eight rabbits with 2-kidney, 1-clip hypertension. Approximate 95% confidence limits are shown by the shaded area surrounding each mean curve. Modified from Thompson JMA and Dickinson CJ [67].

and p-aminohippurate (PAH) are infused during the test so as to permit measurement of, respectively, GFR and plasma flow in each kidney. The classic pattern of disordered function shows, on the affected side, reduced urine flow, reduced clearances of creatinine, inulin, and PAH, and low urine sodium concentration, while the urinary concentrations of creatinine, inulin, and PAH are enhanced. These changes are almost specific for unilateral renal artery stenosis; they also provide a physiological explanation of the pyelographic appearances [10], showing hyperconcentration of dye in the affected side. This is because radio-opaque dye is treated by the kidney similarly to inulin and creatinine.

Techniques designed to assess differential blood flow within the kidney are notoriously difficult and unreliable [69–71]. It was, however, suggested, with a method employing radioactive xenon [69], that in human unilateral renal artery stenosis, the reduction in blood flow on the affected side was mainly at the expense of the cortical circulation. If correct, this implies that the alterations in renal function seen on the affected side reflect the predominant effects of juxtamedullary nephrons that are normally renin poor, but which in this condition are renin rich. These aspects are discussed further in *Chapter 21*. Interestingly, Ladefoged and Munck reported [69] that cortical blood flow appeared to be reduced also in the contralateral kidney. As mentioned above, similar restriction of cortical blood flow has been suggested in the untouched kidney in the rat.

With the administration of an ACE inhibitor, effective renal plasma flow, already low on the affected side, falls further, while it increases via the contralateral kidney [72]; GFR can be very markedly diminished in the affected kidney [73]. These changes are of considerable clinical and diagnostic importance and are discussed in further detail in *Chapters 27* and *88–90*.

EVOLUTION OF CHANGES IN BODY SODIUM CONTENT

Rat

McAreavey *et al* [54] measured total exchangeable sodium (NaE) serially before and during the development of 2-kidney, 1-clip hypertension in the rat and also after relief of the hypertension following removal of the clip (Fig. 55.10). The clipped hypertensive rats at no stage showed significant differences in NaE or in body weight from sham-operated normotensive control rats. On the first day after removal of the clip, NaE was significantly lower in the clipped group than in the sham-operated group, but there were no significant differences between the groups thereafter. Total body sodium additionally was measured at death by

ashing the carcases; the data confirmed the reliability of the NaE measurements, total body sodium being consistently higher than NaE by a mean of 1.25mmol, in hypertensive and control rats alike. These observations of McAreavey *et al* [54] complement the results of Morton and Wallace [20], quoted above, on serial measurements of renin and Ang II in this rat model, and performed in the same laboratory (*Fig. 55.3*). The data show that changes in sodium balance are not a necessary accompaniment of moderate hypertension in the 2-kidney, 1-clip model.

Not all investigators have found such a consistent pattern of body sodium in this form of hypertension in the rat. Swales *et al* [74] reported negative sodium balance in the early phase of hypertension. By contrast, Möhring *et al* [75] described early sodium retention in the same rat model, with the development of negative sodium balance on the later occurrence of severe hypertension. Doyle and Duffy [76], who measured total body sodium by ashing rat carcases 35 days after clipping, found increased values in severely hypertensive animals. Yet again, Tobian *et al* [77] did not detect any changes in NaE. Albertini *et al* [78] distinguished between moderately hypertensive rats with normal NaE and those with severe hypertension in which NaE was increased. It is likely that some of these discordant findings reflect methodological problems. Long-term external balance studies are particularly vulnerable to the cumulative effect of even small daily errors of analysis and computation [54].

Several groups have agreed, nevertheless, that neither dietary sodium restriction [79,80] nor dialysis-induced sodium depletion [81] prevents, in this model, the manifestation of hypertension.

Jackson and Navar [82] found in the rat that administration of 0.9% sodium chloride as a drinking solution for three weeks suppressed PRA and the renin content of the clipped kidney to normal values. The onset of hypertension was delayed, but not its eventual magnitude. The function of the clipped kidneys of saline-drinking rats was enhanced compared with that in water-drinking clipped rats.

Dog

Bianchi *et al* [23] observed that the development of 2-kidney, 1-clip hypertension in the conscious dog was not associated with any detectable change in the equilibrium of sodium balance during the 17 days of their study. Plasma volume was slightly and significantly increased and extracellular fluid volume insignificantly increased 24 hours after renal artery constriction, but by seven days, these measurements had returned towards normal. Bianchi *et al* [23] noted that renal artery constriction in anesthetized dogs caused, by contrast, slight sodium retention; thus, results obtained under anesthesia were, they concluded, less

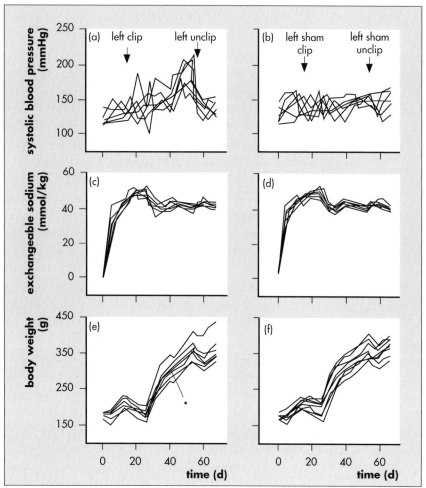

Fig. 55.10 Two-kidney, one-clip hypertension in the rat. Changes in systolic blood pressure, exchangeable sodium, and body weight in individual rats in the clipped (a, c, e) and sham-clipped groups (b, d, f) are shown. The asterisk denotes a rat that died. Modified from McAreavey D *et al* [54].

reliable. These data of Bianchi *et al* [23] accompanied concurrent measurements of PRC mentioned above.

Watson *et al* [83] confirmed that removal of sodium and water by hemodialysis followed by a low dietary intake of sodium for seven days did not prevent the development of hypertension in 2-kidney, 1-clip hypertension in the dog.

Man

McAreavey *et al* [84] measured NaE in 19 hypertensive patients with unilateral renal artery stenosis, without overall renal impairment, and with normal plasma sodium concentrations. Mean NaE for the group, expressed either in relation to body surface area or to leanness index, was normal (Fig. 55.11).

There thus appears to be remarkable concordance between the reports of Bianchi *et al* [23] in 2-kidney, 1-clip hypertension in the dog, and those of McAreavey *et al* [54] and Morton and Wallace *et al* [20] in the same model in the rat. Freeman

et al [85] concur that in neither of these two species does the 2-kidney, 1-clip model require salt or volume expansion for the long-term expression of hypertension. The necessarily more limited data in man [84] are in agreement with the conclusions from studies in rat and dog.

THE HYPONATREMIC HYPERTENSIVE SYNDROME

The hyponatremic hypertensive syndrome requires separate consideration; it is also discussed in some detail in *Chapter 88*.

Occasional patients are encountered in whom a severe unilateral renal artery stenosis or unilateral renal artery occlusion leads to very marked and progressive elevation of peripheral plasma concentrations of active renin and Ang II, with severe hypertension, often entering the malignant phase. There is secondary aldosterone excess, with depression of plasma sodium and potassium concentrations, and usually marked deficits of body sodium and potassium. Plasma Ang II may be sufficiently high

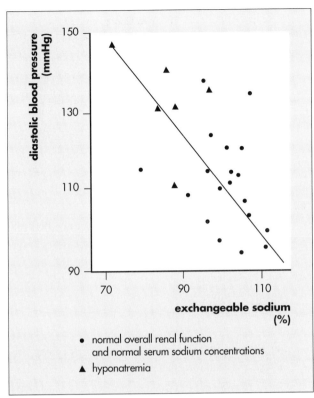

Fig. 55.11 Inverse correlation (r=−0.57; P<0.01) between exchangeable sodium, expressed in terms of body surface area, and diastolic blood pressure, in 25 patients with unilateral renal artery stenosis. Nineteen patients had normal overall renal function and normal serum sodium concentrations. Six patients had hyponatremia (serum sodium ≤ 134mmol/l). One of the hyponatremic patients had azotemia. Modified from McAreavey D et al [84].

to stimulate secretion also of vasopressin (see *Chapter 35*). These patients usually have pronounced symptoms, including thirst, polydipsia, polyuria, and loss of weight [34,35].

This syndrome can be also encountered in experimental animals with 2-kidney, 1-clip hypertension if the renal artery constriction is sufficiently severe; the course of the hyponatremic hypertensive syndrome in phase II of this model is indicated by the dashed lines in *Fig. 55.2*. Masaki *et al* [86] in the dog, and Möhring *et al* [59,75] and Bengis and Coleman [87] in the rat, have reported on detailed experiments. In their terminology, the onset of this syndrome is referred to as 'the development of malignant hypertension'. Fibrinoid arterial necrosis, the hallmark of malignant hypertension (see *Chapter 60*), is indeed very common in the hyponatremic syndrome in these species, as it is also in man (Color Plate 21). Nevertheless, confusion is best avoided, and the terms are preferably distinguished.

The pathogenetic basis of the hyponatremic hypertensive syndrome is as follows. The severe unilateral renal artery stenosis provides an intense stimulus to renin secretion, with consequent elevation of plasma Ang II concentration and severe hypertension (Fig. 55.12). However, because of the severity of the renal artery lesion, systemic blood pressure cannot rise sufficiently to eliminate the intrarenal signal to renin secretion (see *Chapter 24*). The hypertension causes loss of sodium by pressure natriuresis from the contralateral kidney [10,35,66,84] (Fig. 55.12), and the consequent sodium deficiency provides a reinforcing stimulus to the already excessive renin secretion. Even so, the sodium loss, while undoubtedly moderating the pressor effect of Ang II, is insufficient to abrogate it. Secondary aldosterone excess follows, with resulting potassium deficiency, which provides yet another stimulus to renin secretion (see *Chapter 74*). Potassium loss may well moderate the pressor effect of Ang II [88], although in this context, evidently not markedly. The elevated Ang II can cause thirst (see *Chapter 32*) and increased vasopressin secretion (see *Chapter 35*). The hyponatremia thus has multiple causes; these include direct renal actions of Ang II (see *Chapters 26* and *27*), together with Ang II-stimulated thirst and vasopressin secretion.

The abnormalities can be corrected by relief of the renal artery constriction, by removal of the kidney distal to the renal arterial lesion, or by lowering plasma Ang II by the administration of an ACE inhibitor. Indeed, because of the marked

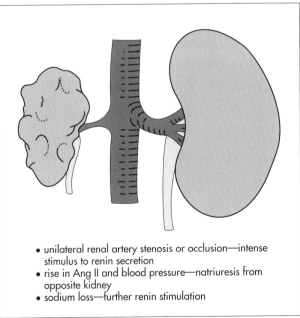

- unilateral renal artery stenosis or occlusion—intense stimulus to renin secretion
- rise in Ang II and blood pressure—natriuresis from opposite kidney
- sodium loss—further renin stimulation

Fig. 55.12 The essential features in the pathogenesis of the hyponatremic hypertensive syndrome. Modifed from Robertson JIS [10].

sodium deficit, the introduction of ACE inhibition will lower blood pressure often precipitously [35,87]. Correction of the sodium deficit can also be therapeutically beneficial [59,75] (see *Chapter 60*).

A very similar syndrome can occur in malignant-phase essential hypertension (see *Chapter 60*), where presumably multiple intrarenal hypertension-induced arterial lesions cause diffuse renal artery stenoses (Color Plates 21 and 22). The hyponatremic syndrome is also encountered in some patients in end-stage renal failure undergoing hemodialysis, and occasionally with intensive diuretic therapy.

The inclusion of patients with the hyponatremic hypertensive syndrome in a series with unilateral renal artery stenosis results in there being, overall, a significant inverse relation between blood pressure and NaE [84] (see *Fig. 55.11*).

It has further been shown in hypertensive patients with unilateral renal artery stenosis that the rate of sodium excretion from the contralateral 'normal' kidney is correlated positively with arterial pressure and negatively with NaE [84].

EFFECT OF POTASSIUM DEPLETION

As described in the preceding section, potassium depletion is one of the features of the hyponatremic hypertensive syndrome, a disorder characterized by severe hypertension.

In other circumstances, potassium depletion may greatly attenuate the severity of 2-kidney, 1-clip hypertension. In a dietary study in rats, Benedetti and Linas [88] found that potassium depletion prevented the development of this form of renovascular hypertension and also reversed it if introduced with established hypertension three weeks after clipping.

In this experiment, potassium depletion elevated PRA while decreasing the vascular sensitivity to Ang II. The latter was considered to be the main effect mediating the antihypertensive action.

THE SYMPATHETIC NERVOUS SYSTEM

The RAS can stimulate the sympathetic nervous system at various levels, as is considered in detail in *Chapter 37*. The evidence from animal experiments for increased sympathetic nervous system activity in renovascular hypertension was reviewed by Zimmerman [89], who concluded that peripheral adrenergic facilitation by Ang II may contribute to the induction of this form of hypertension. However, not all results are consistent.

Rat

DeForrest *et al* [90] observed that guanethidine did not prevent the development of 2-kidney, 1-clip hypertension but did markedly attenuate its appearance if it had been initially prevented by captopril and the captopril then stopped. Thus, both the sympathetic nervous system and the RAS were required for the rise in peripheral resistance and the development of hypertension in this model after prior administration of captopril followed by its withdrawal.

Walker *et al* [91] observed no elevation of plasma norepinephrine either at 4–6 weeks or at more than 16 weeks after clipping in this model in the rat. With unclipping, plasma norepinephrine rose at 4–6 weeks, but was unaltered at more than 16 weeks.

Collis and Vanhoutte [92] isolated and perfused both the clipped and untouched kidneys from hypertensive and sham-operated control rats, 1–104 days postoperatively. Responses to renal nerve stimulation were depressed in clipped kidneys from hypertensive rats at one day after clipping, while these kidneys were observed to be supersensitive to exogenous norepinephrine at 1–31 days when compared with the contralateral organ of the same animal. Similar alterations were found between clipped and contralateral kidneys from sham-operated control rats. There was no difference in responses to renal nerve stimulation or norepinephrine between clipped kidneys from hypertensive and control rats, but clipped kidneys from hypertensive rats were supersensitive to Ang II at 17 and 31 days. Comparison of contralateral kidneys from hypertensive and control rats revealed no change in norepinephrine sensitivity or in responses to renal nerve stimulation, but there was a reduction in the slope of the dose–response curve to norepinephrine and of the maximal effect of the catecholamine at 104 days and a pronounced supersensitivity to Ang II at 17–104 days in the hypertensive rats. The authors concluded that renal nerve function and norepinephrine sensitivity of the isolated renal vasculature are unchanged in renal hypertension, but that clipping partially denervates the kidney, causing depressed nerve function and unilateral norepinephrine supersensitivity, unrelated to hypertension; the prolonged high pressure load on the contralateral kidney may impair the function of the vascular smooth muscle; and bilateral hypersensitivity to Ang II is associated with hypertension but is not solely a consequence of the high pressure.

Kopp and Buckley-Bleiler [93] examined whether the renorenal reflexes were altered in 2-kidney, 1-clip hypertensive rats, in which model it has been suggested that the afferent renal nerves contribute to the enhanced peripheral sympathetic nervous activity. Renal mechanoreceptor and chemoreceptor stimulation of either the untouched or clipped kidney failed to affect ipsilateral afferent renal nerve activity, contralateral efferent renal nerve activity, contralateral urine flow rate, or urinary sodium excretion. Denervation of the untouched kidney increased ipsilateral urinary sodium excretion and decreased contralateral urinary sodium excretion, thus leading to a similar contralateral excitatory renorenal reflex response to that in normotensive rats. However, denervation of the clipped kidney increased both ipsilateral and contralateral urinary sodium excretion. Taken together, these data suggested that the lack of inhibitory renorenal reflexes from the clipped kidney may enhance efferent sympathetic nervous activity and thereby contribute to the hypertension in 2-kidney, 1-clip hypertensive rats.

Dog

Zimmerman [94] examined the roles of the sympathetic nervous system and the RAS in the control of blood pressure and renal blood flow in conscious normotensive and 2-kidney, 1-clip hypertensive dogs. Urapidil, an α-adrenoceptor antagonist, and then captopril, were administered acutely, intravenously. Urapidil decreased mean arterial blood pressure in the hypertensive and normotensive dogs. Contralateral blood flow was unchanged in the hypertensive dogs, but was increased in those that were normotensive. Captopril caused a further fall in the blood pressure of the hypertensives and increased renal blood flow. Blood pressure of the normotensives was further decreased and renal blood flow was increased by captopril. Urapidil increased PRA in the normotensives, but not in the hypertensives, whereas heart rate was increased and renal vascular resistance was decreased in both groups. In 9 of 11 hypertensive dogs, captopril alone had a smaller effect on blood pressure and renal blood flow than when given after α-blockade. These results indicated to Zimmerman [94] that the combined influence of the sympathetic and the renin–angiotensin systems accounts for a major portion of the blood-pressure increase in 2-kidney, 1-clip hypertension, and that their elimination causes profound hypotension and renal vasodilatation.

Man

Izumi *et al* [95] described a single patient with renovascular hypertension and with raised urinary norepinephrine excretion that fell to normal after surgical treatment.

Gordon *et al* [96] assayed venous plasma concentrations of epinephrine, norepinephrine, and dopamine in blood collected simultaneously from three different sites in patients with renovascular hypertension and with essential hypertension. In adrenal venous plasma, levels of catecholamines were increased in renovascular hypertension as compared with essential hypertension. Concentrations were similar within individuals in antecubital and low inferior vena cava plasma, whereas norepinephrine was higher in those with renovascular hypertension. Altered adrenal venous catecholamine levels may, it was concluded, reflect altered sympathetic activity, with renovascular hypertension showing enhanced activity.

Summary

Thus, although agreement is incomplete, a body of evidence in several species suggests that enhanced sympathetic nervous activity can contribute to the raised arterial pressure in the 2-kidney, 1-clip model.

ALTERED BAROREFLEXES

Rat

Berenguer *et al* [97] performed studies of the baroreceptor heart rate reflex in 2-kidney, 1-clip hypertensive rats to evaluate the relative importance of two factors, high blood pressure and high plasma Ang II, on impairment of the baroreflex that is present in the acute phase of this model of hypertension. The sensitivity of the reflex was determined by the slope of the relationship between changes in mean arterial pressure and changes in heart rate in response to injections of phenylephrine and nitroprusside. Bradycardic and tachycardic responses were analyzed separately. In basal conditions, the slope of the blood-pressure–heart rate relationship in hypertensive animals was significantly lower than in control rats, both for tachycardic and bradycardic responses. Lowering of blood pressure with captopril to normotensive levels in the hypertensive rats significantly increased baroreflex gain in bradycardic responses to the level found in normotensive rats. Normalization of blood pressure with nitroprusside did not change baroreflex sensitivity. The infusion of Ang II at a dose that did not change blood pressure, previously normalized with captopril, completely reverted the effect of this agent on baroreflex sensitivity. These authors interpreted their data to indicate that, in 2-kidney, 1-clip hypertensive rats, decreased baroreflex sensitivity is mediated, at least in part, by high circulating Ang II levels. Elevated blood pressure *per se* is of secondary importance.

Dog

These experiments of Berenguer *et al* [97] are of interest in view of the previous work of Cowley and De Clue [98], who performed infusions of Ang II in dogs. The latter data indicated that approximately 35% of the gradual increase in blood pressure over seven days was in large measure a result of baroreceptor resetting (see *Chapter 28*).

INVOLVEMENT OF PROSTANOIDS

The involvement of prostanoids is discussed in detail in *Chapters 38* and *74*, but also warrants brief mention here.

Some prostaglandins (PGE$_2$, PGI$_2$) are known to stimulate renin secretion directly or indirectly. Imanishi *et al* [99] found that PGE$_2$ concentrations in renal venous plasma from the affected kidney in hypertensive patients with unilateral renal artery stenosis were higher than in aortic or contralateral renal venous plasma, and that the renal vein PGE$_2$ ratio correlated with the renal vein renin ratio. The intravenous injection of aspirin DL-lysine lowered acutely both PGE$_2$ and renin levels at all sites and also markedly reduced blood pressure. The data were interpreted as indicating that renal prostaglandins play an important role in the augmented release of renal renin and hence in the pathogenesis of human renovascular hypertension.

Anderson *et al* [100] found that in human renal cortex, the capacity to synthesize thromboxane, and the ratios both of thromboxane:prostacyclin and of thromboxane:PGE$_2$, were enhanced in proportion to the degree of renal ischemia. Unlike the vasodilator PGE$_2$, thromboxane is a potent vasoconstrictor and platelet aggregator. It was postulated that local generation of thromboxane might exacerbate renal ischemia by causing vasospasm and/or platelet aggregation, thereby reinforcing stimuli to renin secretion [101].

EFFECT OF ANTAGONISTS AND INHIBITORS OF THE RENIN–ANGIOTENSIN SYSTEM

Study of the effects of various antagonists and inhibitors of the RAS on hypertension of renovascular origin and especially of the 2-kidney, 1-clip model has helped substantially in the elucidation of pathogenesis. Even so, several aspects remain controversial. Experimental results require to be interpreted cautiously, because there are several potential causes of confusion. Analog antagonists of Ang II, such as saralasin, possess a partial agonistic action (see *Chapter 86*), while ACE inhibitors, although limiting the formation of Ang II, may also prolong the survival of kinins (see *Chapter 87*).

Antagonists of Angiotensin II

Rat: Short-term angiotensin II antagonism

This is an area of considerable disagreement and controversy.

Brunner *et al* [102] studied 2-kidney, 1-clip hypertensive rats at 6 weeks after renal artery constriction. Both an Ang II antiserum and saralasin lowered blood pressure substantially. These authors concluded that Ang II is critically and directly involved, even at this late stage, in sustaining hypertension.

Macdonald *et al* [103,104] reached very different conclusions. They also examined the effect of infusing saralasin briefly into rats with 2-kidney, 1-clip hypertension at times varying from 14 to 79 days after operation. They found that the hypotensive response varied widely, with a continuous spectrum from less than 5mmHg to 55mmHg. Correlations between the blood-pressure fall and the duration from clipping, blood urea, and initial pressure were insignificant. However, the saralasin induced reduction in blood pressure was closely related to the presaralasin level of PRA (Fig. 55.13); this observation accords with the widespread finding in several species and virtually all syndromes studied, that the acute effect on arterial pressure of inhibition of the RAS is directly proportional to the circulating level of renin or Ang II (see *Chapter 86*). Macdonald *et al* [103,104] found that the blood-pressure falls with Ang II blockade were less than those following excision of the clipped kidney, and that this was so even in rats showing marked blood-pressure lowering with saralasin. They concluded that in this model, hypertension is dependent on the RAS only to the extent that PRA is raised; even with high PRA, other factors contribute to the genesis of hypertension.

Bing and Nielsen [105] likewise noted variable responses to infused saralasin in 2-kidney, 1-clip hypertensive rats.

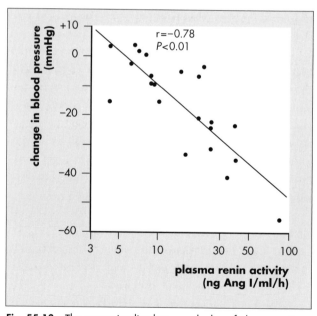

Fig. 55.13 The regression line between the log of plasma renin activity (PRA) and the change in blood pressure during saralasin infusion in 2-kidney, 1-clip rats, showing a highly significant correlation. The line intercepts the zero-change point on the y axis at a PRA of 5.7 ng Ang I/ml/h, almost exactly the mean normal value (5.6ng/ml/h). Modified from Macdonald GJ *et al* [104].

More consistently, Pals *et al* [106] observed a depressor effect with saralasin during the first two weeks after renal artery clipping, but not at four or six weeks; thus, their findings also disagreed with those of Brunner *et al* [102].

Bumpus *et al* [107] administered acutely the Ang II antagonist [Ile^8]Ang II to 2-kidney, 1-clip hypertensive rats six weeks after clipping. Like Brunner *et al* [102] but unlike MacDonald *et al* [103,104], they found a substantial and overall highly significant fall in blood pressure.

Otsuka *et al* [108] gave brief (1–2-hour) intravenous infusions of saralasin into 2-kidney, 1-clip hypertensive rats 12–16 weeks after clipping. They found a spectrum of hypotensive response from zero to 100mmHg, which surprisingly was quite unrelated to PRA; their results yet again thus conflict with those of MacDonald *et al* [103,104].

Clearly, these very divergent reports can not easily be reconciled. Intuitively, the data of MacDonald *et al* [103,104] must be favored because the blood-pressure changes were closely correlated with PRA measurements, which speaks for methodological accuracy. This view is also supported indirectly by concordant observations with saralasin in man, and with ACE inhibition in several species (see later).

Rat: Long-term angiotensin II antagonism

Riegger *et al* [109] studied both the acute and the more prolonged (11-hour) intravenous infusion of saralasin to 2-kidney, 1-clip hypertensive rats between 28 and 60 days (mean 42 days) from clipping. They found a variable small immediate fall in pressure which, as in the studies of Macdonald *et al* [103,104], was significantly correlated with the presaralasin plasma renin level. However, the more prolonged infusion of saralasin gradually returned blood pressure to normal (Fig. 55.14a); the late fall in pressure was not correlated with presaralasin plasma renin. This slow fall in blood pressure was considered to result from antagonism of the slow pressor effect of Ang II (see *Chapter 28*).

Similar 11-hour infusions of saralasin into rats with 2-kidney, 1-clip hypertension, but of more than four months' duration, were made by Thurston *et al* [110]. Unlike Riegger *et al* [109], these workers found saralasin to be quite ineffective.

Bing *et al* [111] extended the latter experiments. They gave 12-hour intravenous infusions of saralasin into rats with 2-kidney 1-clip hypertension of 28–63 days' (mean 44 days) duration, that is, almost exactly comparable to the study of Riegger *et al* [109]. Unlike Riegger *et al* [109], but similar to the observations of Thurston *et al* [110] in rats with more long-standing hypertension, they did not find that saralasin returned blood pressure to normal. Bing *et al* [111] saw the maximal fall in

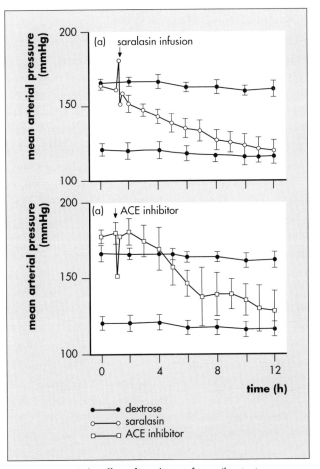

Fig. 55.14 (a) The effect of saralasin infusion (beginning at arrow) in 12 hypertensive rats, compared with dextrose in hypertensive and normal rats. (b) The effect of an ACE inhibitor infusion (beginning at arrow) in hypertensive rats. The controls of dextrose infusion in normal and hypertensive rats were from the study in (a). Data are presented as the mean ± SEM. Modified from Riegger AJG *et al* [109].

blood pressure by 30 minutes, with no change thereafter.

It is again not easy to explain the different results obtained in very similar circumstances in the rat by these two groups of experienced and reputable investigators [109–111]. One suggested possibility [18,112] is that Riegger *et al* [109] performed infusions during the day, when blood pressure in the rat is at the trough of its variation, while Bing *et al* [111] infused during the night, when pressure would be at its highest and could have obscured the effect of saralasin.

Dog

The effects of analog antagonists of Ang II were studied in 2-kidney, 1-clip hypertension in the dog in a series of experiments by Ferrario and his colleagues [86,113]. Intravenous infusions of either [Sar^1–Ile^8]Ang II or [Sar^1–Thr^8]Ang II were given for one hour. Such administration of a competitive Ang II antagonist within 1–5 days of renal artery constriction caused a significant fall in blood pressure which lasted for the duration of the infusion and was associated with a marked diminution in the pressor response to injected Ang II. However, no significant hypotensive effect could be obtained when the Ang II antagonist was given later than one week after renal artery clamping.

Watkins et al [114] similarly found that the short-term infusion of saralasin into dogs with chronic 2-kidney, 1-clip hypertension did not affect arterial pressure.

Man

Short-term incremental infusions of saralasin, to a maximum dose of 10µg/kg/min enjoyed, for a short time, a considerable vogue as a screening or as a diagnostic test for renovascular hypertension, and as a guide to prognosis following surgical intervention. The approach had, however, distinct theoretical, as well as practical, limitations.

There is now little dispute that in man, the early fall in arterial pressure with the administration of saralasin is directly proportional to the presaralasin circulating level of renin or Ang II [115] (see *Chapters 1* and *86*). Thus, the procedure is no more than a surrogate for plasma renin or Ang II assay [10] (see *Figs. 1.13* and *86.4*).

Moreover, there is lack of agreement on the value or otherwise of prior sodium deprivation. Some investigators have advocated furosemide administration and/or sodium restriction before saralasin infusion, claiming that specificity is thereby enhanced [116]. Others have reported contrariwise that such measures obscure the ability of saralasin (or similar drugs) to distinguish renovascular hypertension from other forms of clinical hypertension [11].

A hypotensive response to saralasin was claimed by Brunner et al [117] and by Streeten et al [118] to be an excellent guide to 'true' renovascular hypertension. Other investigators have found, by contrast, appreciable numbers of false-negative and false-positive results [119,120].

The partial agonistic activity of saralasin (see *Chapter 86*) can add a further element of confusion.

Angiotensin-converting enzyme inhibitors

Rat: Short-term angiotensin-converting enzyme inhibition

The short-term administration (from a few minutes up to 3.5 hours) intravascularly of various ACE inhibitors into 2-kidney,

1-clip hypertensive rats from 1–2 days to four weeks after clipping usually had a clear antihypertensive effect [20,121,122] that could be reversed by infusing Ang II or Ang III.

With more prolonged hypertension in this rat model (up to 151 days postclipping), similar brief infusion of an ACE inhibitor was less consistent in lowering arterial pressure [20, 108,109,111]. Irrespective of the duration or severity of the hypertension, Morton and Wallace [20] and Wallace et al [112] found that the fall in blood pressure with such brief ACE inhibition correlated closely with the basal plasma concentration of Ang II. Otsuka et al [108] saw a rather less close relationship between the hypotensive response and the basal PRA. Bing et al [111] by contrast did not find a significant relationship between the acute fall in blood pressure with captopril and the basal PRC.

Despite some variations in emphasis and some inconsistencies, these data appear to agree with those reported by Macdonald et al [103,104], Riegger et al [109], and Bing et al [111] with saralasin. The acute blood-pressure response to antagonism of the RAS with either of these classes of drugs probably reflects immediate elimination of the direct pressor effect of Ang II.

Rat: Long-term angiotensin-converting enzyme inhition

There is less accord on the effects of more prolonged ACE inhibition in the later stages of 2-kidney, 1-clip hypertension in the rat.

Riegger et al [109], studying animals a mean 42 days after clipping, reported that continuous infusion of an ACE inhibitor over 11 hours returned blood pressure to normal, irrespective of the initial hypotensive response (Fig. 55.14b).

While Bing et al [111] agreed that similar 12-hour infusion of captopril often lowered blood pressure substantially at the same chronic stage of hypertension, they saw no difference in the response between 30 minutes and 12 hours — results that are at variance with those of Riegger et al [109]. Bing et al [111] did not find that prolonged captopril administration returned blood pressure to normal.

Thurston et al [110] observed that oral captopril caused a marked fall in blood pressure in rats with 2-kidney, 1-clip hypertension of four months' duration although, as mentioned above, a prolonged infusion of saralasin was quite ineffective.

Bengis and Coleman [87] administered captopril in the drinking water to rats with 2-kidney 1-clip hypertension three weeks after clipping; one week of such treatment reduced blood pressure to normal, although the fall in blood pressure in the first 24 hours was modest in those animals with stable hypertension.

In rats with what Bengis and Coleman [87] term 'malignant' hypertension, which corresponds with the hyponatremic hypertensive syndrome in man (see earlier), a precipitous fall in blood pressure was seen initially, with normotensive values achieved with long-term treatment. This same pattern is seen with ACE inhibition in this syndrome in patients [35].

Wallace *et al* [112] performed what appeared to be a decisive study in this crucial, but thus far contentious, area. Rats with 2-kidney, 1-clip hypertension of duration 5–13 weeks were given a bolus injection of captopril followed by a chronic infusion of either dextrose solution or captopril lasting five days (Fig. 55.15). Following the bolus of captopril, blood pressure fell acutely from a mean of 165mmHg to 138mmHg. By contrast, 12 hours after starting chronic captopril administration, mean arterial pressure fell to a nadir of 112mmHg, significantly lower than that after the acute injection of captopril. Blood pressure remained lower throughout the five days of captopril infusion, whereas it continued to rise in the rats given dextrose. The acute blood-pressure fall with captopril was closely related to the pretreatment plasma Ang II concentration (r=0.87, $P<0.001$). The relationship during long-term captopril was much less close and only occasionally significant. Taken together with their earlier experiments [20], these findings of Wallace *et al* [112] were interpreted as showing that while, in phase II of 2-kidney, 1-clip hypertension in the rat, plasma concentrations of Ang II are low in relationship to those in phase I, they are still elevated compared with normal animals and could indeed be contributing to hypertension by a slower secondary effect. Conversely, chronic administration of captopril, suppressing Ang II formation, can slowly reverse this action.

Rat: Prophylactic angiotensin-converting enzyme inhibition
Even more decisive and gratifyingly uncontroversial are the prophylactic effects of long-term ACE inhibition in this model. Continuous captopril administration, whether started before [123,124] or 12 days after, clipping [125], completely prevented the development of hypertension in studies continued for at least eight weeks. Withdrawal of captopril led to the late appearance of hypertension [90] (Fig. 55.16). Guanethidine did not prevent the development of hypertension, but did limit its late appearance after the withdrawal of captopril. In this model, blockade of the prostaglandin system with indomethacin and of the kallikrein–kinin system with aprotinin had no effect on the antihypertensive action of captopril [90]. Thus, both the RAS and the sympathetic system required to be functional before the blood pressure increased.

Dog
In the dog with 2-kidney, 1-clip hypertension, the brief administration of an ACE inhibitor has been shown to lower systemic

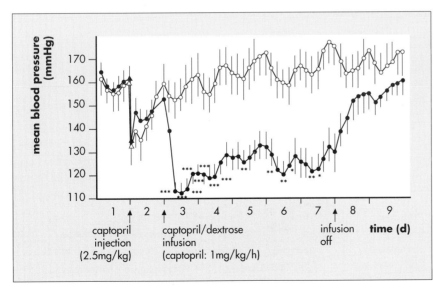

Fig. 55.15 The blood-pressure profile of rats with 2-kidney, 1-clip hypertension given an acute injection of captopril followed by a chronic captopril infusion (closed symbols). The circles represent the four-hour mean of 10-minute measurements starting at 1000 h each day. The triangles represent the mean of ten 1-minute measurements taken before the acute injection of captopril followed by the lowest individual pressure reading obtained after the injection of captopril. A one-tailed Wilcoxon signed rank test for matched pairs was used to compare mean pressures obtained during the chronic infusion of captopril (●) with the lowest pressure obtained after the acute injection of captopril (▲). ***$P<0.005$, **$P<0.025$, *$P<0.01$; bars represent 1 SEM. Modified from Wallace ECH *et al* [112].

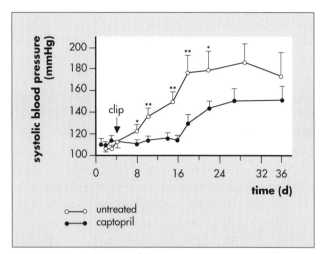

Fig. 55.16 Development of hypertension in two groups of rats with the left renal artery clipped and the contralateral kidney untouched. One group (n = 7) was untreated and the other group (n = 7) was infused continously from days 3–16 with captopril, 80μg/h intraperitoneally. Rats were clipped on day 4. Differences between two groups: *P<0.025, **P<0.01. Modified from Freeman RH *et al* [124].

arterial pressure, whether given immediately after acute renal artery constriction [24], or at intervals from 1–25 days after applying the stenosis [25]. In the latter study, the fall in blood pressure caused by captopril late in the course of the experiment, when peripheral plasma renin was no longer clearly raised, indicated that Ang II was, nevertheless, still constricting resistance arteries at that stage.

Man

In patients with unilateral renal artery stenosis, therapy is inevitably started at a late stage of the disease. With first administration of an ACE inhibitor, the initial fall in blood pressure was shown to be closely proportional to the pretreatment plasma level of renin and Ang II, and to the early fall of Ang II with ACE inhibition [35,72,126]. The fall in pressure is precipitous in the hyponatremic syndrome [35]. These results in man again agree with data in animals presented above. While, with prolonged ACE inhibitor therapy in most patients, there may be further reduction of hypertension, the correlations with components of the RAS become less close and may no longer be statistically significant [72].

Deserving emphasis is that in patients with hypertension and unilateral renal artery stenosis, the blood-pressure response to prolonged ACE inhibition has been reported to predict the

outcome following surgical treatment [127,128] or percutaneous angioplasty [209]. By contrast, the initial blood-pressure response to ACE inhibition is unhelpful.

The clinical aspects of ACE inhibition with renal artery stenosis are presented in greater detail in *Chapters 88–90*.

PATTERNS OF CHANGES IN ACTIVE AND INACTIVE RENIN, AND IN ANGIOTENSIN II, ACROSS THE TWO KIDNEYS

The most detailed studies have been performed in patients with unilateral renal artery stenosis [38,39,129,130]. These matters are discussed further in *Chapter 88*.

As has been described earlier in this chapter, in unilateral renal artery stenosis in man, across the affected kidney, positive venoarterial plasma ratios of active and inactive renin, and of Ang I and Ang II, have been reported, showing net secretion of these substances on the stenotic side. The contralateral kidney shows inhibition of renin secretion and net extraction of Ang II. The renal vein ratio of active renin between the two kidneys has been shown to be more closely related to the reduction of renal plasma flow than to renin secretion rate on the affected side. During long-term ACE inhibition and consequent lowering of peripheral plasma Ang II, active renin concentration is markedly elevated, both in peripheral arterial plasma and in renal venous plasma of the stenotic kidney. However, in these circumstances, despite several potential stimuli to renin secretion, including the lowering of arterial Ang II and of systemic blood pressure, secretion of renin by the contralateral kidney remains suppressed [129], or that kidney may even become a net extractor of renin [38,130].

HEMODYNAMIC EVOLUTION OF THE HYPERTENSION

Very detailed and careful studies have been performed in the dog by several groups, and especially by those of Bianchi, Maxwell, Lupu, Freeman and Anderson [23–25,31,32,131]. From these has emerged a broadly consistent and clear pattern of the main hemodynamic and related events. All are agreed, as already emphasized, on the need to avoid studies under anesthesia, which can disturb the various measurements.

Within the first two hours of unilateral renal artery constriction, there are acute increases in the peripheral plasma levels of renin and Ang II, while the regression of changes in blood pressure on endogenous plasma Ang II match those seen in the same animals during acute pressor infusions of Ang II [22] (*Fig. 55.5*). Graded acute unilateral renal artery stenosis causes graded parallel increases in arterial pressure and plasma renin, with elevated peripheral resistance. After an initial reduction in renal artery pressure and in renal blood flow distal to the applied stenosis, once systemic hypertension has developed, renal blood flow is largely restored [24]. These changes are slight and transient after mild or moderate renal artery stenosis, but are sustained with severe stenosis. Angiotensin-converting enzyme inhibition abolishes the increases in systemic arterial pressure, the contralateral renal vasoconstriction, and the raised peripheral resistance. By contrast, pentolinium administration does not significantly affect the hypertension or contralateral renal vasoconstriction. Thus, circulating Ang II appears to be predominantly responsible for the acute hemodynamic changes, with little or no involvement of the autonomic nervous system. The acute hypertension and raised peripheral resistance with unilateral renal artery stenosis are due to decreased conductance in the stenotic kidney because of the renal artery stenosis (approximately 20%); vasoconstriction in the contralateral kidney (approximately 20%); and vasoconstriction in other systemic vessels (approximately 60%).

With the more prolonged evolution of 2-kidney, 1-clip hypertension in the dog, although increases in cardiac output have been reported by some investigators [131] these are neither consistent nor necessary components [23–25]. There are also no consistent changes in body sodium content or in plasma or extracellular fluid volumes [23–25]. Anderson et al [25] made detailed controlled studies in conscious dogs with unilateral renal artery stenosis for up to 25 days. The above-mentioned prompt and sustained rise in blood pressure was at all stages due to raised peripheral resistance. Thus, raised peripheral resistance was comprised long term of components not greatly different in their quantitative contribution from those seen acutely. The increased peripheral resistance was made up of 25% in the stenotic kidney and was due mainly to the mechanical effect of the stenosis itself; 15% in the contralateral nonstenotic kidney; and 60% in the nonrenal vasculature. Acute administration of captopril lowered both arterial pressure and peripheral resistance, even when peripheral renin levels were no longer elevated, indicating an effect of extracirculatory Ang II. In the stenotic kidney, captopril lowered renal vascular resistance, but did not cause renal blood flow to rise, because of an approximately equal rise in the resistance of the stenosis itself. Autonomic ganglionic blockade with pentolinium had similar hemodynamic effects before and after renal artery stenosis. Thus, at all times, the hypertension was the result of increased peripheral resistance (reduced peripheral conductance), with the two kidneys together responsible for 40% of this change.

EFFECTS OF SURGICAL CORRECTION OF UNILATERAL RENAL ARTERY STENOSIS

The preferred definitive therapy for unilateral renovascular hypertension in man is cure of the hypertension either by surgical or angioplastic relief of the stenosis [10]. While unilateral nephrectomy can also be effective, it is a less desirable procedure because, whereas correction of the stenosis usually improves overall renal function, with nephrectomy, renal function declines [132]. Two groups of investigators [126,128,209] have shown that the long-term preoperative blood-pressure response to ACE inhibition correlates well with the subsequent effect of surgery or angioplasty. These observations are compatible with the notion that the RAS is involved long term with the pathogenesis of renovascular hypertension. However, because the hypotensive effects of ACE inhibitors may involve components additional to lowering of Ang II (see *Chapter 87*), proof is lacking.

While study of the effects of unclipping in experimental 2-kidney, 1-clip hypertension in animals might have been expected to clarify the underlying mechanisms, this problem remains, despite much experimentation, unsolved [53]. The rat model has been observed in extensive detail.

Effects on blood pressure

In the 2-kidney, 1-clip hypertensive rat, unclipping, if performed within the first six weeks after clipping, usually corrects the hypertension within hours. After 16 weeks, some residual hypertension remains, which has been suggested to result from hypertensive damage in the untouched kidney [9,53]. With prolonged hypertension (phase III), there is no longer relief of the hypertension after either unclipping or excision of the clipped kidney. However, if blood pressure does remain elevated after unclipping, it can sometimes be lowered by removal of the untouched kidney [9]. This phenomenon has been attributed to hypertensive vascular damage in the untouched kidney in phase III. A similar sequence has been reported clinically [133].

The renin–angiotensin system

Bing et al [111,134,135] reported that surgical reversal of early (1–3 weeks) or late (four month) 2-kidney, 1-clip hypertension in the rat is associated with a fall in plasma renin and blood pressure. However, as discussed earlier, this group of investigators did not find a consistent effect of either ACE inhibition or Ang II antagonism at the same stage in this model; nor did such maneuvers affect the pattern of fall of blood pressure with unclipping [53,135]. Thus, they reasoned that the response to unclipping is not wholly mediated via the RAS.

Sodium and water balance

Unclipping exposes the clipped kidney suddenly to a much higher arterial pressure, and this might be expected to result in pressure natriuresis and hence a reduction in blood pressure from loss of sodium and intravascular volume. However, balance studies across unclipping in the rat showed that this was associated rather with modest and transient sodium and water retention [54,136,137], while blood volume was unchanged six hours after unclipping. Even when saline was infused so as to maintain positive sodium balance, the extent and course of the blood-pressure fall was unaltered [108].

In man, marked diuresis and natriuresis from the previously stenotic kidney have been seen after surgical relief of the stenosis [138]. However, this could have resulted from ischemic tubular damage rather than from pressure natriuresis.

Prostaglandins

With unclipping, there is little change in the urinary excretion of PGE_2 [139]. Administration of indomethacin before unclipping, with marked reduction in PGE_2 excretion, did not affect the pattern of blood-pressure fall after unclipping [139,140].

Sympathetic nervous activity

As noted earlier, any contribution from the sympathetic nervous system to the pathogenesis of renovascular hypertension remains somewhat controversial. Likewise, there is no agreement on either the pattern of sympathetic activity or its relevance, if any, to relief of hypertension after unclipping [53].

Renal medullary antihypertensive lipids

Two antihypertensive lipids, platelet-activating factor (PAF) and medullipin I, can be extracted from the renal medulla. While these substances may have a role in blood-pressure reduction after unclipping, this at present remains uncertain. Conflicting results have been obtained with various antagonists of PAF [53]. Even less certain is any participation by medullipin I. Nevertheless, Bing et al [141] showed that the fall in arterial pressure after unclipping was less in chemically medullectomized 2-kidney, 1-clip hypertensive rats.

Göthberg et al [142] found evidence of the release of powerful depressor agents from the acutely unclipped kidney in the 2-kidney, 1-clip hypertensive rat. These depressor agents were thought possibly to evoke their hypotensive effects by a central nervous action, because the fall in pressure was not accompanied by reflex tachycardia.

Summary

Much still therefore requires to be learned of the mechanisms underlying the fall of blood pressure after relief of the stenosis in 2-kidney, 1-clip hypertension. The RAS appears to be involved, although not in a clear or straightforward fashion. Renal medullary hypotensive lipids may also participate, although their role, if any, remains even more obscure.

UNCLIPPING WITH RECLIPPING

Skulan et al [143] studied the recurrent development of hypertension after reclipping in rats in which hypertension had been relieved by unclipping in the 2-kidney, 1-clip model. Full hypertensive levels were regained within 1–2 hours after reclipping in rats that had been unclipped for only two days. By contrast, rats that had been unclipped for 21 days did not attain their previous hypertension for at least one week after reclipping. Primary clipping was similarly not accompanied by full hypertensive levels for one week or more. The experiments indicated an increased responsiveness to Ang II concomitant with the development of this form of hypertension.

These results were confirmed and extended by Ten Berg and de Jong [144], who observed an enhanced blood-pressure response to infused renin, Ang II, and norepinephrine similar to that seen after reapplication of the clip.

Aspects of arterial and arteriolar resistance in relation to the pathogenesis of hypertension are discussed in further detail in *Chapters 28* and *96*.

ONE-KIDNEY, ONE-CLIP HYPERTENSION

Study of the pathogenesis and of the effects of treatment of 1-kidney, 1-clip experimental hypertension and of its clinical counterparts is, in theory at least, simpler than that of 2-kidney, 1-clip hypertension, for the obvious reason that only a solitary kidney is present to influence hormonal, metabolic, and excretory events. Even so, as will be shown, many aspects remain obscure.

It is often assumed, with some reason, that the pathogenesis also of 2-kidney, 2-clip hypertension, as well as of that produced experimentally by constricting the aorta above the origins of both renal arteries, follows closely that of the 1-kidney, 1-clip model, and these three forms are therefore considered together here. Experimental aortic constriction is sometimes, erroneously, referred to as 'coarctation', a term which is, in such context, misleading. Etymologically, the word 'coarctation' is of Latin derivation and implies 'constriction'. However, 'coarctation of the aorta' now denotes an abnormality of embryological development of the aortic arch system (see *Chapter 59*).

In some experimental animals, especially if the renal artery constriction is tight, a terminal syndrome of progressively severe hypertension, azotemia, hyperkalemia, and hypothermia can develop in the 1-kidney, 1-clip or the 2-kidney, 2-clip model [113, 145]. This phase has been called 'malignant', although such use of the term differs from the usual clinical definition (see *Chapter 60*). As noted earlier in connection with experimental 2-kidney, 1-clip hypertension, the expression of the hyponatremic hypertensive syndrome in animals has also sometimes been called 'malignant' hypertension [59,87]. This syndrome again is distinct from that seen in the 1-kidney, 1-clip model. Use of the term 'malignant' in connection with either experimental model is potentially confusing, and should be eschewed. Peart *et al* [146, 147] reporting on 121 estimations of blood urea in 82 rabbits with this form of hypertension, found that raised blood pressure was almost invariably associated with azotemia (Fig. 55.17).

The 1-kidney, 1-clip model, and, more commonly, the 2-kidney, 2-clip model, have clinical hypertensive counterparts, athough studies in man are limited.

Some authors have further proposed that there are pathophysiological affinities between 1-kidney, 1-clip hypertension and low-renin essential hypertension (see *Chapters 62* and *63*) [148,149]. However, others [150], while accepting some similarities between these conditions, have cautioned against advancing the analogy in all details (see later).

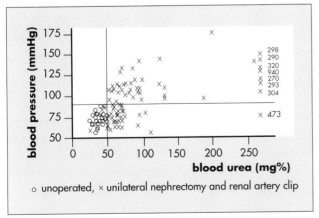

Fig. 55.17 Comparison of blood pressure with blood urea (121 estimations in 82 rabbits) in unoperated animals and those with unilateral nephrectomy and renal artery clip. Modified from Peart WS *et al* [146].

COURSE OF CHANGES IN THE RENIN–ANGIOTENSIN SYSTEM

A broadly consistent and remarkably uncontroversial evolutionary pattern has emerged for the RAS in the 1-kidney, 1-clip model of experimental hypertension, irrespective of species, of which those studied in most detail are rat, rabbit, and dog.

Within 40 minutes of renal artery constriction, possibly earlier, in the dog, and within one hour in the rat, plasma concentrations of active and total renin, of PRA, and of Ang II are increased [4,21,22,151–155]. In the dog, the intravenous infusion of renin [151,156] or of Ang II [22] into control dogs has been shown to lead to increments of arterial pressure in which the regression of PRC and/or Ang II on blood pressure is identical with that in hypertension developing acutely after renal artery constriction.

Thus, this early phase of hypertension, as in the 2-kidney, 1-clip model, appears to be fully explicable by the immediate rise in plasma renin and by the direct pressor action of the consequent increase of plasma Ang II concentration (see *Figs. 55.4–6*). In conformity with the early increased activation of the RAS, there is a parallel transient rise in plasma aldosterone [157,158].

As discussed in the section on 2-kidney, 1-clip hypertension, with enhanced RAS activity, secondary aldosteronism occurs. In the 1-kidney, 1-clip model in the dog, Watkins *et al* [152] found that hypertension developed after adrenalectomy and with constant hormone replacement. Thus, hypersecretion of mineralocorticoids during the early high-renin phase is not necessary for the development of chronic hypertension. Within two days in the rat [21,154,155] and some 7–10 days in the dog [151,152,159], plasma concentrations of active and total renin, PRA, and Ang II return to control values, although hypertension persists. There is general agreement on data from rat [21,154, 155,160], rabbit [146,161–164], and dog [145,152,159,165] that in these later chronic stable stages of 1-kidney, 1-clip hypertension, there is usually no longer evidence of activation of the peripheral plasma RAS.

In rabbits with this form of hypertension, 1–4 weeks after clipping, Lever and Robertson [166] found plasma total renin concentration to be distinctly higher (*P*<0.001) than in control, clipped, normotensive rabbits. However, the assay required the removal of large blood samples, and thus hemorrhage itself could have been responsible for the differences between the two groups. Nevertheless, the study emphasizes the more readily stimulated release of renin when the sole kidney bears a renal artery clip.

A distinction requires to be made also in the case of those animals (see above) that develop terminal severe hypertension, azotemia, and hyperkalemia, and who are, often loosely, described as having 'malignant' hypertension [87,113,145]. With the onset of this complication, the RAS can again become hyperactive.

CHANGES IN BODY SODIUM CONTENT AND FLUID COMPARTMENTS

In this connection, the distorting effect of anesthesia during animal experiments [23,151], already mentioned earlier in this chapter, requires attention; the most reliable data have consequently been obtained in the absence of anesthesia.

With the above proviso, and with only minor inconsistencies, there is general agreement amongst data obtained in rat and dog, on early, sometimes transient but more usually sustained, increases in body sodium, plasma volume, extracellular fluid volume, and total body water [149,151,154,157,167–172,200].

McAreavey *et al* [154] found stable expansion of exchangeable body sodium in rats for up to six weeks after clipping the artery to the sole remaining kidney (Fig. 55.18). In this study, progressively severe hypertension developed despite the fixed increase in body sodium and although plasma active renin concentration had returned to basal values. Thus, these investigators, like others earlier working with dogs [151], could not explain the pathogenesis of the hypertension simply in terms of the observed changes of the plasma RAS and concurrent sodium status, considered either separately or together.

Furthermore, numerous investigators have shown that 1-kidney, 1-clip hypertension, in several species, can develop despite sodium restriction [149]. Considerable hypertension can indeed be sustained in this model even with depletion of sodium [149,153], although its severity may then be abated [81].

CHANGES IN ATRIAL NATRIURETIC FACTOR

Alterations in ANF are largely as would be expected from the pattern of changes in body sodium content described.

In the rat, Garcia *et al* [173] found plasma ANF to be elevated at 1, 2, 4, 6, and 8 weeks after constriction of one renal artery plus removal of the contralateral kidney; plasma ANF was correlated with blood pressure (r=0.56; *P*<0.001). After unclipping, blood pressure returned to normal within six hours; plasma ANF also fell by six hours, but remained higher than in controls. There were no differences in plasma ANF between previously hypertensive and control rats on the 9th and 13th days after unclipping.

Garcia *et al* [174] further showed that with unclipping, there was an increase in glomerular ANF-receptor density and

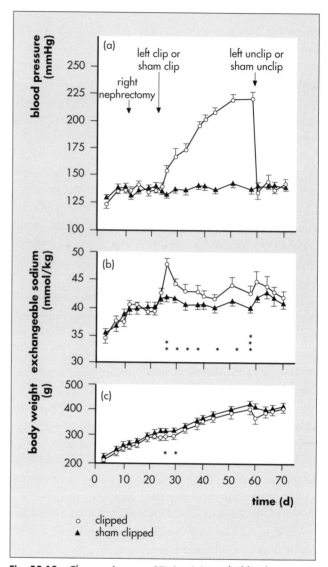

Fig. 55.18 Changes (mean ± SEM) in (a) systolic blood pressure, (b) exchangeable sodium, and (c) body weight in clipped and sham-clipped animals. Significance of differences between clipped and sham-clipped rats. *P<0.05; **P<0.01; ***P<0.001. Modified from McAreavey D *et al* [154].

affinity concomitant with the fall in plasma ANF concentration. They proposed that early after clip removal, pressure natriuresis is predominant in causing sodium loss; later, upregulation of glomerular ANF receptors may become the main mechanism underlying natriuresis.

These workers [175] found evidence in 1-kidney, 1-clip hypertension in the rat that infusion of ANF caused increased natriuresis, associated with lowering of initially elevated epinephrine and norepinephrine, and increased excretion of dopamine metabolites. Thus, ANF appears to act to modulate and suppress increased sympathetic activity in this model of experimental hypertension.

In the dog with 1-kidney, 1-clip hypertension, Verburg *et al* [176] observed elevated plasma ANF in association with raised PRA and aldosterone and hypertension at the third day after renal artery constriction. The raised arterial pressure stabilized at 35–40mmHg above baseline for the four weeks of the study. In this period, PRA and aldosterone returned to control values. Although plasma ANF also fell substantially from the 3rd to the 28th day after clipping, it remained significantly elevated at the end of this time.

THE SYMPATHETIC NERVOUS SYSTEM

Walker *et al* [91] found plasma norepinephrine to be elevated in 1-kidney, 1-clip hypertension in the rat.

Similarly, as mentioned earlier, Debinski *et al* [175] reported elevated urinary excretion rates of norepinephrine and epinephrine in this model in the rat.

EFFECT OF ANTAGONISTS OF THE RENIN–ANGIOTENSIN SYSTEM

In the initial phase of 1-kidney, 1-clip hypertension, when there is undoubted activation of the peripheral RAS, the administration of Ang II antagonists, ACE inhibitors, or renin inhibitors, lowers arterial pressure acutely [21,152,159,165,177,178]. Prior administration of these agents, moreover, prevents the development of early hypertension after constriction of the artery to the solitary kidney.

However, in the rat, Freeman *et al* [124] found that infusion of captopril prevented a rise in blood pressure until the eighth day after clipping; hypertension then developed despite ACE inhibition continuing for a further four days (Fig. 55.19). Watkins *et al* [159] showed that in the dog likewise, blockade of the RAS started 1–2 days before and continued for 6–7 days after, constricting the artery to a sole kidney, using either the Ang II antagonist saralasin or the ACE inhibitor teprotide, delayed the onset of hypertension, but did not prevent its appearance by day 7–8. Long-term saralasin administration can cause a slow pressure rise [179], and thus the significance of this aspect of the study is uncertain. The observations with teprotide, nevertheless, demonstrate that chronic 1-kidney, 1-clip hypertension can develop and be sustained, despite complete or nearly complete antagonism of the RAS during the initial high-renin phase. This is an important point of difference from the 2-kidney, 1-clip model [123–125].

The short-term administration of Ang II antagonists or ACE inhibitors in the chronic phase of hypertension in this

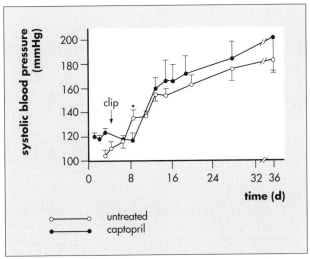

Fig. 55.19 Development of hypertension in two groups of rats with the left renal artery clipped and right nephrectomy. One group was untreated (n = 6) and the other group (n = 6) was infused continuously from days 3–16 with captopril, 80μg/h intraperitoneally. Rats were clipped on day four. Differences between the two groups: *P<0.025. Modified from Freeman RH *et al* [124].

model, when the RAS is not activated, not surprisingly does not lower arterial pressure appreciably either in the rat or dog [87,107,145,180]. Bengis and Coleman [87] noted that the administration of oral captopril over seven days in rats with stable 1-kidney, 1-clip hypertension did reduce the hypertension, but only slightly (Fig. 55.20).

However, the combination of sodium restriction with blockade of the RAS can, during this chronic stable phase of 1-kidney, 1-clip hypertension, lower blood pressure substantially [180, 181].

With supervention of severe late hypertension, uremia, and a secondary rise in plasma renin and Ang II (so-called 'malignant' hypertension), both in the rat and the dog, antagonism of the RAS is again effective in lowering arterial pressure [87,113, 145], but, not surprisingly, is poorly tolerated and usually leads to uremia and death.

INTRARENAL EFFECTS OF ANGIOTENSIN II

Anderson and his colleagues [182–184,198] have studied in detail the intrarenal effects of Ang II in the 1-kidney, 1-clip model in the dog.

In the case of experimental mild renal artery stenosis that is not sufficiently severe to cause systemic hypertension, they showed, by administration of an ACE inhibitor or an Ang II

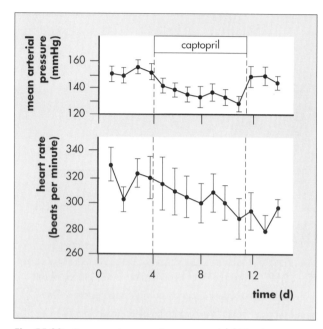

Fig. 55.20 Response to converting enzyme inhibition in seven 1-kidney, 1-clip Goldblatt rats. Data are presented as group mean result ± SEM. Modified from Bengis RG and Coleman TG *et al* [87].

antagonist, that increases in endogenous Ang II restored renal artery pressure distal to the stenosis towards prestenosis values and also maintained GFR. With blockade of the RAS, distal renal artery pressure and GFR fell steeply. Angiotensin II could maintain renal function in this way even when peripheral plasma renin and Ang II were normal, indicating that the Ang II responsible for the compensatory changes in renal function was formed intrarenally. The most likely intrarenal target of action of Ang II in producing these effects is efferent glomerular arterioles, which are differentially sensitive to Ang II; the glomerular mesangium is an additional possibility (see *Chapter 26*). Also probable in these circumstances is that the restricted renal blood flow is then routed mainly via juxtamedullary nephrons, with important functional consequences (see *Chapters 21* and *26*).

With more marked stenosis, there is greater stimulation of the RAS, peripheral plasma levels of renin and Ang II are clearly increased, as described above, and the dependence of renal function, albeit now distinctly impaired, on the RAS, is even bigger.

Anderson *et al* [182–184] confirmed the findings, presented earlier, that over the first few days, sodium, potassium, and water are retained. Surprisingly, however, such fluid and electrolyte retention at this phase was little altered if an ACE inhibitor

was administered. This observation may be relevant to the data of Watkins *et al* [159], mentioned above, which showed that chronic hypertension in this model in the dog can develop even though the RAS is blocked before, and for up to one week after, renal artery constriction.

In the later, chronic stable phase of hypertension in the dog, when peripheral plasma renin and Ang II have reverted to normal, the intrarenal actions of Ang II still remain crucial in the preservation, at least partly, of renal function [182–184,198]. As with mild, nonhypertensive renal artery stenosis, the intrarenal action of locally generated Ang II appears to be responsible.

In summary, in this 1-kidney, 1-clip model, a renal 'barostat'-mediated increase in RAS activity appears, with mild renal artery stenosis, to be the principal mechanism restoring distal renal artery pressure. With more severe stenosis, systemic hypertension makes a substantial contribution towards the correction of distal renal artery pressure [182–184].

THE ROLE OF TRANSFORMED RENIN

Skeggs and his colleagues [161,185] noted the paradox that although there is little evidence of systemic involvement of the RAS in the chronic stable phase of 1-kidney, 1-clip hypertension, direct immunization with purified pig kidney renin lowered the blood pressure of rabbits with this form of hypertension. They postulated that renin is converted into a form that is present most conspicuously in arterial and arteriolar smooth muscle, and that it then acts there to promote vasoconstriction. This transformed renin was suggested as exhibiting new antigenic sites, and eliciting a second antihypertensive antibody. Skeggs *et al* [161,185] found that such an antibody, when free of antirenin, could lower the blood pressure of 1-kidney, 1-clip hypertensive rabbits.

These investigators concluded that plasma renin may enter the cytoplasm of vascular smooth-muscle cells, where it becomes complexed with a very high molecular-weight substance in a mainly perinuclear distribution, and becomes antigenic. This complex antigen is a critical part of the pathogenesis of 1-kidney, 1-clip hypertension in the rabbit; its neutralization corrects the raised blood pressure.

HEMODYNAMIC CHANGES

In the first three days after constricting the artery to a single kidney in conscious dogs, Anderson *et al* [183] did not find a significant rise in cardiac output. There was evidence of an Ang II-mediated vasoconstriction of nonrenal vascular beds which was responsible for approximately two-thirds of the rise in blood pressure. The resistance due to the renal artery stenosis itself was the cause of the remaining one-third of the diminution of peripheral conductance.

Both in the rat and the dog, an increase in cardiac output has been noted, occurring not immediately after renal artery constriction, but, in the dog for example, within 2–7 days [85,151, 169,183,186–189]. The raised cardiac output is held to promote an increase in peripheral resistance [149]. Subsequently, cardiac output reverts to, or towards, normal [149].

Factors that have been invoked as responsible for the increase in cardiac output [149] include a rise in mean circulatory filling pressure [189–191], which in turn might result from the early sodium and water retention already described above. A further contributor could be increased tone and/or diminished compliance in capacitance vessels [189,191–194]. Another possible factor leading to a rise in cardiac output is an enhanced myocardial contractility not attributable to Ang II [195]. Elevated sympathetic activity [175] also may participate.

With the establishment of chronic stable hypertension, increased peripheral resistance develops, with normal or near-normal cardiac output. The mechanisms of this evolution are not agreed; the hypothesis has been advanced that a main reason is microcirculatory autoregulation, perhaps attributable to a rise in tissue oxygen availability, which tends to exceed demand [149, 196].

The studies of Simon [193] in this model in the rat led to the conclusion that in chronic stable hypertension, the contribution of any vascular wall 'waterlogging' either to increased structural arterial resistance or to decreased structural venous capacity was at most minor.

Imig and Anderson [197], also in the rat, observed that small arteries upstream from the microcirculation make a major contribution to the chronically increased peripheral resistance [198].

BAROREFLEXES

Machado et al [199] measured heart rate continuously by electrocardiogram during the development of 1-kidney, 1-clip hypertension in the rat. There was a progressive rise in heart rate in parallel with the increase in blood pressure over the initial seven days following clipping. After the first week, heart rate decreased, although blood pressure continued to rise. These experiments were interpreted as indicating transiently impaired baroreflex control in the initial stages of this model of hypertension.

In the dog, Liard et al [158] demonstrated that the increase in arterial pressure in the first hour was much greater in baroreceptor denervated dogs than in intact animals.

EFFECTS OF UNCLIPPING

The kidney beyond a renal artery stenosis is protected from the adverse vascular effects of systemic hypertension; thus, relief of the stenosis is especially beneficial in restoring renal function. This is a particularly important consideration in the rather uncommon clinical counterpart of 1-kidney, 1-clip hypertension [10]. Furthermore, in this model, relief of the stenosis of the single renal artery immediately, directly, and substantially, increases peripheral conductance.

Removal of the clip thus almost invariably, and promptly, restores blood pressure to normal and corrects the expansion of body sodium [154] (*Fig. 55.18*). The elevated plasma ANF also reverts to normal [173,174] (see earlier). The detailed mechanisms involved have been reviewed extensively [53,149,173, 174]. A highly significant correlation was found in rats between the fall in arterial pressure over the first six hours after unclipping and enhanced sodium excretion [200]; when saline was infused following unclipping, the time taken for blood pressure to return to normal increased from 3 hours to 15 hours [201]. When the body fluid volume was kept constant after unclipping, the fall in blood pressure over the first hour was much diminished [160]. A much-quoted experiment [202] showed that simultaneous clip removal and ureterocaval anastomosis was as effective as clip removal alone in abolishing the hypertension within 24 hours in this model in the rat, and was taken as evidence that external fluid loss is not necessary for the hypotensive process. However, it may be questioned whether the intravenous infusion of large volumes of urine permits ready interpretation of the cause of changes in blood pressure. Even so, ureterocaval anastomosis delays the fall in blood pressure after unclipping similarly to the less crude replacement of lost fluid by saline infusion [149,201]. Therefore, it appears that a substantial, if not a mandatory, component of blood-pressure reduction after unclipping comprises early sodium and fluid loss.

Akahoshi and Carretero [160] showed that removal of the clip in the chronic stable phase of 1-kidney, 1-clip hypertension in the rat was followed by an average fall in systemic blood pressure of 27mmHg, even if very high doses of Ang II were infused; when the Ang II administration was then stopped, blood pressure fell by an additional average 44mmHg. Taken with their concurrent data on fluid balance quoted above, the observations led these investigators to conclude that volume factors, rather than the RAS, are predominant in relation to hypertension in the chronic stable phase.

Unclipping in this model does not usually affect plasma renin [53].

The possible involvement of renal medullary hypotensive

factors has been discussed earlier in this chapter in connection with 2-kidney, 1-clip hypertension. It is possible that increased release of such factors could be in part responsible for lowering blood pressure after unclipping also in the 1-kidney model [149, 203]; so far, however, these aspects remain unclear.

Pamnani et al [204] found decreased myocardial microsomal Na/K ATPase activity, arterial wall ouabain-sensitive rubidium uptake and arterial smooth muscle cell membrane potentials, together with increased plasma Na/K pump inhibitory activity at the fifth week of 1-kidney, 1-clip hypertension in rats. After unclipping, while blood pressure returned to normal within three hours, the various abnormalities under study remained for more than three days. Thus, these changes were not causally involved in the acute blood-pressure reduction with unclipping.

Walker et al [91] observed a slight, but insignificant, fall in plasma norepinephrine on unclipping in this model in the rat. While, as mentioned earlier, hypertension is accompanied by increased plasma norepinephrine, the fall in blood pressure on unclipping does not seem to be mediated via reduced sympathetic activity.

RENAL CELLOPHANE WRAP HYPERTENSION AND THE RENIN–ANGIOTENSIN SYSTEM

Denton and Anderson [205] examined the role of the RAS in the development of hypertension produced in rabbits by bilateral renal cellophane wrap. Sham-operated rabbits served as controls. Half of the animals in each group received enalapril throughout. Four weeks after renal wrapping, mean arterial pressure had risen by 48 ± 5 mmHg in untreated rabbits, but by only 25 ± 4 mmHg in enalapril-treated rabbits ($P<0.01$). Similar differences were also measured six weeks after wrapping. In untreated rabbits, PRA had increased four-fold four and six weeks after renal wrapping. There were no significant changes in blood pressure or PRA following sham operation. Compared with that in sham-operated rabbits, renal blood flow was reduced by 60% in the untreated rabbits four weeks after wrapping but by only 30% in the enalapril-treated wrapped rabbits ($P<0.05$). Renal wrapping did not alter filtration fraction in untreated rabbits, but markedly reduced it in enalapril-treated rabbits.

These results suggested to the authors that Ang II had two major effects in rabbits after bilateral renal wrapping: it contributed substantially to the increase in blood pressure and caused renal vasoconstriction, primarily at a postglomerular site.

Freeman et al [32] made dogs hypertensive by wrapping the left kidney in cellophane and removing the contralateral kidney three weeks later. One week before the nephrectomy, the dogs were fed a diet very low in sodium and were also administered diuretic for three days. The superimposed sodium depletion raised PRA 3–5 times but did not change arterial pressure. Within two days of nephrectomy, which did not further affect PRA, there was a highly significant rise in blood pressure, which remained elevated throughout an additional four weeks during which time sodium depletion was enforced. These investigators concluded that initial blood volume expansion, with such possible consequences as elevated cardiac output, are not necessary for the development of experimental renal hypertension. The results cast doubt in this context of the theory of whole body autoregulation in pathogenesis.

Ferrario et al [113] studied dogs with long-standing cellophane wrap hypertension, the contralateral kidney having been removed. With hypertension of 2–7 months' duration, plasma renin levels were entirely normal. Infusion of analog antagonists of Ang II for 5–48 hours raised arterial pressure further, again emphasizing, as in the experiments of Brown et al [179] in the rat, the agonistic effects of agents of this class (see Chapter 86).

EXPERIMENTAL HYPERTENSION CAUSED BY DIETARY SODIUM RESTRICTION: ROLE OF THE RENIN–ANGIOTENSIN SYSTEM

Several studies quoted earlier in this chapter have made clear that, in a number of different species, variously 2-kidney, 1-clip; 1-kidney, 1-clip; and renal wrap hypertension do not require sodium retention for their expression. Indeed, in the 2-kidney, 1-clip model, excessive sodium loss from the contralateral 'untouched' kidney can, while causing frank sodium depletion, lead to gross elevation of plasma renin and Ang II and very severe, often malignant, hypertension. This is the 'hyponatremic hypertensive syndrome' described in detail above [18,35,59,75].

It is therefore relevant to emphasize that dietary sodium restriction can in the intact, normal rat, cause hypertension, together with elevation of plasma renin and impairment of growth. Such hypertension is held to be more severe with unilateral nephrectomy [206,207].

Vari et al [208], studying sodium-restricted rats with only one kidney, found that renal norepinephrine content was reduced by 96% after renal denervation. If contralateral renal denervation was performed at the time of nephrectomy, this significantly attenuated the rise in PRA, while preventing the subsequent development of hypertension.

Thus, the pressor contribution of the renal nerves in this experimental model appears to involve, at least in part, activation of the RAS.

CONCLUSIONS

As this chapter has re-emphasized, study of the various experimental Goldblatt models of hypertension and of their clinical counterparts, has provided a vast quantity of published data. Central to these investigations has been the consideration of the RAS. Inevitably, many inconsistencies exist between the different accounts, and numerous controversies remain. As always, methodological variations and frailties underlie some, at least, of these conflicts.

It has been possible to survey only a proportion of the voluminous work on the subject in this chapter. Thus, the selection inevitably reflects personal bias and prejudice, albeit an attempt has been made to put forward a fair review of this complex and difficult topic. Even so, the present abbreviated account remains extensive, and thus it may be useful to conclude with an even more succinct, if necessarily arbitrary, summary.

The 2-kidney, 1-clip and 1-kidney, 1-clip models appear to be pathophysiologically distinct, and hence are better considered separately.

TWO-KIDNEY, ONE-CLIP HYPERTENSION

In the clinically more frequently relevant 2-kidney, 1-clip model, the initiation of hypertension is due to increased renin release from the clipped kidney and thus to the immediate direct pressor effect of the elevated peripheral plasma Ang II concentration. Continued exposure to elevated Ang II, even if the increase is only modest, results in an upward shift of the Ang II/pressor dose–response curve. This has been clearly demonstrated experimentally by Ang II infusion, and clinically by study of patients with renin-secreting tumor. Thus, in the second phase, blood pressure is disproportionately elevated in relation to Ang II as compared with phase I.

Hypertension in the 2-kidney, 1-clip model can be prevented by prolonged administration of inhibitors of the RAS and can be corrected, even in phase II, by extended treatment with these agents. While there must remain reservations about the specificity of analog Ang II antagonists and ACE inhibitors in this context, these concerns should be resolved by the use of more specific renin inhibitors and of nonpeptide Ang II antagonists.

This form of hypertension can develop in the absence of changes in sodium balance and is not prevented by sodium restriction. Indeed, with severe unilateral renal artery stenosis or occlusion, frank and progressive sodium depletion can develop, with consequent ever-higher plasma renin and Ang II concentrations, and worsening, often malignant, hypertension (the hyponatremic hypertensive syndrome). Sodium repletion can be therapeutically helpful in lowering blood pressure when this complication has supervened.

Potassium restriction can prevent or correct experimental 2-kidney, 1-clip hypertension, probably by attenuating the pressor action of Ang II. However, potassium depletion, which is one of the features of the hyponatremic hypertensive syndrome, is not in these circumstances sufficient to alleviate severe hypertension.

ONE-KIDNEY, ONE-CLIP HYPERTENSION

Application of the renal artery constriction in the 1-kidney, 1-clip hypertension model is followed by an immediate, though transient, rise in peripheral plasma renin and Ang II. In this brief phase, the high blood pressure is directly attributable to the pressor action of the elevated plasma Ang II. Thereafter, plasma renin and Ang II return to normal and usually remain so, even though arterial pressure can continue to rise. Antagonism of the RAS through this initial brief phase of its stimulation prevents the initial rise of blood pressure. However, such prolonged antagonism of the RAS does not hinder the later development of hypertension; thus, established hypertension in this model does not require the initial transient elevation of circulating Ang II.

With severe renal artery constriction in this model, there can be progression to a terminal phase of severe hypertension and uremia, with a secondary increase in plasma renin and Ang II. Administration of an antagonist of the RAS in this phase will usually cause profound hypotension, worsening uremia, and early death.

One-kidney, one-clip hypertension throughout its stable phase is accompanied by modest, constant expansion of body sodium content, even though the hypertension can be progressively severe. Relief of the stenosis promptly returns body sodium and blood pressure to normal, while plasma renin is unaltered.

Combined sodium restriction and antagonism of the RAS will usually correct hypertension in this model, although prolonged treatment of this kind will further impair renal function.

We should be grateful for the partly serendipitous but nonetheless classical experiments of Goldblatt et al in 1934 [1]. These revived interest in the RAS as well as initiating study of the fascinating, if still partly elusive, problems of renovascular hypertension. Both directly and indirectly, Goldblatt's work stimulated virtually all of the research reviewed in the two volumes of this book.

REFERENCES

1. Goldblatt H, Lynch J, Hanzal RF, Summerville WW. Studies on experimental hypertension. 1. The production of persistent elevation of systolic blood pressure by means of renal ischemia. *Journal of Experimental Medicine* 1934;**59**:347–79.

2. Goldblatt PJ. The Goldblatt experiment: A conceptual paradigm. In: Laragh JH, Brenner BM, eds. *Hypertension: Pathophysiology, diagnosis and management.* New York: Raven Press, 1990:21–32.

3. Tigerstedt R, Bergman PG. Niere und Kreislauf. *Skandinavisches Archiv für Physiologie* 1898;**8**:223–71.

4. Pickering GW, Prinzmetal M. Experimental hypertension of renal origin in the rabbit. *Clinical Science* 1938;**3**:357–68.

5. Braun-Menendez E, Fasciolo JC, Leloir LF, Munoz JM, Taquini AC. *Renal hypertension, translated by Dexter L.* Springfield, Illinois: Charles C Thomas 1946.

6. Page IH, McCubbin JW. *Renal hypertension.* Year Book Medical Publishers: Chicago, 1968.

7. Leadbetter WF, Burkland CE. Hypertension in unilateral renal disease. *Journal of Urology* 1938;**39**:611–26.

8. Peart WS. Renin–angiotensin system in hypertensive disease. In: Fisher JW, ed. *Kidney hormones.* London: Academic Press, 1971:217–42.

9. Floyer MA. Role of the kidney in experimental hypertension. *British Medical Bulletin* 1957;**13**:29–32.

10. Robertson JIS. Unilateral renal disease in hypertension. In: Robertson JIS, ed. *Clinical hypertension. Handbook of hypertension, Volume 15.* Amsterdam: Elsevier 1992:chapter 10.

11. Mackay A, Brown JJ, Lever AF, Morton JJ, Robertson JIS. Unilateral renal disease in hypertension. In: Robertson JIS, ed. *Handbook of hypertension, volume 2: Clinical aspects of secondary hypertension.* Amsterdam: Elsevier 1983:33–79.

12. Page IH. The production of persistent arterial hypertension by cellophane perinephritis. *Journal of the American Medical Association* 1939;**113**:2046–8.

13. Weinberger MH, Grim CE, Donohue JP. A rare but curable form of hypertension: The 'Page kidney'. In: New MI, Levine LS, eds. *Juvenile hypertension.* New York: Raven Press, 1977:133.

14. Grollman A. A simplified procedure for inducing chronic hypertension in the mammal. *Proceedings of the Society for Experimental Biology and Medicine* 1944;**57**:102–4.

15. Oelkers W, Brown JJ, Fraser R, Lever AF, Morton JJ, Robertson JIS. Sensitization of the adrenal cortex to angiotensin II in sodium-deplete man. *Circulation Research* 1974;**34**:69–77.

16. Brown JJ, Davies DL, Lever AF, Parker RA, Robertson JIS. The assay of renin in single glomeruli and the appearance of the juxtaglomerular apparatus in the rabbit following renal artery constriction. *Clinical Science* 1966;**30**:223–35.

17. Brown JJ, Cuesta V, Davies DL, Lever AF, Morton JJ, Padfield PL, Robertson JIS, Trust P. Mechanism of renal hypertension. *Lancet* 1976;**i**:1219–21.

18. Robertson JIS, Morton JJ, Tillman DM, Lever AF. The pathophysiology of renovascular hypertension. *Journal of Hypertension* 1986;**4** (suppl 4):95–103.

19. McAllister RG, Michelakis AM, Oates JA, Foster JH. Malignant hypertension due to renal artery stenosis: Greater renin release from the non-stenotic kidney. *Journal of the American Medical Association* 1972;**221**:865–8.

20. Morton JJ, Wallace ECH. The importance of the renin angiotensin system in the development and maintenance of hypertension in the two-kidney one-clip hypertensive rat. *Clinical Science* 1983;**64**:359–70.

21. Hutchinson JS, Mathews PG, Dax E, Johnston CI. Plasma renin and angiotensin levels in experimental hypertension in the rat. *Clinical and Experimental Pharmacology and Physiology* 1975;(suppl 2):83–8.

22. Caravaggi AM, Bianchi G, Brown JJ, Lever AF, Morton JJ, Powell-Jackson JD, Robertson JIS, Semple PF. Blood pressure and plasma angiotensin II concentration after renal artery constriction and angiotensin infusion in the dog: [5-Isoleucine] angiotensin II and its breakdown fragments in dog blood. *Circulation Research* 1976;**38**:315–21.

23. Bianchi G, Baldoli E, Lucca R, Barbin P. Pathogenesis of arterial hypertension after constriction of the renal artery leaving the opposite kidney intact both in the anaesthetized and the conscious dog. *Clinical Science* 1972;**42**:651–64.

24. Anderson WP, Kline RL, Woods RL. Systemic and hemodynamic changes during acute unilateral renal artery stenosis. *American Journal of Physiology* 1985;**249**: H956–67.

25. Anderson WP, Ramsey DE, Takata M. Development of hypertension from unilateral renal artery stenosis in conscious dogs. *Hypertension* 1990;**16**:441–51.

26. Brown JJ, Casals-Stenzel J, Cumming AMM, Davies DL, Fraser R, Lever AF, Morton JJ, Semple PF, Tree M, Robertson JIS. Angiotensin II, aldosterone and arterial pressure: A quantitative approach. Arthur C Corcoran Memorial Lecture. *Hypertension* 1979;**1**:159–79.

27. Brown JJ, Fraser R, Lever AF, Morton JJ, Robertson JIS, Tree M, Bell PRF, Davidson JK, Ruthven IS. Hypertension and secondary hyperaldosteronism associated with a renin-secreting renal juxtaglomerular cell tumour. *Lancet* 1973;**ii**:1228–32.

28. Dickinson CJ, Lawrence JR. A slowly developing pressor response to small concentrations of angiotensin: Its bearing on the pathogenesis of chronic renal hypertension. *Lancet* 1963;**i**:1354–6.

29. Bean BL, Brown JJ, Casals-Stenzel J, Fraser R, Millar JA, Morton JJ, Petch B, Riegger AJG, Robertson JIS, Tree M. The relation of arterial pressure and plasma angiotensin II concentration: A change produced by prolonged infusion of angiotensin II in the conscious dog. *Circulation Research* 1979;**44**:452–8.

30. Fernandez LA, Caride VJ, Twickler J, Galardy RE. Renin–angiotensin and development of collateral circulation after renal ischemia. *American Journal of Physiology* 1982;**243**:H869–75.

31. Maxwell MH, Lupu AN, Viskoper RJ, Aravena LA, Waks UA. Mechanisms of hypertension during the acute and intermediate phases of the one-clip, two-kidney model in the dog. *Circulation Research* 1977;**40** (suppl I):I-24–8.

32. Freeman RH, Davis JO, Watkins BE. Development of chronic perinephritic hypertension in dogs without volume expansion. *American Journal of Physiology* 1977;**233**:F278–81.

33. Freeman RH, Davis JO, Watkins BE, Lohmeier TE. Mechanisms involved in two-kidney renal hypertension induced by constriction of one renal artery. *Circulation Research* 1977;**40** (suppl I):I-29–35.

34. Brown JJ, Davies DL, Lever AF, Robertson JIS. Renin and angiotensin: A survey of some aspects. *Postgraduate Medical Journal* 1966;**42**:153–76.

35. Atkinson AB, Brown JJ, Davies DL, Fraser R, Leckie B, Lever AF, Morton JJ, Robertson JIS. Hyponatraemic hypertensive syndrome with renal artery occlusion corrected by captopril. *Lancet* 1979;**ii**:606–9.

36. Brown JJ, Davies DL, Parker RA, Lever AF, Robertson JIS. Assay of renin in single glomeruli: Renin distribution in normal rabbit kidney. *Lancet* 1963;**ii**: 668–9.

37. Brown JJ, Davies DL, Lever AF, Parker RA, Robertson JIS. Assay of renin in single glomeruli of the normal rabbit and the appearance of the juxtaglomerular apparatus. *Journal of Physiology* 1965;**176**:418–28.

38. Webb DJ, Cumming AMM, Adams FC, Hodsman GP, Leckie BJ, Morton JJ, Murray GD, Lever AF, Robertson JIS. Changes in active and inactive renin and in angiotensin II across the kidney in essential hypertension and renal artery stenosis. *Journal of Hypertension* 1984;**2**:605–14.

39. Admiraal PJJ, Derkx FHM, Danser AHJ, Pieterman H, Schalekamp MADH. Intrarenal *de novo* production of angiotensin I in subjects with renal artery stenosis. *Hypertension* 1990;**16**:555–63.

40. Judson WE, Helmer OM. Diagnostic and prognostic values of renin activity in renal venous plasma in renovascular hypertension. *Hypertension: Proceedings of the Council for High Blood Pressure Research, American Heart Association* 1965;**13**: 79–89.

41. Seldinger SI. Catheter replacement of the needle in percutaneous arteriography. *Acta Radiologica* 1953;**39**:368–76.

42. Semple PF, Cumming AMM, Millar JA, Angiotensin I and II in renal vein blood. *Kidney International* 1979;**15**:276–82.

43. Mannick JA, Huvos A, Hollander WE. Post-hydralazine renin release in the diagnosis of renovascular hypertension. *Annals of Surgery* 1979;**170**:409–15.

44. Cohen EL, Rovner DR, Conn JW. Postural augmentation of plasma renin activity: Importance in diagnosis of renovascular hypertension. *Journal of the American Medical Association* 1966;**197**:973–8.

45. Strong CG, Hunt JC, Sheps SG. Renal venous renin activity: Enhancement of sensitivity of lateralization by sodium depletion. *American Journal of Cardiology* 1971;**27**:602–11.

46. Delin K, Aurell M, Granerus G. Acute stimulation of renin release in the diagnosis of renal hypertension. In: Glorioso N, Laragh JH, Rapelli A, eds. *Renovascular hypertension.* New York: Raven Press, 1987:341–50.

47. Brown JJ, Lever AF, Robertson JIS. Renal hypertension: Aetiology, diagnosis, and treatment. In: Black D, Jones NF, eds. *Renal disease 4th edition.* Oxford: Blackwell, 1979:731–65.

48. Stockigt JR, Collins RD, Noakes CA, Schambelan M, Biglieri EG. Renal vein renin in various forms of renal hypertension. *Lancet* 1972;**i**:1194–8.

49. Meignan M, Ménard J, Bonvalet JP, de Rouffignac C. Renin uptake by the right kidney in the rat following partial clamping of the left renal artery. *European Journal of Clinical Investigation* 1980;**10**:407–11.

50. Gauquelin G, Schiffrin EL, Cantin M, Garcia R. Atrial natriuretic factor: Specific binding to renal glomeruli during the development of two-kidney, one-clip hypertension in the rat. *Journal of Hypertension* 1988;**6**:587–92.

51. Paul RV. Renal atrial peptide receptors and natriuresis in two-kidney, one-clip hypertension. *Hypertension* 1991;**18**:535–42.

52. Garcia R, Gauquelin G, Cantin M, Schiffrin EL. Glomerular and vascular atrial natriuretic factor receptors in saralasin-sensitive and resistant two-kidney one-clip hypertensive rats. *Circulation Research* 1988;**63**:563–71.

53. Edmunds ME, Russell GI, Bing RF. Reversal of experimental renovascular hypertension. *Journal of Hypertension* 1991;**9**:289–301.

54. McAreavey D, Brown WB, Robertson JIS. Exchangeable sodium in rats with Goldblatt two-kidney one-clip hypertension. *Clinical Science* 1982;**63**:271–4.

55. Larochelle P, Cusson JR, Gutkowska J, Schiffrin EL, Hamet P, Kuchel O, Genest J, Cantin M. Plasma atrial natriuretic factor concentrations in essential and renovascular hypertension. *British Medical Journal* 1987;**294**:1249–52.

56. Richards AM, Tonolo G, Tree M, Robertson JIS, Montorsi P, Leckie BJ, Robertson JIS. Atrial natriuretic peptides and renin release. *American Journal of Medicine* 1988;**84** (3A):112–8.

57. Padfield PL, Brown JJ, Lever AF, Morton JJ, Robertson JIS. Blood pressure in acute and chronic vasopressin excess: Studies of malignant hypertension and the syndrome of inappropriate antidiuretic hormone secretion. *New England Journal of Medicine* 1981;**304**:1067–70.

58. Woods RL, Johnston CI. Role of vasopressin in hypertension: Studies using the Brattleboro rat. *American Journal of Physiology* 1982;**242**:F727–32.

59. Möhring J, Möhring B, Petri M, Haack D. Plasma vasopressin concentrations and effects of vasopressin antiserum on blood pressure in rats with malignant two-kidney Goldblatt hypertension. *Circulation Research* 1978;**42**:17–22.

60. Rabito SF, Carretero OA, Scicli AG. Evidence against a role of vasopressin in the maintenance of high blood pressure in mineralocorticoid and renovascular hypertension. *Hypertension* 1981;**3**:34–8.

61. Filep J, Frölich JC, Fejes-Toth G. Effect of vasopressin blockade on blood pressure in conscious rats with malignant two-kidney Goldblatt hypertension. *Clinical and Experimental Hypertension. Part A, Theory and Practice* 1985;**A7**:1007–14.

62. Ben LK, Maselli J, Keil LC, Reid IA. Role of the renin–angiotensin system in the control of vasopressin and ACTH secretion during the development of renal hypertension in dogs. *Hypertension* 1984;**6**:35–41.

63. Ploth DW, Roy RN, Huang W-C, Navar LG. Impaired autoregulatory responses in contralateral kidneys of two-kidney, one-clip hypertensive rats. *Clinical Science* 1980;**59** (suppl):381–4,

64. Ploth DW, Roy RN, Huang W-C, Navar LG. Impaired renal blood flow and cortical pressure autoregulation in contralateral kidneys of Goldblatt hypertensive rats. *Hypertension* 1981;**3**:67–74.

65. Ploth DW. Angiotensin-dependent renal mechanisms in two-kidney one-clip renal vascular hypertension. *American Journal of Physiology* 1983;**245**:F131–41.

66. Mackenzie HS, Morrill AL, Ploth DW. Pressure dependence of exaggerated natriuresis in two-kidney, one-clip Goldblatt hypertensive rats. *Kidney International* 1985;**27**:731–8.

67. Thompson JMA, Dickinson CJ. Relation between pressure and sodium excretion in perfused kidneys from rabbits with experimental hypertension. *Lancet* 1973;**ii**:1362–3.

68. De Forrest JM, Davis JO, Freeman RH, Watkins BE, Stephens GA. Separate renal function studies in conscious dogs with renovascular hypertension. *American Journal of Physiology* 1978;**235**:F310–6.

69. Ladefoged J, Munck O. Distribution of blood flow in the kidney. In: Fisher JW, ed. *Kidney hormones.* London: Academic Press, 1971:31–58.

70. Ledingham JGG. Overview: Physiology I. *Kidney International* 1987;**31** (suppl 20):49–50.

71. Britton KE. The measurement of intrarenal blood flow distribution in man. *Clinical Science* 1979;**56**:101–4.

72. Hodsman GP, Brown JJ, Cumming AMM, Davies DL, East BW, Lever AF, Morton JJ, Murray GD, Robertson JIS. Enalapril in treatment of hypertension with renal artery stenosis: Changes in blood pressure, renin, angiotensin I and II, renal function, and body composition. *American Journal of Medicine* 1984;**77** (2A):52–60.

73. Wenting GJ, Derkx FHM, Tan-Tjiong LH, Van Seyen AJ, Man in't Veld AJ, Schalekamp MADH. Risks of angiotensin converting enzyme inhibition in renal artery stenosis. *Kidney International* 1987;**31** (suppl 20):180–3.

74. Swales JD, Thurston H, Queiroz FP, Medina A. Sodium balance during the development of experimental hypertension. *Journal of Labortory and Clinical Medicine* 1972;**80**:539–47.

75. Möhring J, Möhring B, Naumann H-J, Philippi A, Homsy E, Orth H, Dauda G, Kazda S, Gross F. Salt and water balance and renin activity in renal hypertension in rats. *American Journal of Physiology* 1975;**228**:1847–55.

76. Doyle AE, Duffy SG. Sodium balance and plasma renin activity during the development of two-kidney Goldblatt hypertension in rats. *Clinical and Experimental Pharmacology and Physiology* 1980;**7**:293–304.

77. Tobian L, Coffee K, McCrea P. Contrasting exchangeable sodium in rats with different types of Goldblatt hypertension. *American Journal of Physiology* 1969;**217**:458–60.

78. Albertini R, Binia A, Otsuka Y, Carretero OA. Exchangeable sodium in angiotensinogenic and non-angiotensinogenic renovascular hypertension. *Hypertension* 1979;**1**:624–30.

79. Swales JD, Thurston H. Sodium restriction and inhibition of the renin–angiotensin system in renovascular hypertension in the rat. *Clinical Science* 1977;**52**:371–5.

80. Munoz-Ramirez H, Chatelain RE, Bumpus FM, Khairallah PA. Development of two-kidney Goldblatt hypertension in rats under dietary sodium restriction. *American Journal of Physiology* 1980;**238**:H889–94.

81. Swales JD, Tange JD. The influence of acute sodium depletion on experimental hypertension in the rat. *Journal of Laboratory and Clinical Medicine* 1971;**78**:369–79.

82. Jackson CA, Navar LG. Arterial pressure and renal function in two-kidney, one-clip Goldblatt hypertensive rars maintained on a high-salt intake. *Journal of Hypertension* 1986;**4**:215–21.

83. Watson ML, McCormick J, Thom A, Whelpdale P, Ungar A. Effects of salt and water depletion on the early phase of hypertension in Goldblatt two-kidney hypertensive dogs. *Clinical Science* 1981;**60**:625–31.

84. McAreavey D, Brown JJ, Cumming AMM, Davies DL, Fraser R, Lever AF, Mackay A, Morton JJ, Robertson JIS. Inverse relation of exchangeable sodium and blood pressure in hypertensive patients with renal artery stenosis. *Journal of Hypertension* 1983;**1**:297–302.

85. Freeman RH, Davis JO, Seymour AA. Volume and vasoconstriction in experimental renovascular hypertension. *Federation Proceedings* 1982;41:2409–14.

86. Masaki Z, Ferrario CM, Bumpus FM, Bravo EL, Khosla MC. The course of arterial pressure and the effect of Sar1-Thr8-angiotensin II in a new model of two-kidney hypertension in dogs. *Clinical Science* 1977;52:163–70.

87. Bengis RG, Coleman TG. Antihypertensive effect of prolonged blockade of angiotensin formation in benign and malignant, one-and two-kidney Goldblatt hypertensive rats. *Clinical Science* 1979;57:63–62.

88. Benedetti RG, Linas SL. Effect of potassium depletion on two-kidney, one-clip renovascular hypertension in the rat. *Kidney International* 1985;28:621–8.

89. Zimmerman BG. Adrenergic facilitation by angiotensin: Does it serve a physiological function? *Clinical Science* 1981;60:343–8.

90. De Forrest JM, Creekmore JS, Ferrone RA. Hypertension after ending captopril administration: Pathogenesis in 2-kidney, 1-clip rat. *American Journal of Physiology* 1984;247:H946–51.

91. Walker SM, Bing RF, Swales JD, Thurston H. Plasma noradrenaline in Goldblatt models of renovascular hypertension in the rat, before and after surgical reversal. *Clinical Science* 1986;71:199–204.

92. Collis MG, Vanhoutte PM. Increased renal vascular reactivity to angiotensin II but not nerve stimulation or exogenous norephinephrine in renal hypertensive rats. *Circulation Research* 1978;43:544–52.

93. Kopp UC, Buckley-Bleiler RL. Impaired renorenal reflexes in two-kidney, one-clip hypertensive rats. *Hypertension* 1989;14:445–52.

94. Zimmerman BG. Determination of role of sympathetic and renin–angiotensin systems in Goldblatt hypertension with urapidil and captopril. *Journal of Hypertension* 1984;2:485–91.

95. Izumi Y, Honda M, Shiratsuchi T, Hatano M. A case of renovascular hypertension with high urinary noradrenaline excretion. *Japanese Circulation Journal* 1980;44:893–8.

96. Gordon RD, Bachmann AW, Jackson RV, Saar N. Increased sympathetic activity in renovascular hypertension in man. *Clinical and Experimental Pharmacology and Physiology* 1982;9:277–81.

97. Berenguer LM, Garcia-Estan J, Ubeda M, Ortiz AJ, Quesada T. Role of renin–angiotensin system in the impairment of baroreflex control of heart rate in renovascular hypertension. *Journal of Hypertension* 1991;9:1127–33.

98. Cowley AW, De Clue JW. Quantification of baroreceptor influence on arterial pressure changes seen in primary angiotensin-induced hypertension in dogs. *Circulation Research* 1976;39:779–87.

99. Imanishi M, Kawamura M, Akabane S, Matsushima Y, Kuramochi M, Ito K, Ohta M, Kimura K, Takamiya M, Omae T. Aspirin lowers blood pressure in patients with renovascular hypertension. *Hypertension* 1989;14:461–8.

100. Anderson CB, Tanenbaum JS, Sicard GA, Etheredge EE. Renal thromboxane synthesis in excised kidney distal to renovascular lesions. *Journal of the American Medical Association* 1984;251:3118–20.

101. Fitzgerald GA, Fitzgerald DJ. Biosynthesis of thromboxane A₂ in renovascular hypertension. *Journal of the American Medical Association* 1984;251:3121–222.

102. Brunner HR, Kirschman JD, Sealey JE, Laragh JH. Hypertension of renal origin: Evidence for two different mechanisms. *Science* 1971;174:1344–6.

103. Macdonald GJ, Boyd GW, Peart WS. The effect of an angiotensin blocker, sarcosyl1-alanyl8-angiotensin II (P113) on two kidney hypertension in the rat. *Clinical and Experimental Pharmacology and Physiology* 1975;(suppl 2):89–91.

104. Macdonald GJ, Boyd GW, Peart WS. Effect of the angiotensin II blocker 1-Sar-8-Ala-angiotensin II on renal artery clip hypertension in the rat. *Circulation Research* 1975;37:640–6.

105. Bing J, Nielsen K. Role of the renin-system in normo- and hypertension: Effect of angiotensin inhibitor (1-Sar-8-Ala-angiotensin II) on the blood pressure of conscious or anaesthetized normal, nephrectomized and renal hypertensive rats. *Acta Pathologica et Microbiologica Scandinavica (A):*1973;81:254–62.

106. Pals DT, Masucci FD, Denning GS, Sipos F, Fessler DC. Role of the pressor action of angiotensin II in experimental hypertension. *Circulation Research* 1971;29:673–81.

107. Bumpus FM, Sen S, Smeby RR, Sweet C, Ferrario CM, Khosla MC. Use of angiotensin II antagonists in experimental hypertension. *Circulation Research* 1973;32 & 33 (suppl I):150–8.

108. Otsuka Y, Carretero OA, Albertini R, Binia A. Angiotensin and sodium balance: Their role in chronic two-kidney Goldblatt hypertension. *Hypertension* 1979;1:389–96.

109. Riegger AJG, Lever AF, Millar JA, Morton JJ, Slack B. Correction of renal hypertension in the rat by prolonged administration of angiotensin inhibitors. *Lancet* 1977;ii:1317–9.

110. Thurston H, Bing RF, Marks ES, Swales JD. Response of chronic renovascular hypertension to surgical correction or prolonged blockade of the renin–angiotensin system by two inhibitors in the rat. *Clinical Science* 1980;58:15–20.

111. Bing RF, Russell GI, Swales JD, Thurston H. Effect of 12-hour infusions of saralasin or captopril on blood pressure in hypertensive conscious rats. *Journal of Laboratory and Clinical Medicine* 1981;98:302–10.

112. Wallace ECH, Balmforth AJ, Morton JJ. Effect of acute and chronic captopril infusion on blood pressure on the two-kidney, one-clip hypertensive rat. *Journal of Hypertension* 1985;3:607–12.

113. Ferrario CM, Bumpus FM, Masaki Z, Khosla MC, McCubbin JW. Effects of angiotensin antagonists in various forms of experimental arterial hypertension. *Progress in Biochemical Pharmacology* 1976;12:86–97.

114. Watkins BE, Davis JO, Hanson RC, Lohmeier TE, Freeman RH. Incidence and pathophysiological changes in chronic two-kidney hypertension in the dog. *American Journal of Physiology* 1976;231:954–60.

115. Brown JJ, Brown WCB, Fraser R, Lever AF, Morton JJ, Robertson JIS, Agabiti-Rosei E, Trust PM. The effects of the angiotensin II antagonist saralasin on blood pressure and plasma aldosterone in man in relation to the prevailing plasma angiotensin II concentration. *Progress in Biochemical Pharmacology* 1976;12:230–41.

116. Frohlich ED, Maxwell MH, Baer L, Gavras H, Hollifield JW, Krakoff LR, Lischitz MD, Logan A, Poutasse E, Streeten DH. Use of saralasin as a diagnostic test in hypertension. *Archives of Internal Medicine* 1982;142:1437–40.

117. Brunner HR, Gavras H, Laragh JH, Keenan R. Angiotensin II blockade in man by Sar1-Ala8-angiotensin II for understanding and treatment of high blood pressure. *Lancet* 1973;ii:1045–8.

118. Streeten DHP, Anderson GH, Freiberg JM, Dalakos TG. Use of angiotensin II antagonist (saralasin) in the recognition of 'angiotensinogenic' hypertension *New England Journal of Medicine* 1975;292:657–62.

119. Krakoff LB, Ribeiro AB, Gorkin JV, Felton KR. Saralasin infusion in screening patients for renovascular hypertension. *American Journal of Cardiology* 1980;45:609–13.

120. Mackay A, Boyle P, Brown JJ, Lever AF, Robertson JIS. The decision on surgery in renal artery stenosis. *Quarterly Journal of Medicine* 1983;52:363–81.

121. Huang W-C, Ploth DW, Bell PD, Work J, Navar LG. Bilateral renal function responses to converting enzyme inhibitor (SQ20881) in two-kidney, one clip Goldblatt hpertensive rats. *Hypertension* 1981;3:285–93.

122. Ding Y-A, Chang S-T, Shieh S-M, Huang W-C. Antihypertensive and renal effects of cilazapril and their reversal by angiotensin in renovascular hypertensive rats. *Clinical Science* 1988;74:365–72.

123. De Forrest JM, Knappenberger RC, Antonaccio MJ, Ferrone RA, Creekmore JS. Angiotensin II is a necessary component for the development of hypertension in the two-kidney, one-clip rat. *American Journal of Cardiology* 1982;49:1515–7.

124. Freeman RH, Davis JO, Watkins BE, Stephens GA, De Forrest JM. Effects of continuous converting enzyme blockade on renovascular hypertension in the rat. *American Journal of Physiology* 1979;236:F21–4.

125. Wallace ECH, Morton JJ. Chronic captopril infusion in two-kidney, one-clip rats with normal plasma renin concentration. *Journal of Hypertension* 1984;2:285–9.

126. Atkinson AB, Brown JJ, Davies DL, Leckie B, Lever AF, Morton JJ, Robertson JIS. Renal artery stenosis with normal angiotensin II values: Relationship between angiotensin II and body sodium and potassium on correction of hypertension by captopril and subsequent surgery. *Hypertension* 1981;3:53–8.

127. Atkinson AB, Brown JJ, Cumming AMM, Fraser R, Lever AF, Leckie BJ, Morton JJ, Robertson JIS, Davies DL. Captopril in the management of hypertension with renal artery stenosis: Its long-term effect as a predictor of surgical outcome. *American Journal of Cardiology* 1982;49:1460–66.

128. Staessen J, Fagard R, Lijnen P, Amery A, Bulpitt CJ. Long-term converting enzyme inhibition as a guide to surgical curability of hypertension associated with renal artery disease. *American Journal of Cardiology* 1983;**51**:1317–22.

129. Derkx FHM, de Wind AE, Lipovsky MM, Stroes ESG, Pieterman H, Van den Meiracker AH, Wenting GJ, Man in't Veld AJ, Schalekamp MADH. Renal vein renin lateralisation is not improved by captopril treatment. In: MacGregor GA, Sever PS, Caldwell ADS, eds. *Current advances in ACE inhibition, volume II.* Edinburgh: Churchill-Livingstone, 1991:213–7.

130. Malatino LS, Cumming AMM, Hodsman GP, Leckie BJ, Lever AF, Tillman DM, Webb DJ, Morton JJ, Robertson JIS. Factors affecting renal vein renin ratio in renal artery stenosis: Secretion of inactive renin. *Nephron* 1986;**44** (suppl 1):68–72.

131. Lupu AN, Maxwell MH, Kaufman J. Mechanisms of hypertension during the chronic phase of the one-clip, two-kidney model in the dog. *Circulation Research* 1977;**40** (suppl I):I57–61.

132. Mackay A, Brown JJ, Lever AF, Robertson JIS. Reconstructive surgery versus nephrectomy in renal artery stenosis: Comparison of effects on total and divided renal function and on blood pressure. *British Medical Journal* 1980;**281**:1313–5.

133. Thal AP, Grage TB, Vernier RL. Function of the contralateral kidney in renal hypertension due to renal artery stenosis. *Circulation* 1963;**27**:36–43.

134. Russell GI, Bing RF, Swales JD, Thurston H. Hemodynamic changes induced by reversal of early and late renovascular hypertension. *American Journal of Physiology* 1983;**245**:H734–40.

135. Russell GI, Bing RF, Thurston H, Swales JD. Surgical reversal of two-kidney, one-clip hypertension during inhibition of the renin–angiotensin system. *Hypertension* 1982;**4**:69–76.

136. Ten Berg RGM, Leenen FHH, De Jong W. Plasma renin activity and sodium, potassium and water excretion during reversal of hypertension in the one-clip, two-kidney hypertensive rat. *Clinical Science* 1979;**57**:47–52.

137. Thurston H, Bing RF, Swales JD. Reversal of two-kidney, one-clip hypertension in the rat. *Hypertension* 1980;**2**:256–65.

138. Peart WS. Hypertension and the kidney I. Clinical, pathological and functional disorders, especially in man. *British Medical Journal* 1959;**ii**:1353–9.

139. Vandongen R, O'Dwyer J, Barden A. Release of prostaglandins during the reversal of one-kidney, but not two-kidney, one-clip hypertension in the rat. *Journal of Hypertension* 1983;**1**:177–82.

140. Russell GI, Bing RF, Swales JD, Thurston H. Indomethacin or aprotonin infusion effect on the reversal of chronic two-kidney, one-clip hypertension in the conscious rat. *Clinical Science* 1983;**62**:361–6.

141. Bing RF, Russell GI, Swales JD, Thurston H, Fletcher A. Chemical medullectomy: Effect upon reversal of two-kidney, one-clip hypertension in the rat. *Clinical Science* 1981;**61** (suppl):335–8.

142. Göthberg G, Lundin S, Folkow B. Acute vasodepressor effect in normotensive rats following extracorporeal perfusion of the declipped kidney of two-kidney, one-clip hypertensive rats. *Hypertension* 1982;**4** (suppl II):101–5.

143. Skulan TW, Brousseau AC, Leonard KA. Accelerated induction of two-kidney hypertension in rats and renin–angiotensin sensitivity. *Circulation Research* 1974;**35**:734–41.

144. Ten Berg R, de Jong W. Mechanisms of enhanced blood pressure rise after reclipping following removal of a renal artery clip in rats. *Hypertension* 1980;**2**:4–13.

145. Johnson JA, Davis JO, Spielman WS, Freeman RH. The role of the renin–angiotensin system in experimental renal hypertension in dogs. *Proceedings of the Society for Experimental Biology and Medicine* 1974;**147**:387–91.

146. Peart WS, Robertson JIS, Grahame-Smith DG. Examination of the relationship of renin release to hypertension produced in the rabbit by renal artery constriction. *Circulation Research* 1961;**9**:1171–84.

147. Peart WS. Hypertension and the kidney. II. Experimental basis of renal hypertension. *British Medical Journal* 1959;**ii**:1421–9.

148. Laragh JH. On the mechanisms and clinical relevance of one-kidney, one-clip hypertension. *American Journal of Hypertension* 1991;**4** (suppl):541–5.

149. Ledingham JM, Sodium retention and volume expansion as mechanisms. *American Journal of Hypertension* 1991;**4** (suppl):534–40.

150. Hall JE. Renal function in one-kidney, one-clip hypertension and low renin essential hypertension. *American Journal of Hypertension* 1991;**4** (suppl):523–33.

151. Bianchi G, Tilde Tenconi L, Lucca R. Effect in the conscious dog of constriction of the renal artery to a sole remaining kidney on haemodynamics, sodium balance, body fluid volumes, plasma renin concentration and pressor responsiveness to angiotensin. *Clinical Science* 1970;**38**:741–66.

152. Watkins BE, Davis JO, Freeman RH, Stephens GA. Production of renal hypertension in adrenalectomised dogs on constant hormone replacement therapy. *Proceedings of the Society for Experimetnal Biology and Medicine* 1978;**157**:116–20.

153. Stephens GA, Davis JO, Freeman RH, De Forrest JM, Early DM. Hemodynamic, fluid, and electrolyte changes in sodium-depleted, one-kidney renal hypertensive dogs. *Circulation Research* 1979;**44**:316–21.

154. McAreavey D, Brown WB, Murray GD, Robertson JIS. Exchangeable sodium in Goldblatt one-kidney one-clip hypertension in the rat. *Clinical Science* 1984;**66**: 545–9.

155. Mourant AJ. Determinants of high blood pressure in salt-deprived renal hypertensive rats: Role of changes in plasma volume, extracellular fluid volume and plasma angiotensin II. *Clinical Science* 1978;**55**:81–7.

156. Bianchi G, Brown JJ, Lever AF, Robertson JIS, Roth N. Changes of plasma renin concentration during pressor infusions of renin in the conscious dog: The influence of dietary sodium intake. *Clinical Science* 1968;**34**:303–14.

157. Blair-West JR, Coghlan JP, Denton DA, Orchard E, Scoggins BA, Wright PD. Renin–angiotensin–aldosterone system and sodium balance in experimental renal hypertension. *Endocrinology* 1968;**83**:1199–209.

158. Liard J-F, Cowley AW, McCaa RE, McCaa CS, Guyton AC. Renin–aldosterone, body fluid volumes, and the baroreceptor reflex in the development and reversal of hypertension in conscious dogs. *Circulation Research* 1974;**34**:549–60.

159. Watkins BE, Davis JO, Freeman RH, De Forrest JM, Stephens GA. Continuous angiotensin II blockade throughout the acute phase of one-kidney hypertension in the dog. *Circulation Research* 1978;**42**:813–21.

160. Akahoshi M, Carretero OA. Body fluid volume and angiotensin II in maintenance of one-kidney, one-clip hypertension. *Hypertension* 1989;**14**:269–73.

161. Skeggs LT, Dorer FE, Lentz KE, Kahn JR, Emancipator SN. A new mechanism in one-kidney, one-clip hypertension. *Hypertension* 1985;**7**:72–80.

162. Johnson JA, Davis JO, Braverman B. Role of angiotensin II in experimental renal hypertension in the rabbit. *American Journal of Physiology* 1975;**288**:11–16.

163. Johnson JA, Stubbs DH, Stanton M, Payne C, Ichikawa S, Keitzer WF. Effect of sodium depletion and angiotensin II antagonism in renal hypertensive rabbits. *American Journal of Physiology* 1977;**233**:H514–9.

164. Romero JC, Lazar JD, Hoobler SW. Effect of renal artery constriction and subsequent contralateral nephrectomy on the blood pressure, plasma renin activity, and plasma renin substrate concentration in rabbits. *Laboratory Investigation* 1970;**22**:581–7.

165. Miller ED, Samuels AI, Haber E, Barger AC, Inhibition of angiotensin conversion and prevention of renal hypertension. *American Journal of Physiology* 1975;**288**:448–53.

166. Lever AF, Robertson JIS. Renin in the plasma of normal and hypertensive rabbits. *Journal of Physiology* 1964;**170**:212–8.

167. Ferrario CM. Contribution of cardiac output and peripheral resistance to experimental renal hypertension. *American Journal of Physiology* 1974;**226**:611–7.

168. Kurihara H, Tanaka T, Terasana F. Differences in changes in plasma volume in two types of Goldblatt hypertension. *Tohoku Journal of Experimental Medicine* 1976;**118**:113–25.

169. Trippodo NC, Walsh GM, Ferrone RA, Duncan RC. Fluid partition and cardiac output in volume-depleted Goldblatt hypertensive rats. *American Journal of Physiology* 1979;**237**:H18–24.

170. Trippodo NC, Ziegler LP. Blood volume and interstitial fluid pressure in the development and reversal of renal hypertension in rats. *Clinical Science* 1980;**59** (suppl):153–6.

171. Kunes J, Jelinek J. Extra-cellular fluid distribution in rats with chronic one-and two-kidney Goldblatt hypertension. *Clinical and Experimental Physiology and Pharmacology* 1979;**6**:507–13.

172. Lucas J, Floyer MA. Changes in body fluid volume distribution and interstitial tissue compliance during the development and reversal of experimental renal hypertension in the rat. *Clinical Science* 1974;47:1–11.

173. Garcia R, Cantin M, Gutkowska J, Thibault G, Atrial natriuretic factor during the development and reversal of one-kidney, one-clip hypertension. *Hypertension* 1987;9:144–9.

174. Garcia R, Gauquelin G, Cantin M, Schiffrin EL. Renal glomerular atrial natriuretic factor receptors in one-kidney, one-clip rats. *Hypertension* 1988;11:185–90.

175. Debinski W, Kuchel O, Garcia R, Buu NT, Racz K, Cantin M, Genest J. Atrial natriuretic factor inhibits the sympathetic nervous activity in one-kidney, one-clip hypertension in the rat. *Proceedings of the Society for Experimental Biology and Medicine* 1986;181:173–7.

176. Verburg KM, Freeman RH, Villareal D, Brands MW. Atrial natriuretic factor in dogs with one-kidney, one-clip Goldblatt hypertension. *American Journal of Physiology* 1987;253:H1623–7.

177. Burton J, Cody RJ, Herd JA, Haber E. Specific inhibition of renin by an angiotensinogen analog: Studies in sodium depletion and renin-dependent hypertension. *Proceedings of the National Academy of Sciences of the USA* 1980;77:5476–9.

178. Miller ED, Haber E, Barger AC. Inhibition of angiotensin conversion in experimental renovascular hypertension. *Science* 1972;177:1108–9.

179. Brown AJ, Clark SA, Lever AF. Slow rise and diurnal change of blood pressure with saralasin and angiotensin II in rats. *American Journal of Physiology* 1983;244:F84–8.

180. Gavras H, Brunner HR, Vaughan ED, Laragh JH. Angiotensin–sodium interaction in blood pressure maintenance of renal hypertensive and normotensive rats. *Science* 1973;180:1369–72.

181. Seymour AA, Davis JO, Freeman RH, De Forrest JM, Rowe BP, Stephens GA, Williams GM. Sodium and angiotensin in the pathogenesis of experimental renovascular hypertension. *American Journal of Physiology* 1981;240:H788–92.

182. Anderson WP, Korner PI, Johnston CI. Acute angiotensin II mediated restoration of distal renal artery pressure in renal artery stenosis and its relationship to the development of sustained one-kidney hyertension in conscious dogs. *Hypertension* 1979;1:292–8.

183. Anderson WP, Selig SE,Korner PI. Role of angiotensin II in the hypertension induced by renal artery stenosis. *Clinical and Experimental Hypertension* 1984;A6:299–314.

184. Anderson WP, Woods RL. Intrarenal effects of angiotensin II in renal artery stenosis. *Kidney International* 1987;31 (suppl 20):157–67.

185. Skeggs LT. On the role of renin in one-kidney, one-clip hypertension. *American Journal of Hypertension* 1991;4 (suppl):578–83.

186. Davis JO, Stephens GA, Freeman RH, De Forrest JM. Changes in cardiac output during the development of renal hypertension in sodium-depleted dogs. *Clinical Science* 1978;55 (suppl):221–3.

187. Ledingham JM, Cohen RD. The role of the heart in the pathogenesis of renal hypertension. *Lancet* 1963;ii:979–81.

188. Ledingham JM, Pelling D. Cardiac output and peripheral resistance in experimental renal hypertension. *Circulation Research* 1967;20 & 21 (suppl II):187–99.

189. Ferrario CM, Page IH, McCubbin JW. Increased cardiac output as a contributory factor in experimental renal hypertension in dogs. *Circulation Research* 1970;27:799–810.

190. Richardson TQ, Fermoso JD, Guyton AC. Increase in mean circulatory pressure in Goldblatt hypertension. *American Journal of Physiology* 1964;207:751–2.

191. Yamamoto J, Trippodo NC, Ishise S, Frohlich ED. Altered pressure/volume in one-kidney Goldblatt hypertensive rats. *Federation Proceedings* 1979;38:1258.

192. Simon G. Altered venous function in hypertensive rats. *Circulation Research* 1976;38:412–8.

193. Simon G. Reversibility of arterial and venous changes in renal hypertensive rats. *Hypertension* 1980;2:192–7.

194. Ackerman U, Tatemichi SR. Regional vascular capacitance in rabbit one-kidney, one-clip hypertension. *Hypertension* 1983;5:712–21.

195. Hawthorne EW, Hinds JE, Crawford WJ, Tearney RJ. Left ventricular myocardial contractility during the first week of renal hypertension in conscious instrumented dogs. *Circulation Research* 1974;34 & 35 (suppl I):223–34.

196. Lombard JH, Cowley AW. Hemodynamic and microcirculatory alterations in reduced renal mass hypertension. *Hypertension* 1989;13:128–38.

197. Imig JD, Anderson G. Small artery resistance increases during the development of renal hypertension. *Hypertension* 1991;17:317–22.

198. Woods RL, Anderson WP, Korner PI. Renal and systemic effects of enalapril in chronic one-kidney hypertension. *Hypertension* 1986;8:109–16.

199. Machado BH, Salgado HC, Krieger EM. Tachycardic responses during the development of renal hypertension. *Hypertension* 1983;5 (suppl V):122–7.

200. Liard JF, Peters G. Mechanism of fall in blood pressure after 'unclamping' in rats with Goldblatt-type hypertension. *Experientia* 1970;26:743–5.

201. Muirhead EE, Brooks B. Reversal of one-kidney, one-clip hypertension by unclipping: The renal, sodium-volume relationship re-examined. *Proceedings of the Society for Experimental Biology and Medicine* 1980;163:540–6.

202. Floyer MA. Further studies on the mechanism of experimental hypertension in the rat. *Clinical Science* 1955;14:163–81.

203. Muirhead EE. Renomedullary system of blood pressure control. *Hypertension* 1986;8 (suppl I):38–46.

204. Pamnani MB, Bryant JH, Clough DL, Haddy FJ. Reversal of one-kidney, one-clip hypertension in rats: Effects on myocardial Na+, K+–ATPase, arterial Na+–K+pump, arterial membrane potential, and plasma Na+–K+pump inhibitory activity. *American Journal of Hypertension* 1991;4 (suppl):546–5.

205. Denton KM, Anderson WP. Role of angiotensin II in renal wrap hypertension. *Hypertension* 1985;7:893–8.

206. Seymour AA, Davis JO, Freeman RH, De Forrest JM, Rowe BP, Stephens GA, Williams GM. Hypertension produced by sodium depletion and unilateral nephrectomy: A new experimental model. *Hypertension* 1980;2:125–9.

207. Webb DJ, Clark SA, Brown WB, Fraser R, Lever AF, Murray GD, Robertson JIS. Dietary sodium deprivation raises blood pressure in the rat but does not produce irreversible hyperaldosteronism. *Journal of Hypertension* 1987;5:525–31.

208. Vari RC, Freeman RH, Davis JO, Sweet WD. Role of renal nerves in rats with low-sodium, one-kidney hypertension. *American Journal of Physiology* 1986;250:H189–94.

209. Staessen J, Wilms G, Baert A, Fagard R, Lijnen P, Say R, Amery A. Blood pressure during longterm converting enzyme inhibition predicts the curability of renovascular hypertension by angioplasty. *American Journal of Hypertension* 1988;1:208–14.

56 RENIN IN ACUTE AND CHRONIC RENAL FAILURE: IMPLICATIONS FOR TREATMENT

GEORGE L BAKRIS AND HARALAMBOS GAVRAS

INTRODUCTION

A central role of the RAS in man is to maintain circulatory and electrolytic homeostasis [1–3] (see *Chapter 74*). Any of the numerous circumstances that either directly or indirectly affect this homeostasis will lead to a perturbation in the system. As one component of this series of homeostatic functions, activation of the RAS is an important compensatory mechanism helping to preserve glomerular filtration rate (GFR) and urea excretion when renal blood flow is lowered [4] (see *Chapters 21* and *26*). However, if this process advances too far, the renal circulation shuts down almost completely [5,6]. Administration of large doses of exogenous Ang II can cause functional and structural damage to the kidney [7,8] (see *Chapter 40*). Alterations in intrarenal hemodynamics or renal excretory capacity can impair the autoregulatory control of the RAS and result in further abnormal perfusion and damage to individual nephrons, creating a vicious circle. Thus, in various syndromes of acute and chronic renal failure, the RAS can be influenced in diverse ways, and can, in different circumstances, either ameliorate or exacerbate the severity of renal impairment.

Hypertension is a frequent occurrence in acute and chronic renal failure [9,10]. In acute renal failure, major alterations responsible for changes in arterial pressure, that is, activation of the RAS and disturbance of sodium balance, are also related to altered volume homeostasis [11]. In chronic renal disease, the major changes seen in the RAS are far more complicated than in acute renal failure. Activation of the RAS in long-standing renal disease is modulated in part by kinins, prostaglandins, vasopressin, and other vasopressor and depressor influences [12–17] (see *Chapter 38*). The RAS directly or via its interaction with other factors is often an important contributory mechanism in the hypertension of chronic renal failure. Chronic renal disease with renal functional impairment is the most common cause of secondary hypertension [18]. However, in many of these patients, the RAS is not the predominant cause of high blood pressure, and in some, it is irrelevant.

This chapter addresses both normal physiology and pathophysiological alterations of the intrarenal RAS in various forms of renal failure. It is concerned with both acute and chronic adaptive changes, as well as with mechanisms by which the RAS is affected by, and in turn contributes to, renal damage. The localization of the components of the RAS, the interrelation of the RAS with other biochemical and hormonal systems, and varied activation or suppression of the RAS in the numerous and diverse conditions of concern here, are dealt with in detail in other chapters of this book. Some aspects are briefly recapitulated in this chapter as they relate to various syndromes of renal failure.

RENAL LOCALIZATION OF THE RENIN–ANGIOTENSIN SYSTEM

Various intrarenal tissues have the genetic capability to synthesize renin and Ang II. These include cells of the glomerular mesangium; the brush border of the proximal tubules; afferent and efferent arterioles, and especially the juxtaglomerular apparatus in the area of the distal tubules; and all endothelium [19–21] (see Color Plates 5–11,13,39). At the cellular level, the RAS modulates growth and repair in these tissues. Intrarenal Ang II is found in plasma, lymph, and interstitium. It arrives as a blood-borne hormone, or arises as the product of Ang I locally converted by ACE or as a locally generated autacoid.

The renin content of individual glomeruli displays great variability in response to physiological and pathophysiological stimuli. Normally, superficial glomeruli have greater quantities of renin than have deep glomerui [22–24] (see *Chapter 21*); this gradient can persist even when the overall glomerular renin content is enhanced, for example by sodium depletion [17], or with renal artery stenosis [25]. As noted in detail in *Chapter 25*, Ang II receptors have been observed in various renal structures, with a particularly high density in cortical glomeruli and in the inner zone of the outer medulla [26].

Studies *in vitro* suggest that alterations in extracellular glucose concentration, as well as the presence of growth factors such as insulin and endothelin, stimulate the RAS. In diabetic states, these hormonal interactions result in abnormal production of Ang II by both endothelial and mesangial cells [14,19], and may thus contribute to diabetic nephropathy and renal failure (see *Chapters 75 and 92*). These processes are interrupted by giving ACE inhibitors [27].

The renal localization of the RAS is also discussed in *Chapters 18–21*.

REGULATION OF RENAL RENIN RELEASE

The regulation of renin secretion from the kidney is discussed in detail in *Chapters 24 and 74*; some major influences are summarized in Fig. 56.1.

One of the most potent regulators of renin release from the juxtaglomerular apparatus is delivery of sodium and chloride to the macula densa [28]. Other contributory factors include hypovolemia and/or hypotension, direct or indirect sympathetic activation, and tubular injury [29]. Renin release is dependent on the serum concentrations of potassium and calcium, and is also influenced by circulating or locally produced hormones, including insulin, vasopressin, and Ang II itself [19,30,31]. Profound lowering of serum calcium concentration, as may be seen in untreated chronic renal failure, or the administration of β-adrenoceptor blocking agents, can lead to decreases in plasma renin concentration (PRC) regardless of sodium delivery to the distal renal tubules [19,30,31] (see *Chapter 84*).

---

increase renin

prostaglandins E and I series
renal sympathetic stimulation
  (β-adrenergic receptor, intrarenal)
  (baroreceptor stimulation)
catecholamines
hypotension, hypovolemia
sodium depletion

inhibit renin

arginine vasopressin
potassium
calcium (low)
Ang II
β-adrenergic receptor antagonists
histamine
adenosine
parathyroid hormone
sodium loading

Fig. 56.1 Factors affecting renin release.

Some of the highest plasma levels of renin and Ang II in man have been reported in disorders that affect the microvasculature and result in rapidly progressive renal failure; for example, in malignant hypertension, scleroderma, collagen diseases, and other forms of vasculitis [32–35] (see *Color Plates 18, 19, 21*). Extremely high plasma concentrations of renin and Ang II have been found in some patients in end-stage renal failure on hemodialysis [36,37]. Glomerular and tubular lesions are less likely to yield high levels of renin, with the possible exception of nephrotic syndrome with minimal change renal disease [38] (see *Chapter 58*). The lowest levels of circulating renin in renal disease are seen in chronic tubulointerstitial processes [12,39,40]. These various conditions and their relationships with arterial pressure and plasma renin are summarized in Fig. 56.2.

INTRARENAL EFFECTS OF ANGIOTENSIN II: ACTIONS AND INTERACTIONS IN RENAL FAILURE

The renal vasculature is especially sensitive to the vasoconstrictor action of Ang II [41], as is confirmed by the marked increase in renal blood flow that occurs after blockade of the RAS despite a concurrent fall in systemic blood pressure [42,43]. Of particular relevance is the effect of Ang II on intrarenal hemodynamics, namely, that it generally constricts efferent arterioles more than afferent arterioles, thus tending to raise the glomerular capillary pressure and filtration fraction (see *Chapter 26*). These changes are important adaptive mechanisms aimed at maintaining glomerular filtration in the face of reduced renal blood flow, diminished perfusion pressure, or reduced renal mass. Concurrently, Ang II-mediated enhancement of countercurrent renal medullary mechanisms sustains urea excretion, medullary osmolality, and urinary concentration when renal function is threatened in these ways [4] (see *Chapters 21 and 26*). These important compensatory mechanisms are lost with ACE inhibition.

The foregoing processes are to be contrasted with the detrimental effects of renal overperfusion. Studies using renal ablation, or experimental diabetic models, have shown convincingly that increased glomerular capillary pressure with hyperfiltration is maladaptive in the long term and leads to glomerular sclerosis and destruction [44]. Conversely, maneuvers that decrease the glomerular filtration pressure, such as dietary protein restriction, or ACE inhibition, which lowers the arteriolar tone more in the efferent than in the afferent arterioles, seem in these circumstances to protect the glomerulus from further damage [45–53].

Disease	Plasma renin	Blood pressure
I microvascular processes	↑ ↑ ↑	↑ ↑ ↑
a) scleroderma		
b) vasculitides		
II glomerular processes	↑ or ↔	↑ ↑
*a) focal glomerulosclerosis		
*b) membranoproliferative glomerulonephritis		
*c) diabetes mellitus		
*d) membranous glomerulonephritis		
*e) minimal change disease†	(↑ ↑)	(↔ or ↑)
f) IgA nephropathy		
III polycystic disease	↑ or ↔	↑ ↑
IV chronic interstitial nephritis		↔ or ↑
V reflux nephropathy (Plates 26–28)	↑ or ↔	↔ or ↑
VI end-stage renal disease‡ (dialysis)	↑ or ↔	↑ ↑

* >3.5g proteinuria/d
†minimal change disease has been reported to have much higher levels of circulating renin than other causes of nephrotic syndrome [38].
‡although renin may be 'normal', it is believed to be inappropriately high in relation to the elevated exchangeable sodium [58–60,64].

Fig. 56.2 Renin status of various chronic renal diseases.

A number of animal studies that have used partial nephrectomy as a model of renal failure have shown a marked increase in GFR in surviving, intact, glomeruli [11]. This is due, in part, to significant increases in locally generated Ang II, which contribute to differential constriction of efferent arterioles in the remaining intact nephrons [11]. The result is an increase in glomerular capillary pressure which maintains overall intrarenal GFR, albeit at much higher pressure levels than are normal for individual nephrons. This hyperfiltration, although beneficial for preservation of renal excretory capacity in the early stages of chronic renal disease, is detrimental to renal function as a long-standing process, ultimately leading to cellular scarring and tissue destruction, and to end-stage renal disease [11,44,54].

In addition to its several intrarenal vasoconstrictor actions, Ang II can directly stimulate reabsorption of sodium at proximal renal tubules [55,56] (see *Chapters 26* and *27*). Abnormal renal sodium handling contributes importantly to the hypertension of chronic renal failure. Although sodium retention is associated with some suppression of the RAS in the majority of patients with chronic renal failure, by contrast, those with microvascular disorders such as collagen vascular diseases or vasculitides, as mentioned earlier (see *Chapter 79*), tend to present with systemic hyperreninemia even in the presence of body sodium overload.

INTERRELATIONSHIPS OF THE RENIN–ANGIOTENSIN SYSTEM WITH SODIUM BALANCE IN RENAL FAILURE

In normotensive patients with chronic renal failure, the relationship between plasma Ang II and exchangeable body sodium is normal (Fig. 56.3). By contrast, the majority of hypertensive patients with end-stage renal disease are salt sensitive. In these subjects, plasma renin and Ang II levels are often within the overall normal range, but appear to be inappropriately elevated in relation to exchangeable sodium (*Fig. 56.3*). In other words, this abnormal relationship reflects more a raised exchangeable sodium rather than high levels of Ang II [57–60]. These patients usually achieve adequate blood-pressure control with attainment of dry body weight during dialysis [13,37,57,61–63], when the RAS is not stimulated unduly by the sodium loss, and the relationship between plasma Ang II and body sodium content is thus normalized (Figs. 56.3 and 56.4). However, 10–20% of long-term dialysis patients clearly have a predominantly renin-dependent hypertension [64,65]. These patients respond to salt subtraction at dialysis, with a marked reactive increase in plasma renin and Ang II, and the abnormal relationship between high Ang II and concurrent body sodium content is exacerbated (see *Figs. 56.3* and *56.4*). In consequence, there is a further rise in

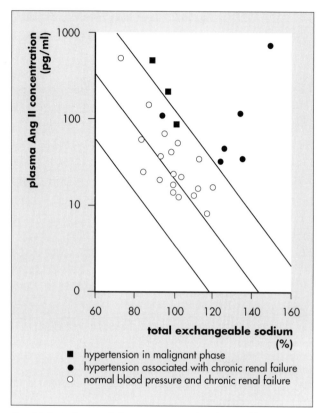

Fig. 56.3 Relation of plasma Ang II and exchangeable sodium (expressed as a percentage of the predicted normal value), in patients whose untreated hypertension was in the malignant phase or was associated with chronic renal failure. Patients with normal blood pressure and chronic renal failure are shown for comparison. The lines represent mean ± 2SD of the normal mean. Modified from Davies DL *et al* [58].

blood pressure, while there may be other features of gross Ang II excess such as extreme thirst [36,37,59] (see *Chapter 32*). In this subset, moreover, there is then a significant positive relationship between arterial pressure and plasma renin activity (PRA) [14]. The predominant role of RAS activation in this subpopulation is evidenced by a number of studies that have demonstrated marked reductions of arterial pressure and relief of thirst on lowering of circulating Ang II, either following bilateral nephrectomy [36,37] (*Fig. 56.4*), or with ACE inhibition [59,66–68,151].

Thus, a stimulated RAS contributes to hypertension in chronic renal failure via at least two direct mechanisms: Ang II-mediated vasoconstriction and Ang II-mediated reduction in renal tubular sodium excretion. In addition, there is evidence which indicates that intrarenal Ang II may have a growth-enhancing and mitogenic effect that tends to promote hypertrophy and/or hyperplasia of arteriolar myocytes and mesangial cells [69,70] (see *Chapter 31*). Proliferation of cellular elements is part of the picture of glomerulopathy and nephrosclerosis [71].

By contrast, in other circumstances, stimulation of the RAS can protect against renal functional impairment when the kidney is underperfused, for example in renal artery stenosis or cardiac failure. In these latter conditions, renal function sometimes deteriorates with ACE inhibition [72–77] (see *Chapters 88* and *93*).

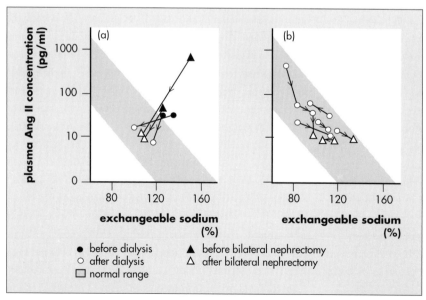

Fig. 56.4 Relationship between plasma Ang II concentration and exchangeable sodium (expressed as a percentage of the predicted normal value) in hypertensive (a) and normotensive (b) patients with chronic renal failure responding to dialysis treatment alone (before and after treatment) or to bilateral nephrectomy (before and after). Modified from Schalekamp MA *et al* [60].

PROSTAGLANDIN MODULATION OF THE RENIN–ANGIOTENSIN SYSTEM

Angiotensin II and its 2–8 heptapeptide derivative, Ang III, are known to increase production of prostaglandins, especially those of the E series [11,78] (see *Chapter 38*). Teleologically, this increase in vasodilatory prostaglandins may be to balance the vasoconstricting effects of Ang peptides and thereby to maintain renal perfusion. In support of this view are observations from studies in models of renal failure, where nonsteroidal antiinflammatory agents increase renal vascular resistance and reduce GFR [79]. Such data suggest that locally generated prostaglandins antagonize the effects of vasoconstrictors such as Ang II. In this connection, it is also probably relevant that the administration of aspirin consistently exacerbates the worsening of renal function observed when ACE inhibitors are given to patients with cardiac failure [77].

In renal parenchymal disease, the possible interaction of the RAS with renal prostaglandins, the renal kallikrein–kinin system, and perhaps with renomedullary vasodepressor lipids in the pathogenesis of hypertension, is still uncertain. Evidence of diminished renal prostacyclin synthesis has been reported in patients with chronic glomerulonephritis [80]. Decreased urinary kallikrein excretion has also been observed in some hypertensives with renal parenchymal disease [81], while urinary prostaglandin E_2 excretion is said to be normal [82]. Experimental studies have suggested that loss of vasodepressor and natriuretic substances of renomedullary origin [83] may also play a role, but the clinical significance of these observations remains unknown. Nevertheless, it is believed that the activity of the RAS is closely interrelated with those of the renal kallikrein–kinin and prostaglandin systems [84] (see *Chapter 38*). This complex relationship is illustrated by the fact that a reduction in blood pressure through inhibition of ACE, a procedure which also potentiates the vasodilator effects of bradykinin, can be partly reversed with bradykinin antagonists, but only if prostaglandin synthesis is also inhibited [85].

THE SYMPATHETIC NERVOUS SYSTEM AND THE RENIN–ANGIOTENSIN SYSTEM IN RENAL FAILURE

Most of the hemodynamic and hormonal changes described above tend to enhance the tubular reabsorption of sodium and thereby diminish renal sodium excretion. Salt retention with extracellular fluid volume expansion can increase activity of the sympathetic nervous sytem, which in turn promotes further sodium retention. These changes would be expected to raise cardiac output and total peripheral resistance, both of which are indeed usually enhanced in end-stage renal disease [14,86,87]. As previously noted, heightened activity of the sympathetic nervous system also stimulates the RAS. Angiotensin-converting enzyme inhibitors can interrupt the positive feedback loop between these two systems as shown by the fact that under some circumstances they lower the level of sympathetic activity [88], a subject that is discussed in detail in *Chapter 37*.

TUBULOGLOMERULAR FEEDBACK IN RENAL FAILURE

The tubuloglomerular feedback system is a critical autoregulatory mechanism that determines GFR and depends upon the concentration and delivery of sodium and chloride to the macula densa [28,29] (see *Chapter 26*). Defective sodium reabsorption at proximal tubules, which is present in acute renal failure, has been postulated as a mechanism that leads to increased tubuloglomerular feedback and ultimately decreases GFR [28,29]. Experiments have demonstrated that obstruction proximal to the macula densa for 24 hours appears to reduce glomerular capillary pressure and, hence, GFR [89].

Activation of tubuloglomerular feedback in acute renal failure has thus been viewed as a powerful volume-conserving mechanism designed to turn off glomerular filtration in order to prevent massive urinary losses in the face of impaired tubular reabsorption. Some studies support the concept of regulation of tubuloglomerular feedback by the RAS in acute renal failure [29,90]. Other factors such as adenosine and intracellular calcium, probably also have critical roles in the modulation of this system [91,92].

THE RENIN–ANGIOTENSIN SYSTEM IN RENAL FAILURE

ACUTE CIRCULATORY RENAL FAILURE

Conditions leading to excessive renal underperfusion and/or ischemia can cause renal circulatory shutdown and acute renal failure. This can result from systemic hypotension due to hemorrhage, from sodium and volume depletion, from severe injuries ('crush syndrome'), after extensive surgery, or in cardiac failure. In some of these situations, renal circulatory failure may be just one component of multiple organ failure [93–94]. Acute circulatory renal failure can alternatively be due to local problems such as renal artery stenosis or obstruction, which again lead to diminished renal perfusion (see *Chapter 88*). As described earlier, in all these situations, the initial stimulation of the RAS is a compensatory response, which helps to preserve GFR, urea excretion, and the ability to concentrate urine [4–6] (see *Chapter 21*). However, if these processes develop too far, the response of the renin system is excessive, and the renal circulation shuts down [5,6]. In severe renal ischemia, as well as in other animal models of acute circulatory renal failure, renin has been shown to be increased in the juxtaglomerular apparatus, renal vein, and systemic circulation [11,95,96]. This intense stimulation of the RAS tends to divert the already reduced blood flow away from cortical nephrons. Renal renin content and PRC do not always move in parallel; in acute circulatory renal failure induced by glycerol administration in the rabbit, Brown *et al* found PRC to be significantly raised, while renal renin content was initially depressed [97], the latter presumably because of marked renin secretion.

The hypothesis that excessive activation of the renal RAS, by causing vasoconstriction and renal ischemia, might be involved in the pathogenesis of acute renal failure was first proposed by Goormaghtigh in the early 1940s [93]. However, the prevailing theory at the time was that renal tubular necrosis and disruption were the primary pathogenetic events. The ischemic theory was revived in the late 1960s and early 1970s, when methods were developed to measure regional intrarenal perfusion and components of the RAS. It was then shown that preferential renal cortical ischemia could diminish glomerular filtration to a degree sufficient to cause acute renal failure even if overall renal blood flow appeared to be only moderately impaired [94]; that infusions of exogenous Ang II sufficient to produce blood levels similar to those found in pathologic states could lead to acute tubular necrosis and renal failure [7,8,98] (Plate 53, see Color Plate Section); and that various maneuvers that induced activation of the endogenous renal RAS to the same extent produced the same pathologic effects in the kidneys of experimental animals [97,99]. The alterations that occur in the RAS in acute circulatory renal failure are demonstrated schematically in Fig. 56.5.

In man, excessive circulating levels of renin, angiotensinogen, Ang II, and (less consistently) aldosterone were found in the early stages of acute circulatory renal failure [98,100–105], whereas during the second and third weeks, the values decreased towards normal often despite persistent uremia (Fig. 56.6). On the basis of these data, it was proposed that intense renal vasoconstriction due to high levels of Ang II might be the primary pathogenetic event leading to acute renal failure [98,104,106]. The excessive amounts of Ang II could be either blood-borne or generated locally (within the renal circulation, or in the extravascular space of the kidney by locally existing ACE, or both [107]).

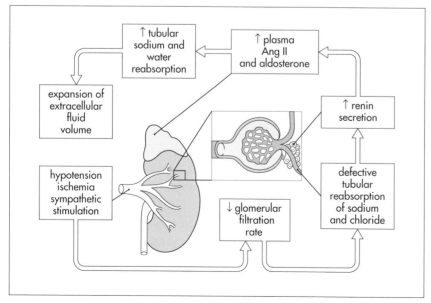

Fig. 56.5 Participation of the RAS in acute circulatory renal failure.

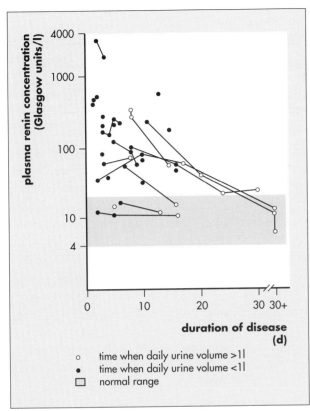

Fig. 56.6 Estimations (47) of plasma renin concentrations in 25 patients with acute renal failure. The lines join estimates from the same patient. Modified from Brown JJ *et al* [102].

However, efforts to protect against experimentally induced acute circulatory renal failure by suppressing renin, by blocking Ang II with antibodies or specific receptor antagonists, or by limiting Ang II formation with ACE inhibitors, have given conflicting results. Some studies did show improvement [96,108–112]; for example, in one experiment, antibodies against Ang II were administered and fully prevented renal impairment, although leaving the histological abnormalities unchanged [109]. In the analogous terminal phase of cardiac failure in which there is grossly excessive activation of the RAS, renal circulatory shutdown, and rapidly progressive renal failure with hyponatremia, ACE inhibitors can reverse these adverse processes, at least temporarily [113]. Even so, many attempts to modify the course of circulatory renal failure by antagonizing the RAS failed [114–119]. In this respect, it has been suggested that the activated RAS, although being adverse early in the disease, may later, in recovery, protect renal cells from reperfusion injury in the postischemic phase, including prevention of cellular calcium overload and tissue damage by oxygen-free radicals [120]. In such a case, inhibition of Ang II in the recovery phase may be detrimental to the ability of cells to recover from ischemia and may actually hasten the development of acute tubular necrosis [120].

It has also been pointed out that many animal models of acute renal failure are associated with acute volume depletion, and some of the Ang II-inhibiting maneuvers also used plasma volume expansion [104,108,109]. Since volume restoration *per se* is associated with improved renal perfusion and renin suppression, it is difficult to define the benefits resulting separately from each of these mechanisms, if indeed they are separable. Moreover, during recovery from acute circulatory renal failure, there is a diuretic phase in which the kidney produces large quantities of dilute urine. Maintenance of fluid and electrolyte balance is critical in this diuretic phase.

In short, most pathophysiologic circumstances that lead to acute circulatory renal failure generally involve significant alterations in arterial pressure and volume homeostasis. Regardless of the original triggering event, the RAS is generally activated in these circumstances to help preserve GFR, urea excretion, and urine concentration, and to maintain volume homeostasis and arterial pressure. There can be little doubt that excessive activation of the RAS in these circumstances could sometimes cause renal damage and failure. However, detailed elucidation of the role of the RAS in the pathogenetic processes of acute circulatory renal failure is as yet incomplete. Any therapeutic benefits from inhibition of the RAS are so far only fragmentary and inconsistent, and require to be further examined and defined.

ACUTE TOXIC RENAL FAILURE

A contrasting form of acute renal failure can be caused by the administration of agents such as cephaloridine. Toxic renal failure of this kind is characterized histologically by extensive necrosis localized to proximal renal tubules [8].

In this syndrome, only minor and inconsistent increases in peripheral plasma concentrations of renin and Ang II have been observed, occurring often some 24–48 hours into the disease course [8,98] (Fig. 56.7). In contrast to acute circulatory renal failure, it does not seem that the RAS is important pathogenically.

ACUTE GLOMERULONEPHRITIS

Acute glomerulonephritis is seen most often in a child or young adult who has suffered a recent streptococcal infection (group A, β-hemolytic), typically of the throat or skin. Antibodies to the streptococci are formed, and antigen–antibody complexes lodge within the glomerular capillary tuft. The clinical features include oliguria, hematuria, proteinuria, and facial edema. Granular,

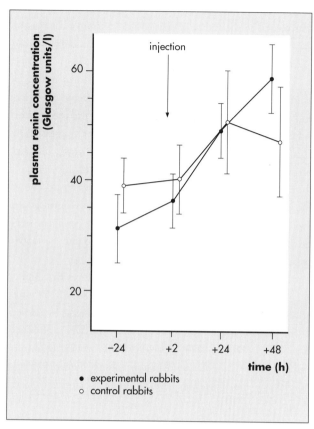

Fig. 56.7 Plasma renin concentration before and after acute toxic renal failure produced by an injection of cephaloridine, and in control rabbits injected with dextrose. The values are shown as mean ± SEM. Modified from Brown JJ *et al* [98].

leukocyte, and red-cell casts appear in the urine. There is variable impairment of renal function. Hypertension is a frequent feature, and occasionally, may enter the malignant phase. The disease is usually self-limiting, the hypertension subsiding within days or weeks. In most cases, hematuria and proteinuria clear within months at most [71,121].

In a detailed study of two patients, Birkenhäger *et al* [122] showed that PRC was disproportionately high for the state of fluid balance, with consequent increased total peripheral resistance (Fig. 56.8). They attributed the hypertension to this inappropriate stimulation of the RAS. In accordance with this view, captopril treatment was reported by Parra *et al* [123] to be effective in controlling hypertension in a series of nine patients, even though pretreatment PRA was in some instances in the overall normal range. Dietary salt and water restriction are also traditionally applied, and may well be of value. With more severe renal failure and hypertension, dialysis may be needed.

CHRONIC RENAL FAILURE

Hypertension is both an important cause and an important consequence of chronic renal failure. Hypertension exists in virtually all patients with end-stage renal disease regardless of the underlying etiology, and is the cause of end-stage renal disease in approximately 25% of cases [124].

The status of the RAS and blood pressure in chronic renal failure of various causes is summarized in *Fig. 56.2*. It is clear that the RAS is only one of several hormonal systems involved in the pathogenesis of this condition. In hypertension associated with chronic renal insufficiency, there is a complex and very variable interaction amongst pressor factors such as endothelin, vasopressin, and catecholamines; and depressor substances such as kinins, atrial natriuretic factor, and prostaglandins, to modulate activity of the RAS and the level of arterial pressure [14,82,86,87,125,126]. Moreover, sodium and volume status, which greatly influences the pressor effect of Ang II, also can vary substantially [58,60,127]. Unlike acute renal failure states, which are largely dependent on systemic and local hemodynamic perturbations that may be induced by, and in turn may modulate, the RAS, the slow progressive decline of renal function in chronic renal failure has multiple etiologies, including inflammatory, mechanical, and other injuries, which lead to destruction of nephrons.

Hypertension as a cause of chronic renal failure

Untreated malignant (accelerated) hypertension leads inexorably and quickly to progressive renal failure. While stimulation of the RAS is not a requisite component of malignant hypertension, many, probably most, cases are associated with activation of the RAS (see *Chapter 60*] (see Color Plates 21 and 22). Rapid deterioration may be attributable in part to the adverse vascular effects of Ang II [128–130] (see *Chapters 40* and *60*). Effective blood-pressure control by virtually any means will arrest or reverse the malignant phase [131–133]; the fact that blockade of the RAS can be particularly successful in promoting or accelerating healing, at least in those patients with a hyperactive RAS, has been suggested but is not proven [33].

Chronic mild essential hypertension has also been proposed as a cause of renal failure, although this remains debatable. At present, there appears to be no clear causal relationship between the degree of blood-pressure control and the occurrence of renal disease [134]. Even authors who have reported a relationship between the level of blood pressure and an accelerated rate of decline in renal function with age [135] have been unable to conclude whether hypertension was the cause of this phenomenon

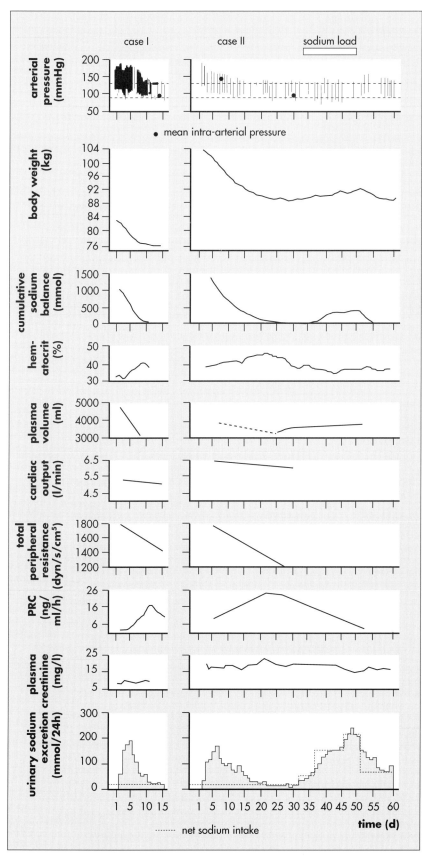

Fig. 56.8 Observations in two cases of acute glomerulonephritis. Case I received a salt-poor diet. The same regimen was applied in case II up to a period of deliberate salt loading. 'Net' sodium intake (intake minus loss from extrarenal sources) was considered to be equal to the mean urinary sodium excretion during equilibrium (constancy of urinary sodium excretion and flattening of the body-weight curve). From the net sodium intake, a retrograde cumulative sodium balance was constructed. The accumulation of sodium, which was purposely induced later in case 2, was calculated from the period of equilibrium onwards. PRC = plasma renin concentration. Modified from Birkenhäger WH *et al* [122].

or whether renal microvascular or parenchymal pathology was the reason for the hypertension. Indeed, many investigators believe that factors such as race [136,137], or underlying subclinical metabolic or renal disease, may be more important determinants of the development of chronic renal failure than the prevailing levels of blood pressure alone. Nevertheless, aggressive antihypertensive treatment may, in some cases, retard further deterioration of existing renal insufficiency [138,139], and early trials such as the Veterans Administration study [140,141] did show a slowing of the progression of renal failure in actively treated versus placebo-treated patients.

Microvascular processes: Scleroderma and vasculitides

Scleroderma and vasculitides are discussed in detail in *Chapter 79* (see Color Plates 18 and 19). Blood pressure can often be very high, with supervention of retinal and other features of the malignant phase [142,143]. There is some evidence that drugs blocking the RAS can be particularly effective [33], but controlled trials are, for obvious reasons, difficult to mount.

Glomerular diseases

Most glomerular diseases can sometimes be accompanied by heavy proteinuria, and the nephrotic syndrome may ensue. The nephrotic syndrome, and its involvement with the RAS, is considered in detail in *Chapter 58*. Relapses and remissions of nephrotic syndrome can occur largely independently of renal failure, the latter being the concern in this chapter.

There is some evidence, discussed again in more detail in *Chapter 58*, that stimulation of the RAS can be more marked in 'minimal change' disease than in the other conditions in this group [28].

In diabetic nephropathy (see Color Plate 31), there is good evidence that aggressive antihypertensive drug treatment can limit the progressive decline of renal function [144,145] (see *Chapter 92*).

Polycystic kidney disease

Hypertension is common in adult polycystic disease and can antedate the onset of renal failure (see *Chapter 57*). While there are reasons to suggest that stimulation of the RAS is responsible for hypertension in these early stages of the disease process, this has been difficult to establish and remains controversial (see *Chapter 57*) (see Color Plates 23–25).

Chronic interstitial nephritis

Chronic interstitial nephritis, a form of progressive renal disease, is not usually accompanied by stimulation of the RAS.

End-stage renal disease

End-stage renal disease, the eventual outcome of progressive renal disease of any of the aforementioned etiologies (see *Fig. 56.2*), requires to be treated by dialysis and/or renal transplantation.

Untreated, this syndrome is characterized by expansion of body sodium content, and plasma renin and Ang II tend to be disproportionately high for concurrent exchangeable (or total body) sodium [58,60] (see *Figs. 56.3* and *56.4*; Color Plates 27 and 28). As discussed earlier, in the majority of patients, blood pressure can be controlled, with or without the addition of antihypertensive drugs, by the removal of salt and water at dialysis, which returns the Ang II/body sodium relationship to normal [37]. In a minority of patients, by contrast, the nature of the intrarenal lesion is such that these attempts simply stimulate more marked renin secretion, resulting in very high plasma Ang II concentrations, persistent or worsening hypertension, and often the addition of other Ang II-induced features such as extreme thirst [36,37] (see *Chapter 32*). In cases of this kind, control of blood pressure is achieved only by lowering plasma Ang II, either by bilateral nephrectomy or by administering an ACE inhibitor.

THERAPEUTIC INTERVENTIONS DIRECTED AT THE RENIN–ANGIOTENSIN SYSTEM: CONCLUSIONS

The diversity of conditions considered in this chapter, and the very varied role of the RAS in different diseases and at several stages even of the same disease, preclude any simple generalization concerning treatment directed at the RAS. Even so, a number of human studies have demonstrated clear benefits to the course of chronic renal failure from ACE inhibition. This is particularly true in patients who have microvascular disorders generally associated with extreme activation of the RAS, such as connective tissue disease and scleroderma [33] (see *Chapter 79*). Furthermore, several reports have documented attenuation in the progression of renal failure in patients with other renoparenchymal disease processes associated with abnormal intrarenal hemodynamics, such as diabetic nephropathy [48,146,147] (see *Chapter 92*) or loss of renal mass on treatment with an ACE inhibitor. It is clear from animal studies that ACE inhibitors given at the appropriate time (that is, early in the course of diseases that otherwise lead eventually to chronic renal failure), can preserve renal function. This benefit appears to result from a lowering of intraglomerular pressure as well as of systemic arterial pressure.

As mentioned earlier, patients with end-stage renal disease have multiple factors in addition to the RAS, which contribute to elevation of arterial pressure. Thus, ACE inhibition alone may not be sufficient to control blood pressure in this population [147–149]. Combination therapy with loop diuretics, sympatholytic agents, or calcium antagonists is frequently needed to counteract volume expansion and activation of the sympathetic nervous system and other neurohumoral vasopressor mechanisms [59,66–68].

While the pathogenic involvement of the RAS in acute circulatory renal failure seems evident, early attempts, circa 1970, to prevent or correct this condition by abrogating the RAS, gave conflicting results [98,109,150]. The more recent availability of drugs that more effectively attack the RAS, such as ACE inhibitors, renin inhibitors (see *Chapter 85*), and nonpeptide Ang II antagonists (see *Chapter 86*), together with a clearer perception of reperfusion injury and the means of its minimization, should reopen this topic. Progress in this field would facilitate therapy over a range of problems from acute circulatory multiple organ failure to renal transplantation.

REFERENCES

1. Catt KJ, Cain MD, Coghlan JP, Zimmet PZ, Cran E, Best JB. Metabolism and blood levels of angiotensin II in normal subjects, renal disease and essential hypertension. *Circulation Research* 1970;26–27 (suppl II):177–83.

2. Navar LG. Renal regulation of body fluid balance. In: Straub NC, Taylor AE, eds. *Edema. 1st edition.* New York: Raven Press, 1984:335–52.

3. Koomans HA, Roos JC, Boer P, Geyskes GG, Dorhout Mees EJ. Salt sensitivity of blood pressure in chronic renal failure. Evidence for renal control of body fluid distribution in man. *Hypertension* 1982;4:190–5.

4. Brown JJ, Davies DL, Johnson VW, Lever AF, Robertson JIS. Renin relationships in congestive cardiac failure, treated and untreated. *American Heart Journal* 1970;80:329–42.

5. Robertson JIS, Richards AM. Converting enzyme inhibitors and renal function in cardiac failure. *Kidney International* 1987;31 (suppl 20):216–9.

6. Robertson JIS, Richards AM. Cardiac failure, the kidney, renin and atrial peptides. *European Heart Journal* 1988;9 (suppl H):11–4.

7. Gavras H, Brown JJ, Lever AF, Macadam RF, Robertson JIS. Acute renal failure, tubular necrosis and myocardial infarction induced in the rabbit by intravenous angiotensin II. *Lancet* 1971;ii:19–22.

8. Gavras H, Kremer D, Brown JJ, Gray B, Lever AF, MacAdam RF, Medina A, Morton JJ, Robertson JIS. Angiotensin- and norepinephrine-induced myocardial lesions: Experimental and clinical studies in rabbits and man. *American Heart Journal* 1975;89:321–32.

9. Baldwin DS, Neugarten J. Hypertension and renal diseases. *American Journal of Kidney Diseases* 1987;10:186–93.

10. Acosta JH. Hypertension in chronic renal disease. *Kidney International* 1982;22:702–13.

11. Smith MC, Dunn MJ. Renovascular and renal parenchymal hypertension. In: Brenner BM, Rector FC Jr, eds. *The kidney.* Philadelphia: WB Saunders, 1986:1221–53.

12. Blythe WB. Natural history of hypertension in renal parenchymal disease. *American Journal of Kidney Diseases* 1985;5:A50–7.

13. Schultze G, Piefke S, Malzahn M. Blood pressure in terminal renal failure: Fluid spaces and the renin–angiotensin system. *Nephron* 1980;25:15–24.

14. Textor SC, Gavras H, Tifft CP, Bernard DB, Idelson B, Brunner HR. Norepinephrine and renin activity in chronic renal failure. Evidence for interacting roles in hemodialysis hypertension. *Hypertension* 1981;3:294–301.

15. Zucchelli P, Zuccola A, Degli Esporti E, Santoro A, Sturani A. Pathophysiology and management of hypertension in hemodialysis patients. *Contributions to Nephrology* 1987;54:209–16.

16. Papadoliopoulou-Diamandopoulou N, Papagalanis N, Gavras I, Gavras H. Vasopressin in end stage renal disease: Relationship to salt, catecholamines and renin activity. *Clinical and Experimental Hypertension. Part A, Theory and Practice* 1987;A9:1197–205.

17. Weidmann P. Pathogenesis of hypertension associated with chronic renal failure. *Contributions to Nephrology* 1984;41:47–53.

18. Sinclair AM, Isles CG, Brown I, Cameron H, Murray BD, Robertson JWK. Secondary hypertension in a blood pressure clinic. *Archives of Internal Medicine* 1987;147:1289–94.

19. Dzau VJ, Kreisberg J. Cultured glomerular mesangial cells contain renin: Influence of calcium and isoproterenol. *Journal of Cardiovascular Pharmacology* 1986;8 (suppl 10): S6–10.

20. Baumbach L, Skott T. Isolated glomeruli *in vitro*: An approach to the macula densa mediated renin release. *Kidney International* 1982;12 (suppl):S73–8.

21. Lilly LS, Pratt RE, Alexander RW, Larson DM, Ellison KE, Gimbrone MA Jr, Dzau VJ. Renin expression by vascular endothelial cells in culture. *Circulation Research* 1985;57:312–8.

22. Brown JJ, Davies DL, Lever AF, Parker RA, Robertson JIS. Assay of renin in single glomeruli: Renin distribution in the normal rabbit kidney. *Lancet* 1963;ii:668.

23. Brown JJ, Davies DL, Lever AF, Parker RA, Robertson JIS. The assay of renin in single glomeruli in the normal rabbit and the appearance of the juxtaglomerular apparatus. *Journal of Physiology* 1965;176:418–28.

24. Gavras H, Brown JJ, Lever AF, Robertson JIS. Changes of renin in individual glomeruli in response to variation of sodium intake in the rabbit. *Clinical Science* 1970;38:409–14.

25. Brown JJ, Davies DL, Lever AF, Parker RA, Robertson JIS. The assay of renin in single glomeruli and the appearance of the juxtaglomerular apparatus in the rabbit following renal artery constriction. *Clinical Science* 1966;30:223–35.

26. Mendelsohn FAO, Dunbar M, Allen A, Chou ST, Millan MA, Aguilera G, Catt KJ. Angiotensin II receptors in the kidney. *Federation Proceedings* 1986;45:1420–7.

27. Bakris GL, Akerstrom V, Re RN. Insulin, angiotensin II antagonism and converting enzyme inhibition: Effect on human mesangial cell mitogenicity and endothelin [Abstract]. *Hypertension* 1990;16:326.

28. Thurau K, Gruner A, Mason J, Dahlhein H. Tubular signal for the renin activity in the juxtaglomerular apparatus. *Kidney International* 1982;22:S55–63.

29. Bell PD, Navar LG. Intrarenal feedback control of glomerular filtration rate. *Seminars in Nephrology* 1982;2:289–301.

30. Weber MA, Drayer JIM. Renal effects of beta-adrenoceptor blockade. *Kidney International* 1980;18:685–701.

31. Lindner A, Douglas SW, Adamson JW. Propranolol effects in long-term hemodialysis patients with renin-dependent hypertension. *Annals of Internal Medicine* 1978;88:457–62.

32. Gavras H, Gavras I, Cannon PJ, Brunner HR, Laragh JH. Is elevated plasma renin activity of prognostic importance in progressive systemic sclerosis? *Archives of Internal Medicine* 1977;137:1554–62.

33. Lopez-Ovejero JS, Sall SD, D'Angelo WA, Cheigh JS, Stenzel KH, Laragh JH. Reversal of vascular and renal crisis of scleroderma by oral angiotensin converting enzyme blockade. *New England Journal of Medicine* 1979;**300**: 1417–23.

34. Stockigt JR, Topliss RJ, Hewett MJ. High-renin hypertension in necrotizing vasculitis. *New England Journal of Medicine* 1979;**300**:1218–25.

35. Brown JJ, Casals-Stenzel J, Cumming AMM, Davies DL, Fraser R, Lever AF, Morton JJ, Semple PF, Tree M, Robertson JIS. Angiotensin II, aldosterone and arterial pressure: A quantitative approach. Arthur C Corcoran Memorial Lecture. *Hypertension* 1979;**1**:159–79.

36. Brown JJ, Curtis JR, Lever AF, Robertson JIS, de Wardener HE, Wing AJ. Plasma renin concentration and the control of blood pressure on maintenance haemodialysis. *Nephron* 1969;**6**:329–49.

37. Brown JJ, Düsterdieck GO, Fraser R, Lever AF, Robertson JIS, Tree M, Weir RJ. Hypertension and chronic renal failure. *British Medical Bulletin* 1971;**27**:128–35.

38. Hammond TG, Whitworth JA, Saines D, Thatcher R, Andrews J, Kincaid-Smith P. Renin–angiotensin aldosterone system in nephrotic syndrome. *American Journal of Kidney Diseases* 1984;**4**:18–26.

39. Danielson H, Kornerup HJ, Olsen S, Posborg V. Arterial hypertension in chronic glomerulonephritis. An analysis of 310 cases. *Clinical Nephrology* 1983;**19**:284–94.

40. Orofino L, Quereda C, Lamas S, Orte L, Gonzalo A, Mampaso F, Ortuno J. Hypertension in primary chronic glomerulonephritis: Analysis of 288 biopsied patients. *Nephron* 1987;**45**:22–6.

41. Hollenberg NK, Solomon HS, Adams DF. Renal vascular response to angiotensin and norepinephrine in normal man: Effect of salt intake. *Circulation Research* 1972;**31**:750–62.

42. Liang C, Gavras H, Hood WB Jr. Renin–angiotensin system inhibition in conscious sodium-depleted dogs: Effects on systemic and coronary hemodynamics. *Journal of Clinical Investigation* 1978;**61**:874–81.

43. Gavras H, Liang C, Brunner HR. Redistribution of regional blood flow after inhibition of the angiotensin converting enzyme. *Circulation Research* 1978; **43** (suppl 1):59–68.

44. Anderson S, Brenner BM. Progressive renal disease: A disorder of adaptation. *Quarterly Journal of Medicine* 1989;**70**:185–9.

45. Hostetter TH, Olson JL, Rennke HG, Venkatachalam MA, Brenner BM. Hyperfiltration in remnant nephrons: A potentially adverse response to renal ablation. *American Journal of Physiology* 1981;**241**:F85–93.

46. Hostetter TH, Troy JL, Brenner BM. Glomerular hemodynamics in experimental diabetes mellitus. *Kidney International* 1980;**19**:410–5.

47. Zatz R, Meyer TW, Rennke GH, Brenner BM. Predominance of hemodynamic rather than metabolic factors in the pathogenesis of diabetic glomerulopathy. *Proceedings of the National Academy of Sciences of the USA* 1985;**82**:5963–7.

48. Hostetter TH, Rennke HG, Brenner BM. The case for intrarenal hypertension in the initiation and progression of diabetic and other glomerulopathies. *American Journal of Medicine* 1982;**72**:375–83.

49. El-Nahas AM, Paraskevakou H, Zoob S, Rees AJ, Evans DJ. Effect of dietary protein restriction on the development of renal failure after subtotal nephrectomy in rats. *Clinical Science* 1983;**65**:399–406.

50. Anderson S, Meyer TW, Rennke HG, Brenner BM. Control of glomerular hypertension limits glomerular injury in rats with reduced renal mass. *Journal of Clinical Investigation* 1985;**76**:612–9.

51. Zatz R, Dunn BR, Meyer TW, Anderson S, Rennke HG, Brenner BM. Prevention of diabetic glomerulopathy by pharmacological amelioration of glomerular capillary hypertension. *Journal of Clinical Investigation* 1986;**77**: 1925–30.

52. Zatz R, Anderson S, Meyer TW, Dunn BR, Rennke HG, Brenner BM. Lowering of arterial blood pressure limits glomerular sclerosis in rats with renal ablation and in experimental diabetes. *Kidney International* 1987;**31** (suppl 20):S123–9.

53. Nahas AE, Wight JP. The management of chronic renal failure: Ten unanswered questions. *Quarterly Journal of Medicine* 1991;**81**:799–809.

54. Anderson S, Rennke HG, Brenner BM. Therapeutic advantage of converting enzyme inhibitors in arresting progressive renal disease associated with systemic hypertension in the rat. *Journal of Clinical Investigation* 1986;**77**: 1993–2000.

55. Hall JE. Intrarenal actions of converting enzyme inhibitors. *American Journal of Hypertension* 1989;**2**:875–84.

56. Laragh JH. Nephron heterogeneity: Clue to the pathogenesis of essential hypertension and effectiveness of angiotensin-converting enzyme inhibitor treatment. *American Journal of Medicine* 1989;**87** (suppl 6B):2–13S.

57. Wilkinson R, Scott DF, Udall PR, Kerr DNS, Swinney J. Plasma renin and exchangeable sodium in the hypertension of chronic renal failure. *Quarterly Journal of Medicine* 1970;**39**:377–96.

58. Davies DL, Beevers DG, Briggs JD, Medina AM, Robertson JIS, Schalekamp MADH, Brown JJ, Lever AF, Morton JJ, Tree M. Abnormal relationship between exchangeable sodium and the renin–angiotensin system in malignant hypertension and in hypertension with chronic renal failure. *Lancet* 1973;**i**: 683–6.

59. Brunner HR, Waeber B, Wauters JP, Turini GA, McKinstry DN, Gavras H. Inappropriate renin secretion unmasked by captopril (SQ 14,225) in hypertension of chronic renal failure. *Lancet* 1979;**ii**:705–6.

60. Schalekamp MA, Beevers DG, Briggs JD, Brown JJ, Davies DL, Fraser R, Lebel M, Lever AF, Medina A, Morton JJ, Robertson JIS, Tree M. Hypertension in chronic renal failure. An abnormal relation between sodium and the renin–angiotensin system. *American Journal of Medicine* 1973;**55**:379–90.

61. Hull AR, Long DL, Prati RC, Pettinger WA, Parker TF. The control of hypertension in patients undergoing regular maintenance hemodialysis. *Kidney International* 1975;**2**:S184–93.

62. Maiorca R, Scolari F, Cancarini G, Brunori G, Camerini C. Management of hypertension in chronic renal failure. *Contributions to Nephrology* 1987;**54**: 190–201.

63. Kim KE, Onesti G, DelGuercio ET, Greco J, Fernandes M, Eidelson B, Swartz C. Sequential hemodynamic changes in end-stage renal disease and anephric state during volume expansion. *Hypertension* 1980;**2**:102–10.

64. Stokes GS, Mani MK, Stewart JH. Relevance of salt, water and renin to hypertension in chronic renal failure. *British Medical Journal* 1970;**3**:126–31.

65. Weidmann P, Maxwell MH, Lupu AN, Lewin AJ, Massry SG. Plasma renin activity and blood pressure in terminal renal failure. *New England Journal of Medicine* 1971;**285**:757–63.

66. Lifschitz MD, Kirschenbaum MA, Rosenblatt SG, Gibney R. Effect of saralasin in hypertensive patients on chronic hemodialysis. *Annals of Internal Medicine* 1978;**88**:23–9.

67. Wauters JP, Waeber B, Brunner HR, Guignard JP, Turini GA, Gavras H. Uncontrollable hypertension in patients on hemodialysis: Long-term treatment with captopril and salt subtraction. *Clinical Nephrology* 1981;**16**:86–92.

68. Ledingham JGG. Effects of angiotensin II and angiotensin converting enzyme inhibition in chronic renal failure. *Kidney International* 1987;**31** (suppl 20): 112–6.

69. Gibbons GH, Pratt RE, Dzau VJ. Angiotensin II (ANG II) is a bifunctional vascular smooth muscle cell (VSMC) growth factor [Abstract]. *Hypertension* 1989;**14**:358.

70. Bhandarn S, Bakris GL. Effects of vasoactive peptides on mesangial cell growth in the presence and absence of high glucose and insulin [Abstract]. *Journal of the American Society of Nephrology* 1991;**2**:314.

71. Fischbach H, Mackensen S, Grund K-E, Kellner A, Bohle A. Relationship between glomerular lesions, serum creatinine and interstitial volume in membrane-proliferative glomerulonephritis. *Klinische Wochenschrift* 1977;**55**:603–8.

72. Hodsman GP, Brown JJ, Cumming AMM, Davies DL, East BW, Lever AF, Morton JJ, Murray GD, Robertson JIS. Enalapril in treatment of hypertension with renal artery stenosis: Changes in blood pressure, renin, angiotensin I and II, renal function, and body composition. *American Journal of Medicine* 1984;**77** (2A):52–60.

73. Cleland JGF, Dargie HJ, Hodsman GP, Ball SG, Robertson JIS, Morton JJ, East BW, Robertson I, Murray GD, Gillen G. Captopril in heart failure: A double blind controlled trial. *British Heart Journal* 1984;**52**:530–45.

74. Cleland JGF, Dargie HJ, Ball SG, Gillen G, Hodsman GP, Morton JJ, East BW, Robertson I, Ford I, Robertson JIS. Effects of enalapril in heart failure: A study on exercise performance, renal function, hormones, and metabolic state. *British Heart Journal* 1985;**54**:305–12.

75. The SOLVD Investigators. Effect of enalapril on survival in patients with reduced left ventricular ejection fractions and congestive heart failure. *New England Journal of Medicine* 1991;**325**:293–302.

76. Cohn JN, Johnson G, Ziesche S, Cobb F, Francis G, Tristani F, Smith R, Dunkman WB, Loeb H, Wong M, Bhat G, Goldman S, Fletcher RD, Doherty J, Hughes CV, Carson P, Cintron G, Shabetai R, Haakenson CS. A comparison of enalapril with hydralazine-isosorbide dinitrate in the treatment of chronic congestive heart failure. *New England Journal of Medicine* 1991;**325**:303–10.

77. Dietz R, Osterziel K-J, Nagel F, Pöschke C, Kübler W. Impairment of renal function during treatment of heart failure with ACE inhibitors: Role of aspirin. *Circulation* 1990;**84** (suppl 2):471.

78. Smith MC, Dunn MJ. The role of prostaglandins in human hypertension. *American Journal of Kidney Diseases* 1985;**5**:A32–41.

79. Ichikawa I, Brenner BM. Local intra-renal vasoconstrictor–vasodilator interaction in mild partial ureteral obstruction. *American Journal of Physiology* 1979;**236**:F131–42.

80. Ciabattoni G, Cinotti GA, Pierucci A, Simonetti BM, Manzi M, Pugliese F, Barsotti P, Pecci G, Taggi F, Patrono C. Effects of sulindac and ibuprofen in patients with chronic glomerular disease. Evidence for the dependence of renal function on prostacyclin. *New England Journal of Medicine* 1984;**310**:279–86.

81. Mitas JA, Levy SB, Holle R, Frigon RP, Stone RA. Urinary kallikrein in the hypertension of renal parenchymal disease. *New England Journal of Medicine* 1978;**299**:162–71.

82. Ruilope L, Robles RG, Bernis C, Barrientos A, Alcazar J, Tresguerras JAF, Sancho J, Rodicio JL. Role of renal prostaglandin E₂ in chronic renal disease hypertension. *Nephron* 1982;**32**:202–6.

83. Muirhead EE. Vasodepressor renal medullary lipids. In: Dunn MJ, ed. *Renal endocrinology*. Baltimore: Williams and Wilkins, 1983:75–95.

84. Smith MC, Dunn MJ. Renal kallikrein, kinins and prostaglandins in hypertension. In: Brenner BM, Stein JH, eds. *Contemporary issues in nephrology: Hypertension*. New York: Churchill Livingstone, 1981:168–93.

85. Mulinari R, Gavras I, Franco R, Gavras H. Bradykinin antagonism and prostaglandins in blood pressure regulation. *Hypertension* 1989;**13**:960–7.

86. DeQuattro V, Miura Y. Neurogenic factors in human hypertension; mechanism or myth? *American Journal of Medicine* 1973;**55**:362–9.

87. Levitan D, Massry SG, Romoff M, Campese V. Plasma catecholamines and autonomic nervous system function in patients with early renal insufficiency and hypertension: Effect of clonidine. *Nephron* 1984;**36**:24–31.

88. Kohlmann O, Bresnahan M, Gavras H. Central and peripheral indices of sympathetic activity following blood pressure lowering with enalapril (MK-421) or hydralazine in normotensive rats. *Hypertension* 1984;**6** (suppl 1):1–7.

89. Tanner GA. Nephron obstruction and tubuloglomerular feedback. *Kidney International* 1982;**22**:S213–9.

90. Ploth DW, Roy RN, McLean C. Renin angiotensin influences on tubuloglomerular feedback activity in the rat. *Kidney International* 1982;**22**:S114–9.

91. Oswald H, Hermes HH, Nabakowski G. Role of adenosine in signal transmission of tubuloglomerular feedback. *Kidney International* 1982;**22**:S136–42.

92. Bell P. Luminal and cellular mechanisms for the mediation of tubuloglomerular feedback responses. *Kidney International* 1982;**22**:S97–103.

93. Goormaghtigh N. Vascular and circulatory changes in the anuria crush syndrome. *Proceedings of the Society for Experimental Biology and Medicine* 1945;**59**:303–8.

94. Hollenberg NK, Epstein M, Rosen SM, Basch RI, Oken DE, Merrill JP. Acute oliguric renal failure in man: Evidence for preferential renal cortical ischemia. *Medicine* 1968;**47**:455–74.

95. Thurau K, Vogt C, Dahlheim H. Renin activity in the juxtaglomerular apparatus of the rat kidney post-ischemic acute renal failure. *Kidney International* 1976;**10**:S177–84.

96. Iaina A, Solomon S, Eliahou HE. Reduction in severity of acute renal failure in rats by beta-adrenergic blockade. *Lancet* 1975;**ii**:157–60.

97. Brown WC, Brown JJ, Gavras H, Jackson A, Lever AF, McGregor J, MacAdam RF, Robertson JIS. Renin and acute circulatory renal failure in the rabbit. *Circulation Research* 1971;**30**:114–22.

98. Brown JJ, Gavras H, Leckie B, Lever AF, Macadam R, Morton JJ, Robertson JIS. Acute circulatory renal failure: A probable manifestation of excess renin release. In: Assaykeen TA, ed. *Control of renin secretion*. New York: Plenum Publishing Co, 1972:263–85.

99. DiBona GF, Sawin LL. The renin–angiotensin system in acute renal failure in the rat. *Labortory Investigation* 1971;**25**:528–39.

100. Massani ZM, Finkielman S, Worcel M, Agrest A, Paladini AC. Angiotensin blood levels in hypertensive and non-hypertensive disease. *Clinical Science* 1966;**30**:473–83.

101. Kokot F, Kuska J. Plasma renin activity in acute renal insufficiency. *Nephron* 1969;**6**:115–21.

102. Brown JJ, Gleadle RI, Lawson DH, Lever AF, Linton AL, Macadam RF, Prentice E, Tree M, Robertson JIS. Renin and acute renal failure: Studies in man. *British Medical Journal* 1970;**1**:253–8.

103. Ochoa E, Finkielman S, Agrest A. Angiotensin blood levels during the evolution of acute renal failure. *Clinical Science* 1970;**38**:225–32.

104. Hollenberg NK, Wilkes BM, Schulman G. The renin–angiotensin system in acute renal failure. In: Brenner BM, Lazarus JM, eds. *Acute renal failure*. Philadelphia: Saunders, 1983:137–62.

105. Paton AM, Lever AF, Oliver NWJ, Medina A, Briggs JD, Morton JJ, Brown JJ, Fraser R, Robertson JIS, Tree M, Gavras H. Plasma angiotensin II, renin, renin-substrate and aldosterone concentrations in acute renal failure in man. *Clinical Nephrology* 1975;**3**:18–23.

106. Hollenberg NK, Adams DF, Oken DE, Abrams HL, Merrill JP. Acute renal failure due to nephrotoxins: Renal hemodynamic and angiographic studies in man. *New England Journal of Medicine* 1970;**282**:1329–34.

107. Brown JJ, Gavras H, Kremer D, Lever AF, Macgregor J, Powell-Jackson JD, Robertson JIS. Renin and acute renal failure. *Proceedings of the conference on acute renal failure. Dept of Health, Education and Welfare, Publication No. (NIH) 74–608, Washington DC*, 1973:57–69.

108. McDonald FD, Thiel G, Wilson DR, DiBona GF, Oken DE. The prevention of acute renal failure in the rat by long-term saline loading: A possible role of the renin–angiotensin axis. *Proceedings of the Society for Experimental Biology and Medicine* 1969;**131**:610-8.

109. Powell-Jackson JD, Brown JJ, Lever AF, MacGregor J, Macadam RF, Titterington DM, Robertson JIS, Waite MA. Protection against acute renal failure in rats by passive immunization against angiotensin II. *Lancet* 1972;**i**:774–6.

110. Schor N, Ichikawa I, Rennke HG, Troy JL, Brenner BM. Pathophysiology of altered glomerular function in aminoglycoside-treated rats. *Kidney International* 1981;**19**:288–96.

111. Lindner A, Cutler RE. Attenuation of acute renal failure in the dog by angiotensin converting enzyme inhibitor [Abstract]. *Tel Aviv Satellite Symposium on Acute Renal Failure*, 1981:94.

112. Magnusson MO, Rybka SJ, Stowe NT, Novick AC, Stratton RA. Enhancement of recovery in post-ischemic acute renal failure with captopril. *Kidney International* 1983;**24** (suppl 16):324–6.

113. Montgomery AJ, Shepherd AN, Emslie-Smith B. Severe hyponatraemia and cardiac failure successfully treated with captopril. *British Medical Journal* 1982;**284**:1085–6.

114. Flamenbaum W, Kotchen TA, Oken DE. Effect of renin immunization on mercuric chloride and glycerol induced renal failure. *Kidney International* 1972;1:406–13.

115. Mathews PG, Morgan TU, Johnston CI. The renin–angiotensin system in acute renal failure in rats. *Clinical Science* 1974;47:79–86.

116. Baranowski RL, O'Connor GJ, Kurtzman NA. The effect of 1-sarcosine, 8-leucyl angiotensin II on glycerol-induced acute renal failure. *Proceedings of the American Society of Nephrology* 1973;6:7–13.

117. Shapira J, Iaina A, Eliahou HE, Solomon S. High renin activity accompanying angiotensin inhibition in rats with ischemic renal failure. *Israel Journal of Medical Sciences* 1976;12:124–31.

118. Ichikawa I, Hollenberg NK. Pharmacologic interruption of the renin–angiotensin system in myohemoglobinuric acute renal failure. *Kidney International* 1976;10:S183–9.

119. Munda R, Alexander JW. Failure of saralasin in preventing renal failure in ischemic transplanted kidneys. *American Surgeon* 1980;46:637–9.

120. Burke TJ, Schrier RW. Angiotensin converting enzyme inhibition and acute tubular necrosis. *Kidney International* 1987;31 (suppl 20):143–7.

121. Schacht RG, Gall GR, Gluck MC, Iqbal MS, Baldwin DS. Irreversible disease following acute poststreptococcal glomerulonephritis in children. *Journal of Chronic Diseases* 1979;32:515–24.

122. Birkenhäger WH, Schalekamp MADH, Schalekamp-Kuyken MPA, Kolsters G, Krauss XH. Inter-relations between arterial pressure, fluid volumes, and plasma-renin concentration in the course of acute glomerulorephritis. *Lancet* 1970;i:1086–7.

123. Parra G, Rodriguez-Iturbe B, Colina-Chourio J, Garcia R. Short-term treatment with captopril in hypertension due to acute glomerulonephritis. *Clinical Nephrology* 1988;29:58–62.

124. US Renal Data System. *USRDS 1989 Annual Report, National Institutes of Health, National Institute of Diabetes and Digestive and Kidney Diseases, Bethesda, Maryland,* 1989.

125. Beretta-Piccoli C, Weidmann P, Schiffl H, Cottier C, Reubi FC. Enhanced cardiovascular pressor reactivity to norepinephrine in mild renal parenchymal disease. *Kidney International* 1982;22:297–303.

126. Ishii M, Ikeda T, Takagi M, Sugimoto T, Atarashi K, Igari T, Uehara Y, Matsuoka H, Hirata Y, Kimura K, Takeda T, Murao S. Elevated plasma catecholamines in hypertensives with primary glomerular diseases. *Hypertension* 1983;5:545–51.

127. Cangiano JL, Ramirez-Muxo O, Ramirez-Gonzales R, Trevino A, Campos JA. Normal renin uremic hypertension. Study of cardiac hemodynamics, plasma volume, extracellular fluid volume and the renin angiotensin system. *Archives of Internal Medicine* 1976;136:17–24.

128. Kincaid-Smith P, McMichael J, Murphy EA. The clinical course and pathology of hypertension with papilloedema (malignant hypertension). *Quarterly Journal of Medicine* 1958;27:117–29.

129. Giese J. Acute vascular disease caused by severe renal ischemia. *Acta Pathologica et Microbiologica Scandinavica* 1962;56:399–411.

130. Gavras H, Brunner HR, Laragh JH. Renin and aldosterone and the pathogenesis of hypertensive vascular damage. *Progress in Cardiovascular Diseases* 1974;28:39–46.

131. Moyer JH, Heider C, Pevey K, Ford RV. The effect of treatment on the vascular deterioration associated with hypertension with particular emphasis on renal function. *American Journal of Medicine* 1958;24:177–83.

132. Woods JW, Blythe WB, Huffines WD. Management of malignant hypertension complicated by renal insufficiency — a follow up study. *New England Journal of Medicine* 1974;291:10–7.

133. Ledingham JGG. Management of hypertensive crises. *Hypertension* 1983;5 (suppl III):114–20.

134. Rostand SG, Brown G, Kirk KA, Dustan HP. Renal insufficiency in treated essential hypertension. *New England Journal of Medicine* 1989;320:684–8.

135. Lindemann RD, Tobin JD, Schock NW. Association between blood pressure and the rate of decline in renal function with age. *Kidney International* 1984;26:861–8.

136. Rostand SG, Kirk KA, Rutsky EA, Pate BA. Racial differences in the incidence of treatment for end-stage renal disease. *New England Journal of Medicine* 1982;306:1276–9.

137. Cowie CC, Port FK, Wolfe RA, Savage PJ, Moll PP, Hawthorne VM. Disparities in incidence of diabetic end-stage renal disease according to race and type of diabetes. *New England Journal of Medicine* 1989;321:1074–9.

138. Taverner D, Bing RF, Heagerty A, Russell GI, Pohl JEF, Swales JD, Thurston H. Improvement of renal function during long-term treatment with minoxidil. *Quarterly Journal of Medicine* 1983;206:280–8.

139. Mitchell HC, Graham RM, Pettinger WA. Renal function during long-term treatment of hypertension with minoxidil. *Annals of Internal Medicine* 1980;93:676–81.

140. Veterans Administration Cooperative Study Group on Antihypertensive Agents. Effects of treatment on morbidity in hypertension. I Results in patients with diastolic blood pressure averaging 115 through 129mmHg. *Journal of the American Medical Association* 1967;202:1028–34.

141. Veterans Administration Cooperative Study Group on Antihypertensive Agents. Effects of treatment on morbidity in hypertension. II Results in patients with diastolic blood pressures averaging 90 through 114mmHg. *Journal of the American Medical Association* 1970;213:1143–52.

142. Adu D, Howie AJ, Scott DGI, Bacon PA, McGonigle RJS, Michael J. Polyarteritis and the kidney. *Quarterly Journal of Medicine* 1987;62:221–3.

143. Serra A, Cameron JS, Turner DR, Hartley B, Ogg CS, Neild GH, Williams DG, Tauber D, Brown CB, Hicks JA. Vasculitis affecting the kidney: Presentation histopathology and long-term outcome. *Quarterly Journal of Medicine* 1984;53:181–207.

144. Mogensen CE. Long-term antihypertensive treatment inhibiting progression of diabetic nephropathy. *British Medical Journal* 1982;285:685–9.

145. Parving H-H, Smidt UM, Andersen AR, Svendsen PA. Early aggressive antihypertensive treatment reduces rate of decline in kidney function in diabetic nephropathy. *Lancet* 1983;i:1175–8.

146. Hollenberg NK, Swartz SL, Passan DR, Williams GH. Increased glomerular filtration rate after converting enzyme inhibition in essential hypertension. *New England Journal of Medicine* 1979;301:9–15.

147. Anderson S, Rennke HG, Garcia DL, Brenner BM. Short and long term effects of antihypertensive therapy in the diabetic rat. *Kidney International* 1989;36:526–34.

148. Sulkova S, Valek A. Role of antihypertensive drugs in the therapy of patients on regular dialysis treatment. *Kidney International* 1988;34 (suppl 25):198–200.

149. Maggiore Q, Zoccali C, Monzani G, Contini C. Chronic hemodynamic effects of propranolol treatment in dialysis-refractory hypertension. *Nephron* 1978;22:391–9.

150. Robertson JIS. Overview: Renal disease and ACE inhibition: II. *Kidney International* 1987;31 (suppl 20):130–1.

151. Yamamoto T, Shimizu M, Morioka M, Kitano M, Wakabayashi H, Aizawa N. Role of angiotensin II in the pathogenesis of hyperdipsia in chronic renal failure. *Journal of the American Medical Association* 1986;256:604–8.

57 POLYCYSTIC KIDNEY DISEASE AND THE RENIN SYSTEM

J IAN S ROBERTSON

INTRODUCTION

Adult polycystic kidney disease is transmitted as an autosomal dominant condition. It has been estimated that approximately 1 in 1,000 people carries a mutant gene for this malady, which is responsible for between 5 and 10% of cases of end-stage renal failure in Europe and North America [1–6]. Davies *et al* [3] noted that in south Wales, the clinical prevalence of end-stage renal disease was less than half the supposed gene frequency, indicating that many undiagnosed cases of polycystic renal disease may exist, and carry a benign prognosis. Kimberling *et al* [7] found evidence that there may be two genetically distinct forms of the disease.

RENAL AND EXTRARENAL LESIONS

In addition to the prominent renal lesions that characterize this condition (see Color Plate 23), extrarenal manifestations include liver cysts [8], colonic diverticulosis [9], aortic aneurysms [10], annuloaortic ectasia [11], mitral valve prolapse [12], and intracranial berry aneurysms [13–15]. These extrarenal lesions indicate that the disease involves a generalized connective tissue disorder. The intracranial aneurysms can predispose to subarachnoid hemorrhage [15,16], especially if there is concomitant hypertension.

PREVALENCE OF HYPERTENSION

Hypertension is a very frequent accompaniment of polycystic kidney disease, with a prevalence probably as much as 75% [8,17–19]. The fact that high blood pressure accompanies renal failure is unremarkable; these aspects and their relationships with the RAS are discussed in *Chapter 56*. However, hypertension can also occur with polycystic kidney disease in the absence of perceptible overall renal functional impairment. The possible involvement of the RAS in pathogenesis in the latter circumstances is addressed in this chapter.

INDIRECT EVIDENCE OF INVOLVEMENT OF THE RENIN SYSTEM

There are good reasons to suppose that stimulation of the RAS might be involved in the pathogenesis of hypertension in polycystic renal disease in the absence of renal impairment. Angiography has indicated that the renal cysts can cause intrarenal arterial attenuation [20,21]; immunohistochemical studies of the renal juxtaglomerular apparatus have shown increased numbers of

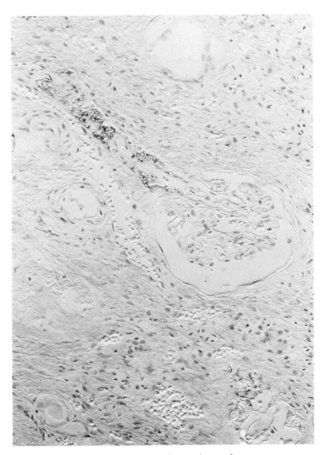

Fig. 57.1 A glomerulus showing hyperplasia of renin-containing cells at the juxtaglomerular apparatus, with extension along the afferent arteriole. (Autopsy kidney; renin PAP; interference contrast x 200.) Reproduced with permission of Graham PC and Lindop GBM [22].

57.1

renin-secreting granules [22] (*Chapter 19*) (Fig. 57.1, Color Plates 24 and 25); and cyst decompression can alleviate hypertension [23,24]. Thus, raised arterial pressure may be due to mechanisms akin to those with renal artery stenosis (*Chapter 55*).

CLINICAL STUDIES OF THE RENIN SYSTEM IN NONAZOTEMIC POLYCYSTIC KIDNEY DISEASE

Despite the apparent probability of such a conjunction, however, not all studies have demonstrated clearly increased activity of the RAS in these circumstances [18,25–31]. Some of the reports merit more detailed description.

Anderson *et al* [25] compared data obtained in 15 hypertensive patients having polycystic disease with those in seven patients with unilateral renal artery stenosis (Fig. 57.2). Overall, renal function was similar in the two groups. Diastolic pressure was lowered to less than 90mmHg after surgical correction of the lesion in all seven patients with renal artery stenosis, indicating that these were cases of genuine renovascular hypertension. The subjects with renovascular hypertension had significantly higher values for plasma renin activity (PRA) and aldosterone than did those with polycystic disease; moreover, infusion of the Ang II antagonist, saralasin, lowered blood pressure only in the patients with renovascular disease. These authors concluded therefore that the RAS did not play a pathogenic role in the maintenance of hypertension in this series of cases of nonazotemic polycystic kidney disease.

Danielsen *et al* [26] studied 8 normotensive and 10 hypertensive patients with polycystic kidney disease, and 11 normotensive control subjects. Plasma Ang II, aldosterone, and vasopressin

Group	Mean age (years)	Males (%)	2-h upright plasma renin activity (ng/ml/h)	2-h upright plasma aldosterone (pg/ml)	24-h urinary sodium excretion at time of PRA and plasma aldosterone (mmol/24h)	24-h endogenous creatinine clearance (ml/min)	Blood pressure response to saralasin (mm Hg) Systolic		Diastolic	
polycystic disease	35.1 ± 2.0 (NS)	80 (NS)	2.2 ± 0.4 (<0.005)	213 ± 36 (<0.001)	144 ± 21 (NS)	93 ± 9 (NS)	135 ± 3 (NS)	140 ± 4	99 ± 2 (NS)	101 ± 3
renovascular hypertension	39.1 ± 5.0	75	10.6 ± 2.6	548 ± 46	131 ± 24	90 ± 10	169 ± 9 (<0.05)	149 ± 8	114 ± 5 (<0.02)	99 ± 6

Fig. 57.2 Plasma renin activity (PRA) and blood pressure response to saralasin in hypertensive patients with polycystic kidney disease or renovascular hypertension. Data are means ± SEM; probabilities are given in parentheses; NS = not significant. Modified from Anderson RJ *et al* [25].

	Polycystic patients		Controls	
	Low	High	Low	High
mean arterial pressure (mmHg)	107.2 ± 3.4†	111.2 ± 2.9*§	92.7 ± 2.7	91.9 ± 2.5
Ang II concentration (fmol/ml)	22.2 ± 3.8	5.7 ± 0.6*	28.1 ± 6.8	7.9 ± 1.1*
Ang II receptors (sites/platelet)	1.5 ± 0.47	3.4 ± 0.49*	2.7 ± 0.98	6.1 ± 2.19*
K_D (10^{-12}mol/l)	163 ± 11	178 ± 17	155 ± 19	177 ± 24
atrial natriuretic factor (fmol/ml)	42.6 ± 10.6	252 ± 85*§	14.7 ± 4.2	23.5 ± 7.0
inulin clearance (ml/min/1.73m²)	88 ± 11	91 ± 10	106 ± 5	109 ± 5
para-aminohippurate clearance (ml/min/1.73m²)	410 ± 64	413 ± 61	556 ± 34	583 ± 37
fractional sodium excretion (%)	0.22 ± 0.06	1.92 ± 0.25*	0.12 ± 0.03	1.38 ± 0.06*

K_D = apparent affinity constant; *$P<0.02$ versus low sodium intake; †$P<0.05$, §$P<0.02$, versus respective controls; high sodium intake 200mmol/d; low sodium intake 20mmol/d.

Fig. 57.3 Hormonal and renal changes on a low or high sodium intake. Data are means ± SEM. Modified from Schmid M *et al* [31].

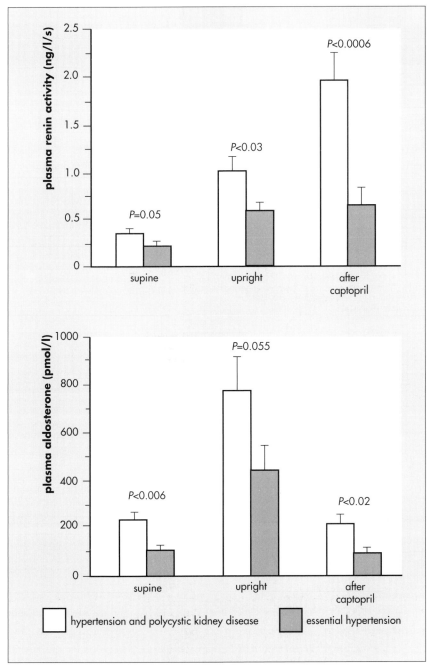

Fig. 57.4 Mean (± SEM) plasma renin activity and plasma aldosterone concentrations in 14 patients with hypertension and polycystic kidney disease and in nine patients with essential hypertension. The patients were studied in the supine and upright positions and one hour after oral administration of 50mg captopril. *P* values were determined by rank-sum analysis. Modified from Chapman AB *et al* [18].

concentrations were elevated in the hypertensive patients, while blood volume and extracellular fluid volume were similar in all three groups. Plasma Ang II and vasopressin concentrations were positively correlated with blood pressure and were believed to be possibly involved in pathogenesis. This analysis, however, included some polycystic patients with demonstrable renal impairment.

Schmid *et al* [31] studied nine patients with autosomal dominant polycystic kidney disease and hypertension, and nine normotensive healthy probands, under standardized conditions of both high (200mmol/d) and low (20mmol/d) sodium diet (Fig. 57.3). Average renal function was similar in the two groups. Plasma Ang II concentrations were comparable in both groups under both dietary circumstances, as were Ang II binding sites on platelets, the latter reflecting pressor sensitivity to Ang II [32]. In hypertensive patients, plasma atrial natriuretic factor concentrations were higher at baseline and showed an exaggerated response to sodium loading. The hypertensive subjects had an enhanced pressor sensitivity to sodium which might well have been pathogenically relevant.

Chapman et al [18] compared PRA and plasma aldosterone, and their responses to orthostasis, in 14 hypertensive and 11 normotensive nonazotemic patients with polycystic kidney disease; 13 normal subjects; and 9 patients with essential hypertension. Both immediate and long-term (six weeks) responses to ACE inhibition were also examined in the two hypertensive groups. Plasma renin activity and aldosterone, and their responses to orthostasis, were closely similar in both the hypertensive and normotensive groups with polycystic disease and in the normal subjects. Under both postural conditions, PRA and aldosterone were lower in the patients with essential hypertension (Fig. 57.4), as is well established (see *Chapter 62*). The absolute increase in PRA one hour after giving captopril was substantially greater in the hypertensive polycystic patients than in those with essential hypertension (Fig. 57.4). Longerterm ACE inhibition with enalapril led to increases in renal plasma flow and decreases in renal vascular resistance and filtration fraction in the hypertensive patients with polycystic disease, but not in those with essential hypertension. The interpretation of their data by these authors [18] was that increased renin release probably contributes to the early development of hypertension in polycystic renal disease.

Chapman et al [33] subsequently supported their view by demonstrating, in five patients with polycystic kidney disease, reversible deterioration of renal function with ACE inhibition. Such reversible renal impairment is well recognized with ACE inhibition in renovascular hypertension (see *Chapters 55* and *88–90*) and indicates compensatory dependence of renal function on an intrarenal action of the RAS [34]. Nevertheless, the conclusions of Chapman et al [18] were criticized as perhaps wrongly invoking the RAS in pathogenesis [35].

Bell *et al* [30] found that captopril administration stimulated the RAS to a greater extent in hypertensive than in normotensive patients with polycystic disease, all of whom had normal renal function.

Harrap and colleagues measured renal function and activity of the RAS in 19 affected and 20 unaffected offspring from families with polycystic disease. Compared with unaffected offspring, those with polycystic disease had similar glomerular filtration rates but reduced effective renal plasma flow rates and elevated plasma renin and plasma aldosterone levels [34]. This was despite the fact that both arterial pressure and total exchangeable sodium were higher in the affected offspring. On the basis of these data, the authors proposed that reduced renal blood flow, activation of the RAS, and increased body sodium may play a central role in the genesis of hypertension in this disorder. They also raised the possibility that the renin system might contribute to the rate at which the renal cysts grow [34], since earlier studies showed that growth of experimental cysts was enhanced when the RAS was activated and reduced when it was suppressed [36].

CONCLUSIONS

In conclusion therefore, although there appear good grounds for expecting the RAS to be involved in the pathogenesis of hypertension in nonazotemic polycystic renal disease, and strong circumstantial evidence exists in favor of such a mechanism, no such involvement has been unequivocally revealed despite several careful studies. While the notion has its advocates [18,37], their arguments appear to several workers to be, on the presently available evidence, tenuous. Nevertheless, it should be borne in mind that in the second phase of 2-kidney, 1-clip renovascular hypertension, a condition in which the RAS is almost certainly involved pathogenically, and which is postulated to be analogous in some respects to early polycystic disease, plasma renin and Ang II may return to the normal range (see *Chapter 55*). For the present, the issue remains open.

REFERENCES

1. Parfrey PS, Bear JC, Morgan J, Cramer BC, McManamon PJ, Gault MH, Churchill DN, Singh M, Hewitt R, Somlo S, Reeders ST. The diagnosis and prognosis of autosomal dominant polycystic kidney disease. *New England Journal of Medicine* 1990;**323**:1085–90.

2. Reeders ST. Autosomal dominant polycystic kidney disease. *Quarterly Journal of Medicine* 1991;**79**:459–60.

3. Davies F, Coles GA, Harper PS, Williams AJ, Evans C, Cochlin D. Polycystic kidney disease re-evaluated: A population-based study. *Quarterly Journal of Medicine* 1991;**79**:477–85.

4. Watson ML, Macnicol AM, Wright AF. Adult polycystic kidney disease. *British Medical Journal* 1990;**300**:62–3.

5. Ravine D, Walker RG, Gibson RN, Sheffield LJ, Kincaid-Smith P, Danks DM. Treatable complications in undiagnosed cases of autosomal dominant polycystic kidney disease. *Lancet* 1991;**337**:127–9.

6. Grantham JJ. Polycystic kidney disease — an old problem in a new context. *New England Journal of Medicine* 1988;**319**:944–6.

7. Kimberling WJ, Fain PR, Kenyon JB, Goldgar D, Sujansky E, Gabow PA. Linkage heterogeneity of autosomal dominant polycystic kidney disease. *New England Journal of Medicine* 1988;**319**:913–8.

8. Dalgaard OZ. Bilateral polycystic disease of the kidneys: A follow-up of two hundred and eighty-four patients and their families. *Acta Medica Scandinavica* 1957;(suppl 158):1–251.

9. Scheff RT, Zuckerman G, Harter H, Delmez J, Koehler R. Diverticular disease in patients with chronic renal failure due to polycystic disease. *Annals of Internal Medicine* 1980;**92**:202–4.

10. Montoliu J, Torras A, Revert L. Polycystic kidneys and abdominal aortic aneurysms. *Lancet* 1980;**i**:1133–4.

11. Nuñez L, O'Connor LF, Pinto AG, Gil-Aguado M, Gutierrez M. Annuloaortic ectasia and adult polycystic kidney: A frequent association. *Chest* 1986;**90**:299–300.

12. Hossack KF, Leddy CL, Johnson AM, Schrier RW, Gabow PA. Echocardiographic findings in autosomal dominant polycystic kidney disease. *New England Journal of Medicine* 1988;**319**:907–12.

13. Bigelow NH. The association of polycystic kidneys with intracranial aneurysms and other related disorders. *American Journal of the Medical Sciences* 1953;**225**:485–94.

14. Crompton MR. The pathogenesis of cerebral aneurysms. *Brain* 1966;**89**:797–801.

15. Chauveau D, Sirieix M-E, Schillinger F, Legendre C, Grünfeld JP. Recurrent rupture of intracranial aneurysms in autosomal dominant polycystic kidney disease. *British Medical Journal* 1990;**301**:966–7.

16. Graham DI, Lee WR, Cumming AMM, Robertson JIS, Jones JV. Hypertension and the intracranial and ocular circulations: Effects of antihypertensive treatment. In: Robertson JIS, ed. *Handbook of hypertension, vol. 1: Clinical aspects of essential hypertension.* Amsterdam: Elsevier Science Publishers BV, 1983:174–201.

17. Goddard DH, Pearce VR, Boyle RM, Hamilton M. Hypertension in polycystic renal disease. *Journal of the Royal College of Physicians of London* 1980;**14**:218–20.

18. Chapman AB, Johnson A, Gabow PA, Schrier RW. The renin–angiotensin–aldosterone system and autosomal dominant polycystic kidney disease. *New England Journal of Medicine* 1990;**323**:1091–6.

19. Hansson L, Karlander LE, Lundgren W, Peterson LE. Hypertension in polycystic kidney disease. *Scandinavian Journal of Urology and Nephrology* 1974;**8**:203–5.

20. Ettinger A, Kahn PC, Wise HM. The importance of selective angiography in the diagnosis of polycystic disease. *Journal of Urology* 1969;**102**:156–61.

21. Cornell SH. Angiography in polycystic disease of the kidneys. *Journal of Urology* 1970;**103**:24–6.

22. Graham PC, Lindop GBM. The anatomy of the renin-secreting cell in adult polycystic kidney disease. *Kidney International* 1988;**33**:1084–90.

23. Bennett WM, Elzinga L, Golper TA, Barry JM. Reduction of cyst volume for symptomatic management of autosomal dominant polycystic kidney disease. *Journal of Urology* 1987;**137**:620–2.

24. Frang D, Czvalinga 1, Polyak L. A new approach to the treatment of polycystic kidneys. *International Urology and Nephrology* 1988;**20**:13–21.

25. Anderson RJ, Miller PD, Linas SL, Katz FH, Holmes JH. Role of the renin–angiotensin system in hypertension of polycystic kidney disease. *Mineral and Electrolyte Metabolism* 1979;**2**:137–41.

26. Danielsen H, Pedersen EB, Nielsen AH, Herlevsen P, Kornerup HJ, Posborg V. Expansion of extracellular volume in early polycystic kidney disease. *Acta Medica Scandinavica* 1986;**219**:399–405.

27. Valvo E, Gammaro L, Tessitore N, Panzetta G, Lupo A, Loschiavo C, Oldrizzi L, Fabris A, Rugiu C, Ortalda V, Maschio G. Hypertension of polycystic kidney disease: Mechanisms and hemodynamic alterations. *American Journal of Nephrology* 1985;**5**:176–81.

28. Brod J, Bahlmann J, Cachovan M, Hubrich W, Pretschner PD. Mechanisms for the elevation of blood pressure in human renal disease. *Hypertension* 1982;**4**:839–44.

29. Nash DA. Hypertension in polycystic kidney disease without renal failure. *Archives of Internal Medicine* 1977;**137**:1571–5.

30. Bell PE, Hossack KF, Gabow PA, Durr JA, Johnson AM, Schrier RW. Hypertension in autosomal dominant polycystic kidney disease. *Kidney International* 1988;**34**:683–90.

31. Schmid M, Mann JFE, Stein G, Herter M, Nussberger J, Klingbeil A, Ritz E. Natriuresis-pressure relationship in polycystic kidney disease. *Journal of Hypertension* 1990;**8**:277–83.

32. Mann JFE, Leidig M, Ritz E. Human angiotensin II receptors are regulated by angiotensin II. *Clinical and Experimental Hypertension. Part A, Theory and Practice* 1988;**A10**:151–68.

33. Chapman AB, Johnson AM, Gabow PA, Schrier RW. Reversible renal failure associated with angiotensin-converting enzyme inhibitors in polycystic kidney disease. *Annals of Internal Medicine* 1991;**115**:769–73.

34. Harrap SB, Davies DL, Macnicol AM, Dominiczak AF, Fraser R, Wright AF, Watson ML, Briggs JD. Renal, cardiovascular and hormonal characteristics of young adults with autosomal dominant polycystic kidney disease. *Kidney International* 1991;**40**:501–8.

35. Del Castello Caba D, Martin-Malo A, Calderon RP. The renin–angiotensin system and polycystic kidney disease. *New England Journal of Medicine* 1991;**324**:775–6.

36. Torres VE, Berndt TJ, Okamura M, Nesbit JW, Holley KE, Carone FA, Knox FG, Romero JC. Mechanisms affecting the development of renal cystic disease induced by diphenylthiazole. *Kidney International* 1988;**33**:1130–9.

37. Chapman AB, Johnson AM, Gabow PA, Schrier RW. The renin–angiotensin system and polycystic kidney disease. *New England Journal of Medicine* 1991;**324**:776.

58

RENIN AND THE NEPHROTIC SYNDROME

J IAN S ROBERTSON

INTRODUCTION

The nephrotic syndrome comprises severe proteinuria, hypoproteinemia, sodium and water retention, edema, and hyperlipidemia. The RAS can be involved in three distinct ways. First, marked stimulation of renin secretion, as with a severe renal artery stenosis or occlusion, or accompanying a renin-secreting tumor, can cause heavy proteinuria, and hence lead to the nephrotic syndrome. In the case of renal artery stenosis, the proteinuria is largely, but not necessarily exclusively, from the contralateral kidney. Second, a primary intrinsic lesion of the kidney can result in proteinuria and thus the nephrotic syndrome, with consequent pathophysiological changes in the RAS. It has been disputed whether such secondary changes in the RAS may in turn promote worsening of the nephrotic syndrome in some clinical circumstances. Third, rare instances have been reported where large doses of sulfhydryl-containing ACE inhibitors have precipitated severe proteinuria and nephrotic syndrome.

These three forms of the disease will be considered separately.

RENIN, RENAL ARTERY STENOSIS, RENIN-SECRETING TUMOR, AND NEPHROTIC SYNDROME

CLINICAL OBSERVATIONS

An uncommon, but regularly reported, mode of presentation of renal artery stenosis is of severe proteinuria, progressing to frank nephrotic syndrome with hypoalbuminemia and peripheral edema [1–6]. The syndrome can be corrected severally by renal artery reconstruction, by unilateral nephrectomy, or by treatment with ACE inhibitors (see *Chapters 55* and *88*). Severe proteinuria has similarly been reported accompanying marked excess of circulating renin (and hence of Ang II) in a patient with renin-secreting tumor [7] (see *Chapter 54*).

Administration of large doses of renin or of Ang II to animals has been shown to cause proteinuria, and the proposed mechanism of the clinical syndrome is thus similar [8] (see *Chapter 22*). With renovascular disease, gross excess of renin and hence of Ang II originating in the kidney distal to the renal artery stenosis or occlusion leads to severe proteinuria. The protein loss is probably mainly from the kidney contralateral to the renal arterial lesion, and has, for example, been reported with unilateral renal artery occlusion, where the affected kidney was not producing urine [5]. In the patient of Eiser *et al* [3], unilateral nephrectomy relieved both hypertension and proteinuria, although the latter resolved only gradually after nephrectomy, again indicating the contralateral kidney as the source of protein loss. However, fusion of glomerular foot processes in the nephrectomy specimen in this case suggested that the excised kidney also might *in vivo* have contributed to the proteinuria (see later). In the patient of Holman *et al* [6], the proteinuria cleared with administration of an ACE inhibitor, where other antihypertensive agents, although controlling blood pressure, were ineffective.

In the case of renin-secreting tumor, the associations are more straight forward. Proteinuria resolves with removal of the tumor [7].

PATHOPHYSIOLOGICAL BASIS

Administration of renin or Ang II causes proteinuria in various animals, including rabbits [9–13], rats [14–17], and dogs [18]. This effect has been demonstrated in a rabbit kidney perfused with whole blood from an artificial heart–lung preparation [19]. The excreted protein consists of all components of serum proteins [20]. The proteinuria is due at least in part to increased glomerular permeability [20–23]. It is enhanced by pretreatment with deoxycorticosterone or cortisone [24], but is impaired by adrenalectomy or hypophysectomy [25–28]. In man, renin [10] or Ang II [29,30] do not, however, consistently produce proteinuria. The ability of Ang II to cause proteinuria is probably species dependent, with the rat and man representing the two extremes [8]. Thus, the occurrence of nephrotic syndrome with renal lesions in man usually requires very marked elevation of renin and Ang II, perhaps in concert with a high renal artery pressure, as has been emphasized [3].

It has been suggested that the proteinuria represents the local effect of a generalized increase in permeability of the vascular bed [31] (see *Chapters 22, 27,* and *40*). A possibility other than a direct effect on membrane permeability is that Ang II, by acting on pre- and postcapillary vessels, would cause changes in capillary pressure [32]. This would agree with the view of Giese [33] that increased permeability is not a specific effect of Ang II but represents the result of abnormal and focal vascular reactions. The reported differential tonic effect of Ang II on efferent glomerular arterioles would enhance the tendency for protein to enter the glomerular filtrate [34–36]. An increase in intraglomerular pressure could result in stretching of a small proportion of the total pore area. The absence of a similar response after adrenalectomy has been attributed to the severe reduction of glomerular filtration rate and renal plasma flow with infusion of renin or Ang II in these circumstances [28]. Any tubular action of Ang II limiting reabsorption of filtered protein would worsen the proteinuria.

Electron microscopic studies made at the time of maximal proteinuria show a focal flattening and fusion of epithelial foot processes, as well as swelling and vesicle formation in endothelial and epithelial cells of the glomeruli [27,28,37]. These could be a cause or the consequence, or both, of enhanced protein filtration.

NEPHROTIC SYNDROME DUE TO AN INTRINSIC RENAL LESION

MEASUREMENTS OF COMPONENTS OF THE SYSTEM

Medina *et al* [38] reported a detailed study, performed under controlled conditions, of the RAS in patients with the nephrotic syndrome, in comparison with healthy subjects. All seven patients were men, aged 25–42 years, having a plasma albumin concentration of 3g/100ml or less, and a 24-hour urinary protein excretion of 3g or more. Renal biopsy showed proliferative glomerulonephritis (three cases), membranous glomerulonephritis (two cases), and 'no light microscopy change' (one case). A biopsy was not obtained in the remaining patient. All had a history of chronic relapsing edema, and each patient had peripheral edema at the onset of the study. None had received drug therapy in the four weeks before the investigations. The subjects were given a diet of known sodium and potassium content (between 40 and 60mmol of each cation per day, held

constant for each patient). Between 9 and 10am on the fourth day of this regime, all patients having fasted and remained recumbent for at least 10 hours, blood samples were taken from an arm vein for measurement of the plasma concentrations of renin (PRC), renin substrate, Ang II, and aldosterone. An overnight urine sample was also obtained. The patients were then allowed out of bed and encouraged to remain ambulant for three hours, at which time further blood samples were obtained. The three-hour urine specimen was collected. In one patient, the whole procedure was repeated on two further occasions. Control data were obtained under similar conditions from five apparently healthy male subjects aged 27–44.

The mean PRC was significantly elevated in the nephrotic patients as compared with the controls (Fig. 58.1), both in recumbency and after ambulation ($P<0.01$ and $P<0.05$). There was a significant increase in PRC with change of posture in both groups ($P<0.05$ for each). Plasma renin substrate (angiotensinogen) was below the normal male range in five estimations from four of the nephrotic patients. No significant changes in substrate level occurred after three hours of ambulation in either control or nephrotic groups. There was no significant difference in plasma Ang II concentrations between the nephrotic subjects and the controls either in recumbency or after ambulation (Fig. 58.1). A significant increase occurred on ambulation in the patients, but was marginal in the controls ($P<0.001$ and $P<0.1$, respectively). Despite the reduced sodium intake, recumbent plasma aldosterone concentrations (Fig. 58.1) were not particularly high in either group (nephrotic patients, mean 12.8, range 3.4–32.8ng/100ml; controls, mean 2.8, range 1.5–4.7ng/100ml). Mean plasma aldosterone in the nephrotic group was higher than in the control group ($P<0.02$). A rise in plasma aldosterone occurred on standing both in the patients ($P<0.01$) and in the controls ($P<0.001$). This postural increase was significantly greater in the controls than in the nephrotics ($P<0.001$), but there was no difference in the mean plasma aldosterone concentration between the groups when ambulant. Both in the nephrotic patients and in the controls, a marked fall in the urinary Na/K ratio occurred on ambulation. Plasma renin concentration was significantly related to the concurrent plasma Ang II level in the nephrotics (r=+0.59, n=18, $P<0.01$) and in the control subjects (r=+0.67, n=10, $P<0.05$). The regression lines for these two sets of data differed significantly in slope, however ($P<0.05$) (Fig. 58.2), with plasma Ang II being systematically lower for a given PRC in the patients than in the controls. This was interpreted as being a consequence of the lower angiotensinogen values in the patients. Thus, in this study, while PRC was frequently elevated, angiotensinogen was

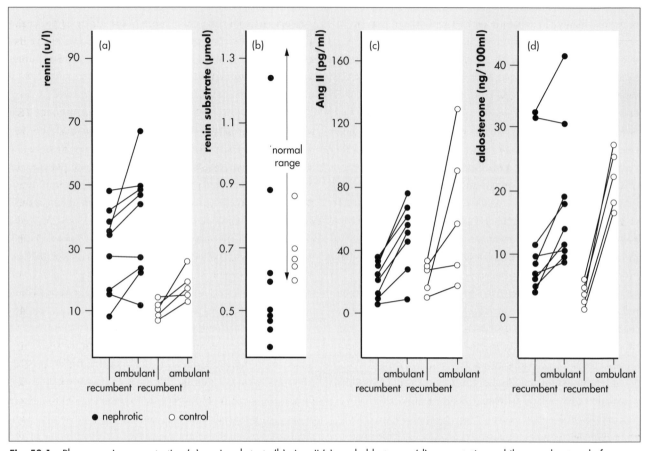

Fig. 58.1 Plasma renin concentration (a), renin substrate (b), Ang II (c), and aldosterone (d) concentations while recumbent and after being ambulant for three hours. Modified from Medina A *et al* [38].

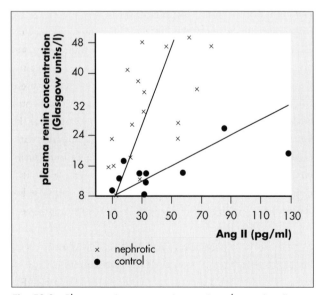

Fig. 58.2 Plasma renin concentration against plasma Ang II concentration for nephrotic patients (r=+0.59, n=18, *P*<0.01) and control subjects (r=+0.67, n=10, *P*<0.05). Modified from Medina A *et al* [38].

lowered in several patients, and plasma Ang II and aldosterone concentrations were generally within the normal range.

Boer *et al* [39] studied plasma renin activity (PRA) and angiotensinogen in 27 episodes of the nephrotic syndrome in 24 patients suffering various renal lesions; 10 of these were investigated further after remission. During the nephrotic phase, angiotensinogen was low in 8%, normal in 44%, and elevated in 48%, while PRA was low in 41%, normal in 48%, and elevated in 11%. After remission, angiotensinogen rose in 50% and fell in 20%, while PRA increased in 70% of patients. These authors thus confirmed the findings of Medina *et al* [38], that in the nephrotic syndrome, large changes in angiotensinogen concentrations can markedly influence Ang II and PRA values. Boer *et al* [39] further concluded that low angiotensinogen and high PRA are not always characteristic of the nephrotic syndrome.

THE RENIN SYSTEM AND ETIOLOGY

Hammond *et al* [40] evaluated the RAS in relation to the underlying renal lesion. They compared PRC, plasma aldosterone, and plasma volume in three groups: five nephrotic patients with 'minimal change' disease on renal biopsy; seven nephrotic patients with other renal histopathology; and eight patients having glomerulonephritis but with no past or present nephrosis.

Plasma volume was found to be similar in all three groups. However, both PRC and aldosterone were significantly higher in the nephrotic subjects with minimal change on biopsy, compared with the two groups with other histopathology.

These authors concluded that high PRC and aldosterone are, in the nephrotic syndrome, markers for 'minimal change' disease.

THE RENIN SYSTEM AND EXACERBATIONS OF SODIUM RETENTION

Brown and her colleagues have made a detailed series of investigations into the involvement of the RAS in exacerbations and remissions of the disease. They first studied patients on controlled sodium intake while retaining sodium and gaining weight [41,42]. Approximately 50% of the subjects had elevated PRA, with high plasma aldosterone values; blood volume was less than the predicted normal value. In the remainder, PRA and aldosterone were normal or low, and blood volume tended to be expanded. There was a significant inverse correlation between PRA and plasma albumin level. Thus, these investigators found that the RAS is not stimulated in many patients during spontaneous sodium retention, and they proposed that there is an overriding mechanism causing sodium retention which is largely independent of the RAS and blood volume; this mechanism might be related to the underlying renal process and was considered probably to be intrarenal. Stimulation of the RAS in some patients was thought possibly to be compensatory to reduced plasma albumin and contracted blood volume.

Kutyrina et al [43] confirmed that PRA did not correlate with the degree of sodium retention.

Brown et al [44] proceeded to studies during steroid-induced remission. At the onset of natriuresis, blood volume and plasma albumin were low and did not change; PRA and aldosterone were initially high and fell during the natriuresis. After natriuresis, when patients had lost their edema, PRA and aldosterone rose to high values, while plasma albumin and blood volume remained low, although sodium was no longer being retained and sodium balance was restored. It was proposed that the natriuresis of remission is due to correction of an intrarenal abnormality causing sodium retention.

These workers performed a trial of oral captopril during 10 separate episodes of sodium retention in the nephrotic syndrome, in seven of which the RAS showed enhanced activity [45]. Despite a marked fall in plasma aldosterone with captopril, all

patients continued to retain sodium and water and to gain weight (Fig. 58.3). These results provided further evidence of the independence of sodium retention in this disease from stimulation of the RAS.

EXPERIMENTAL NEPHROTIC SYNDROME IN RATS

Many of the clinical data have been supported by studies in rats in which nephrotic syndrome has been induced by the administration of puromycin aminonucleoside [46–48]. Nephrotic rats developed proteinuria, hypoproteinemia, edema, ascites, hypercholesterolemia, and hypertriglyceridemia. Plasma renin concentration, PRA, aldosterone, and serum ACE activity increased with the onset of disease, while plasma angiotensinogen fell. The temporal evolution of these various changes did not indicate that the sodium retention was a consequence of proteinuria or of hypoproteinemia, or that it was due to increases in plasma renin; as in the clinical studies of Brown and her colleagues [41,42,44], the renal lesion *per se* was invoked as the cause.

In the rats, as in man, administration of captopril, while increasing PRC and lowering aldosterone, had no beneficial effect on the course of the disease. Indeed, mortality was higher (37%) in nephrotic rats given captopril than in untreated nephrotic rats (13%) [48]. These experiments thus further support the contention that sodium retention in the disease can be largely independent of the prominence of the RAS.

RENIN AND VASOPRESSIN IN THE NEPHROTIC SYNDROME

Schrier and Howard [49] have implicated nonosmotic stimulation of secretion of vasopressin in the water retention of various clinical disorders, including the nephrotic syndrome. Activation of the sympathetic nervous system and the RAS have been invoked in this connection. It is probable that in some patients, at certain stages of the disease, peripheral plasma Ang II concentrations could be sufficiently raised [38] to stimulate secretion of vasopressin [50] (see *Chapter 35*). Such increases in vasopressin might then contribute to the disorder. However, the evidence summarized earlier suggests that this is unlikely to be a necessary or consistent component of the nephrotic syndrome.

RENIN AND ATRIAL NATRIURETIC FACTOR IN THE NEPHROTIC SYNDROME

Pedersen et al [51] assayed plasma atrial natriuretic factor (ANF), Ang II, and aldosterone during basal conditions in 17 patients with the nephrotic syndrome and in 20 control subjects. Additionally, six of the patients were studied after seven remissions.

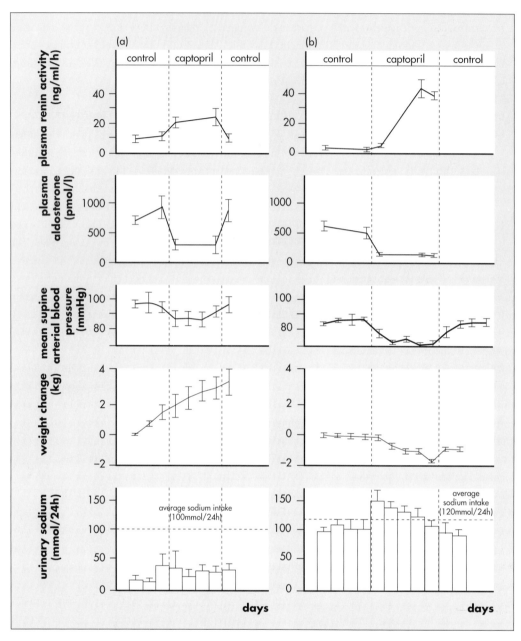

Fig. 58.3 Contrasting effects of captopril on sodium excretion, blood pressure, plasma renin activity and plasma aldosterone in patients with nephrotic syndrome (n=6) (a) who were spontaneously retaining sodium, and in normal subjects (n=8) (b). Modified from Brown EA et al [42].

While Ang II and aldosterone values were similar in the patients and controls, plasma ANF was significantly higher in the patients. Following remission, plasma ANF was significantly lower than before, whereas Ang II and aldosterone were unchanged. Atrial natriuretic factor values were not correlated with either Ang II or aldosterone.

The elevated ANF in nephrotic syndrome is therefore independent of the RAS and seems to represent a response to retention of sodium and water.

RENIN AND KALLIKREIN IN THE NEPHROTIC SYNDROME

Cumming et al [52] observed that virtually all patients with nephrotic syndrome excrete supranormal amounts of urinary kallikrein. They studied the relationship between urinary kallikrein output and PRA in 16 subjects with the disease. Plasma renin activity was high in eight and normal in eight of these. Urinary kallikrein was elevated in both groups, but significantly more so in those with increased PRA.

Class	Description
I	no abnormal proteinuria prior to therapy.
	discontinuation of drug associated with resolution of proteinuria
	no relapse of proteinuria unless therapy is repeated
II	no abnormal proteinuria prior to therapy
	resolution of proteinuria occurs despite continuation of drug
III	abnormal proteinuria documented prior to therapy
	proteinuria worsens with therapy and returns to baseline when drug discontinued
IV	administration of the drug associated with increased urine protein excretion
	discontinuation of drug associated with resolution of proteinuria
	one or more relapses of proteinuria is later documented in absence of therapy
V	onset of proteinuria documented during a therapeutic trial
	however, patient is receiving placebo and not drug being tested

Fig. 58.4 Classification of drug-associated membranous glomerulonephritis. Modified from Lewis EJ [58].

Cumming *et al* [52] interpreted these results as being consistent with a functional link between the RAS and the renal kallikrein–kinin system (see *Chapter 38*), but as indicative also of activation of the kallikrein–kinin system in some nephrotic patients independently of the RAS.

NEPHROTIC SYNDROME DUE TO CAPTOPRIL THERAPY

In the early days of clinical use of the ACE inhibitor captopril, doses up to 450mg daily, and sometimes higher, were employed. At these doses, proteinuria was reported in a proportion of cases [53]. Heel *et al* [54] estimated in 1980 that proteinuria occurred in 2% of patients given captopril for 18 months or more. Since captopril contains a sulfhydryl group, and since penicillamine, which also possesses a sulfhydryl group, has been shown similarly to cause proteinuria [55,56], this chemical moiety was suspected of being responsible for the complication with both drugs

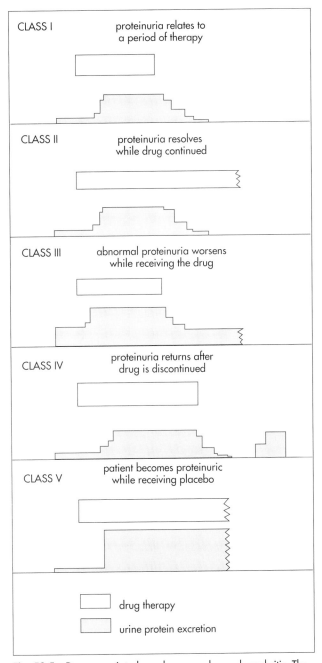

Fig. 58.5 Drug-associated membranous glomerulonephritis. The definition of patients entering into each class is given in Fig. 58.4. The likelihood of a drug causing the glomerular lesion is greatest in class I, and of diminishing probability in class II and class III. Patients entered into class IV appear likely to have a drug-associated lesion. These patients more probably are exhibiting a relapsing course of idiopathic membranous glomerulopathy. The existence of class V underscores the observation that proteinuria and membranous glomerulonephritis exist in the hypertensive population and can be unrelated to drug therapy. Modified from Lewis EJ [58].

[57,58]. Like penicillamine, captopril has been implicated as inducing IgA deficiency [59].

In 1979, Prins *et al* [60] reported the appearance of nephrotic syndrome, with proteinuria of 5g/24h, in a patient taking captopril 50mg three times daily. Renal biopsy showed evidence of membranous glomerulopathy. Several reports of nephrotic syndrome with captopril use followed [61–64]; the early incidence was 7 of 34 patients when captopril was introduced with pre-existent proteinuria [54]. Membranous glomerulopathy was detected in a number of captopril-treated patients undergoing renal biopsy [53,61,62,65,66] but not in all [67].

While the data were strongly suggestive of a causal relationship of captopril therapy with nephrotic syndrome, unimpeachable evidence of such was found in only approximately half of the cases [65]. More detailed evaluation revealed that many of the glomerular abnormalities attributed to captopril were already present in the hypertensive population irrespective of the administration of a particular drug [57,58,68]. It has been emphasized that drug-associated proteinuria requires to be critically evaluated in relation to drug intake and the stage of the disease before a causal involvement is established (Figs. 58.4 and 58.5). Lewis [58] has stated that, nevertheless, in 7 of a series of 17 cases, captopril was likely to be the cause.

Webb and Atkinson [64] reported on a 40-year-old woman with a 10-year history of hypertension and with urine protein excretion in the range 0.6–1.5g/24h. Due to poor blood-pressure control on a combination of furosemide, labetalol, and hydralazine, treatment was altered to captopril 450mg daily with furosemide 80mg daily. Although blood pressure became well-controlled, she developed nephrotic syndrome, with edema, hypoalbuminuria, and protein excretion of 7–18g/24h. There was no evidence of renal arterial disease, and renal venography was also normal. The regimen was changed to enalapril 20mg daily with furosemide 500mg daily plus atenolol 100mg daily. Over the next 20 months, blood pressure remained well controlled and urinary protein output fell to around 1g daily. This case is thus strongly suggestive of a causal relationship of nephrotic syndrome with captopril, not seen with an alternative nonsulfhydryl-containing ACE inhibitor.

Despite its interest, nephrotic syndrome due to captopril is now of negligible clinical importance. All the reported cases received high or very high doses of the drug, and such dosage is no longer extant [57,58]. Moreover, captopril-induced nephrotic syndrome has seldom led to irreversible deterioration in renal function [57].

REFERENCES

1. Berlyne GM, Tavill AS, Baker SB de C. Renal artery stenosis and the nephrotic syndrome. *Quarterly Journal of Medicine* 1964;33:325–35.

2. Kumar A, Shapiro AP. Proteinuria and nephrotic syndrome induced by renin in patients with renal artery stenosis. *Archives of Internal Medicine* 1980;140:1631–4.

3. Eiser AR, Katz SM, Swartz C. Reversible nephrotic range proteinuria with renal artery stenosis: A clinical example of renin-associated proteinuria. *Nephron* 1982;30:374–7.

4. Gephardt GN, Tubbs RR, Novick AC, McMahon JT, Pohl MA. Renal artery stenosis, nephrotic-range proteinuria, and focal and segmental renal artery stenosis. *Cleveland Clinic Quarterly* 1984;51:371–6.

5. Takeda R, Morimoto S, Uchida K, Kigoshi T, Sumitani T, Matsubare F. Effects of captopril on both hypertension and proteinuria: Report of a case of renovascular hypertension associated with nephrotic syndrome. *Archives of Internal Medicine* 1980;140:1531–3.

6. Holman ND, Donker AJ, Van Der Meer J. Disappearance of renin-induced proteinuria by treatment with an ACE inhibitor: A case report. *Clinical Nephrology* 1990;34:70–1.

7. Baruch D, Corvol P, Alhenc-Gelas F, Dufloux MA, Guyenne TT, Gaux JD, Raymond A, Brisset JM, Duclos JM, Menard J. Diagnosis and treatment of renin secreting tumors. Report of three cases. *Hypertension* 1984;6:760–6.

8. Bock KD, Brown JJ, Lever AF, Robertson JIS. Effects of renin and angiotensin on excretion and distribution of water and salts. In: Page IH, McCubbin JW, eds. *Renal hypertension*. Chicago: Year Book Medical Publishers, 1968:184–203.

9. Pickering GW, Prinzmetal M. The effect of renin on urine formation. *Journal of Physiology* 1940;98:314–35.

10. Schales O, Hoobler SW, Haynes FW. Cardiovascular effects of renin. *Proceedings of the Society for Experimental Biology and Medicine* 1941;48:720–3.

11. Brandt JL, Gruhn JG. Effect of renin on proteinuria and PAH clearance at low plasma levels. *American Journal of Physiology* 1948;153:458–64.

12. Hughes-Jones NC, Pickering GW, Sanderson PH, Scarborough H, Vandenbroucke J. The nature of the action of renin and hypertensin on renal function in the rabbit. *Journal of Physiology* 1949;109:288–307.

13. Rosenfeld S, Sellers AL, Marmorston J, Eliasch H. Effect of renin on renal function. *American Journal of Physiology* 1954;179:177–80.

14. Addis T, Barrett E, Boyd RL, Ureen HJ. Renin proteinuria in the rat. *Journal of Experimental Medicine* 1949;89:131–40.

15. Addis T, Marmorston J, Goodman HC, Sellers AL, Smith M. Effect of adrenalectomy on spontaneous and induced proteinuria in the rat. *Proceedings of the Society for Experimental Biology and Medicine* 1950;74:43–6.

16. Masson GMC, Corcoran AC, Page IH. Some effects of chronic treatment of rats with renin. *American Journal of Physiology* 1950;162:379–84.

17. Sellers AL, Smith S, Marmorston J, Goodman HC. Studies on the mechanism of experimental proteinuria. *Journal of Experimental Medicine* 1952;96:643–51.

18. Coye RD, Maude DL, Dibble RF, Yuile CL. Experimental proteinuria: An electrophoretic study of three different types in dogs. *Archives of Pathology* 1955;60:548–55.

19. Rosenfeld S, Kraus R, McCullen A. Effect of renin, ischemia, and plasma protein loading on the isolated perfused kidney. *American Journal of Physiology* 1965;209:835–43.

20. Sellers AL, Roberts S, Rask I, Smith S, Marmorston J, Goodman HC. An electrophoretic study of urinary protein in the rat. *Journal of Experimental Medicine* 1952;95:465–72.

21. Lippman RW, Ureen HJ, Oliver J. Mechanism of proteinuria. IV. Effect of renin on hemoglobin excretion. *Journal of Experimental Medicine* 1951;**93**:605–13.

22. Paldino RL, Hyman C. Mechanism whereby renin increases the rate of T-1824 disappearance from the circulation of rabbits. *American Journal of Physiology* 1954;**179**:599–600.

23. Sellers AL, Marmorston J. Mechanism of renin proteinuria. *American Journal of Physiology* 1955;**183**:299-301.

24. Lewis LA, Masson GMC, Corcoran AC, Page IH. Effects of renin on serum and urinary proteins in desoxycorticosterone or cortisone-treated rats. *American Journal of Physiology* 1955;**180**:331–6.

25. Croxatto L, Barnafi L, Passi J. Effect of renin on diuresis in rats. *Science* 1952;**116**:507–10.

26. Masson GMC, Del Greco F, Corcoran AC, Page IH. Factors influencing renin diuresis and proteinuria. *Proceedings of the Society for Experimental Biology and Medicine* 1953;**83**:631–6.

27. Deodhar SD, Cuppage FE, Gableman E. Studies of the mechanism of experimental proteinuria induced by renin. *Journal of Experimental Medicine* 1964;**120**:677–90.

28. Pessina AC, Hulme B, Peart WS. Renin induced proteinuria and the effects of adrenalectomy II. Morphology in relation to function. *Proceedings of the Royal Society of London, Series B: Biological Sciences* 1972;**180**:61–71.

29. Bock KD, Krecke HJ. Synthetisches hypertensin II auf die PAH- und inulin-clearance. *Klinische Wochenschrift* 1958;**36**:69–74.

30. Bock KD, Krecke HJ, Kuhn HM. Wirkung von synthetischem hypertensin II. *Klinische Wochenschrift* 1958;**36**:254–61.

31. Masson GMC, Corcoran AC, Page IH. Renal and vascular lesions elicited by renin in rats with desoxycorticosterone hypertension. *Archives of Pathology* 1952;**53**:217–25.

32. Bock KD. *Angiotensin: Pharmakologie und klinische anwendung.* Heidelberg: Huttig, 1966.

33. Giese J. Renin, angiotensin and hypertensive vascular damage: A review. In: Laragh JH, ed. *Hypertension manual.* New York: Dun-Donnelly, 1973:371–403.

34. Myers BD, Deen WM, Brenner BM. Effects of norepinephrine and angiotensin II on the determinants of glomerular ultrafiltration and proximal tubule reabsorption in the rat. *Circulation Research* 1975;**37**:101–10.

35. Blantz RC, Konnen KS, Tucker BJ. Angiotensin II effects upon the glomerular microcirculation and ultrafiltration coefficient in the rat. *Journal of Clinical Investigation* 1976;**57**:419–34.

36. Steinhausen M, Sterzel RB, Fleming JT, Kühn R, Weis S. Acute and chronic effects of angiotensin II on the vessels of the split hydronephrotic kidney. *Kidney International* 1987;**31** (suppl. 20):64–73.

37. Fisher ER, Masson GMC. Renal lesions in renin proteinuria. *Archives of Pathology* 1961;**71**:480–4.

38. Medina A, Davies DL, Brown JJ, Fraser R, Lever AF, Mallick NP, Morton JJ, Robertson JIS, Tree M. A study of the renin–angiotensin system in the nephrotic syndrome. *Nephron* 1974;**12**:233-40.

39. Boer P, Roos JC, Dorhout-Mees ET. Observations on plasma renin substrate in the nephrotic syndrome. *Nephron* 1980;**26**:121–5.

40. Hammond TG, Whitworth JA, Saines D, Thatcher R, Andrews J, Kincaid-Smith P. Renin–angiotensin–aldosterone system in nephrotic syndrome. *American Journal of Kidney Diseases* 1984;**4**:18–23.

41. Brown EA, Markandu ND, Roulston JE, Jones BE, Squires M, MacGregor GA. Is the renin–angiotensin system involved in the sodium retention in the nephrotic syndrome? *Nephron* 1982;**32**:102–7.

42. Brown EA, Markandu ND, Sagnella GA, Squires M, Jones BE, MacGregor GA. Evidence that some mechanism other than the renin system causes sodium retention in nephrotic syndrome. *Lancet* 1982;**ii**:1237–40.

43. Kutyrina IM, Klepikov PV, Tareeva IE. O roli renin–angiotenzinovoi sistemy v patogeneze nefroticheskogo sindroma. *Terapevticheskii Arkhiv* 1988;**60**:32–4.

44. Brown EA, Markandu N, Sagnella GA, Jones BE, MacGregor GA. Sodium retention in nephrotic syndrome is due to an intrarenal defect: Evidence from steroid-induced remission. *Nephron* 1985;**39**:290–5.

45. Brown EA, Markandu ND, Sagnella GA, Jones BE, MacGregor GA. Lack of effect of captopril on the sodium retention of the nephrotic syndrome. *Nephron* 1984;**37**:43–8.

46. Pedraza-Chaverri J, Cruz C, Ibarra-Rubio ME, Chavez MT, Calleja C, Tapia E, del-Carmen-Uribe M, Romero L, Pena JC. Pathophysiology of experimental nephrotic syndrome induced by puromycin aminonucleoside in rats. I. The role of proteinuria, hypoproteinemia and the renin–angiotensin–aldosterone system on sodium retention. *Revista de Investigacion Clinica* 1990;**42**:29–38.

47. Pedraza-Chaverri J, Cruz C, Chavez MT, Lopez A, Ibarra-Rubio ME, Tapia E, Pena JC. Pathophysiology of experimental nephrotic syndrome induced by puromycin aminonucleoside in rats. II. *In vitro* release of renin, angiotensinogen, and aldosterone. *Revista de Investigacion Clinica* 1990;**42**:120–6.

48. Pedraza-Chaverri J, Cruz C, Chavez MT, Ibarra-Rubio ME, Tapia E, Pena JC. Pathophysiology of experimental nephrotic syndrome induced by puromycin aminonucleoside in rats. III. Effects of captopril, an angiotensin converting enzyme inhibitor, on proteinuria and sodium retention. *Revista de Investigacion Clinica* 1990;**42**:210–6 .

49. Schrier RW, Howard RL. Pathophysiology of vasopressin in edematous disorders. *Nippon Naibunpi Gakkai Zasshi. Folia Endocrinologica Japonica* 1989;**65**:1311–27.

50. Padfield PL, Morton JJ. Effects of angiotensin II on arginine-vasopressin in physiological and pathological situations in man. *Journal of Endocrinology* 1977;**74**:251–9.

51. Pedersen EB, Danielsen H, Eiskjaer H, Jespersen B, Sorensen SS. Increased atrial natriuretic peptide in the nephrotic syndrome: relationship to renal function and the renin–angiotensin–aldosterone system. *Scandinavian Journal of Clinical and Laboratory Investigation* 1988;**48**:141–7.

52. Cumming AD, Jeffrey S, Lambie AT, Robson JS. The kallikrein–kinin and renin–angiotensin systems in nephrotic syndrome. *Nephron* 1989;**51**:185–91.

53. Case DB, Atlas SA, Mouradian JA, Fishman RA, Sherman RL, Laragh JH. Proteinuria during long-term captopril therapy. *Journal of the American Medical Association* 1980;**244**:346–9.

54. Heel RC, Brogden RN, Speight TM, Avery GS. Captopril: A preliminary review of its pharmacological properties and therapeutic efficacy. *Drugs* 1980;**20**:409–52.

55. Bacon PA, Tribe CR, MacKenzie JC, Verrier JJ, Cumming RN, Amer B. Penicillamine nephropathy in rheumatoid arthritis: A clinical pathological and immunological study. *Quarterly Journal of Medicine* 1976;**45**:661–84.

56. Jaffe IA, Treser G, Suzuki Y, Ehrenech T. Nephropathy induced by d-penicillamine. *Annals of Internal Medicine* 1968;**69**:549–56.

57. Donker AJM. Nephrotoxicity of angiotensin converting enzyme inhibition. *Kidney International* 1987;**31** (suppl. 20) :132–7.

58. Lewis EJ. Glomerular abnormalities in patients receiving angiotensin converting enzyme inhibitor therapy. *Kidney International* 1987;**31** (suppl. 20):138–42.

59. Hammarström L, Smith CIE, Berg U. Captopril-induced IgA deficiency. *Lancet* 1991;**337**:436.

60. Prins EJL, Hoorntje SJ, Weening JJ, Donker AJM. Nephrotic syndrome in patient on captopril. *Lancet* 1979 ;**ii**:306–7.

61. Textor SC, Gephardt GN, Bravo EL, Tarazi RC, Fouad FM, Tubbs R, McMahon JT. Membranous glomerulopathy associated with captopril therapy. *American Journal of Medicine* 1983;**74**:705–12.

62. Rosendorff C, Milne FJ, Levy H, Ninin DT, Lewin JR. Nephrotic syndrome during captopril therapy. *South African Medical Journal* 1980;**58**:172–3.

63. Seedat YK. Nephrotic syndrome from captopril. *South African Medical Journal* 1980;**57**:390.

64. Webb DJ, Atkinson AB. Enalapril following captopril-induced nephrotic syndrome. *Scottish Medical Journal* 1986;**31**:30–2.

65. Hoorntje SJ, Weening JJ, The TH, Kallenberg CGM, Donker AJM, Hoedemaeker PH. Immune-complex glomerulopathy in patients treated with captopril. *Lancet* 1980;**i**:1212–5.

66. Smith AJ, Hoorntje SJ, Weening JJ, Donker AJM, Hoedemaeker PJ. Unilateral membranous glomerulopathy during captopril therapy. *Netherlands Journal of Medicine* 1985;**28**:23–7.

67. Kincaid-Smith P, Whitworth JA, Walter NMA, Dowling JP. Immune complex glomerulopathy and captopril. *Lancet* 1980;**ii**:37.

68. Captopril Collaborative Study Group. Does captopril cause renal damage in hypertensive patients? *Lancet* 1982;**i**:988–90 .

59

RENIN AND AORTIC COARCTATION

J IAN S ROBERTSON

INTRODUCTION

Coarctation of the aorta results from an abnormality of embryological development of the aortic arch system, such that there persists a structural narrowing of the aorta, usually in its descending intrathoracic course [1]. An extensive collateral arterial system develops so as to circumvent the coarctation and thus to supply blood to the lower part of the body. Hypertension, readily detected in the upper limbs, is a characteristic feature; although the malignant phase (*Chapter 60*) is very rare, it has been reported [2].

Transient exacerbation of hypertension (so-called 'paradoxical' hypertension) can also occur immediately following surgical reconstruction of the coarctation. Closely related to paradoxical hypertension are the gastrointestinal symptoms of so-called postcoarctectomy syndrome (mesenteric arteritis), which occurs in 2–28% of patients after coarctation repair [3,4]. Since this syndrome is almost always accompanied by paradoxical hypertension, it is considered by several investigators that the pathogenesis of both entities may be the same [4]. Typically, the onset of abdominal symptoms occurs on approximately the third postoperative day and is characterized by abdominal pain and tenderness, ileus, vomiting, fever, melena, leukocytosis, and paradoxical hypertension. Progressive bowel necrosis and death can occur. It has been proposed that the change to a more pulsatile blood flow after repair of the coarctation leads to increased mesenteric intra-arterial wall tension, resulting in intimal damage and thrombosis and in secondary necrotizing arteritis [5]. The mesenteric arteries may, it is suggested, be more susceptible to these changes because of the lack of surrounding supporting tissue and their fragility resulting from their previous exposure to subnormal pulse pressure before coarctation repair [3]. The arterial histopathology in this syndrome (see Color Plate 21) is very similar, if not identical, to that of malignant-phase hypertension. As is discussed in more detail in *Chapters 40* and *60*, exposure to severe, and especially sudden, arterial hypertension, is probably the main pathogenic influence causing

malignant hypertension. However, superadded high plasma renin, and hence Ang II, possibly exacerbate its onset.

In common with most forms of secondary hypertension [6], arterial pressure, although often corrected, can remain above normal following operative reconstruction [7] (Fig. 59.1).

The possible involvement of the RAS will be considered in these clinical circumstances. Several animal models, intended to mimic genuine embryological aortic coarctation, have been developed. Although these are of uncertain relevance to the clinical disease, they will also be considered briefly in this chapter in relation to the RAS.

RENIN AND PATHOGENESIS OF THE HYPERTENSION BEFORE AORTIC RECONSTRUCTION

EVIDENCE OF INVOLVEMENT OF THE RENIN–ANGIOTENSIN SYSTEM

In a very early study, Morris *et al* [8] found Ang II to be detectable in arterial blood of nine patients with aortic coarctation. In

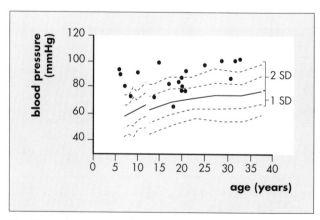

Fig. 59.1 The average values for diastolic pressure after repair of aortic coarctation, related to the values found in a sample of the general population. Values are postoperative mean diastolic pressures. Readings of arterial pressure obtained in the first month after operation have been excluded. Modified from Counihan TB [7].

this respect, the patients with coarctation resembled hypertensive patients with renal ischemia. By contrast, Ang II was not detectable by their methodology in arterial blood of patients with essential hypertension.

Pickens [9] assayed plasma renin activity (PRA) in peripheral venous blood in a youth with aortic coarctation, before and after operation; plasma samples were also obtained after a fall in arterial pressure induced by intravenous nitroprusside. Before operation PRA appeared inappropriately high when related to pressure in the arm, but appropriate to the pressure distal to the coarctation. PRA fell after surgical repair (Fig. 59.2).

Van Way et al [10] assayed PRA in four patients with aortic coarctation, supine, standing, and during and after treadmill exercise. The PRA increase was enhanced in response to posture and exercise in three of the four patients, as compared with that after correction of the coarctation. The authors, like Pickens [9], interpreted their data cautiously, concluding that, despite the apparent hyperactivity of the RAS, this was not the primary cause of the hypertension.

Ribeiro and Krakoff [11] observed that two patients with coarctation showed a significant decrease in blood pressure, accompanied by a hyperactive increase in PRA, in response to the Ang II antagonist saralasin, as compared with 10 subjects with essential hypertension. They concluded that their results constituted direct evidence of the participation of the RAS in the pathogenesis of hypertension with coarctation of the aorta.

Lardoux et al [12] made a detailed study of the RAS in seven hypertensive patients with pure isthmic coarctation of the aorta. Plasma volume was also measured, and the pressure drop across the site of coarctation was assessed by intra-aortic catheter. Plasma volume was found to be expanded in five of these seven patients. While on normal sodium intake, and standing, PRA was raised in five patients and normal in two. Following moderate salt depletion, administration of the Ang II antagonist saralasin caused, overall, a significant fall in blood pressure, with an accompanying rise in PRA; two patients did not show a drop in blood pressure with saralasin. The cardioselective β-blocker acebutolol, given during normal sodium intake, had a modest antihypertensive effect, while also lowering PRA; there was no significant correlation between the blood-pressure fall and the fall in PRA with acebutolol. No correlations could be seen, moreover, between the various measurements of PRA, plasma volume, and either the systolic or diastolic gradient in pressure across the coarctation. The authors did not find interpretation of their results to be easy. However, the responsiveness of the arterial pressure under the conditions of testing to saralasin, coupled with the increase in plasma volume, led them to liken

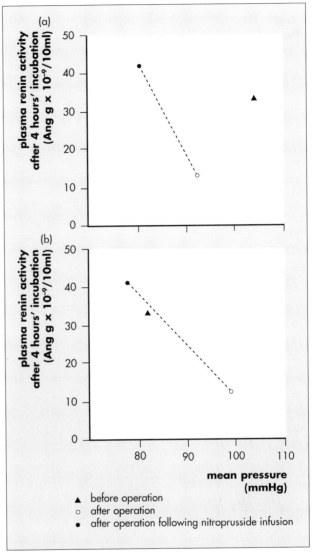

Fig. 59.2 Relation of plasma renin activity to mean pressure in the arm (a) and in the leg (b) before operation, after operation, and after operation following nitroprusside infusion. Modified from Pickens PT [9].

pathogenesis to that seen in Goldblatt 1-kidney, 1-clip experimental hypertension (see *Chapter 55*), in which the pressor effect of the RAS is apparently enhanced by concurrent volume expansion.

Alpert et al [13] reached rather similar conclusions to those of Lardoux et al [12]. Twenty hypertensive patients with coarctation of the aorta were studied during normal and low sodium intake and after diuresis with furosemide. Eight patients with essential hypertension and 13 control subjects were similarly studied. Plasma renin activity values in patients with coarctation were similar to those in patients with essential hypertension and in controls during normal and low sodium diets. However, after the administration of furosemide, PRA values were significantly higher in the patients with coarctation than in the other two groups. The values for urinary aldosterone, plasma volume, and extracellular fluid volume were increased in patients with coarctation during both normal and low sodium intake. These renin and aldosterone responses, and the expanded body fluid spaces in patients with coarctation, suggested to these authors also that the hypertension resembles that in 1-kidney, 1-clip experimental renal hypertension.

Parker *et al* [14] measured PRA in eight children before and again 32-51 months after surgical correction of aortic coarctation, on each occasion while the patients were taking a low salt diet together with a diuretic. Mean PRA was four-fold lower after operation, a finding that was interpreted by these authors as indicating possibly relevant enhanced activity of the RAS in coarctation.

These same investigators [15] further compared the effect of the Ang II antagonist saralasin in a group of patients with aortic coarctation before operation with that in normal subjects. Both groups were studied after salt restriction and diuresis. Saralasin lowered blood pressure acutely to a more marked extent in the patients with coarctation. This again was interpreted as indicating excessive activity of the RAS in coarctation.

Warren *et al* [16] made a detailed investigation of the responses of the RAS to high and low sodium intake, to orthostasis, and to saralasin infusion, before and after surgical correction of aortic coarctation in a 27-year-old man. Before operation, PRA levels were high and responded sluggishly, severally to changes in dietary sodium, to standing, and to infusion of saralasin. The heart-rate responses to the Valsalva maneuver and to standing were also abnormal before operation. After operation, the renin responsiveness and cardiovascular reflexes returned to normal. The authors interpreted these data cautiously as indicating a high level of sympathetic activity in aortic coarctation and as demonstrating the importance of factors other than the RAS in the pathogenesis of hypertension.

Fallo *et al* [17] compared data obtained in eight patients with hypertension and coarctation of the aorta with those in 14 patients with essential hypertension, before, and again 90 minutes after, a single oral dose of 25mg captopril. There were no significant differences in mean arterial pressure, PRA, or plasma aldosterone concentration between the two groups under baseline conditions. After captopril administration, blood pressure and plasma aldosterone concentration fell distinctly in both groups, while PRA, which remained unchanged in those with

essential hypertension, increased markedly in those with aortic coarctation. The findings were interpreted as supporting the view that in coarctation, the systemic hypertension is mediated in part via the RAS.

In a further study, Fallo *et al* [18] treated two patients with aortic coarctation with captopril for 12 weeks, using increasing doses. After an early fall in aterial pressure, hypertension returned and was accompanied by restoration of plasma aldosterone to elevated levels similar to those seen before treatment (Fig. 59.3). This loss of control of hypertension was thought to be due to the appearance of secondary mechanisms leading to excessive secretion of renin.

Pelech *et al* [19] studied the responses to exercise in 15 children with aortic coarctation before, and at intervals up to six months after, surgical repair. Exercise PRA was elevated before

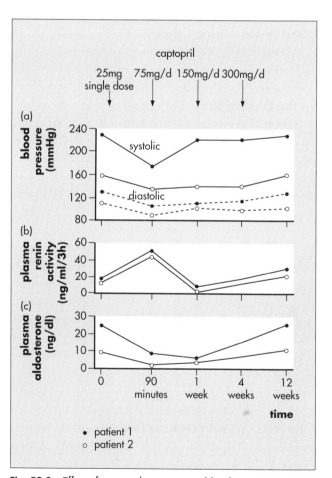

Fig. 59.3 Effect of captopril treatment on blood pressure (a), plasma renin activity (b), and plasma aldosterone (c) in two patients with coarctation of the aorta. Modified from Fallo F *et al* [18].

operation but was normal after surgery. No significant difference in plasma catecholamines at rest or on exercise was seen before and after surgery. Preoperatively, 11 children had systolic hypertension at rest and 12 after exercise. Following operation, only one child had mild systolic hypertension at rest, although exercise-induced hypertension persisted in five.

The various suggestions from the studies summarized above were interpreted, albeit often in muted fashion, as providing support for a contribution of the RAS to the pathogenesis of hypertension in coarctation.

EVIDENCE AGAINST INVOLVEMENT OF THE RENIN–ANGIOTENSIN SYSTEM

Brown *et al* [20] found peripheral venous plasma renin concentration (PRC) in four patients with hypertension and coarctation of the aorta to be in the normal range (Fig. 59.4). A further estimation made in one of these patients four months after surgical correction of the lesion, with consequent reduction of the arterial pressure, showed no marked change.

Amsterdam *et al* [21] studied peripheral venous PRA in 16 children aged 2–13 years with aortic coarctation, and in 11 normal children. There was no significant difference in PRA between the two groups (Fig. 59.5).

Werning *et al* [22] made a study of 10 patients with coarctation of the aorta. Plasma renin activity was measured after recumbency and orthostasis, in peripheral venous blood and, in some cases, in renal venous blood also. In nine of these patients, basal plasma renin values and those obtained under

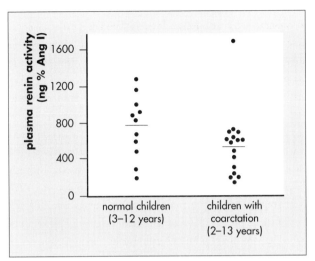

Fig. 59.5 The values for peripheral plasma renin activity in children with coarctation of the aorta, contrasted with the values in a group of control children (all subjects in a fasting state and supine position). The difference between the mean plasma renin value in the children with coarctation and that for the corresponding control subjects is not significant. Modified from Amsterdam EA *et al* [21].

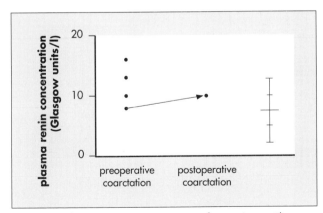

Fig. 59.4 Plasma renin concentrations in four patients with coarctation of the aorta. In one patient, a further estimation is shown which was made four months after surgical correction of the coarctation and relief of hypertension. The normal mean ± 1 and ± 2 SD is indicated. Modified from Brown JJ *et al* [20].

stimulatory conditions lay within the normal range, and only in one patient were the values elevated. However, since this patient displayed the smallest gradient of mean arterial blood pressure across the stenosis, it was regarded as improbable that the elevation in PRA was caused by the coarctation. Plasma renin activity in the renal venous blood of both kidneys, which was measured in three patients, showed no elevation. These investigators concluded that the RAS was not important in the pathogenesis of hypertension in aortic coarctation.

Rocchini *et al* [23] found no difference in peripheral venous PRA between seven children with coarctation of the aorta and a group of five acyanotic children undergoing elective cardiac surgery.

Similar findings and conclusions were reported by Strong *et al* [24]. Fifteen patients (aged 4–21 years) with coarctation of the aorta were studied. In 10, both peripheral and renal vein PRA were measured. Twelve patients were operated upon and peripheral PRA was measured preoperatively and during the acute (postoperative day 0–10) and long-term (mean 112 days) postoperative period. Three patients who were deprived of sodium showed borderline to moderately elevated peripheral and renal vein PRA, suggesting that the renin secretory apparatus responded to appropriate stimulation. The peripheral PRA was within the range of normal both preoperatively and longterm postoperatively. During the acute postoperative period, each patient had a transient elevation of peripheral PRA. There was no correlation between peripheral PRA and blood-pressure levels in the postoperative period. It was concluded that the RAS does not play a significant role in maintaining the chronic hypertension that is associated with coarctation of the aorta.

Markiewicz *et al* [25] measured PRA in 11 cases of coarctation of the aorta before and after operation. The values of PRA in the recumbent position before operation were significantly lower than in the control group (Fig. 59.6). After surgery, PRA rose to normal levels. There was no correlation between PRA and arterial blood pressure. It was concluded that the RAS seems not to participate directly in the maintenance of hypertension in patients with aortic coarctation.

Involvement of the RAS in the pathogenesis of hypertension in aortic coarctation was also not supported by the paper of Sehested *et al* [26]. These workers investigated a group of 12 patients having an average age of 21 years with uncomplicated aortic coarctation, before, and a mean of 204 days after, surgery. Following operation, both resting and exercise upper limb blood

pressures were lowered, although 6 of the 11 patients still had abnormally high blood pressures on exercise as compared with a normal control group of six people. No significant differences in plasma aldosterone, catecholamines, or PRA were seen before and after operation, or between the patients and the control subjects. Sehested *et al* [26] concluded that the RAS does not have a major role in the pathogenesis of hypertension in coarctation of the aorta.

RENIN AND TRANSIENT ('PARADOXICAL') HYPERTENSION FOLLOWING REPAIR OF COARCTATION

Rocchini *et al* [23] studied the course and pathogenesis of paradoxical hypertension in seven hypertensive children undergoing repair of aortic coarctation. A comparison was made with five normotensive 'control' children undergoing elective cardiovascular surgery. Peripheral venous PRA levels before operation did not differ between the groups. During the first 24 hours after

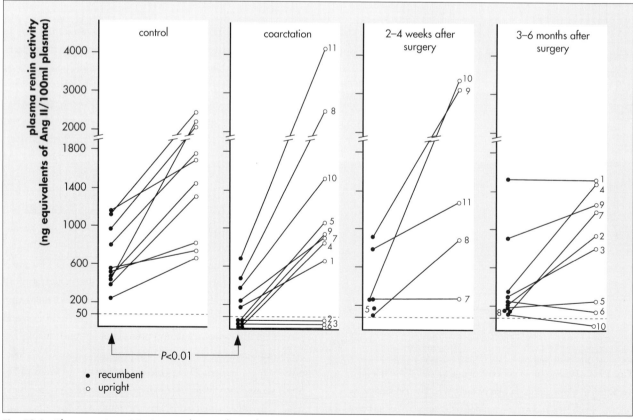

Fig. 59.6 Plasma renin activity in recumbent and upright positions in a series of 11 patients with coarctation before and at intervals after surgery, and in 10 control subjects. The numerals denote individual patients. Modified from Markiewicz A *et al* [25].

59.5

surgery, all coarctation patients demonstrated a rise in systolic blood pressure (35 ± 15.5mmHg; $P<0.001$), a significant depression in cold pressor test response, and only a slight elevation in PRA (Figs. 59.7 and 59.8). In the next 24–72 hours, coarctation patients developed a rise in diastolic blood pressure (26.8 ± 10.6mmHg: $P<0.0001$) and PRA (22.9 ± 10.2/ml/h; $P<0.001$), and fluid retention. By contrast, control patients had no significant postoperative changes. Abdominal pain occurred in five coarctation patients during the period of maximal PRA. The data suggested that the sympathetic nervous system may be responsible for the initial phase of hypertension after coarctation resection and that the RAS plays a major role in the second phase of hypertension and in the pathogenesis of mesenteric arteritis.

Fox *et al* [3] noted that in a series of 25 patients undergoing surgical repair of coarctation, paradoxical hypertension occurred in 56% in the immediate postoperative period. These workers proposed, on the basis of analyses of animal experiments, that stimulation of sympathetic nerve fibers in the aortic isthmus could release norepinephrine, while simultaneously there could be reflex hypersecretion of renal renin. Both of these mechanisms were held to be possibly relevant to the pathogenesis of the paradoxical hypertension.

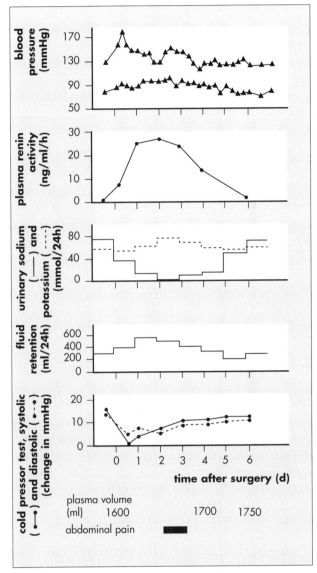

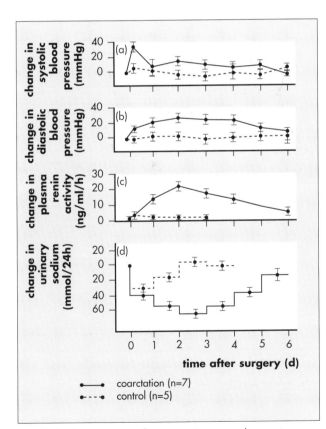

Fig. 59.7 A comparison of postoperative mean changes in systolic (a) and diastolic (b) blood pressure, plasma renin activity (c), and urinary sodium excretion (d) in seven patients with coarctation and in a control group of patients. Data are presented as mean ± SEM. Modified from Rocchini AP *et al* [23].

Fig. 59.8 The postoperative clinical course of a patient with coarctation. Note the rise in systolic blood pressure during the first postoperative day, with a more gradual increase in diastolic pressure peaking in days 2–4. Cold pressor test response is most suppressed at the initial phase. Plasma renin activity (PRA) increases markedly after surgery, reaches a maximum at days 2–4, and is accompanied by increased retention of fluid and sodium. Abdominal pain coincides with peak PRA level. Modified from Rocchini AP *et al* [23].

Parker *et al* [15] found in man, a marked hypotensive effect of saralasin during the appearance of postoperative paradoxical hypertension, which they interpreted as indicating increased circulating Ang II during this phenomenon.

A more direct approach to the issue was made by Gidding *et al* [27]. Seven children undergoing surgical repair of coarctation were randomly assigned to receive propranolol for two weeks before surgery and throughout the first postoperative week, while seven others received only standard postoperative care. In response to surgery, both groups had a similar significant rise in plasma norepinephrine. However, the administration of propranolol significantly attenuated the postoperative rise in PRA, while also lowering both systolic and diastolic blood pressures.

Choy *et al* [28] studied postoperative paradoxical hypertension in seven children undergoing surgical repair of aortic coarctation and in eight children having balloon dilatation. Both procedures resulted in a significant diminution in the pressure drop across the coarctation. In the immediate postoperative period, both systolic and diastolic blood pressures increased after surgical repair, whereas systolic pressures decreased and diastolic pressures remained unchanged, after balloon angioplasty. Following surgical repair, but not after balloon angioplasty, plasma catecholamines and PRA were increased in the first two days after intervention (Fig. 59.9).

Thus, there exists a consistent, albeit limited, body of evidence that the paradoxical postoperative hypertension in coarctation is associated with a transient rise in PRA and catecholamines; that the sudden rise in mesenteric arterial pressure, perhaps with the additional influence of increased plasma Ang II concentrations, can cause mesenteric arteritis, that this is more likely to occur after surgical repair than balloon angioplasty, that Ang II antagonists can correct the hypertension, and that suppression of the rise in PRA can prevent the phenomenon.

PERSISTENT LONG-TERM HYPERTENSION AFTER OPERATIVE REPAIR OF COARCTATION

Pelech *et al* [19] observed that although exercise-induced increases in PRA were elevated in children with coarctation before operation, these increases were abolished by reconstructive surgery. Nevertheless, exercise-induced enhanced rises in arm blood pressure persisted in one-third of children, who tended to

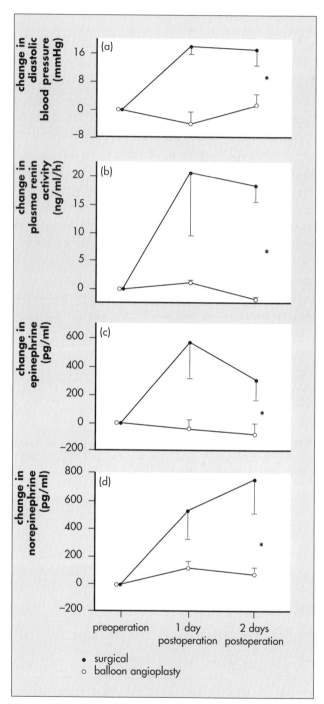

Fig. 59.9 The changes in diastolic blood pressure (a), plasma renin activity (b), plasma epinephrine (c), and plasma norepinephrine (d) after relief of coarctation of the aorta. A significant difference (*P*<0.05) in the responses of patients in the surgical and balloon angioplasty groups (profile analysis) is indicated by the asterisks. Modified from Choy M *et al* [28].

be older than those who did not show this phenomenon (Fig. 59.10). Likewise, left ventricular hypertrophy regressed in younger, but less readily in older, children with exercise-induced hypertension. These workers considered that structural changes in arterial walls above the site of the coarctation, and which had become more prominent in older patients, were mainly responsible for persistent postoperative hypertension.

Simsolo *et al* [29] measured PRA, plasma aldosterone, epinephrine, and norepinephrine under basal conditions and in response to standing and treadmill exercise in 24 normal children, 7 children with essential hypertension, 16 children normotensive after surgical correction of aortic coarctation, and 8 children who remained hypertensive after coarctation repair. Of the children normotensive at rest after operative correction of coarctation, 20% showed an excessive rise in blood pressure on exercise. Exercise caused a greater rise in systolic pressure in the children with hypertension, yet the changes in PRA, aldosterone, epinephrine, and norepinephrine were similar in all four groups. Orthostasis led to a significant rise in plasma norepinephrine in normotensive, but not in hypertensive, children. Neither at rest nor on exercise was persistent postoperative hypertension attributable to an excessive increase in catecholamines or in the RAS. These authors concluded that, alternatively, the persistent hypertension could be related to primary baroreceptor alterations or to structural changes in arterial walls, or to both.

EXPERIMENTAL ANIMAL STUDIES OF AORTIC COARCTATION

Several experimental animal models intended to mimic coarctation have been studied. Data provided by these models should, however, be interpreted with some caution in relation to coarctation of the aorta in man, where the abnormality is one of embryological development.

EXPERIMENTS IN DOGS

Bagby and her colleagues [30] performed aortic banding in six neonatal dogs, while seven littermates served as controls. Measurements of PRC, PRA, and angiotensinogen were made serially over 1–12 months under conditions of varied sodium intake. At no time and under no dietary circumstances were differences seen in any of these biochemical measurements between the two groups, although the animals with aortic narrowing developed higher blood pressures.

In further studies [31], these investigators extended their observations to dogs two years of age. They found that some animals with experimental neonatally applied aortic constriction showed hyperresponsiveness of PRA to the combination of low sodium intake plus furosemide administration, at 18 and 24 months of age. This difference could not be attributed to a disproportionate body sodium deficit. The PRA hyperresponsiveness was a variable feature, occurring late in development,

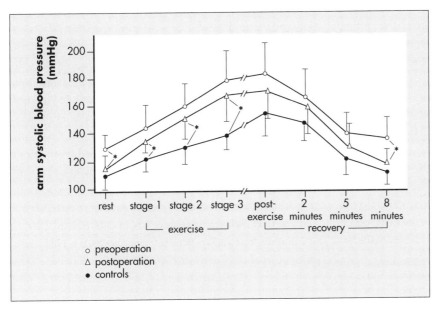

Fig. 59.10 Arm systolic blood pressure at rest and during and after exercise in 15 control subjects and in 15 patients before and after coarctectomy. Bars indicate ± 1 SD. *P<0.01 postoperative versus control values. Modified from Pelech AN *et el* [19].

reproducible for a given animal, and irrespective of the severity of hypertension.

Liard and Spadone [32,33] obtained results in some respects at variance with those of Bagby et al [30,31]. Conscious dogs were studied at various times up to 28 days after the creation of stenosis of the descending thoracic aorta. Mean arterial pressure increased proximal to the stenosis; distally, arterial pressure fell acutely below control values and then returned gradually over 28 days. Plasma renin activity increased six-fold at one and six hours after aortic constriction, and remained elevated for four days. Blood volume did not change significantly. Regional blood flows, estimated using radioactive microspheres, showed initial increases in some of the vascular beds subjected to increased arterial pressures, mainly the myocardium, brain, skeletal muscles, and bones. At 28 days, however, blood flows had become significantly reduced in most tissues exposed to the proximal pressure. Several vascular beds perfused at distal arterial pressure also showed a significant fall in blood flow at 28 days; they included those in small intestine, skin, skeletal muscle, and bones. Thus, a transient rise in PRA could contribute early to the hypertension. Later, a generalized increase in vascular resistance was observed, involving some tissues never exposed to increased arterial pressure.

Langdon et al [34] constricted the aorta experimentally in dogs within one week of birth. Eighteen months later, these animals all underwent surgical repair of the aortic constriction; in a subgroup, following repair, an occluder was placed on the aorta to maintain distal aortic pulse pressure at its diminished preoperative value. Normal dogs undergoing aortic transection with immediate reanastomosis served as controls; these dogs had a further sham operation at 18 months. Plasma renin activity and proximal blood pressure were elevated and distal pulse pressure was diminished before operation at 18 months in the dogs with aortic narrowing. Plasma renin activity increased significantly after operation in the dogs having correction of the aortic stenosis and in those sham operated alike.

Early changes following experimental aortic constriction with a pneumatic cuff were studied by Whitlow and Katholi [35] in chronically instrumented conscious dogs. Hypertension developed within 48 hours and was associated with a rise in PRA, with sodium retention, and with an exaggerated blood-pressure fall when a competitive Ang II antagonist was given. Concurrently, plasma norepinephrine fell with the development of hypertension, and the α-adrenergic blocker phentolamine had a diminished depressor effect.

In order to study the relationship between renal and other factors associated with coarctation of the aorta, Ferguson et al [36] created thoracic aortic strictures in two groups of adult dogs. In one of these groups (group B), a prosthetic vascular graft was inserted proximal to the aortic constriction and anastomosed to an isolated segment of the abdominal aorta containing both renal arteries. The kidneys remained in situ with normal venous and ureteral drainage. Thus, in group B, the renal aspects of the aortic constriction were minimized. Those dogs with aortic constriction only (group A) developed progressive generalized hypertension, while the others, with the renal blood supply maintained (group B), developed hypertension confined to the arteries proximal to the constriction (Fig. 59.11). Peripheral PRA was not significantly different between the groups. These experiments were interpreted as demonstrating a mechanical influence responsible for hypertension proximal to the aortic constriction and manifest as localized hypertension in the dogs of group B with the aortorenal conduit. In group A, there was an additional, but unidentified, renal factor, causing progressive, generalized hypertension.

Wickre et al [37] studied hemodynamic changes with surgical correction of neonatally applied aortic constriction in comparison with data in sham-operated littermate controls. Excision of the tight aortic band with aortic reanastomosis abolished the pressure drop across the previously constricted aorta. After this corrective operation, there was an early transient fall in systemic blood pressure, followed by a return to preoperative hypertensive levels similar to those seen proximal to the aortic constriction before corrective surgery. This postoperative hypertension was sustained for 2–4 weeks before subsiding to normal values. Although femoral artery (and hence renal perfusion) pressure rose following the corrective operation, there was expansion of extracellular fluid volume, which reached a maximum coincident with the postcoarctectomy blood-pressure elevation. There was also, after corrective surgery, a transient rise in heart rate. Sham-operated control animals showed no hypertension, no tachycardia, and no changes in exchangeable body sodium. There were at no stage significant differences between the control and postcoarctectomy dogs in PRA, or in blood losses or fluid administration. It was postulated that postcoarctation baroreceptor stimulation resulted in sympathetically mediated renal sodium retention, preventing a pressure diuresis. As PRA was not concomitantly suppressed, the transient postoperative hypertension might in part have been due to disproportion between PRA and the temporary volume expansion.

Tarkka et al [38] induced constriction of the thoracic aorta in eight-week-old dogs. After seven months, a corrective operation with a venous patch was performed, and the dogs were observed for a further 12 months. With removal of the aortic

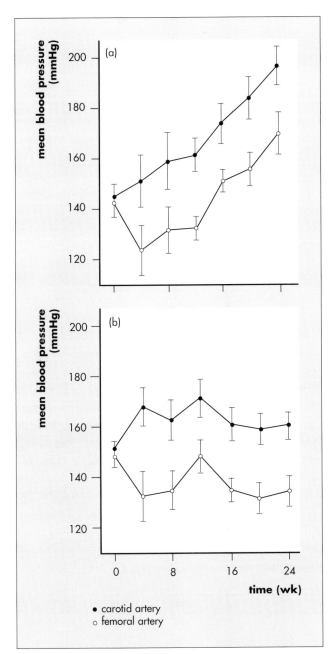

Fig. 59.11 Comparison of the changes in arterial pressure between two groups of dogs with experimental thoracic aortic constriction. Those of group B (b) had a conduit inserted from above the constriction to the renal arteries. Note the progressive rise in pressure proximal and distal to the coarctation in group A (a). The pressure changes in group B remained relatively constant. Data are presented as mean ± SEM. Modified from Ferguson JC et al [36].

constriction, PRA rose on the day after operation, subsequently subsiding to preoperative values. Although these experiments were not adequately controlled, the data were interpreted as supporting the notion of a contribution of increased PRA to the transient paradoxical hypertension seen after correction of aortic coarctation.

EXPERIMENTS IN RATS

Bailie *et al* [39] applied aortic constriction above the renal arteries in rats. The development of sustained hypertension was accompanied by an increase in PRA within 24 hours. Plasma renin activity had returned to control values, despite maintenance of hypertension, within five days. When captopril was introduced 10 days after aortic constriction, there was no effect on blood pressure. These authors considered that their data suggested that the RAS is important in the early development, but not in the maintenance, of this form of experimental hypertension.

Mercadier *et al* [40] studied a similar model of suprarenal aortic constriction in the rat, in which there was a progressive rise of aortic blood pressure and left ventricular mass up to 30 days after operation. Plasma renin concentration was markedly elevated at day 4, although by day 30, with stable hypertension, PRC had returned to control values. Plasma atrial natriuretic factor (ANF) remained elevated at 30 days. There was evidence of ventricular activation of the ANF gene, which appeared to be dependent severally on the development of hypertension, of left ventricular hypertrophy, and on left ventricular end-diastolic pressure. The data suggested to Mercadier *et al* [40] that ANF production by the overloaded myocardium may help in the regulation of cardiac preload.

INTERPRETATION OF ANIMAL EXPERIMENTS

Interpretation of the animal experimental data is not easy. In the studies of Bagby *et al* [30,31], which probably approximate most closely to clinical coarctation of the aorta, no evidence was found of a contribution of the RAS to the pathogenesis of established hypertension, while variable PRA hyperresponsiveness, unrelated to the severity of the hypertension, was seen [31]. Several groups [32–35,39,40] observed transient enhancement of the RAS after the experimental application of aortic constriction, both in the dog and the rat. These data seem more akin to experimental renovascular hypertension than to human aortic coarctation (see *Chapter 55*); nevertheless, it is possible that there are affinities between the pathogenesis of the hypertension in aortic coarctation and that in the 1-kidney, 1-clip Goldblatt model.

A transient increase in circulating renin and Ang II might well, moreover, contribute to 'paradoxical' hypertension following surgical correction of aortic constriction in the dog [3,34,38].

CONCLUSIONS

In sustained hypertension in human aortic coarctation before surgery, there is evidence from some centers of enhanced activity of the RAS in response to several stimuli [9,11,12,14–19]; of concomitant expansion of plasma and extracellular fluid volume in some patients [12,13]; of brief, but not sustained, falls in arterial pressure with administration of antagonists of the RAS [11,12,15–19]; and of a reduction in plasma renin after corrective surgery [14]. However, other investigators [20,24–26] could not confirm this last observation. The data are not entirely consistent, but are compatible with there being a contribution to the hypertension of aortic coarctation from the RAS, at least in some patients. Any such participation is at most partial, and does not fully explain the raised arterial pressure.

If the RAS is relevant to the pathogenesis of hypertension in aortic coarctation, the site of the lesion in relation to the kidneys would indicate that the experimental model most likely to show similarities would be Goldblatt 1-kidney, 1-clip, or, more strictly, 2-kidney, 2-clip, hypertension. In that model, which is discussed in more detail in *Chapter 55*, there is usually only transient elevation of the RAS. Concomitantly, there is sustained expansion of body sodium content and of body fluid spaces. Neither the transient elevation of renin, nor the expansion of body sodium, separately or together, provide a satisfactory explanation for the raised arterial pressure. The RAS is readily, and often markedly, activated upon sodium depletion in this model.

Several of the preceding accounts of both clinical and experimental coarctation show points of similarity to 1-kidney, 1-clip experimental hypertension.

It should be noted that supervention of the malignant phase is extremely rare, although not unreported [2] preoperatively in patients with coarctation of the aorta. As is discussed in greater detail in *Chapters 40* and *60*, while raised plasma renin and Ang II values are not an absolute requirement for transition to malignant-phase hypertension, they may, if present, predispose to that progression. To the extent that this perhaps tenuous argument is valid, the rarity of the malignant phase in coarctation of the aorta suggests that the RAS is not prominent in the pathogenesis of the hypertension.

The animal experiments that probably most closely mimic human coarctation [30,31] are not strongly supportive of a contribution from the RAS.

Both in patients [3,15,23,27,28] and in the dog [3,34,38] there is more convincing evidence of a transient enhancement of the RAS following correction of human coarctation or experimental aortic constriction, and that this may be involved in postoperative paradoxical hypertension. The mesenteric arteritis that frequently accompanies postoperative paradoxical hypertension may be caused by a combination of a sudden increase in pressure in fragile arteries not previously exposed to high pressure, plus the effects of transiently raised plasma Ang II concentrations.

There is little to suggest that the RAS contributes to any hypertension that may persist longterm after surgical correction of the coarctation [7]. Structural changes in arterial walls above the site of the previous aortic lesion are considered to be largely responsible in these circumstances [19,29].

REFERENCES

1. de Leeuw PW, Birkenhäger WH. Coarctation of the aorta. In: Robertson JIS, ed. *Handbook of hypertension, volume 15. Clinical aspects of hypertension*. Amsterdam: Elsevier, 1992:chapter 9.

2. Cleland WP, Counihan TB, Goodwin JF, Steiner R. Coarctation of the aorta. *British Medical Journal* 1956;2:379–84.

3. Fox S, Pierce WS, Waldhausen JA. Pathogenesis of paradoxical hypertension after coarctation repair. *Annals of Thoracic Surgery* 1980;29:135–41.

4. Sealy WC. Coarctation of the aorta and hypertension. *Annals of Thoracic Surgery* 1967;3:15–28.

5. Mays ET, Sergeant CK. Postcoarctectomy syndrome. *Archives of Surgery* 1965;91: 58–66.

6. Pickering GW. *High blood pressure, 2nd edition*. London: J and A Churchill, 1968.

7. Counihan TB. Changes in blood pressure following resection of coarctation of the aorta. *Clinical Science* 1956;15:149–59.

8. Morris RE, Robinson PR, Scheele GA. The relationship of angiotensin to renal hypertension. *Canadian Medical Association Journal* 1964;90:272–6.

9. Pickens PT. Relation of plasma renin to blood pressure in a patient with coarctation. *British Heart Journal* 1967;29:135–6.

10. Van Way CW, Michelakis AM, Anderson WJ, Manlove A, Oates JA. Studies of plasma renin activity in coarctation of the aorta. *Annals of Surgery* 1976;183: 229–38.

11. Ribeiro AB, Krakoff LR. Angiotensin blockade in coarctation of the aorta. *New England Journal of Medicine* 1976;295:148–50.

12. Lardoux H, Corvol P, Kreft C, Lancelin B, Ménard J, Pauly-Laubry C, Guermonprez JL, Maurice P. Rôle du système rénine–angiotensine dans l'hypertension artérielle de la coarctation aortique de l'adulte jeune. *Archives des Maladies du Coeur et des Vaisseaux* 1980;73:246–53.

13. Alpert BS, Bain HH, Balfe JW, Kidd BSL, Olley PM. Role of the renin–angiotensin–aldosterone system in hypertensive children with coarctation of the aorta. *American Journal of Cardiology* 1979;43:828–34.

14. Parker FB, Streeten DHP, Farrell B, Blackman MS, Sondheimer HM, Anderson GH. Preoperative and postoperative renin levels in coarctation of the aorta. *Circulation* 1982;66:513–4.

15. Parker FB, Farrell B, Streeten DHP, Blackman MS, Sondheimer HM, Anderson GH. Hypertensive mechanisms in coarctation of the aorta: Further studies of the renin–angiotensin system. *Journal of Thoracic and Cardiovascular Surgery* 1980;80: 568–73.

16. Warren DJ, Smith RS, Naik RB. Inappropriate renin secretion and abnormal cardiovascular reflexes in coarctation of the aorta. *British Heart Journal* 1981;45:733–6.

17. Fallo F, Maragno I, Meroda P, Mantero F. Effect of captopril on blood pressure and on the renin–angiotensin–aldosterone system in coarctation of the aorta. *Clinical and Experimental Hypertension. Part A, Theory and Practice* 1983;A5: 321–8.

18. Fallo F, Maragno I, Mantero F. Resistance to captopril in hypertension of coarctation of the aorta. *International Journal of Cardiology* 1985;9:111–3.

19. Pelech AN, Katodihardjo W, Balfe JA, Balfe JW, Olley PM, Leenen FHH. Exercise in children before and after coarctectomy: Hemodynamic, echocardiographic, and biochemical assessment. *American Heart Journal* 1986;112:1263–70.

20. Brown JJ, Davies DL, Lever AF, Robertson JIS. Plasma renin concentration in human hypertension. II: Renin in relation to aetiology. *British Medical Journal* 1965;2:1215–9.

21. Amsterdam EA, Albers WH, Christlieb AR, Morgan CL, Nadas AS, Hickler RB. Plasma renin activity in children with coarctation of the aorta. *American Journal of Cardiology* 1969;23:396–9.

22. Werning C, Schönbeck M, Weidmann P, Baumann K, Gysling E, Wirz P, Siegenthaler W. Plasma renin activity in patients with coarctation of the aorta: A comment on the pathogenesis of prestenotic hypertension. *Circulation* 1969;40:731–7.

23. Rocchini AP, Rosenthal A, Barger AC, Castaneda AR, Nadas AS. Pathogenesis of paradoxical hypertension after coarctation resection. *Circulation* 1976;54: 382–7.

24. Strong WB, Botti RE, Silbert DR, Liebman J. Peripheral and renal vein plasma renin activity in coarctation of the aorta. *Pediatrics* 1970;45:254–9.

25. Markiewicz A, Wojczuk D, Kokot F, Cicha A. Plasma renin activity in coarctation of the aorta before and after surgery. *British Heart Journal* 1975;37:721–5.

26. Sehested J, Kornerup HJ, Pedersen EB, Christensen NJ. Effects of exercise on plasma renin, aldosterone, and catecholamines before and after surgery for aortic coarctation. *European Heart Journal* 1983;4:52–8.

27. Gidding SS, Rocchini AP, Beekman R, Szpuner CA, Moorehead C, Behrendt D, Rosenthal A. Therapeutic effect of propranolol on paradoxical hypertension after repair of coarctation of the aorta. *New England Journal of Medicine* 1985;312: 1224–8.

28. Choy M, Rocchini AP, Beekman RH, Rosenthal A, Dick M, Crowley D, Behrendt D, Snider AR. Paradoxical hypertension after repair of coarctation of the aorta in children: Balloon angioplasty versus surgical repair. *Circulation* 1987;75:1186–91.

29. Simsolo R, Grunfeld B, Gimenez M, Lopez M, Berri G, Becu L, Barontini M. Long-term systemic hypertension in children after successful repair of coarctation of the aorta. *American Heart Journal* 1988;115:1268–73.

30. Bagby SP, McDonald WJ, Gray DK. *In vitro* determinants of plasma renin activity in serially-studied inbred dogs with neonatally-induced coarctation hypertension: Renin reactivity, renin substrate, and renin concentration. *Clinical and Experimental Hypertension. Part A, Theory and Practice* 1981;3:455–75.

31. Bagby SP, Baur GM, Gray DK. Canine neonatally induced coarctation hypertension in the second year: Variably hyper-responsive plasma renin activity. *Hypertension* 1983;5:328–35.

32. Liard JF, Spadone JC. Changes in regional vascular resistance in canine aortic coarctation. *Journal of Hypertension* 1984;2 (suppl. 3):375–7.

33. Liard JF, Spadone JC. Regional circulations in experimental coarctation of the aorta in conscious dogs. *Journal of Hypertension* 1985;3:281–91.

34. Langdon TJ, Boerboom LE, Olinger GN, Declusin RJ, Bonchek Ll, Liu TZ. Operative factors, not hemodynamics, modify hormones in repair of coarctation. *Journal of Surgical Research* 1989;47:144–8.

35. Whitlow PL, Katholi RE. Neurohumoral mechanisms in acute aortic coarctation in conscious and anesthetized dogs. *American Journal of Physiology* 1983;244: H614–21.

36. Ferguson JC, Barrie WW, Schenk WG. Hypertension of aortic coarctation: The role of renal and other factors. *Annals of Surgery* 1977;185:423–8.

37. Wickre CG, Baur GM, Wong J, Woodruff J, Bagby S. Extracellular volume expansion and delayed resolution of hypertension after canine aortic coarctectomy. *Life Sciences* 1983;32:1197–206.

38. Tarkka M, Uhari M, Heikkila J, Pakarinen A. Decreased renal perfusion after correction of experimental coarctation. *Pediatric Research* 1987;22:445–8.

39. Bailie MD, Donoso VS, Gonzalez NC. Role of the renin–angiotensin system in hypertension after coarctation of the aorta. *Journal of Laboratory and Clinical Medicine* 1984;104:553–62.

40. Mercadier JJ, Samuel JL, Michel JB, Zongazo MA, de la Bastie D, Lompre AM, Wisnewsky C, Rappaport L, Levy B, Schwartz K. Atrial natriuretic factor gene expression in rat ventricle during experimental hypertension. *American Journal of Physiology* 1989;257:H979–87.

60

RENIN AND MALIGNANT HYPERTENSION

J IAN S ROBERTSON

THE NATURE OF MALIGNANT HYPERTENSION

Malignant hypertension (or 'accelerated hypertension'—the terms are now taken as synonyms [1,2]) is defined as severe elevation of arterial pressure accompanied by a characteristic vascular lesion, fibrinoid arterial or arteriolar necrosis (Plates 21 and 22, see Color Plate Section). Fibrinoid necrosis occurs especially in small arteries in the kidney, while those of the brain, retina, pancreas, adrenal, heart, and gut are also susceptible [3]. The renal lesions are reflected in variable proteinuria, hematuria, and granular casts. Clinically, the most striking features are retinal hemorrhages, which may be flame shaped or circular; exudates, either fluffy ('cotton wool') or circumscribed ('hard'); and papilledema. Papilledema was once reegarded as an absolute requirement for the clinical diagnosis of the malignant phase [3]. It is now, however, recognized that renal arteriolar fibrinoid necrosis may be extensive with accompanying retinal hemorrhages and exudates but in the absence of papilledema [4],while prognosis is similar whether or not papilledema is added. Thus, papilledema is no longer an absolute criterion for the diagnosis [1,2,4–6].

Microangiopathic hemolytic anemia is frequently associated with both experimental and clinical malignant-phase hypertension, and has been considered to be either a consequence of malignant hypertension or a contributory factor in its pathogenesis [7–9].

The term 'malignant' is appropriate; in the absence of effective antihypertensive therapy, the condition is rapidly and invariably fatal.

The traditional view of the etiology of the malignant phase is that it is a direct adverse consequence of very high arterial pressure, compounded by the speed of pressure increase [3]. The latter factor has been taken by some workers to explain, for example, the appearance of fibrinoid arterial and retinal lesions with only modest blood pressure elevation in pregnancy-induced hypertension [10]. Other authors [11], however, prefer to distinguish the syndrome in pregnancy from genuine malignant hypertension. Conversely, the very chronic elevation of pressure in aortic coarctation could explain the extreme rarity (but not absence [12]) of the malignant phase in that disease. The malignant phase is rare, but nevertheless well recognized [4,13–17], with hypertension accompanying aldosterone-secreting adenoma, a syndrome in which plasma renin and Ang II are characteristically low (see *Chapter 63*). By contrast, the malignant phase is frequent in hypertensive syndromes with secondary forms of aldosterone excess [18]. This latter observation led to the further hypothesis, which antedated reliable renin assays, that elevation of plasma renin, and hence of Ang II, together with increased plasma aldosterone, was needed for the development of the arteriolar fibrinoid necrosis of the malignant phase [19,20]. The latter notions were supported by evidence of arterial lesions induced experimentally by administering Ang II [21,22] (see *Chapter 40*). The fact that lesions of the fundus oculi, closely similar in appearance to those of malignant hypertension, can complicate severe hemorrhage [23]—a circumstance in which renin and Ang II are markedly elevated (see *Chapter 71*)—also lent some credence to the idea. The hypothesis has been espoused by a much more recent reviewer [8].

This chapter examines changes in various components of the RAS in the malignant phase and the effect of control of hypertension. It also considers to what extent elevation of plasma renin and hence of Ang II may contribute to the development of clinical malignant-phase hypertension.

EARLY REPORTS

Early papers indicated that plasma renin and Ang were elevated in many, but not in all, patients with malignant-phase hypertension. Few of these were systematic studies, and the assay methods used would now be regarded as often crude. Nevertheless, a fairly consistent pattern was suggested.

Kahn *et al* [24], employing one of the very first assays for Ang, reported a significant increase in peripheral blood in malignant hypertension. Using different Ang II assay methods, neither Genest *et al* [25] nor Morris *et al* [26] could confirm this. Massani *et al* [27] did, however, find Ang blood levels to be high in the malignant phase.

Plasma renin activity (PRA) was stated to be increased in a proportion of cases of malignant hypertension by several groups [25,28–32]. The paper by Genest *et al* [25] presented some difficulties, since it reported increased PRA in the absence of a comparable elevation of Ang II.

PLASMA RENIN CONCENTRATION

Brown *et al* [4] published results of plasma total renin concentration (PRC) measurements in a series of 82 patients with malignant hypertension. These findings will be described in some detail since they served to clarify several relevant issues, and interpretation has not changed markedly with later studies and the subsequent development of improved methods for the assay of renin and Ang II. In the paper by Brown *et al* [4], malignant hypertension was defined and diagnosed by the presence of bilateral retinal hemorrhages and exudates, whether or not there was concomitant papilledema; and/or on the histological demonstration of fibrinoid arteriolar necrosis. In no case of the series was an explanation other than arterial hypertension present for the retinal or histological lesions. This publication [4] was, parenthetically, one of the earliest to justify the clinical diagnosis of malignant-phase hypertension on the basis of bilateral retinal hemorrhages and exudates in the absence of papilledema; the authors quote data of their own of renal histology, almost exclusively on biopsy specimens, in 104 hypertensive patients. Renal fibrinoid arteriolar necroses were found in 11 of 16 cases with bilateral retinal hemorrhages and exudates plus papilledema; in 8 of 19 with bilateral hemorrhages and exudates in the absence of papilledema; and in 7 of 69 without any of these ocular lesions.

MALIGNANT HYPERTENSIVE RETINOPATHY WITHOUT ANGIOGRAPHIC RENAL ARTERY STENOSIS

Of the series, 53 had ophthalmoscopic evidence of the malignant phase, while renal arteriography had shown no stenotic lesion. Peripheral venous PRC values ranged from abnormally low to 10 times the upper limit of normal (highest value 240 Glasgow units/l) (Fig. 60.1a). In none of these 53 patients was hypertension under effective control at the time of sampling. Of the 53 patients, 12 were strictly untreated; in these 12, PRC

values, as in the whole group, ranged from abnormally low to abnormally high.

MALIGNANT HYPERTENSIVE RETINOPATHY WITH RENAL ARTERY STENOSIS

Of the patients, 25 had retinal lesions of malignant hypertension together with renal artery stenosis on the evidence of both arteriography and ureteric catheterization studies [33]. In every one of these patients, PRC was abnormally high, ranging from just above the upper limit of normal, to values a hundred times higher, with the highest being 1,920 Glasgow units/l (Fig. 60.1b). Patients with the most severe renal artery stenoses tended to have the most markedly elevated renin values.

FIBRINOID ARTERIAL LESIONS WITHOUT RETINOPATHY

Of the series, seven hypertensive patients had fibrinoid renal or adrenal arteriolar lesions but did not have malignant hypertensive retinopathy. Of these, three were patients with aldosterone-secreting adenomata. Two others were in chronic renal failure, due respectively to polycystic disease and glomerulonephritis. In all of these seven, PRC was either normal or abnormally low (mean 6.4 ± 1.8 SEM Glasgow units/l).

In emphasizing that the malignant phase can supervene in the absence of elevated PRC, these authors [4] pointed out that depression of plasma renin could well occur in hypertensive patients if there were sodium overload, to which subjects with renal or cardiac impairment would be particularly susceptible. It was stressed that the series, nevertheless, showed instances of patients having retinal and/or histological evidence of malignant hypertension, with normal or subnormal PRC, in the absence of evidence of cardiac or renal failure.

PLASMA RENIN ACTIVITY

McAllister *et al* [34] studied 22 patients with malignant hypertension on first admission to hospital, whenever possible before drug treatment, and then again under strictly controlled metabolic circumstances, in balance while ingesting a diet containing 100mmol of sodium daily, with body posture also regulated at blood sampling. Entry criteria were strict: all had a diastolic pressure of at least 120mmHg, and all had marked retinopathy, including papilledema; none had severe elevation of blood urea. Patients with evidence of renal artery stenosis, pheochromocytoma, or cortisol hypersecretion were excluded.

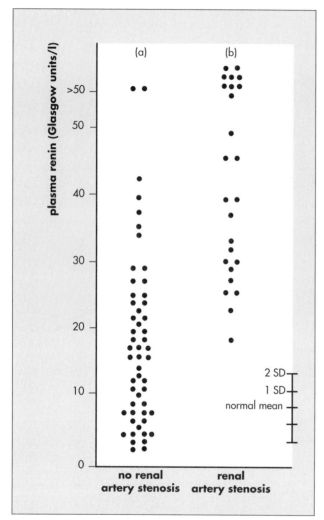

Fig. 60.1 (a) Plasma renin concentrations (PRC) in Glasgow units/l in 53 patients with malignant-phase hypertension without renal artery stenosis. The PRC ranged from abnormally low to very high (from 2.5–240 units/l). (b) Plasma renin concentrations in Glasgow units/l in 25 patients with malignant hypertension and renal artery stenosis. All values were abnormally high (from 19–1,920 units/l). All samples are from peripheral venous blood. See text for further details. Modified from Brown JJ *et al* [4].

Therapy with a range of antihypertensive drugs had been necessary before the metabolic balance studies were performed.

Of the eight patients who had blood sampled on admission to hospital, and before drug therapy was initiated, five had elevated, and three normal, PRA. When measurements were performed during metabolic balance conditions, 7 had elevated, and 15 normal, PRA values. Thus, PRA was found to be not invariably increased in the malignant phase.

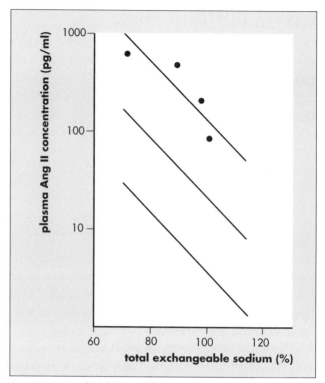

Fig. 60.2 Peripheral venous plasma Ang II concentrations in relation to concurrent total exchangeable sodium in four patients with untreated malignant hypertension. Total exchangeable sodium is expressed as a percentage of that predicted for a normal person of the same leanness index [37]. Diagonal lines indicate mean ± 2 SD of the relationship between Ang II and exchangeable sodium in normal subjects. In all four patients, Ang II is elevated (normal range 5–35pg/ml), and disproportionately so for the concurrent exchangeable sodium. Data from Davies DL *et al* [37] and Atkinson AB *et al* [42].

ANGIOTENSIN II

Consistent with the foregoing observations on plasma renin, several groups of investigators have reported elevation of plasma Ang II in a majority, but not in all, patients in the malignant phase of hypertension [35–37]. Davies *et al* [37] noted that in several patients in the malignant phase, not only was plasma Ang II elevated, but also that it was disproportionately high for the concurrent value of total exchangeable body sodium; they emphasized that this disproportionate elevation of plasma Ang II almost certainly was a factor contributing to the very high arterial pressure (Fig. 60.2).

ALDOSTERONE

Aldosterone secretion or excretion rates have similarly been reported by several workers to be elevated in many, but not all, patients in the malignant phase of hypertension [18,25,38,39]. These were observations which suggested to some writers that the malignant phase may, perhaps invariably, be a condition of secondary aldosterone excess [8,19,20].

Nevertheless, the careful metabolic studies of McAllister *et al* [34], already mentioned above, make it clear that the situation is not uniform. Of the series of 22 patients with malignant hypertension studied by them, three had both PRA and aldosterone secretion rate within the normal range. While 86% of patients in this series had elevated aldosterone secretion rates, only 36% had concomitantly elevated PRA. The authors' observations led them to conclude that in the malignant phase, a hormone additional to Ang II may be at least partly responsible for the increased secretion rate of aldosterone, a possibility hinted at earlier by Genest *et al* [25]. An alternative, which was considered both by Brown *et al* [40] and McAllister *et al* [34], is that prolonged and excessive stimulation of aldosterone by Ang II could lead to persistent hyperfunction of the adrenocortical cells responsible for secreting aldosterone.

EFFECT OF THERAPY ON THE RENIN–ANGIOTENSIN SYSTEM AND ALDOSTERONE

Occasional reports [38,39] of hyperaldosteronism in the malignant phase, which was reversed by drug treatment that controlled the high blood pressure, indicated that in some way the aldosterone excess was a consequence, rather than a proximate cause, of the severe hypertension.

Brown *et al* [41] (Fig. 60.3) took measurements of PRC in 12 patients with malignant hypertension before and after treatment. In all cases, the retinal lesions had cleared by the time of the second sample. Renal artery stenosis was present in seven of the eight patients initially with elevated renin; in five of these seven, the hypertension was corrected and the retinopathy cleared following surgical repair of the renal arterial lesion or after nephrectomy. Hypotensive drugs alone were effective in one patient with renal artery stenosis, and also in the single case of the eight with elevated PRC who did not have renal artery stenosis. Surgical treatment was combined with drug therapy in the remaining patient with a renal artery lesion. Plasma renin concentration fell with control of the hypertension and resolution of the

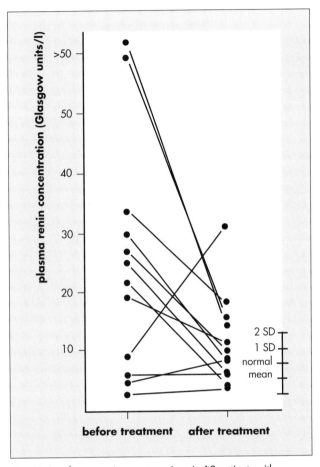

Fig. 60.3 Plasma renin concentrations in 12 patients with malignant hypertension before and after treatment. In all cases, the retinal lesions had cleared by the time of the second sample. Renal artery stenosis was present in seven of the eight patients initially with elevated renin; in five of these, the hypertension was corrected and the retinopathy cleared following surgical repair of the lesion or nephrectomy. Hypotensive drugs alone were effective in one patient with renal artery stenosis and in the single case of the eight patients who did not have renal artery stenosis. Surgical treatment was combined with drug therapy in the remaining patient with a renal artery lesion. Hypotensive drugs only were used in the four patients in whom renin was initially normal or low; the one case showing a marked rise in the renin had received thiazides. Additional details are given in the text. The range of plasma renin in normals is also indicated. Modified from Brown JJ *et al* [41].

malignant phase in all eight patients in whom it was initially elevated. Hypotensive drugs alone were used in the four patients in whom PRC was initially normal or low; in three of these there was little change with treatment. The one patient who showed a marked rise in PRC with clearing of retinopathy (Fig. 60.3) received a thiazide diuretic.

Atkinson *et al* [42] reported in detail on a patient with unilateral renal artery occlusion, severe malignant-phase hypertension, hyponatremia, hypokalemia, depletion of body sodium and potassium, and elevated blood concentrations of active renin, Ang I, Ang II, aldosterone, and vasopressin. As in the patients earlier reported by Davies *et al* [37] (see *Fig. 60.2*), Ang II was disproportionately high in relation to exchangeable body sodium. Captopril, by inhibiting conversion of Ang I to Ang II, further elevated blood levels of renin and Ang I, but corrected the hypertension and all other biochemical abnormalities. Unilateral nephrectomy was subsequently curative.

McAllister *et al* [34], as mentioned earlier, studied a series of patients with essential hypertension during a period of controlled dietary sodium intake, first while in the malignant phase and then at intervals during long-term follow-up on pharmacological treatment. Plasma renin activity returned to the normal range in almost 90% of these patients after drug therapy. Aldosterone secretion rate fell to normal with treatment in six patients; in all of these there was, however, a period during the postmalignant phase in which aldosterone secretion rate remained elevated although PRA was normal or low. In all but two of the remaining patients with raised aldosterone secretion rate initially, there were periods when aldosterone secretion was high but when PRA was not. These authors emphasize that reduction in PRA with treatment in several of their patients could not have been due to correction of a sodium deficit, since the studies were performed with the subjects in balance on a fixed sodium diet. Moreover, the fall in PRA was unlikely to be a specific direct inhibiting effect of antihypertensive drugs on renin secretion, because several of the patients were treated with guanethidine, an agent which does not lower plasma renin in uncomplicated essential hypertension. These workers considered that the reduction in renin correlated best with healing of renal arteriolar lesions.

The possibility that depletion of body sodium is a necessary trigger to the development of malignant hypertension under some circumstances receives support from observations that saline drinking can reverse, at least temporarily, all changes characteristic of malignant hypertension in rats with unilateral renal artery stenosis [43]. An early report by Hilden [44] and a more detailed study in one patient by Kaneda *et al* [45], suggest that both the hypertension and gross activation of the RAS may be reduced by saline administration (Fig. 60.4).

Several conclusions can be drawn from these extensive studies. First, not surprisingly, when the malignant phase accompanies renovascular hypertension, relief of the renal artery stenosis, unilateral nephrectomy, or the administration of an ACE inhibitor can correct the hypertension and return plasma Ang II and aldosterone to normal, with accompanying resolution of the malignant phase. Second, antihypertensive treatment with agents that do not affect renin secretion directly can lead to resolution of the malignant phase, with associated falls of renin, Ang II, and aldosterone. Third, PRA and aldosterone do not always move together, either in the malignant phase or during its correction; thus, factors additional to the RAS can contribute to the regulation of aldosterone secretion, both in the malignant phase and while it is healing. Fourth, while sodium deficiency can in some patients be one stimulus to renin secretion, a stimulus that is relieved with correction of the malignant phase, it is not ubiquitous. Fifth, and not withstanding the fourth conclusion, saline administration can reduce arterial pressure, renin, and aldosterone levels in at least some patients who show gross volume depletion and extreme activation of the RAS. Sixth, the malignant phase can resolve while plasma renin is rising, especially when diuretics are given.

MALIGNANT PHASE IN PATIENTS WITH RENIN-SECRETING TUMORS OR WITH ALDOSTERONE-SECRETING ADENOMA

The two hypertensive syndromes, renin-secreting tumors and aldosterone-secreting adenoma, deserve separate mention in the present connection, because patients with renin-secreting tumors have very high plasma renin and Ang II values (see *Chapter 54*), while, by contrast, patients with an aldosterone-secreting adenoma of the adrenal cortex are characterized by high aldosterone secretion rates accompanied by low plasma values of renin and Ang II [16,17,19,34] (see *Chapter 63*).

In subjects harboring a renin-secreting tumor, the malignant phase is not particularly prevalent, although it has been reported [46]. Segmental renal infarction can result in malignant hypertension, presumably through a 'primary' excess of renin secretion akin to the situation with renin-secreting tumor. The hypertension resolves in such patients when renin levels decline spontaneously or with surgery [47,48].

Supervention of the malignant phase is unusual in patients with aldosterone-secreting adenoma, and the rarity of the event was central to the hypothesis that elevated levels of renin, Ang II, and aldosterone might be prerequisites for progression to malignant hypertension [8,19,20]. Nevertheless, although uncommon, the malignant phase has repeatedly been described in patients with primary aldosterone excess. Retinal hemorrhages, exudates and papilledema, and fibrinoid arterial necrosis have all

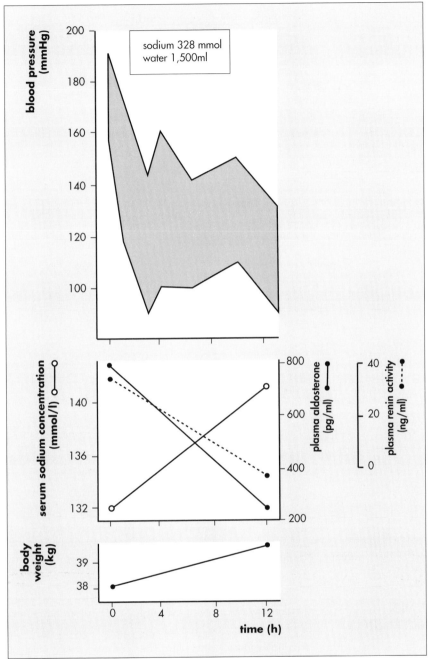

Fig. 60.4 Effects of infusion of sodium chloride over 12 hours in a patient with essential hypertension who entered the malignant phase. Plasma renin activity and plasma aldosterone levels declined. Modified from Kaneda H *et al* [45].

been recorded [13–17,34,49–51,59–61] (Fig. 60.5). In the patient reported by McAllister *et al* [34], manifestations of hyper-aldosteronism antedated the development of malignant hypertension. These observations, together with a report that malignant hypertension developed in a patient with systemic lupus erythematosus while taking the ACE inhibitor, captopril [52], clearly show that elevated plasma values of renin and/or

Ang II are not obligatory for the transition to the malignant phase. Nevertheless, the report by Ideishi *et al* [53] of a patient with high plasma renin levels in malignant hypertension secondary to an aldosterone-secreting adenoma, indicate that when the malignant phase has supervened in this syndrome, vascular renal lesions can, as in malignant hypertension from other causes, then lead to hypersecretion of renin.

Reference	Age (years)	Sex	Optic fundi	Renal histology
17	36	F	bilateral papilledema, hemorrhages and exudates	fibrinoid necrosis
	59	F	no papilledema, hemorrhages or exudates	fibrinoid necrosis
	33	M	no papilledema, hemorrhages or exudates	fibrinoid necrosis
13	28	M	bilateral hemorrhages and exudates; no papilledema	not reported
49	41	M	bilateral hemorrhages and exudates; no papilledema	no fibrinoid necrosis
14	42	M	bilateral papilledema and exudates; one hemorrhage	no fibrinoid necrosis
34	56	M	bilateral papilledema, exudates and hemorrhages	not reported
15	37	F	bilateral papilledema, exudates and hemorrhages	no fibrinoid necrosis
51	23	F	bilateral papilledema, one hemorrhage	not reported
59	18	M	bilateral papilledema with widespread fresh hemorrhages and exudates	severe small vessel changes consistent with malignant hypertension
60	21	F	no papilledema, hemorrhages or exudates	changes of malignant hypertension with obliterative intimal arteriolar lesions

Fig. 60.5 Examples of eleven patients with aldosterone-secreting adenoma and malignant-phase hypertension.

THE INVOLVEMENT OF THE RENIN SYSTEM IN MALIGNANT HYPERTENSION

The data reviewed herein have demonstrated that an increase in circulating renin and/or Ang II is not an absolute requirement for progression to the malignant phase of hypertension. Arteriolar fibrinoid necrosis, bilateral retinal hemorrhages and exudates, and papilledema have all been observed in hypertensive patients in whom plasma renin levels were not elevated or even were low. Moreover, the malignant phase can resolve while plasma renin is rising.

Nevertheless, it is also apparent that when the malignant phase has supervened in patients with renal artery stenosis, plasma renin is almost invariably elevated, in proportion to the severity of the stenosis. Extremely high renin and Ang II values may be seen in the hyponatremic hypertensive syndrome [42] (see *Chapter 55*), a condition which is most often a result of a very severe unilateral renal artery stenosis or occlusion (Fig. 60.6). The malignant phase is an almost constant accompaniment of this syndrome.

Once the malignant phase has developed in a case of hypertension, then the kidneys will (except when distal to aortic coarctation or renal artery stenosis, which are protective against the high systemic arterial pressure [33]) usually suffer extensively from arteriolar fibrinoid necroses. These intrarenal lesions, while leading to progressive renal impairment, can often act also as multiple intrarenal arterial stenoses. Thus, such intrarenal lesions may provide a mechanism stimulating even greater secretion of renin [33,54]. A further probable instance of this phenomenon is the

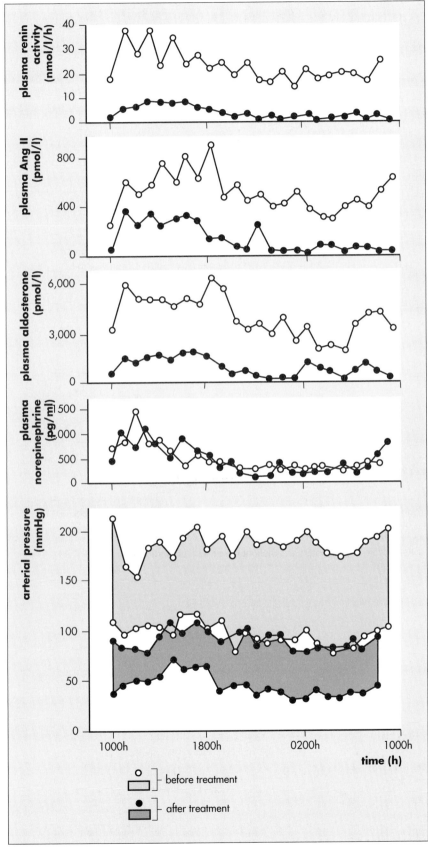

Fig. 60.6 Plasma renin activity, Ang II, aldosterone, and norepinephrine levels, together with hourly mean arterial pressures (from continuous intra-arterial monitoring) in a 68-year-old woman with the hyponatremic hypertensive syndrome due to occlusion of the left renal artery. The woman had retinal hemorrhages but no papilledema. Results are shown before treatment and three months after uninephrectomy. Modified from Maslowski AH *et al* [58].

patient described by Hodsman et al [55]. A young woman developed malignant hypertension as a result of oral contraceptive therapy. After withdrawal of oral contraceptives and control of the hypertension, intravenous urography, renal vein renin measurements, and ureteric catheterization studies all showed evidence of unilateral renal ischemia, although no main renal arterial stenosis was visible at arteriography. Almost certainly in this patient, the renal ischemia was a result of predominantly unilateral intrarenal small arterial lesions, initially the consequences of malignant hypertension.

In conclusion, while it is thus evident that elevated plasma renin or Ang II are not necessary for transition to malignant hypertension, the data do not exclude the possibility that a direct adverse effect of Ang II on small arteries could, independently of high blood pressure as such, in some instances promote and aggravate the progression of the malignant phase. Moreover, such a sequence of events could cause peripheral Ang II to increase to

values sufficiently high to stimulate secretion of vasopressin [42,56] (see Chapter 35), which in turn may then also directly exacerbate vascular lesions [57]. Thus, while a high circulating Ang II concentration appears not to be an absolute requirement for the development of malignant hypertension, once elevation of plasma Ang II has been attained, it probably can, both directly and indirectly, accelerate the baleful advance of the disease. A corollary is that blood pressure reduction, by promoting healing of intrarenal arteriolar lesions, will thus lead to a reduction in renin secretion and will facilitate resolution of the malignant phase [34].

One final point deserves mention. Prorenin and probably renin are synthesized locally in the eye [62,63] (Chapters 6 and 7), and this intraocular RAS could promote retinopathy. It has been suggested that blockade of this local system could have favorable effects on retinal vascular lesions [64].

REFERENCES

1. World Health Organization. Arterial Hypertension. Technical Report Series No 628. Geneva 1978:57.

2. Gross FH, Robertson JIS. Arterial hypertension. London: Pitman Medical 1979.

3. Pickering GW. High blood pressure, 2nd edition. London: J and A Churchill, 1968.

4. Brown JJ, Davies DL, Lever AF, Robertson JIS. Plasma renin concentration in human hypertension III: Renin in relation to complications of hypertension. British Medical Journal 1966;1:505–8.

5. McGregor E, Isles CG, Jay JL, Lever AF, Murray GD. Retinal changes in malignant hypertension. British Medical Journal 1986;292:233–4.

6. Ahmed MEK, Walker JM, Beevers DG, Beevers M. Lack of difference between malignant and accelerated hypertension. British Medical Journal 1986;292:235–7.

7. Gavras H, Brown WCB, Brown JJ, Lever AF, Linton AL, MacAdam RF, NcNicol GP, Robertson JIS, Wardrop C. Microangiopathic hemolytic anemia and the development of the malignant phase of hypertension. Circulation Research 1971;28 and 29 (suppl II):127–41.

8. Kincaid-Smith P. Malignant hypertension. Journal of Hypertension 1991;9:893–9.

9. Gavras H, Oliver N, Aitchison J, Begg C, Briggs JD, Brown JJ, Horton PW, Lee F, Lever AF, Prentice C, Robertson JIS. Abnormalities of coagulation and the development of the malignant phase of hypertension. Kidney International 1975;8 (suppl 5):254–63.

10. Spence JD, Arnold JMO, Gilbert JJ. Consequences of hypertension and effects of antihypertensive therapy. In: Robertson JIS, ed. Handbook of hypertension, volume 15. Clinical aspects of hypertension. Amsterdam: Elsevier, 1992:chapter 23.

11. Redman C. Hypertension in pregnancy. In: Ginsburg J, ed. The circulation in the female: From the cradle to the grave. New Jersey: Parthenon Press, 1989:63–77.

12. Cleland WP, Counihan TB, Goodwin JF, Steiner RE. Coarctation of the aorta. British Medical Journal 1956;2:379–90.

13. Brill GC, Creamer B, Mills IH, Pullan JM. Hyperaldosteronism: Report of a case. British Medical Journal 1960;2:990–1.

14. Kaplan NM. Primary aldosteronism with malignant hypertension. New England Journal of Medicine 1963;269:1282–6.

15. Del Greco F, Dolkart R, Skom J, Method H. Association of accelerated (malignant) hypertension in a patient with primary aldosteronism. Journal of Clinical Endocrinology and Metabolism 1966;26:808–14.

16. Brown JJ, Davies DL, Lever AF, Peart WS, Robertson JIS. Plasma concentration of renin in a patient with Conn's syndrome with fibrinoid lesions of the renal arterioles: The effect of treatment with spironolactone. Journal of Endocrinology 1965;33:279–93.

17. Beevers DG, Brown JJ, Ferriss JB, Fraser R, Lever AF, Robertson JIS, Tree M. Renal abnormalities and vascular complications in primary hyperaldosteronism: Evidence on tertiary hyperaldosteronism. Quarterly Journal of Medicine 1976;45:401–10.

18. Laragh JH, Ulick S, Januszewicz V, Kelly WG, Lieberman S. Electrolyte metabolism and aldosterone secretion in benign and malignant hypertension. Annals of Internal Medicine 1960;53:259–72.

19. Conn JW, Knopf RF, Nesbit RM. Primary aldosteronism: Present evaluation of its clinical characteristics and of the result of surgery. In: Baulieu EE, Robel P, eds. Aldosterone. Oxford: Blackwell Scientific Publications, 1964:327–52.

20. Laragh JH, Cannon PJ, Ames RP. Aldosterone in man: The control of its secretion, its interaction with sodium balance and angiotensin activity. In: Baulieu EE, Robel P, eds. Aldosterone. Oxford: Blackwell Scientific Publications, 1964:427–48.

21. Giese J. Renin, angiotensin and hypertensive vascular damage: A review. In: Laragh JH, ed. Hypertension manual. New York: Dun-Donnelley, 1973:371–403.

22. Goldby FS, Beilin LJ. How an acute rise in arterial pressure damages arterioles: Electron microscopic changes during angiotensin infusion. Cardiovascular Research 1972;6:569–84.

23. Pears MA, Pickering GW. Changes in the fundus oculi after haemorrhage. Quarterly Journal of Medicine 1960;29:153–78.

24. Kahn JR, Skeggs LT, Shumway NP, Wisenbaugh PE. The assay of hypertensin from the blood of normotensive and hypertensive human beings. Journal of Experimental Medicine 1952;95:523–9.

25. Genest J, Boucher R, de Champlain J, Veyrat R, Chrétien M, Biron P, Tremblay G, Roy P, Cartier P. Studies on the renin–angiotensin system in hypertensive patients. Canadian Medical Association Journal 1964;90:263–8.

26. Morris RE, Robinson PE, Scheele GA. The relationship of angiotensin to renal hypertension. Canadian Medical Association Journal 1964;90:272–6.

27. Massani ZM, Finkielman S, Worcel M, Agrest A, Paladini AC. Angiotensin blood levels in hypertensive and non-hypertensive diseases. *Clinical Science* 1966;**30**:473–83.

28. Yoshinaga K, Aida M, Maebashi M, Sato T, Abe K, Miwa I. Assay of renin in peripheral blood: A modification of Helmer's method for the estimation of circulating renin. *Tohoku Journal of Experimental Medicine* 1963;**80**:32–41.

29. Helmer OM. Renin activity in blood from patients with hypertension. *Canadian Medical Association Journal* 1964;**90**:221–5.

30. Fitz AE, Armstrong ML. Plasma vasoconstrictor activity in patients with renal, malignant and primary hypertension. *Circulation* 1964;**29**:409.

31. Kirkendall WM, Fitz A, Armstrong ML. Hypokalemia and the diagnosis of hypertension. *Diseases of the Chest* 1964;**45**:337–44.

32. Fasciolo JC, de Vito E, Romero JC, Cucchi JN. The renin content of the blood of humans and dogs under several conditions. *Canadian Medical Association Journal* 1964;**90**:206–9.

33. Brown JJ, Owen K, Peart WS, Robertson JIS, Sutton D. The diagnosis and treatment of renal artery stenosis. *British Medical Journal* 1960;**2**:327–38.

34. McAllister RG, Van Way CW, Dayani K, Anderson WJ, Temple E, Michelakis AM, Coppage WS, Oates JA. Malignant hypertension: Effect of therapy on renin and aldosterone. *Circulation Research* 1971;**28 and 29** (suppl 2):160–73.

35. Catt KJ, Cain MD, Coghlan JP, Zimmet PZ, Cran E, Best JB. Metabolism and blood levels of angiotensin II in normal subjects, renal disease and essential hypertension. *Circulation Research* 1970;**26 and 27** (suppl 2):177–93.

36. Catt KJ, Cran E, Zimmet PZ, Best JB, Cain MD, Coghlan JP. Angiotensin II blood levels in human hypertension. *Lancet* 1971;**i**:459–64.

37. Davies DL, Schalekamp MA, Beevers DG, Brown JJ, Briggs JD, Lever AF, Medina AM, Morton JJ, Robertson JIS, Tree M. Abnormal relationship between exchangeable sodium and the renin–angiotensin system in malignant hypertension and in hypertension with chronic renal failure. *Lancet* 1973;**i**:683–7.

38. Sambhi MA, Beck JC, Venning EH. Malignant hypertension and aldosterone secretion. *American Journal of Medicine* 1963;**35**:251–6.

39. Gill JR, George JM, Solomon A, Bartter FC. Hyperaldosteronism and sodium loss reversed by drug treatment for malignant hypertension. *New England Journal of Medicine* 1964;**270**:1088–92.

40. Brown JJ, Davies DL, Lever AF, Robertson JIS. Variations in plasma renin concentration in several physiological and pathological states. *Canadian Medical Association Journal* 1964;**90**:201–6.

41. Brown JJ, Davies DL, Lever AF, Robertson JIS. Plasma renin concentration in human hypertension IV: Renin in relation to treatment and prognosis. *British Medical Journal* 1965;**2**:268–71.

42. Atkinson AB, Brown JJ, Davies DL, Fraser R, Leckie B, Lever AF, Morton JJ, Robertson JIS. Hyponatraemic hypertensive syndrome with renal-artery occlusion corrected by captopril. *Lancet* 1979;**ii**:606–9.

43. Möhring J, Petri M, Szokol M, Haack D, Möhring B. Effects of saline drinking on malignant course of renal hypertension in rats. *American Journal of Physiology* 1976;**230**:849–57.

44. Hilden T. Hypertensive encephalopathy associated with hypochloremia. *Acta Medica Scandinavica* 1950;**76**:199–202.

45. Kaneda H, Yamauchi T, Murata T, Matsumoto J, Haruyama T. Treatment of malignant hypertension with infusion of sodium chloride; a case report and a review. *Tohoku Journal of Experimental Medicine* 1980;**132**:179–86.

46. Corvol P, Pinet F, Galen FX, Plouin PF, Chatellier G, Pagny JY, Bruneval P, Camilleri JP, Ménard J. Primary reninism. In: Laragh JH, Brenner BM, eds. *Hypertension: Pathophysiology, diagnosis and management.* New York: Raven Press, 1990:1573–82.

47. Lifschitz MD, Cody T. Spontaneous remission of accelerated (malignant) hypertension in renal infarction. *Archives of Internal Medicine* 1977;**137**:1079–81.

48. Elkik F, Corvol P, Idatte J–M, Ménard J. Renal segmental infarction: A cause of reversible malignant hypertension. *Journal of Hypertension* 1984;**2**:149–56.

49. Luetscher JA. Primary aldosteronism: Observations in six cases and review of diagnostic procedures. *Medicine (Baltimore)* 1964;**43**:437–57.

50. Delorme P, Genest J. Primary aldosteronism. *Canadian Medical Association Journal* 1959;**81**:893–902.

51. Aloia JF, Beutow G. Malignant hypertension with aldosterone-producing adenoma. *American Journal of the Medical Sciences* 1974;**268**:241–5.

52. Bailey RR. Malignant hypertension developing while on captopril. *New Zealand Medical Journal* 1980;**92**:31.

53. Ideishi M, Ishikawa K, Kinoshita A, Sasaguri M, Ikeda M, Takebayashi S. High-renin malignant hypertension secondary to an aldosterone-producing adenoma. *Nephron* 1990;**54**:259–62.

54. McAllister RG, Michelakis AM, Oates JA, Foster JH. Malignant hypertension due to renal artery stenosis: Greater renin release from the nonstenotic kidney. *Journal of the American Medical Association* 1972;**221**:865–68.

55. Hodsman GP, Robertson JIS, Semple PF, Mackay A. Malignant hypertension and oral contraceptives: Four cases, with two due to the 30μg oestrogen pill. *European Heart Journal* 1982;**3**:255–9.

56. Padfield PL, Morton JJ. Effects of angiotensin II on arginine-vasopressin in physiological and pathological situations in man. *Journal of Endocrinology* 1977;**74**:251–9.

57. Möhring J. Neurohypophysical vasopressor principle: Vasopressor hormone as well as antidiuretic hormone? *Klinische Wochenschrift* 1978;**56** (suppl 1):71–9.

58. Maslowski AH, Nicholls MG, Espiner EA, Ikram H, Bones PJ. Mechanisms in human renovascular hypertension. *Hypertension* 1983;**5**:597–602.

59. Murphy BF, Whitworth JA, Kincaid-Smith P. Malignant hypertension due to an aldosterone-producing adrenal adenoma. *Clinical and Experimental Hypertension.* 1985;**A7**:939–50.

60. Sunman W, Rothwell M, Sever PS. Case report: Conn's syndrome can cause malignant hypertension. *Journal of Human Hypertension* 1992;**6**:75–6.

61. Bravo EL, Tarazi RC, Dustan HP, Fouad FM, Textor SC, Gifford RW, Vidt DG. The changing clinical spectrum of primary aldosteronism. *American Journal of Medicine* 1983;**74**:641–51.

62. Danser AHJ, Dorpel MA van den, Deinum J, Derkx FHM, Peperkamp E, de Jong PTVM, Schalekamp MADH. Renin, prorenin and immunoreactive renin in vitreous fluid from eyes with and without diabetic retinopathy. *Journal of Clinical Endocrinology and Metabolism* 1989;**68**:160–7.

63. Deinum J, Derkx FHM, Danser AHJ, Schalekamp MADH. Identification and quantification of renin and prorenin in the bovine eye. *Endocrinology* 1990;**126**:1673–82.

64. Dahlöf B, Stenkula S, Hansson L. Hypertensive retinal vascular changes: Relationship to left ventricular hypertrophy and arteriolar changes before and after treatment. *Blood Pressure* 1992;**1**:1–10.

61 GENETICS OF ESSENTIAL (PRIMARY) HYPERTENSION: THE CONTRIBUTION OF RENIN — STUDIES IN RAT AND MAN

DANIELE CUSI AND GIUSEPPE BIANCHI

HYPERTENSION AS A COMPLEX PHENOTYPIC TRAIT

There is general agreement that human essential hypertension is at least partly under genetic control. From the many studies published so far, the heritability of blood pressure may account for as much as 30% of total variability [1–7]. In some surveys, nearly 60–70% of total blood-pressure variability is apparently the result of genetic effects [7], with as yet unidentified major genes playing a major role. Unfortunately, in spite of persistent attempts to perform a genetic analysis, there is still no clear and consistent interpretation of the mode of inheritance of hypertension, and further progress in the analysis may never be made if only the phenotype 'blood-pressure level' and its distribution in families or in samples of the general population are studied. Human essential hypertension, in fact, is a typical example of a complex phenotypic trait where many body-control systems at different levels of organization are involved so that the effect of a mutation in a single gene will be diluted by the other mechanisms that control blood-pressure level, and where different major pathogenetic mchanisms may lead to the same final phenotype of high blood pressure with elevated peripheral resistances.

MAJOR GENES VERSUS POLYGENES

A major gene is one whose allelic mutation exerts a major quantitative effect on the final phenotype, as for instance an average increase of blood pressure of 20mmHg, whereas a polygene is one whose allelic mutation has only very small quantitative effects on the final phenotype. A polygene acts additively with other genes, and the more the number of alleles that increase blood pressure which are present simultaneously, the higher the blood pressure of the individual will be.

A phenotype determined by a major gene is transmitted to the progeny according to the classical rules of Mendelian inheritance, with the affected and nonaffected individuals clearly identified.

For this reason, a bimodal distribution of the phenotype in the population is generally considered good evidence that the character under investigation is determined by a major gene, though this is not always the case, as exemplified by the polymorphism of erythrocyte acid-phosphatase activity in the general population [8]. Erythrocytes of different individuals contain one or two of three electrophoretically distinguishable acid-phosphatase isoenzymes controlled by three alleles (A, B, C) at a single locus. Each of the six resulting genotypes has a different phenotypic mean, with specific variance for acid-phosphatase activity. The frequency distribution of acid-phosphatase activity of the five most common genotypes (the very rare CC homozygote was not considered) is plotted in Fig. 61.1, superimposed on acid-phosphatase activity measured in a sample of the general population. It is evident from Fig. 61.1 that phenotypes A and B (corresponding to genotypes AA and BB) hardly overlap at all, whereas phenotypes A and BA show great overlap in their relative distribution. The distribution of acid-phosphatase activity in the general population, however, which corresponds to the sum of the activities of the individual phenotypes, is clearly unimodal. Considering only

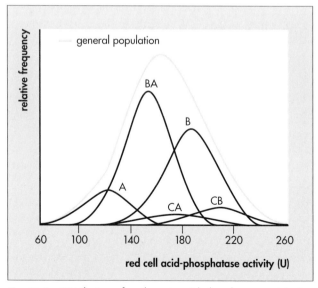

Fig. 61.1 Distribution of erythrocyte acid-phosphatase activity in the general population and in the separate phenotypes.

the acid-phosphatase activity phenotype in the general population, it could be postulated that its variation is not due to major gene effects. On the contrary, continuing the analysis by computing the ratio of the variance of the means of the five most common phenotypes to the total variance shows that at least two-thirds of the total variation in acid-phosphatase activity is due to the factors determined by one major gene with three alleles.

A phenotype determined by polygenes is transmitted to the progeny according to the rules of polygenic inheritance, with the mating of individuals with the highest phenotypic values producing offspring of the highest phenotypic value, and the mating of individuals with the lowest phenotypic values producing offspring of the lowest phenotypic value. Conversely, the mating of one individual with the highest phenotypic value with one individual with the lowest phenotypic value, as well as the mating of two individuals with intermediate phenotypic values, will produce offspring with intermediate phenotypic values. Since polygenes are distributed randomly; the distribution of such a phenotype in the population should resemble a normal gaussian one.

It is unlikely that the genetic component of human essential hypertension is due to a unique effect of a major gene. Two other, not necessarily conflicting, possibilities exist. Human essential hypertension may be a *multiple unilocus disease*, and hence the final phenotypic expression of several different, unrelated pathogenetic mechanisms determined by allelic mutation of different major genes; or alternatively, it may be a *polygenic disease* determined by the additive effect of many polygenes and for which the final phenotypic value depends on the algebraic sum of polygenes that tend to increase and those that tend to prevent the increase of blood pressure. The lack of a clear bimodality of blood-pressure distribution in the population seems to support the second hypothesis. A similar distribution, however, may be found in the case of a multiple unilocus disease, particularly if polygenes and/or the environment also have a quantitative effect on blood-pressure level; for example, some patients may develop mild hypertension because they are homozygous for a recessive mutation (plus unmeasurable polygenic and environmental effects), whereas others may develop more severe hypertension since they are homozygous for the same mutation (again plus unmeasurable polygenic and environmental effects) but have also inherited some other major factor(s) or susceptibility to peculiar environmental effects that determine a further increase in blood pressure. The same may be true for individuals that become hypertensive with a different pathogenic mechanism. They may be either heterozygous or homozygous for another major gene. If the pathologic allele is dominant, mild hypertension results. Should another major gene have a pathologic allele, there may be an additive

effect, causing more severe hypertension. The simple hypothesis of three major factors, with different degrees of penetrance, plus the polygenes, makes analysis of the distribution of the blood-pressure phenotype completely useless for the purpose of understanding the mechanism of inheritance of blood pressure. This should be self-evident, since despite over 50 years of genetic analysis of blood pressure, it is still known only that hypertension is probably transmitted by polygenic inheritance with some degree of dominance [2,7,9–13].

If the hypothesis that hypertension is a multiple unilocus disease is accepted, it may be assumed that there must be different groups of patients with essential hypertension which tend to cluster into groups with similar pathogenetic differences and also that each particular subtype of essential hypertension is determined by the association of an allelic mutation of a major gene with each individual's polygenic background and the environment. The additive effect of the major gene to a polygenic background produces intermediate phenotypes that are independently modulated by the environment at all the different levels of organization. Both polygenes and major genes may influence the phenotypic expression at each intermediate level, so that the paths connecting each intermediate step may be extremely complex.

A classical example of dissection of a complex phenotypic trait is represented by the different phenotypic markers of phenylketonuria described by Penrose [15], although in the case of hypertension, the situation is much more complex. Findings subsequent to Penrose's original description have complicated today's picture of the molecular genetics of phenylketonuria, but we will follow it since it provides guidelines in the dissection of a qualitative character from an apparently quantitative phenotype.

Phenylketonuria affects homozygotes for a recessive mutant allele at the locus controlling the enzyme, phenylalanine-hydroxylase, which converts phenylalanine to tyrosine [16]. Figure 61.2 reports the distribution of some quantitatively measurable phenotypes in a group of affected and one of nonaffected subjects. Measurement of the serum concentration does not show overlap between cases and controls. Qualitative differences, however, can be found only at the molecular level as differences in the restriction fragment-length polymorphism (RFLP) pattern or DNA sequence for the gene phenylalanine hydroxylase. Moreover, the distribution of phenylalanine serum concentration around its mean is relatively wide, particularly in affected individuals, ranging from 13 to 45mg/dl (the abscissa is in log scale). Since the accumulation of phenylalanine in infancy and childhood causes a severe mental defect, measurements of intelligence will identify two discrete subpopulations, affected and nonaffected. In this case, some overlap exists, but interestingly, the variances increase substantially, indicating that the farther we go from the first gene products, the greater is the influence of both the environment and other genes on the intermediate phenotype under study. Furthermore, the distributions of head size and hair colour clearly indicate that, on average, patients with phenylketonuria tend to have smaller heads and blonder hair, but considerable overlap exists between affected and nonaffected subjects so that it is not possible to use these as distinguishing characters. As one proceeds from phenylalanine blood level to hair colour, the difference between the means of the distributions tends to disappear while the variances increase. This is a good example of how extension of the analysis from a not well-selected 'final phenotype' (hair colour or head size, for example) to an intermediate phenotype more closely related to the genetic defect (phenylalanine serum levels) can reveal a qualitative genetic difference that contributes to the determination of hair colour, head size, or intelligence quotient in phenylketonuric patients, over an apparently complex polygenic background. In addition, the variation around the means in phenylalanine levels observed in both subjects with phenylketonuria and normals is the result of genetic and environmental (for example, dietary) factors, but homozygosity for the phenylketonuria gene clearly has a greater effect on phenylalanine levels than has any other common genetic or environmental factor.

HUMAN ESSENTIAL HYPERTENSION

Due to its genetic heterogeneity, it is highly likely that in man, the final phenotype 'essential hypertension' also develops through multiple genetic mechanisms. As in rats, however, the study of intermediate phenotypes may be of help in finding homogeneous subgroups of human subjects which become hypertensive with similar pathogenetic mechanisms.

It has long been recognized that patients with essential hypertension present differences, at least clinical ones. One of the first postulated subtypes of essential hypertension was 'low-renin' hypertension. Some sodium-replete patients with essential hypertension ('nonmodulators') have abnormal adrenal and renal vascular responses to Ang II infusion [17]. The state of being a 'nonmodulator' is heritable [18] and associated with elevated erythrocyte lithium–sodium countertransport values [19], another intermediate phenotype present only in a subset of patients. Patients with elevated sodium–potassium–chloride (Na-K-Cl) cotransport and low plasma renin activity (PRA) respond selectively to potassium canrenoate, whereas those with normal or high PRA and low or normal Na-K-Cl cotransport respond selectively to ACE inhibitors, to β-blockers [20], or to hydrochlorothiazide [21]. If the differences among subgroups of patients are due to the multigenic component of hypertension, this would justify efforts to identify the effect of the individual genes on the final expression of the phenotype 'hypertension'. Such efforts will probably be fruitless if the genetic component of blood pressure is determined only by additively acting polygenes, but fruitful if some major gene is present. If the final phenotype depends partly on a polygenic background associated with some major genes that make a substantial contribution to the phenotypic expression by allelic variation on single loci (plus the random effect of the environment), the closer we will be able to get to the primary gene products, the greater will be the separation between affected and nonaffected individuals, and the higher will be the power of resolution of our analysis. Note that in this case, we are dealing only with hypertensive subjects and that 'affected' and 'nonaffected' refer only to hypertensive subjects bearing or not bearing the specific gene (mutation) that is under investigation.

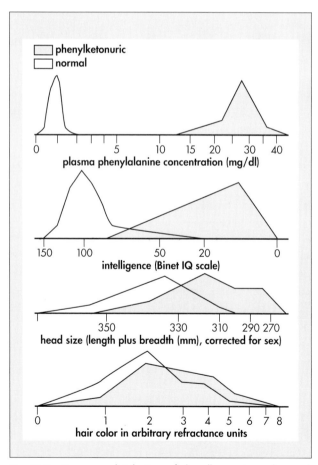

Fig. 61.2 Frequency distributions of phenylketonurics and normal subjects for plasma phenylalanine and the different intermediate phenotypes under study.

Penrose's example shows the approach that should be followed in studying the genetic mechanisms involved in the pathogenesis of hypertension. So far, only the final phenotype 'high blood pressure' has been considered, which might be viewed as similar to hair colour in phenylketonuric patients; Fig. 61.3 summarizes this concept by analogy with the dissection of the phenylketonuric trait. On the right of the figure, the increase in complexity is indicated from the bottom with a schematic representation of qualitative differences in RFLP patterns between hypertensives and controls (indicated with the arrows). There is a progressively greater overlap to the top of the figure, indicating the distribution of the phenotypic values at the different levels of organization. The broadening of the distribution is caused by the influence of the polygenic background and the environment (which both vary from one individual to another) on the effect of the major gene. Some of the major genes considered as 'candidate genes', that is, genes that are presumably relevant to hypertension, have recently been cloned, whereas others have not yet been identified [22].

RAT MODELS OF GENETIC HYPERTENSION

The fact that human essential hypertension is a complex disease with different pathogenetic mechanisms all leading to the final phenotype 'high blood pressure' is supported by studies on genetically hypertensive rat strains. Such studies have clearly shown that several independent pathogenic mechanisms may produce similar final phenotypes (hypertension), acting through very different intermediate phenotypes. An example is the difference between the development of hypertension in Milan hypertensive strain (MHS) rats and spontaneously hypertensive rats (SHR). Both strains develop a form of hypertension that is transplantable with the kidney, so a genetically inherited abnormality of kidney function must be present in both strains to produce hypertension [23–27].

When continuing the dissection of the phenotype 'kidney-function abnormality', some differences are found between MHS rats and SHR. Before and during the development of hypertension, MHS rats have a much more positive sodium balance

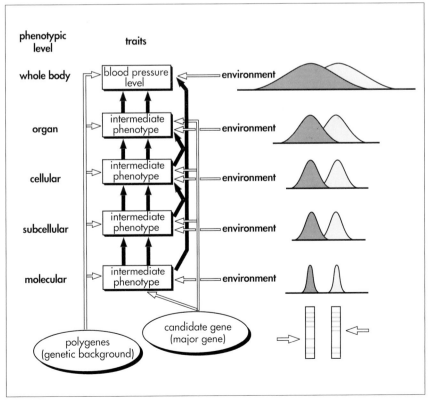

Fig. 61.3 Example of dissection of a complex phenotypic trait.

than have rats of the Milan normotensive strain (MNS), with concomitant reduction of PRA (probably secondary to increased body-fluid volumes) [28]. Tubuloglomerular feedback is blunted before and hyperactivated after the development of hypertension in MHS rats [29]. Isolated perfused prehypertensive kidneys from four-week-old MHS animals have a faster glomerular filtration rate (GFR) and greater sodium resorption than have controls [30]. They show increased sensitivity to furosemide, the selective inhibitor of Na-K-Cl cotransport, indicating that more sodium is reabsorbed through Na–K–Cl cotransport in MHS than in MNS rats [31]. It was then proposed that MHS rats become hypertensive through an increase of kidney tubular resorption, which involves an increase of Na-K-Cl cotransport [32,33]. Different changes have been reported in SHR including reduced total kidney as well as single nephron filtration rate and renal plasma flow in six-week-old animals [34].

Data on PRA are somewhat difficult to interpret, since some authors have found high, but others low, PRA levels in SHR compared with Wistar–Kyoto (WKY) rats. It must be noted that SHR have increased sympathetic acitivity [35] and that renin secretion is largely dependent on this. When PRA was measured in SHR with sympathetic activation carefully avoided, it was found to be reduced also in this strain [36]. Moreover, renin release is low in isolated perfused SHR kidneys [37] as well as in SHR kidney slices [38]. Tubuloglomerular feedback is hyperactive in young (five-week-old) SHR, as compared with WKY rats, but the difference tends to disappear in young-adult animals with fully

developed hypertension [39]. The SHR have low erythrocyte Na-K-Cl cotransport [40,41] (though not all authors agree on this [42]), and less sensitivity to furosemide in the isolated perfused kidney [43]. This observation is compatible with the hypothesis that the primary abnormality is an increase of preglomerular resistances or a decrease of ultrafiltration coefficient. Hypertension seems to compensate for this abnormality since the decrease in filtration rate tends to disappear in adult (12–16-week-old) SHR [44]. Some caution is needed, however, in interpreting the data on SHR. Some heterogeneities have been shown in SHR and WKY rat strains from different sources [45,46]. Figure 61.4 summarizes the differences at the final and intermediate phenotypic levels so far described for MHS rats and SHR compared with their respective controls. The figure suggests several points that are relevant for the way human essential hypertension should be viewed and studied: the methods of collecting data are of extreme importance, as exemplified by the values of PRA and Na-K-Cl cotransport reported in SHR by different investigators using different techniques; the timing of the study of the phenotypic value of the intermediate phenotype is critical, as exemplified by the dynamic changes of GFR and tubuloglomerular feedback sensitivity before and after the development of hypertension; and similar final phenotypic levels (blood pressure, effect of the transplanted kidney on the recipient's blood pressure, and PRA) present different intermediate phenotypes at a lesser level of complexity (GFR and flow, Na-K-Cl cotransport and furosemide sensitivity).

Phenotypic level		Milan hypertensive strain rats	Spontaneously hypertensive rats
final	blood pressure	↑	↑
whole body	blood pressure in the recipient of hypertensive kidney	↑	↑
whole body	plasma renin activity	↓	↓ (=, ↑)
organ	glomerular filtration rate (prehypertensive state)	↑	↓
organ	glomerular filtration rate (adult)	↑ =	=
organ	renal plasma flow (prehypertensive state)	=	↓
cell	furosemide inhibition of tubular sodium resorption	↑	↓
cell	tubuloglomerular feedback sensitivity (prehypertensive state)	↓	↑
cell	tubuloglomerular feedback sensitivity (adult)	↑	=
subcellular	Na-K-Cl cotransport	↑	↓ (↑)

Fig. 61.4 Differences between Milan hypertensive strain and spontaneously hypertensive rats at different phenotypic levels. The arrows indicate higher (↑), lower (↓), or equal (=) phenotypic value of the respective controls (Milan normotensive strain rats or Wistar–Kyoto rats).

A final note of caution must be added. The SHR strains are genetically inbred animals, and some criteria must be satisfied before any observed difference in intermediate phenotype between the hypertensive strain and its control may be proposed as relevant for the pathogenesis of hypertension in that particular strain. Rapp proposed three criteria (a paradigm) to show whether a given intermediate phenotype is relevant in explaining a blood-pressure difference between two strains of rats. First, the phenotype must be different in hypertensive and normotensive animals. Second, it must cosegregate with a significant increment of blood pressure in the F_2 generation produced by mating F_1 animals that resulted from crossing the parental strains (hypertensive x normotensive). The blood pressure distribution of F_2 will be very wide, ranging from normotensive to hypertensive values, due to the random assortment of the other genes influencing blood pressure which produces a wide range of new genotypes. Third, some logical biochemical or physiological link must be present between the intermediate phenotype and blood pressure [47].

Two alternative approaches can be followed in the search for genes whose allelic mutation is responsible for the development of a disease. If we have no idea which genes have a major effect in the 'final phenotype', we can try to identify some 'intermediate phenotypes' that are more closely related to the genetic defect. This approach may be called 'TOP-DOWN', since it starts from the peak of complexity, the final phenotype, and tries to analyze hypertension descending downwards to the primary genetic (molecular) defect. The second approach, which may be called by analogy, 'BOTTOM-UP', has recently received a great impetus from the techniques of molecular biology and from the availability of many genes that are believed to be relevant in blood-pressure control. It studies the genetic or molecular difference of the genes or primary gene products and tries to establish whether any polymorphism among hypertensive and normotensive subjects and families is relevant for the pathogenesis of hypertension.

THE 'BOTTOM-UP' APPROACH — MOLECULAR BIOLOGY OF THE RENIN GENE

Among the influences that play a major role in the control of blood pressure and volume homeostasis, the RAS is a major candidate for molecular biological studies. In fact, though circulating plasma renin levels are not substantially different in hypertensive and normotensive individuals, and apparently do not play a major role in the hypertension of genetically hypertensive rat strains, some observations suggest a possible role of local tissue renin–angiotensin

systems in blood-pressure control in several experimental conditions. As already recalled, the nonmodulator state is inheritable and associated with normal or high levels of PRA; Ang II infusion does not decrease renal plasma flow or increase aldosterone secretion adequately in these patients [48]. Moreover, ACE inhibition tends to normalize the modulation response selectively in the nonmodulators. This suggests that intrarenal Ang II concentration is abnormal in these patients, in spite of relatively normal circulating levels [49]. Indeed, renal renin or prorenin generation, which may well be under genetic control, might elevate blood pressure by increasing local Ang II concentration and hence shifting the pressure-natriuresis curve to the right [50,51] with no measurable concomitant change in PRA. Furthermore, ACE inhibitors injected directly into the cerebroventricular space, selectively reduce blood pressure in a stroke-prone substrain of SHR (SHR-SP) [52]. This is confirmed by the finding that the cerebrospinal fluid Ang II concentration is elevated, in spite of normal peripheral circulating levels, in SHR-SP [53] and also in some patients with essential hypertension [54]. All these observations justify the study of the genetics and molecular biology of the RAS in this connection.

The molecular biology of the RAS has been extensively reviewed [55,56], and is also surveyed elsewhere in this book (see *Chapter 3*). Human [57–59], rat [60], and mouse [61,62] renin genes have been cloned and homologies between species studied [63]. Mouse fibroblasts or pituitary tumors have been transfected with the human renin gene, showing the existence of different pathways of human renin secretion [64]. Data on transgenic animals are difficult to interpret. In order to produce hypertension in a transgenic mouse, both rat renin and angiotensinogen genes have to be present simultaneously in the same animal, whereas transgenic mice bearing only one transgene remain normotensive [65]. Finally, the transgenic mice bearing both transgenes have higher plasma levels of serum angiotensinogen and their blood pressure can be normalized by treatment with the ACE inhibitor, captopril. The opposite experiment performed by Mullins *et al* consisted of producing transgenic rats bearing mouse Ren-2 renin gene [66]. They introduced the mouse Ren-2 renin gene into the rat genome and thus caused severe hypertension. These transgenic animals represent a model for hypertension in which the genetic basis for the disease is known. Interestingly, transgenic animals do not overexpress active renin in the kidney and have low levels of active renin in their plasma, providing a new model for low-renin hypertension.

Furthermore, the influence of external factors (dietary sodium or other experimental conditions) on renin mRNA has been studied. Angiotensin II infusion increased liver angiotensinogen mRNA levels and decreased kidney renin mRNA levels, whereas enalapril treatment had the opposite effect, suggesting that Ang II is one of the factors that regulates angiotensinogen mRNA levels in the liver and renin mRNA levels in the kidney [67]. Desoxycorticosterone acetate (DOCA) plus salt treatment of rats suppresses the production of renin mRNA in the kidney, as compared with control rats receiving 0.4% NaCl in their diet; clipping of the left renal artery caused a three-fold increase in the steady-state level of renin mRNA in the ischemic kidney and a 0.5-fold decrease in the contralateral one. A high protein diet increases plasma renin as well as kidney renin mRNA, whereas liver or kidney angiotensinogen mRNA remains unchanged [68]. Lutwig *et al* treated rats by adrenalectomy, by ACE inhibition, or by a low salt diet plus furosemide and observed a parallel increase in both PRA and submandibular gland renin mRNA [69]. This indicates that expression of the renin gene *in vivo* is regulated by blood pressure as well as by other stimuli known to control peripheral renin levels [70], at least in some experimental conditions. Similar results were obtained in transgenic animals, with a two-fold reduction in renin mRNA in the kidneys of one-gene, two-gene, and transgenic mouse strains with a high NaCl diet compared with low NaCl diets. Moreover, it was shown that renin mRNAs derived from the different renin gene alleles are all NaCl responsive [71].

Although the level of renin gene mRNA seems responsive to normal stimuli in parallel with renin secretion, its regulation, however, seems different in normotensive and hypertensive animals. Samani *et al* reported higher renin mRNA levels (indicating increased renin-gene expression) in the kidneys, livers, brains, adrenals, and hearts of young (five-week-old) SHR, compared with WKY rats [72]. In older (12-week-old) animals, the renin level in the kidney became the same in the two strains whereas the levels in the heart and aorta were lower in SHR than in WKY rats, indicating a widespread abnormality of renin-gene expression in the SHR, modulated in some tissues by the development of hypertension [73]. Moreover, when SHR and WKY rats were treated with a low sodium diet and furosemide, or with captopril, a similar rise was observed in peripheral PRA in both strains, whereas levels of kidney renin mRNA of SHR were greater than those of the corresponding WKY rats [74]. These results indicate an enhanced expression of the renin gene in the kidney of SHR compared with WKY rats in response to stimuli that increase renin release. Although it is not clear whether the difference between SHR and WKY rats in mRNA content of the various organs has pathophysiological relevance, three facts need to be pointed out: first, peripheral PRA has not yet been demonstrated to have a clear role in the pathogenesis of hypertension in SHR,

since PRA was found to be normal or reduced in SHR; second, it is not clearly established that an increase in renin mRNA levels in a specific organ leads to increased renin secretion from that organ, since there are many steps between the translation process and the actual secretion; and third, the parallel increase of renin mRNA levels observed after stimuli that normally increase renin secretion seems to suggest, though does not prove, a difference in intrarenal generation of renin between SHR and WKY rats at different ages.

The most consistent result of the studies on the molecular structure of the renin gene in rats is a major polymorphism in its first intron (noncoding region). Samani *et al* found that the rat renin gene is polymorphic in its first intron, probably due to a variation of the number of copies of a 38-base-pair tandem-repeated sequence in the intron [75]. A 650-base-pair deletion of a tandem-repeat sequence was observed in the first intron in the SHR compared with their normotensive control WKY rats [72]. Studies in genetically hypertensive rats, however, have to be interpreted with caution, first because of the known heterogeneity of WKY rats and SHR from different sources [45,46], and second, because chance fixation of contrasting alleles in the homozygous state in the contrasting inbred strain due to genetic drift cannot be excluded *a priori*. This latter possibility found some support when the same analysis was repeated using an oligonucleotide probe complementary to the tandem-repeat sequence on two other spontaneously hypertensive strains (Lyon hypertensive (LH) and MHS); and also in comparison with several strains of Sprague–Dawley rats, with different results [76]. In the Milan rats, no difference was found in the size of the fragment enclosing the tandem-repeat region between MHS and MNS rats. In the Lyon rats, a difference of approximately 1.1kb was observed. The hypertensive (LH) and hypotensive (LL) Lyon strains are missing the same 1.1-kb fragment, which corresponds to 28 copies of the 38-base-pair tandem-repeat sequence, when compared with the normotensive (LN) strain. The finding of an identical deletion of part of the repeat sequence in the first intron of renin gene in rats with high and low blood pressure seems to suggest that the polymorphism of the first intron is not a major cause of the blood-pressure difference between LH and LN strains, and that the difference is due to chance fixation, although a small effect on blood pressure, masked by other genes, cannot be excluded. Finally, a study on Sprague–Dawley rats, from which the Lyon strain was derived, showed that the same kind of polymorphism as that of the Lyon strain segregates randomly in this population, with no relation to blood pressure.

Ongoing human studies are attempting to identify differences between hypertensive and normotensive individuals, but, although the human renin gene is also polymorphic, no evidence of cosegregation of renin-gene polymorphism with hypertension has been found for any of the restriction enzymes so far tested [77–79].

MOLECULAR BIOLOGY OF THE RENIN GENE: ITS RELATIONSHIP WITH BLOOD PRESSURE

So far, cosegregation of renin alleles and blood pressure have been studied in different rat strains by three groups of workers who reached very different conclusions. The first published reports by Rapp *et al* were on substrains (SS/Jr and SR/Jr) of Dahl rats and will be described in more detail [80]. Dahl rats are two substrains of genetically inbred animals. One (SS/Jr) develops a genetic form of severe hypertension when fed a high NaCl (8%) diet at weaning. The other (SR/Jr) shows little change in blood pressure if challenged with the same sodium load. Eight of 28 tested restriction enzymes gave different RFLP patterns for SS/Jr and SR/Jr rats [81]. This finding was interpreted as an important gene rearrangement in one of the strains. The study of genomic DNA demonstrated a 1.2-kb insertion/deletion mutation in the first intron of the renin gene [82]. The RFLP pattern of the SR/Jr rat was named Ren^r/Ren^r, and that of the SS/r, Ren^s/Ren^s. In both strains, the RFLP pattern was homozygous. Cosegregation analysis of renin-gene alleles and blood pressure was performed. All F_2 were genotyped and the distribution of the three possible genotypes (Ren^r/Ren^r, Ren^r/Ren^s, and Ren^s/Ren^s) was no different from the expected Mendelian ratio of 1:2:1. All F_2 were maintained on the standard high NaCl diet to produce the differences in blood pressure. The mean blood pressure values of the male individuals with the three different genotypes were highly significantly different and were 148.7mmHg for the Ren^r/Ren^r, 165.6mmHg for the Ren^r/Ren^s, and 171mmHg for the Ren^s/Ren^s [80]. This experiment indicates that the renin gene itself either is responsible for the observed blood-pressure differences or is closely linked genetically to some other as yet unknown genetic locus whose alleles are responsible for the blood-pressure rise in SS/Jr. The association between blood pressure and the Ren^s/Ren^s genotype, as well as the blood-pressure difference between this genotype and the Ren^r/Ren^r genotype, give an idea of the magnitude of this effect. In this case, one single abnormality in the renin gene accounted for a blood-pressure difference of 20mmHg between SS/Jr and SR/Jr since the other polygenes influencing blood pressure are by definition, distributed randomly in the F_2 generation. The remaining mean blood-pressure difference of approximately 60mmHg between the parental SS/Jr and SR/Jr strains depends on other as yet unidentified genes. Moreover,

since the renin-gene abnormality was found in the first intron, that is, a noncoding region of the genome, and since regulatory sites are believed to be located mostly in the first intron, it is reasonable to suppose that the difference in renin between SS/Jr and SR/Jr was not qualitative but quantitative, since its regulation or expression could be altered. The biochemical or physiological link between the observed genetic abnormality and blood pressure is less clear. Although renin levels are much lower in SS/Jr than in SR/Jr, and SS/Jr has been proposed as a model of the low-renin form of human hypertension, it is not clear how a genetically low or depressed production of renin should lead to high blood pressure, although transgenic rats, which develop a form of fulminating hypertension when they receive a graft of mouse renin Ren-2 gene, have surprisingly low levels of PRA [66].

Similar results were obtained in SHR by Kurtz *et al* [83]. Since WKY rats are not genetically homogeneous, Lewis rats, a strain of normotensive inbred rats, were used for crossbreeding experiments. As in Rapp's design for SS/Jr and SS/Jr crossbreeding, mean arterial pressures of the F_2 crosses with the different genotypes were compared. The blood pressure of the rats heterozygous for the renin allele (one from Lewis and one from SHR) was significantly higher (+8mmHg) than the blood pressure of the rats homozygous for the Lewis allele. Although slightly higher, the blood pressure of the F_2 homozygous for the SHR allele (5mmHg), was not sig-nificantly different from that of the F_2 homozygous for the Lewis allele.

Opposite results were reported by Lindpaintner *et al* on the F_2 produced by mating rats from SHR-SP and WKY. Again, a deletion of approximately 700 base pairs was reported in the first intron of SHR-SP, but no cosegregation of blood-pressure level or other phenotypical variables (heart rate, ventricular hypertrophy, absolute and relative magnitude of changes in blood pressure induced by stress or dietary sodium, PRA) was observed [84]. No explanation for these opposite findings is yet available.

In conclusion, only part of the difference in blood pressure between hypertensive and normotensive rat strains can be attributed to polymorphism of the renin gene or some other closely linked, as yet unknown, genes. Although the mechanisms underlying an allelic variation in the renin or closely linked genes are unknown, however, the use of molecular biology techniques is starting to provide useful information in this regard. Although the results so far obtained are inconsistent in different rat strains and negative in man, it is possible that a strong effect of the renin gene in a few patients, or a small effect in many patients, may have been missed, due to the polymorphic nature of human essential hypertension and the longstanding controversy over the classification of patients. Further studies, which possibly consider other genetic markers of hypertension, need to be performed on larger population samples.

REFERENCES

1. Miall WE, Henage P, Khosal T, Lovell HG, Moore P. Factors influencing the degree of resemblance in arterial pressure of close relatives. *Clinical Science* 1967;**33**:271–83.

2. Longini IM, Higgins MW, Minton PC, Moll PP, Keller JB. Environmental and genetic sources of familial aggregation of blood pressure in Tecumseh, Michigan. *American Journal of Epidemiology* 1984;**120**:131–44.

3. Havlik RJ, Garrison RJ, Feinleib M, Kannel WB, Castelli WP, McNamara PM. Blood pressure aggregation in families. *American Journal of Epidemiology* 1979;**110**:304–12.

4. Wolanski N. An approach to the problem of inheritance of systolic and diastolic blood pressure. *Genetica Polonica* 1969;**10**:263–8.

5. Hayes CG, Tyroler HA, Cassel CJ. Family aggregation of blood pressure in Evans County, Georgia. *Archives of Internal Medicine* 1971;**128**:965–75.

6. Shull WJ, Harburg E, Erfurt JC, Schork MA, Rice RA. A family set method for estimating heredity and stress: II. Preliminary results of the genetic methodology in a pilot survey of Negro blood pressure, Detroit 1966–67. *Journal of Chronic Diseases* 1970;**23**:83–92.

7. Cavalli Sforza LL, Bodmer WF. *The genetics of human populations*. New York: Freeman, 1973.

8. Harris H. Enzyme polymorphism in man. *Proceedings of the Royal Society (Series B)* 1966;**164**:298–310.

9. Williams RR, Dadone M, Hunt SC, *et al.* The genetic epidemiology of hypertension: A review of past studies and current results for 948 persons in 48 Utah pedigrees. In: Rao DC, Elston RC, Kuller LH, *et al*, eds. *Genetic epidemiology of coronary heart disease: Past, present and future.* New York: Alan R Liss, 1984; 419–44.

10. Weinberg R, Shear CL, Avet LM Frerichs RR, Fox M. Path analysis of environmental and genetic influences on blood pressure. *American Journal of Epidemiology* 1979;**109**:588–96.

11. Morton NE, Gulbrandsen Cl, Rao DC, Rhoads CG, Kagan A. Determinants of blood pressure in Japanese–American families. *Human Genetics* 1980;**53**:261–6.

12. Krieger H, Morton NE, Rao DC, Azevedo E. Familial determinants of blood pressure in northeastern Brazil. *Human Genetics* 1980;**53**:415–8.

13. Moll PP, Harburg E, Burns TL, Schork MA, Ozgoren F. Heredity, stress and blood pressure, a family set approach: The Detroit project revisited. *Journal of Chronic Diseases* 1983;**36**:317–28.

14. Longini IM, Higgins MW, Hinton PC, Moll PP, Keller JB. Environmental and genetic sources of familial aggregation of blood pressure in Tecumseh, Michigan. *American Journal of Epidemiology* 1984;**120**:131–44.

15. Penrose LS. Measurement of pleiotropic effect in phenylketonuria. *Annals of Eugenics* 1952;**16**:134–41.

16. Ledley FD, Levy HL, Woo SLC. Molecular analysis of the inheritance of phenylketonuria and mild phenylalaninemia in families with both disorders. *New England Journal of Medicine* 1986;**314**:1276–80.

17. Hollenberg NK, Moore T, Shoback D, Redgrave J, Rainbowe S, Williams GH. Abnormal renal sodium handling in essential hypertension. Relation to failure of renal and adrenal modulation of responses to angiotensin II. *American Journal of Medicine* 1986;**81**:412–8.

18. Dluhy RG, Hopkins P, Hollenberg NK, Williams GH. Heritable abnormalities of the renin–angiotensin–aldosterone system in essential hypertension. *Journal of Cardiovascular Pharmacology* 1988;**12** (suppl 3):s145–54.

19. Redgrave J, Canessa M, Gleason R, Hollenberg NK, Williams GH. Red blood cell lithium–sodium countertransport of non-modulating essential hypertension. *Hypertension* 1989;**13**:721–6.

20. Niutta E, Cusi D, Colombo R, Pellizzoni M, Cesana B, Barlassina C, Soldati L, Bianchi G. Predicting interindividual variations in antihypertensive therapy: The role of sodium transport systems and renin. *Journal of Hypertension* 1990;**8** (suppl 4):s53–8.

21. Manunta P, Melis MG, Niutta E, Cusi D, Colombo R, Barlassina C, Melis MG, Pellizzoni M, Glorioso N, Bianchi G. Variation in the individual response to antihypertensive drugs. *13th Scientific Meeting of the International Society of Hypertension, Montreal* 1990:Abstract.

22. Sing CF, Boerwinkle E, Turner ST. Genetics of primary hypertension. *Clinical and Experimental Hypertension* 1986;[A]**8**:623–51.

23. Rettig R, Stauss H, Floberth D, Ganten D, Waldherr R, Unger T. Hypertension transmitted by kidneys from stroke-prone spontaneously hypertensive rats. *American Journal of Physiology* 1989;**257**:F197–203.

24. Rettig R, Folberth C, Stauss H, Kopf D, Waldherr R, Unger T. Role of the kidney in primary hypertension. A renal transplantation study in rats. *American Journal of Physiology* 1990;**258**:F606-61.

25. Rettig R, Kopf D, Unger T. Posttransplantation hypertension in recipients of renal grafts from prehypertensive SHR donors. *Journal of Hypertension* 1990;**8** (suppl 3): s21.

26. Bianchi G, Fox U, Di Francesco GF, Giovannetti AM, Pagetti D. Blood pressure changes produced by kidney cross-transplantation between spontaneously hypertensive and normotensive rats. *Clinical Science and Molecular Medicine* 1974;**47**:435–48.

27. Fox U, Bianchi G. The primary role of the kidney in causing the blood pressure differences in the Milan hypertensive strain (MHS) and normotensive rats. *Clinical and Experimental Pharmacology and Physiology* 1976;suppl **3**:71–4.

28. Bianchi G, Baer PG, Fox U, Duzzi L, Pagetti D, Giovannetti AM. Changes in renin, water balance and sodium balance during development of high blood pressure in genetically hypertensive rats. *Circulation Research* 1975;**36–37** (suppl 1):153–61.

29. Boberg U, Persson EG. Increased tubulo-glomerular feed-back activity in Milan hypertensive rats. *American Journal of Physiology* 1986;**250**:F967–74.

30. Salvati P, Pinciroli GP, Bianchi G. Renal function of isolated perfused kidneys from hypertensive (MHS) and normotensive (MNS) rats of the Milan strain at different ages. *Journal of Hypertension* 1984;**2** (suppl 3):s351–3.

31. Salvati P, Ferrario RG, Bianchi G. Diuretic effect of bumetanide in isolated perfused kidneys of Milan hypertensive rats. *Kidney International* 1990;**37**: 1084–9.

32. Bianchi G, Ferrari P, Trizio D, Ferrandi M, Torielli L, Barber BR, Polli E. Red blood cell abnormalities and spontaneous hypertension in the rat. *Hypertension* 1985;**7**:319–25.

33. Ferrandi M, Salardi S, Parenti P, Ferrari P, Bianchi G, Braw R, Karlish JD. Na, K, Cl co-transport mediated by Rb fluxes in membrane vesicles from kidneys of normotensive and hypertensive rats. *Biochemica et Biophysica Acta* 1990;**1021**: 13–20.

34. Dilley JR, Stier CT, Arendshorst WJ. Abnormalities in glomerular function in rats developing spontaneous hypertension. *American Journal of Physiology* 1984;**246**:F12–20.

35. De Wardener HE. The primary role of the kidney and salt intake in the aetiology of hypertension: Part I. *Clinical Science* 1990;**79**:193–200.

36. Shiono K, Sokabe H. Renin–angiotensin system in spontaneously hypertensive rats. *American Journal of Physiology* 1976;**231**:1295–9.

37. Tobian L, Johnson MA, Lange J, Magraw S. Effect of varying perfusion pressures on the output of sodium and renin and the vascular resistance in kidneys of rats with 'post-salt' hypertension and Kyoto spontaneous hypertension. *Circulation Research* 1975;**36&37** (suppl 1):162–70.

38. Watanabe M, Nishikawa T, Takagi T, Kamiyama Y, Tamura Y, Kumagay A. Mechanism of suppressed renin–angiotensin system in spontaneously hypertensive rat. *Clinical and Experimental Hypertension. Part A, Theory and Practice* 1983;A**5**:49–70.

39. Dilley JR, Arendshorst WJ. Enhanced tubuloglomerular feed-back activity in rats developing spontaneous hypertension. *American Journal of Physiology* 1984;**247**:F672–9.

40. De Mendonca M, Knorr A, Grichois ML, Ben-Ishay D, Garay RP, Meyer P. Erythrocytic sodium ion transport systems in primary and secondary hypertension of the rat. *Kidney International* 1982;**21** (suppl 11):s69–75.

41. Rosati C, Meyer P, Garay R. Sodium transport kinetics in erythrocytes from spontaneously hypertensive rats. *Hypertension* 1988;11:41–8.

42. Orlov SN, Postnov IY, Pokudin NI, Kukharenko VY, Postnov YV. Na$^+$–H$^+$ exchange and other ion-transport systems in erythrocytes of essential hypertensive and spontaneously hypertensive rats: A comparative analysis. *Journal of Hypertension* 1989;7:781–8.

43. Raine EAG, Roberts AFC, Ledingham JGG. Resetting of pressure-natriuresis and furosemide sensitivity in spontaneously hypertensive rats. *Journal of Hypertension* 1984;2 (suppl 2):359–61.

44. Azar S, Johnson MA, Scheinman J, Bruno L, Tobian L. Regulation of glomerular capillary pressure and filtration rate in young Kyoto hypertensive rats. *Clinical Science* 1979;56:203–9.

45. Louis WJ, Howes LG. Genealogy of the spontaneously hypertensive rat and Wistar–Kyoto rat strains: Implications for studies of inherited hypertension. *Journal of Cardiovascular Pharmacology* 1990;16 (suppl 7):s1–5.

46. Kurtz TW, Montano M, Chan L, Kabra P. Molecular evidence of genetic heterogeneity in Wistar–Kyoto rats: Implications for research with the spontaneously hypertensive rat. *Hypertension* 1989;13:188–92.

47. Rapp JP. Genetics of experimental and human hypertension. In: Genest J, Kuchel O, Hamet P, Cantin M, eds. *Hypertension: Pathophysiology and treatment. 2nd edition.* New York: McGraw-Hill, 1983;582–98.

48. Williams GH, Hollenberg NK. Abnormal adrenal and renal response to angiotensin II in essential hypertension: Implications for pathogenesis. In: Edwards CRW, Carey RM, eds. *Essential hypertension as an endocrine disease.* London: Butterworth, 1985;479–500.

49. Redgrave JH, Rabinowe SL, Hollenberg NK, Williams GH. Correction of abnormal renal blood flow response to angiotensin II by converting-enzyme inhibition in essential hypertensives. *Journal of Clinical Investigation* 1985;75:1285–90.

50. Sealey JE, Rubattu S. Prorenin and renin as separate mediators of tissue and circulating systems. *American Journal of Hypertension* 1989;2:358–66.

51. Guyton AC. The surprising kidney-fluid mechanism for pressure control — Its infinite gain! *Hypertension* 1990;16:725–30.

52. Unger T, Kaufmann–Beuhler I, Schoelkens BA, Ganten D. Brain converting enzyme inhibition: A possible mechanism for the antihypertensive action of captopril in spontaneously hypertensive rats. *European Journal of Pharmacology* 1981;70:467–78.

53. Deboben A, Inagami T, Ganten D. Tissue renin. In: Genest J, Kuchel O, Hamet P, Cantin M, eds. *Hypertension: Physiopathology and treatment, 2nd edition.* New York: McGraw Hill, 1983:194–209.

54. Eggena P, Ito T, Barrett JD, Villareal H, Sambhi MP. A comparison of human renin substrate in plasma and cerebrospinal fluid. In: Ganten D, Prinz M, Phillips MI, Schoelkens BA, eds. *Experimental Brain research (suppl 4): The renin–angiotensin system in the brain.* New York: Springer–Verlag, 1982:169–177.

55. Dzau VJ, Burt DW, Pratt RE. Molecular biology of the renin – angiotensin system. *American Journal of Physiology.* 1988;255:F563–73.

56. Dzau VJ, Paul M, Nakamura N, Pratt RE, Ingelfinger JR. Role of molecular biology in hypertension research. *EMBO Journal* 1982;11:1461–6.

57. Soubrier F, Panthier JJ, Corvol P, Rougeon F. Molecular cloning of human renin cDNA fragment. *Nucelic Acids Research* 1983;11:7181–90.

58. Hardman JA, Hort YJ, Catanzaro DF, Tellman JT, Baxter JD, Morris BJ, Shine J. Primary structure of human renin gene. *DNA* 1984;3:457–68.

59. Miyazaki H, Fukamizu A, Hirose S, Hayashi T, Hori H, Ohkubo H, Nakanishi S, Murakami K. Structure of the human renin gene. *Proceedings of the National Academy of Sciences of the USA* 1984;81:5999–6003.

60. Burnham CE, Hawelu-Johnson CL, Frank BM, Lynch KR. Molecular cloning of rat renin cDNA and its gene. *Proceedings of the National Academy of Sciences of the USA* 1987;84:5600–9.

61. Mullins DW, Burt DW, Windass DJ, Mc Turk P, George H, Brammar WJ. Molecular cloning of two distinct renin genes from DBA/2 mouse. *EMBO Journal* 1982;11:1461–6.

62. Field LJ, Gross KW. Ren-1 and Ren-2 loci are expressed in mouse kidney. *Proceedings of the National Academy of Sciences of the USA* 1985;82:6196–6200.

63. Soubrier F, Panthier JJ, Houot AM, Rougeon F, Corvol P. Segmental homology between the promoter region of the human renin gene and the mouse Ren 1 and Ren 2 promoter regions. *Gene* 1986;41:85–92.

64. Pratt RE, Flynn JA, Hobart PM, Paul M, Dzau VJ. Different secretory pathways of renin from mouse cells transfected with human renin gene. *Journal of Biological Chemistry* 1988;263:3137–41.

65. Ohkubo H, Kawakami H, Kakehi Y, Takumi T, Arai H, Yokota Y, Iwai M, Tanabe Y, Masu M, Hata J, Iwao H, Okamoto H, Yokoyama M, Nomura T, Katsuki M, Nakanishi S. Generation of transgenic mice with elevated blood pressure by introduction of the rat renin and angiotensinogen genes. *Proceedings of the National Academy of Sciences of the USA* 1990;87:5153–7.

66. Mullins JJ, Peters J, Ganten D. Fulminant hypertension in transgenic rats harbouring the mouse Ren-2 gene. *Nature* 1990;334:541–4.

67. Nakamura A, Iwao H, Fukui K, Kimura S, Tamaki T, Nakanishi S, Abe Y. Regulation of liver angiotensinogen and kidney renin mRNA levels by angiotensin II. *American Journal of Physiology* 1990;258:E1–6.

68. Rosenberg ME, Chmielewski D, Hostetter TH. Effect of dietary protein on rat renin and angiotensinogen gene expression. *Journal of Clinical Investigation* 1990;85:1144–9.

69. Ludwig G, Ganten D, Murakami K, Fasching U, Hackenthal E. Relationship between renin mRNA, and renin secretion in adrenalectomised, salt depleted or converting enzyme inhibitor treated rats. *Molecular and Cellular Endocrinology* 1987;50:223–9.

70. Makrides SC, Mulinari R, Zannis VI, Gavras H. Regulation of renin gene expression in hypertensive rats. *Hypertension* 1988;12:405–10.

71. Miller CCJ, Samani NJ, Carter AT, Brooks JI, Brammar WJ. Modulaton of mouse renin gene expression by dietary sodium chloride intake in one-gene, two-gene and transgenic mice. *Journal of Hypertension* 1989;7:861–3.

72. Samani NJ, Brammar WJ, Swales JD. Renal and extra-renal renin gene expression. Effects of salt intake, hypertension and genetic background [Abstract]. *Journal of Hypertension* 1988;6:940.

73. Samani NJ, Swales JD, Brammar WJ. A widespread abnormality of renin gene expression in the spontaneously hypertensive rat: Modulation in some tissues with the development of hypertension. *Clinical Science* 1989;77:629–34.

74. Kitami Y, Hiwada K, Kokubu T. Kidney renin gene expression in spontaneously hypertensive rats. *Journal of Hypertension* 1989;7:727–31.

75. Samani NJ, Brammar WJ, Swales JD. A major structural abnormality in the renin gene of the spontaneously hypertensive rat. *Journal of Hypertension* 1989;7:249–54.

76. Samani NJ, Vincent M, Sassard J, Henderson IW, Kaiser MA, Brammar WJ, Swales JD. Analysis of the renin gene intron A tandem repeat region of Milan and Lyon hypertensive rat strains. *Journal of Hypertension* 1990;8:805–9.

77. Morris BJ, Griffiths LR. Frequency in hypertensives of alleles for a RFLP associated with the renin gene. *Biochemical and Biophysical Research Communications* 1989;150:219–24.

78. Naftilan AJ, Williams R, Burt D, Paul M, Pratt RE, Hobart P, Chirgwing J, Dzau VJ. A lack of genetic linkage of renin gene restriction fragment length polymorphism with human hypertension. *Hypertension* 1989;14:614–8.

79. Soubrier F, Jeunmaitre X, Rigat B, Houot AM, Cambien F, Corvol P. Similar frequencies of renin gene restriction fragment length polymorphism in hypertensive and normotensive subjects. *Hypertension* 1990;16:712–7.

80. Rapp JP, Wang S-M, Dene H. A genetic polymorphism in the renin gene of Dahl rats cosegregates with blood pressure. *Science* 1989;243:542–4.

81. Dene H, Wang S-M, Rapp JP. Restriction fragment length polymorphism for the renin gene in Dahl rats. *Journal of Hypertension* 1989;7:121–6.

82. Wang S-M, Rapp JP. Structural differences in the renin gene of Dahl salt-sensitive and salt-resistant rats. *Molecular Endocrinology* 1989;3:288–94.

83. Kurtz TW, Simonet L, Kabra PM, Wolfe S, Chan L, Hjelle BL. Cosegregation of renin allele of the spontaneously hypertensive rat with an increase in blood pressure. *Journal of Clinical Investigation* 1990;85:1328–1332.

84. Lindpaintner K, Takahashi S, Ganten D. Structural alterations of the renin gene in stroke-prone spontaneously hypertensive rats: Examination of genotype–phenotype correlations. *Journal of Hypertension* 1990;8:763–73.

62 THE RENIN–ANGIOTENSIN SYSTEM IN ESSENTIAL HYPERTENSION

JOHN D SWALES

INTRODUCTION

The role of a pressor substance derived from the kidneys in hypertension was a source of controversy for many years after the original observation of Tigerstedt and Bergman (see *Chapter 1*). Uncertainty was the result of technical shortcomings on two fronts. Firstly, demonstration and measurement of renin proved difficult in the absence of any knowledge of its properties. Secondly, there was no reproducible model of hypertension.

The development of Goldblatt's model, initially in the dog [1] and subsequently in other species [2], made an enormous contribution to studies of the pathogenesis of hypertension. It is ironic, if by no means unique, in the history of medicine that Goldblatt's starting hypothesis was probably erroneous. Thus, noting the fact that nephrosclerosis was almost always associated with hypertension, he suggested that vascular disease was the cause rather than the effect of high blood pressure in patients with essential hypertension [1]. The Goldblatt model of hypertension was developed as a means of reproducing the effects of human renal vascular changes by constriction of the renal arteries. The unexpected finding that unilateral renal artery constriction could elevate blood pressure led directly to the recognition of renovascular hypertension in man and to its correction by surgery [3]. Goldblatt's concept of essential hypertension being a disease caused by release of a renal pressor substance as a result of renal vascular disease was not generally accepted for two reasons. Firstly, the development of a bioassay for plasma renin failed to demonstrate elevated levels in the majority of patients with essential hypertension [4]. Secondly, renal vascular changes associated with hypertension appeared to be secondary. Thus, increased renal vascular resistance and decreased renal blood flow appear to be features of established, rather than early, hypertension [5–7]. Even more persuasive, however, is the fact that structural changes in the renal vasculature occur in the nonclipped kidney only after blood pressure has become elevated as a result of unilateral renal artery constriction (the Goldblatt 2-kidney, 1-clip model). By contrast, the ischemic kidney 'protected' by a clip does not show vascular thickening [8]. As a result of these observations, the concept that essential hypertension is caused by increased renin secretion as a result of renal vascular disease has been abandoned. Nevertheless, recognition of the RAS as a major factor in blood-pressure regulation has led some groups to suggest that it may participate in the pathogenesis of essential hypertension.

PLASMA RENIN IN ESSENTIAL HYPERTENSION

Strong evidence that essential hypertension is multifactorial [9] suggests that abnormalities of renin secretion may at most, play only a part in blood-pressure elevation. Comparison between small groups of hypertensive individuals and normotensive controls may therefore be insufficient to demonstrate such a role. Furthermore, where control and hypertensive subjects have been selected from different populations, it is possible that differences may be due to confounding factors unrelated to hypertension *per se*. Ideally, therefore, an investigation of plasma renin in essential hypertension should be based upon population studies in which renin is measured in relation to blood-pressure level. Such population studies have been carried out by three groups of investigators.

Lucas *et al* randomly selected 154 men and women from the Stanford Heart Disease Prevention Program [10]. Subjects were classified as hypertensive or normotensive using a blood pressure of 140/90mmHg as the dividing line. There was an inverse relationship between plasma renin activity (PRA) and blood pressure in the normotensive subjects but not in the hypertensive individuals. The authors concluded that renin was inappropriately elevated for blood pressure in subjects with essential hypertension. The concept of the inappropriate is of dubious validity when applied to a variable such as plasma renin, which has multiple determinants. Thus, plasma renin may appear inappropriately high for a given blood pressure, but may be quite appropriate for the state of sodium balance or sympathetic drive to the kidneys [11]. The comparatively small numbers of subjects recruited, and the use of an arbitrary criterion to divide a population into hypertensive and normotensive subjects, limit the value of this study.

Meade *et al* embarked on a much larger population study of 1,999 individuals randomly selected from several working populations in north and west London. No attempt was made to divide subjects into hypertensive and normotensive although 64 (51 men and 13 women) had been diagnosed as hypertensive in the past [12]. Overall, there was an inverse association between systolic (and to a lesser extent, diastolic) blood pressure and PRA such that PRA fell by 8.4% for each increase of one standard deviation in systolic blood pressure in men (Fig. 62.1). The relationship was less obvious for women. In both sexes, however, it was very weak: thus, blood pressure accounted for less than 1% of variance in PRA. Plasma renin activity fell with increasing age, was lower in women than in men, and was considerably lower in blacks of either sex than in whites.

In the most carefully matched comparison, using subjects recruited from the same working population, Thomas *et al* demonstrated reduced PRA in 89 hypertensive patients compared with age- and sex-matched controls [13].

As a group, therefore, essential hypertensives exhibit a modest suppression of plasma renin. Unfortunately, the normal range for plasma renin in normal subjects (particularly in the older age groups) approaches the limit of detectability of many assay methods. It is therefore sometimes difficult to assess the degree of

Stimulus	Number with suppressed renin response	Reference
none	174/600	19
none	6/68	20
low salt + thiazide	12/30	21
low salt + diazoxide	8/25	18
low salt, upright	6/14	22
low salt, upright	16/60	23
	5/24	24
nitroprusside	12/28	25
low salt, upright	12/45	26
sodium restriction and standing	85/300 (63 on 2 occasions)	27
sodium restriction	11/21	28

Fig 62.2 Proportion of essential hypertensives with suppressed renin response to stimulation. Modified from Jose A *et al* [26].

suppression of plasma renin when only basal levels are measured. It is more easy to demonstrate suppression of plasma renin secretion by attempted stimulation with dietary salt depletion (with or without standing) [14], diuretics [13–17], or diazoxide [18]. Under these circumstances, many patients with essential hypertension show a subnormal response (Fig. 62.2). In most cases, results are presented using the response of normotensive controls as a criterion of normality. Usually, results are presented as a percentage of patients exhibiting 'low-renin hypertension'. Since factors such as age, race, and sex are determinants of renin responsiveness, the use of a 'normal range' applied to different populations is open to considerable question. Classification of patients into 'renin subgroups' also presupposes that these groups form discrete biological entities.

RENIN SUBGROUPS

Three studies examined the characteristics of the distribution of plasma renin among patients with essential hypertension. Two reports were based on referred patients [29,30] so that the representative nature of the populations investigated cannot be assumed, although it seems more likely that selective referral would create spurious subgroups within the renin distribution rather than the converse.

Padfield *et al* measured plasma renin concentration in 81 untreated hypertensive patients. Distribution was unimodal with

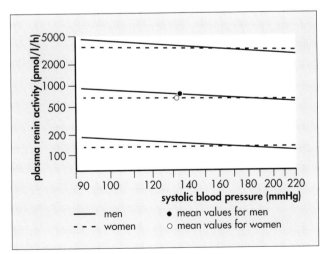

Fig. 62.1 Decrease of renin (measured as plasma renin activity: PRA) with systolic blood pressure (first reading). Fitted regression slopes and 95% population range are shown. Results are adjusted for age. Mean values of plasma renin activity and systolic blood pressure are shown. Modified from Meade TW *et al* [12].

no evidence of a separate subgroup of patients with 'low-renin hypertension' [29]. Exchangeable sodium was not elevated, although exchangeable potassium was reduced in patients at the lower end of the renin distribution. When five hypokalemic patients, however, were excluded, exchangeable potassium was normal in the remaining patients. It seems possible therefore that a small minority of patients had mineralocorticoid excess although the proportion of these patients fell well short of the expected number of patients with 'low-renin hypertension'.

Thurston *et al* measured PRA in 181 patients referred to a hospital outpatient clinic; 15 of these were excluded because of abnormalities of renal function [30]. Plasma renin activity was distributed as a smooth unimodal curve that could be normalized by taking the square root of PRA. After seven days of treatment with bendrofluazide (5mg/d), the percentage rise in PRA was much less than that in age-matched controls (Fig. 62.3). One-third of patients showed a stimulated renin that fell below the range encountered in normotensive-matched subjects treated similarly, although the distribution of stimulated PRA was still smooth and unimodal (Fig. 62.4). Of the patients in this study, 17% had a baseline PRA which lay above the range of values observed in normotensive subjects.

Thomas *et al* [13] investigated PRA in patients and controls derived from the same working population with very similar results to those of Padfield and Thurston and their colleagues. Plasma renin activity after logarithmic transformation was distributed as a smooth unimodal curve. Renin secretion was then stimulated both in normotensive controls and in hypertensive patients by administration of furosemide. The hypertensive group showed a reduced renin response that was not confined to patients whose baseline renin values were at the lower end of the range.

Although the source of patients was different in these three studies, there is unanimity in the conclusion that subdivision of

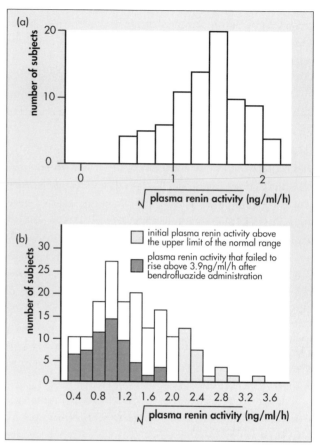

Fig. 62.3 (a) Distribution of square root plasma renin activity (PRA) in 83 normotensive subjects. (b) Distribution of square root PRA in essential hypertensive patients. Modified from Thurston H *et al* [30].

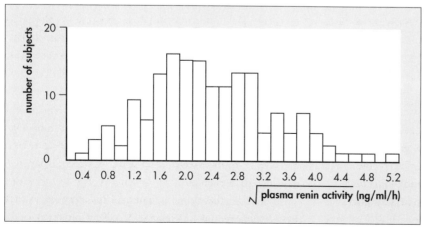

Fig 62.4 Distribution of square root plasma renin activity of hypertensive subjects after bendrofluazide for one week. Modified from Thurston H *et al* [30].

hypertensives into renin subgroups is arbitrary, whether such subdivision is based upon baseline values or upon stimulated values.

REPRODUCIBILITY OF RENIN SUBGROUPS

The absence of any clear dividing line within plasma renin distribution makes it necessary to adopt arbitrary criteria for classification. Not surprisingly, under these circumstances, reproducibility is fairly poor. Thus, restudy results in a reclassification of 20–30% of hypertensives [31]. Furthermore, different stimuli do not identify the same individuals when applied to the same population. In some comparisons, consistency was observed in only 50–80% of cases where different modes of stimulating the RAS were employed [14]. Lastly, treatment can result in reclassification of patients. Thus, prolonged diuretic treatment results in substantial numbers of patients diagnosed initially as having low-renin hypertension, subsequently regaining renin responsiveness to stimulation [32–35].

VOLUME EXPANSION IN LOW-RENIN HYPERTENSION

The absence of bi- or multimodality does not necessarily indicate that suppression of renin secretion in essential hypertension cannot provide a relevant pathogenetic clue. Renin suppression could serve as an indicator of one or a number of pathogenetic factors. Thus, Laragh's group has suggested that the renin subgroup to which a patient belongs has significance for pathogenesis, treatment, and prognosis [36–38]. A rather different criterion is used to distinguish low-renin hypertension and the results therefore are difficult to extrapolate to other clinical series. Plasma renin activity is plotted against 24-hour urinary sodium output, which is used as an index for sodium intake. Since it is argued that, patients with low-renin hypertension have a plasma renin that is low for their salt intake, renin values will lie below the confidence limits for the regression of renin upon 24-hour urinary sodium. Conversely, patients with high-renin hypertension lie above the confidence limits of the regression equation. While this approach has the merit of simplicity, it is difficult to utilize the nomogram when subjects consume conventional sodium intakes. Thus, plasma renin in normal subjects extends almost to the lower level of detectability for the range of sodium intakes commonly encountered (100–200mmol/d), so that low-renin hypertension can only reliably be diagnosed from the 24-hour urinary sodium

nomogram when sodium intake has been restricted to 50mmol/d or less. Confident diagnosis of low-renin hypertension using the nomogram therefore involves a degree of sodium restriction. Laragh's group has usually employed linear axes when constructing this nomogram, which results in the plot having the form of a rectangular hyperbola. It has been pointed out that with logarithmic axes, the relationship becomes rectilinear, greatly facilitating interpretation [104] (see *Chapter 83*).

Using extensive clinic experience based upon the 24-hour nomogram, Laragh has postulated that renin subgrouping provides a clue about the mechanism of hypertension [37,38]. According to this hypothesis, it is suggested that a volume factor predominates in low-renin hypertension and a vasoconstrictor factor in the high-renin group. Since both factors can co-exist and make a graded contribution to hypertension, bimodality would not necessarily be expected.

The hypothesis that renin in low-renin hypertension is suppressed by volume expansion initially proved extremely popular. Thus, there was an obvious analogy between low-renin essential hypertension and primary aldosteronism (*Chapter 63*). Several steroid hormones were targeted as possible candidates for putative volume expansion [39–42]. These included deoxycorticosterone (DOC), 18-hydroxydeoxycorticosterone (18-OH-DOC), 16-β-hydroxydehydroepiandrosterone (16-β-OHDEA), and 16-α-18-dihydrodeoxycorticosterone (16-α-18-diOHDOC). It was not possible to incriminate these steroids either on the grounds of only weak mineralocorticoid activity or because levels were insufficient to cause hypertension. In addition, *in vitro* tests failed to demonstrate an increase in mineralocorticoid activity in the serum of patients with low-renin essential hypertension [43]. Furthermore, plasma aldosterone secretion is usually normal in low-renin essential hypertension whereas it would be expected to be suppressed by excessive levels of other mineralocorticoids [44,45]. The absence of reduced serum potassium is also not consistent with excessive mineralocorticoid activity.

Laragh and colleagues [46] have proposed an alternative explanation of low renin levels in hypertensive patients. They argued that there are two functionally abnormal types of nephrons in patients with essential hypertension. Ischemic nephrons hypersecrete renin, but fail to excrete sodium normally. Secondly, a more numerous group of normal nephrons are in a state of sustained hypernatriuresis as a result of sodium retention. As a consequence, sodium load to distal nephrons is increased and renin suppressed. The hypersecretion of renin by ischemic nephrons tends to attenuate compensatory natriuresis in normal nephrons. The balance of these effects results in maintenance of high blood pressure either by abnormal sodium retention or by inappropriately high plasma renin levels. While ingenious, this hypothesis has been presented in very simple terms of individual nephron structure, renin content, and function. The nephron population by contrast, is remarkably diverse in structure, function, and individual renin content [105,106], while the distribution of renin and single nephron function vary greatly in response to stimuli such as changes in sodium balance or renal ischemia [107,108] (*Chapter 21*). It would be of interest to have the hypothesis developed taking this knowledge into account.

Both the mineralocorticoid hypothesis of low-renin hypertension and the more recent Laragh 'nephron heterogeneity' hypothesis require maintenance of blood pressure by volume expansion in 'low-renin essential hypertension'. Although there were early claims that sodium and fluid retention were responsible for the reduced plasma renin level in low-renin hypertension, more recent studies measuring plasma volume or exchangeable sodium have uniformly failed to demonstrate this [26,47–50]. Julius and co-workers have produced evidence for an alternative explanation, that there is redistribution of blood centrally,

producing a relative increase in cardiopulmonary volume. Thus, venous compliance was reduced in patients with 'low-renin hypertension' [51]. The marked tendency for patients with 'low-renin hypertension' to be older, would suggest that this hemodynamic change, if it is responsible for suppression of renin, is a secondary one. Other indirect evidence has been adduced in favor of volume expansion. Thus low-renin essential hypertensives have been claimed to have a greater reduction in leukocyte ouabain-sensitive sodium efflux than other hypertensives [52]. The relationship between leukocyte sodium-pump activity and volume expansion is, however, controversial [53] and such evidence is unpersuasive. It could be argued by proponents of the volume hypothesis of low-renin hypertension that demonstrable volume expansion is corrected by volume-regulatory homeostatic systems at the stage at which chronic hypertension is present. The tendency, however, in almost all published series for patients with low-renin hypertension to be older than other groups, suggests strongly that suppression of renin secretion is a secondary change. The volume hypothesis of low-renin hypertension has shown

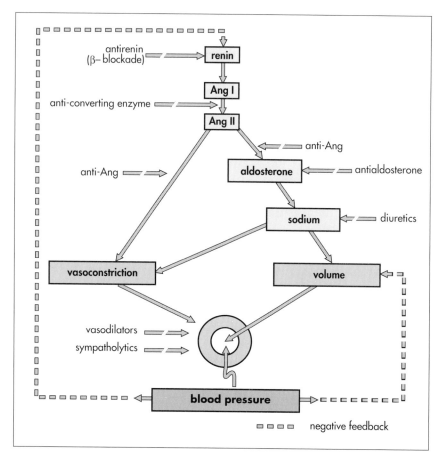

Fig. 62.5 Sites of intervention of various antihypertensive drugs. The proposed modes of treatment are according to Laragh's 'vasoconstriction-volume' hypothesis. Modified from Laragh JH [54].

a remarkable capacity for survival in the literature of essential hypertension despite the singular lack of evidence to support it.

RENIN SUBGROUPS AND THE RESPONSE TO TREATMENT

Laragh's group has suggested that classification of patients into renin subgroups provides guidance for management [37]. It was suggested that patients with low-renin hypertension responded particularly well to diuretics, while patients with high-renin hypertension responded to β-adrenoceptor blockers (Fig. 62.5). Later, the treatment schedule was modified as it was suggested that responsiveness of the two groups was not as sharply demarcated as was originally claimed [54].

Experience from other centers has been mixed. Some groups have found a relationship between initial renin and blood-pressure response to β-blockade or a diuretic [55]. Most groups, however, have not [30, 56–58]. In addition, it is possible to demonstrate the divergent effects upon blood pressure and renin using different β-blockers that have little effect upon renin, but still retain their antihypertensive action [59,60]. The mode of action of β-adrenoceptor blockers may be dose dependent in this respect. Thus, Hollifield et al demonstrated that the antihypertensive action of propranolol was directly related to plasma renin only when small doses of the drug were used. With higher doses, propranolol lowered blood pressure even when patients were classified as having low-renin hypertension [61]. While it seems possible that responsiveness to different agents may differ in the different renin subgroups, in most studies there has been sufficiently great overlap for this to be unhelpful in the management of the individual patient. Even if low-renin hypertension responded preferentially to diuretic therapy, this does not support the concept of a specific volume-expansion mechanism for elevated blood pressure. The protective action of the RAS in maintaining blood pressure is important in the face of volume contraction, and where this mechanism is for any reason impaired, a greater blood-pressure fall would be expected [62,63].

RENIN SUBGROUPS AND PROGNOSIS

Brunner et al [36] demonstrated a lower frequency of heart attacks and strokes in patients with low-renin hypertension in a retrospective clinical study. Other retrospective studies supported this claim [64] while the majority of other workers were unable

to confirm these observations [65–69]. Retrospective clinic studies of this type are fraught with hazard, with the possibility of major differences in unrecognized confounding risk factors and modes of treatment. If, as was suggested in the original work, renin had a vascular toxic action, this would be modified by the drug therapy used, which may either stimulate or suppress plasma renin levels depending upon the class of agent used.

The population-based study of Meade et al [12] observed the opposite effect to that reported by Brunner et al [36], that is, patients with a low renin level had suffered a higher incidence of cardiovascular disease. This is perhaps not surprising as blood pressure was inversely related to plasma renin. In a prospective study, Laragh et al confirmed an association between plasma renin levels and myocardial infarction [70]. The incidence of myocardial infarction per 1,000 patient years was 13 in the high-, 5.3 in the normal-, and 3.3 in the low-renin subgroup, as defined by the Laragh nomogram. The relationship was observed even after correcting for cholesterol level, smoking, ethnic group, age, and blood glucose. In contrast to the earlier study, this relationship was not obtained for strokes. Drug treatment of hypertension was not controlled, so that the relationship between renin and myocardial infarction appears to have been preserved despite drug-induced alterations in plasma renin. Whether renin per se is a factor in ischemic heart disease or, as appears more likely at present, acts as a marker for another risk factor (such perhaps as increased sympathetic nervous system activity), remains to be elucidated. These topics are discussed further in Chapter 40.

RENIN SUBGROUPS AND THE ADRENAL GLAND

Although there is no indication of secretion of a novel mineralocorticoid in low-renin hypertension, there is some evidence for more subtle adrenal abnormalities. Thus, aldosterone levels and secretion are usually normal [44,45] rather than reduced, and aldosterone secretion cannot be suppressed by sodium loading in some patients with essential hypertension [71]. There is also structural evidence for an abnormality of the adrenal glands in essential hypertension. Russell and Masi found 870 patients with adrenal cortical abnormalities during the course of 35,000 autopsies [72]. Of these abnormalities, 690 were adenomata and 180 examples of bilateral hyperplasia.

There was an excessive prevalence of essential hypertension among patients with adrenal cortical abnormalities. The differences between normotensive and hypertensive subjects were not, however, great, and the prevalence of adrenal cortical structural change was much lower than the prevalence of low-renin hypertension in clinical studies. Other smaller clinical studies have also shown a relatively high frequency of adenomata and of hyperplasia among subjects with low-renin hypertension [73]. It seems likely that the category of low-renin hypertension does include a small group of subjects with unrecognized primary aldosteronism although this can only account for a very small minority of cases. Henry and Grim have suggested that low-renin hypertension is a manifestation of the Selye response to stress, that is, a withdrawn and passive attitude [74]. As a result of increased sympathetic drive to the adrenal gland, hyperplasia and a high aldosterone to renin ratio is created. This syndrome is contrasted with high-renin essential hypertension which is a manifestation of Cannon's flight response to stress, with increased sympathetic stimulation of renin rather than mineralocorticoid secretion. This hypothesis is capable of testing by means of appropriate psychological assessment. The only brief study reported so far in 61 hypertensive patients showed evidence of multiple differences in six out of nine clinical rating scales when high-renin hypertensive patients were compared with low-renin hypertensive patients [75]. The former demonstrated more sensitivity, depression, anxiety, hostility, paranoia, and psychotic thought, than did the low-renin subjects.

Ferriss *et al* have also implicated adrenal cortical activity in a specific group of subjects with low plasma renin [76]. Up to one-third of all patients investigated for primary aldosteronism with increased aldosterone levels, low plasma renin, and hypokalemia, do not have an adrenocortical tumor. In this situation, there is diffuse or focal hyperplasia of otherwise normal zona glomerulosa, usually associated with adrenocortical nodules (micronodular hyperplasia). These patients show important physiological differences from patients with an adrenal adenoma causing hyperaldosteronism. Thus, aldosterone secretion is still regulated by circulating Ang II. Plasma levels of renin and Ang II are not as low as in primary aldosteronism, while exchangeable sodium is not as increased, and exchangeable potassium not as reduced. Furthermore, the inverse relationship between plasma renin and age, observed in essential hypertension and in normotensive individuals, is preserved, while in primary aldosteronism, no such relationship can be observed. The authors suggest on this persuasive evidence that idiopathic hyperaldosteronism associated with micronodular hyperplasia is part of the spectrum of essential hypertension. Again, it should be emphasized, however, that the prevalence of idiopathic hyperaldosteronism is much lower than that of low-renin hypertension on all currently used criteria. It seems likely, however, that patients with primary aldosteronism, and those discussed by

Henry and Grim [74] with histological adrenal abnormalities, comprise a small group of hypertensive patients with evidence of mineralocorticoid excess who constitute a very small minority of patients with 'low-renin' essential hypertension conventionally defined. For further discussion see *Chapter 63*.

HIGH-RENIN HYPERTENSION

A small proportion of patients with essential hypertension show plasma renin levels above the range of normotensive controls (on average approximately 15% of hospital outpatients) [30]. In some cases, high renin levels are attributable to the presence of malignant-phase (accelerated) hypertension, but high-renin

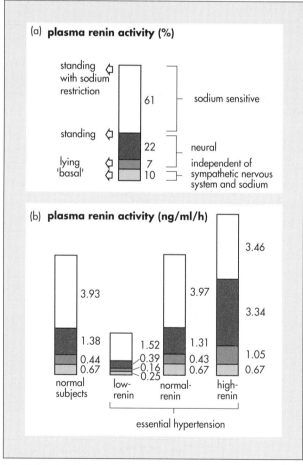

Fig 62.6 Semischematic representation of the mechanisms of renin release under different conditions of testing. (a) Relative contributions of the independent mechanisms of renin release to plasma renin activity (PRA) in normal subjects. (b) The components of PRA in patients with essential hypertension. Modified from Esler M *et al* [78].

hypertension can still be demonstrated in patients with no evidence that hypertension had entered the malignant phase (Fig. 62.6) [30]. In these patients, there is usually evidence for increased sympathetic nervous system activity [77,78]. Thus, in one study, there was a correlation between plasma norepinephrine and PRA, and plasma norepinephrine levels were higher in patients with high-renin hypertension than in the normal- or low-renin hypertension groups [78].

Julius and co-workers have suggested that high renin levels are part of the clinical picture of increased autonomic activity, which they postulate as the early phase of essential hypertension (Fig. 62.7) [79]. Thus, blood pressure can be normalized in patients with 'high-renin hypertension' by parasympathetic and sympathetic blockade [80]. Psychometric testing has demonstrated more frequent suppressed anger in high-renin than in normal-renin essential hypertensives or in normotensive controls

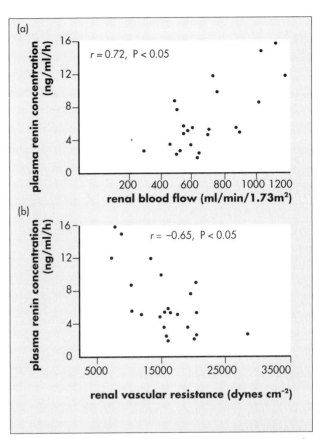

Fig 62.8 Relationships between plasma renin concentration and estimated renal blood flow (a) or renal vascular resistance (b), in 20 hypertensive patients during recumbency. Significance levels are indicated for each relationship. Modified from Schalekamp MADH *et al* [82].

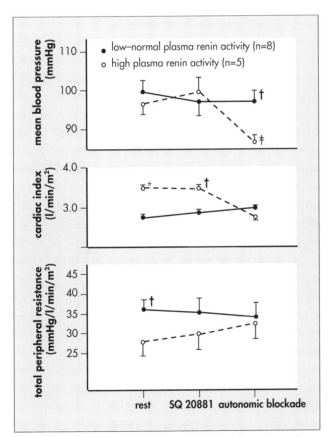

Fig 62.7 Hemodynamic effect after the ACE inhibitor teprotide (SQ 20881) and 'triple autonomic blockade' with atropine, propranolol, and regitine. †*P* < 0.05 and ‡*P* < 0.01 difference between the groups (Student *t* tests), and ‡ denotes *P*<0.05 by paired comparison within the group. Modified from Julius S [79].

[77]. According to this view, as opposed to that of Laragh, high renin levels are an epiphenomenon of the early stage of essential hypertension. In support of this proposal, while high-renin hypertension responded to sympathetic blockade, it did not respond to ACE inhibition [79]. This view is of course diametrically opposed to Laragh's hypothesis that plasma renin levels reflect the predominant pressor factor in the vasoconstrictor end of the volume/vasoconstrictor spectrum [37]. There is, on the other hand, little justification for attributing a pathogenetic role to renin in 'high-renin essential hypertension'. Hemodynamically, it is characterized by high cardiac output [81] as might be expected from the other evidence for elevated sympathetic activity. Furthermore, resistance in one vascular bed, that is the kidney, is inversely, rather than directly correlated with

plasma renin in essential hypertension (Fig. 62.8) [82]. As Conway has pointed out, demonstration of a dominant vasoconstrictor factor requires measurement of peripheral resistance, for which a reliable clinical assessment of cardiac output is mandatory. Such accuracy has so far, in Conway's view, been wanting [109].

THE DETERMINANTS OF PLASMA RENIN IN ESSENTIAL HYPERTENSION

The unimodal distribution of both blood pressure and plasma renin underlines the fact that each has multiple determinants. Plasma renin could either reflect the cause of elevated blood pressure or could be a consequence of elevated blood pressure, or some combination of the two. Several factors may play a role (Fig. 62.9). The relative importance of each is difficult to assess in any individual. Thus, it could be argued that reduced renin secretion is a 'normal' physiological response to increased perfusion pressure. It also seems likely that histological changes in the

renal vascular responsiveness to Ang II is not enhanced by change from low to high salt diet [89,90]

renal blood flow is not increased with salt loading [89,90]

excretion of an acute or chronic sodium load is reduced [91]

adrenal aldosterone response to Ang II is not enhanced by shifting from a high to a low salt diet [90]

suppression of plasma renin activity in response to sodium infusion is delayed [92]

suppression of renin release by Ang II is impaired [93]

Fig. 62.10 Characteristics of nonmodulating essential hypertension.

juxtaglomerular apparatus may be important. Thus, hyaline degeneration is increasingly prevalent in the afferent arterioles of the kidney, and the frequency of benign nephrosclerosis increases with age [83]. Similar experimental lesions can reduce afferent nervous activity from the carotid baroreceptor [84,85]. However, degeneration occurs with much increased frequency in older patients (see Color Plate 20). It seems likely therefore that this lesion may contribute both to the development of low-renin essential hypertension and to the decline in plasma renin with age, which is particularly marked in hypertensive subjects [86]. The role of fibrinoid necrosis (Color Plate 21) in modifying the functional characteristics of the juxtaglomerular apparatus is unknown.

RENAL AND ADRENAL MODULATION AND NONMODULATION

The renal vasoconstrictor response to Ang II is potentiated by a high salt diet; on the other hand, the adrenal aldosterone response to Ang II is enhanced by sodium depletion. The modification of responses of these two tissues to Ang II is described as 'modulation'. Approximately 45% of patients with normal-renin and high-renin hypertension do not show such modulation [87,88]. These abnormalities are linked with other abnormalities of renal and adrenal function (Fig. 62.10), and the defects can be corrected by ACE inhibitor treatment [87]. It has further been claimed that nonmodulators constitute a discrete genetically determined subgroup [88]. The evidence that these comprise a biologically separate group, based as it is upon small numbers of hospital-referred patients, is not especially persuasive. However, the evidence for genetic factors is stronger. Thus, there is a higher frequency of a family history of hypertension in nonmodulators [94], while normotensive relatives of hypertensive subjects have been shown to demonstrate a blunted aldosterone response to

	Low renin	High renin
renal perfusion pressure	raised	—
sodium balance mineralocorticoid	positive excess or abnormal	negative —
renal disease	bilateral or single kidney	—
pressure natriuresis	—	positive
sympathetic nervous activity	reduced	raised
venous compliance (with central volume diversion)	reduced	—
potassium excretion	reduced	—
histological change in juxtaglomerular apparatus	benign nephrosclerosis	fibrinoid necrosis
drug treatment	β-blockers (without sympathomimetic activity) centrally acting agents (methyldopa and clonidine)	diuretics vasodilators ACE inhibitors

Fig. 62.9 Putative mechanisms for alterations in plasma renin in essential hypertension.

Ang II infusion [95]. Lastly, in population studies, there was an increase in the frequency of increased lithium–sodium countertransport among nonmodulators [96]. Lithium–sodium countertransport has been associated with a genetic predisposition to essential hypertension in large family studies, although the relationship is a weak one [97].

The role of nonmodulation in the pathogenesis of essential hypertension is still controversial. Correction of nonmodulation by ACE inhibition suggests that enhanced Ang II generation may be responsible for the phenomenon either through receptor occupancy or receptor downregulation, or a combination of the two. Whether this occurs at the intrarenal and adrenal level, as the authors suggest, still requires demonstration. If so, this phenomenon provides fascinating insight into a genetic abnormality of tissue renin–angiotensin systems in essential hypertension.

TISSUE RENIN–ANGIOTENSIN SYSTEMS IN ESSENTIAL HYPERTENSION

Evidence in the spontaneously hypertensive rat (SHR) for increased expression of the renin gene, despite normal or low circulating renin levels, raises the possibility that a similar phenomenon may occur in essential hypertension [98]. So far there is no evidence for such a phenomenon in man. In the Dahl rat and in the SHR, it has been reported that there is a polymorphism in intron 1 of the renin gene and that the relevant allele cosegregates with blood pressure [99,100]. Examination of human populations in this respect has, however, demonstrated no association [101]. Furthermore, the abnormality can also be demonstrated in some nonhypertensive strains of rat [102]. Transgenic rats with an additional mouse renin-gene construct inserted into the genome, develop severe hypertension despite low circulating renin levels [103]. It still remains possible therefore that the RAS plays a role in blood-pressure elevation in essential hypertension through local tissue-based systems. 'Nonmodulating' essential hypertension provides a possible but speculative example of such a phenomenon. The application of molecular and cellular biology to essential hypertension in man is, however, still in its infancy and it is likely that over the next few years, major new insights will be obtained into the role of tissue renin–angiotensin systems in essential hypertension.

REFERENCES

1. Goldblatt H, Lynch J, Hanzal RF, Summerville WW. Studies on experimental hypertension. 1. The production of persistent elevation of systolic blood pressure by means of renal ischaemia. *Journal of Experimental Medicine* 1934;**59**:347–79.

2. Wilson C, Pickering GW. Acute arterial lesions in rabbits with experimental renal hypertension. *Clinical Science* 1938;**3**:343–51.

3. Beutler AM. Chronic pyelonephritis and arterial hypertension. *Journal of Clinical Investigation* 1937;**16**:889–97.

4. Harris J, Crane MG, Johns VJ. Plasma renin activity in hypertension. *Annals of Internal Medicine* 1967;**66**:1036–7.

5. Goldring W, Chasis H, Ranges HA, Smith HW. Effective renal blood flow in subjects with essential hypertension. *Journal of Clinical Investigation* 1941;**20**:637–53.

6. de Leeuw PW, Birkenhäger WH. The renal circulation in essential hypertension. *Journal of Hypertension* 1983;**1**:321–31.

7. Baer PG, Bianchi G. Renal micropuncture study of normotensive and Milan hypertensive rats before and after development of hypertension. *Kidney International* 1978;**13**:452–66.

8. Byrom FB, Dodson LF. The causation of acute arterial necrosis in hypertensive disease. *Journal of Pathology and Bacteriology* 1948;**60**:357–68.

9. Pickering GW. *High blood pressure*. London: Churchill–Livingstone, 1968.

10. Lucas CP, Holzwarth GJ, Ocoback RW, Stern MP, Haskell WL, Holzworth GJ, Sozen T, Wood PD, Farquhar JW. Disturbed relationship of plasma renin to blood pressure in hypertension. *Lancet* 1974;**ii**:1337.

11. Swales JD. On the inappropriate in hypertension research. *Lancet* 1977;**ii**:702–4.

12. Meade TW, Imeson JD, Gordon D, Peart WS. The epidemiology of plasma renin. *Clinical Science* 1983;**64**:273–80.

13. Thomas GW, Ledingham JGG, Beilin LJ, Stott AN, Yeates KM. Reduced renin activity in essential hypertension: A reappraisal. *Kidney International* 1977;**13**:513–8.

14. Drayer IM, Kloppenborg PWC, Benraad TJ. Detection of low renin hypertension; evaluation of outpatient renin stimulating methods. *Clinical Science and Molecular Medicine* 1975;**48**:91–6.

15. Wallach L, Nyarai I, Dawson KG. Stimulated renin: A screening test for hypertension. *Annals of Internal Medicine* 1975;**82**:27–34.

16. Thurston H, Swales JD. Low renin hypertension; A distinct entity? *Lancet* 1976;**ii**:930–2.

17. Kaplan NM, Kem DC, Holland B, Kramer NJ, Higgins J, Gomez–Sanchez C. The intravenous frusemide test: A simple way to evaluate renin responsiveness. *Annals of Internal Medicine* 1976;**84**:639–45.

18. Kuchel O, Fishman LM, Liddle GW, Michelakis A. Effect of diazoxide on plasma renin activity in hypertensive patients. *Annals of Internal Medicine* 1967;**67**:791–9.

19. Helmer OM. The renin–angiotensin system and its relation to hypertension. *Progress in Cardiovascular Diseases* 1965;**8**:117–28.

20. Ledingham JGG, Bull MB, Laragh JH. The meaning of aldosteronism in hypertensive disease. *Circulation Research* 1967;**20** and **21** (suppl 2):177–86.

21. Creditor MC, Loschky UK. Plasma renin activity in hypertension. *American Journal of Medicine* 1967;**43**:371–82.

22. Weinberger MH, Dowdy AJ, Nokes EW. Plasma renin activity and aldosterone secretion in hypertensive patients during high and low sodium intake and administration of diuretic. *Journal of Endocrinology* 1968;**28**:359–71.

23. Granger P, Boucher R, Genest J. L'aldosteronisme primaire. *Pathologie Biologie* 1968;**16**:511–6.

24. Fischman LM, Kuchel O, Liddle GW. Incidence of primary aldosteronism in uncomplicated 'essential' hypertension. *Journal of the American Medical Association* 1968;**205**:497–502.

25. Taneko Y, Ikado T, Takeda I. Renin release in patients with benign essential hypertension. *Circulation* 1968;**38**:353–62.

26. Jose A, Crout JR, Kaplan NM. Suppressed plasma renin activity in essential hypertension: Roles of plasma volume, blood pressure and sympathetic nervous system. *Annals of Internal Medicine* 1970;**72**:9–16.

27. Coghlan JP, Doyle AE, Jerums G, Scoggins BA. The effect of sodium loading and deprivation on plasma renin and plasma k and urinary aldosterone in hypertension. *Clinical Science* 1972;**42**:15–23.

28. Crane MG, Harris JJ, Varner JJ. Hyporeninaemic hypertension. *American Journal of Medicine* 1972;**52**:457–66.

29. Padfield PL, Brown JJ, Lever AF, Schalekamp MA, Beevers DG, Davies DL, Robertson JIS, Tree M. Is low renin hypertension a stage in the development of essential hypertension or a diagnostic entity? *Lancet* 1975;**i**:548–50.

30. Thurston H, Bing RF, Pohl JEF, Swales JD. Renin sub-groups in essential hypertension: An analysis and critique. *Quarterly Journal of Medicine* 1978;**47**:325–37.

31. Dunn MJ, Tannen RL. Low-renin hypertension. *Kidney International* 1974;**5**:317–25.

32. Lowder SC, Liddle GW. Prolonged alteration of renin responsiveness after spironolactone therapy. A cause of false–negative testing for low-renin hypertension. *New England Journal of Medicine* 1974;**291**:1243–4.

33. Spark RF, O'Hare CM, Regan RM. Low renin hypertension. Restoration of normotension and renin responsiveness. *Archives of Internal Medicine* 1974;**133**:205–11.

34. Swart S, Bing RF, Swales JD, Thurston H. Plasma renin in long term diuretic treatment of hypertension. Effect of discontinuation and restarting therapy. *Clinical Science* 1982;**63**:121–5.

35. Bing RF, Thurston H, Swales JD. Salt intake and diuretic treatment in hypertension. *Lancet* 1979;**ii**:121–3.

36. Brunner HR, Laragh JH, Baer L, Newton MA, Goodwin FT, Krakoff LR, Bard RH, Buhler FR. Essential hypertension: Renin and aldosterone, heart attack and stroke. *New England Journal of Medicine* 1972;**286**:441–9.

37. Laragh JH. Vasoconstriction-volume analysis for understanding and treating hypertension: The use of renin and aldosterone profiles. *American Journal of Medicine* 1973;**55**:261–74.

38. Laragh JH. Renin as a predictor of hypertensive complications: Discussion. *Annals of the New York Academy of Sciences* 1978;**304**:165–77.

39. Melby JC, Dale SL, Wilson TE. 18-hydroxy-deoxycorticosterone in human hypertension. *Circulation Research* 1971;**28** (suppl 2):II-143–50.

40. Brown JJ, Ferriss JB, Fraser R, Lever AF, Love DR, Robertson JIS, Wilson A. Apparently isolated excess deoxycorticosterone in hypertension. A variant of the mineralocorticoid excess syndrome. *Lancet* 1972;**ii**:243–7.

41. Oliver JT, Birmingham MK, Bartova A, Li MP, Chan TH. Hypertensive action of 18-hydroxydeoxycorticosterone. *Science* 1973;**182**:1249–51.

42. Sennett JA, Brown RD, Island DP, Yarbro LR, Watson JT, Slaton PE, Hollifield JW, Liddle GW. Evidence for a new mineralocorticoid in patients with low-renin essential hypertension. *Circulation Research* 1975;**36, 37** (suppl 1):2–9.

43. Baxter JD, Schambelan M, Matulick DT, Spinder BJ, Taylor AA, Bartter FC. Aldosterone receptors and the evaluation of plasma mineralocorticoid activity in normal and hypertensive states. *Journal of Clinical Investigation* 1976;**58**:579–89.

44. Messerli FH, Kuchel DO, Nowaczynski W, Seth K, Honda M, Kubo S, Boucher R, Tolis G, Genest J. Mineralocorticoid secretion in essential hypertension with normal and low plasma renin activity. *Circulation* 1976;**53**:406–10.

45. Brown RD. Aldosterone metabolic clearance is normal in low-renin essential hypertension. *Journal of Clinical Endocrinology and Metabolism* 1976;**42**:661–6.

46. Sealey JE, Blumenfeld JD, Bell GM, Pecker MS, Sommers SC, Laragh JH. On the renal basis for essential hypertension: Nephron heterogeneity with discordant renin secretion and sodium excretion causing a hypertensive vasoconstriction–volume relationship. *Journal of Hypertension* 1988;**6**:763–77.

47. Lebel M, Schalekamp MA, Beevers DG, Brown JJ, Davies DL, Fraser R, Kremer D, Lever AF, Morton JJ, Robertson JIS, Tree M, Wilson A. Sodium and the renin–angiotensin system in essential hypertension and mineralocorticoid excess. *Lancet* 1974;**ii**:308–10.

48. Solheim SB, Sundsfjord JA, Giezendanner L. The effect of spironolactone and methyl dopa in low and normal renin hypertension. *Acta Medica Scandinavica* 1975;**197**:451–6.

49. Hunyor SN, Zweifler AJ, Hansson L. Effect of high-dose spironolactone and cholorthalidone in essential hypertension: Relation to plasma renin activity and plasma volume. *Australian and New Zealand Journal of Medicine* 1975;**5**:17–24.

50. Levenson JA, Safar ME, Sassard JE, Simon AC, Vincent ML, Temmar JL, Alexandre JM. Relationship between renin and extracellular fluid volume in normotensive and hypertensive subjects. *Nephron* 1980;**25**:238–42.

51. Julius S, Esler M. Increased central blood volume: A possible pathological factor in mild low renin essential hypertension. *Clinical Science* 1976;**51** (suppl 3);207–10.

52. Edmonson RPS, MacGregor GA. Leucocyte-cation transport in essential hypertension: Its relation to the renin–angiotensin system. *British Medical Journal* 1981;**282**:1267–9.

53. Heagerty AM, Alton SM, El-Ashry A, Bing RF, Thurston H, Swales JD. Effects of changes in sodium balance on the leucocyte-sodium transport: Qualitative differences in normotensive offspring of hypertensives and matched controls. *Journal of Hypertension* 1986;**4**:333–7.

54. Laragh JH. Modern system for treating high blood pressure based on renin profiling and vasoconstriction volume analysis: A primary role for beta blocking drugs such as propranolol. *American Journal of Medicine* 1976;**61**:797–810.

55. Geyskes GG, Boer P, Vos J, Dorhout Mees EJ. Change in the renin dependency of blood pressure induced by volume depletion and/or propranolol therapy in hypertensive patients. *Clinical Science and Molecular Medicine* 1976;**51** (suppl 3);189–92s.

56. Kaplan NM, Holland OB, Gomez–Sanchez C. Effects of antihypertensive therapy on plasma renin activity. In: Sambhi M, ed. *Systemic effects of antihypertensive agents.* New York: Stratten Publishers, 1976:207–16.

57. Thomas GW, Ledingham JGG, Beilin LJ, Yeates KM. Renin unresponsiveness and the effects of oxprenolol, methyldopa and spironolactone in patients with essential hypertension. *Australian and New Zealand Journal of Medicine* 1976;**6** (suppl 3):44–8.

58. Wyndham RN, Gimenez L, Walker WG, Whelton PK, Russell RP. Influence of renin levels on the treatment of essential hypertension with thiazide diuretics. *Archives of Internal Medicine* 1987;**147**:1021–5.

59. Weber MA, Stokes GS, Gain JM. Comparison of the effects on renin release of beta adrenergic anatagonists with differing properties. *Journal of Clinical Investigation* 1974;**54**:1413–9.

60. Stokes GS, Weber MA, Thornell IR. Beta blockers and plasma renin activity in hypertension. *British Medical Journal* 1974;**1**:60–2.

61. Hollifield JW, Shermman K, Zwagg RV, Shand DG. Proposed mechanisms of propranolol's antihypertensive effect in essential hypertension. *New England Journal of Medicine* 1976;**295**:68–73.

62. Vaughan ED, Carey RM, Peach MJ, Ackerly JA, Ayers CR. The renin response to diuretic therapy: A limitation of antihypertensive potential. *Circulation Research* 1978;**42**:376–81.

63. Cappucio FP, Markandu ND, Sagnella GA, MacGregor GA. Sodium restriction lowers high blood pressure through a decreased response of the renin system — direct evidence using saralasin. *Journal of Hypertension* 1985;**3**:243–7.

64. Christlieb AR, Gleason RE, Hickler RB, Lauler DP. Renin: A risk factor for cardiovascular disease? *Annals of Internal Medicine* 1974;**81**:7–10.

65. Doyle AE, Jerums G, Johnston CI, Louis W. Plasma renin levels and vascular complications in hypertension. *British Medical Journal* 1973;2:206–7.

66. Mroczek WJ, Finnerty FA, Catt KJ. Lack of association between plasma renin and history of heart attack and stroke in patients with essential hypertension. *Lancet* 1973;ii:464–9.

67. Abe K, Irokawa N, Ioyagi H, Memezawa H, Yasujima M, Otsuka Y, Saito T, Yoshinaga K. Circulating renin in essential hypertension: An evaluation of its significance in the Japanese population. *American Heart Journal* 1975;89: 723–30.

68. Kaplan NM. The prognostic implications of plasma renin in essential hypertension. *Journal of the American Medical Association* 1975;231:167–70.

69. Kirkendall WM, Hammond JJ, Overturf ML. Renin as a predictor of hypertensive complications. *Annals of the New York Academy of Sciences* 1978;304:147–54.

70. Alderman M, Madhaven S, Ooi WL, Cohen H, Sealey J, Laragh J. Association of the renin–sodium profile with the risk of myocardial infarction in patients with hypertension. *New England Journal of Medicine* 1991;324:1098–1104.

71. Helber A, Wambach G, Hummerich W, Bonner G, Muerer KA, Kauffmann W. Evidence for a subgroup of essential hypertensives with non-suppressible excretion of aldosterone during sodium loading. *Klinische Wochenschrift* 1980;58:439–47.

72. Russell RP, Masi AT. Significant association of adrenal cortical abnormalities with 'essential hypertension'. *Americal Journal of Medicine* 1973;54:44–51.

73. Gunnells JC Jr, McGuffin WL Jr, Robinson RR, Grim GE, Wells S, Silver D, Glenn JF. Hypertension, adrenal abnormalities and alterations in plasma renin activity. *Annals of Internal Medicine* 1970;73:901–11.

74. Henry JP, Grim CE. Psychosocial mechanisms of primary hypertension. *Journal of Hypertension* 1990;8:783–93.

75. Thailer SH, Friedman R, Harshfield GA, Pickering TG. Psychologic differences between high, normal and low renin hypertensives. *Psychosomatic Medicine* 1985;47:294–7.

76. Ferriss JB, Brown JJ, Fraser R, Lever AF, Robertson JIS. Primary aldosterone excess: Conn's syndrome and similar disorders. In: Birkenhager WH, Reid JL, eds. *Handbook of hypertension. Clinical aspects of secondary hypertension, volume 2*. Ed. Robertson JIS. Amsterdam: Elsevier Press, 1983:132–61.

77. Esler M, Julius S, Zweifler A, Randall O, Harburg E, Gardiner H, de Quattro V. Mild high-renin essential hypertension. *New England Journal of Medicine* 1977;296:405–11.

78. Esler M, Zweifler A, Randall O, Julius S, de Quattro V. The determinants of plasma-renin activity in essential hypertension. *Annals of Internal Medicine* 1978;88:746–52.

79. Julius S. Interaction between renin and the autonomic nervous system in hypertension. *American Heart Journal* 1988;116:611–6.

80. Esler MD, Julius S, Randall DS, Ellis CN, Kashidma T. Relation of renin status to neurogenic vascular resistance in borderline hypertension. *American Journal of Cardiology* 1975;36:708–15.

81. Julius S, Esler MD, Randall DS, Ellis CN. Neurogenic maintenance of peripheral resistance in borderline hypertension. *Acta Physiologica Latino Americana* 1974;24:425–31.

82. Schalekamp MADH, Schalekamp–Kuyken MPA, Birkenhager WH. Abnormal renal haemodynamics and renin suppression in hypertensive patients. *Clinical Science* 1970;38:101–10.

83. Smith P. Hyaline arteriolosclerosis in the kidney. *Journal of Pathology and Bacteriology* 1955;69:147–68.

84. Angell–James JE. Arterial baroreceptor activity in rabbits with experimental atherosclerosis. *Circulation Research* 1974;34:27–39.

85. Angell–James JE, George MJ. Carotid sinus baroreceptor control of the circulation in medial sclerotic and renal hypertensive rabbits and its modification by the aortic baroreceptors. *Circulation Research* 1980;47:890–901.

86. Swales JD. Low renin hypertension: Nephrosclerosis? *Lancet* 1975;i:75–7.

87. Hollenberg NK, Williams GH. Volume control and altered renal and adrenal responsiveness to angiotensin in essential hypertension: Implications for treatment with converting enzyme inhibition. *Journal of Hypertension* 1983;1 (suppl 1);119–28.

88. Guidi E, Hollenberg NK. The kidney in 'essential' hypertension: Evidence from animal models and man. *Journal of Nephrology* 1989;3:165–72.

89. Williams GH, Tuck ML, Sullivan V, Dluhy RG, Hollenberg NK. Parallel adrenal and renal abnormalities in young patients with essential hypertension. *American Journal of Medicine* 1982;72:907–14.

90. Shoback DM, Williams GH, Hollenberg NK, Davies RO, Moore TJ, Dluhy RG. Endogenous angiotensin II as a determinant of sodium modulated changes in tissue responsiveness to angiotensin II in normal man. *Journal of Clinical Endocrinology and Metabolism* 1983;56:764–70.

91. Rydstedt LL, Williams GH, Hollenberg NK. The renal and endocrine response to saline infusion in essential hypertension. *Hypertension* 1986;8:217–22.

92. Rabinowe SL, Redgrave JE, Shoback DM, Podolsky S, Hollenberg NK, Williams GH. Renin suppression by saline is blunted in non-modulating essential hypertension. *Hypertension* 1987;10:404–8.

93. Seely EW, Moore TJ, Rogacz S, Gordon MS, Gleason RE, Hollenberg NK, Williams GH. Angiotensin-mediated renin suppression is altered in non-modulating hypertension. *Hypertension* 1989;13:31–7.

94. Hollenberg NK, Moore T, Shoback D, Redgrave D, Rabinowe S, Williams GH. Abnormal renal sodium handling in essential hypertension: Relation of failure to renal and adrenal modulation of response to angiotensin II. *American Journal of Medicine* 1986;81:412–8.

95. Beretta–Piccoli C, Pusterla C, Stadler P, Weidmann P. Blunted aldosterone responsiveness to angiotensin II in normotensive subjects with familial predisposition to essential hypertension. *Journal of Hypertension* 1988;6:57–61.

96. Redgrave J, Canessa M, Gleason R, Hollenberg NK, Williams GH. Red blood cell lithium–sodium countertransport in non-modulating hypertension. *Hypertension* 1989;13:721–6.

97. Williams RR, Hunt SC, Wu LL, Hasstedt SJ, Hopkins PN, Ash DKO. Genetic and epidemiological studies on electrolyte transport systems in hypertension. *Clinical Physiology and Biochemistry* 1988;6:136–49.

98. Samani NJ, Swales JD, Brammar WJ. A widespread abnormality of renin gene expression in spontaneously hypertensive rats: Modulation in some tissues with the development of hypertension. *Clinical Science* 1989;77:629–36.

99. Rapp JP, Wang S–M, Dene H. A genetic polymorphism in the renin gene of Dahl rat co-segregates with blood pressure. *Science* 1989;243:542–4.

100. Kurtz TW, Simonet L, Kabra PM, Wolfe S, Chan L, Hjelle BL. Cosegregation of the renin allele of the spontaneously hypertensive rat with an increase in blood pressure. *Journal of Clinical Investigation* 1990;85:1328–32.

101. Naftilan AJ, Williams R, Burt D, Paul M, Pratt RE, Hobart P, Chirgwin J, Dzau VJ. A lack of genetic linkage of renin gene restriction fragment length polymorphisms with human restriction. *Hypertension* 1989;14:614–6.

102. Samani NJ, Vincent M, Sassard J, Henderson IW, Kaiser MA, Brammar WJ, Swales JD. Analysis of the renin gene intron A tandem repeat region of Milan and Lyon hypertensive rat strains. *Journal of Hypertension* 1990;8:805–9.

103. Mullins JJ, Peters J, Ganten D. Fulminant hypertension in transgenic rats harbouring the mouse Ren-2 gene. *Nature* 1990;344:541–4.

104. Agabiti Rosei E, Brown JJ, Cumming AM, Fraser R, Semple PF, Morton JJ, Robertson AS, Robertson JIS, Tree M. Is the 'sodium index' a useful way of expressing clinical plasma renin, angiotensin and aldosterone values? *Clinical Endocrinology* 1978;8:141–7.

105. Bankir L, Bouby N, Trinh–Trang–Tan MM. Heterogeneity of nephron anatomy. *Kidney International* 1987;31 (suppl 20):25–39.

106. Brown JJ, Davies DL, Lever AF, Parker RA, Robertson JIS. The assay of renin in single glomeruli of the normal rabbit and the appearance of the juxtaglomerular apparatus. *Journal of Physiology* 1965;176:418–28.

107. Brown JJ, Davies DL, Lever AF, Parker RA, Robertson JIS. The assay of renin in single glomeruli and the appearance of the juxtaglomerular apparatus in the rabbit following renal artery constriction. *Clinical Science* 1966;30:223–35.

108. Gavras H, Brown JJ, Lever AF, Robertson JIS. Changes of renin in individual glomeruli in response to variations of sodium intake in the rabbit. *Clinical Science* 1970;38:409–14.

109. Conway J. Clinical assessment of cardiac output. *European Heart Journal* 1990;11 (suppl I):148–50.

63

MINERALOCORTICOID-INDUCED HYPERTENSION AND THE RENIN–ANGIOTENSIN SYSTEM

PAUL L PADFIELD AND CHRISTOPHER RW EDWARDS

INTRODUCTION

A consideration of the RAS is central to an evaluation of any of the diverse syndromes of mineralocorticoid-induced hypertension. The principal endogenous mineralocorticoid hormone in man, aldosterone, is under important regulatory control by the RAS (see *Chapter 33*). In circumstances in which increased secretion of aldosterone is recruited in the course of homeostatic physiological control, for example with sodium deprivation or hemorrhage (see *Chapters 71, 72*, and *74*), there is activation of the RAS, with resultant secondary aldosteronism. Such secondary aldosteronism is usually mounted as a defence against volume depletion and hypotension, and a raised blood pressure is not a feature. Aldosterone excess secondary to stimulation by the RAS and with accompanying hypertension does occur with renal or renal arterial lesions; these conditions are discussed in detail in *Chapters 55* and *56*.

It follows further, nevertheless, that the RAS is inextricably involved in any form of mineralocorticoid-induced hypertension, whether such primary excess of mineralocorticoid be endogenous or exogenous. Such involvement has important pathophysiological, diagnostic, and conceptual implications. These aspects form the substance of this chapter.

METABOLIC EFFECTS OF MINERALOCORTICOID EXCESS: THE 'ESCAPE' PHENOMENON

The critical action of a mineralocorticoid such as aldosterone, is to promote, at distal renal tubules, sodium reabsorption in exchange for potassium, magnesium, and hydrogen ions. Thus, sodium is retained, while potassium, magnesium, and hydrogen are lost. When there is a physiologically inappropriate excess of such a mineralocorticoid (as for example with an aldosterone-secreting tumor) there is consequent elevation of arterial pressure accompanied by sodium retention, hypernatremia, potassium deficiency, hypokalemia, and extracellular alkalosis [1,2]. With such long-term mineralocorticoid excess there is chronic stable expansion of body sodium content (assessed either as total exchangeable or total body sodium), of plasma volume, of extracellular fluid volume, and of total body water, while body potassium content (assessed as total exchangeable or total body potassium) is deficient.

As is described in detail in *Chapter 24*, these events include several powerful mechanisms inhibiting the secretion of renin; hence, plasma renin and Ang II levels fall [1–4]. One contrary stimulus is the fall in body potassium content and in plasma potassium concentration, which tends to stimulate renin secretion (see *Chapter 74*); this tendency is, however, overwhelmed by the more powerful inhibitory influences. Concurrently, as described in *Chapter 36*, the secretion of atrial natriuretic factor (ANF) is increased and plasma concentrations of ANF rise [5–7].

It is emphasized that these alterations in body composition and related hormones are stable; after an initial period of sodium and water retention when the organism is first exposed to mineralocorticoid excess, equilibrium is re-established and the excretion rates of sodium, potassium, and water return so as to balance intake. The physiological events that enable the re-establishment of metabolic equilibrium, rather misleadingly termed 'mineralocorticoid escape', have attracted considerable attention and investigation.

Nicholls *et al* [8] examined the effects, in six normal male volunteers, of administering the mineralocorticoid substance fludrocortisone orally, 0.5mg 12-hourly, for 10 days. Systolic blood pressure was significantly elevated from the fifth day of fludrocortisone treatment, the mean increment being 10mmHg both lying and standing by the 10th day. Fludrocortisone caused a progressive weight gain over the first six days to a plateau 1.5kg above control values. Urine sodium excretion was initially reduced markedly by fludrocortisone but returned to control values after eight days, when body weight had stabilized (Fig. 63.1). There were converse changes in potassium excretion, and measured total body potassium content fell. There was a progressive lowering of plasma renin concentration from a mean (± SEM) of 133.1 ± 6.4μu/ml (international units) to 56.3 ± 6.6μu/ml over the 10 days of fludrocortisone administration

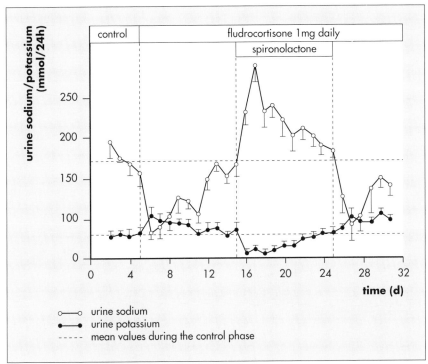

Fig. 63.1 Data on six normal male volunteers taking a diet containing constant amounts of sodium and potassium daily for each individual. No treatment for five days (control) was followed by oral fludrocortisone 1mg daily for 27 days. Spironolactone 50–200mg daily was added on days 16–25. The data are presented as mean ± SEM for 24-hour urinary excretion of sodium and potassium. Modified from Nicholls MG *et al* [8].

($P<0.01$), paralleled by a similar fall in plasma Ang II. When the data from individual subjects in this study were examined, it was seen that 'escape' from the sodium-retaining influence of fludrocortisone was not determined by the quantity of sodium retained, but was closely related to the rise in systolic blood pressure during the first 48 hours of therapy. A more pronounced rise of blood pressure was associated with earlier renal 'escape'. The central importance of arterial pressure (or more strictly renal artery perfusion pressure) in regulating the level of urinary sodium excretion, is discussed in detail in *Chapter 26*.

Nicholls *et al* emphasized the remarkable range of responses to fludrocortisone seen in healthy men [8]. At one extreme, there was a prompt elevation of blood pressure, early renal escape, little weight gain or sodium retention, and a small drop in plasma potassium. At the other, there was a delayed rise in systolic pressure, later escape, considerable weight gain and sodium retention, and marked hypokalemia. It was not possible to relate these different patterns of response to age, body weight, blood pressure, or plasma renin or Ang II concentrations during the control phase, or to the dietary intake of sodium or potassium.

Biollaz *et al* [9] exposed normal volunteers to fludrocortisone 0.6mg daily, with double-blind addition of the ACE inhibitor enalapril 40mg daily or placebo. Plasma Ang II was lower, and plasma renin activity (PRA) higher, in the enalapril phase, while

urinary aldosterone excretion was initially, but not subsequently, more markedly suppressed with enalapril (Fig. 63.2). However, the course of daily urinary excretion of sodium and potassium was not affected by enalapril (Fig. 63.3); the blood pressure increase was likewise closely similar in the two phases. This experiment provided no evidence that in man, suppression of circulating Ang II is causally related to escape from mineralocorticoid excess.

Other studies have implicated rises in glomerular filtration rate [10], renal actions of prostaglandins [11,12] and/or kinins [11,13], and decreased renal adrenergic activity [14] in the mineralocorticoid escape phenomenon.

The study of Nicholls *et al* summarized above [8] antedated recognition of the possible role of ANF in the mechanism of renal escape from the effects of mineralocorticoids. Subsequent reports have shown increases in plasma ANF occurring conversely to the falls in plasma renin and Ang II.

Miyamori *et al* [15] studied escape from the effects of fludrocortisone 0.6mg daily given to healthy volunteers. Plasma ANF concentrations increased exponentially to reach significantly elevated levels on the day before escape, remaining high thereafter (Fig. 63.4). These workers concluded that the increase in ANF made important contributions to the natriuresis and diuresis during escape from mineralocorticoid excess.

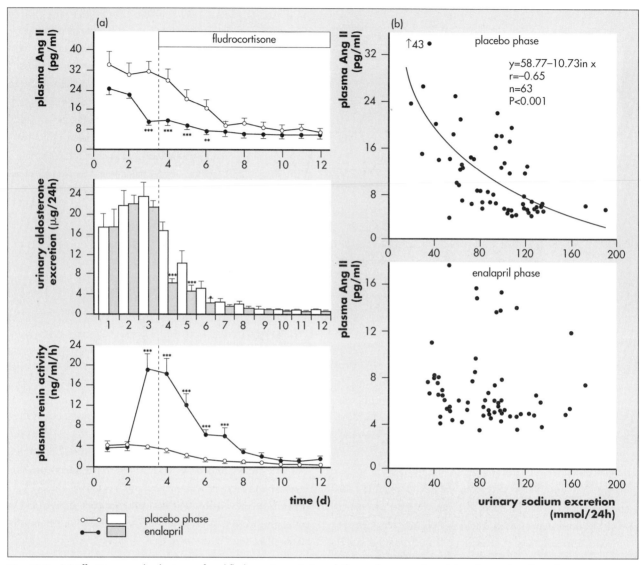

Fig. 63.2 (a) Effect in normal volunteers of oral fludrocortisone 0.6mg daily on plasma renin activity, plasma Ang II, and urinary aldosterone excretion, with the addition, double-blind, of enalapril 40mg daily or placebo. *P<0.05; **P<0.01; ***P<0.001.
(b) Relationship between daily urinary sodium excretion and plasma Ang II in the enalapril and placebo phases. Whereas a significant inverse correlation was observed during the placebo phase, this was absent with enalapril. Modified from Biollaz J *et al* [9].

The findings were confirmed and extended by Gaillard *et al* [16] in volunteers given fludrocortisone 1mg daily. It was found that mineralocorticoid escape was accompanied not only by a rise in plasma ANF, but also by potentiation of its natriuretic effect. It was considered that elevated systemic arterial pressure could be responsible for this enhanced natriuretic effect of ANF during exposure to mineralocorticoid excess.

Concordant observations have been made during the re-establishment of mineralocorticoid hypertension on withdrawing spironolactone treatment in patients with endogenous aldosterone excess due to aldosterone-secreting adenoma [17–19]. In these circumstances also, the restoration of sodium excretion after initial sodium retention is related to a rise in blood pressure.

It seems likely that the interplay of several influences, prominent amongst which are rises in arterial pressure and in plasma ANF, is responsible for the renal escape from mineralocorticoid excess [147] (Fig. 63.5). The RAS is markedly suppressed, and further suppression, for instance by adding an ACE inhibitor, makes no visible additional contribution.

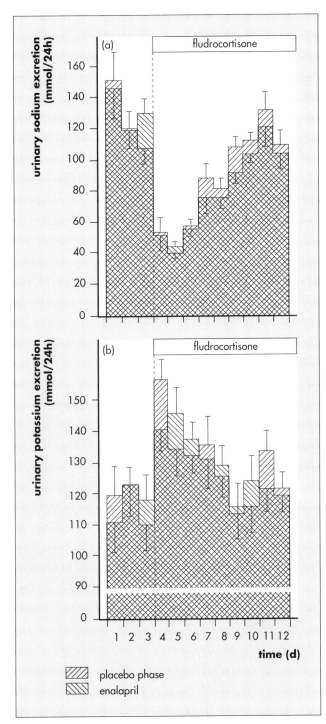

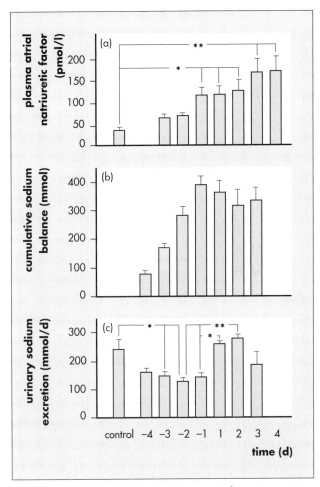

Fig. 63.4 Changes in plasma atrial natriuretic factor (ANF) (a), cumulative sodium balance (b), and urinary sodium excretion (c) under control conditions and before and during escape from the effects of fludrocortisone 0.6mg daily, in normal volunteers. Results are compared using the first day of escape as reference. *P<0.05; **P<0.01. Plasma ANF increased significantly on the day before escape and remained high thereafter. Modified from Miyamori I *et al* [15].

Fig. 63.3 Study of *Fig. 63.2.* showing daily urinary sodium (a) and potassium (b) excretion during the placebo and enalapril phases, respectively. No significant difference between the two phases was observed. The data are presented as mean ± SEM. n=8. Modified from Biollaz J *et al* [9].

MECHANISMS OF BLOOD-PRESSURE ELEVATION WITH PRIMARY MINERALOCORTICOID EXCESS

Primary mineralocorticoid excess has attracted considerable interest over the years because it constitutes a form of hypertension readily studied in man and has appeared to offer the opportunity for the elucidation of the underlying mechanisms responsible for the raised arterial pressure. Investigational approaches have included the administration of mineralocorticoids

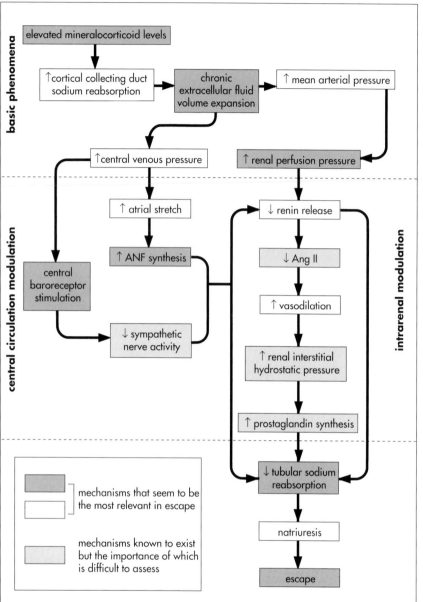

Fig. 63.5 The mechanisms of escape. Mechanisms that seem to be the most relevant in escape and those known to exist in escape but whose importance is difficult to assess, are shown. Modified from Gonzalez-Campoy JM *et al* [147].

to normal man [8,20]; the treatment of patients with primary aldosterone excess by surgery [21] or by employing potassium-conserving diuretics such as spironolactone or amiloride; and the controlled withdrawal of spironolactone in medically treated patients with aldosterone-secreting tumor [17–19].

As mentioned above, in untreated patients with primary mineralocorticoid excess because of an aldosterone-secreting adenoma, there is clear expansion of total exchangeable (and of total body) sodium, of extracellular fluid and plasma volumes,

and of total body water, while total exchangeable and total body potassium are depleted. The height of the blood pressure is proportional to the expansion of body sodium (Fig. 63.6). Correction of the mineralocorticoid excess by excision of the tumor or via abolition of the effects of mineralocorticoid excess by administration of a potassium-conserving diuretic, rectifies these abnormalities of the various body spaces (Figs. 63.6 and 63.7; see also *Fig. 1.12*) [1–4,21].

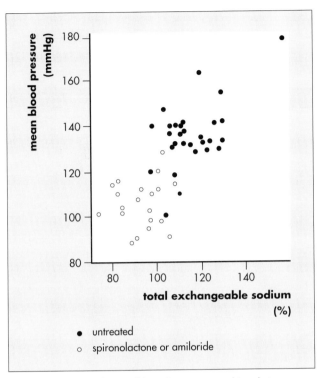

Fig. 63.6 Total exchangeable sodium expressed in relation to leanness index plotted against mean arterial pressure (diastolic + $^1/_3$ pulse pressure) in 29 patients, all of whom were later proved to have an aldosterone-secreting adenoma. Measurements made without treatment and also made in 20 of these patients after at least one month's treatment with either spironolactone or amiloride, are shown. In the untreated patients, mean exchangeable sodium is clearly expanded and there is a significant positive correlation with arterial pressure. During treatment with the potassium-conserving and natriuretic agents, arterial pressure falls in proportion to the fall in exchangeable sodium. Modified from Robertson JIS and Fraser R [65].

In untreated patients with aldosterone-secreting adenoma, which can be taken as the classic model of mineralocorticoid excess, both systolic and diastolic blood pressures have been shown to be significantly and positively correlated with exchangeable or total body sodium, with plasma sodium concentration, with the ratio of body sodium/body potassium, and with the ratio of plasma sodium/plasma potassium; and significantly and negatively correlated with plasma potassium concentration [21].

As noted already, treatment, whether by surgery or by using spironolactone or amiloride, has been seen to lower arterial

pressure in proportion to the reduction in exchangeable body sodium [21] (see *Fig. 63.6* and Fig. 63.7). With such treatment, plasma levels of renin and Ang II increase, while those of ANF fall [5–7].

It is against this factual background that possible hypertensive mechanisms have been considered. Despite the apparent comparative ease of observation, none of the following proposals is certain.

ROLE OF SODIUM RETENTION AND VOLUME EXPANSION

Despite the close quantitative association between the height of the blood pressure and the extent of sodium retention and the accompanying volume expansion in mineralocorticoid-induced hypertension [2–4] (see *Fig. 63.6*), it is unlikely that sodium retention is the immediate cause of the rise in blood pressure. The reasons have been given in detail in the paper by Beretta-Piccoli *et al* [21] and are summarized here.

On withdrawing spironolactone in patients whose blood pressure is controlled by the drug, there is at first marked sodium retention, but blood pressure does not begin to rise for a week or more and when it does rise, sodium excretion increases. Similarly as discussed in the preceding section, when normal subjects are given the mineralocorticoid fludrocortisone, there is sodium retention which is followed after an interval by an increase of blood pressure associated with sodium loss [8,9,12, 15]. This interval suggests that there are intermediate events between the retention of sodium and the rise of blood pressure.

One possibility is whole-body autoregulation. In this, a rise in cardiac output is followed by an increase in peripheral vascular resistance. The sequence of events usually occurs when spironolactone is stopped in patients with aldosterone-secreting tumor [17,19], but this does not establish that it is a necessary step. Nor is it certain that autoregulation is sufficiently slow to account for the long interval between early sodium retention and the eventual rise in blood pressure to its highest point. In some patients, the increase in blood pressure is maintained long-term mainly by increased cardiac output without a secondary rise of peripheral vascular resistance. Moreover, pigs injected with deoxycorticosterone (DOC) sometimes develop hypertension without passing through a phase of increased cardiac output [22,23].

On balance, sodium retention appears to be a necessary step in the sequence of events raising blood pressure, although there are almost certainly other intermediate events. Whole-body autoregulation and structural changes in resistance vessels are two possibilities. Redistribution of sodium is a third (see below).

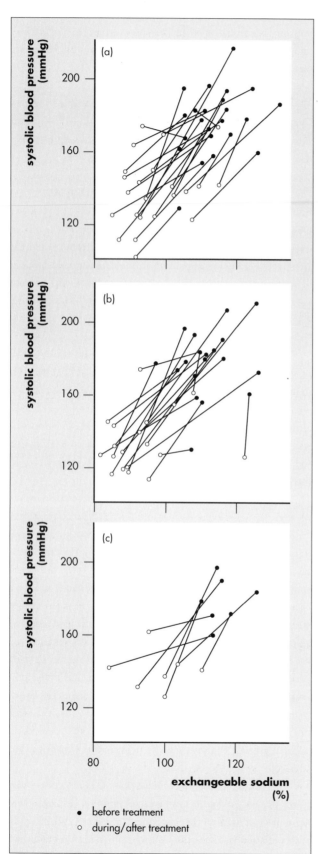

Fig. 63.7 Exchangeable sodium (related to body surface area) and systolic blood pressure in patients with Conn's syndrome (a) before and after surgery, (b) before and during spironolactone, and (c) before and during amiloride. Five of the seven patients having amiloride also had spironolactone, and all patients having these drugs also had surgery. Modified from Beretta-Piccoli C *et al* [21].

STRUCTURAL CHANGES IN RESISTANCE ARTERIES

Another way of explaining the delay in the rise in blood pressure is that structural changes develop in resistance vessels as a result of a small rise of blood pressure and that these amplify the pressor effect of sodium retention, producing a progressive rise in blood pressure [24] (see *Chapters 28* and *96*).

DIRECT PRESSOR ACTION OF MINERALOCORTICOIDS

Mineralocorticoids may also act directly on vascular smooth-muscle cells [25,26]. Thus, aldosterone may increase blood pressure by such an action and, independently, cause sodium retention. Although the data summarized above do not exclude this possibility, it is unlikely. Three methods were used to reduce blood pressure in patients with aldosterone-secreting tumor (Fig. 63.7) and each produced a similar fall in blood pressure and a similar change in the relation of exchangeable sodium and arterial pressure. Surgery reduced aldosterone, spironolactone increased aldosterone slightly, while amiloride, acting by a different mechanism, increased aldosterone more markedly. These changes do not suggest an important direct pressor action of aldosterone independent of sodium balance since blood pressure was more closely related to sodium balance than to plasma aldosterone concentration. Thus, if amiloride raises aldosterone and does not at the same time anatagonize its direct action on smooth muscle, blood pressure should not decrease during treatment with amiloride because aldosterone increases.

THE NERVOUS SYSTEM

There is a large amount of literature, some controversial, on the existence and importance of increased sympathetic nerve activity in mineralocorticoid hypertension [22,27–29].

Gordon *et al* [148] found that in eight patients with aldosterone-secreting adenoma, adrenal venous levels of catecholamines were decreased, indicating diminished sympathetic activity.

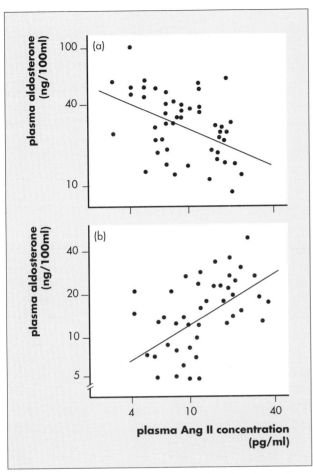

Fig. 63.8 Relationship between concurrent basal early morning plasma concentrations of aldosterone and Ang II in untreated patients with (a) Conn's syndrome (r=−0.43; P<0.01; log scale) and (b) idiopathic hyperaldosteronism (r=+0.46; P<0.01). Modified from Ferriss JB et al [3].

Mineralocorticoids may raise blood pressure by a direct action on the brain [23]. These are important possibilities although it has been clearly shown that blood pressure can fall during treatment of patients with aldosterone-secreting adenoma, which may increase, decrease, or leave unchanged, the plasma concentration of aldosterone [21].

VASOPRESSIN

Vasopressin has also been invoked as a pressor agent in mineralocorticoid hypertension, but in a series of five hypertensive patients with aldosterone-secreting adenoma, plasma vasopressin concentration was found to be normal or low [30]. It is agreed that the plasma concentration of vasopressin is increased

in animals with DOC-induced hypertension, but opinion divides on whether the increase has a pressor effect [31–33]. Considerable evidence suggests that it does not [30,33].

VASOCONSTRICTOR EFFECT OF HYPOKALEMIA

A decrease in extracellular potassium concentration causes vasoconstriction and an increase causes vasodilatation [34,35]. In patients with aldosterone-secreting tumor, there is, before treatment an inverse correlation of plasma potassium concentration and arterial pressure, raising the possibility that hypokalemia contributes in some way to the hypertension [21]. It has been shown, for example, that increasing extracellular potassium produces vasodilation in pigs with DOC hypertension [34]. An effect of this type cannot readily be excluded, though partial regression analysis in the study of Beretta-Piccoli et al [21] suggested that the relation of potassium with blood pressure is secondary to that between body sodium content and blood pressure. Thus, sodium retention may cause potassium loss. If sodium retention raised blood pressure in some as yet unidentified way, a secondary correlation would arise between potassium and blood pressure. It is known, for example, that sodium loading in mineralocorticoid excess lowers the plasma concentration of potassium further [36]. However, a kaliuretic effect of sodium retention is unlikely to be the whole explanation, since aldosterone also produces urinary potassium loss by a direct action that does not depend upon sodium retention [37].

AN INHIBITOR OF SODIUM TRANSPORT

Haddy et al [38] have proposed that volume expansion in mineralocorticoid hypertension stimulates release of an inhibitor of sodium transport with a digitalis-like action. One of its supposed effects is to counteract the volume expansion by causing natriuresis, while another is to increase the sodium content of vascular smooth muscle, thereby causing vasoconstriction and hypertension. A report that antibodies to digitalis lower blood pressure in DOC-hypertensive rats lends some support for the idea [39]. At present, there is little or no evidence that the correlation of blood pressure with body sodium in mineralocorticoid hypertension arises more from intracellular sodium than from extracellular sodium.

ROLE OF ANGIOTENSIN II AND ATRIAL NATRIURETIC FACTOR

It should be reiterated that plasma Ang II is suppressed [3,4], while ANF is increased [5–7], in subjects with mineralocorticoid-induced hypertension. As Ang II is pressor, while ANF is depressor, these changes will tend to moderate the severity of any accompanying hypertension. However, sodium loading, a central feature of mineralocorticoid hypertension, enhances the pressor action of circulating Ang II [40]. Thus, the sodium expansion will, to an extent, offset the antihypertensive effect of the reduction in plasma Ang II concentration.

SUMMARY

In summary, several mechanisms have been proposed to explain the increase of arterial pressure in mineralocorticoid hypertension: a direct vasoconstrictor effect of hypokalemia, increased vasopressin, a direct action of the mineralocorticoid on vascular smooth muscle, and sodium retention acting either though whole-body autoregulation or by its stimulant effect on a sodium transport inhibitor. These mechanisms are not mutually exclusive. Some of them could be different steps in a sequence linking excess mineralocorticoid and hypertension. It is fairly clear that abnormal sodium retention is one of the necessary components and that hypokalemia and the action of aldosterone are relatively unimportant [21].

PRIMARY EXCESS OF ALDOSTERONE: CONN'S SYNDROME

The classic clinical model of aldosterone excess, and one that has been studied in most detail, is that of the patient suffering from aldosterone-secreting adrenocortical adenoma. The first detailed description of this condition was provided by Conn [41], although it appears that his 1955 paper was antedated by earlier accounts [42,43].

In this syndrome, chronic excessive secretion of aldosterone from the tumor leads to hypertension with expansion of body sodium content (whether measured as total exchangeable or as total body sodium); hypernatremia; increased plasma and extracellular fluid volumes; increased total body water; contraction of body potassium content; hypokalemia; and extracellular alkalosis [1–4].

As is discussed in detail in *Chapter 33*, the RAS is one of the principal regulators of normal aldosterone secretion. Thus, when there is uncontrolled aldosterone secretion from an adrenocortical adenoma, the RAS is suppressed; hence the very characteristic combination of hypertension associated with aldosterone excess and subnormal plasma renin and Ang II levels [1–4,44–46]. The extent of the suppression of the RAS is in proportion to the magnitude of the aldosterone excess; as shown by Ferriss *et al* [3], in untreated patients, there is a significant, though statistically weak, inverse correlation between concurrent measurements of plasma aldosterone and plasma Ang II concentrations (Fig. 63.8). It has further been observed that while plasma concentrations of active renin are low, plasma levels of inactive renin are very low in this syndrome [47]; this interesting observation is discussed further in *Chapters 6* and *7*.

The biosynthetic pathway of aldosterone is dependent to an extent on potassium. In the presence of severe potassium deficiency in this syndrome, the biosynthesis may not proceed beyond 18-hydroxycorticosterone, which then becomes the predominant excessive mineralocorticoid, while aldosterone is no longer superabundant [48]. Correction of the potassium deficiency in this situation restores aldosterone excess.

Treatment of Conn's syndrome, either by surgical removal of the tumor (Plate 54, see Color Plate Section) or by the administration of potassium-conserving agents such as spironolactone or amiloride, corrects the various abnormalities of body spaces described above, when the depressed plasma renin and Ang II (Fig. 63.9), and the elevated plasma ANF, return to normal [1–7,49,149].

The plasma RAS is corrected irrespectively of whether medical or surgical treatment is employed. Thus, it is clear that renin secretion is regulated directly or indirectly by the changes in sodium balance (see *Chapter 24*) and not by plasma aldosterone, because aldosterone falls to normal following surgery, but is unchanged, or even further increased, with therapy employing spironolactone or amiloride [21]. Moreover, the RAS remains suppressed in patients who, because of gross potassium depletion, do not synthesize an excess of aldosterone [48]. While potassium loss, which is a central feature of aldosterone excess, tends to stimulate renin secretion (see *Chapter 24*), this is a weak influence in comparison with the contrary effect of sodium retention, and hence is overwhelmed.

Administration of ANF, even so as to cause only modest increases in its plasma concentration, which remain within the normal range, can markedly lower plasma renin and Ang II in healthy volunteers [50] (see *Chapter 36*). Thus, the raised plasma ANF in untreated cases, and the fall of ANF to normal with therapy, could be important influences causing the reciprocal changes in renin and Ang II. Even so, infusion of exogenous ANF in patients with aldosterone-secreting adenoma can cause natriuresis and a slight fall in blood pressure, while renin remains suppressed and the elevated plasma aldosterone concentration is unchanged [7,51,52].

A crucial observation in patients with aldosterone-secreting adenoma is that increasing the very low plasma Ang II concentrations acutely by the infusion of exogenous Ang II does not affect plasma aldosterone concentration (see *Fig. 33.11*). This is in

	Before treatment	During spironolactone	Number of pairs	t	P
systolic blood pressure (mmHg)	198.6 (2.45)	148.1 (2.82)	95	−20.45	<0.001
diastolic blood pressure (mmHg)	121.5 (1.12)	97.3 (1.50)	95	−17.96	<0.001
plasma sodium (mmol/l)	142.4 (0.27)	138.2 (0.31)	83	−10.61	<0.001
plasma potassium (mmol/l)	3.2 (0.07)	4.6 (0.05)	85	15.91	<0.001
plasma T_{CO_2} (mmol/l)	28.6 (0.40)	23.9 (0.33)	74	−11.2	<0.001
blood urea (mg/100ml)	33.4 (1.2)	48.6 (2.1)	80	11	<0.001
plasma renin (μu/ml)	26.8 (1.4)	129.5 (16.9)	45	6.12	<0.001
plasma Ang II (pg/ml)	10.2 (.075)	57.4 (19.2)	16	2.49	<0.05
plasma aldosterone (ng/100ml)	31.2 (5.0)	41.7 (5.0)	19	1.67	0.2>P>0.1
exchangeable sodium (mmol)	2969.4 (82.7)	2464.9 (72.7)	36	−10.55	<0.001
exchangeable sodium (mmol/kg body weight)	44.5 (1.0)	37.9 (0.9)	36	−8.18	<0.001
exchangeable potassium (mmol)	2347.0 (107.5)	2551.2 (107.1)	36	2.95	<0.01
exchangeable postassium (mmol/kg body weight)	35.1 (1.4)	39.4 (1.3)	36	4.65	<0.001
total body water (l)	38.5 (1.3)	35.9 (1.4)	28	−4.73	<0.001
extracellular fluid (l)	19.3 (0.79)	16.6 (0.82)	13	−4.31	<0.01
plasma volume (l)	3.07 (0.21)	2.80 (0.24)	10	−2.27	<0.05

Fig. 63.9 Comparison of variables before and during treatment with spironolactone in patients with aldosterone-secreting adenoma (paired *t*-test). Data are means; Values in parentheses are SEMs. Modified from Ferriss JB *et al* [149].

marked contrast to normal subjects or to patients with essential hypertension, in whom Ang II administration causes a prompt rise in aldosterone [53] (see *Fig. 33.11*). As ANF is one factor that can inhibit the stimulant action of Ang II on aldosterone secretion (see *Chapter 36*), the elevated ANF in Conn's syndrome could be one reason for the characteristic lack of Ang II effect.

As discussed in more detail in *Chapter 60*, despite the low circulating levels of renin and Ang II in Conn's syndrome, the malignant phase of hypertension, while uncommon, is well described [54,55]. Such evidence is critical in demonstrating that increased plasma concentrations of Ang II are not necessary for progression to malignant hypertension.

As described earlier, surgical removal of the adenoma, or medical therapy with a potassium-conserving diuretic such as spironolactone or amiloride, corrects the metabolic abnormalities, while restoring the subnormal plasma renin and Ang II values and the elevated ANF to the normal range. Blood pressure is lowered, but, as in most forms of secondary hypertension [56], returns to the normal range only in approximately 50% of patients [4,49]. The preoperative long-term response to a potassium-conserving diuretic can predict reasonably accurately the subsequent response to surgery [3,4,49]. Those patients with evidence of renal functional impairment tend to have less satisfactory blood-pressure reduction with either form of therapy [3,4,49].

As would be expected in a disease characterized by low circulating levels of renin and Ang II, blood pressure does not fall with acute infusion of an analog antagonist of Ang II such as saralasin; indeed, the partial agonistic effect of saralasin may lead in these circumstances to a slight further increase in blood pressure [57]. Angiotensin-converting enzyme inhibitors likewise are not effective in monotherapy in this disease [58,59]. However, as mentioned earlier, treatment with amiloride or spironolactone leads to elevation of plasma renin and hence Ang II, which will then have an influence on arterial pressure. If, in these circumstances, the control of arterial pressure remains inadequate, addition of an ACE inhibitor can therefore be worthwhile. Atkinson et al [60] reported the case of a 26-year-old man with Conn's syndrome, who had hypertension and renal functional impairment (Fig. 63.10). Exchangeable body sodium was expanded and total body potassium contracted; there were hypernatremia, hypokalemia, low plasma concentrations of active renin and Ang II, and aldosterone excess. Oral spironolactone 400mg daily for six weeks reduced total exchangeable sodium while expanding total body potassium and correcting serum electrolyte abnormalities. Plasma concentrations of active renin and of Ang II increased concomitantly, while the already elevated plasma aldosterone concentration rose further. However, creatinine clearance fell and, as is usual with spironolactone, there were further increases in serum urea and creatinine. Arterial pressure remained high. A decision was made to use captopril in addition to spironolactone. Captopril was given in an initial dose of 25mg, increasing to a total of 450mg daily. Circulating Ang II fell at once to undetectable levels, while active renin and Ang I concentrations increased. After two months on this combined therapy, blood-pressure control was greatly improved, although values were still slightly elevated for a man of his age. Plasma Ang II remained suppressed, while there was continued elevation of both active renin and Ang I. Plasma aldosterone

concentrations were approximately twice pretreatment values, but less than those seen on spironolactone alone. Total exchangeable sodium remained substantially below, and total body potassium above, untreated values. No adverse effects of captopril treatment were observed.

OTHER FORMS OF PRIMARY ALDOSTERONE EXCESS

Several clinical syndromes of apparently primary excess of aldosterone other than classical Conn's syndrome due to an adrenocortical adenoma require mention.

ANGIOTENSIN-RESPONSIVE ALDOSTERONE-PRODUCING ADENOMA

As described above, in the classical form of Conn's syndrome, the elevated plasma concentrations of aldosterone remain unchanged with the intravenous infusion of Ang II (see *Fig. 33.11*).

Gordon et al [61] have identified a subgroup of patients with aldosterone-secreting adrenocortical adenoma in whom, by contrast, plasma aldosterone does increase further with Ang II infusion. They found that plasma renin levels were not as completely suppressed in this Ang II-responsive subgroup as in the more usual form of the disease, while plasma ANF was, correspondingly less elevated. If indeed the raised ANF is important in inhibiting the aldosterone-stimulating effect of Ang II in classical Conn's syndrome, this less marked increase of ANF might partly explain the persistent effect of Ang II in this variant. Urinary 18-oxocortisol levels were normal in this subgroup and elevated in the more typical Ang II-unresponsive patients, raising the possibility of a biosynthetic abnormality in the former.

Since these Ang II-responsive cases respond just as well to surgery as do those with Ang II-unresponsive tumors, Gordon et al [61] emphasize the need to recognize them, and especially to distinguish them from patients with low-renin essential hypertension or so-called 'idiopathic hyperaldosteronism' (see later).

Irony et al have also described a form of aldosterone excess associated with suppressed plasma renin levels, which is biochemically similar to Conn's syndrome (aldosterone unresponsive to infused Ang II) but which is caused by unilateral (or occasionally bilateral) 'primary adrenal hyperplasia' [62]; again surgery may be curative [62].

ALDOSTERONE-SECRETING CARCINOMA

A carcinoma of the adrenal cortex or, more rarely, of the ovary, can secrete predominantly, an excess of aldosterone [3,4].

Date	Treatment	Supine blood pressure (mmHg)	Plasma active renin (μu/ml) (5–50)*	Blood Ang I (pmol/l) (8–60)*	Plasma Ang II (pmol/l) (5–35)*	Plasma aldosterone (pmol/l) (<500)*	Serum sodium (mmol/l)	Serum potassium (mmol/l)	Serum urea (mmol/l) (2.5–7.5)*	Serum creatinine (μmol/l) (35–130)*	Creatinine clearance (ml/1.73m²/min)	Exchangeable sodium (mmol) and per cent expected normal value	Total body potassium (mmol)
12 June 1979	—	242/136	10	—	12	554	145	2.8	7.6	—	—	3,978 (117%)	4,139
13 June 1979	—	236/134	9	—	10	500	144	2.6	8.3	152	76		
14 June 1979	—	212/138	16	—	13	526	144	2.7	7.6	—	—		
13 December 1979 Basal (09:30)	spironolactone 400mg daily	184/132	119	15	22	1,468	139	4.5	10.4	165	44	3,309 (96%)	4,358
Basal (10:00)	spironolactone 400mg daily	186/136	78	12	21	1,717	—	—	—	—	—		
2 h after captopril (12:00)	spironolactone 400mg daily + captopril 25mg	168/124	193	36	0	1,800	—	—	—	—	—		
18 December 1979 10:00	spironolactone 400mg + captopril 450mg daily	150/104	268	66	3	1,191	136	4.8	16.5	203	39	—	—
12:00		142/106	320	130	0	1,800	—	—	—	—	—		
16:00		142/98	475	89	0	1,994	—	—	—	—	—		
11 February 1980 10:00	spironolactone 400mg + captopril 450mg daily	140/92	260	78	3	1,108	141	5.3	9.5	225	44	3,178 (95%)	4,606
12:00		156/112	360	113	0	1,108	—	—	—	—	—		
16:00		148/96	330	99	0	1,191	—	—	—	—	—		

* normal ranges

Fig. 63.10 Blood pressure and other measurements made in a patient with unoperated aldosterone-secreting adenoma when untreated (June 1979), after six weeks of spironolactone orally daily (December 1979), and at intervals after the addition of captopril. The various normal ranges are shown. Plasma Ang II concentrations less than 2pmol/l are undetectable and shown as zero. Modified from Atkinson AB et al [60].

	Patient 1		Patient 2	
	Untreated	**Treated**	**Untreated**	**Treated**
blood pressure (mmHg)	210/112	134/84	160/106	132/86
serum potassium (mmol/l)	3.3	4.2	3.5	4.2
total body potassium (mmol)	3,995	4,384	4,355	4,655
serum sodium (mmol/l)	142	139	141	139
total body sodium (mmol)	4,029	3,656 (−373)	3,817	3,494 (−323)
plasma active renin (μu/ml)	<3	68	<3	49
plasma aldosterone (ng/dl)	27	4	20	2
plasma cortisol (μg/dl)	15	<1	13	<1
plasma deoxycorticosterone (ng/dl)	19	1	21	1

Fig. 63.11 Data on two patients with glucocorticoid-suppressible aldosterone excess, untreated and after dexamethasone 2mg daily for four weeks. Modified from Robertson JIS and Fraser R [65].

GLUCOCORTICOID-SUPPRESSIBLE ALDOSTERONE EXCESS

Glucocorticoid-suppressible aldosterone excess, a rare variant of primary aldosterone excesss, was first described by Sutherland *et al* in 1966 [63,150]. The diagnosis is based on the usual criteria for primary hyperaldosteronism, that is, high plasma aldosterone concentration or aldosterone secretion rate, low plasma renin, and hypokalemia, as well as the special criterion for this disease — sustained correction of blood pressure and of biochemical abnormalities by administration of the synthetic glucocorticoid dexamethasone. Dexamethasone suppresses adrenocorticotropic hormone (ACTH) secretion; aldosterone secretion, which is supersensitive to ACTH infusion in this condition, is also suppressed. As the condition is inherited as an autosomal dominant factor, other members of the family are likely to be affected. The adrenal cortices usually show bilateral nodular hyperplasia.

There is evidence that the genetic defect in this condition involves a mutation whereby the 5′ regulatory region of 11β-hydroxylase is fused to the coding sequences of aldosterone synthetase on chromosome 8 [151]. This unequal crossing over allows the expression of aldosterone synthetase in the zona fasciculata so that aldosterone can then be produced under continuing ACTH control [150,151].

Some details of studies performed in two hypertensive brothers aged 24 and 29, suffering from this malady, are shown in Fig. 63.11. When untreated, plasma aldosterone concentrations were high (upper limit of normal, 18ng/dl) and plasma active renin concentration low (normal, 10–50μu/l) in both cases [64,65]. Plasma cortisol concentration was normal, suggesting normal ACTH secretion, but interestingly, plasma DOC, another mineralocorticoid, was slightly raised (normal range, 4–16ng/dl). Hypokalemia was apparent, while serum sodium concentration was normal. Total body sodium and potassium were measured before and after the administration of 2mg of dexamethasone (0.5mg four times daily) for four weeks. The fall in plasma cortisol concentration to undetectable levels with dexamethasone indicated suppression of ACTH secretion to subnormal during treatment. This decrease in cortisol occurred concurrently with a decrease in the concentration of plasma aldosterone to low–normal and a slight fall in serum sodium concentration. Total body potassium increased and in each patient, total body sodium fell by more than 300mmol. The decrease in body sodium was accompanied by a return of blood pressure to the normal range. The biochemical abnormalities and hypertension recurred within four weeks after dexamethasone was withdrawn.

Infusion of ACTH while the patients were untreated gave dose–response curves for aldosterone and DOC that were steeper than normal, whereas the curve for cortisol was normal. The dose–response curve for aldosterone was unaffected by dexamethasone treatment.

In one patient, the side effects of dexamethasone were unacceptable and the patient was subsequently treated successfully with amiloride. The second patient remained well controlled long term on a low dose of dexamethasone (0.25mg/d).

The ability of the adrenal gland to hydroxylate cortisol in position 18 (18-hydroxylation) in this condition was put to diagnostic use in this department following the development of a specific radioimmunoassay [152]. Plasma and urinary levels of 18-hydroxycortisol are extremely high both in glucocorticoid-suppressible aldosteronism and in Conn's syndrome (Fig. 63.12).

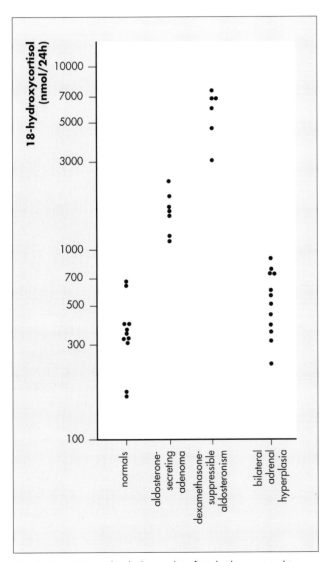

Fig. 63.12 Urinary levels (log-scale) of 18-hydroxycortisol in patients with low-renin hyperaldosteronism (bilateral adrenal hyperplasia), aldosterone-secreting adenoma, dexamethasone-suppressible aldosteronism and normal controls. Modified from Corrie JET et al [152].

HYPERTENSION DUE TO EXCESS OF MINERALOCORTICOIDS OTHER THAN ALDOSTERONE

In a variety of conditions, hypertension, with suppression of the RAS, results from excess of endogenous or exogenous mineralocorticoids other than aldosterone. Nearly always, in this range of conditions, plasma aldosterone is subnormal. In most other respects, the patterns of changes in body spaces, and their relation to the RAS, are closely similar to those described above for patients with aldosterone-secreting adenoma. However, in several of these disorders, some of which are rare, the detailed changes are much less fully elucidated than they are in Conn's syndrome.

17α-HYDROXYLASE DEFICIENCY
Congenital deficiency of the enzyme 17α-hydroxylase leads to defective steroid biosynthesis in both the adrenal cortex and the gonads [66]. The site of the enzyme defect is indicated in Fig. 63.13 [153].

Due to the impaired biosynthesis of androgens and estrogens, genetic males appear as pseudohermaphrodites, while genetic females fail to develop secondary sexual characteristics.

An accompanying defective biosynthesis of cortisol (Fig. 63.13) leads to the mineralocorticoid excess, to hypertension, and to suppression of the RAS. Since cortisol secretion is defective, there is excessive secretion of ACTH, which causes a gross increase in a range of ACTH-sensitive mineralocorticoids, including DOC, 18-hydroxy-DOC, corticosterone, and 18-hydroxycorticosterone [67]. In consequence, there is hypertension, which can be severe, accompanying the pattern of distorted electrolytes and of body compartments typical of mineralocorticoid excess and already described in detail for patients with Conn's syndrome. Thus, there is hypernatremia and hypokalemia, with extracellular alkalosis and with expansion of body sodium and contraction of body potassium content. Plasma levels of renin and Ang II are low, as also is plasma aldosterone.

Treatment with dexamethasone leads to correction of the excessive secretion of ACTH; the various superabundant ACTH-dependent corticosteroids revert to normal, the distorted pattern of electrolytes and of body compartments is rectified, and blood pressure falls [67] (Figs. 63.14 and 63.15). With correction of the previously expanded body sodium content, plasma levels of renin, Ang II, and hence of aldosterone return from subnormal into the normal range (Figs. 63.14 and 63.15).

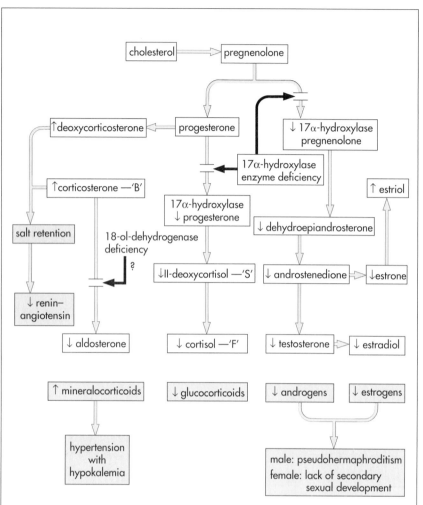

Fig. 63.13 Defect in adrenal steroid synthesis in the syndrome of congenital adrenal hyperplasia, caused by a deficiency of the 17-hydroxylase and, perhaps, the 18-ol-dehydroxygenase, enzymes. Modified from Kaplan NM [153].

	Untreated	On dexamethasone (0.5mg/bid)
sodium (mmol/l)	146	136
potassium (mmol/l)	2.8	4.4
bicarbonate (mmol/l)	32	28
exchangeable sodium (mmol)	2,801	2,258
(per kg)	43.6	34.3
exchangeable potassium (mmol)	2,110	2,489
(per kg)	32.8	37.8
blood pressure (mmHg)	250/165	136/94

Fig. 63.14 Plasma sodium, potassium, and bicarbonate, exchangeable body sodium and potassium, and blood pressure in a 29-year-old genetic female with 17α-hydroxylase deficiency, untreated and during treatment with dexamethasone 0.5mg twice daily.

This correction of the RAS and of aldosterone with dexamethasone treatment establishes a critical point of pathogenesis. The consistent finding of low values of aldosterone in untreated patients [67,68], in the presence of excessive amounts of the biosynthetic precursors of aldosterone, namely DOC and corticosterone, previously raised the possibility [69] that, in addition to the deficiency of 17α-hydroxylase, there was an associated deficiency of the enzyme 18-ol-dehydrogenase that is needed to convert corticosterone to aldosterone (see *Fig. 63.13*). However, the demonstration that with correction of the ACTH excess and of the associated mineralocorticoid-induced sodium expansion, plasma renin, Ang II, and aldosterone can rise into the normal range, makes it clear that 18-ol-dehydrogenase is not lacking. In the untreated state, the aldosterone deficiency is a consequence of the very low levels of Ang II, together with possibly the effects of potassium deficiency and high plasma levels of ANF on aldosterone biosynthesis. When these are corrected, aldosterone levels rise to normal [67,70].

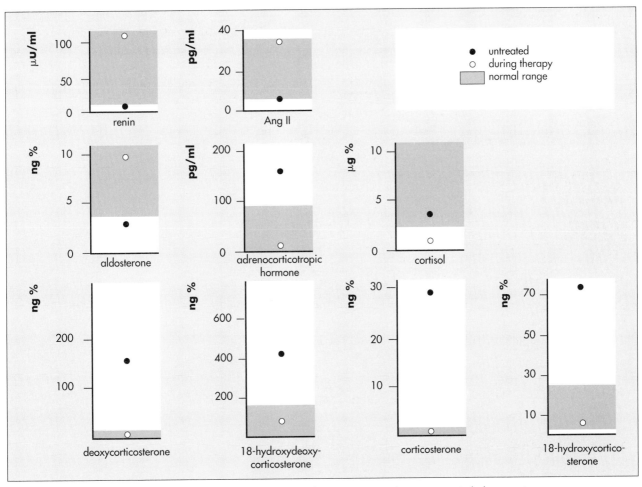

Fig. 63.15   Plasma concentrations of renin, Ang II, aldosterone, adrenocorticotropic hormone, cortisol, deoxycorticosterone, 18-hydroxydeoxycorticosterone, corticosterone, and 18-hydroxycorticosterone, untreated and during therapy with dexamethasone 0.5mg twice daily in a patient with 17α-hydroxylase deficiency (same patient as Fig. 63.14). Modified from Fraser R *et al* [67].

11β-HYDROXYLASE DEFICIENCY

Congenital deficiency of the enzyme 11β-hydroxylase interferes with corticosteroid biosynthesis as shown in Fig. 63.16 [66]. It can be seen that the biosynthetic defect leads to excessive secretion of androgens, such that male children evince precocious sexual development, while females are virilized.

Deficiency of cortisol leads to oversecretion of ACTH and hence consequent excessive production of ACTH-sensitive mineralocorticoids, notably DOC, with resultant hypertension accompanying hypokalemia, hypernatremia, expanded body sodium and contracted body potassium content. The RAS is suppressed. Since the corticosteroid biosynthetic pathway is interrupted proximal to corticosterone, neither corticosterone nor aldosterone can be synthesized adequately.

Treatment with dexamethasone, by lowering ACTH, will correct the mineralocorticoid excess and the hypertension and relieve the suppression of the RAS. However, in this disease return of Ang II to normal cannot correct the hypoaldosteronism, and sodium wasting may occur after treatment is started [71].

APPARENTLY IDIOPATHIC DEOXYCORTICOSTERONE EXCESS

Occasional patients with hypertension and low plasma renin values have been described in whom circulating levels of the mineralocorticoid DOC were present [72]. Other stigmata of mineralocorticoid excess such as hypokalemia were usually lacking. Demonstrable excess of a mineralocorticoid hormone is otherwise unusual in low-renin essential hypertension (see below and *Chapter 62*).

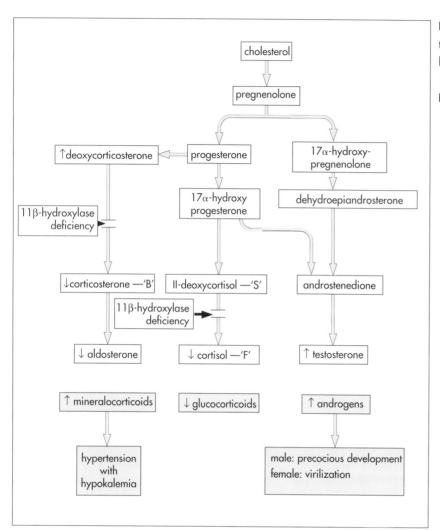

Fig. 63.16 Defect in adrenal synthesis in the syndrome of congenital adrenal hyperplasia caused by a deficiency of the 11-hydroxylase enzyme. Modified from Kaplan NM [153].

CARCINOMA SECRETING DEOXYCORTICOSTERONE OR CORTICOSTERONE

Rare cases of patients have been reported with carcinomata secreting excessive quantities of DOC [73] or of corticosterone [74]. These patients can show the typical features of mineralocorticoid excess, including hypertension, hypokalemia, and suppression of the RAS.

11β-HYDROXYSTEROID DEHYDROGENASE DEFICIENCY (THE 'APPARENT MINERALOCORTICOID EXCESS' SYNDROME)

The extremely rare deficiency of the enzyme 11β-hydroxysteroid dehydrogenase (11β-OHSD) was first described by Werder *et al* [75], who studied a three-year-old girl with severe hypertension and hypokalemia. Plasma renin activity was undetectable but

plasma aldosterone levels were low. Most cases described have been children although an adult case has been studied in detail [76] in this department.

A 21-year-old man presented with clear-cut biochemical evidence of mineralocorticoid-induced hypertension while both PRA and plasma aldosterone levels were suppressed [76]. Investigations revealed a much prolonged half-life of administered 11α[^{3}H]cortisol with high urinary free cortisol levels despite normal plasma levels of ACTH and cortisol. These data, together with a marked increase in urinary cortisol metabolites (for example, tetrahydrocortisol) and a decrease in urinary cortisone metabolites (for example, tetrahydrocortisone) confirmed the diagnosis. Infusion of physiological amounts of cortisol after biochemical correction with dexamethasone confirmed the mineralocorticoid action of cortisol in this syndrome (Fig. 63.17).

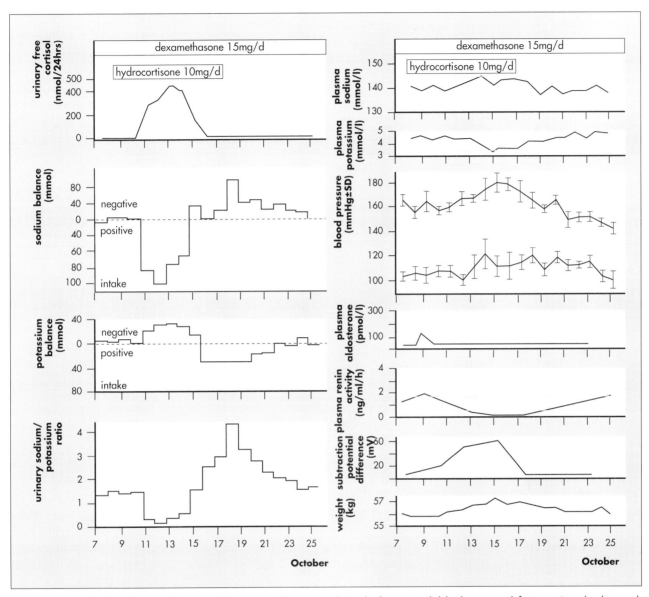

Fig. 63.17 Metabolic balance study in an adult patient with congenital 11β-hydroxysteroid dehydrogenase deficiency. On a background of dexamethasone suppression, a physiological dose of infused hydrocortisone caused clear mineralocorticoid effects, including sodium retention, kaliuresis, and raised blood pressure; a mineralocorticoid effect on rectal potential difference was also noted. Modified from Stewart PM *et al* [76].

The features of the disease have been highlighted in a review by Walker and Edwards [77] and include:

- Normal circulating levels of cortisol but a reduced cortisol production rate.
- Elevation of the ratio of urinary metabolites of cortisol (tetrahydrocortisol and allotetrahydrocortisol) to those of cortisone (tetrahydrocortisone).
- Prolongation of the half-life of 11α-^{3}H cortisol (which is acted on by 11β-OHSD to produce tritiated water and unlabeled cortisone).

- Intact ability to convert orally administered cortisone to cortisol.
- Excess mineralocorticoid activity in kidney (as judged by suppression of renin and aldosterone, hypokalemia, and a very low urinary sodium/potassium ratio), which can be reversed with dexamethasone and reproduced by physiological doses of hydrocortisone.
- No demonstrable excess of any other mineralocorticoid.

The congenital variety of this condition is thus established as being a result of a deficiency of the enzyme 11β-OHSD

[78,79]. 11β-hydroxysteroid dehydrogenase regulates the conversion of cortisol to cortisone [76].

It is known that mineralocorticoids and glucocorticoids have remarkable structural homology [80] and also similar patterns of steroid binding *in vitro* [81]. As the levels of circulating free cortisol are approximately 100-fold higher than those of aldosterone, it is evident that some mechanism is required to prevent the activation of the mineralocorticoid receptor by cortisol. It is now clear that this protection is effected via the local action of 11β-OHSD, which converts cortisol to cortisone and thus prevents access to the type I mineralocorticoid receptor [75,82]. Treatment with a glucocorticoid such as dexamethasone, which is not subject to metabolism by renal 11β-OHSD, represents effective therapy for these patients.

INGESTION OF LICORICE OR CARBENOXOLONE

Extracts of licorice, a substance prepared from the root of the plant *Glycyrrhiza glabra*, contain glycyrrhetinic acid, a compound with mineralocorticoid activity *in vivo*. Carbenoxolone, the semisynthetic hemisuccinate derivative of glycyrrhetinic acid, is a drug used to speed the healing of peptic ulcers.

People who ingest large quantities of licorice-containing sweets or beverages, and susceptible individuals taking carbenoxolone or licorice, may develop mineralocorticoid hypertension [20,83,84]. Some patients may be especially sensitive to the biochemical changes and to the blood-pressure increases. More generally, it has been found that 300mg/d of carbenoxolone regularly induces metabolic and blood-presssure changes, whereas 20mg/d does not.

The initial hypothesis that glycyrrhetinic acid bound directly to the mineralocorticoid receptor [85] was untenable in that hypertension was reversible with dexamethasone [86] and absent in patients without intact adrenal glands [87]. Again, it is now clear that glycyrrhetinic acid inhibits 11β-OHSD, allowing free access of cortisol to the mineralocorticoid receptor [88–90]. It has been demonstrated that the mineralocorticoid effects of licorice, in normal volunteers, are associated with evidence of inhibition of 11β-OHSD [88] (Fig. 63.18). It has also been shown that carbenoxolone induces mineralocorticoid hypertension in a similar fashion [91].

The pattern and biochemical accompaniments of this condition closely resemble those of an aldosterone-secreting tumor, except that aldosterone secretion and plasma aldosterone concentrations are low. The raised blood pressure is characteristically associated with hypernatremia; hypokalemia; increased body sodium and diminished body potassium content; and depression of plasma renin, Ang II, and aldosterone [83,84,92]. The

Subject	THF + allo-THF:THE			Allo-THF:THF		
	Day −1	Day 4	Day 10	Day −1	Day 4	Day 10
1	0.96	0.97	1.30	0.51	0.57	0.53
2	0.60	0.71	0.70	0.26	0.32	0.26
3	0.95	1.03	1.08	0.76	0.77	0.98
4	1.17	1.50	1.47	0.89	1.24	1.20
5	0.91	1.05	1.04	0.72	0.80	0.57
6	0.84	0.91	1.05	0.62	0.71	0.86
7	1.04	1.52	1.61	0.97	0.99	1.47
mean	0.92	1.10	1.18**	0.67	0.77	0.84
SEM	0.07	0.11*	0.12	0.09	0.11	0.16

[1] For comparison with value on day −1:*P<0.05; **P<0.01.

[2] THF = tetrahydrocortisol, THE = tetrahydrocortisone

Fig. 63.18 Effect on steroid metabolism of 10 days of oral licorice (200g/d) in seven healthy volunteers. The increased ratio of cortisol metabolites to those of cortisone is diagnostic of 11β-hydroxysteroid dehydrogenase deficiency. Modified from Stewart PM *et al* [88].

hypokalemia may be accompanied by muscular weakness, paresthesiae, polyuria, cardiac arrhythmias and, occasionally, red urine because of the presence of myoglobin.

Any patient with hypertension, especially if this is associated with hypokalemia, should be questioned concerning possible ingestion of licorice or carbenoxolone If these substances are being taken, they should be discontinued and the patient reassessed initially after 3–4 weeks. It may take 6–8 weeks before the biochemical abnormalities and the hypertension are corrected.

GLUCOCORTICOID RESISTANCE

A very rare abnormality in which hypertension is associated with glucocorticoid resistance was first reported by Vingerhoeds *et al* [93]. In this account, a father and son were found to have hypertension with low renin, low aldosterone, and hypokalemia. There were no clinical features of Cushing's syndrome, although cortisol secretion rates and plasma free cortisol levels were high.

This appears to be an ACTH-driven phenomenon, with consequent high levels of DOC and corticosterone causing mineralocorticoid hypertension. Abnormalities of the affinity of the receptor have been found, and high-dose dexamethasone (3mg/d) appears to be an effective therapy [94].

LIDDLE'S SYNDROME

Liddle's syndrome, first described by Liddle in 1963 [95], has all the clinical and biochemical features of mineralocorticoid hypertension with sodium retention and hypokalemia, although no responsible mineralocorticoid has ever been discovered. In its complete form, hypertension does not, in this disorder, respond to spironolactone therapy but it does to amiloride, implying that that there is a tubular transport abnormality in the kidney rather than excess of any circulating mineralocorticoid substance. It is possible that some of the cases reported in the literature will represent examples of 11β-OHSD deficiency but clearly this would not explain the defect in the patients with no hypotensive response to spironolactone.

Liddle's syndrome is described in more detail in *Chapter 66*.

ESSENTIAL HYPERTENSION WITH LOW PLASMA RENIN

The development of quantitative methods for the assay of plasma renin in man in the early 1960s revealed that a substantial proportion of patients with essential hypertension had low levels of renin [96,97]. Interpretation of this partial suppression of the RAS in essential hypertension has subsequently been a subject of considerable debate. The matter is discussed here because of its possible relevance to mineralocorticoid-induced hypertension; further analysis is given in *Chapter 62*.

While several investigators over the years have proposed that low-renin, apparent essential, hypertension represents a form of mineralocorticoid excess [98], the evidence in favor is elusive [99–101]. Beretta-Piccoli *et al* [102] made a detailed study of body composition in untreated patients with essential hypertension in comparison with normal subjects. Body sodium content was measured both by isotope dilution (exchangeable sodium) and by activation analysis (total body sodium). Body sodium content was higher with age in hypertensive subjects but not in normotensive subjects. Body sodium was not related to arterial pressure in normal subjects, but in hypertensive patients there was a significant positive correlation of arterial pressure with body sodium content which was not explained by an influence of age. However, mean body sodium was not different in normal and hypertensive subjects provided the two groups were matched for leanness index. In hypertensive patients aged less than 36 years, mean body sodium was significantly subnormal (Fig. 63.19) [103,104]; thus, essential hypertension in young patients does not appear to involve sodium retention.

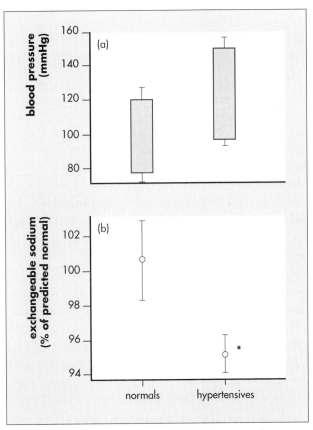

Fig. 63.19 Systolic and diastolic blood pressure (a) and exchangeable sodium (b) (expressed as a percentage of predicted normal value) in 20 normal subjects and 20 young hypertensives matched for age, sex, and leanness index. The data are presented as mean ± SD. Exchangeable sodium is significantly reduced in the hypertensives (*$P<0.05$). Modified from Robertson JIS [103].

Although arterial pressure and body sodium content were progressively higher with age in essential hypertension while plasma renin is well known to fall with age [105], in this series, mean body sodium was not significantly different in patients with essential hypertension whether they had low or normal renin [102]. An alternative proposed explanation for lowering of plasma renin with age and increasing blood pressure in essential hypertension is progressive sclerosis of afferent renal glomerular arterioles, thus leading to diminished renin release [101]. If the latter explanation is correct, it would appear to be more dominant than the effects of expansion of body sodium content.

Plasma ANF has been found to be raised in essential hypertension [105,106], including the elderly [107]. Weak correlations, positive with age and inverse with the RAS, have also been noted [105].

In essential hypertension, aldosterone secretion likewise tends to diminish progressively with age; however, the stimulant effect of Ang II on aldosterone secretion is concurrently enhanced (see *Chapter 33*). In patients with essential hypertension, the increase of plasma aldosterone when Ang II is infused is much brisker than normal and is in marked contrast to the lack of response in Conn's syndrome [53] (see *Fig. 33.11*).

In the series of patients with essential hypertension studied by Beretta Piccoli *et al* [102], those with low renin showed little or no evidence of mineralocorticoid excess. Neither plasma sodium nor aldosterone concentrations were increased; body potassium content and plasma potassium were not decreased; and, both with and without matching for age and leanness index, body sodium was found to be similar in patients with normal or low plasma renin.

Thus, although increased plasma concentrations of DOC have been reported in occasional patients with low plasma renin and apparent essential hypertension [72], the great majority of low-renin essential hypertensives do not appear to be examples of mineralocorticoid excess.

It has been known for many years that dexamethasone lowers blood pressure in patients with essential hypertension [108], and there has been speculation that a defect in the enzyme 11β-OHSD) might be relevant in this condition [77]. Clearly, the majority of patients with essential hypertension do not manifest features of mineralocorticoid hypertension, but direct local actions of cortisol at the vascular wall could still result in hypertension without having a systemic effect [77].

IDIOPATHIC ALDOSTERONISM/NON-TUMOROUS ALDOSTERONISM/PSEUDOPRIMARY ALDOSTERONISM

Approximately 25% of patients with hypertension, aldosterone excess, and low plasma renin do not harbor an adrenocortical adenoma, but instead are found to have, usually bilaterally, nodular or simple hyperplasia of the zona glomerulosa or, in a few instances, normal adrenocortical histology [109,110]. This condition has been termed variously 'idiopathic aldosteronism' 'non-tumorous aldosteronism', or pseudoprimary aldosteronism' [111–113].

Initially the disorder was considered to be a variant of Conn's syndrome (aldosterone-secreting adenoma; see above) [111–113]; however, important differences soon became apparent.

Aldosterone secretion is more readily suppressed in patients

without adenoma when exogenous mineralocorticoids or saline are administered. Patients with aldosterone-secreting tumors do not, as a rule, show the normal postural increase in plasma aldosterone, whereas this tends to be preserved in the nonadenomatous cases [110,114,115]. The biochemical abnormalities (but not the severity of the hypertension) are generally more striking in the patients with adenoma [99,111,112]; this observation is the basis for statistical methods of differential diagnosis such as quadric analysis [116,117], multiple logistic analysis [118], and linear discriminant analysis [68], and for use of the Mahalanobis distance [119].

Aldosterone is abnormally high in relation to plasma renin or Ang II in essential hypertension, particularly in low-renin essential hypertension; thus, the distinction from Conn's syndrome proper on this basis tends to be blurred. The aldosterone response to administered Ang II, while suppressed in Conn's syndrome, is enhanced in both low-renin essential hypertension, and in idiopathic aldosteronism [53]. The relation between plasma aldosterone and Ang II is negative in Conn's syndrome, insignificantly positive in essential hypertension, and significantly positive in idiopathic aldosteronism [3,4] (see *Fig. 63.8*). Plasma renin, Ang II, and aldosterone values are continuously distributed when data from patients with idiopathic aldosteronism and essential hypertension are pooled; by contrast, data from patients with Conn's syndrome are discontinuous with those from the other groups [120]. Age is inversely related to plasma renin essential hypertension [121] and in idiopathic aldosteronism [109], but the two are unrelated in Conn's syndrome [3,4,109].

Plasma ANF is markedly increased in Conn's syndrome [5–7]; while it is much more modestly raised, in proportion to age, in essential hypertension [105]. If as suggested above, the raised plasma ANF of Conn's syndrome is partly responsible for the inhibition of the action of Ang II on aldosterone, the slight increase of ANF in essential hypertension has no such evident action.

Exchangeable sodium and total body sodium are expanded and negatively related to plasma renin in Conn's syndrome but are not expanded and are unrelated to aldosterone or renin in essential hypertension and idiopathic aldosteronism [3,4,21,99,102,109,120,122]. Exchangeable and total body potassium are contracted and inversely related to plasma aldosterone in Conn's syndrome but are normal and unrelated to aldosterone in essential hypertension and idiopathic aldosteronism [3,4,21,99,102,120,122]. Conn's syndrome is characterized by an adrenocortical adenoma, whereas both in essential hypertension and idiopathic aldosteronism, zona glomerulosa hyperplasia, nodules, or even normal histology are variously found [109,110,120].

These several observations led to the proposal [120,121, 123], that while Conn's syndrome is a distinct entity, essential hypertension, low-renin hypertension and idiopathic aldosteronism comprise a continuum within which artificial diagnostic distinctions have been created by overrigid application of arbitrary 'normal' limits. This concept is strongly supported by the application of the statistical technique of Mahalanobis distances to data from the three conditions [119]. This shows that while essential hypertension and idiopathic aldosteronism are closely akin, possibly being the same disorder, Conn's syndrome is a distinctly different disease (Fig. 63.20).

Differentiation between these various conditions has considerable practical, as well as theoretical, interest. Many workers have reported that, in Conn's syndrome proper, excision of the adrenocortical adenoma substantially lowers arterial pressure, to normal values in 50–60% of cases. By contrast, in idiopathic

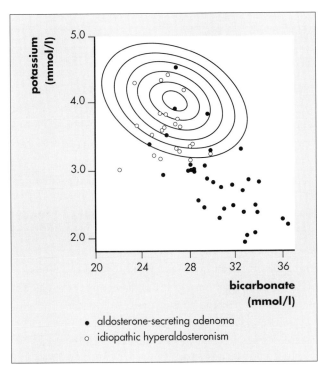

Fig. 63.20 Mahalanobis distances derived from serum potassium and bicarbonate estimations. Concentric ellipses indicate distribution for patients with essential hypertension, the center point corresponding to potassium 4.08mmol/l and bicarbonate 26.7mmol/l. Values for individual patients later proved to have aldosterone-secreting adenoma and for patients with idiopathic hyperaldosteronism are shown. The distribution for idiopathic hyperaldosteronism more closely resembles essential hypertension than Conn's syndrome. Modified from McAreavey D *et al* [119].

aldosteronism, subtotal or total adrenalectomy, with the often consequent adrenocortical deficiency, is needed, while the antihypertensive effect of such surgery is less effective [49,62]. Long-term treatment with potassium-conserving diuretics such as spironolactone or amiloride is now preferred in this latter disease although these drugs too are less effective in idiopathic aldosteronism than in Conn's syndrome [3,4]. This further supports the view of a fundamental difference between the two conditions.

CUSHING'S SYNDROME

Although cortisol is only a weak mineralocorticoid hormone, there is normally a much greater production of cortisol than of aldosterone. This disproportion is exaggerated in patients with Cushing's syndrome.

Ritchie *et al* [124,125] found, however, no alteration in the RAS and no expansion of total exchangeable sodium in a group of patients with Cushing's disease. There was no correlation between blood pressure and exchangeable sodium, while serum potassium was normal. Thus, it has been concluded that in most patients with hypercortisolism, hypertension is not sodium-dependent and that the features are not those of mineralocorticoid excess [126].

The relationships between ACTH, cortisol, and the RAS in Cushing's syndrome and under other circumstances, are discussed further in *Chapter 34*.

ACROMEGALY

Administration of growth hormone can cause sodium and water retention variously in normal, adrenalectomized, and hypophysectomized animals and man. Acromegalics show, consistently, marked elevation of body sodium, nitrogen, chloride, phosphorus, and calcium [127,128]. Body potassium content is also, it should be emphasized, increased, in contrast to classical forms of mineralocorticoid excess where it is low. Plasma and extracellular fluid volumes are consistently raised in acromegaly. These changes correlate with growth hormone levels [129], are corrected when treatment reduces growth hormone secretion [130], and can be induced in animals by administration of growth hormone [131]. Such an abnormal sodium-fluid status should have predictable effects both on the basal activity of the RAS and on its sensitivity to various stimuli. Thus, plasma renin might be expected to be severely suppressed as it is, for example, in primary hyperaldosteronism, and the response to upright posture or to moderate sodium depletion might be expected to be blunted compared with normal. Similarly, plasma aldosterone concentration or aldosterone secretion should be subnormal in acromegaly since aldosterone biosynthesis is largely controlled by the RAS and responses to agonists such as Ang II or ACTH should be attenuated [40,132].

In fact, the situation in acromegaly is less clear cut, in part because the inadequacies of control series and the heterogeneity of patient groups (in respect to age, stage of disease, and treatment) make interpretation and comparison between reports difficult [127]. However, it is probably valid to conclude that, although basal plasma renin levels are usually low [133–136] or low–normal [137,138], they are not as suppressed as would be expected from the concurrent sodium and potassium status, nor is there any obvious relationship between the degree of suppression of the RAS and the severity of hypertension [133,134,138]. However, subnormal renin responses to upright posture [133], to diuretics [138,139], or to restriction of sodium intake [137, 138] are more consistent findings. Cain et al [138] found a normal renin response to the diuretic furosemide, but their patients had already been subject to several days of sodium restriction. If plasma Ang II is indeed inadequately suppressed for the degree of sodium expansion, this could contribute to a rise in blood pressure.

Aldosterone levels are normal or slightly suppressed [133, 135,138,139] but show subnormal responses to dietary sodium restriction [137], diuretic use [138], upright posture [134], and ACTH [140]. The normal aldosterone response to ACTH reported by Cain et al [138] was again obtained in sodium-restricted patients. In a few cases, high plasma aldosterone concentrations in acromegaly have been traced to co-existing primary hyperaldosteronism [128,136]. Acute infusion of growth hormone does not alter either plasma renin [141] or aldosterone concentration [142] in normal subjects, but more prolonged administration may cause increases in both substances after 3–5 days [143–144].

A surprising, and probably very relevant, finding is that plasma ANF is, despite the sodium retention, normal [145,146]. The renal and hypotensive responses to exogenous ANF are greater in active acromegaly. Davies et al [128] have speculated on likely reasons for the lack of rise in plasma ANF in acromegaly despite the sodium and water retention. Among possible explanations are the fact that acromegalic atrial hypertrophy may modify atrial compliance with alterations in the effects of transmural pressure and atrial stretch, and that growth hormone may modify parasympathetic and sympathetic tone,

with consequent impairment of ANF release. The lack of the expected rise of ANF in acromegaly could well be one factor mediating hypertension.

In summary, the long-term pressor mechanisms in acromegaly are complex and imperfectly elucidated. Acromegaly does not conform to the classic pattern of mineralocorticoid-induced hypertension.

CONCLUSIONS

A consistent feature of all forms of mineralocorticoid-induced hypertension is suppression of the circulating RAS. This suppression occurs predominantly as a result of sodium retention, although other factors such as a rise in circulating ANF or an increase in blood pressure itself may contribute. Conversely, a suppressed plasma renin or Ang II level does not necessarily imply sodium retention but may reflect an enhanced adrenal responsiveness to Ang II such as is seen in low-renin hypertension (or in patients with idiopathic hyperaldosteronism).

Blood-pressure elevation in mineralocorticoid-induced hypertension is critically dependent upon sodium retention; indeed, blood pressure is closely correlated with body sodium content in patients with Conn's syndrome. However, the evidence suggests that other factors must play a part both in the initial development and in the established phases of mineralocorticoid-induced hypertension, and has been outlined above.

The organism defends itself vigorously against sodium retention. Various mechanisms, which have been discussed in detail, are activated to this end. In this chapter, the diverse clinical conditions that result in mineralocorticoid-induced hypertension have been described, and the varied biochemical and genetic abnormalities that make up the rich tapestry of this area of clinical medicine have been enumerated. The pathogenesis of certain disorders such as glucocorticoid-suppressible hyperaldosteronism and licorice-induced hypertension are well understood. Other diseases, such as some of the subgroups of 'primary hyperaldosteronism' continue to mystify.

The enigmatic relationship between low-renin hypertension and the condition known as idiopathic hyperaldosteronism — an area of debate for 20 years — has been reviewed. Again, however, we remain unclear as to the reason or reasons for the increased stimulant effects of Ang II on the adrenal gland in these states.

Finally, both Cushing's syndrome and acromegaly, two endocrine disorders long thought to be related to sodium balance, have been examined. While acromegalic patients do retain sodium, the RAS is not proportionately suppressed and true mineralocorticoid-induced hypertension does not exist.

Cortisol is a mineralocorticoid substance and binds to the mineralocorticoid receptors with equal affinity to that of aldosterone. The absence of evidence of mineralocorticoid effects in Cushing's syndrome is thus a remarkable testament to the kidney's ability to protect itself against such a potent steroid.

We have come a long way since Conn's description of an aldosterone-secreting adenoma [41] but, as is so often the case, the more we discover, the more questions arise. Many of the answers remain tantalizingly beyond our reach.

REFERENCES

1. Brown JJ, Davies DL, Lever AF, Peart WS, Robertson JIS. Plasma renin in a case of Conn's syndrome with fibrinoid lesions: Use of spironolactone in treatment. *British Medical Journal* 1964;2:1636–7.

2. Brown JJ, Davies DL, Lever AF, Peart WS, Robertson JIS. Plasma concentration of renin in a patient with Conn's syndrome with fibrinoid lesions of the renal arterioles: The effect of treatment with spironolactone. *Journal of Endocrinology* 1965;33:279–93.

3. Ferriss JB, Brown JJ, Fraser R, Lever AF, Robertson JIS. Primary aldosterone excess: Conn's syndrome and similar disorders. In: Robertson JIS, ed. *Handbook of hypertension, volume 2. Clinical aspects of secondary hypertension.* Amsterdam: Elsevier, 1983:132–61.

4. Ferriss JB. Primary hyperaldosteronism: Conn's syndrome and similar disorders. In: Robertson JIS, ed. *Handbook of hypertension, volume 15. Clinical aspects of hypertension.* Amsterdam: Elsevier, 1992:chapter 12.

5. Yamaji T, Ishibashi M, Sekihara H, Takaku F, Nakaoka H, Fujii J. Plasma levels of atrial natriuretic peptide in primary aldosteronism and essential hypertension. *Journal of Clinical Endocrinology and Metabolism* 1986;63:815–8.

6. Tunny TG, Higgins BA, Gordon RD. Plasma levels of atrial natriuretic peptide in primary aldosteronism, Gordon's syndrome, and Bartter's syndrome. *Clinical and Experimental Pharmacology and Physiology* 1986;13:341–85.

7. Rocco S, Opocher G, Carpene G, Mantero F. Atrial natriuretic peptide infusion in primary aldosteronism: Renal, hemodynamic, and hormonal effects. *American Journal of Hypertension* 1990;3:668–73.

8. Nicholls MG, Ramsay LE, Boddy K, Fraser R, Morton JJ, Robertson JIS. Mineralocorticoid-induced blood pressure, electrolyte and hormone changes, and reversal with spironolactone, in healthy men. *Metabolism* 1979;28:584–93.

9. Biollaz J, Dürr J, Brunner HR, Porchet M, Gavras H. Escape from mineralocorticoid excess: The role of angiotensin II. *Journal of Clinical Endocrinology and Metabolism* 1982;54:1187–93.

10. Sonnenberg H. Proximal and distal tubular function in salt-deprived and salt-loaded deoxycorticosterone acetate-escaped rats. *Journal of Clinical Investigation* 1973;52:263–73.

11. Zipser RD, Zia RA, Stone RA, Horton R. The prostaglandin and kallikrein–kinin system in mineralocorticoid escape. *Journal of Clinical Endocrinology and Metabolism* 1978;37:996–1001.

12. Durr J, Favre L, Gaillard R, Riondel AM, Valloton MB. Mineralocorticoid escape in man: Role of renal prostaglandins. *Acta Endocrinologica (Copenhagen)* 1982;99:474–80.

13. Overlack A, Backer-Kreutz E, Ressel C, Muller HMR, Kolloch R, Stumpe KO. Mineralocorticoid escape during kallikrein inhibition. *Clinical Science* 1986;70:13–7.

14. Lungqvist A. The effect of angiotensin infusion, sodium loading and sodium restriction on the renal and cardiac adrenergic nerves. *Acta Pathologica et Microbiologica Scandinavica* 1975;83:661–8.

15. Miyamori I, Ikeda M. Matsubara T, Okamoto S, Koshida H, Morise T, Takeda R. Human atrial natriuretic polypeptide during escape from mineralocorticoid excess in man. *Clinical Science* 1987;73:431–6.

16. Gaillard CA, Koomans HA, Rabelink TJ, Braam B, Boer P, Dorhout Mees EJ. Enhanced natriuretic effect of atrial natriuretic factor during mineralocorticoid escape in humans. *Hypertension* 1988;12:450–6.

17. Schalekamp MA, Wenting GJ, Man in't Veld AJ. Pathogenesis of mineralocorticoid hypertension. *Clinics in Endocrinology and Metabolism* 1981;10:397–418.

18. Wenting GJ, Man in't Veld AJ, Derkx FHM, Schalekamp MA. Recurrence of hypertension in primary aldosteronism after discontinuation of spironolactone. *Clinical and Experimental Hypertension. Part A, Theory and Practice* 1982;A4:1727–48.

19. Distler A, Just HJ, Philipp TH. Studies on the mechanism of aldosterone-induced hypertension in man. *Clinical Science* 1973;45:743–50.

20. Molhuysen JA, Gerbrandy J, De Vries LA, De Jong JC, Lenstra JB, Turner KP, Borst JGG. A liquorice extract with deoxycortone-like action. *Lancet* 1950;ii:381–6.

21. Beretta-Piccoli C, Davies DL, Brown JJ, Ferriss JB, Fraser R, Lasaridis A, Lever AF, Morton JJ, Robertson JIS, Semple PF, Watt R. Relation of blood pressure with body and plasma electrolytes in Conn's syndrome. *Journal of Hypertension* 1983;1:197–205.

22. Miller AW, Bohr DF, Schork AM, Terris JM. Hemodynamic responses to DOCA in young pigs. *Hypertension* 1979;1:591–7.

23. Bohr DF. What makes the pressure go up? A hypothesis. *Hypertension* 1981;3 (suppl II):160–5.

24. Folkow B. Physiological aspects of primary hypertension. *Physiological Reviews* 1982;62:347–504.

25. Kornel L, Ramsay C, Kanamarlapudi N, Travers T, Packer W. Evidence for the presence in arterial walls of intracellular–molecular mechanisms for action of mineralocorticoids. *Clinical and Experimental Hypertension. Part A, Theory and Practice* 1982;A4:1561–82.

26. Berecek KH, Murray RD, Gross F, Brody MJ. Vasopressin and vascular activity in development of DOCA hypertension in rats with hereditary diabetes insipidus. *Hypertension* 1982;4:3–12.

27. Takeda K, Bunag R. Augmented sympathetic nerve activity and pressor responsiveness in DOCA hypertensive rats. *Hypertension* 1980;2:97–101.

28. Nicholls MG, Julius S, Zweifler AJ. Withdrawal of endogenous sympathetic drive lowers blood pressure in primary aldosteronism. *Clinical Endocrinology* 1981;15:253–8.

29. Lewis PJ, Dargie HJ, Dollery CT. Role of saline consumption in the prevention of deoxycorticosterone hypertension in rats having control 6-hydroxydopamine. *Clinical Science* 1975;48:327–30.

30. Padfield PL. Vasopressin in hypertension. *American Heart Journal* 1977;94:327–30.

31. Rabito SF, Carretero OA, Scicli AG. Evidence against a role of vasopressin in the maintenance of blood pressure in mineralocorticoid and renovascular hypertension. *Hypertension* 1981;3:34–8.

32. Crofton JT, Share L, Shade RE, Lee-Kwon WJ, Manning M, Sawyer WH. The importance of vasopressin in the development and maintenance of DOC-salt hypertension in the rat. *Hypertension* 1979;1:31–8.

33. Morton JJ, Garcia del Rio C, Hughes MJ. Effect of acute vasopressin infusion on blood pressure and plasma angiotensin II in normotensive and DOCA-salt hypertensive rats. *Clinical Science* 1982;**62**:143–9.

34. Webb RC. Potassium relaxation of vascular smooth muscle from DOCA hypertensive pigs. *Hypertension* 1982;**4**:609–19

35. Blaustein M. Sodium ions, calcium ions, blood pressure regulation and hypertension: A reassessment and a hypothesis. *American Journal of Physiology* 1977;**132**:C165–73.

36. George JM, Wright L, Bell NH, Bartter FC. The syndrome of primary aldosteronism. *American Journal of Medicine* 1970;**48**:323–36.

37. Barger AC, Berlin RD, Tulenko JF. Infusion of aldosterone, 9-α-fluorohydrocortisone and antidiuretic hormone into the renal artery of normal and adrenalectomised dogs: Effect on water and electrolyte excretion. *Endocrinology* 1958;**62**:804–15.

38. Haddy F, Pamnani M, Clough D. The sodium–potassium pump in volume-expanded hypertension. *Clinical and Experimental Hypertension* 1978;**1**:295–336.

39. Kojima I, Yoshihara S, Ogata E. Involvement of endogenous digitalis-like substance in the genesis of deoxycorticosterone-salt hypertension. *Life Sciences* 1982;**30**:1775–81.

40. Oelkers W, Brown JJ, Fraser R, Lever AF, Morton JJ, Robertson JIS. Sensitization of the adrenal cortex to angiotensin II in sodium-deplete man. *Circulation Research* 1974;**34**:69–77.

41. Conn JW. Primary aldosteronism: A new clinical syndrome. *Journal of Laboratory and Clinical Medicine* 1955;**45**:3–7.

42. Kucharz EJ. Forgotten description of primary hyperaldosteronism. *Lancet* 1991;**337**:1490.

43. Berlin R. Before Conn's classic paper. *Lancet* 1991;**338**:198.

44. Kirkendall WM, Fitz AE, Armstrong ML. Hypokalemia and the diagnosis of hypertension. *Diseases of the Chest* 1964;**45**:337–45.

45. Conn JW, Cohen EL, Rovner DR. Suppression of plasma renin activity in primary aldosteronism. *Journal of the American Medical Association* 1964;**190**:222–5.

46. Williams ED, Boddy K, Brown JJ, Cumming AMM, Davies DL, Harvey IR, Haywood JK, Lever AF, Robertson JIS. Body elemental composition, with particular reference to total and exchangeable sodium and potassium and total chlorine, in untreated and treated primary hyperaldosteronism. *Journal of Hypertension* 1984;**2**:171–6.

47. Sealy JE, Atlas SA, Laragh JH. Prorenin and other large molecular weight renins. *Endocrine Reviews* 1980;**1**:365–91.

48. Biglieri EH, Schambelan M. The significance of elevated levels of plasma 18-hydroxy-corticosterone in patients with primary aldosteronism. *Journal of Clinical Endocrinology and Metabolism* 1979;**49**:87–91.

49. Brown JJ, Davies DL, Ferriss JB, Fraser R, Haywood E, Lever AF, Robertson JIS. Comparison of surgery with prolonged spironolactone therapy in patients with hypertension, aldosterone excess, and low plasma renin. *British Medical Journal* 1972;**2**:729–34.

50. Richards AM, Tonolo G, Tree M, Robertson JIS, Montorsi P, Leckie BJ, Polonia J. Atrial natriuretic peptides and renin release. *American Journal of Medicine* 1988;**84** (3A):112–8.

51. Pedrinelli R, Bruschi G, Graziadei L, Taddei S, Paranace G, Orlandini G, Natali A, Borghetti A, Salvetti A. Dietary sodium change in primary aldosteronism: Atrial natriuretic factor, hormonal and vascular responses. *Hypertension* 1988;**12**:192–8.

52. Pedrinelli R, Paranace G, Spessot M, Taddei S, Favilla S, Graziadei L, Lucarini A, Salvetti A. Low dose atrial natriuretic factor in primary aldosteronism: Renal, hemodynamic, and vascular effects. *Hypertension* 1989;**14**:156–63.

53. Fraser R, Beretta-Piccoli C, Brown JJ, Cumming AMM, Lever AF, Mason PA, Morton JJ, Robertson JIS. Response of aldosterone and 18-hydroxycorticosterone to angiotensin II in normal subjects and patients with essential hypertension, Conn's syndrome, and non-tumorous hyperaldosteronism. *Hypertension* 1981;**3** (suppl 1):I-87–92.

54. Beevers DG, Brown JJ, Ferriss JB, Fraser R, Lever AF, Robertson JIS, Tree M. Renal abnormalities and vascular complications in primary hyperaldosteronism. *Quarterly Journal of Medicine* 1976;**45**:401–10.

55. Murphy BF, Whitworth JA, Kincaid-Smith P. Malignant hypertension due to an aldosterone-producing adrenal adenoma. *Clinical and Experimental Hypertension. Part A, Theory and Practice* 1985;**A7**:939–50.

56. Pickering GW. High blood pressure. London: J and A Churchill, 1955.

57. Brown JJ, Brown WCB, Fraser R, Lever AF, Morton JJ, Robertson JIS, Rosei EA, Trust PM. The effects of the angiotensin II antagonist saralasin on blood pressure and plasma aldosterone in man in relation to the prevailing plasma angiotensin II concentration. *Progress in Biochemical Pharmacology* 1976;**12**:230–41.

58. Unger T, Gohlke P, Gruber M-G. Converting enzyme inhibitors. In: Ganten D, Mulrow P, eds. *Pharmacology of antihypertensive therapeutics*. Berlin: Springer-Verlag, 1990:377–481.

59. Muratani H, Abe I, Tomita Y, Ueno M, Kawazoe N, Kimura Y, Tsuchihashi T, Takishita S, Uezona K, Kawasaki T. Is single oral administration of captopril beneficial in screening for primary aldosteronism? *American Heart Journal* 1986;**112**:361–7.

60. Atkinson AB, Brown JJ, Davies DL, Lever AF, Robertson JIS. Combined captopril and spironolactone treatment in Conn's syndrome with refractory hypertension. *Clinical Endocrinology* 1981;**14**:105–8.

61. Gordon RD, Gomez-Sanchez CE, Hamlet SM, Tunny TJ, Klemm SA. Angiotensin-responsive aldosterone-producing adenoma masquerades as idiopathic hyperaldosteronism (IHA: adrenal hyperplasia) or low-renin essential hypertension. *Journal of Hypertension* 1987;**5** (suppl 5):103–6.

62. Irony I, Kater CE, Biglieri EG, Shackleton CHL. Correctable subsets of primary aldosteronism: Primary adrenal hyperplasia and renin responsive adenoma. *American Journal of Hypertension* 1990;**3**:576–82.

63. Sutherland DJA, Ruse JL, Laidlaw JC. Hypertension, increased aldosterone secretion and low plasma renin activity relieved by dexamethasone. *Canadian Medical Association Journal* 1966;**95**:1109–19.

64. Connell JMC, Kenyon CJ, Corrie JET, Fraser R, Watt R, Lever AF. Dexamethasone-suppressible hyperaldosteronism: Adrenal transition cell hyperplasia? *Hypertension* 1986;**8**:669–76.

65. Robertson JIS, Fraser R. Salt, volume and hypertension: Causation or correlation? *Kidney International* 1987;**32**:590–602.

66. Fraser R. Inborn errors of corticosteroid biosynthesis and metabolism. In: Robertson JIS, ed. *Handbook of hypertension, volume 15. Clinical aspects of hypertension*. Amsterdam: Elsevier, 1992:chapter 14.

67. Fraser R, Brown JJ, Mason PA, Morton JJ, Lever AF, Robertson JIS, Lee HA, Miller H. Severe hypertension with absent secondary sex characteristics due to partial deficiency of steroid 17 α-hydroxylase activity. *Journal of Human Hypertension* 1987;**1**:53–8.

68. Biglieri EG, Stockigt JR, Schambelan M. Adrenal mineralocorticoids causing hypertension. *American Journal of Medicine* 1972;**52**:623–32.

69. Waldhäusl W, Herkner K, Nowotny P, Bratusch-Marrain P. Combined 17α-and 18-hydroxylase deficiency associated with complete male pseudohermaphroditism hypoaldosteronism. *Journal of Clinical Endocrinology and Metabolism* 1978;**46**:236–46.

70. Kater CE, Biglieri EG, Rost CR, Schambelan M, Hirai J, Chang BCF, Brust N. The constant plasma 18-hydroxycorticosterone to aldosterone ratio: An expression of the efficacy of corticosterone methyloxidase type II activity in disorders with variable aldosterone production. *Journal of Clinical Endocrinology and Metabolism* 1985;**60**:225–8.

71. Zadik Z, Kahana L, Kaufman H, Benderli A, Hochberg Z. Comments: Salt loss in hypertensive form of congenital adrenal hyperplasia (11-β-hydroxylase deficiency). *Journal of Clinical Endocrinology and Metabolism* 1984;**58**:384–7.

72. Brown JJ, Ferriss JB, Fraser R, Lever AF, Love DR, Robertson JIS, Wilson A. Apparently isolated excess deoxycorticosterone in hypertension: A variant of the mineralocorticoid excess syndrome. *Lancet* 1972;**ii**:243–7.

73. Powell-Jackson JD, Calin A, Fraser R, Grahame R, Mason P, Missen GAK, Powell-Jackson PR, Wilson A. Excess deoxycorticosterone secretion from adrenocortical carcinoma. *British Medical Journal* 1974;2:32–3.

74. Fraser R, James VHT, Landon J, Peart WS, Rawson A, Giles CA, McKay AM. Clinical and biochemical studies of a patient with a corticosterone-secreting adrenocortical tumour. *Lancet* 1968;ii:1116–20.

75. Werder E, Zachmann M, Vollmin JA. Unusual steroid excretion in a child with low renin hypertension. *Research Steroids* 1974;6:385–9

76. Stewart PM, Corrie JET, Shackleton CHL, Edwards CRW. The syndrome of apparent mineralocorticoid excess: A defect in the cortisol: cortisone shuttle. *Journal of Clinical Investigation* 1988;82:340–9.

77. Walker BR, Edwards CRW. 11β-hydroxysteroid dehydrogenase and enzyme mediated receptor protection: Life after liquorice? *Clinical Endocrinology* 1991;35:281–9.

78. Ulick S, Levine LS, Gunczler P, Zaaconato G, Ramirez LC, Rauh W, Rosler A, Bradlow HL, New MI. A syndrome of apparent mineralocorticoid excess associated with defects in the peripheral metabolism of cortisol. *Journal of Clinical Endocrinology and Metabolism* 1979;49:757–64.

79. Ulick S. Two uncommon causes of mineralocorticoid excess. *Endocrinology and Metabolism Clinics of North America* 1991;20:269–77.

80. Arriza JL, Weinberger C, Cerelli G, Glaser TM, Handelin BL, Housman DE, Evans RM. Cloning of human mineralocorticoid receptor complementary DNA: Structural and functional kinship with the glucocorticoid receptor. *Science* 1987;237:268–75.

81. Krozowski ZS, Funder JW. Renal mineralocorticoid receptors and hippocampal corticosterone-binding species have identical intrinsic steroid specificity. *Proceedings of the National Academy of Sciences of the USA* 1983;80:6056–60.

82. Edwards CRW. Renal 11β-hydroxysteroid dehydrogenase: A mechanism ensuring mineralocorticoid specificity. *Hormone Research* 1990;34:114–7.

83. Nicholls MG, Espiner EA. Liquorice, carbenoxolone and hypertension. In: Robertson JIS, ed. *Handbook of hypertension, volume 2. Clinical aspects of secondary hypertension.* Amsterdam: Elsevier, 1983:l89–95.

84. Nicholls MG, Richards AM, Lai KN. Drug-induced hypertension. In: Robertson JIS, ed. *Handbook of hypertension, volume 15. Clinical aspects of hypertension.* Amsterdam: Elsevier, 1992:chapter 8.

85. Armanini D, Karbowiak I, Funder JW. Affinity of liquorice derivatives for mineralocorticoid and glucocorticoid receptors. *Clinical Endocrinology* 1983;19:609–12.

86. Hoefnagels WHL, Kloppenborg PWC. Antimineralocorticoid effects of dexamethasone in subjects treated with glycyrrhetinic acid. *Journal of Hypertension* 1983:1 (suppl 2):313–5.

87. Borst JGG, Ten Holt SP, DeVries LA. Synergistic action of liquorice and cortisone in Addison's and Simmonds' disease. *Lancet* 1953;i:657–63.

88. Stewart PM, Valentino R, Wallace AM, Burt D, Shackleton CHL, Edwards CRW. Mineralocorticoid activity of liquorice 11β-hydroxysteroid dehydrogenase deficiency comes of age. *Lancet* 1987;ii:821–4.

89. MacKenzie MA, Hoefnagels WHL, Jansen RWMM, Benraad TJ, Kloppenborg PWC. The influence of glycyrrhetinic acid on plasma and cortisone in healthy young volunteers. *Journal of Clinical Endocrinology and Metabolism* 1990;70:1637–43.

90. Edwards CRW. Lessons from licorice. *New England Journal of Medicine* 1991;325:1242–3.

91. Stewart PM, Wallace AM, Atherden SM, Shearing CH, Edwards CRW. Mineralocorticoid activity of carbenoxolone: Contrasting effects of carbenoxolone and liquorice on 11β-hydroxysteroid dehydrogenase activity in man. *Clinical Science* 1990;78:49–54.

92. Beretta-Piccoli C, Salvade G, Crivelli PL, Weidmann P. Body-sodium and blood volume in a patient with licorice-induced hypertension. *Journal of Hypertension* 1985;3:19–23.

93. Vingerhoeds ACM, Thijssen JHH, Schwartz F. Spontaneous hypercortisolism without Cushing's syndrome. *Journal of Clinical Endocrinology and Metabolism* 1976;43:1128–33.

94. Lipsett MB, Tomitta M, Brandon DD, De Vroede MM, Loriaux DL, Chrousos GP. Cortisol resistance in man. *Advances in Experimental Medicine and Biology* 1986;196:97–101.

95. Liddle GW, Bledsoe T, Coppage WS. A familial renal disorder simulating primary aldosteronism but with negligible aldosterone secretion. In: Baulieu EE, Robel P, eds. *Aldosterone.* Oxford: Blackwell Scientific Publications, 1964: 353–75.

96. Helmer OM. Renin activity in blood from patients with hypertension. *Canadian Medical Association Journal* 1964;90:221–5.

97. Brown JJ, Davies DL, Lever AF, Robertson JIS. Variations in plasma renin concentration in several physiological and pathological states. *Canadian Medical Association Journal* 1964;90:201–6.

98. Spark RF, Melby JC. Hypertension and low plasma renin activity: Presumptive evidence for mineralocorticoid excess. *Annals of Internal Medicine* 1971;75:831–6.

99. Ferriss JB, Beevers DG, Brown JJ, Fraser R, Lever AF, Padfield PL, Robertson JIS. Low-renin ('primary') hyperaldosteronism. *American Heart Journal* 1978;95:641–58.

100. Padfield PL, Beevers DG, Brown JJ, Davies DL, Lever AF, Robertson JIS, Tree M. Is low-renin hypertension a stage in the development of essential hypertension or a diagnostic entity? *Lancet* 1975;i:548–50.

101. Thurston H, Bing RF, Pohl JEF, Swales JD. Renin subgroups in essential hypertension: An analysis and critique. *Quarterly Journal of Medicine* 1978;47: 325–37.

102. Beretta-Piccoli C, Davies DL, Boddy K, Brown JJ, Cumming AMM, East BW, Fraser R, Lever AF, Padfield PL, Semple PF, Robertson JIS, Weidmann P, Williams ED. Relation of arterial pressure with body sodium, body potassium, and plasma potassium in essential hypertension. *Clinical Science* 1982;63:257–70.

103. Robertson JIS. The renin–aldosterone connection: Past, present and future. The Franz Gross Memorial Lecture. *Journal of Hypertension* 1984;2 (suppl 3):1–14.

104. Thomas GW, Ledingham JGG, Beilin LJ, Stott AN. Reduced plasma renin activity in essential hypertension: Effects of blood pressure, age and sodium. *Clinical Science* 1976;51 (suppl):185–8.

105. Montorsi P, Tonolo G, Polonia J, Hepburn D, Richards AM. Correlates of plasma atrial natriuretic factor in health and hypertension. *Hypertension* 1987;10:570–6.

106. Hollister AS, Inagami T. Atrial natriuretic factor and hypertension: A review and meta-analysis. *American Journal of Hypertension* 1991;4:850–65.

107. Sumimoto T, Murakami E, Hiwada K. Plasma atrial natriuretic factor in isolated systolic hypertension in the elderly: Response to hypertonic saline infusion. *Journal of Human Hypertension* 1991;5:411–5.

108. Hamilton BP, Zadik Z, Edwin CM, Hamilton JH, Kowarski AA. Effect of adrenal suppression with dexamethasone in essential hypertension. *Journal of Clinical Endocrinology and Metabolism* 1979;48:848–53.

109. Ferriss JB, Beevers DG, Brown JJ, Davies DL, Fraser R, Lever AF, Mason P, Neville AW, Robertson JIS. Clinical, biochemical and pathological features of low-renin ('primary') hyperaldosteronism. *American Heart Journal* 1978;95: 375–88.

110. Weinberger MH, Grim CE, Hollifield JW, Kem DH, Ganguly A, Kramer NJ, Yune HY, Wellman H, Donohue JP. Primary aldosteronism: Diagnosis, localization, and treatment. *Annals of Internal Medicine* 1979;90:386–95.

111. Baer L, Sommers SC, Krakoff LR, Newton MA, Laragh JH. Pseudoprimary aldosteronism: An entity distinct from true primary aldosteronism. *Circulation Research* 1970;26/27 (suppl 1):203–16.

112. Liddle GW. In discussion. *Transactions of the Association of American Physicians* 1967;80:182.

113. Biglieri EG, Schambelan M, Slaton PE, Stockigt JR. The intercurrent hypertension of primary aldosteronism. *Circulation Research* 1970;26/27 (suppl 1):195–202

114. Ganguly A, Melada GA, Luetscher JA, Dowdy AJ. Control of plasma aldosterone in primary aldosteronism: Distinction between adenoma and hyperplasia. *Journal of Clinical Endocrinology and Metabolism* 1973;37:765–75.

115. Schambelan M, Brust NL, Chang BCF, Slater KL, Biglieri EG. Circadian rhythm and effect of posture on plasma aldosterone concentration in primary aldosteronism. *Journal of Clinical Endocrinology and Metabolism* 1976;43:115–31.

116. Ferriss JB, Brown JJ, Fraser R, Kay AW, Lever AF, Neville AM, O'Muircheartaigh IG, Symington T, Robertson JIS. Hypertension with aldosterone excess and low plasma renin: Pre-operative distinction between patients with and without adrenocortical tumour. *Lancet* 1970;ii:995–1000.

117. Aitchison J, Brown JJ, Fraser R, Haywood E, Davies DL, Kay AW, Lever AF, Neville AM, Symington T, Robertson JIS. Quadric analysis in the pre-operative distinction between patients with and without adrenocortical tumours in patients with aldosterone excess and low plasma renin. *American Heart Journal* 1971;82:660–71.

118. Luetscher JA, Ganguly A, Malada GA, Dowdy AJ. Pre-operative differentiation of adrenal adenoma from idiopathic adrenal hyperplasia in primary aldosteronism. *Circulation Research* 1974;34 & 35 (suppl 1):175–82.

119. McAreavey D, Murray GD, Lever AF, Robertson JIS. Similarity of idiopathic aldosteronism and essential hypertension: A statistical comparison. *Hypertension* 1983;5:116–21.

120. Davies DL, Beevers DG, Brown JJ, Cumming AMM, Fraser R, Lever AF, Mason PA, Morton JJ, Robertson JIS, Titterington M, Tree M. Aldosterone and its stimuli in normal and hypertensive man: Are essential hypertension and primary hyperaldosteronism without tumour the same condition? *Journal of Endocrinology* 1979;81:79–91P.

121. Padfield PL, Brown JJ, Davies D, Fraser R, Lever AF, Morton JJ, Robertson JIS. The myth of idiopathic hyperaldosteronism. *Lancet* 1981;ii:83–4.

122. Lasaridis A, Brown JJ, Davies DL, Fraser R, Robertson JIS, Lever AF. Arterial blood pressure and plasma and body electrolytes in idiopathic hyperaldosteronism: A comparison with primary hyperaldosteronism (Conn's syndrome) and essential hypertension. *Journal of Hypertension* 1984;2:329–36.

123. Editorial. Idiopathic aldosteronism: A diagnostic artifact? *Lancet* 1979;ii: 1221–2.

124. Ritchie CM, Hadden DR, Kennedy L, Sheridan B, Riddell J, Atkinson AB. Pathogenesis of hypertension in Cushing's disease. *Journal of Hypertension* 1987;5 (suppl 5):497–9.

125. Ritchie CM, Sheridan B, Fraser R, Hadden DR, Kennedy AL, Riddell J, Atkinson AB. Studies on the pathogenesis of hypertension in Cushing's disease and acromegaly. *Quarterly Journal of Medicine* 1990;76:855–67.

126. Atkinson AB. Cushing's syndrome. In: Robertson JIS, ed. *Handbook of hypertension, volume 15. Clinical aspects of hypertension.* Amsterdam: Elsevier, 1992: chapter 13.

127. Fraser R, Davies DL, Connell JMC. Hormones and hypertension. *Clinical Endocrinology* 1989;31:701–46.

128. Davies DL, Connell JMC, Reid R, Fraser R. Acromegaly: The effects of growth hormone on blood vessels, sodium homeostasis and blood pressure In: Robertson JIS, ed. *Handbook of hypertension, volume 15. Clinical aspects of hypertension.* Amsterdam: Elsevier, 1992:chapter 17.

129. Snow MH, Piercy DA, Robson V, Wilkinson R. An investigation into the pathogenesis of hypertension in acromegaly. *Clinical Science* 1977;53:87–91.

130. McLellan AR, Connell JMC, Beastall GH, Teasdale G, Davies DL. Growth hormone, body composition and somatomedin C after treatment of acromegaly. *Quarterly Journal of Medicine* 1988;69:997–1008.

131. Batts AA, Bennett LL, Garcia J, Stein J. The effect of growth hormone on muscle potassium and on extracellular fluid. *Endocrinology* 1954;55:456–65.

132. Gordon RD, Nicholls MG, Tree M, Fraser R, Robertson JIS. Influence of sodium balance on ACTH/adrenal corticosteroid dose–response curves in the dog. *American Journal of Physiology* 1980;238:E543–51.

133. Kraatz C, Benker G, Weber F, Ludecke D, Hirche H, Reinwein D. Acromegaly and hypertension: Prevalence and relationship to the renin–angiotensin–aldosterone system. *Klinische Wochenschrift* 1990;68:583–7.

134. Slowinska-Srednicka J, Zgliczynski S, Pucilowska J. Studies on the pathogenesis of arterial hypertension in acromegaly. I. The renin–angiotensin–aldosterone system. *Polskie Archiwum Medycyny Wewnetrznej* 1983;69:129–36.

135. Ogihara T, Hata T, Muruyama A, Mikami H, Nakamaru M, Okada Y, Kumahara Y. Blood pressure response to an angiotensin antagonist in patients with acromegaly. *Journal of Clinical Endocrinology and Metabolism* 1979;48: 159–62.

136. Dluhy RG, Williams GH. Primary aldosteronism in a hypertensive acromegalic patient. *Journal of Clinical Endocrinology and Metabolism* 1969;29:1319–24.

137. Moore TJ, Thein-Wai W, Dluhy RG, Dawson-Hughes BP, Hollenberg NK, Williams GH. Abnormal adrenal and vascular responses to angiotensin II and an angiotensin antagonist in acromegaly. *Journal of Clinical Endocrinology and Metabolism* 1980;51:215–22.

138. Cain JP, Williams GH, Dluhy RG. Plasma renin activity and aldosterone secretion in patients with acromegaly. *Journal of Clinical Endocrinology and Metabolism* 1972;34:73–81.

139. Mantero F, Opocher G, Arminini D, Paviotti G, Boscaro M, Muggeo M. Plasma renin activity and urinary aldosterone in acromegaly. *Journal of Endocrinological Investigation* 1979;2:13–8.

140. Slowinska-Srzednicka J, Pucilowska J, Zgliczynski S. Arterial hypertension in acromegaly: Altered dopaminergic control of aldosterone secretion. *Clinical and Experimental Hypertension. Part A, Theory and Practice* 1987;A9:1843–58.

141. Epstein S, Roith DLe, Rabkin R. The effect of different preparations of human growth hormone on plasma renin activity in normal males. *Journal of Clinical Endocrinology and Metabolism* 1976;42:390–2.

142. Birkhäuser M, Gaillard R, Riondel AM, Zahnd GR. Influence of acute administration of human growth hormone and alpha-MSH on plasma concentrations of aldosterone, cortisol, corticosterone and growth hormone in man. *Acta Endocrinologica (Copenhagen)* 1975;79:16–24.

143. Moller J, Jorgensen JOL, Hansen KW, Pedersen EB, Christiansen JS. Expansion of extracellular volume and suppression of atrial natriuretic peptide after growth hormone administration in normal man. *Journal of Clinical Endocrinology and Metabolism* 1991;72:768–72.

144. Ho KY, Weissberger AJ. The antinatriuretic action of biosynthetic human growth hormone in man involves activation of the renin angiotensin system. *Metabolism* 1990;39:133–7.

145. McKnight JA, McCance DR, Hadden DR, Kennedy L, Roberts G, Sheridan B, Atkinson AB. Basal and stimulated levels of atrial natriuretic peptide in acromegaly. *Journal of Endocrinology* 1988;117 (suppl):58.

146. McKnight JA, McCance DR, Hadden DR, Kennedy L, Roberts G, Sheridan B, Atkinson AB. Basal and saline-stimulated levels of plasma atrial natriuretic factor in acromegaly. *Clinical Endocrinology* 1989;31:431–8.

147. Gonzalez-Campoy JM, Romero JC, Knox FG. Escape from the sodium-retaining effects of mineralocorticoids: Role of ANF and intrarenal hormone systems. *Kidney International* 1989;35:767–77.

148. Gordon RD, Bachmann AW, Jackson RV, Saar N. Increased sympathetic activity in renovascular hypertension in man. *Clinical and Experimental Pharmacology and Physiology* 1982;9:277–81.

149. Ferriss JB, Beevers DG, Boddy K, Brown JJ, Davies DL, Fraser R, Kremer D, Lever AF, Robertson JIS. The treatment of low-renin ('primary') hyperaldosteronism. *American Heart Journal* 1978;96:97–109.

150. Editorial: Glucocorticoid-suppressible hyperaldosteronism. *Lancet* 1992;339: 1024–5.

151. Lifton RP, Dluhy RG, Powers M, Rich GM, Cook S, Ulick S, Lalouel J-M. A chimaeric 11β-hydroxylase/aldosterone synthase gene causes glucocorticoid-remediable aldosteronism and human hypertension. *Nature* 1992;355:262–5.

152. Corrie JET, Edwards CRW, Budd PS. A radioimmunoassay for 18- hydroxycortisol in plasma and urine. *Clinical Chemistry* 1985;31:849–52

153. Kaplan NM. *Clinical hypertension, 5th edition.* Baltimore: Williams and Wilkins, 1990.

64 RENIN IN BARTTER'S SYNDROME

RICHARD D GORDON, SHELLEY A KLEMM, AND
TERRY J TUNNY

INTRODUCTION

Bartter's syndrome is characterized by severe hypokalemic alkalosis, hyperreninemia, pressor insensitivity to Ang II, and normal or low values of plasma sodium, plasma chloride, and blood pressure. When the electrolyte disturbance is severe, growth failure can occur. Chronic renal sodium and potassium wasting are invariably present, although the initiating cause may vary

(Fig. 64.1). Many of the clinical features and biochemical abnormalities appear to be secondary to chronic hypokalemia (Figs. 64.1 and 64.2).

Bartter's syndrome is often congenital, and sometimes familial. It can also result from chloride-deficient diets [1,2], from renal complications of chemotherapy [3] and, rarely, from cystic fibrosis [4] (see *Fig. 64.1*). A syndrome biochemically indistinguishable from Bartter's syndrome can result from surreptitious diuretic abuse [5,6] (see *Chapter 72*); exclusion of this condition depends on the availability of reliable assays for a variety of diuretics, and a high index of suspicion [7]. Bulimia, anorexia nervosa, and laxative abuse [8–10] are additional causes of a syndrome that resembles Bartter's syndrome biochemically,

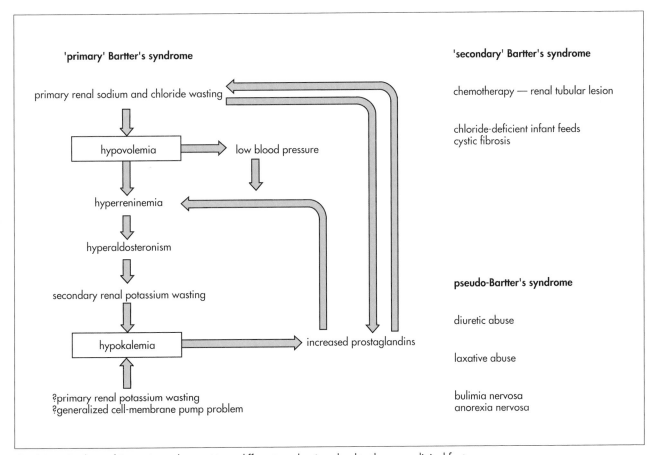

Fig. 64.1 Etiology of Bartter's syndrome. Many different mechanisms lead to the same clinical features.

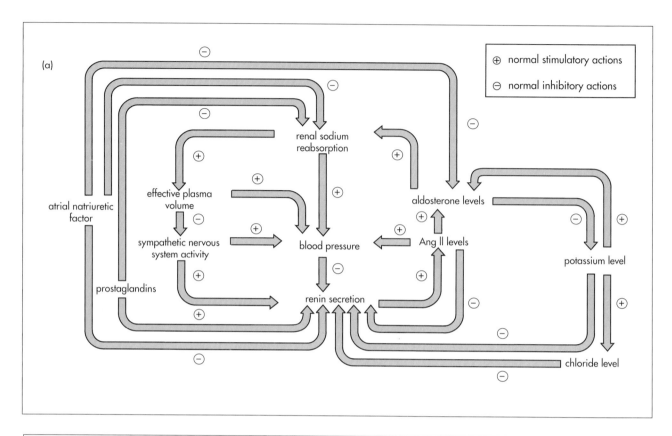

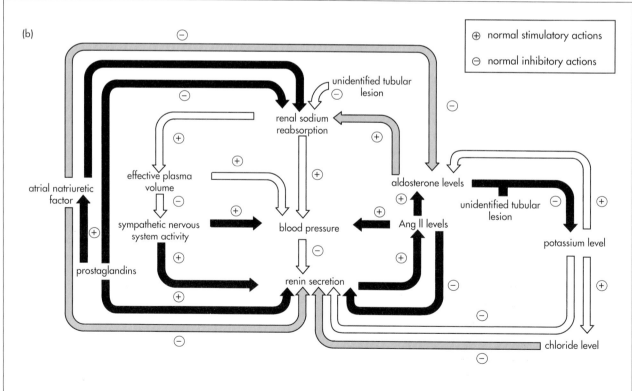

Fig. 64.2 (a) Normal influences (positive or negative) on renin secretion. (b) Altered levels of activity in the directions indicated by the plus and minus signs in Bartter's syndrome, are shown by black arrows (increased) or open arrows (decreased).

except that urinary potassium and chloride are low [11]. These conditions may, however, lead to diagnostic confusion on first presentation. Anorexia nervosa, bulimia nervosa, purgative abuse, and diuretic abuse are considered in detail in *Chapter 72*. A number of 'variants' of classical Bartter's syndrome have been reported, sometimes associated with less prominent hyperreninemia and juxtaglomerular hyperplasia, and sometimes with additional features such as hypomagnesemia. Thus, Bartter's syndrome can occasionally be associated with hypercalciuria, nephrocalcinosis, and nephrolithiasis [12]. Rarely, severe Bartter's syndrome in infancy has been associated with progressive nephritis leading to renal failure and death [13]. Gullner *et al* [14] described a sibship with a condition almost identical to Bartter's syndrome, except for histological changes in the proximal renal tubules and uncharacteristically normal distal fractional chloride reabsorption. Others have described familial potassium-wasting disorders which they believed should be distinguished from Bartter's syndrome [15–17], while sharing common clinical and biochemical features.

Renal histology has been quite variable, depending on the cause and the course, but marked juxtaglomerular hyperplasia, reflecting hypersecretion of renin, has frequently been present. (Plate 29, see Color Plate Section). Juxtaglomerular hyperplasia was a feature of the first two patients reported by Bartter *et al* [18], and some authors have suggested that demonstration of this is essential for the diagnosis of Bartter's syndrome. There are several problems, however. First, this presupposes that it is appropriate, even necessary, to subject patients with clinical and biochemical criteria of Bartter's syndrome to a renal biopsy, an often uncomfortable procedure not without risk. Second, the management of the patient will not, in most circumstances, be altered by the presence or absence of definite juxtaglomerular hyperplasia. Third, the recognition of juxtaglomerular hyperplasia is influenced by the angle at which sampled glomeruli are cut, the number of glomeruli in the specimen, and the anatomical position of glomeruli in the inner or outer cortex. Fourth, histological assessment of juxtaglomerular hyperplasia would not be expected to be closely correlated with function as manifested in circulating renin levels, which are a better pathophysiological index. Fifth, juxtaglomerular hyperplasia appears to become more pronounced with time and reflects the duration as well as the degree of renin hypersecretion. Sixth, juxtaglomerular hyperplasia has been documented in disorders that mimic Bartter's syndrome; thus a diagnosis cannot rest upon this finding on renal biopsy.

Bartter's syndrome may occur sporadically or in families. Familial Bartter's syndrome affects only one generation, except in the case of consanguinous marriages. This speaks in favor of a recessive mode of inheritance [19].

Since high plasma renin levels (often extremely high and only exceeded in such conditions as malignant hypertension, untreated Addison's disease, and uncontrolled diabetes insipidus) are consistently present in Bartter's syndrome, they are an essential diagnostic feature. The mechanisms of production and the effects of these very high plasma renin levels are explored in this chapter.

HISTORICAL BACKGROUND

In 1962, Bartter and associates reported a newly recognized syndrome in two patients with severe hypokalemia and retardation of growth [18]. The findings in one of these patients had been briefly reported earlier [20]. Other features were normal blood pressure despite high levels of renin and aldosterone, hyperplasia of the juxtaglomerular apparatus, and a markedly reduced pressor responsiveness to infused Ang II. This led to a hypothesis, since discarded by most reviewers, that vascular resistance to Ang II was the initiating mechanism. It was the then-recent availability of reliable measurements of plasma renin activity (PRA) and urinary aldosterone which permitted the formulation of this hypothesis and made the 1962 report a seminal paper. Earlier accounts of spontaneous hypokalemia [21–23] may well have been of the same syndrome, but lack of proven hyperreninemia does not permit a firm diagnosis. By 1980, Gill was able to draw on approximately 100 published cases in order to write his excellent review [24], and by 1990, at least 300 patients had been described in reasonable detail. If normal or low blood pressure, elevated renin, and severe hypokalemia are accepted as the minimal diagnostic features, it has long been clear that Bartter's syndrome is a heterogeneous disorder with a variety of etiologies, as has been well discussed by Stein [25] (see *Fig. 64.1*).

In 1976, several workers [26–29] drew attention to the high levels of vasodilator, natriuretic prostaglandins in Bartter's syndrome, and to the beneficial effects of inhibition of prostaglandin synthesis. This led to the short-lived idea that the basic pathophysiological mechanism responsible for Bartter's syndrome had been identified. Unfortunately, prostaglandin inhibition appears incapable of correcting completely the hypokalemia of Bartter's syndrome.

In 1969, Imai *et al* [30] suggested that Bartter's syndrome might be caused by excessive action of a natriuretic factor. In 1979, Grekin and co-workers [31] hypothesized that Bartter's syndrome might be due to excessive secretion of a putative 'chloriuretic hormone'. In 1986, Gordon and co-workers described inappropriately high levels of atrial natriuretic factor (ANF), which fell to normal with prostaglandin inhibition, in their patients with Bartter's syndrome [32,33]. They later showed that this occurred despite concomitant increases in right atrial pressure [34]. Elevated levels of ANF were also reported in a Japanese patient with Bartter's syndrome [35], but also in pseudo-Bartter's syndrome due to diuretic abuse [36]. Others have, however, reported low levels of ANF in Bartter's syndrome [37,38], again attesting to the heterogeneity of this disorder. While inappro-priately high levels of ANF in at least some patients with Bartter's syndrome suggest an abnormality in ANF production or action as a possible etiological mechanism, Graham *et al* in a family study, could find no evidence for involvement of the gene coding for ANF in Bartter's syndrome [39]. Levels of ANF were not, however, reported in affected and unaffected members of that large kindred, and Graham *et al* [39] pointed out that abnormalities in ANF release, metabolism, or action were not excluded in their study. Since, as has already been discussed, there may be several different etiologies resulting in the clinical manifestations of Bartter's syndrome, these would presumably involve different genotypic abnormalities in affected families. Thus, there could be multiple alleles at the same locus, or at several different loci. Furthermore, environmental (for example, dietary) differences could affect expression of the genetic abnormality.

ETIOLOGY OF PRIMARY BARTTER'S SYNDROME

In the most common variety of Bartter's syndrome ('primary'), the etiology is still unclear. There has, in some patients, been evidence for defective chloride reabsorption in the ascending limbs of the loops of Henle [40,41] and pure chloride depletion can cause hypokalemic alkalosis [42,43]. Indeed, this was believed to be the mechanism of production of a pseudo-Bartter's syndrome ('secondary') in infants fed a chloride-deficient dietary formula (see *Fig. 64.1*). This was reversible on substitution of a diet containing adequate chloride [3,4,]. If, however, the proximal tubules were the major site of wastage of chloride and sodium, phosphaturia, glycosuria, and aminoaciduria might be expected, but are not seen. Decreased chloride transport in the loops of Henle may affect the signal at the macula densa which regulates renin secretion (see *Chapter 24*), and together with hypovolemia from salt loss, lead to hyperreninemic hyperaldosteronism and hypokalemia. Conversely, it has been suggested that potassium depletion can lead to decreased chloride transport in Henle's loops [44], and that severe hypokalemia, however induced, might be the initiating event in Bartter's syndrome.

Whatever the cause of renal sodium and chloride wasting, and of hypokalemia, there is good evidence for renal overproduction of the prostanoids PGE_2, PGF_2, and 6-keto PGF_1 in Bartter's syndrome. As discussed in detail by Dunn [45], this is probably secondary to the high levels of Ang II. Prostaglandins can, however, stimulate renin and Ang II production, and it is unclear as to which comes first — prostaglandins stimulating renin secretion or Ang II stimulating prostaglandin production.

With hyperreninemia and hypokalemia as the constant features, the most likely candidates for a primary mechanism are a chloride reabsorption defect in the thick renal tubular ascending limbs, provoking hyperreninemia by stimulation of the macula densa and through hypovolemia, with both secondary hyperaldosteronism and increased distal delivery of sodium explaining hypokalemia; a primary sodium reabsorptive defect in the proximal tubules, where inappropriately high levels of ANF could be involved; a primary potassium oversecretion in the distal tubules, which might involve hypersensitivity to aldosterone, for example due to a more complete block of reabsorption of chloride in the distal tubules than usually exists — such a mechanism would be the mirror image of that proposed by Schambelan *et al* [46] to explain Gordon's syndrome; a primary defect of potassium reabsorption, which would presumably be in the proximal tubules and which could complement any of the other mechanisms; or a generalized cell-membrane electrolyte-transport defect, discussed later.

In addition, increased levels of plasma bradykinin, secondary to raised renal kallikrein production [47] due to the actions of aldosterone and Ang II, may contribute to the low blood pressure.

The failure of bilateral adrenalectomy to cure hypokalemia in one patient with Bartter's syndrome [48] is an oft-quoted argument against the hypokalemia being solely due to secondary hyperaldosteronism. Furthermore, reduction of aldosterone to normal levels by subtotal adrenalectomy [49], aminoglutethimide [50], or albumin infusion [50,51] also failed to prevent persistent hypokalemia, although aminoglutethimide did permit maintenance of normal plasma potassium in another patient while on a high potassium diet (130mmol/d), [52]. Thus, in at least some patients, there appears to be a second mechanism leading to hypokalemia. If this depends on renal potassium wasting, the location is presumably either in the proximal tubules or at the site where aldosterone acts, but independent of aldosterone. Alternatively, the fault could be a defective transmembrane regulator affecting all cells.

Since the detailed renal actions of ANF are still controversial, the significance of the observations that ANF can be inappropriately normal or raised in Bartter's syndrome [32–36] is

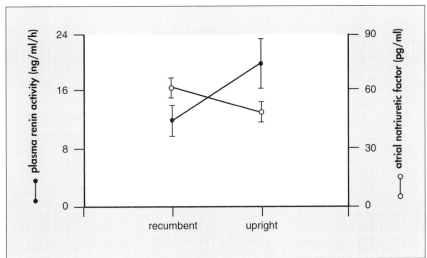

Fig. 64.3 Opposite effects of upright posture on plasma renin activity and atrial natriuretic factor in five patients with Bartter's syndrome (mean ± SEM), consistent with a chronic effect of prostaglandins on Ang II overridden by an acute effect of posture mediated by central blood volume and atrial stretch. (Unpublished data).

unclear. Like the elevated prostaglandins, unexpectedly normal or raised ANF levels could be a secondary phenomenon, with high levels of prostaglandins [53] or of Ang II [32–34, 54] being responsible. The fact that ANF and PRA move in opposite directions in response to postural changes in Bartter's syndrome (Fig. 64.3) suggests that Ang II is not the major acute regulator of ANF in this disorder, but either prostaglandins or Ang II (or both) may contribute to steady-state ANF levels in the long term.

Some workers have found evidence for a generalized cell-membrane defect in Bartter's syndrome, which could explain the failure to correct hypokalemia by therapeutic methods that should be successful in a purely renal tubular disorder. Thus, Gall et al [55] found increased erythrocyte intracellular sodium concentrations and increased active sodium transport in a patient with Bartter's syndrome, and Gardner et al [56] confirmed that erythrocyte sodium concentrations were raised in six of eight patients with Bartter's syndrome and in some of their relatives as well. It has been suggested that these abnormalities may be secondary manifestations of potassium deficiency, which disappear with potassium repletion [57]. Delaporte et al [58], however, measured muscle electrolytes in six children with Bartter's syndrome and found increased intracellular sodium which fell with correction of hypokalemia, but not to normal. There was a negative relationship between intracellular sodium and potassium. Intracellular potassium increased with correction of plasma potassium, but never reached normal, even in the bilaterally nephrectomized (previously hypokalemic) sister of one of the children with Bartter's syndrome.

While the methodology in this area is difficult, and the results are frequently conflicting, the evidence overall is suggestive of an inherited membrane-transport dysregulation in Bartter's syndrome, affecting sodium and potassium transfer. Garrick et al [59] have suggested that a generalized increase in cell sodium permeability in Bartter's syndrome stimulates sodium–potassium–ATPase activity through raised intracellular sodium, and that the activity of this process in the distal nephrons explains potassium wasting which continues despite suppression of renin and aldosterone.

It will perhaps be only when the molecular genetics of familial Bartter's syndrome have been worked out in detail, with the abnormal genes, their protein products, and resultant alterations in actions clearly displayed, that this perplexing syndrome will be understood.

CLINICAL FEATURES

The clinical features of Bartter's syndrome are manifestations of the two major pathophysiological and biochemical abnormalities: sodium chloride wasting with hypovolemia and hypokalemic alkalosis. The first leads to salt craving, low–normal to frankly low blood pressure, with symptoms of lethargy, dizziness and, occasionally, syncope, as well as thirst and polyuria. The second leads to muscle weakness, tetany, and further polyuria and polydipsia because of secondary renal tubular resistance to vasopressin resulting from the chronic hypokalemia. There is evidence that chronic electrolyte disturbance, as in Bartter's syndrome, can lead to personality disorders [60].

Some early authors alluded to characteristic triangular-shaped facies in Bartter's syndrome [61]. Many patients with severe hypokalemia have been of short stature during early childhood, with a tendency to achieve normal size during later childhood and adolescence, provided plasma potassium levels are maintained at 2.5mmol/l or more [12].

BIOCHEMICAL FEATURES

The biochemical features already described in the introduction include hypokalemic alkalosis, hypochloremia and, occasionally, hyponatremia. Urinary sodium, potassium, and chloride are inappropriately high considering prevailing plasma values. Renin and Ang II levels are invariably elevated, but because of the hypokalemia, aldosterone may not be raised and can be normal or even low. Low levels of magnesium and calcium are sometimes seen in Bartter's syndrome [62,63] because of renal wastage. Magnesium levels are more often in the low–normal range than frankly depressed, but attempts to raise them with oral supplements can do more harm than good, due to ensuing diarrhea which exacerbates potassium depletion (see later).

Occasionally, plasma levels of enzymes such as creatine phosphokinase are raised in patients with severe hypokalemia [64,65], but these return to normal on correction of the low plasma potassium.

DIAGNOSIS AND DIFFERENTIAL DIAGNOSIS

The diagnosis of Bartter's syndrome depends first on finding hypokalemia unprovoked by diuretics, vomiting, anorexia, or purgation; since these aberrations are often indulged secretly [9] (see *Chapter 72*), this can sometimes be difficult. The next step is to demonstrate inappropriate urinary potassium loss in the face of hypokalemia, that is, a 24-hour urinary potassium excretion of 20mmol/d or more. This should be associated with normal or increased urinary chloride excretion despite a low–normal or a low plasma chloride value. Plasma renin activity or concentration, or Ang II, should be clearly elevated, while plasma aldosterone may be high, normal, or low, depending on the prevailing potassium level. Systolic blood pressure should be in the low–normal range (95–110mmHg) or reduced (75–95mmHg). Postural hypotension may be present, because of hypovolemia and poor responsiveness of resistance vessels to sympathetic activation, due perhaps to low sodium and potassium in the vessel wall. Pressor responsiveness to Ang II is always reduced [18,24,29,66], and that to norepinephrine is also usually diminished. The pressor hyporesponsiveness to Ang II is corrected by inhibition of prostaglandins [67]; a similar qualitative change in pressor responsiveness to Ang II is seen in normal subjects and in patients taking a diuretic [102] when given indomethacin (Fig. 64.4).

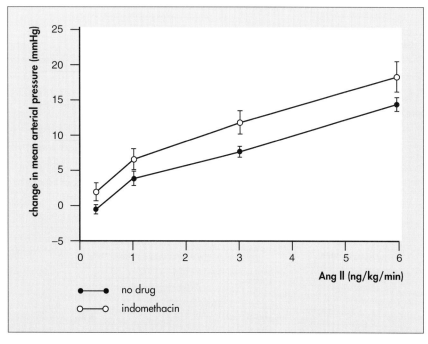

Fig. 64.4 Pressor responsiveness to Ang II infusion (mean ± SEM) in 12 normal subjects. This is altered by 48 hours of indomethacin, 50mg/tid. (Unpublished data).

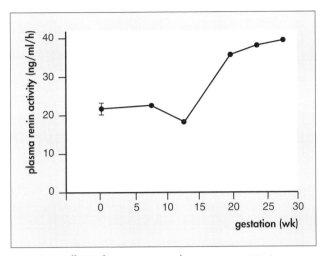

Fig. 64.5 Effects of pregnancy on plasma renin activity in a patient with Bartter's syndrome. (Unpublished data).

Juxtaglomerular hyperplasia on renal biopsy is best not considered an essential diagnostic feature as discussed in the introduction. With the wide availability of accurate biochemical measurements, use of this imprecise and risky tool is no longer justified.

Renal tubular acidosis can occasionally be confused with Bartter's syndrome [68,69] because of common features of muscle weakness, polyuria, polydipsia, salt craving, growth failure, hypokalemia, increased PRA, pressor insensitivity to Ang II, and juxtaglomerular hyperplasia. This disorder, however, is associated with acidosis and a low plasma bicarbonate value, bicarbonaturia, and inability to excrete an acid urine, whereas Bartter's syndrome is associated with alkalosis, reflected in a high plasma bicarbonate level.

Loss of potassium and chloride from the gut due to laxative abuse or chronic diarrhea is reflected in low urinary levels of these ions; thus, differentiation from Bartter's syndrome is not difficult, once suspected [11]. Surreptitious diuretic abuse is harder to diagnose, particularly if it is intermittent, unless the unprescribed diuretic can be measured in a blood or urine sample [5–7].

PREGNANCY IN BARTTER'S SYNDROME

Pregnancy is normally associated with high levels of renin, Ang II, and aldosterone (see *Chapter 50*), so the occurrence of pregnancy in Bartter's syndrome is of great interest. Few observations, however, appear to have been made. Klaus *et al* [70] reported apparent amelioration of hyperreninemia and hypokalemia during pregnancy in one patient with Bartter's syndrome. Another subject

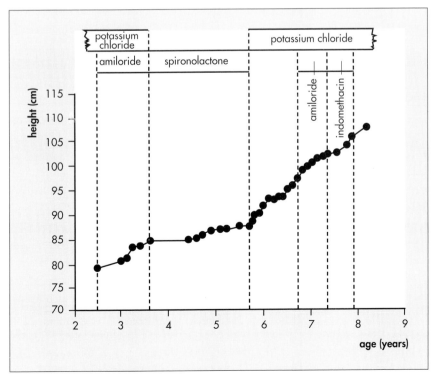

Fig. 64.6 Slowing in the rate of growth of a girl with Bartter's syndrome during administration of spironolactone. Throughout the period of observation, her growth remained below the third percentile. (Unpublished data).

described by Stokes et al [65] presented for the first time with marked muscle weakness at 12 weeks of gestation, and had severe hypokalemia (2.2mmol/l). Elevation of serum potassium only to 2.7mmol/l with supplemental potassium chloride (135mmol/d) was accompanied by disappearance of symptomatic weakness. As pregnancy progressed and with continued potassium supplementation of 135mmol/d, serum potassium rose to 3.8–4.2mmol/l, suggesting amelioration of renal potassium wasting later in pregnancy. In contrast, Almeida and Spinnato [71] found increasing requirements for potassium supplements and of amiloride during pregnancy in their patient with Bartter's syndrome. Ross and Weber [72] also described a patient who developed marked proximal muscle weakness for the first time when two months pregnant. Her hypokalemic sister also developed similar symptoms for the first time during pregnancy. Overall, these reports suggest worsening hypokalemia in early pregnancy, perhaps due to the increase in potassium requirements.

We have also observed increased needs of potassium chloride along with rising levels of renin (Fig. 64.5) and aldosterone in the first two trimesters of pregnancy in a patient with Bartter's syndrome who had been treated for five years. We avoided adding potassium-sparing diuretics to supplemental potassium chloride in this patient, because Almeida and Spinnato [71] reported intra-uterine growth retardation in their pregnant patient who had received amiloride. We had earlier noted cessation of growth in a 10-year-old girl with Bartter's syndrome during treatment with spironolactone (Fig. 64.6), despite the achievement of normal potassium levels, but in the presence of hyponatremia.

BASAL ACTIVITY OF THE RENIN–ANGIOTENSIN SYSTEM IN BARTTER'S SYNDROME

Levels of PRA, plasma renin concentration, and Ang II are invariably raised, and sometimes to very high levels (2–200 times normal). Renal cortical tissue obtained at necrosopy from two patients with Bartter's syndrome was found to have a 50–200-fold increase in renin content [73]. The normal diurnal variation of PRA [74] has been shown to persist in Bartter's syndrome [75]. Low levels of circulating renin substrate (angiotensinogen) have been reported [30,76]. Plasma concentrations of inactive renin appear to vary inversely with active renin [77], being therefore low but capable of elevation by addition of exogenous substrate [78,79]. Angiotensin II levels are raised as expected [49,80], and the striking pressor insensitivity to infused Ang II reflects presumably, the very high levels of endogenous Ang II, the

hypovolemia, and the low sodium and potassium content in the walls of resistance vessels. The dose of Ang II required to raise diastolic blood pressure by 20mmHg can be as great as 70 times normal, and is corrected by measures that lower endogenous Ang II and expand blood volume, such as saline infusion [52] or inhibition of prostaglandin synthesis [67]. It has been proposed that very high Ang II levels can be nephrotoxic (see Chapter 40) [81], and this might explain the glomerulosclerosis seen in some patients with Bartter's syndrome [13,49].

Presumably, the markedly raised basal renin levels are the result of, first, hypovolemia and a tendency to hypotension causing baroreceptor-activated stimulation of the sympathetic nervous system, including the renal nerves, although circulating catecholamine levels have been reported to be normal; and second, markedly elevated prostaglandin levels as evidenced by the large falls in renin following administration of prostaglandin inhibitors [27,29,32–34] (Fig. 64.7), notwithstanding the fact that prostaglandin inhibitors also cause sodium and water retention and volume expansion and tend to lower renin by this mechanism as well.

DYNAMIC CHANGES IN RENIN

The elevated renin levels of Bartter's syndrome are usually responsive to upright posture [26,28,75,82,83], although Norby et al [52] found no posture-related change in renin in their patient. We observed consistent increases in PRA with upright posture in our patients (see Fig. 64.3). A number of workers [50,84] have described further increments in PRA with dietary salt restriction and converse suppression with saline [84–87] or albumin infusion [50,88,89]. We saw suppression of both plasma renin and aldosterone by dietary salt loading (Fig. 64.8) and of renin by saline infusion (see Fig. 64.7), even when basal levels had been already lowered by inhibition of prostaglandins. These data are consistent with there being two independent mechanisms underlying the high levels of renin of Bartter's syndrome.

Norby et al [52] observed the expected changes in PRA following changes in plasma potassium, that is, a rise in renin when potassium levels were reduced, and a fall when potassium levels were raised. This could, however, be either a direct [90,91] or an indirect effect of potassium acting through aldosterone, sodium retention, and volume expansion [91,92].

Is renin secretion in Bartter's syndrome subject to the normal 'negative feedback' effect of Ang II (see Chapter 24)? Godard et al [93] and Sann et al [94] found that PRA fell with

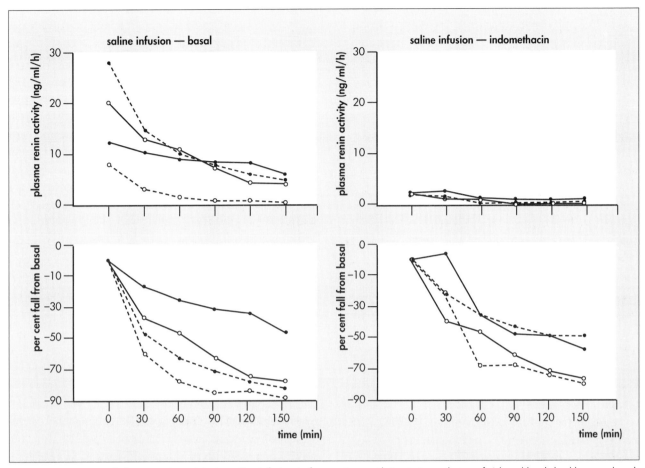

Fig. 64.7 Lowering of plasma renin activity by saline infusion in four patients with Bartter's syndrome after basal levels had been reduced by prostaglandin inhibition with indomethacin, indicating the independent effects of volume and prostaglandins on renin secretion. (Unpublished data).

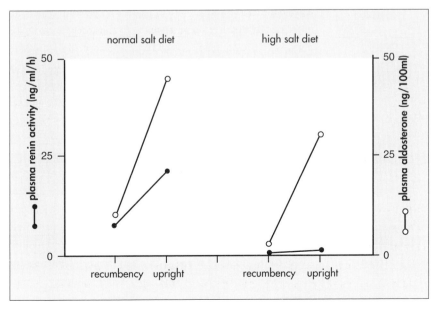

Fig. 64.8 Lowering of plasma renin activity (PRA) and aldosterone by dietary salt loading (180mmol sodium supplement daily) in a 45-year-old woman with Bartter's syndrome. Both PRA and aldosterone respond to the postural change from overnight recumbency to two hours upright (standing, sitting, or walking), both on normal and high salt diets (PRA levels on high salt diet, 0.5 recumbency, and 1.1ng/ml/h upright. (Unpublished data).

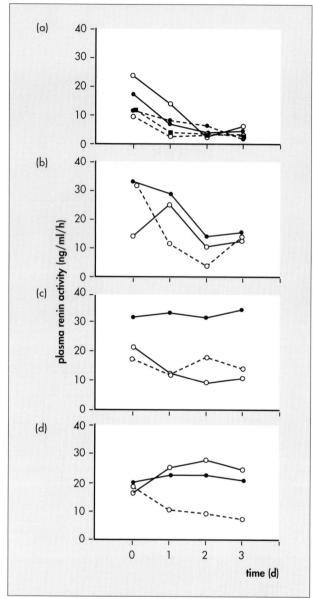

Fig. 64.9 Responses in plasma renin activity (PRA) to administration of various prostaglandin inhibitors: (a) indomethacin 50mg tid, (b) piroxicam 10mg bid, (c) sulindac 50mg tid, (d) aspirin 600mg tid in individual patients with Bartter's syndrome. Indomethacin gave the most consistent responses. (Unpublished data).

Ang II infusion, as expected. Thus, the inhibitory effect of very high endogenous levels of Ang II on renin release were not maximal. Furthermore, an Ang II antagonist was found to elevate further, endogenous PRA levels, again proving functional adequacy of this inhibitory mechanism [95].

A variety of drugs lower renin levels in Bartter's syndrome. These include the β-adrenoceptor blocker, propranolol [86], the false transmitter and peripheral α-adrenoceptor blocker, methyldopa [83], and of course, various inhibitors of prostaglandin synthesis [27,29,32,82,96,97]. Indomethacin has, in our experience, been the most consistently effective agent in this regard (Fig. 64.9).

It thus appears that renin is normally responsive to the known stimulators and inhibitors of its secretion, but has a high basal set point, presumably as a result of hypovolemia/relative hypotension/sympathetic stimulation, on the one hand, and high levels of stimulatory prostaglandins, on the other. Sudan *et al* [98] considered hypovolemia to be more important than prostaglandins in regulating renin in this disease.

ACTIONS OF RENIN IN BARTTER'S SYNDROME

Bartter's original contention, that unresponsiveness to Ang II was the basic defect in Bartter's syndrome, was based on pressor unresponsiveness, but this is difficult to sustain since lowering of endogenous renin and Ang II or volume expansion corrects this abnormality and the blood vessels can then respond clearly to Ang II. Endogenous plasma Ang II concentrations are now known to be very high in Bartter's syndrome, and it is therefore inevitable that the pressor responsiveness to administered Ang II will be proportionately diminished. Since, as already discussed, endogenous Ang II is also capable of inhibiting renin secretion, there is no reason to suspect that in this respect, the actions of renin and of the Ang II it generates are abnormal in Bartter's syndrome. As was noted earlier, however, angiotensinogen values are reported to be low [30,76], despite high Ang II, which normally stimulates angiotensinogen production (see *Chapter 8*). The consistently parallel movements of Ang II and aldosterone in a variety of circumstances suggest that the action of Ang II on the adrenal glomerulosa to stimulate aldosterone is normal in Bartter's syndrome, although the response is modified of course by hypokalemia. We have observed (Fig. 64.10) that plasma aldosterone rises in response to pressor doses of Ang II but not to the smaller doses (2ng/kg/min) which consistently stimulate aldosterone secretion in normal subjects. This is presumably explained by the already elevated endogenous levels of Ang II and again, the hypokalemia. The responsiveness of aldosterone to adrenocorticotropic hormone (ACTH) in Bartter's syndrome has not, to our knowledge, been examined systematically. In one

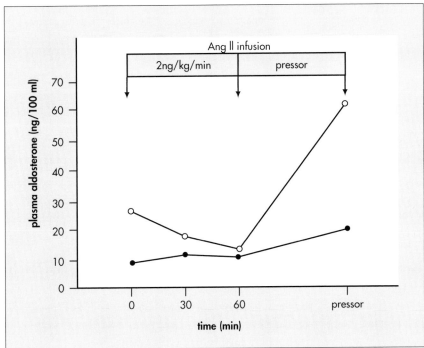

Fig. 64.10 Plasma aldosterone response to subpressor (2ng/kg/min) and pressor (increase in diastolic blood pressure, 20mmHg) Ang II infusion in two patients with Bartter's syndrome. Aldosterone increased in one patient from 9.1 to 19.6ng/100ml and in the other from 26 to 61ng/100ml with the pressor infusion (30 and 25ng/kg/min, respectively). (Unpublished data).

patient, Norby *et al* [52] reported a decline in aldosterone levels between 8am and noon, at a time when the patient was upright and ACTH was falling; they also noted suppression of aldosterone secretion by dexamethasone administration. In one of our own studies in a patient with Bartter's syndrome on a constant metabolic diet, aldosterone was strikingly responsive to ACTH.

The presence of polycythemia in a few patients with Bartter's syndrome [103,104] raises the possibility that erythropoietin production might be enhanced through activation of the RAS. This question is discussed further in *Chapter 39*.

EFFECTS OF TREATMENT ON RENIN LEVELS

As already discussed, inhibitors of prostaglandin synthesis are very effective in lowering renin in Bartter's syndrome. Methyldopa [83] and propranolol [75] have been used in an attempt to diminish renin levels, but are less potent than are prostaglandin inhibitors. Norby *et al* [52] observed a reduction of plasma renin during potassium supplementation.

TREATMENT OF BARTTER'S SYNDROME

POTASSIUM SUPPLEMENTATION

The mainstay of treatment is potassium chloride supplementation. Potassium is administered preferably in a slow-release form such as a sugar-coated honeycomb wax matrix impregnated with 8mmol potassium as potassium chloride, which minimizes irritation and ulceration of the esophagus, stomach, and small bowel. Alkaline preparations, for example those containing bicarbonate in order to produce an effervescent elixir, are best avoided as they aggravate the alkalosis and are relatively ineffective in correcting the hypokalemia. Use of an oral magnesium salt in an attempt to correct hypomagnesemia is best avoided, since any tendency to diarrhea will lower magnesium and potassium levels further. Patients with Bartter's syndrome tolerate chronic hypokalemia (down to 2.5–2.8mmol/l) very well. Indeed, it is often difficult to demonstrate clinical improvement associated with return of potassium levels from 2.8 to 3.5mmol/l and above. In any case, it is hard to maintain potassium levels above 3.0mmol/l in most patients, no matter how high the dose of potassium supplements, or whether other methods of treatment are added [99]. Very high doses of supplemental potassium chloride used alone are well tolerated in the form of slow-release tablets, and our patients routinely take 8–15 of these tablets three times daily with meals, giving a total of 192–360mmol supplemental potassium daily.

SODIUM CHLORIDE SUPPLEMENTATION

Logically, since salt wasting is a constant feature of Bartter's syndrome, salt supplements should be helpful, especially as hypovolemia is probably invariable and symptomatic hypotension can be a problem. In practice, there are difficulties with this because of the tendency of oral sodium chloride to cause nausea. This can usually be overcome if given in a slow-release form (10mmol sodium per tablet), in a dose of 2–4 tablets three times daily with meals. All patients with Bartter's syndrome should be encouraged to add salt to their food liberally, and, indeed, many have a spontaneous craving for salt (see *Chapter 32*). An adverse effect of salt supplements results from the further increase in the load of sodium reaching the distal nephron, which augments the kaliuresis and may therefore exacerbate hypokalemia. This will depend on the extent to which hypovolemia has been corrected and whether the high endogenous levels of renin and aldosterone have been reduced.

The decision whether or not to use supplemental sodium chloride should depend on the relative magnitude of hypotensive versus hypokalemic symptoms. This distinction often requires careful monitoring of blood pressure, with the patient ambulant, since the lethargy produced by hypotension is usually indistinguishable from that due to hypokalemia. Nerve conduction studies may be helpful in quantifying the contribution of hypokalemia to muscle weakness.

ANGIOTENSIN-CONVERTING ENZYME INHIBITORS

The ACE inhibitor, captopril, has been given in order to inhibit Ang II production [105], but whereas this may induce some rise in plasma potassium levels, worsening of hypotension can result.

POTASSIUM-SPARING DIURETICS

Potassium-sparing diuretics (spironolactone, amiloride, or triamterene) raise potassium and magnesium levels but, by inducing natriuresis, can exacerbate the hypovolemia and further stimu-late renin and aldosterone secretion, thus limiting their effectiveness. Since they aggravate hypovolemia, they should not be used in patients with prominent symptoms of low blood pressure.

Hyponatremia, which can be initiated or aggravated by potassium-sparing diuretics, may be just as serious an electrolyte disturbance as hypokalemia. As already noted (see *Fig. 64.6*), we observed cessation of growth in a child with Bartter's syndrome after introduction of spironolactone in doses which corrected hypokalemia more completely than did other therapies, but which also caused hyponatremia. Almeida and Spinnato observed retardation of intrauterine growth when amiloride was used during pregnancy [71]. Fanconi *et al* [12], however, observed acceleration of growth during administration of spironolactone. Amiloride, a weaker natriuretic agent than spironolactone, may be preferable, provided that blood pressure and plasma sodium, as well as potassium levels, are monitored.

PROSTAGLANDIN INHIBITION

The use of nonsteroidal anti-inflammatory drugs (NSAIDs) in Bartter's syndrome was initially hailed both as a therapeutic breakthrough and as an important clue to the underlying pathophysiology [26–28,82]. With further experience, however, it became clear that prostaglandin inhibition did not usually correct the hypokalemia completely, even when used in conjunction with oral potassium supplements. Furthermore, the chronic use of NSAIDs in Bartter's syndrome carries the same potentially life-threatening risks of upper gastrointestinal tract ulceration, hemorrhage, and perforation seen in patients given these drugs for other reasons. Furthermore, 'pseudotumor cerebri', with headache and papilledema as clinical features of raised intracranial pressure, and presumably due to salt and water retention, has been reported during treatment with both indomethacin [100] and ketoprofen [101] in Bartter's syndrome. Hence, the use of prostaglandin inhibitors must be cautious, and the patient kept under careful surveillance for gastrointestinal symptoms or asymptomatic ulceration leading, for example, to chronic blood loss and anemia.

FUTURE DIRECTIONS

Atrial natriuretic factor has been studied for only a decade, and its role in disease states has not been fully clarified. The therapeutic effects in hypertension and heart failure of increased endogenous levels of ANF induced by inhibition of its destruction by atriopeptidases is under examination. In the search for hormone agonists, antagonists are often discovered. Such an ANF antagonist could be useful in Bartter's syndrome where ANF levels are in some cases inappropriately high.

Since Bartter's syndrome can be mimicked by abuse of thiazide or loop diuretics, it is theoretically possible that an endogenous agent that acts on the same receptors is produced in excess in Bartter's syndrome. Examination of this hypothesis would involve isolation of appropriate receptors and the development of suitable probes. By analogy with morphine, morphine receptors, and the discovery of endorphins, such developments are entirely possible. Deficiency of an endogenous agent of this kind might then by contrast, account for Gordon's syndrome (see *Chapter 65*).

Finally, the eventual unraveling of the molecular genetic basis of all inherited (familial) conditions can now be confidently expected with the development of new technology. Many of the unanswered questions discussed in this chapter should then be answered.

CONCLUSIONS

The etiology of primary Bartter's syndrome remains obscure, although hyperreninemia and hypokalemia are constant features. The failure to correct hypokalemia completely despite massive oral supplementation with potassium, with or without almost complete suppression of renin by prostaglandin inhibitors, remains an enigma, but must constitute a clue to the pathophysiology. Renin appears to be regulated qualitatively in Bartter's syndrome in the normal way.

Failure to understand the pathophysiology means that treatment remains empirical. Importantly, these patients tolerate chronic hypokalemia (down to 2.8mmol/l) very well, and overstrenuous attempts to normalize plasma potassium can result in serious side effects from medications, and a reduced, rather than an enhanced, quality of life.

Bartter's syndrome and Gordon's syndrome (see *Chapter 65*) are biochemically, and perhaps pathophysiologically, mirror images of each other. Careful, persistent clinical investigation, complemented by rapid advances in molecular genetics, will one day solve the puzzle of both, bringing better understanding of normal renal potassium handling and of renin regulation. A treatment for both Bartter's and Gordon's syndromes should then be achieved.

ACKNOWLEDGMENT

We gratefully acknowledge the support of the National Health and Medical Research Council of Australia for our Research Project, *Volume-regulatory hormones in congenital disorders of sodium balance in man*.

REFERENCES

1. Kallen RJ, Aronson DG. Metabolic alkalosis in identical twins receiving a low-chloride formula (Pseudo-Bartter's syndrome). *Canadian Medical Association Journal* 1980;**123**:527–30.

2. Roy S, Arant BS. Alkalosis from chloride-deficient neo-mull-soy. *New England Journal of Medicine* 1979;**301**:615.

3. Lieber IH, Stoneburner SD, Floyd M, McGuffin NL. Potassium-wasting nephropathy secondary to chemotherapy simulating Bartter's syndrome. *Cancer* 1984;**54**:808–10.

4. Davison AG, Snodgrass GJAI. Cystic fibrosis mimicking Bartter's syndrome. *Acta Pediatrica Scandinavica* 1983;**72**:781–3.

5. Katz FH, Eckert RC, Gebott MD. Hypokalemia caused by surreptitious self-administration of diuretics. *Annals of Internal Medicine* 1972;**76**:85–90.

6. Rosenblum M, Simpson DP, Evenson M. Factitious Bartter's syndrome. *Archives of Internal Medicine* 1977;**137**:1244–5.

7. Jamieson RL, Ross JC, Kempson RL, Sufit CR, Parker TE. Surreptitious diuretic ingestion and pseudo-Bartter's syndrome. *American Journal of Medicine* 1982;**73**:142–7.

8. Ramos E, Hall–Craggs M, Demers LM. Surreptitious habitual vomiting simulating Bartter's syndrome. *Journal of the American Medical Association* 1980;**243**:1070–2.

9. Wolff HP, Vecsei PK, Kruck F, Roscher S, Brown JJ, Düsterdieck GO, Lever AF, Robertson JIS. Psychiatric disturbance leading to potassium depletion, sodium depletion, raised plasma-renin concentration and secondary hyperaldosteronism. *Lancet* 1968;**i**:257–61.

10. Fleischer N, Brown H, Graham DY, Delena S. Chronic laxative-induced hyperaldosteronism and hypokalemia simulating Bartter's syndrome. *Annals of Internal Medicine* 1969;**70**:791–8.

11. Ooi TC, Poznanski WJ, Ooi DS. The value of urinary chloride measurement in distinguishing surreptitious vomiting from Bartter's syndrome. *Clinical Biochemistry* 1983;**16**:263–5.

12. Fanconi A, Schachenmann G, Nussli R, Prader A. Chronic hypokalaemia with growth retardation, normotensive hyperrenin–hyperaldosteronism ('Bartter's syndrome'), and hypercalciuria. *Acta Helvetica Paediatrica* 1971;**2**:144–63.

13. Arant BS, Brackett NC, Young RB, Still WJS. Case studies of siblings with juxtaglomerular hyperplasia and secondary aldosteronism associated with severe azotemia and renal rickets — Bartter's syndrome or disease? *Pediatrics* 1970;**46**:344–61.

14. Gullner HG, Gill JR, Bartter FC, Chan JCM, Dickman PS. A familial disorder with hypokalemic alkalosis, hyperreninemia, aldosteronism, high urinary prostaglandins and normal blood pressure that is not 'Bartter's syndrome'. *Transactions of the American Association of Physicians* 1979;**92**:175–88.

15. McCredie DA, Blair–West JR, Scoggins BA, Shipman R. Potassium-losing nephropathy of childhood. *Medical Journal of Australia* 1971;**1**:129–35.

16. Desmit EM, Cost WS, Brown JJ, Fraser R, Lever AF, Robertson JIS. An unusual type of hypokalaemic alkalosis with a disturbance of renin and aldosterone. *Acta Endocrinologica* 1970;**64**:75–94.

17. Seyberth HW, Roscher W, Schneer H, Kuhl PG, Mehls O, Scharer K. Congenital hypokalaemia with hypercalciuria in preterm infants: A hypoprostaglandin uric tubular syndrome different from Bartter's syndrome. *Journal of Pediatrics* 1985;**107**:694–701.

18. Bartter FC, Pronove P, Gill JR, MacCardle RC. Hyperplasia of the juxtaglomerular complex with hyperaldosteronism and hypokalemic alkalosis. *American Journal of Medicine* 1962;**33**:811–28.

19. Delaney VB, Oliver JF, Sims M, Costello J, Bourke E. Bartter's syndrome: Physiologic and pharmacologic studies. *Quarterly Journal of Medicine* 1981;**198**:213–32.

20. Pronove P, MacCardle RC, Bartter FC. Aldosteronism, hypokalemia and a unique lesion in a four year old boy. *Acta Endocrinologica* 1960;**34** (suppl 51):167.

21. Earle DP, Sherry S, Eichna LW, Conan NJ. Low potassium syndrome due to defective renal tubular mechanisms for handling potassium. *American Journal of Medicine* 1951;**11**:283–301.

22. Slater RJ, Azzopardi P, Slater PE, Chute AL. An unusual case of chronic hypokalemia associated with renal tubular degeneration. *American Journal of Diseases in Childhood* 1958;**96**:469–71.

23. Borst JR, Smith PA. Chronic hypopotassaemia, refractory to potassium treatment, and tetany in a girl aged 14 years. *Acta Medica Scandinavica* 1958;**161**:207–13.

24. Gill JR. Bartter's syndrome. *Annual Reviews in Medicine* 1980;**31**:405–19.

25. Stein JH. The pathogenetic spectrum of Bartter's syndrome. *Kidney International* 1985;**28**:85–93.

26. Fichman MP, Telfer N, Zia P, Speckart P, Golub M, Rude R. Role of prostaglandins in the pathogenesis of Bartter's syndrome. *American Journal of Medicine* 1976;**60**:785–97.

27. Verberckmoes R, Van Damme B, Clement J, Amery A, Michielsen P. Bartter's syndrome with hyperplasia of renomedullary cells. Successful treatment with indomethacin. *Kidney International* 1976;**9**:302–7.

28. Gill JR, Frolich JC, Bowden RE, Taylor AA, Keiser HR, Seyberth HW, Oates JA, Bartter FC. Bartter's syndrome. A disorder characterized by high urinary prostaglandins and a dependence of hyperreninemia on prostaglandin synthesis. *American Journal of Medicine* 1976;**61**:43–51.

29. Norby L, Lentz R, Flamenbaum W, Ramwell P. Prostaglandins and aspirin therapy in Bartter's syndrome. *Lancet* 1976;**ii**:604–6.

30. Imai M, Yabuta K, Marata H, Takita S, Ohbe Y, Sokabe H. A case of Bartter's syndrome with abnormal renin response to salt loading. *Journal of Pediatrics* 1969;**74**:738–49.

31. Grekin RJ, Nicholls MG, Padfield PL. Disorders of chloriuretic hormone secretion. *Lancet* 1979;**i**:1116–8.

32. Gordon RD, Tunny TJ, Klemm SA. Indomethacin and atrial natriuretic peptide in Bartter's syndrome. *New England Journal of Medicine* 1986;**315**:459.

33. Gordon RD, Tunny TJ, Klemm SA, Hamlet SM. Elevated levels of plasma atrial natriuretic peptide in Bartter's syndrome fall to normal with indomethacin: Implications for atrial natriuretic peptide regulation in man. *Journal of Hypertension* 1986;**4** (suppl 6):S555–8.

34. Klemm SA, Gordon RD, Tunny TJ, Hawkins PG, Finn WL, Hamlet SM, Kewal NK, Purton KJ. Levels of atrial natriuretic peptide are not always consistent with atrial pressure: Is there alternative regulation as evidenced in Gordon's and Bartter's syndrome. *Clinical and Experimental Pharmacology and Physiology* 1989;**16**:269–74.

35. Yamada K, Tajima K, Moriwaki K, Tarui S, Miyata A, Kangawa K, Matsuo H. Atrial natriuretic peptide in Bartter's syndrome. *Lancet* 1986;**i**:273.

36. Sasaki H, Okumura M, Kawasaki T, Kangawa K, Matsuo H. Indomethacin and atrial natriuretic peptide in pseudo-Bartter's syndrome. *New England Journal of Medicine* 1987;**316**:167.

37. Doorenbos CJ, Daha MR, Buhler FR, Van Brummelen P. Effects of posture and saline infusion on atrial natriuretic peptide and haemodynamics in patients with Bartter's syndrome and healthy controls. *European Journal of Clinical Investigation* 1988;**18**:369–74.

38. Soupart A, Unger J, Debieve MF, Decaux G. Bartter's syndrome with a salt reabsorption defect in the cortical part of Henle's loop. *American Journal of Nephrology* 1988;**8**:309–15.

39. Graham RM, Bloch KD, Delaney VB, Bourke E, Seidman JG. Bartter's syndrome and the atrial natriuretic factor gene. *Hypertension* 1986;**8**:549–51.

40. Gill JR, Bartter FC. Evidence for a prostaglandin independent defect in chloride reabsorption in the loop of Henle as a proximal cause of Bartter's syndrome. *American Journal of Medicine* 1978;**65**:766–72.

41. Kurtzman NA, Gutierrez LF. The pathophysiology of Bartter's syndrome. *Journal of the American Medical Association* 1975;**234**:758–9.

42. Kassirer JP, Berkman PM, Lawrenz DR, Schwartz WB. The critical role of chloride in the correction of hypokalemic alkalosis in man. *American Journal of Medicine* 1965;**38**:172–89.

43. Kassirer JP, Schwartz WB. Correction of metabolic alkalosis in man without repair of potassium deficiency. *American Journal of Medicine* 1966;**40**:19–26.

44. Kotchen TA, Galla JH, Guthrie GP, Luke RG. Regulation of renin release by chloride. *Cardiovascular Medicine* 1979;**4**:479–96.

45. Dunn MJ. Prostaglandins and Bartter's syndrome. *Kidney International* 1981;**19**:86–102.

46. Schambelan M, Sebastian A, Rector FC. Mineralocorticoid-resistant renal hyperkalemia without salt wasting (type II pseudohypoaldosteronism): Role of increased renal chloride reabsorption. *Kidney International* 1981;**19**: 716–27.

47. Vinci JM, Gill JR, Bowden RE, Pisano JJ, Izzo JL, Radfar N, Taylor AA, Zusman RM, Bartter FC, Keiser HR. The kallikrein–kinin system in Bartter's syndrome and its response to prostaglandin synthetase inhibition. *Journal of Clinical Investigation* 1978;**61**:1671–82.

48. Trygstad CW, Mangos JA, Bloodworth JMB, Lobeck CC. A sibship with Bartter's syndrome: Failure of total adrenalectomy to correct the potassium wasting. *Pediatrics* 1969;**44**:234–42.

49. Bryan GT, MacCardle RD, Bartter FC. Hyperaldosteronism, hyperplasia of the juxtaglomerular complex, normal blood pressure and dwarfism: Report of a case. *Pediatrics* 1966;**37**:43–50.

50. Goodman AD, Vagnucci AH, Hartroft PM. Pathogenesis of Bartter's syndrome. *New England Journal of Medicine* 1969;**281**:1435–9.

51. Brackett NC, Coppel M, Randall RE, Nixon WP. Hyperplasia of the juxtaglomerular complex with secondary aldosteronism without hypertension (Bartter's syndrome) *American Journal of Medicine* 1968;**44**:803–19.

52. Norby L, Mark AL, Kaloyanides GJ. On the pathogenesis of Bartter's syndrome: Report of studies in a patient with this disorder. *Clinical Nephrology* 1976;**6**: 404–13.

53. Gardner DG, Schultz HD. Prostaglandins regulate the synthesis and secretion of the atrial natriuretic peptide. *Journal of Clinical Investigation* 1990;**86**:52–9.

54. Tunny TJ, Klemm SA, Gordon RD. Effects of angiotensin and noradrenaline on atrial natriuretic peptide levels in man. *Clinical and Experimental Pharmacology and Physiology* 1987;**14**:221–5.

55. Gall G, Vaitukaitis J, Haddow JE, Klein R. Erythrocyte Na flux in a patient with Bartter's syndrome. *Journal of Clinical Endocrinology and Metabolism* 1971;**32**:562–7.

56. Gardner JD, Simopolous AP, Lapey A, Shibolet S. Altered membrane sodium transport in Bartter's syndrome. *Journal of Clinical Investigation* 1972;**51**: 1565–71.

57. Korff JM, Siebens AW, Gill JR. Correction of hypokalemia corrects the abnormalities in erythrocyte sodium transport in Bartter's syndrome. *Journal of Clinical Investigation* 1984;**74**:1724–9.

58. Delaporte C, Stulzaft J, Loirat C, Broyer M. Muscle electrolytes and fluid compartments in six children with Bartter's syndrome. *Clinical Science and Molecular Medicine* 1978;**54**:223–31.

59. Garrick R, Ziyadeh FN, Jorkasky D, Goldfarb S. Bartter's syndrome: A unifying hypothesis. *American Journal of Nephrology* 1985;**5**:379–84.

60. Lucas A, Didisheim R. Secondary hyperaldosteronism (Bartter's syndrome) mimicking psychiatric illness. *Journal of the American Academy of Child Psychiatry* 1974;**12**:509–23.

61. James T, Holland NH, Preston D. Bartter's syndrome. Typical facies and normal plasma volume. *Clinical Journal of Diseases of Childhood* 1975;**129**:1205–7.

62. Cushner HM, Peller TP, Fried T, Delea CS. Does magnesium play a role in the hypokalemia of Bartter's syndrome? *American Journal of Kidney Diseases* 1990;**16**:495–500.

63. McCredie DA, Rotenberg E, Williams AL. Hypercalciuria in potassium-losing nephropathy: A variant of Bartter's syndrome. *Australian Pediatric Journal* 1974;10:286–95.

64. Knochel JP, Schlein EM. On the mechanism of rhabdomyolysis in potassium depletion. *Journal of Clinical Investigation* 1972;51:1750–8.

65. Stokes GS, Andrews BS, Hagon E, Thornell IR, Palmer AA, Posen S. Bartter's syndrome presenting during pregnancy. *Medical Journal of Australia* 1974;2:360–5.

66. Takayasu H, Aso Y, Nakauchi K, Kawabe K. A case of Bartter's syndrome with surgical treatment followed for four years. *Journal of Clinical Endocrinology and Metabolism* 1971;32:842–5.

67. Richards CJ, Mark AL, VanOrden DE, Kaloyanides GJ. Effects of indomethacin on the vascular abnormalities of Bartter's syndrome. *Circulation* 1978;58:544–9.

68. Rodriquez–Soriano J, Vallo A, Oliveros R. Bartter's syndrome presenting with features resembling renal tubular acidosis. *Helvetica Paediatrica Acta* 1978;33:141–51.

69. Lamabadusuriya SP, Goonaratna C De FW. Renal tubular acidosis or Bartter's syndrome? *Ceylon Medical Journal* 1977;22:55–60.

70. Klaus D, Klumpp F, Roessler R. Einfluss der Schwangerschaft auf das Bartter-syndrome. *Klinische Wochenschrift* 1972;49:1280–5.

71. Almeida OD, Spinnato JA. Maternal Bartter's syndrome and pregnancy. *American Journal of Obstetrics and Gynecology* 1989;160:1225–6.

72. Ross D, Weber HP. Bartter's syndrome. *Journal of the Kansas Medical Society* 1976;77:378–82.

73. Sutherland LE, Hartroft P, Balis JU, Bailey JD, Lynch MJ. Bartter's syndrome. A report of four cases in three in one sibship, with comparative histologic evaluation of the juxtaglomerular apparatuses and glomeruli. *Acta Pediatrica Scandinavica* 1970;201 (suppl 1):2–24.

74. Gordon RD, Wolfe LK, Island DP, Liddle GW. A diurnal rhythm in plasma renin activity in man. *Journal of Clinical Investigation* 1966;45:1587–92.

75. Modlinger RS, Nicolis GL, Krakoff LR, Gabrilove JL. Some observations on the pathogenesis of Bartter's syndrome. *New England Journal of Medicine* 1973;289:1022–4.

76. Cannon PJ, Leeming JM, Sommers SC. Juxtaglomerular hyperplasia and secondary hyperaldosteronism (Bartter's syndrome): A reevaluation of the pathophysiology. *Medicine* 1968;47:107–31.

77. Chan LL, Osmond DH, Balfe JW, Halperin ML. Plasma 'prorenin'–renin in Bartter's syndrome, cystic fibrosis, and chloride deficiency, and the effect of prostaglandin synthetase inhibition. *Journal of Laboratory and Clinical Medicine* 1981;97:785–90.

78. Nagai H, Matsunaga M, Ogawa K, Kuwahara T, Kanatsu K, Pak CH, Hara A, Tamura T, Kono T, Kawai C. High level of plasma inactive renin in Bartter's syndrome. *Japanese Circulation Journal* 1984;48:633–7.

79. McKenzie IM, Heiman D, Winter JSD, McKenzie JK. Inactive renin and aldosterone in Bartter's syndrome. *Clinical and Investigative Medicine* 1987;10:303–8.

80. Nakada T, Momose G, Yoshida T, Tateno Y, Shigematsu H, Saito T. Renin–angiotensin–aldosterone system of a woman with Bartter's syndrome: Juxtaglomerular cell hyperplasia without hypertension. *Journal of Urology* 1974;112:293–8.

81. Laragh JH, Baer L, Brunner HR, Bühler FR, Sealey JE, Vaughan ED Jr. Renin, angiotensin and aldosterone system in the pathogenesis and management of hypertensive vascular disease. *American Journal of Medicine* 1972;52:633–52.

82. Bartter FC, Gill JR, Frolich JC, Bowden RE, Hollifield JW, Radfar N, Keiser HR, Oates JA, Seyberth H, Taylor AA. Prostaglandins are overproduced by the kidneys and mediate hyperreninemia in Bartter's syndrome. *Transactions of the American Association of Physicians* 1976;89:77–90.

83. Strauss RG, Mohammed S, Loggie JMH, Schubert WK, Fasola AF, Gaffney TE. The effect of methyldopa on plasma renin activity in a child with Bartter's syndrome. *Journal of Pediatrics* 1970;77:1071–4.

84. Beilen LJ, Schiffman N, Crane M, Nelson DH. Hypokalaemic alkalosis and hyperplasia of the juxtaglomerular apparatus without hypertension or oedema. *British Medical Journal* 1967;4:327–31.

85. White MG. Bartter's syndrome. *Archives of Internal Medicine* 1972;129:41–7.

86. Solomon RJ, Brown RS. Bartter's syndrome. *American Journal of Medicine* 1975;59:575–83.

87. Tomko DJ, Yeh BPY, Falls WF. Bartter's syndrome: Study of a 52 year old man with evidence for a defect in proximal tubular sodium reabsorption and comments on therapy. *American Journal of Medicine* 1976;61:111–8.

88. Fujita T, Sakaguchi H, Shibagaki M, Fukui T, Nomura M, Sekiguchi S. The pathogenesis of Bartter's syndrome. Functional and histologic studies. *American Journal of Medicine* 1977;63:467–74.

89. Wald NK, Perrimen R, Bolande PR. Bartter's syndrome in early infancy. *Pediatrics* 1971;47:254–63.

90. Brunner HR, Baer L, Sealey JE, Ledingham JGG, Laragh JH. The influence of potassium administration and of potassium deprivation on plasma renin in normal and hypertensive subjects. *Journal of Clinical Investigation* 1970;49:2128–38.

91. Himathongkam T, Dluhy RG, Williams GH. Potassium–aldosterone–renin interrelationships. *Journal of Clinical Endocrinology and Metabolism* 1975;41:153–9.

92. Dluhy RG, Greenfield M, Williams GH. Effect of simultaneous potassium and saline loading on plasma aldosterone levels. *Journal of Clinical Endocrinology and Metabolism* 1977;45:141–6.

93. Godard C, Vallotton MB, Broyer M, Royer P. A study of the inhibition of the renin–angiotensin system in potassium wasting syndromes, including Bartter's syndrome. *Helvetica Pediatrica Acta* 1972;27:495–511.

94. Sann L, David M, Richard P, Floret D, Sassard J, Bizollon CA, Francois R. Effect of sodium restriction and angiotensin II infusion in Bartter's syndrome. *Pediatric Research* 1976;10:971–7.

95. Sasaki H, Okumura M, Asano T, Arakawa K, Kawasaki T. Responses to angiotensin II antagonist before and after treatment with indomethacin in Bartter's syndrome. *British Medical Journal* 1977;ii:995–6.

96. Littlewood JM, Lee MR, Meadow SR. Treatment of Bartter's syndrome in early childhood with prostaglandin synthetase inhibitors. *Archives of Disease in Childhood* 1978;53:43–8.

97. Bowden RE, Gill JR, Radfar N, Taylor AA, Keiser HR. Prostaglandin synthetase inhibitors in Bartter's syndrome. Effect on immunoreactive prostaglandin E excretion. *Journal of the American Medical Association* 1978;239:117–21.

98. Sudan M, Stacey WK, Falls WF. Analysis of factors influencing the renin–aldosterone system in a patient with Bartter's syndrome. *Southern Medical Journal* 1979;72:779–82.

99. Simopolous AP, Bartter FC. Growth characteristics and factors influencing growth in Bartter's syndrome. *Journal of Pediatrics* 1972;81:56–65.

100. Konomi H, Imai M, Nihea K, Kamoshita S, Tada H. Indomethacin causing pseudotumor cerebri in Bartter's syndrome. *New England Journal of Medicine* 1978;298:855.

101. Larizza D, Colombo A, Lorini R, Severi F. Ketoprofen causing pseudotumor cerebri in Bartter's syndrome. *New England Journal of Medicine* 1979;300:796.

102. Padfield PL, Grekin RJ, Nicholls MG. Clinical syndromes associated with disorders of renal tubular chloride transport: Excess and deficiency of a circulating factor? *Medical Hypotheses* 1984;14:387–400.

103. Jepson J, McGarry EE. Polycythemia and increased erythropoietin production in a patient with hypertrophy of the juxtaglomerular apparatus. *Blood* 1968;32:370–5.

104. Erkelens DW, Van Eps LWS. Bartter's syndrome and erythrocytosis. *American Journal of Medicine* 1973;55:711–9.

105. Jest P, Pederson KE, Klitgaard NA, Thomsen N, Kjaer K, Simons E. Angiotensin-converting enzyme inhibition as a therapeutic principle in Bartter's syndrome. *European Journal of Clinical Pharmacology* 1991;41:303–5.

65

RENIN IN GORDON'S SYNDROME

RICHARD D GORDON, SHELLEY A KLEMM,
AND TERRY J TUNNY

INTRODUCTION

Gordon's syndrome [1-6] is a congenital, often familial, condition with hyperkalemic, hyperchloremic acidosis in the presence of normal renal glomerular function as its unique, characteristic feature. The cause is chronic renal sodium and potassium retention, but the underlying abnormality is so far, incompletely explained. The fully developed syndrome includes hypertension [1,4,7–25], muscle weakness due to hyperkalemia [1,7,21,26,27], growth failure due to hyperkalemia and acidemia [1,13,15, 16,19,28–31], and intellectual impairment due to hyperkalemia and acidemia [1,19].

A characteristic of untreated Gordon's syndrome is low renin levels, the causes and consequences of which are explored in this chapter.

HISTORY

In 1964, Paver and Pauline described the clinical and routine biochemical findings in a 15-year-old Australian boy who presented seeking a medical certificate of fitness to commence factory work [7]. At the time, he had no symptoms, but subsequently complained of muscle weakness [8]. He had severe hypertension, hyperreactivity to cold pressor testing, severe hyperkalemia, and hyperchloremia. Serum creatinine, an intravenous pyelogram, renal angiography, and renal biopsy were normal. Renin and aldosterone measurements were unavailable, but Paver and Pauline [7] speculated that hyperaldosteronism, driven by hyperkalemia, might be causing sodium retention and hypertension. This left the hyperkalemia unexplained. Normal acidification of the urine, a kaliuresis during treatment with a carbonic-anhydrase inhibitor, and negligible effects from the administration of spironolactone led them later to discount either a primary distal renal tubular defect or aldosterone excess. The same patient was restudied with renin and aldosterone measurements [8, 32] but meanwhile had received diuretics, which are now known to alter basal renin and aldosterone levels for long periods [3,5]. In spite of this, plasma renin and aldosterone remained low, leading to speculation that suppressed renin was due to hyperkalemia [32]. Arnold and Healy [8] concluded that the boy had chronic renal potassium retention, and demonstrated kaliuresis with mineralocorticoid administration during restriction of dietary salt.

Gordon et al [1] in 1970, reported their detailed studies in a previously untreated 10-year-old unrelated Australian girl presenting with short stature, hypertension, and hyperkalemia (8.5mmol/l). She complained of muscle weakness, particularly after meals or exercise, and had impaired intellect. Plasma renin activity (PRA) was undetectable and aldosterone excretion low–normal, falling to very low levels when hyperkalemia was corrected using a cation-exchange resin. Gordon and co-workers [1] proposed a primary renal tubular defect leading to excessive sodium reabsorption proximal to the site of action of aldosterone. Volume expansion would then explain hypertension and, through suppressed renin, inadequate levels of aldosterone could account for insufficient excretion of potassium by distal renal tubules. As a consequence of hyperkalemia, aldosterone secretion should rise towards or to normal, but may still prove insufficient to maintain potassium balance in the presence of a suppressed RAS. Gordon et al [1] hypothesized that if the above mechanisms were correct, all abnormalities should be correctable by a low sodium diet alone. This indeed proved to be the case, and was later confirmed in two Australian brothers from another family, who were among seven affected members in two generations [33].

Habitual salt intake was high in the case reported by Gordon et al [1]. Hypertension and pressor hyperreactivity to cold, Ang II, and norepinephrine were corrected by restriction of dietary salt. Long-term dietary sodium restriction (20mmol/d) increased renin and aldosterone levels and reduced plasma potassium to normal. Correction of hyperchloremia and acidemia followed. Long-term treatment consisted of a moderately restricted sodium diet and a thiazide diuretic. With this treatment, muscle weakness disappeared, linear growth increased, plasma renin and aldosterone levels ranged from normal to high, and plasma potassium levels ranged from normal to low [1].

Case	Age (years)	Sex	Plasma or serum potassium (mmol/l)	Plasma renin activity (ng/ml/h)		Plasma aldosterone (ng/dl)		Urinary aldosterone (μg/d)	Dietary or urinary sodium		Reference
				Rec	Up	Rec	Up		(mmol/ 24h)	(mmol/kg/ 24h)	
1	10	F	6.3–8.5	<0.07	<0.07			2.2–3.2	150	3.1	1
2	52	M	5.8–6.2	UD	UD				170	3.0	10
3	28	F	5.8		0.3		16.2				10
4	23	F	5.9		0.9		47.1				10
5	21	M	6.2	0.2	1.1	3.5	5.5	20.0	140		9
6	33	M	5.8–7.6		<0.1		2.2–6.9	23.4	100	1.2	11
7	17	F	5.0–5.9		0.06			13.7	10		12
8	3	M	9.6		0.6		2.0		46	3.9	26
9	54	M	5.2		0.2		13.5				13
10	52	M	5.3		0.8		15.6				13
11	23	M	5.3–6.0	0.4±0.1	0.5±0.1	14.3±4.2	37.5±4.6	23.8±5.0	120		14
12	15	F	5.2–6.4	0.2–0.4		20.7–32.4		6.1–7.3	normal		17
13	16	F	6.8–7.4		0.3				250	8.5	19
14	22	M	5.3–6.9		<0.1		32.0–100.0		120–170	2.3	20
15	12	F	6.0–7.0	0.4		13.0			80	3.4	31
16	14	M	6.5–7.9		0.3		<2.0		175	3.2	21
17	13	M	6.8	UD	0.1	5.0	21.0		normal		30
18	35	F	6.6		0.43		25.6		150	2.8	45
19	40	M	5.8–7.5		0.2–0.7		6.8–35.0		85	1.3	4
20	9	F	5.9–7.9		0.3–0.6		4.8–36.8		78	2.2	4
21	38	M	5.1–7.1		0.4–1.5		6.5–38.2		85	1.0	4
22	6	F	6.0–6.8		0.3–1.3		8.1–73.8		20	0.7	4
23	5	M	6.0–7.7		0.4–1.6		11.4–44.0		59	2.0	4
24	37	F	5.6–5.7		0.6		59.2		normal		4
25	18	M	5.3	1.7	4.3	12.3	24.2	20.2	94–106	2.0	22
26	50	M	5.7–6.8		<0.04		6.8	5.8	85		24
27	24	M	6.2–8.1		<0.04		2.2	8.6	85		24
28	21	F	6.3–7.6		<0.04		6.4	13.7	85		24
29	39	F	5.5–6.0	<0.1	0.5	7.3	17.9		135	2.6	25
30	43	M	5.8–6.1	0.3	0.1	23.4	21.8		135	1.8	25
31	33	F	5.6–6.0	0.2	0.5	2.9	50.8		135	2.2	25

Rec = recumbent; Up = upright; UD = undetectable.

Fig. 65.1 Plasma renin activity in previously untreated patients with Gordon's syndrome.

In 1973, de Wardener [2] included Gordon's syndrome with Liddle's syndrome and Bartter's syndrome as disorders resulting from congenital defects of renal tubular function. There have now been over 50 well-described patients with hyperkalemia and hyperchloremia despite normal glomerular function [3,5,6] (Fig. 65.1). Values of renin have been reported in many of them.

BASAL ACTIVITY OF THE RENIN–ANGIOTENSIN SYSTEM IN GORDON'S SYNDROME

Levels of PRA in untreated Gordon's syndrome have been consistently low (Fig. 65.1) and often markedly suppressed. In interpreting reported values for renin, it is important to note whether or not there had been prior treatment with a diuretic, and if so, how much time had elapsed since treatment ceased. Renin levels rise, often briskly, in Gordon's syndrome in response to diuretics, and do not immediately return to low levels when the drug is withdrawn. For this reason, Fig. 65.1 includes only previously untreated patients, and renin levels were uniformly low.

Major factors known or believed to influence the secretion of renin in man are shown in Fig. 65.2. Sodium balance is a powerful influence, acting via blood volume, blood pressure, sympathetic nervous system activity, and perhaps also directly through plasma and tubular sodium and chloride [34]. In Gordon's syndrome, sodium-chloride overload and hypertension are potent inhibitors

of renin secretion. Urinary and plasma catecholamines have been reported as normal in Gordon's syndrome [5,7,14,18] but it is often difficult to distinguish normal from low levels. Reduced sympathetic stimulation of renin release might be expected in the volume-expanded state, although in the DOCA-salt hypertensive rat model, sympathetic activity is reportedly increased [35]. Prostaglandins (especially those which are vasodilator and natriuretic, whether locally produced or circulating) can stimulate renin release. In Gordon's syndrome, prostaglandin levels are reduced [24,36,37], and this may contribute to suppression of renin. Levels of atrial natriuretic factor (ANF) have been reported to be inappropriately normal in Gordon's syndrome

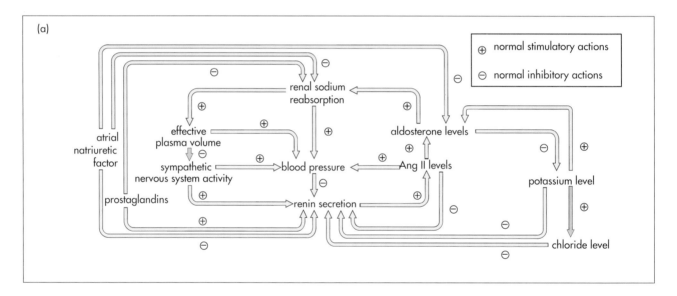

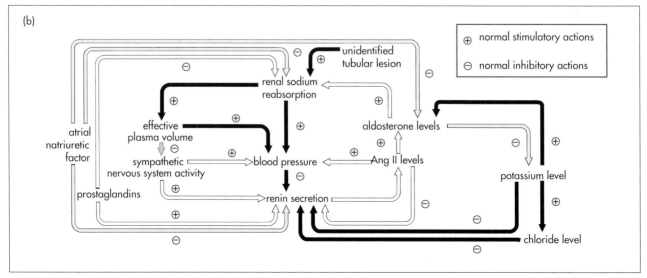

Fig. 65.2 (a) Factors influencing renin secretion in normal man. (b) Altered regulation of renin in Gordon's syndrome is indicated by black (increased) or in open (decreased) arrows. Normal stimulatory or inhibitory actions are shown as + and − respectively.

[4,5,21–24,38] rather than clearly elevated as they should be in a volume-expanded condition causing hypertension, such as primary aldosteronism [38] (see *Chapter 63*). In keeping with this, the ANF responses to saline infusion and Ang II infusion have been subnormal in some patients with Gordon's syndrome [4,5,22,38]. Thus, while ANF is capable of inhibiting renin release [39], this effect is probably not exaggerated in Gordon's syndrome, as it might be in other volume-expanded states.

A negative feedback of generated Ang II on renin release has been long recognized [40] although its importance under physiological conditions is speculative (see *Chapter 24*). This effect should be minimal in Gordon's syndrome where circulating levels of AngII are low. There is evidence, somewhat inconsistent, that hyperkalemia lowers renin levels [41,42] (see *Chapter 74*). In Gordon's syndrome, there is often remarkable hyperkalemia which may contribute to renin suppression. However, when plasma potassium was reduced to normal by a cation-exchange resin in patients with this syndrome, renin remained low [1,10,14]. Raising plasma calcium levels can reduce renin [43] (see *Chapter 24*), but in Gordon's syndrome, there is no evidence for abnormalities in calcium balance or levels.

Thus, in Gordon's syndrome, likely determinants of low basal renin levels are renal sodium retention, hypertension, reduced activity of the sympathetic nervous system, hyperkalemia, hyperchloremia, and low prostaglandins (Fig. 65.2).

DYNAMIC CHANGES IN RENIN LEVELS IN GORDON'S SYNDROME

Are the low basal renin levels in Gordon's syndrome capable of being stimulated or suppressed by normal physiological mechanisms? All the evidence suggests that they are, and indeed are capable of reaching supraphysiological levels.

When the effect of upright posture was studied, there was usually an increase in renin, even if absolute levels were low (see *Fig. 65.1*). Further, when levels of PRA are viewed in relation to dietary sodium and to treatment with diuretics, the expected relationship holds. Levels achieved on a low salt diet and on diuretics are often higher than in an unmedicated population on an unrestricted diet (Fig. 65.3). When we infused Ang II at 2ng/kg/min in our patients with Gordon's syndrome (Fig. 65.4), levels of PRA fell appropriately, suggesting normal negative feedback regulation. Note that basal PRA levels were significantly higher on sodium-restricted diets.

When PRA is viewed in relation to concomitant ANF levels during various dietary regimens (Fig. 65.5), a curvilinear

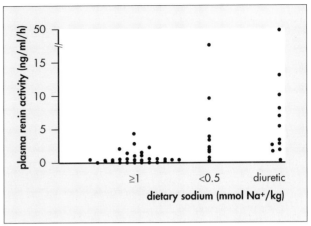

Fig. 65.3 Plasma renin activity in patients with Gordon's syndrome in relation to dietary sodium and diuretic therapy. All samples were taken between 1000 and 1100 hours after 2–3 hours of ambulation: from 52 published observations in 25 patients.

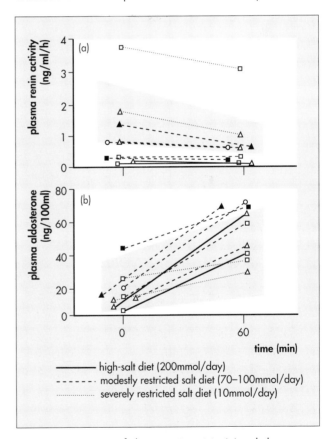

Fig. 65.4 Responses of plasma renin activity (a) and plasma aldosterone (b) to 60-minute infusions of Ang II (2ng/kg/min) in five related patients with Gordon's syndrome on a high salt diet (200mmol/d), a modestly restricted salt diet (70–100mmol/d), and a severely restricted salt diet (10mmol/d). The shaded area represents the range of responses in normal subjects taking an unrestricted diet. Gordon RD, unpublished data.

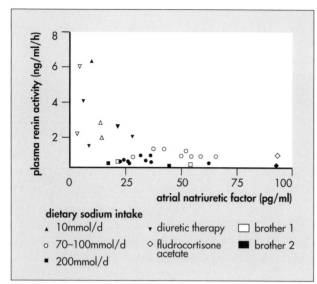

Fig. 65.5 Relationship between atrial natriuretic factor and plasma renin activity at different levels of dietary sodium intake (10mmol/day; 70–100mmol/d; 200mmol/d) and on therapy (diuretic therapy; fludrocortisone acetate) in two brothers with Gordon's syndrome. Gordon RD, unpublished data.

relationship (fourth order, r=0.73, P<0.001) is apparent. This is consistent with ANF having a suppressive effect on renin production, but is also consistent with plasma volume or blood pressure affecting each of them independently (see *Chapter 36*).

EFFECTS OF THE RENIN–ANGIOTENSIN SYSTEM IN GORDON'S SYNDROME

Given that renin levels are low in Gordon's syndrome but can respond vigorously to a low salt diet and to diuretics, does the RAS exert its expected effects? Available evidence suggests that the answer is yes. Infused Ang II has its usual actions, suppressing renin while stimulating aldosterone secretion (see *Fig. 65.4*) [9,10,25,44] (see *Chapter 33*).

Activity of the RAS as measured by PRA was positively correlated (r=0.49, P<0.001) with plasma aldosterone in pooled observations from six related patients with Gordon's syndrome in various states of sodium balance induced by dietary changes or diuretics (Fig. 65.6). While there was no significant correlation between potassium and aldosterone (r=0.1), factoring PRA for potassium levels (PRA×K⁺) improved the renin/aldosterone relationship further (r=0.73). This suggests that in Gordon's syndrome the RAS is the dominant regulator of aldosterone

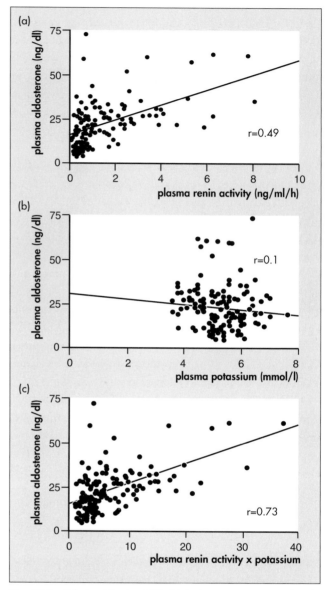

Fig. 65.6 Relationships (n=137) of (a) plasma renin activity (PRA) (b) plasma potassium (K⁺), and (c) both PRA and K⁺ with plasma aldosterone in six patients with Gordon's syndrome in various states of sodium balance (dietary sodium 200, 70–100, 10mmol/d, and 70–100mmol/d plus chlorothiazide 500mg daily). Gordon RD, unpublished data.

secretion, whereas potassium is of lesser importance, as has been demonstrated in normal human subjects [45] and in dogs [46].

Further clarification regarding the relative importance of potassium and renin comes from measurements of renin, potassium, and aldosterone levels when diuretics are introduced or withdrawn in Gordon's syndrome. Aldosterone decreased in parallel with renin levels, despite rising plasma potassium, when a thiazide diuretic was withdrawn in one patient [18]. On the other hand, elevated potassium levels are believed to explain the normal or even raised aldosterone levels sometimes seen in Gordon's syndrome, despite suppression of renin (see *Fig. 65.1*). Due to hyperkalemia and its independent effects on aldosterone, a higher than normal aldosterone/renin ratio would be expected. In this regard, Isenring *et al* [25] noted an exaggerated rise in plasma aldosterone during intravenous Ang II infusion in three patients with Gordon's syndrome.

The RAS should play a significant role in blood-pressure regulation in Gordon's syndrome, since pressor responsiveness to Ang II is increased [1, 4, 8, 9, 25]. This increase in responsiveness, however, disappears when dietary sodium is lowered [1], and the RAS may only influence blood pressure slightly once treatment with a low salt diet or diuretic is introduced.

EFFECTS OF TREATMENT ON RENIN IN GORDON'S SYNDROME

Dietary sodium restriction and diuretic therapy in Gordon's syndrome remove the suppressant effect of sodium-volume overload, so that renin levels rise into or above the normal range [1,9,10,13–16,19,21,25,33]. If the hyperkalemia is corrected using either fludrocortisone acetate or polystyrene sulfonate cation-exchange resin without correction of volume expansion, renin remains suppressed [1,4,10,14,23].

FURTHER COMMENTS AND CONCLUSIONS

Plasma renin is suppressed to low levels in untreated Gordon's syndrome, but as noted above, it is capable of responding to stimuli such as volume depletion (low salt diet or diuretics), or to sympathetic activation (change from recumbency to upright posture). Hence, renin levels at any time reflect not only the disease state but also recent dietary sodium intake and drug treatment, especially with diuretics.

Some patients with Gordon's syndrome are very sensitive to standard doses of thiazide diuretics. They may show dramatic falls in plasma potassium and blood pressure, with vigorous stimulation of the RAS. It is reasonable to assume that under these circumstances, normal or supranormal levels of renin and aldosterone represent an appropriate response to a fall in plasma volume. Hypokalemia, which is sometimes observed with diuretic therapy, results from secondary hyperaldosteronism and is in stark contrast to hyperkalemia which is a hallmark of untreated Gordon's syndrome. The fact that such wide variations in plasma

potassium can occur, points to a normal capability of potassium excretory mechanisms in the distal nephron (distal renal tubules and collecting ducts) in this disorder.

Renin in Gordon's syndrome exercises, through Ang II, normal stimulation of aldosterone secretion as evidenced by normal or exaggerated aldosterone responsiveness to infused Ang II. In the untreated state, and during treatment that alters both renin and potassium, the prevailing plasma concentration of aldosterone reflects levels of both renin and potassium but particularly the former. When account is taken of the ever-present effects of potassium on the adrenal zona glomerulosa, Gordon's syndrome is a state of true hypoaldosteronism secondary to hyporeninism. Stimulation of renin causes stimulation of aldosterone and thus, eventually, correction of hyperkalemia.

In most, but not all, reported cases of Gordon's syndrome, the aldosterone-sensitive distal nephron has been shown to be responsive to synthetic mineralocorticoids such as fludrocortisone acetate, or to endogenous (or infused) aldosterone, with an ensuing kaliuresis [3,5]. In the remaining minority, there may be partial or complete tubular resistance to aldosterone, perhaps secondary to an inability to reabsorb sodium without chloride, the putative mechanism for generation of an electrochemical gradient that encourages excretion of potassium and hydrogen ions in the distal nephron.

The sodium and water retention of untreated Gordon's syndrome would be satisfactorily explained by a deficiency of a natriuretic or chloriuretic hormone such as ANF [12]. Resting plasma levels of ANF in Gordon's syndrome have generally been in the normal range, although one can question whether they are lower than expected in the presence of volume expansion. They are indeed lower than the significantly raised levels in primary aldosteronism (see *Chapter 63*). Furthermore, in some patients with Gordon's syndrome, ANF levels are not responsive to stimulatory maneuvers such as saline infusion. Atrial natriuretic factor in Gordon's syndrome should exert a suppressor effect on renin production, and may counter to a greater or lesser extent, the aldosterone-stimulating effect of hyperkalemia.

Gordon's syndrome is unique in being the only condition in which a normal glomerular filtration rate is associated with hyperkalemia. When hypoaldosteronism results from adrenocortical insufficiency (isolated analdosteronism, Addison's disease, or bilateral adrenalectomy), the salt wasting and resulting volume contraction reduce renal perfusion and glomerular filtration.

Eicosanoids, in particular prostaglandins I_2 and E_2, are believed to be important in renin regulation. In untreated Gordon's syndrome, vasodilator prostaglandin levels are reduced, but increase in parallel with renin in response to a low salt diet or to diuretic administration. Whether a causal relationship exists between prostaglandins and renin under these circumstances, or whether each is responding independently to change in sodium or volume status, is not yet clear.

FUTURE DIRECTIONS

Careful measurements of factors known to regulate renin secretion, both in the basal state before exposure to treatment and during dietary and pharmacological manipulations, are needed; for example, comparison of renin responses to various diuretic agents (dose–response curves) with different sites of action in the nephron, would be very useful. Similarly, the definition of relationships between renal prostaglandins and renin and between ANF and renin during various maneuvers would assist in clarifying whether these factors play primary, as opposed to coincidental, roles in the suppression of renin which is characteristic of Gordon's syndrome. Whether a switch in the intrarenal synthesis of prostaglandins from E_2 to F_2 could contribute to low renin levels [47], should also be considered.

Studies aimed at further elucidation of the site of excessive sodium reabsorption in the renal tubules would clarify the pathophysiology of this rare syndrome, including its hyporeninemia. Studies on lithium clearance have in some patients suggested proximal renal tubular sites for excessive sodium reabsorption [48], as have observations of raised plasma phosphate levels in some patients [8,11,28,29]. Demonstration of an appropriate kaliuresis following infusion of sodium chloride when aldosterone secretion has been stimulated by dietary sodium restriction [8,15,33], suggests that the basic abnormality is not in the late distal tubules and collecting ducts where aldosterone acts. In other patients, lack of a kaliuresis following infusion of sodium chloride is suggestive of excessive sodium chloride reabsorption in the distal renal tubules and collecting ducts perhaps as the primary lesion [14,24]. Careful performance of similar studies in additional patients may establish whether Gordon's syndrome, like Bartter's syndrome (*Chapter 64*), is heterogeneous pathophysiologically and biochemically.

The sympathetic nervous system is normally very important in determining the level of renin secretion [49,50]. Since measurements of plasma or urinary norepinephrine are not sufficiently sensitive to define accurately underactivity of the sympathetic system, additional indices, and especially measurements of muscle sympathetic activity [51], would be of great interest before and after treatment in patients with Gordon's syndrome. As well, administration of agents that block either the formation or actions of Ang II to untreated patients, should elucidate the role of the RAS in the pathophysiology of this disorder.

Finally, elucidation of the molecular genetics of this often familial disorder will identify the responsible gene or genes and their abnormal products, and thus explain the primary pathophysiology.

ACKNOWLEDGMENT

We gratefully acknowledge the support of the National Health and Medical Research Council of Australia for our Research Project, *Volume-regulatory hormones in congenital disorders of sodium balance in man.*

REFERENCES

1. Gordon RD, Geddes RA, Pawsey CGK, O'Halloran MW. Hypertension and severe hyperkalaemia associated with suppression of renin and aldosterone and completely reversed by dietary sodium restriction. *Australasian Annals of Medicine* 1970;19:287–94.

2. De Wardener HE. Selective defects of tubular function. *The kidney: An outline of normal and abnormal structure and function, 4th edition.* London: Churchill–Livingstone, 1973:230–43.

3. Gordon RD. Syndrome of hypertension and hyperkalemia with normal glomerular filtration rate: Gordon's syndrome. *Hypertension* 1986;8:93–102.

4. Gordon RD, Ravenscroft PJ, Klemm SA, Tunny TJ, Hamlet SM. A new Australian kindred with the syndrome of hypertension and hyperkalemia have dysregulation of atrial natriuretic peptide. *Journal of Hypertension* 1988;6 (suppl 4):S323–6.

5. Gordon RD, Tunny TJ, Klemm SA, Hamlet SM. The syndrome of hypertension with hyperkalemia and normal glomerular filtration rate. In: Laragh JH, Brenner BM, eds. *Hypertension: Pathophysiology, diagnosis and management,* New York Raven Press, 1990:1625–38.

6. Gordon RD, Klemm SA, Tunny TJ. Gordon's syndrome and Liddle's syndrome. In: Robertson JIS, ed. *Handbook of hypertension, volume 15.* Amsterdam: Elsevier, 1992:chapter 15.

7. Paver WKA, Pauline GJ. Hypertension and hyperpotassaemia without renal disease in a young male. *Medical Journal of Australia* 1964;2:305–6.

8. Arnold JE, Healy JK. Hyperkalemia, hypertension and systemic acidosis without renal failure associated with a tubular defect in potassium excretion. *American Journal of Medicine* 1969;47:461–72.

9. Farfel Z, Iaina A, Rosenthal T, Waks U, Shibolet S, Gafni J. Familial hyperpotassemia and hypertension accompanied by normal plasma aldosterone levels: Possible hereditary cell membrane defect. *Archives of Internal Medicine* 1978;138;1828–32.

10. Brautbar N, Levi J, Rosler A, Leitesdorf E, Djaldeti M, Epstein M, Kleeman CR. Familial hyperkalemia, hypertension and hyporeninemia with normal aldosterone levels: A tubular defect in potassium handling. *Archives of Internal Medicine* 1978;138:607–10.

11. Lee MR, Ball SG, Thomas TH, Morgan DB. Hypertension and hyperkalemia responding to bendrofluazide. *Quarterly Journal of Medicine* 1979;48:245–58.

12. Grekin RJ, Nicholls MG, Padfield PL. Disorders of chloriuretic hormone secretion. *Lancet* 1979;i:1116–7.

13. Bravo E, Textor S, Mujais S, Cotton D. Chronic hyperkalemia in siblings associated with enhanced renal chloride absorption [Abstract]. *Clinical Research* 1980;28:782A.

14. Schambelan M, Sebastian A, Rector FC. Mineralocorticoid-resistant renal hyperkalemia without salt wasting (type II pseudohypoaldosteronism): Role of increased renal chloride reabsorption. *Kidney International* 1981;19:716–27.

15. Sanjad SA, Mansour FM, Hernandez RH, Hill LL. Severe hypertension, hyperkalemia and renal tubular acidosis responding to dietary sodium restriction. *Pediatrics* 1982;69:317–24.

16. Licht JH, Amundson D, Hsueh WA, Lombardo JV. Familial hyperkalemic acidosis. *Quarterly Journal of Medicine* 1985;54:161–76.

17. Soppi E, Viikari J, Seppala P, Lehtonen A, Saarinen R, Miilunpalo S. Unusual association of hyperkalemia and hypertension. *Hypertension* 1986;8:174–7.

18. Gordon RD, Hodsman GP. The syndrome of hypertension and hyperkalaemia without renal failure: Long term correction by thiazide diuretic. *Scottish Medical Journal* 1986;31:43–4.

19. Wayne VS, Stockigt JR, Jennings GL. Treatment of mineralocorticoid resistant renal hyperkalemia with hypertension (type II pseudohypoaldosteronism). *Australian and New Zealand Journal of Medicine* 1986;16:221–3.

20. Nahum H, Paillard M, Pridgent A, Leviel F, Bichara M, Gardin J, Idatte JDAVP. Pseudohypoaldosteronism type II: Proximal renal tubular acidosis and dDVAP-sensitive renal hyperkalaemia. *American Journal of Nephrology* 1986;6:253–62.

21. Semmekrot B, Monnens L, Theelen BGA, Rascher W, Gabreels F, Willems J. The syndrome of hypertension and hyperkalemia with normal glomerular function (Gordon's syndrome). A pathophysiological study. *Pediatric Nephrology* 1987;1:473–8.

22. Valimaki M, Pelkonin R, Tikkanen I, Fyhrquist F. A deficient response of atrial natriuretic peptide to volume overload in Gordon's syndrome. *Acta Endocrinologica* 1989;120:331–6.

23. Ader JL, Waeber E, Suc JM, Brunner HR, Tran–van T, Durand D, Praddaude F. Syndrome of arterial hypertension, hyperkalemia, renal tubular acidosis with normal renal function: Gordon's syndrome and/or type II pseudohypoaldosteronism? *Archives des Maladies du Coeur et des Vaisseaux* 1988;81:193–7.

24. Take C, Ikeda K, Kurasawa T, Kurokawa K. Increased chloride reabsorption as an inherited renal tubular defect in familial type II pseudohypoaldosteronism. *New England Journal of Medicine* 1991;324:472–6.

25. Isenring P, Lebel M, Grose JH. Endocrine sodium and volume regulation in familial hyperkalemia with hypertension. *Hypertension* 1992;19:371–7.

26. Iitaka K, Watanabe N, Asakura A, Kasai N, Sakai T. Familial hyperkalemia, metabolic acidosis and short stature with normal renin and aldosterone levels. *International Journal of Pediatrics and Nephrology* 1980;1:242–5.

27. Pasman JW, Gabreels FJM, Semmekrot B, Renier WO, Monnens LAH. Hyperkalemic periodic paralysis in Gordon's syndrome: A possible defect in atrial natriuretic peptide function. *Annals of Neurology* 1989;26:392–5.

28. Spitzer A, Edelmann CM, Goldberg LD, Henneman PH. Short stature, hyperkalemia and acidosis: A defect in renal transport of potassium. *Kidney International* 1973;3:251–7.

29. Weinstein SF, Allan DME, Mendoza SA. Hyperkalemia, acidosis and short stature associated with a defect in renal potassium excretion. *Journal of Pediatrics* 1974;85:355–8.

30. Sauder SE, Kelch RP, Grekin RJ, Kelsch RC. Suppression of plasma renin activity in a boy with chronic hyperkalemia. *American Journal of Diseases in Childhood* 1987;141:922–7.

31. Margolis BL, Lifschitz MD. The Spitzer–Weinstein syndrome: One form of type IV renal tubular acidosis and its response to hydrochlorothiazide. *American Journal of Kidney Diseases* 1986;7:241–4.

32. Stokes GS, Gentle JL, Edwards KDG, Stewart JH, Scoggins BA, Coghlan JP. Syndrome of idiopathic hyperkalaemia and hypertension with decreased plasma renin activity: Effects on plasma renin and aldosterone of reducing the serum potassium level. *Medical Journal of Australia* 1968;2:1050–3.

33. Klemm SA, Gordon RD, Tunny TJ, Finn WL. Biochemical correction in the syndrome of hypertension and hyperkalaemia by severe dietary salt restriction suggests renin–aldosterone suppression critical in pathophysiology. *Clinical and Experimental Pharmacology and Physiology* 1990;17:191–5.

34. Kirchner KA, Kotchen TA, Galla JM, Luke RG. Importance of chloride for acute inhibition of renin by sodium chloride. *American Journal of Physiology* 1978;235:F444–50.

35. de Champlain J, Farley L, Cousineau D, van Ameringen M–R. Circulating catecholamine levels in human and experimental hypertension. *Journal of Neurochemistry* 1973;21:61–7.

36. Sanjad SA, Keenan BS, Hill LL. Renal hypoprostaglandism, hypertension and type IV renal tubular acidosis reversed by furosemide. *Annals of Internal Medicine* 1983;99:624–7.

37. Klemm SA, Hornych A, Tunny TJ, Gordon RD. The syndrome of hypertension and hyperkalaemia with normal glomerular filtration rate: Is there a deficiency in vasodilator prostaglandins? *Clinical and Experimental Pharmacology and Physiology* 1991;18:309–14.

38. Tunny TJ, Gordon RD. Plasma atrial natriuretic peptide in primary aldosteronism (before and after treatment) and in Bartter's and Gordon's syndromes. *Lancet* 1986;i:272–3.

39. Richards AM, MacDonald D, Fitzpatrick MA, Nicholls MG, Espiner EA, Ikram H, Jans S, Grant S, Yandle T. Atrial natriuretic hormone has biological effects in man at physiological plasma concentrations. *Journal of Clinical Endocrinology and Metabolism* 1988;67:1134–9.

40. Blair–West JR, Coghlan JP, Denton DA. Inhibition of renin secretion by systemic and intrarenal angiotensin infusion. *American Journal of Physiology* 1971;220:1309–15.

41. Brunner HR, Baer L, Sealey JE, Ledingham JGG, Laragh JH. The influence of potassium administration and of potassium deprivation on plasma renin in normal and hypertensive subjects. *Journal of Clinical Investigation* 1970;49:2128–38.

42. Himathongkam T, Dluhy RG, Willams GH. Potassium–aldosterone–renin interrelationships. *Journal of Clinical Endocrinology and Metabolism* 1975;41:153–9.

43. Kotchen TA, Mauli KI, Luke R, Rees D, Flamenbaum W. Effect of acute and chronic calcium administration on plasma renin. *Journal of Clinical Investigation* 1974;54:1279–86.

44. Ito K, Yamada K, Hasunuma K, Shiina T, Ebata T, Kikuno K, Yoshida S, Tamura Y, Yoshida S. A case of mineralocorticoid-resistant renal hyperkalemia without sodium wasting (Type II pseudohypoaldosteronism). *Japanese Journal of Medicine* 1988;77:425–9.

45. Dluhy RG, Greenfield M, Williams GH. Effect of simultaneous potassium and saline loading on plasma aldosterone levels. *Journal of Clinical Endocrinology and Metabolism* 1977;45:141–6.

46. Pratt JH. Role of angiotensin II in potassium-mediated stimulation of aldosterone secretion in the dog. *Journal of Clinical Investigation* 1982;70:667–72.

47. Tormey WP, Morgan DB. Etiological considerations in Gordon's syndrome: Possible role of prostaglandins. *Prostaglandins and Medicine* 1980;4:107–12.

48. Klemm SA, Gordon RD, Tunny TJ, Thompson RE. The syndrome of hypertension and hyperkalemia with normal GFR (Gordon's syndrome): Is there increased proximal sodium reabsorption? *Clinical and Investigative Medicine* 1991;14:551–8.

49. Vander AJ. Control of renin release. *Physiological Reviews* 1967;47:359–82.

50. Gordon RD, Wolfe LK, Island DP, Liddle GW. A diurnal rhythm in plasma renin activity. *Journal of Clinical Investigation* 1966;45:1587–92.

51. Wallin BG, Sundlof G. A quantitative study of muscle nerve sympathetic activity in resting normotensive and hypertensive subjects. *Hypertension* 1979;1:67–77.

66

RENIN IN LIDDLE'S SYNDROME AND IN THE SYNDROME OF APPARENT MINERALOCORTICOID EXCESS

RICHARD D GORDON, SHELLEY A KLEMM,
AND TERRY J TUNNY

INTRODUCTION

LIDDLE'S SYNDROME

Liddle's syndrome [1] is a congenital disorder affecting renal sodium and potassium transport and which possibly also involves abnormalities in sodium transport in other body cells (Fig. 66.1). The clinical syndrome mimics primary hyperaldosteronism due to an aldosterone-producing adenoma (see *Chapter 63*), and the kidney behaves as if it were under the influence of supranormal levels of aldosterone; hence the term 'pseudohyperaldosteronism' has been used, but the disorder must be distinguished from the 'pseudo-hyperaldosteronism' seen in neonates due to tubular resistance to the action of aldosterone and which is usually transient. Liddle's syndrome by contrast, is probably a lifelong disorder.

In the pseudohyperaldosteronism described by Liddle, the renal tubule is capable of responding to aldosterone, but so little aldosterone is present in the untreated state that blockade of its receptors with spironolactone effects no change in urinary or plasma electrolytes. Since the tubule is, however, responsive to both exogenous (infused) and endogenous aldosterone, spironolactone does have an effect when aldosterone levels are normal or high.

The hypertension of Liddle's syndrome is associated with hypokalemic alkalosis which is often severe (Fig 66.2a). The symptoms are therefore those of hypertension (headache, left ventricular failure, stroke, and so on) and hypokalemia (muscle weakness, polyuria, and occasionally short stature). The condition is readily distinguished biochemically from primary hyperaldosteronism because aldosterone levels are low, even after hypokalemia is corrected. Aldosterone is suppressed because of low renin levels (which result from sodium retention) and hypokalemia.

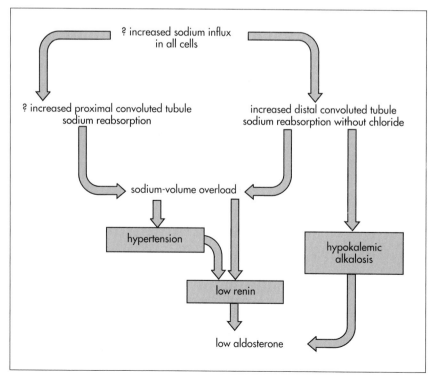

Fig. 66.1 Pathophysiology of Liddle's syndrome. Increased renal sodium reabsorption, probably by cells of both the proximal and distal convoluted tubules, leads to sodium-volume overload. This suppresses renin through mechanisms which may include reduced sympathetic nervous system activity and hypertension. Distal nephron sodium reabsorption without chloride leads to loss of potassium and hydrogen ions and hypokalemic alkalosis. Low renin and low potassium combine to produce very low aldosterone levels.

Case	Age (year)	Sex	K+ (mmol/l)	Cl- (mmol/l)	HCO₃⁻ (mmol/l)	Plasma renin activity (ng/ml/h)		Plasma aldosterone (ng/dl)		Urine aldosterone (μg/d)	Reference
						Rec	Up	Rec	Up		
(a) Liddle's syndrome											
1	14	F	2.4–3.0	96		0.05	0.1		17.3	6.8	5
2	16	M	2.1–2.8	94		0.06	0.09		2.8	11.1	5
3	2	M	1.8	106	32		0.02			<2.5	6
4	12	M	3.4	100	27		0.06		4.4	1.4	30
5	0.8	F	3.2	78			0.001		0.5	0.5	27
6	22	M	2.6	99			0.1		3.0		8
7	18	F	2.8	103	33		0.1		3.0		40
(b) Syndrome of apparent mineralocorticoid excess											
1	3	F	2.8				UD		1.9		13
2	4	F	2.0–3.3	88–102	23–38	0.4	0.3	1.0	2.5	2.6	33
3	3	F	2.3				<0.5			<2.0	38
4	1.6	M	1.8–2.0	105	26		0.3		0.6	0.7	35
5	2.8	F	2.5–2.8	79	31		UD		UD		35
6	9	M	2.0–2.6				low		<1.0	<0.5	14
7	2	M	2.2	105	36		0.013		<1.3		19
8	1.8	M	2.6–3.0	104–108	25–28		0.4		3.0		32
9	0.4	M	1.8		29		0.02		1.1		39
10	8	M	1.9–3.3				0.25			UD	17
11	21	M	1.7		32	0.1		<3.6			18

K+ = plasma potassium; Cl⁻ = plasma chloride; HCO₃⁻ = plasma bicarbonate; Up = upright; Rec = recumbent; UD = undetectable.

Fig. 66.2 Plasma renin activity in previously untreated patients with Liddle's syndrome and the syndrome of apparent mineralocorticoid excess.

APPARENT MINERALOCORTICOID EXCESS

Another condition associated with hypertension and hypokalemia is the syndrome of 'apparent mineralocorticoid excess' (Figs. 66.2b and 66.3). This disorder can be distinguished from Liddle's syndrome because the biochemical abnormalities are corrected by blocking mineralocorticoid activity with spironolactone or by suppressing endogenous adrenocorticotropic hormone (ACTH) secretion with dexamethasone. Failure of conversion of cortisol (which has high affinity for the aldosterone receptor) to cortisone (which does not) within the kidneys (see *Chapter 63*) is one possible cause of this syndrome, while another is excessive secretion of one or more unidentified mineralocorticoids. Some patients, however, do not fit easily into either category.

This chapter discusses renin levels in previously untreated patients with Liddle's syndrome, in an attempt to explain the regulation of renin and its contribution to the pathophysiology. It also refers to renin levels in the syndrome of apparent mineralocorticoid excess.

HISTORY

LIDDLE'S SYNDROME

In 1963, Liddle [1] presented details of a family with hypertension and hypokalemia presenting as, but not explained by, aldosterone excess; in fact, aldosterone levels were very low. The renal tubule behaved as though it was exposed to excessive mineralocorticoid, except that spironolactone, a competitive receptor antagonist of aldosterone, was ineffective. Administration of the nonsteroidal potassium-retaining diuretic, triamterene, increased potassium levels, but failed to lower blood pressure to normal unless combined with dietary sodium restriction. Renin levels were found to be low despite moderate sodium restriction and administration of triamterene, but were noted to be responsive to severe dietary sodium restriction and to high-dose triamterene when measured some three years later (Gordon RD, Wolfe LK, Liddle GW, unpublished data). In subsequent reports of untreated patients with Liddle's syndrome (Fig. 66.2(a)), renin and aldosterone levels have generally been very low.

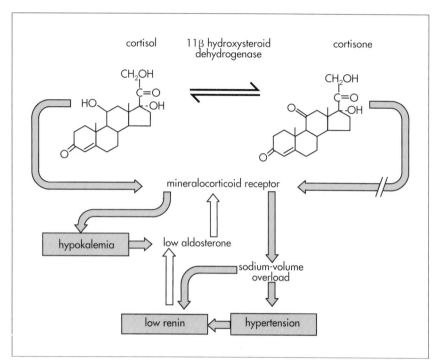

Fig. 66.3 Pathophysiology of the syndrome of apparent mineralocorticoid excess. Failure of metabolic inactivation of cortisol in the renal parenchyma leads to excessive stimulation of the mineralocorticoid receptor with resulting sodium retention, hypertension, and hypokalemia and low levels of renin and aldosterone. In some patients, unidentified steroids with mineralocorticoid activity may be involved. Open arrows indicate decreased stimulation, shaded arrows increased stimulation.

It is likely that a brief report by Ross in 1959 [2] was also of a patient with Liddle's syndrome. Aldosterone secretion was low, and bilateral adrenalectomy did not cure the hypertension or the hypokalemia. For a steroid to be involved therefore, its production would need to be extra-adrenal.

Following on Liddle's detailed description of the syndrome, reports of new cases have ensued slowly. Wang and co-workers [3] carefully investigated a patient with features of Liddle's syndrome and found that a combination of restriction of dietary salt and administration of triamterene was required to correct all measured abnormalities. In none of the patients with Liddle's syndrome were the biochemical abnormalities influenced by suppression of endogenous ACTH with dexamethasone [3–9].

Most patients with Liddle's syndrome reported before 1976 were familial, whereas most since then have been sporadic. Helbock and Reynolds in 1970 [10] drew attention to increased red-cell sodium influx in Liddle's syndrome, and this was later confirmed by several workers [6,11,12]. There are, however, inconsistencies in this area.

APPARENT MINERALOCORTICOID EXCESS

Since 1974, when Werder and co-workers [13] reported a three-year-old girl with hypertension, hypokalemic alkalosis, and low renin and aldosterone, all corrected with dexamethasone, at least 23 patients, mostly young children, have been described with the syndrome of apparent mineralocorticoid excess. The mean age at diagnosis (9 ± 1.7 SEM years) is significantly ($P<0.01$) less than in Liddle's syndrome (17.1 ± 3.4 years). This may be because the hypokalemia is more severe, causing earlier presentation. Although all such patients are not easily categorized, the syndrome usually can be distinguished from Liddle's syndrome by its dependence on ACTH and hence correction by ACTH suppression using dexamethasone. Moreover, spironolactone blocks the mineralocorticoid activity (which is too low in Liddle's syndrome for an observable effect), and the salivary sodium/potassium ratio is low, as expected in mineralocorticoid excess syndromes (not so in Liddle's syndrome).

In at least some cases, the offending mineralocorticoid appears to be cortisol, which accumulates in all tissues including the kidney due to partial deficiency of 11β-hydroxysteroid dehydrogenase [14–18], and possibly also of 5β-steroid reductase enzymes [17,19], leading to an increased half-life for cortisol [17,18,20] and a low tetrahydrocortisone/tetrahydrocortisol ratio in urine [20,21]. Cortisol has a similar affinity for renal mineralocorticoid receptors to aldosterone [22] but is, of course, present in much larger amounts.

In 1988, the first adult case of apparent mineralocorticoid excess was reported in detail [18]. In 1989, Ulick [23] pointed out that there could be a number of mechanisms underlying a reduction in the metabolic inactivation of cortisol, all resulting in a longer plasma and tissue half-life for cortisol [23]. Thus, the syndrome can be explained if aldosterone specificity for mineralocorticoid-sensitive tissues is dependent on the conversion of abundant glucocorticoids to their 11-keto analogs (which have a low affinity for mineralocorticoid receptors) by microsomal 11β-hydroxysteroid dehydrogenase [24].

The syndrome of apparent mineralocorticoid excess has been reviewed by Shackleton and Stewart [25].

BASAL ACTIVITY OF THE RENIN–ANGIOTENSIN SYSTEM

LIDDLE'S SYNDROME

In patients with untreated Liddle's syndrome (see *Fig. 66.2a*), plasma renin activity (PRA) is low or very low. The factors known or believed to influence renin levels in man are shown in Fig. 66.4. In Liddle's syndrome, sodium reabsorption both proximally and distally (where it promotes potassium excretion) is probably excessive, leading to sodium and volume overload. This in turn leads to hypertension, suppression of sympathetic nervous system activity through effect on arterial baroreceptors and venous volume receptors, and possibly an increase in plasma sodium levels, all of which would tend to reduce renin secretion. An increase in sodium and chloride flux across the macula densa cells might also contribute to the suppression of renin secretion. Catecholamine levels in Liddle's syndrome have been reported as normal [3,8,9,12,26,27], but it is often difficult to distinguish low from normal levels.

We are not aware of reports of prostaglandin, vasopressin, or atrial natriuretic factor (ANF) levels in Liddle's syndrome. Due to hypervolemia, prostaglandin levels would be expected to be low and ANF levels high, both of which would lower renin levels. In conditions of mineralocorticoid excess, urinary kallikrein is usually raised [28,29] but it is low in Liddle's syndrome [7,30], as might be expected in states of sodium retention which are not the result of mineralocorticoid overactivity. Although the effect of potassium on renin secretion is not a powerful or consistent one (see *Chapter 74*), the very low potassium levels seen in this syndrome would tend to stimulate renin secretion. Circulating calcium levels may affect renin secretion [31] but are normal in Liddle's syndrome [5,9,12,26,30]. High chloride levels and delivery rates to the macula densa are believed to lower renin levels [31], but chloride levels are low in some patients with Liddle's syndrome [5,27]. The well-described negative feedback effect of Ang II on renin secretion would have little impact in Liddle's syndrome.

The important determinants of suppressed basal renin levels are presumably sodium-volume overload, reduced sympathetic stimulation of the juxtaglomerular apparatus, and hypertension. Other less certain, but possibly important, influences are raised ANF levels and increased sodium flux at the macula densa.

APPARENT MINERALOCORTICOID EXCESS

Plasma renin activity levels in previously untreated patients with apparent mineralocorticoid excess are uniformly low (see *Fig. 66.2b*), as are aldosterone levels. The explanation for the suppressed renin and aldosterone values in most patients is presumably the same as for Liddle's syndrome. Fiselier [32] reported elevated levels of prostaglandin E_2 in the syndrome of apparent mineralocorticoid excess, but any stimulatory action on renin must be overcome by the inhibitory factors listed above.

DYNAMIC CHANGES IN RENIN

LIDDLE'S SYNDROME

The effect of upright posture on plasma renin has been examined in only a few instances [3,5] and clear effects were sometimes apparent only after stimulation with either triamterene [7,30] or dietary salt restriction [3,5–7,30]. As previously mentioned, PRA remained low after two years on an unrestricted sodium diet and triamterene treatment in Liddle's two index patients, but rose to normal on a severely restricted diet (10mmol/d) alone, and to supranormal levels with moderate sodium restriction (30mmol/d) plus triamterene 100mg daily (Gordon RD, Wolfe LK, Liddle GW, unpublished data). In the patient reported by Wang *et al* [3], PRA increased to above normal during treatment with triamterene 150mg/d. There seems no reason to doubt that the juxtaglomerular apparatus in Liddle's syndrome is capable of responding normally to the major stimuli of volume depletion and activation of the sympathetic nervous system.

APPARENT MINERALOCORTICOID EXCESS

There have been several reports of normal or even increased plasma renin during dietary sodium restriction [13,20] and with chronic treatment with dexamethasone [18,33,34], triamterene [19,33,35], or spironolactone [21,33,36], each of which ultimately corrects the characteristic volume expansion. Cortisol administration, however, leads to further suppression of renin [20,18,36] presumably via its effects on mineralocorticoid receptors. Whereas dietary salt restriction is dependent on obligatory urinary and fecal losses to achieve a negative sodium balance, the pharmacological agents work either by suppression of mineralocorticoid production, or by noncompetitive or competitive inhibition of distal tubular sodium reabsorption (without

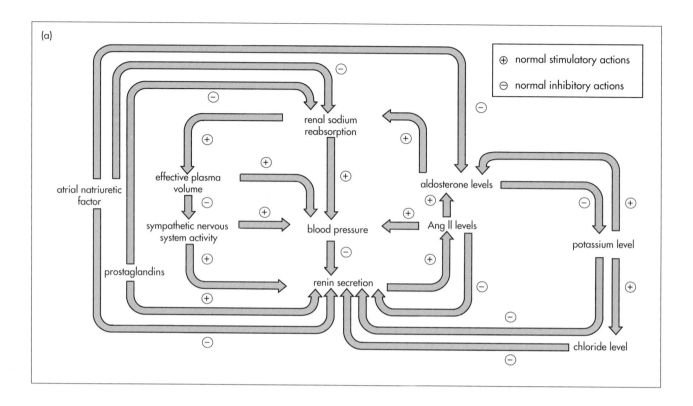

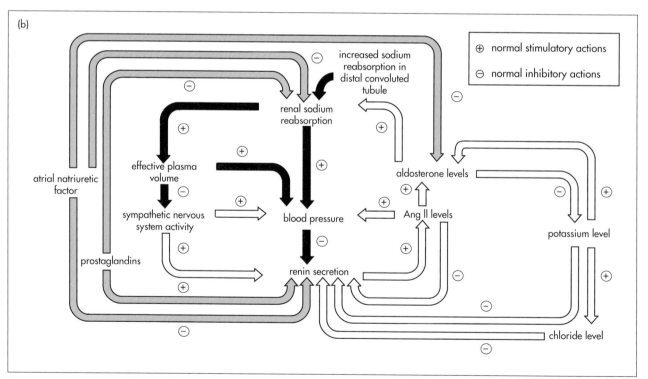

Fig. 66.4 (a) Factors which normally influence renin secretion. (b) Alterations in these factors which influence renin secretion in Liddle's syndrome and in the syndrome of apparent mineralocorticoid excess are shown in black arrows (increased) or open arrows (decreased).

chloride). Once renin is unsuppressed, it appears capable of responding to upright posture [32], presumably through the normal mechanism of sympathetic stimulation of the juxtaglomerular apparatus (see *Chapters 24* and *74*).

EFFECTS OF RENIN

In general, any changes in renin are accompanied by parallel changes in aldosterone in these two syndromes. We are, however, not aware of any studies which document aldosterone and arterial pressure responsiveness to Ang II infusion in Liddle's syndrome or in the syndrome of apparent mineralocorticoid excess. Due to severe hypokalemia in both diseases, the aldosterone/renin ratio might be expected to be low, but renin levels are in general so suppressed before treatment that this is in fact not the case.

EFFECTS OF TREATMENT ON RENIN

In both conditions, severe dietary sodium restriction [3,5–7, 13,20,30], high-dose triamterene alone [7,19,30,33,35], high-dose amiloride [30,37], or a potassium-sparing diuretic and low sodium diet in combination [32] have all led to stimulation of renin secretion. A failure of renin to respond can generally be explained by the brevity of the studies or uncertain compliance.

Renin levels are unresponsive to spironolactone monotherapy in previously untreated Liddle's syndrome [3,7–9,12,30] but are responsive in the syndrome of apparent mineralocorticoid excess [33,35,36,38] because spironolactone blocks the mineralocorticoid receptor regardless of whether the pathogenetic hormone is aldosterone, cortisol, or some unidentified mineralocorticoid.

Renin levels in Liddle's syndrome are unaffected by administration of dexamethasone in doses which are sufficient to suppress endogenous ACTH secretion [3,6,7,9] but are responsive in most patients with the syndrome of apparent mineralocorticoid excess, provided dexamethasone is given for a sufficient period of time [18,34,38].

FURTHER COMMENTS AND CONCLUSIONS

Liddle's syndrome is a very rare congenital renal tubular disorder [1–12,26,27,37,39,40] recognized less frequently than Gordon's syndrome and much less frequently than Bartter's syndrome (see *Chapters 64* and *65*). It is more often sporadic than familial, and is probably the result of changes in a recessive gene or genes with poor penetrance.

The syndrome of apparent mineralocorticoid excess is reported with ever-increasing frequency, especially in young children [13–21,23,32–36,38,39, 41]. It is possible that the underlying enzyme deficiencies are sometimes transient, as in pseudohypoaldosteronism (renal tubular resistance to aldosterone in the neonate). On the other hand, the enzyme deficiency is sometimes very severe, leading to early death [39].

While it is difficult to find a classification which will accommodate all reported patients with the syndrome of hypertension, hypokalemic alkalosis, and suppressed renin, the subgroups shown in Fig. 66.5 encompass most of them. In the untreated state, careful examination of electrolyte, renin, and hormone responses to spironolactone and to dexamethasone is critical.

The disorders described in Fig. 66.5 as pseudohyperaldosteronism are all characterized by sodium-volume overload, suppressed renin and aldosterone, and hypertension which is dependent upon the level of habitual salt intake. Unless the source of mineralocorticoid activity is an inoperable tumor, they are all amenable to successful treatment. In Liddle's syndrome, a combination of strict dietary sodium restriction with triamterene or amiloride is very effective. For the syndrome of apparent mineralocorticoid excess, chronic suppression of endogenous ACTH with dexamethasone, or competitive inhibition of cortisol (or other steroids) at the level of the mineralocorticoid receptor, is effective.

In the syndrome of apparent mineralocorticoid excess, the cellular mechanisms controlling transport of sodium and potassium across cell membranes appear to be intact, but need to be studied in detail. This is an area where confidence in the interpretation of results is lacking.

Since micropuncture studies involving renal tubules are not possible in intact human subjects, it is difficult to imagine how the renal defect in Liddle's syndrome will be finally localized and characterized. However, the fact that blood pressure and renin levels return towards normal with thiazide diuretics suggests there is an underlying disorder in distal renal tubular sodium reabsorption [7]. Studies of membrane transport in accessible cells such as the erythrocyte have given inconsistent results, since a number have suggested increased sodium influx [6,10–12] whereas at least one has suggested increased efflux [11]. Levin has pointed out [42] that potassium depletion itself, regardless of its cause, can result in increased sodium influx. At present,

(1) Hyperaldosteronism
    (a) aldosterone-producing adrenocortical adenoma (Conns' syndrome)
    (b) nontumorous hyperaldosteronism not suppressible with glucocorticoid ('idiopathic' hyperaldosteronism)
    (c) glucocorticoid-suppressible hyperaldosteronism
    (d) adrenocortical carcinoma
(2) Excessive production of mineralocorticoid other than aldosterone — **pseudohyperaldosteronism type I**
    (a) DOC–secreting adrenal cortical adenomas or carcinomas
    (b) congenital adrenal hyperplasia due to relative deficiency of 11β-hydroxylase or 17α-hydroxylase
    (c) ectopic adrenocorticotropic hormone secretion by tumors causing excessive secretion of DOC and cortisol
    (d) administration of excessive cortisol, prednisone, 9α-fluoro-hydrocortisone, etc, orally or transdermally
(3) Failed conversion of cortisol to cortisone — syndrome of apparent mineralocorticoid excess — **pseudohyperaldosteronism type II**
    (a) sporadic or familial, congenital partial deficiency of 11β-hydroxysteroid dehydrogenase and/or of 5β-steroid reductase
    (b) enzyme block as in (a) due to ingestion of glycyrrhyzinic acid in licorice or peptic ulcer remedies
(4) Congenital overactivity of sodium reabsorption without chloride in the distal nephron not due to mineralocorticoid activity — Liddle's syndrome — **pseudohyperaldosteronism type III**

Fig. 66.5 Hypertension and hypokalemic alkalosis with suppressed renin: a classification based on mineralocorticoid activity (see *Chapter 63*).

no firm conclusions can be drawn as to whether the disordered electrolyte transport in Liddle's syndrome is confined to the kidney or affects all cells.

Regardless of the underlying abnormality, the RAS is severely suppressed but is capable of responding to normal stimuli, and is probably potentially able to exert its normal actions in these syndromes.

FUTURE DIRECTIONS

It is essential to make careful observations of basal hormone and electrolyte levels before commencing treatment in all patients in whom a diagnosis of one of these rare disorders (Fig. 66.5) is suspected. Confident interpretation of data is complicated by the effects of therapy. Evaluation of responses to treatment such as severe dietary salt restriction, spironolactone, triamterene, amiloride, or dexamethasone should be carried out in hospital under strict supervision in order to ensure compliance. Patients with these diseases are rare, and improved understanding of their disordered physiology holds the key to better insight into normal adrenocortical, renal, and cardiovascular physiology.

Careful measurements of prostaglandins, ANF, and vasopressin are needed to clarify their role in the pathophysiology of these rare disorders. Localization of the underlying renal lesion in both syndromes, however, is critical. The painstaking

accumulation of evidence for a role for cortisol as a mineralocorticoid hormone [14,16,18,19,25,38,41] is of great potential significance and has many important implications for normal physiological functioning. The recent clarification of the pathophysiology in at least some patients with the syndrome of apparent mineralocorticoid excess emphasizes the value of careful observation and intuitive reasoning when faced by puzzling experiments of nature. Too often, the 'conventional wisdom' derived from observations that are no longer questioned, but which were made under conditions of great technical difficulty and uncertainty, limits our understanding.

The syndrome of apparent mineralocorticoid excess will continue to raise questions, to excite and to stimulate studies which expand our knowledge. The painstaking studies of Liddle and co-workers 30 years ago have established a pathophysiological entity. The question of whether the abnormality in transcellular sodium transport is localized to the kidney or is general, remains as alive as ever.

ACKNOWLEDGMENT

We gratefully acknowledge the support of the National Health and Medical Research Council of Australia for our Research Project, *Volume-regulatory hormones in congenital disorders of sodium balance in man.*

REFERENCES

1. Liddle GW, Bledsoe T, Coppage WS. A familial renal disorder simulating primary aldosteronism but with negligible aldosterone secretion. *Transactions of the Association of American Physicians* 1963;26:199–213.

2. Ross EJ. Hypertension and hypokalaemia associated with hypoaldosteronism. *Proceedings of the Royal Society of Medicine* 1959;52:1056.

3. Wang C, Chan TK, Yeung RTT, Coghlan JP, Scoggins BA, Stockigt JR. The effect of triamterene and sodium intake on renin, aldosterone, and erythrocyte sodium transport in Liddle's syndrome. *Journal of Clinical Endocrinology and Metabolism* 1981;52:1027–32.

4. Milora R, Vagnucci A, Goodman AD. A syndrome resembling primary aldosteronism but without mineralocorticoid excess (MCE). *Clinical Research* 1967:15:482A.

5. Ohno F, Harada H, Komatsu K, Saijo K, Miyoshi K. Two cases of pseudoaldosteronism (Liddle's syndrome) in siblings. *Endocrinological Reviews* 1975;22:163–7.

6. Hyman PE, Sha'afi RI, Tan SY, Hintz R. Liddle's syndrome. *Journal of Pediatrics* 1979;95:77–8.

7. Sakamoto N, Uda M, Kojima S, Tsuchiya M, Ito K, Ogino K, Ikeda M, Watabe R. Hypertension, hypokalemia and hypoaldosteronism with suppressed renin: A clinical study of a patient with Liddle's syndrome. *Endocrinologia Japonica* 1981;28:357–62.

8. Mutoh S, Hirayama H, Ueda S, Tsuruta K, Imafuji M, Ikegami K. Pseudohyperaldosteronism (Liddle's syndrome): A case report. *Journal of Urology* 1986;135:557–8.

9. Takeuchi K, Abe K, Sato M, Yasujima M, Omata K, Murakami O, Yoshinaga K. Plasma aldosterone level in a female case of pseudohyperaldosteronism (Liddle's syndrome). *Endocrinologia Japonica* 1989;36:167–73.

10. Helbock HJ, Reynolds JW. Pseudoaldosteronism (Liddle's syndrome): Evidence for increased cell membrane permeability to Na⁺. *Pediatric Research* 1970;4:455.

11. Gardner JD, Lapey A, Simopoulos AR, Bravo EL. Abnormal membrane sodium transport in Liddle's syndrome. *Journal of Clinical Investigation* 1971;50:2253–8.

12. Nakada T, Koike H, Akiya T, Katayama T, Kawamata S, Takaya K, Shigematsu H. Liddle's syndrome, an uncommon form of hyporeninemic hypoaldosteronism: Functional and histopathological studies. *Journal of Urology* 1987;137:636–40.

13. Werder E, Zachmann M, Vollmin JA, Veyrat R, Prader A. Unusual steroid excretion in a child with low renin hypertension. *Research in Steroids* 1974;6:385–9.

14. Ulick S, Levine LS, Gunczler P, Zanconato G, Ramirez LC, Rauh W, Rosler A, Bradlow HL, New MI. A syndrome of apparent mineralocorticoid excess associated with defects in the peripheral metabolism of cortisol. *Journal of Clinical Endocrinology and Metabolism* 1979;49:757–64.

15. Harinck HIJ, van Brummelen P, van Seters AP, Moolenaar AJ. Apparent mineralocorticoid excess and deficient 11β-oxidation of cortisol in a young female. *Clinical Endocrinology* 1984;21:505–14.

16. Shackleton CHL, Rodriguez J, Arteaga E, Lopez JM, Winter JSD. Congenital 11β-hydroxysteroid dehydrogenase deficiency associated with juvenile hypertension: Corticosteroid metabolite profiles of four patients and their families. *Clinical Endocrinology* 1985;22:701–12.

17. Monder C, Shackleton CHL, Bradlow HL, New MI, Stoner E, Iohan F, Lakshmi V. The syndrome of apparent mineralocorticoid excess: Its association with 11β-dehydrogenase and 5β-reductase deficiency and some consequences for corticosteroid metabolism. *Journal of Clinical Endocrinology and Metabolism* 1986;63:550–7.

18. Stewart PM, Corrie JET, Shackleton CHL, Edwards CRW. Syndrome of apparent mineralocorticoid excess: A defect in the cortisol–cortisone shuttle. *Journal of Clinical Investigation* 1988;82:340–9.

19. Shackleton CHL, Honour JW, Dillon MJ, Chantler C, Jones RWA. Hypertension in a four-year old child: Gas chromotographic and mass spectrometric evidence for deficient hepatic metabolism of steroids. *Journal of Clinical Endocrinology and Metabolism* 1980;50:786–92.

20. Dimartino–Nardi J, Stoner E, Martin K, Balfe JW, Jose PA, New MI. New findings in apparent mineralocorticoid excess. *Clinical Endocrinology* 1987;27:49–62.

21. Batista M, Mendonca BB, Kater CE, Amhold IJP, Rocha A, Nicolau W, Blosie W. Spironolactone-reversible rickets associated with 11β-hydroxysteroid dehydrogenase deficiency syndrome. *Journal of Pediatrics* 1986;109:989–93.

22. Lan NC, Matulich DT, Stockigt JR, Biglieri EG, New MI, Winter JSD, McKenzie JK, Baxter JD. Radioreceptor assay of plasma mineralocorticoid activity: Role of aldosterone, cortisol, and deoxycorticosterone in various mineralocorticoid-excess states. *Circulation Research* 1980;46 (suppl 1): I-94–100.

23. Ulick S, Chan CK, Rao KN, Edassery J, Mantero F. A new form of the syndrome of apparent mineralocorticoid excess. *Journal of Steroid Biochemistry* 1989;32:209–12.

24. Funder JW. How can aldosterone act as a mineralocorticoid? *Endocrine Reviews* 1989;15:227–38.

25. Shackleton CHL, Stewart PM. The hypertension of apparent mineralocorticoid excess (AME) syndrome. In: Biglieri EG, Melby JC, eds. *Endocrine hypertension.* New York: Raven Press, 1990:155–73.

26. Aaskog D, Stoa KF, Thorsen T, Wefring KW. Hypertension and hypokalemic alkalosis associated with underproduction of aldosterone. *Pediatrics* 1967;39:884–90.

27. Signoretti A, Bacchetta V, Cugini P, Di Erasmo A, Lombari MR, Imperato C. Liddle's syndrome: Diagnosis and treatment in a 10 months old female. *Minerva Pediatrica* 1981;33:1013–20.

28. Holland OB, Clud JM, Braunstein H. Urinary kallikrein excretion in essential and mineralocorticoid hypertension. *Journal of Clinical Investigation* 1980;65:347–56.

29. Margolius HS, Chao J, Kaizu T. The effects of aldactone and spironolactone on renal kallikrein in the rat. *Clinical Science and Molecular Medicine,* 1976;51 (suppl 3):279–82s.

30. Rodriguez JA, Biglieri EG, Schambelan M. Pseudohyperaldosteronism with renal tubular resistance to mineralocorticoid hormones. *Transactions of the Association of American Physicians* 1981;94:172–82.

31. Kotchen TA, Mauli KI, Luke R, Rees D, Flamenbaum W. Effect of acute and chronic calcium administration on plasma renin. *Journal of Clinical Investigation* 1974;54:1279–86.

32. Fiselier TJW, Otten BJ, Monnens LAH, Honour JW, Munster PJJ. Low-renin, low-aldosterone hypertension and abnormal cortisol metabolism in a 19-month-old child. *Hormone Research* 1982;16:107–14.

33. Sann L, Revol A, Zachmann M, Legrand JC, Bethenod M. Unusual low plasma renin hypertension in a child. *Journal of Clinical Endocrinology and Metabolism* 1975;43:265–71.

34. Hoefnagels WHL, Hofman JA, Smals AGH, Drayer JIM, Kloppenborg PWC, Benrad TJ. Dexamethasone-responsive hypertension in young women with suppressed renin and aldosterone. *Lancet* 1979;i:741–3.

35. Winter JS, McKenzie JK. A syndrome of low-renin hypertension in children. In: New MI, Levine LS, eds. *Juvenile hypertension.* New York: Raven Press, 1977:123–31.

36. Oberfield SE, Levine LS, Carey RM, Greig F, Ulick S, New MI. Metabolic and blood pressure responses to hydrocortisone in the syndrome of apparent mineralocorticoid excess. *Journal of Clinical Endocrincology and Metabolism* 1983;56:332–9.

37. Lopez–Uriarte A, Ojeda–Duran S, Vargas–Rosendo R. Liddle's syndrome. *Boletin Médico del Hospital Infantil de Mexico* 1984;41:281–3.

38. New MI, Levine LS, Biglieri EG, Pareira J, Ulick S. Evidence for an unidentified steroid in a child with apparent mineralocorticoid hypertension. *Journal of Clinical Endocrinology and Metabolism* 1977;44:924–33.

39. Honour JW, Dillon MJ, Levin M, Shah V. Fatal, low renin hypertension associated with a disturbance of cortisol metabolism. *Archives of Disease in Childhood* 1983;53:1018–20.

40. Fukutake N, Kawashima S, Matsumoto T, Ryo K, Mitani Y, Iwasaki T. A case of Liddle's syndrome with familial occurrence. *Journal of Japanese Society of Internal Medicine* 1988;77:441–2.

41. Ulick S, Ramirez LC, New MI. An abnormality in steroid reductive metabolism in a hypertensive syndrome. *Journal of Clinical Endocrinology and Metabolism* 1977;44:799–802.

42. Levin ML, Rector FC, Seldin DW. The effects of chronic hypokalemia, hyponatraemia, and acid–base alterations on erythrocyte Na⁺ transport. *Clinical Science* 1972:43:251–63.

67

PHEOCHROMOCYTOMA AND THE RENIN SYSTEM

J IAN S ROBERTSON

INTRODUCTION

There have been numerous reports of enhanced activity of the RAS in patients with pheochromocytoma [1–7].

Maebashi *et al* [2] found plasma renin to be elevated in patients in whom norepinephrine was secreted to excess, whereas Vetter *et al* observed plasma renin activity (PRA) to be elevated in subjects with excessive excretion of epinephrine [3]. Maebashi *et al* [2] observed that plasma renin returned within the normal range following excision of the pheochrome tumors. These early studies prompted more detailed investigation.

CONTROLLED CLINICAL STUDIES

Plouin and colleagues [8] made a very detailed investigation of the association between pheochromocytoma and the RAS. These

workers measured PRA and plasma catecholamines in 26 untreated patients with pheochromocytoma, in 18 untreated patients with essential ('primary') hypertension, and in 10 normal volunteers. They observed that PRA, measured severally with the subjects supine, standing, and after one hour of ambulation, was higher in the patients with pheochrome tumors than in those with essential hypertension or the normal control subjects ($P<0.001$) (Fig. 67.1). In all three circumstances of blood sampling, PRA was correlated with concurrent plasma norepinephrine in the patients with pheochromocytoma (r=0.545, 0.600, and 0.739; $P<0.01$) but these correlations were not seen in normal subjects or in essential hypertension. In the patients with pheochromocytoma, PRA and plasma epinephrine were significantly correlated only after standing for five minutes. Administration of the cardioselective β-adrenoceptor blocking agent acebutolol to seven of the patients with pheochromocytoma (Fig. 67.2) reduced PRA by an average of 89%, and heart rate and mean blood pressure by averages of 20% and 12%, respectively. The ACE inhibitor captopril was given acutely

	Normal controls	Patients with essential hypertension	Patients with pheochromocytoma
plasma renin activity (ng/ml/h)†			
supine	0.85 ± 0.62	1.01 ± 0.74	2.54 ± 2.16
standing	1.07 ± 0.64	1.14 ± 0.84	3.83 ± 3.97*
walking one hour	1.53 ± 0.75*	1.89 ± 1.72*	6.23 ± 4.89*
norepinephrine (pg/ml)‡			
supine	358 ± 149	284 ± 195	5104 ± 7982
standing	800 ± 360*	465 ± 187*	5425 ± 7487
walking one hour	578 ± 97*	600 ± 217*	6197 ± 7420*
epinephrine (pg/ml)§			
supine	38 ± 31	104 ± 72	979 ± 1197
standing	65 ± 42	136 ± 131	779 ± 711
walking one hour	53 ± 17	146 ± 116	880 ± 872

*$P<0.05$ versus supine value (Wilcoxon test). Conversion of SI units to traditional units: norepinephrine 1nmol/1 = 169pg/ml; epinephrine 1nmol/l = 183pg/ml. †Group effect: F = 9, $P<0.001$; position effect: F = 35, $P<0.001$; group x position: F = 4.8, not significant. ‡ Group effect: F = 47, $P<0.001$; position effect: F = 29, $P<0.001$; group x position: F = 4.8, $P<0.01$. §Group effect: F = 46, $P<0.001$; position effect: F = 3, $P=0.05$; group x position: not significant.

Fig. 67.1 Plasma renin activity and plasma epinephrine and norepinephrine concentrations (mean ± SD) after one hour in the supine position, five minutes of standing, and one hour of walking. Intergroup variance analysis and intragroup paired comparisons have been made. Modified from Plouin P-F *et al* [8].

Patient	Heart rate (beats/min)		Blood pressure (mmHg)		Plasma renin activity (ng/ml/h)	
	Before acebutolol	On acebutolol	Before acebutolol	On acebutolol	Before acebutolol	On acebutolol
1	72	51	159/90	144/65	0.86	0.50
2	78	64	172/92	142/82	1.60	0.50
3	111	76	179/135	152/125	4.60	0.40
4	80	64	147/95	128/90	0.79	0.08
5	72	61	202/129	182/123	1.89	0.32
6	75	68	146/103	128/89	1.80	0.10
7	82	70	190/110	168/103	10.80	0.55
average	81.4	64.9*	171/108	149/97*	3.19	0.35*
standard deviation	13.6	7.8	21/18	20/22	3.59	0.19

*$P=0.02$ by Wilcoxon test compared to 'before' values

Fig. 67.2 Effects of β-blockade with 800mg/d acebutolol for three days, on supine heart rate, blood pressure, and plasma renin activity, in seven patients with pheochromocytoma. Modified from Plouin P-F et al [8].

Patient	Mean blood pressure (mmHg)		Plasma renin activity (ng/ml/h)	
	Before captopril	On captopril	Before captopril	On captopril
A	86	74	1.6	9.1
B	100	89	0.5	1.3
C	102	81	3.0	15.7
D	85	78	0.3	0.8
E	108	84	0.7	1.6
F	144	112	2.8	19.2
G	100	73	3.0	3.4
H	89	62	2.8	14.8
I	102	87	1.0	3.6
average	101.8	82.2*	1.74	7.72*
standard deviation	17.8	13.9	1.16	7.16

*$P=0.008$ by Wilcoxon test compared to 'before' values

Fig. 67.3 Acute effects of 1mg/kg oral captopril on mean blood pressure and plasma renin activity. Modified from Plouin P-F et al [8].

to nine patients with pheochromocytoma and lowered mean blood pressure similarly, by an average of 19% (Fig. 67.3).

Plouin *et al* [8] proposed that high plasma concentrations of norepinephrine, released from the pheochromocytomata, directly affect the adrenergic receptors of the renal juxtaglomerular apparatus, stimulating release of renin. The consequent enhanced activity of the RAS then contributes, via Ang II, to the systemic blood-pressure elevation. The antihypertensive response to both β-blockade and ACE inhibition was taken as indirect support for this possibility.

Richards and colleagues measured PRA, Ang II, and plasma catecholamine levels hourly for 24 hours in two patients with pheochromocytoma before surgery and again three months after successful removal of the tumor [9]. Dietary electrolyte intake and body posture were identical in both studies. In both patients, PRA and Ang II (and aldosterone) levels were above the normal range initially, but fell within the normal range three months after removal of the tumor. As in the study of Plouin *et al* [8], Richards and colleagues observed a positive and statistically significant correlation between concurrent PRA and plasma norepinephrine levels prior to surgery [9].

LOCAL ADRENAL RENIN SYSTEM IN PHEOCHROMOCYTOMA

Measurements of components of the RAS and of catecholamines in peripheral blood may not provide a full account of the inter-relationships of these systems in pheochromocytoma. The presence of renin activity in human adrenal glands [10] (see *Chapter 44*), the finding of renin, Ang II, and converting enzyme activity in neuroblastoma and glioma cells [11,12], and the generation of angiotensins in cultured pheochromocytoma cells [13], raised the possibility of an active RAS in mammalian adrenal medulla [14]. The normal human adrenal gland was found to contain binding sites for both Ang II and ACE in the medulla and zona glomerulosa [14]. However, in pheochromocytomata, while

ACE binding was homogeneously distributed, no Ang II binding could be detected [14]. These authors [14] emphasize the highly variable pattern and extent of catecholamine release in patients with pheochromocytoma, and thus the likelihood that these local changes in adrenal medullary tissue could have very different effects from case to case. They point out, moreover, that ACE is a nonspecific enzyme and could well affect the formation and/or metabolism of other peptides than Ang II.

CARDIOMYOPATHY IN PHEOCHROMOCYTOMA

A further aspect of pheochromocytoma where there may be important interactions between catecholamines and the RAS is cardiomyopathy. The administration of large doses of various catecholamines, including epinephrine and norepinephrine, to experimental animals produces multifocal ventricular myocardial necrosis; apparently identical cardiac lesions can result also from the administration of Ang II [15,16] (see *Chapter 40*). The catecholamine-induced cardiac lesions can be ameliorated in part by prior administration of α- or β-blockers, and more completely by combined α- and β-blockade [17]. These same cardiomyopathic abnormalities are found both in patients with pheochrome tumors [18,19] and in subjects with very high plasma Ang II concentrations [16]. The recognition of enhanced activity of the RAS in patients with pheochromocytoma raises the possibility that the clinical cardiac lesions may be a consequence of the combined activity of the two biochemical systems.

RENAL ARTERY STENOSIS IN PHEOCHROMOCYTOMA

Although rare, the combination of pheochromocytoma and renal artery stenosis is well known. Hill and colleagues in 1982 described one such patient and noted reports of 36 others [20]. Pheochromocytoma may be associated with renal artery stenosis by several mechanisms including direct compression of the renal artery or one of its branches in the hilum of the kidney [21] (Fig. 67.4); angulation or constriction of the renal artery by fibrous tissue from the tumor; intense vasoconstriction of renal vessels by high circulating levels of catecholamines [20,22]; or the presence of atherosclerotic narrowing of the renal artery [20,23]. Since stenosis or occlusion of a renal artery can stimulate renin release (see *Chapter 55*), this may be an additional mechanism contributing to the level of arterial pressure in the

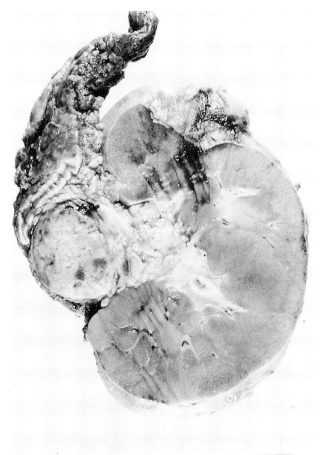

Fig. 67.4 Operation specimen of a left kidney with spherical pheochromocytoma lying in the hilum. The tumor involved the renal arteries; note the scarring at the upper pole of the kidney. The normal left adrenal gland lies above the pheochromocytoma. For details, see [21].

rare patient with both pheochromocytoma and renal artery stenosis.

MALIGNANT HYPERTENSION IN PHEOCHROMOCYTOMA

Malignant hypertension with extreme activation of the RAS has been reported in a patient with pheochromocytoma in the absence of an organic renal vascular lesion [24], and in a patient with both pheochromocytoma and renal artery occlusion [23], although renin levels were not measured in the latter case. Under such unusual circumstances, it is likely that the blood-pressure level is determined in part by the RAS.

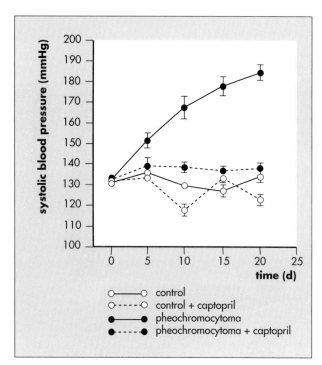

Fig. 67.5 Systolic blood pressures in captopril-treated or untreated rats harboring pheochromocytoma (n=16) and in captopril-treated or untreated implanted control rats (n=16). Systolic blood pressures were significantly elevated in untreated rats with pheochromocytoma at day 10 and later. Results are expressed as mean ± SEM. Modified from Hu Z-W *et al* [26].

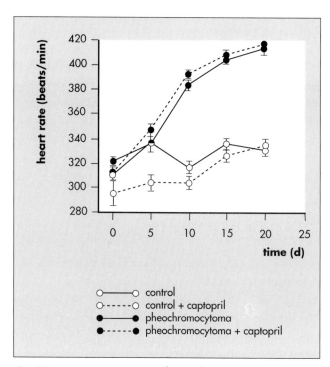

Fig. 67.6 Heart rate in captopril-treated or untreated rats harboring pheochromocytoma and unimplanted control rats. Heart rate increased in rats harboring pheochromocytoma but captopril did not suppress this increase in heart rate. Modified from Hu Z-W *et al* [26].

MECHANISMS OF ACTIVATION OF THE RENIN–ANGIOTENSIN SYSTEM IN PHEOCHROMOCYTOMA

Possible mechanisms whereby the RAS could be activated in patients with pheochromocytoma, and alluded to above, include stimulation by circulating catecholamines of renal adrenoceptors [8,9], and/or catecholamine-mediated renal arterial constriction [20,22]. Further possibilities are severe hypotension, which can follow an attack in which catecholamines are paroxysmally secreted to excess, or postural hypotension [25].

RATS WITH PHEOCHROMOCYTOMA IMPLANTS

Several of these aspects have been explored in rats implanted with pheochromocytoma [26]. In such animals, plasma norepinephrine is markedly elevated, although, in contrast to the various clinical accounts [1–9], PRA was found to be slightly lower than in unimplanted control rats. Rats with implanted pheochromocytoma suffer the typical cardiomyopathic lesions, which can be ameliorated, along with the hypertension, by giving α- and β-adrenoceptor antagonists [26,27]. Hu *et al* [26] further observed that in rats with pheochromocytoma, the ACE inhibitor captopril could both prevent and correct the systemic hypertension (Fig. 67.5) and attenuate the cardiomyopathy, without lowering the very high plasma norepinephrine concentrations or correcting tachycardia (Fig. 67.6). In some respects, the observations and conclusions of Hu *et al* [26] differ from those in the clinical studies of Plouin *et al* [8]. Hu *et al* [26] did not regard the antihypertensive action of captopril in the implanted rats to be due to a fall in circulating Ang II, because PRA was not elevated before treatment. They did, however, consider the possibility that the benefical effects of captopril might reflect inhibition of local renin–angiotensin sytems.

In this regard, competitive Ang II blockers and ACE inhibitors have been shown to reduce arterial pressure in patients with pheochromocytoma [8,28].

CONCLUSIONS

Although there are minor inconsistencies between several of the papers cited herein, and undoubtedly many aspects await clarification, it is evident both clinically and experimentally that there are, in patients or animals with pheochromocytoma, important interactions with the RAS. These interactions appear relevant to the pathogenesis both of hypertension and the cardiomyopathy, as well as to drug therapy in this disease.

REFERENCES

1. Meyer P, Alexandre JM, Devaux C, Leroux-Robert C, Milliez P. Détermination de l'activité rénine plasmatique chez 261 hypertendus. *Presse Medicale* 1966;**40**:2025–30.

2. Maebashi M, Miura Y, Yoshinaga K, Sato K. Plasma renin activity in pheochromocytoma. *Japanese Circulation Journal* 1968;**32**:1427–32.

3. Vetter H, Vetter W, Warnholz C, Bayer JM, Kaser H, Vielhaber K, Kruk F. Renin and aldosterone secretion in pheochromocytoma. *American Journal of Medicine* 1976;**60**:866–71.

4. Ganguly A, Weinberger MH, Grim CE. The renin–angiotensin–aldosterone system in Cushing's syndrome and pheochromocytoma. *Hormone Research* 1983;**17**:1–10.

5. Bravo EL, Tarazi RC, Fouad F, Textor SC, Gifford RW, Vidt DG. Blood pressure regulation in pheochromocytoma. *Hypertension* 1982;**4** (suppl 2):193–9.

6. Hung W, August GP. Hyperreninemia and secondary hyperaldosteronism in pheochromocytoma. *Journal of Pediatrics* 1979;**94**:215–7.

7. Muratani H, Kawasaki T, Kawano Y, Abe I, Kumamoto K, Omae T. Activation of renin–angiotensin system in maintenance of high blood pressure in uncomplicated pheochromocytoma. *Japanese Journal of Medicine* 1983;**22**:227–30.

8. Plouin P-F, Chatellier G, Rougeot M-A, Comoy E, Ménard J, Corvol P. Plasma renin activity in phaeochromocytoma: Effects of beta-blockade and converting enzyme inhibition. *Journal of Hypertension* 1988;**6**:579–85.

9. Richards AM, Nicholls MG, Espiner EA, Ikram H, Hamilton E, Maslowski AH. Arterial pressure and hormone relationships in phaeochromocytoma. *Journal of Hypertension* 1983;**1**:373–9.

10. Naruse M, Sussman CR, Naruse K, Jackson RV, Inagami T. Renin exists in human adrenal tissue. *Journal of Clinical Endocrinology and Metabolism* 1983;**57**:482–7.

11. Fishman MC, Zimmerman EA, Slater EE. Renin and angiotensins: The complete system within the neuroblastoma–glioma cell. *Science* 1981;**214**:921–3.

12. Okamura T, Clemens DL, Inagami T. Renin, angiotensins and angiotensin converting enzyme in neuroblastoma cells: Evidence for intracellular formation of angiotensins. *Proceedings of the National Academy of Sciences of the USA* 1981;**78**:6940–3.

13. Okamura T, Clemens DL, Inagami T. Generation of angiotensins in cultured pheochromocytoma cells. *Neuroscience Letters* 1984;**46**:151–6.

14. Gonzalez-Garcia C, Keiser HR. Angiotensin II and angiotensin converting enzyme binding in human adrenal gland and phaeochromocytomas. *Journal of Hypertension* 1990;**8**:433–41.

15. Rona G. Catecholamine cardiotoxicity. *Journal of Molecular and Cellular Cardiology* 1985;**17**:291–306.

16. Gavras H, Kremer D, Brown JJ, Gray B, Lever AF, MacAdam RF, Medina A, Morton JJ, Robertson JIS. Angiotensin- and norepinephrine-induced myocardial lesions: Experimental and clinical studies in rabbits and man. *American Heart Journal* 1975;**89**:321–32.

17. Van Belle H. *In vivo* effects of inhibitors of adenosine uptake. In: Paton DM, ed. *Adenosine and adenine nucleotides: Physiology and pharmacology*. London: Taylor and Francis 1988:251–8.

18. Kline IK. Myocardial alterations associated with pheochromocytomas. *American Journal of Pathology* 1961;**38**:539–43.

19. Sardesai SH, Mourant AJ, Sivathandon Y, Farrow R, Gibbons DO. Phaeochromocytoma and catecholamine-induced cardiomyopathy presenting as heart failure. *British Heart Journal* 1990;**63**:234–7.

20. Hill FS, Jander HP, Murad T, Diethelm AG. The coexistence of renal artery stenosis and pheochromocytoma. *Annals of Surgery* 1983;**197**:484–90.

21. Agabiti-Rosei E, Brown JJ, Lever AF, Robertson AS, Robertson JIS, Trust PM. Treatment of phaeochromocytoma and of clonidine withdrawal hypertension with labetalol. *British Journal of Clinical Pharmacology* 1976;**3** (suppl 3):809–15.

22. Brewster DC, Jensen SR, Novelline RA. Reversible renal artery stenosis with pheochromocytoma. *Journal of the American Medical Association* 1982;**248**:1094–6.

23. Stern Z, Gross DJ, Cotev S, Eliakim M. Coexistence of pheochromocytoma and renal artery occlusion in a patient with malignant hypertension. *Israel Journal of Medical Science* 1981;**17**:372–4.

24. Harrison TS, Birbari A, Seaton JF. Malignant hypertension in pheochromocytoma: Correlation with plasma renin activity. *Johns Hopkins Medical Journal* 1972;**130**:329–32.

25. Ball SG. Pheochromocytoma. In: Robertson JIS, ed. *Handbook of hypertension, volume 2: Clinical aspects of secondary hypertension*. Amsterdam: Elsevier, 1983: 238–75.

26. Hu Z-W, Billingham M, Tuck M, Hoffman BB. Captopril improves hypertension and cardiomyopathy in rats with pheochromocytoma. *Hypertension* 1990;**15**:210–5.

27. Hoffman BB. Observations in New England Deaconess Hospital rats harboring pheochromocytoma. *Clinical and Investigative Medicine* 1987;**10**:555–60.

28. van Hoogdalem P, Donker AJM, Brentjens JRH, van der Hem GK, Oosterhuis JW. Partial correlation of hypertension by angiotensin II blockade in a patient with phaeochromocytoma. *Acta Medica Scandinavica* 1977;**201**:395–9.

68 THE RENIN–ANGIOTENSIN SYSTEM IN ADRENAL INSUFFICIENCY

JAN R STOCKIGT

INTRODUCTION

A relationship between the RAS and adrenal insufficiency had already been established long before Ang II was recognized as an adrenotrophic hormone. In 1942, Houssay *et al* [1] and Lewis and Goldblatt [2] showed that angiotensinogen ('preangiotonin') became depleted in dogs 48 hours after adrenalectomy, resulting in a reduced pressor response to exogenous renin, without alteration in the response to Ang II [1,2]. The importance of these findings, which suggested a key influence of adrenocortical hormones on angiotensinogen, tended to be forgotten after the feedback relationship between aldosterone and Ang II became the major focus of attention.

The suggestion by Gross in 1958 [3], that renin was elevated after adrenalectomy, was one of the vital clues which related the RAS to the control of aldosterone secretion. When renin assays became established in the 1960s, it was shown that the negative sodium balance associated with spontaneous or experimental adrenocortical insufficiency was associated with markedly increased plasma renin and that plasma renin fell when corticosteroids were replaced [4–6]. It is notable that these reports were of plasma renin concentration (PRC) rather than plasma renin activity (PRA), so that the influence of changes in angiotensinogen deficiency would not have been detected. Some later papers have identified divergent changes amongst PRC, PRA, and Ang II in adrenal insufficiency, discrepancies which reflect the role of glucocorticoids in preventing angiotensinogen depletion in the face of renin excess.

This chapter focuses on the effects of adrenocortical hormone deficiency on various components of the RAS, as well as the importance of this system in circulatory homeostasis when adrenal corticosteroid production fails. The value of renin measurement in assessing optimal replacement therapy is also considered.

EFFECTS OF ADRENOCORTICAL INSUFFICIENCY

RENIN

Before clinically reliable renin assays had been developed, it was already known that hypertrophy and hyperplasia of the juxtaglomerular apparatus occurred in experimental adrenocortical insufficiency and that these changes could be prevented with mineralocorticoid [7]. Marked hypertrophy and hyperplasia of the juxtaglomerular apparatus was reported in 1968 in 15 fatal cases of Addison's disease (see Color Plate 30) [8]. Gross *et al* [5] found that experimental adrenal insufficiency in rats was associated with a marked increase in both plasma renin and renal renin content. From the 1960s, when assays became widely available, it was shown that circulating renin excess occurred in both experimental and clinical adrenal failure [4–6,9]. The detailed findings depend on whether PRA or PRC was measured (see below).

Also relevant is that adrenocorticotropic hormone (ACTH) may directly stimulate renin release in normal subjects, even in the face of sodium retention [10] (see *Chapter 34*). The effect is not due to higher levels of angiotensinogen [10] or to changes in the ratio of active to inactive renin [11].

The presence or absence of the adrenal medulla may also influence renin responses in adrenal insufficiency. Peytremann *et al* [12] noted a lack of the normal renin response to intracellular hypoglycemia induced by 2-deoxyglucose in Addison's disease of tuberculous origin. Surprisingly, it has not been established whether there is a difference in the renin response to stimuli such as upright posture and volume depletion, between subjects with idiopathic Addison's disease and those with total adrenal destruction, or after bilateral adrenalectomy.

ANGIOTENSINOGEN

Reid *et al* [9] showed that adrenalectomy in dogs was associated with a marked decrease in plasma angiotensinogen in the face of marked excess in PRC; the increase in PRA was less marked. Angiotensinogen was restored by the administration of dexamethasone but not by aldosterone (Fig. 68.1).

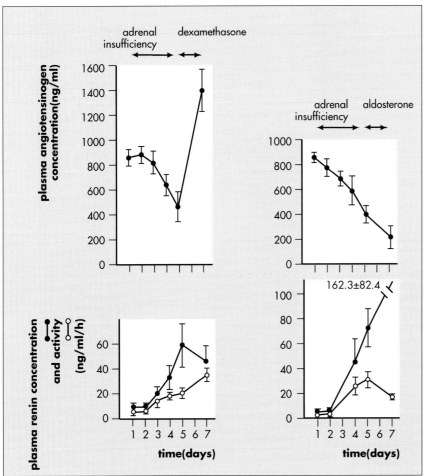

Fig 68.1 Effect of adrenal insufficiency on plasma angiotensinogen, plasma renin activity, and renin concentration (mean ± SEM) in dogs, showing the contrasting effects of dexamethasone and aldosterone replacement. Modified from Reid IA *et al* [9].

In most states of marked renin excess, there is usually no tendency for angiotensinogen to become depleted in the face of high plasma renin levels. Increased hepatic production of angiotensinogen occurs in response to circulating Ang II [13,14], but this response fails in the absence of normal glucocorticoid levels [15], thereby allowing the plasma level of angiotensinogen to run down as a result of increased utilization. It is notable that depletion of angiotensinogen has also been reported during long-term administration of converting-enzyme inhibitors [16], an effect attributed by some, but not all, workers (*Chapter 23*) to failure of positive feedback of Ang II on angiotensinogen secretion [16].

In man, glucocorticoid excess can elevate angiotensinogen [17], but the crucial hepatic response to Ang II which prevents substrate depletion in high renin states appears to be glucocorticoid dependent (that is, a permissive effect), rather than directly glucocorticoid mediated [15]. In contrast to the glucocorticoid dependence of increased substrate production in high renin states, the response to estrogens in rats appears to be independent of glucocorticoids [18].

Angiotensinogen levels are reported to increase in response to glucocorticoid excess, either endogenous in Cushing's syndrome, or exogenous, but the aldosterone excess of Conn's syndrome does not produce this effect [17]. Further details are given in *Chapter 8*.

ANGIOTENSIN-CONVERTING ENZYME

Several observations indicate that ACE may be influenced by adrenocortical hormones, although the physiological importance of these changes remains uncertain (see also *Chapters 10* and *16*). Mendelsohn *et al* [19] demonstrated that dexamethasone increased cell ACE content in cultured bovine endothelial cells and rat lung cells. Furthermore, glucocorticoids, but not mineralocorticoids, reversed the subnormal pulmonary ACE content found in adrenalectomized rats, although serum ACE did not change [19]. In contrast, increased serum ACE levels that returned to normal with replacement therapy, have been reported in patients with untreated adrenal insufficiency [20].

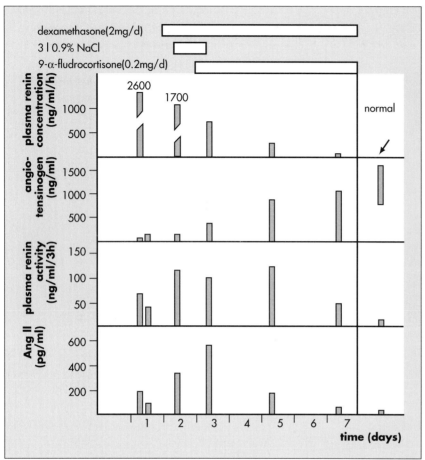

Fig. 68.2 Effect of treatment of a patient with severe adrenocortical failure on plasma renin concentration (PRC), angiotensinogen, renin activity, and circulating Ang II. Urinary aldosterone excretion was <1μg/24h on days 2, 3, and 4, and plasma cortisol was unresponsive to adrenocorticotrophic hormone on days 1 and 3. The normal range for PRC is 4–12ng/ml/h. Modified from Stockigt JR *et al* [21].

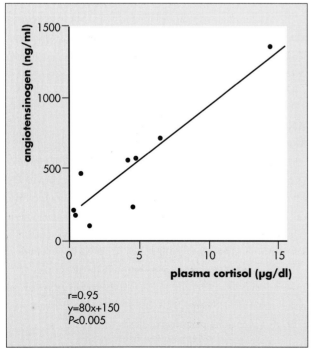

Fig. 68.3 Relationship between pretreatment values of plasma cortisol and angiotensinogen in patients with untreated Addison's disease. Modified from Stockigt JR *et al* [21].

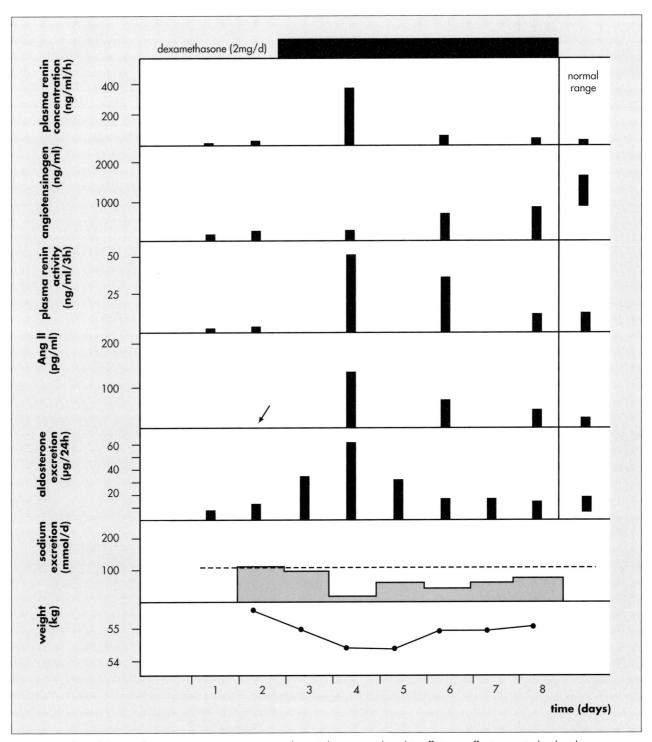

Fig. 68.4 Effect of dexamethasone treatment in a patient with partial primary adrenal insufficiency affecting cortisol rather than aldosterone production. Dexamethasone treatment was associated with water diuresis and weight loss with increase in renin, Ang II, and aldosterone, followed by eventual return of angiotensinogen to normal. In response to six hours of adrenocorticotropic hormone infusion, plasma cortisol remained below 2.5μg/dl (70nmol/l). Modified from Stockigt JR *et al* [21].

DISSOCIATION BETWEEN GLUCOCORTICOID AND MINERALOCORTICOID EFFECTS

In a study of PRC, PRA, and angiotensinogen in patients with newly diagnosed, untreated Addison's disease, who showed varying degrees of aldosterone and cortisol deficiency, Stockigt *et al* [21], showed that there was dissociation between the effects of lack of glucocorticoid and lack of mineralocorticoid. Severe untreated adrenocortical failure, affecting both aldosterone and cortisol, resulted in renin substrate levels falling to less than 10% of mean normal values (Fig. 68.2), associated with gross increase in PRC. Note that the method for the measurement of PRC used here [22] and in the earlier studies of experimental adrenal insufficiency [9] omits the preliminary plasma acidification step previously used to inactivate endogenous angiotensinases and angiotensinogen [23]; acidification was later also shown to activate prorenin [24]. Hence, the difference between PRC and PRA in these studies does not reflect an imbalance between prorenin and active renin [25] (*Chapters* 6 and 7).

When angiotensinogen depletion was severe, renin excess was reflected poorly by measurements of PRA or Ang II. Angiotensinogen deficiency is related closely to the extent of cortisol deficiency (Fig. 68.3). In contrast, severe glucocorticoid deficiency, with preservation of normal aldosterone secretion, resulted in very low angiotensinogen levels without renin excess, suggesting that severe substrate depletion can occur without excessive utilization (Fig. 68.4). With marked renin excess in predominant mineralocorticoid deficiency and in untreated diabetic ketoacidosis, angiotensinogen remained normal, indicating that renin excess *per se* does not lead to depletion of its substrate. These findings suggest that while mineralocorticoid failure stimulates renin release, adequate glucocorticoid production is crucial in preventing angiotensinogen depletion. These distinct effects of adrenocortical failure are summarized in Fig. 68.5.

There are several reports of apparent hyporeninemic hypoaldosteronism (based on measurements of PRA) in patients with hypopituitarism or isolated corticotrophin deficiency [26–28]. In some instances, hyporeninemia was reversed by glucocorticoid replacement alone [26,27]. This sequence remains unexplained, but correction of glucocorticoid deficiency could, by restoring angiotensinogen levels towards normal, lead to reversal of low PRA. It is not yet established whether there is dissociation between PRA and PRC before glucocorticoid replacement in such instances of hypopituitarism.

ROLE OF THE RENIN–ANGIOTENSIN SYSTEM IN CIRCULATORY HOMEOSTASIS IN ADRENAL INSUFFICIENCY

The competitive antagonist, 1-sarcosine, 8-glycine Ang II, has been used to assess the importance of Ang II in maintaining circulatory homeostasis in dogs with experimental adrenal insufficiency [29]. After 5 days' withdrawal of either mineralocorticoid or glucocorticoid replacement, the increase in basal PRA and the hypotensive response to the Ang II antagonist were greater in mineralocorticoid than in glucocorticoid deficiency [29] (Fig. 68.6). Since PRC and angiotensinogen were not assessed separately, the effect of glucocorticoid deficiency may have been underestimated after only five days of glucocorticoid withdrawal, as the half-life of angiotensinogen in dogs has been estimated to be 2–4 days [9]. In man, the dependence of blood pressure in untreated Addison's disease on Ang II has also been confirmed by infusion of a competitive antagonist [30].

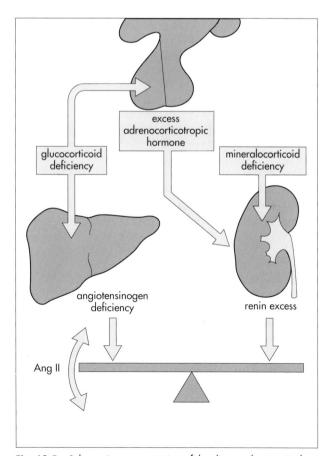

Fig. 68.5 Schematic representation of the diverse changes in the RAS in adrenocortical failure.

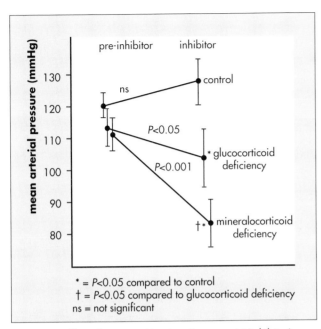

Fig. 68.6 Effect of a competitive Ang II antagonist (inhibitor) on mean arterial blood pressure in adrenalectomized dogs after withdrawal of glucocorticoid or mineralocorticoid replacement. Data are mean ± SEM. Modified from Berns AS *et al* [29].

One may speculate that the angiotensinogen depletion of severe glucocorticoid deficiency is an important factor in the circulatory collapse of very severe untreated adrenocortical failure. With increasing severity of sodium depletion and increasing dependence of blood pressure on circulating Ang II [31], the failure of Ang II production, due to angiotensinogen deficiency, may ultimately be catastrophic.

MONITORING OF ADRENAL REPLACEMENT THERAPY

Measurement of PRA has become well established in monitoring the effectiveness of long-term adrenocortical replacement, particularly when hypertension, cardiac failure, or renal insufficiency co-exist with deficiency of adrenocortical hormones, and in congenital adrenal hyperplasia where suppression of ACTH-dependent adrenal androgen excess is required with the minimum dose of glucocorticoid.

In congenital adrenal hyperplasia, whether associated with an obvious clinical problem of sodium chloride loss or not, there is now good evidence that adequate mineralocorticoid replacement, precisely monitored by measurement of PRA, can improve growth rate and reduce the requirement for glucocorticoid [32,33].

Measurement of PRA rather than of ACTH appears to be preferable as an index of replacement, because the latter may show wide fluctuations, depending on the time interval between glucocorticoid dosage and blood sampling [34].

Oelkers and L'age [35] studied the effects of treatment with various combinations of glucocorticoid and mineralocorticoid in seven patients with established Addison's disease on a free diet. Each regimen was given for two weeks. On dexamethasone, 2mg/d only, PRA was markedly elevated, with progressive reduction as mineralocorticoid was added (Fig. 68.7). Angiotensin II levels correlated closely with PRA in this study.

It remains controversial whether plasma renin should routinely be returned completely to normal in treating Addison's disease. It is of interest to reflect that in the first report of elevated plasma renin in Addison's disease [4], steroid replacement that was judged on clinical grounds to be adequate lowered PRC substantially, but not to within the normal range. On the basis of a study in which fludrocortisone, 0.05–0.1mg/d was first withdrawn and then resumed at a higher than usual dose (0.3mg/d) in adults with Addison's disease, Smith *et al* [36] have inferred that the standard dose of fludrocortisone is probably less than optimal in many patients, even for a sodium intake of approximately 150mmol/d. They demonstrated normalization of PRA, associated with increased wellbeing with higher doses. The follow-up period of three months in the study was, however, too short for the beneficial effects of sodium retention to be balanced against possible long-term adverse effects on blood pressure. In this context, it should be noted that Wenting *et al* [37] demonstrated that fludrocortisone, 0.5mg/d, increased the mean blood pressure of dexamethasone-treated subjects with adrenal insufficiency by approximately 10mmHg after 6–9 weeks. Jadoul *et al* [38] have argued against routinely using doses of fludrocortisone which completely normalize PRA because of the adverse effect of this drug on blood pressure.

Oelkers & Bähr studied the effect of fludrocortisone withdrawal in eight hydrocortisone-treated patients with established Addison's disease [39]. Within a week, PRA and Ang II levels had increased 2- to 3-fold; these changes were reversed by adding 120mmol sodium chloride/d to the normal diet. It was notable that in some patients, plasma potassium increased by up to 2.5mmol/l during the period of mineralocorticoid deficiency, without an increase in circulating Ang II, suggesting that both potassium and renin should be monitored when inadequate adrenocortical replacement is suspected.

Assessment of adrenocortical replacement with measurements of PRA is especially indicated where compliance is in doubt, or where other medications may alter replacement needs.

Lithium [40] has been shown to increase mineralocorticoid replacement requirements, while 2,2-bis(2-chlorophenyl-4-chlorophenyl)-1,1-dichloroethane (o,p'-DDD) increases the clearance of numerous corticoids [41]. An increased dose of fludrocortisone may be needed with both of these drugs. It should be noted that the use of nonsteroidal anti-inflammatory agents, together with fludrocortisone, may aggravate fluid retention and any tendency to hypertension [42].

If PRA is used to monitor adrenal replacement in pregnancy [43] or during oral-contraceptive use, results need to be compared with the appropriate reference ranges. Normal values are certainly higher in pregnancy, but some results suggest that there is no consistent rise during oral contraceptive use [44] (see also *Chapter 53*). If active renin is measured in the presence of excess substrate (PRC), reference values are higher in pregnancy, but may be lower during oral-contraceptive use [44]. Methods that allow activation

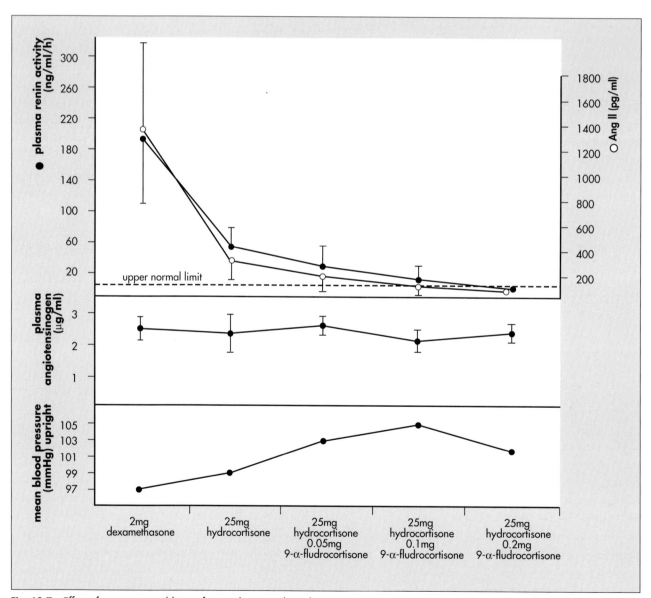

Fig. 68.7 Effect of progressive addition of mineralocorticoid on plasma renin activity, Ang II, angiotensinogen, and mean blood pressure in seven patients with established Addison's disease. Each regimen was given for two weeks on a free diet. Data are mean ± SEM. Modified from Oelkers W and L'age M [35].

of prorenin by acid or trypsin [24], will show extremely high values in normal pregnancy [44] (*Chapters* 7 and 50).

Where heart failure develops in a patient with adrenal insufficiency, assessment of the need for diuretics poses a difficult problem. Firm therapeutic guidelines are lacking, but monitoring of PRA may be valuable in achieving a balance between volume overload and depletion. The value of renin measurement is of course lost if ACE inhibitors are used.

Due to the divergent effects of glucocorticoid and mineralocorticoid deficiency [9,21], no single measurement can give an adequate assessment of the RAS in adrenocortical failure. Plasma renin concentration may not reflect concurrent Ang II levels; conversely, PRA and Ang II levels may underestimate renal renin secretion in the face of substrate deficiency. The extent of this divergence will depend on the duration of *in vitro* incubation in each assay for PRA and also on the degree of renin excess. The higher the PRC and the longer the incubation, the greater the discrepancy. Nevertheless, measurement of PRA generally correlates well with circulating Ang II and gives a useful index of physiologically appropriate mineralocorticoid activity.

REFERENCES

1. Houssay BA, Dexter L. The sensitivity to hypertensin, adrenalin and renin of unanesthetized normal adrenalectomized, hypophysectomized and nephrectomized dogs. *Annals of Internal Medicine* 1942;17:451–60.

2. Lewis HA, Goldblatt H. Studies on experimental hypertension XVIII. Experimental observations on the humoral mechanism of hypertension. *The Bulletin of the New York Academy of Medicine* 1942;18:459–87.

3. Gross F. Renin und Hypertensin, physiologische oder pathologische Wirkstoffe? *Klinische Wochenschrift* 1958;36:693–706.

4. Brown JJ, Davies DL, Lever AF, Robertson JIS. Variations in plasma renin concentration in several physiological and pathological states. *Canadian Medical Association Journal* 1964;90:201–6.

5. Gross F, Brunner H, Ziegler M. Renin–angiotensin system, aldosterone, and sodium balance. *Recent Progress in Hormone Research* 1965;21:119–77.

6. Brown JJ, Fraser R, Lever AF, Robertson JIS, James VHT, McCusker J, Wynn V. Renin, angiotensin, corticosteroids, and electrolyte balance in Addison's disease. *Quarterly Journal of Medicine* 1968;145:97–118.

7. Dunihue FW. The effect of adrenal insufficiency and of desoxycorticosterone acetate on the juxtaglomerular apparatus. *American Association of Anatomists* 1949;103:442–3.

8. Alexander F. The juxtaglomerular apparatus in Addison's disease. *Journal of Pathology and Bacteriology* 1968;96:27–32.

9. Reid IA, Tu WH, Otsuka K, Assaykeen TA, Ganong WF. Studies concerning the regulation and importance of plasma angiotensinogen concentration in the dog. *Endocrinology* 1973;93:107–14.

10. Oelkers W, Köhler A, Belkien L, Fuchs–Hammoser R, Maiga M, Scherer B, Weber PC. Studies on the mechanism by which ACTH stimulates renin activity and angiotensin II formation in man. *Acta Endocrinologica* 1982;100:573–80.

11. Belkien L, Exner P, Oelkers W. Active and inactive renin in primary and secondary adrenal insufficiency and during ACTH infusion. *Acta Endocrinologica* 1983;102:265–70.

12. Peytremann A, Favre L, Vallotton MB. Effect of cold pressure test and 2-deoxy-D-glucose infusion on plasma renin activity in man. *European Journal of Clinical Investigation* 1972;2:432–8.

13. Khayyall M, MacGregor J, Brown JJ, Lever AF, Robertson JIS. Increase of plasma renin-substrate concentration after infusion of angiotensin in the rat. *Clinical Science* 1973;44:87–90.

14. Beaty III O, Sloop CH, Schmid Jr HE, Buckalew Jr VM. Renin response and angiotensinogen control during graded hemorrhage and shock in the dog. *American Journal of Physiology* 1976;231:1300–7.

15. Reid IA. Effect of angiotensin II and glucocorticoids on plasma angiotensinogen concentration in the dog. *American Journal of Physiology* 1977;232:E234–6.

16. Rasmussen S, Damkjaer Nielsen M, Giese J. Captopril combined with thiazide lowers renin substrate concentration: Implications for methodology in renin assays. *Clinical Science* 1981;60:591–3.

17. Krakoff LR. Measurement of plasma renin substrate by radioimmunoassay of angiotensin I: Concentration in syndromes associated with steroid excess. *Journal of Clinical Endocrinology and Metabolism* 1973;37:110–7.

18. Krakoff LR, Eisenfeld AJ. Hormonal control of plasma renin substrate (angiotensinogen). *Circulation Research* 1977;41(suppl II):II-43–8.

19. Mendelsohn FAO, Lloyd CJ, Kachel C, Funder JW. Induction by glucocorticoids of angiotensin converting enzyme production from bovine endothelial cells in culture and rat lung *in vivo*. *Journal of Clinical Investigation* 1982;70:684–92.

20. Falezza G, Santonastaso CL, Parisi T, Muggeo M. High serum levels of angiotensin-converting enzyme in untreated Addison's disease. *Journal of Clinical Endocrinology and Metabolism* 1985;61:496–8.

21. Stockigt JR, Hewett MJ, Topliss DJ, Higgs EJ, Taft P. Renin and renin substrate in primary adrenal insufficiency. Contrasting effects of glucocorticoid and mineralocorticoid deficiency. *American Journal of Medicine* 1979;66:915–22.

22. Stockigt JR, Collins RD, Biglieri EG. Determination of plasma renin concentration by angiotensin I immunoassay. *Circulation Research* 1971;28 & 29(suppl II):II-175–89.

23. Skinner SL. Improved assay methods for renin 'concentration' and 'activity' in human plasma. *Circulation Research* 1967;20:391–402.

24. Hsueh WA, Luetscher JA, Carlson EJ, Grislis G. Inactive renin of high molecular weight (big renin) in normal human plasma. *Hypertension* 1980;2:750–6.

25. Franken AAM, Derkx FHM, Man in't Veld AJ, Hop WCJ, van Rens GH, Peperkamp E, de Jong PTVM, Schalekamp MADH. High plasma prorenin in diabetes mellitus and its correlation with some complications. *Journal of Clinical Endocrinology and Metabolism* 1990;71:1008–15.

26. Major P, Kuchel O, Boucher R, Nowaczynski W, Genest J. Selective hypopituitarism with severe hyponatremia and secondary hyporeninism. *Journal of Clinical Endocrinology and Metabolism* 1978;46:15–9.

27. Merriam GR, Baer L. Adrenocorticotropin deficiency: Correction of hyponatremia and hypoaldosteronism with chronic glucocorticoid therapy. *Journal of Clinical Endocrinology and Metabolism* 1980;50:10–4.

28. Manser TJ, Estep H. Pseudo-Addison's disease. Isolated corticotropin deficiency associated with hyporeninemic hypoaldosteronism. *Archives of Internal Medicine* 1986;146:996–7.

29. Berns AS, Pluss RG, Erickson AL, Anderson RJ, McDonald KM, Schrier RW. Renin–angiotensin system and cardiovascular homeostasis in adrenal insufficiency. *American Journal of Physiology* 1977;233:F509–13.

30. Ogihara T, Hata T, Nakamaru M, Mikami H, Maruyama A, Oakada Y, Kumahara Y. Decreased blood pressure in response to an angiotensin II antagonist in Addison's disease. *Clinical Endocrinology* 1979;10:377–81.

31. Sancho J, Re R, Burton J, Barger AC, Haber E. The role of the renin–angiotensin–aldosterone system in cardiovascular homeostasis in normal human subjects. *Circulation* 1976;53:400–5.

32. Kuhnle U, Rösler A, Pareira JA, Gunzcler P, Levine LS, New MI. The effects of long-term normalization of sodium balance on linear growth in disorders with aldosterone deficiency. *Acta Endocrinologica* 1983;102:577–82.

33. Rösler A, Levine LS, Schneider B, Novogroder M, New MI. The interrelationship of sodium balance, plasma renin activity and ACTH in congenital adrenal hyperplasia. *Journal of Clinical Endocrinology and Metabolism* 1977;45:500–12.

34. Khalid BAK, Burke CW, Hurley DM, Funder JW, Stockigt JR. Steroid replacement in Addison's disease and in subjects adrenalectomized for Cushing's disease: Comparison of various glucocorticoids. *Journal of Clinical Endocrinology and Metabolism* 1982;55:551–9.

35. Oelkers W, L'age M. Control of mineralocorticoid substitution in Addison's disease by plasma renin measurement. *Klinische Wochenschrift* 1976;54:607–12.

36. Smith SJ, MacGregor GA, Markandu ND, Bayliss J, Banks RA, Prentice MG, Dorrington–Ward P, Wise P. Evidence that patients with Addison's disease are undertreated with fludrocortisone. *Lancet* 1984;i:11–4.

37. Wenting GJ, Man in't Veld AJ, Schalekamp M. Time course of vascular resistance changes in mineralocorticoid hypertension in man. *Clinical Science* 1981;61 (suppl):97–100.

38. Jadoul M, Ferrant A, De Plaen JF, Crabbé J. Mineralocorticoids in the management of primary adrenocortical insufficiency. *Journal of Endocrinological Investigation* 1991;14:87–91.

39. Oelkers W, Bähr V. Effects of fludrocortisone withdrawal on plasma angiotensin II, ACTH, vasopressin, and potassium in patients with Addison's disease. *Acta Endocrinologica* 1987;115:325–30.

40. Stewart PM, Grieve J, Nairn IM, Padfield PL, Edwards CRW. Lithium inhibits the action of fludrocortisone on the kidney. *Clinical Endocrinology* 1987;27:63–8.

41. Robinson BG, Hales IB, Henniker AJ, Ho K, Luttrell BM, Smee IR, Stiel JN. The effect of o,p'-DDD on adrenal steroid replacement therapy requirements. *Clinical Endocrinology* 1987;27:437–44.

42. Martin K, Zipser R, Horton R. Effect of prostaglandin inhibition on the hypertensive action of sodium-retaining steroids. *Hypertension* 1981;3:622–8.

43. Symonds EM, Craven DJ. Plasma renin and aldosterone in pregnancy complicated by adrenal insufficiency. *British Journal of Obstetrics and Gynaecology* 1977;84:191–6.

44. Derkx FHM, Stuenkel C, Schalekamp MPA, Visser W, Huisveld IH, Schalekamp MADH. Immunoreactive renin, prorenin, and enzymatically active renin in plasma during pregnancy and in women taking oral contraceptives. *Journal of Clinical Endocrinology and Metabolism* 1986;63:1008–15.

69 HYPERRENINEMIC SELECTIVE HYPOALDOSTERONISM

GERHARD H SCHOLZ AND JAN R STOCKIGT

The combination of renin excess and aldosterone deficiency occurs most commonly as an appropriate physiologic response to impaired production of aldosterone, due either to a biosynthetic defect or to adrenal destruction. The common forms of adrenocortical insufficiency, and especially Addison's disease, are described in detail in *Chapter 68*. Features of selective aldosterone deficiency, such as hyperkalemia and metabolic acidosis, and a tendency towards sodium loss and volume depletion, are usually present in most of the causes of hyperreninemic hypoaldosteronism which are listed in Fig. 69.1. Of the conditions shown in Fig. 69.1, those that are clearly understood from the physiologic, if not the molecular point of view, are not considered in detail here.

This brief review focuses on reports of selective aldosterone deficiency (usually associated with marked cortisol excess) which appears to be due to acquired transient failure of the adrenal zona glomerulosa to respond to Ang II [1–3]. In contrast to the other types of hypoaldosteronism, clinical and biochemical features of mineralocorticoid deficiency are usually absent. This recently recognized entity is of particular interest because it may demonstrate how the aldosterone response to trophic influences can be modified by acute or chronic disease. Most cases have been reported during critical illness and appear to be distinct from those with aldosterone deficiency and hyperreninemia as a stage of progressive autoimmune adrenocortical failure [4], adrenal replacement, infiltration, or destruction [5–7].

Pseudohypoaldosteronism, type 1 [8], in which aldosterone receptors are defective or absent, is included in the classification shown in Fig. 69.1; in this condition features of aldosterone deficiency are most marked in infancy, and are associated with excess circulating renin and aldosterone.

The definition of hyperreninemia depends on the method used to assess the state of the renin–angiotensin axis (see *Chapters 13* and *15*); for example, renin concentration will be high, but renin activity may not show an equivalent increase if angiotensinogen is depleted, as in marked glucocorticoid deficiency [9] or during chronic treatment with ACE inhibitors [10]. In the face of acute inhibition or deficiency of converting enzyme, high renin concentration and activity will not be reflected by the level of circulating Ang II [11], although circulating Ang II levels may sometimes be close to normal during chronic treatment with ACE inhibitors [12].

Deficiency of angiotensinogen
    converting-enzyme inhibition [10]
    hereditary? [38]
    severe glucocorticoid deficiency [9]

Inhibition or deficiency of converting enzyme
    pharmacologic [11]
    endogenous inhibitors? [14]
    plasma exchange [33]
    hypoxia [34]
    sepsis [35]

Impaired adrenal stimulation
    interleukin I, tumor necrosis factor [29,30]
    adrenocorticotropic hormone excess [27]
    pharmacological
        heparin [19], chlorbutol [22],
        cyclosporin A [20], dopamine [21]
    atrial natriuretic factor [39]
    other effects of critical illness [?]

Biosynthetic defects
    21-hydroxylase deficiency
    corticosterone methyl-oxidase deficiency, types I and II

Adrenal destruction (partial)

Defective aldosterone action (receptor defect)
    pseudohypoaldosteronism, type I [8]

Fig. 69.1 Classification of selective hyperreninemic hypoaldosteronism

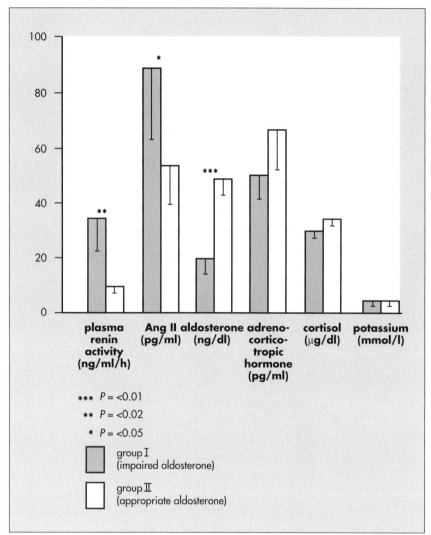

Fig. 69.2 Data from 59 critically ill patients classified according to the ratio of plasma aldosterone to plasma renin activity (group I <2, group II >2). Aldosterone was lower in group I, despite much higher levels of both renin activity and Ang II. Cortisol was markedly increased in both groups. Reference normal ranges were renin activity <3ng/ml/h, Ang II <18pg/ml, plasma aldosterone 5–15ng/dl, adrenocorticotropic hormone 20–80pg/ml, and cortisol 5–18μg/dl. Reference ranges are as given in reference [14]. Modified from Findling JW et al [3].

THE CLINICAL ENTITY

In 1981, Zipser et al [1] found hyperreninemic hypoaldosteronism in 18 of 28 severely ill hypotensive, normokalemic patients under intensive care, in whom plasma renin activity, cortisol, and 18-hydroxycorticosterone (18OHB) were elevated; paradoxically, aldosterone levels were low and showed little response to exogenous adrenocorticotropic hormone (ACTH) and Ang II. Increased aldosterone clearance and suppression by exogenous dopamine were ruled out. Plasma ACE activity was slightly reduced; Ang II was not directly measured. Ten years later, the pathogenesis of this condition remains uncertain.

Davenport and Zipser [2] and Findling et al [3] subsequently reported similar findings in approximately 20% of critically ill patients and showed that the abnormally low ratio of aldosterone to renin activity could revert to normal after recovery. As shown in Fig. 69.2, aldosterone was markedly reduced in relation to renin activity and circulating Ang II [3], usually in association with marked cortisol excess [1–3]. In patients who died, there was no consistent evidence of adrenocortical ischemia or infarction at necropsy. Stern et al [13] found that basal corticosterone and 18OHB levels were lower in eight patients with hyperreninemic hypoaldosteronism than in other patients under intensive care with comparable renin excess but without hypoaldosteronism. In response to a single pharmacological dose of synthetic 1–24-α-ACTH, the mean values for 18OHB, corticosterone, and cortisol were 6%, 28%, and 95%, respectively, of the values found in critically ill patients without impairment of aldosterone synthesis. On the basis of this impaired corticosterone response to ACTH, the authors inferred the presence of a generalized defect of zona glomerulosa function affecting both early and late steps in aldosterone biosynthesis.

Detailed reports of single cases that apparently correspond to this entity have shown diverse findings, variously suggestive of an endogenous inhibitor of Ang II production or inhibition of aldosterone secretion. Suggested causes include atrial natriuretic factor [14], a generalized defect in zona glomerulosa function [15], an acquired defect of corticosterone methyloxidase, type II [16], or a dual defect in both aldosterone production and renal tubular responsiveness to exogenous mineralocorticoids [17,18]. At present, it is not possible to reconcile these reports with a single causal abnormality.

EFFECT OF MEDICATIONS

Medications must be included amongst the factors that could contribute to the pathogenesis of this syndrome. Those that can selectively impair the aldosterone response to Ang II include heparin [19], cyclosporin A [20], and dopamine [21]. It is of interest to note that the preservative chlorbutol, which is included in many parenteral drug formulations, has been shown to have a selective inhibitory effect on both basal and Ang II-stimulated aldosterone production by isolated bovine zona glomerulosa cells [22]. The possible blocking effects of such preservatives, amongst the multiple medications given to critically ill patients, have not yet been thoroughly evaluated.

Apart from these medications, speculations on the pathogenesis of this disorder include the influence of stress-induced ACTH excess; an effect of cytokines on zona glomerulosa function; and the effects of hypoxia, sepsis, or plasma exchange on ACE. Such mechanisms are not mutually exclusive when associated with critical illness.

EXCESS OF ADRENOCORTICOTROPIC HORMONE

It is well known that chronic high doses of ACTH may impair aldosterone synthesis [23,24], the fall in aldosterone often being most marked after cessation of high-dose exogenous ACTH [23]. Prolonged ACTH administration to rats decreases the number of Ang II receptors in zona glomerulosa cell suspensions [25] and prolonged administration of ACTH to sheep causes cell separation and disruption of cords in the zona glomerulosa [26]. Braley *et al* demonstrated that treatment of bovine zona glomerulosa cells

with high-dose ACTH inhibited their subsequent aldosterone response to Ang II but augmented the cortisol response to ACTH [27]. These authors suggested that the chronic ACTH excess of critical illness may induce 17-α-hydroxylase activity in the zona glomerulosa, with a shift in steroid production from aldosterone to cortisol, thus inducing the changes of hyperreninemic hypoaldosteronism. Although it remains uncertain whether endogenous ACTH levels during critical illness are sufficiently high to exert an inhibitory effect on aldosterone production, this hypothesis merits further detailed study.

CYTOKINES

The possible role of interleukin 1 (IL-1) and tumor necrosis factor (TNF) in the pathogenesis of hyperreninemic hypoaldosteronism has recently been the subject of speculation. During activation of the immune system, and in severe infection, these cytokines activate the pituitary–adrenal axis and stimulate renal renin release [28]. In contrast, both of these compounds exert a dose-dependent inhibitory effect on Ang II-induced aldosterone synthesis by isolated rat adrenal zona glomerulosa cells [29]; an inhibitory effect was seen with picomolar concentrations of recombinant IL-1β [29]. It has been suggested that such effects could reproduce the changes of hyperreninemic hypoaldosteronism.

LIPOXYGENASE PRODUCTS

In several studies by Natarajan *et al* [29] and Stern *et al* [30], a possible relationship has been postulated between selective aldosterone deficiency and alterations in intra-adrenal arachidonic-acid metabolism. In rat zona glomerulosa cells, the 12-lipoxygenase product, 12-hydroxyeicosatetraenoic acid (12-HETE), reversed the TNF-induced blockade of Ang II-induced stimulation of aldosterone production [29]. The production of 12-HETE was inhibited by the 5-lipoxygenase product, 5-HETE [30], which can originate either from neutrophils [31] or from the adrenal zona fasiculata after ACTH stimulation [32]. These studies suggest the possibility that the intra-adrenal 5-lipoxygenase and 12-lipoxygenase pathways may exert inverse modulatory effects on adrenal zona glomerulosa responsiveness to Ang II, but it remains to be established whether these interactions are relevant to the pathogenesis of hyperreninemic hypoaldosteronism.

OTHER FACTORS

The studies of Fourrier et al [33] suggest several ways in which decreased ACE activity could lead to the changes of hyperreninemic hypoaldosteronism. These workers demonstrated profound decreases in the levels of ACE activity after repeated plasma exchange, partly due to enzyme removal and partly due to inhibition of the enzyme by the synthetic plasma substitute, polygelin [33]. Decreases in serum levels of ACE activity have also been described during hypoxia [34], endotoxin shock [35], and adult respiratory distress syndrome [36], suggesting a possible role for these changes in the pathogenesis of hyperreninemic hypoaldosteronism. Although the levels of Ang II have been elevated in some reports of hyperreninemic hypoaldosteronism [3,18], this peptide has not been measured in most cases, thus leaving open the possibility that a transient deficiency of ACE may be important.

CLINICAL EVALUATION

In evaluating critically ill patients with confirmed severe hyperkalemia, it is often not possible to rule out generalized adrenal insufficiency, which may be acute in onset if due to adrenal hemorrhage, infarction, or infiltration. Short-term glucocorticoid replacement may be appropriate, preferably after samples have been taken for measurements of ACTH, cortisol, aldosterone, and renin activity, and after an assessment has been made of the acute corticosteroid response to ACTH. If glucocorticoid function is shown to be normal in the face of aldosterone deficiency, replacement therapy is probably inappropriate. Severely ill patients with hyperreninemic hypoaldosteronism almost invariably show marked cortisol excess [1–7,14–18]. From radioreceptor studies of specific mineralocorticoid binding sites in various tissues, it has been estimated that such cortisol levels would result in high occupancy of mineralocorticoid receptors [37]; this 'crossover' probably accounts for the absence of features of mineralocorticoid deficiency in most critically ill patients who show selective hyperreninemic hypoaldosteronism.

REFERENCES

1. Zipser RD, Davenport MW, Martin KL, Tuck ML, Warner NE, Swinney RL, Davis CL, Horton R. Hyperreninemic hypoaldosteronism in the critically ill: A new entity. *Journal of Clinical Endocrinology and Metabolism* 1981;**53**: 867–73.

2. Davenport MW, Zipser RD. Association of hypotension with hyperreninemic hypoaldosteronism in the critically ill patient. *Archives of Internal Medicine* 1983;**143**:735–7.

3. Findling JW, Waters VO, Raff H. The dissociation of renin and aldosterone during critical illness. *Journal of Clinical Endocrinology and Metabolism* 1987;**64**:592–5.

4. Saenger P, Levine LS, Irvine WJ, Gottesdiener K, Rauh W, Sonino N, Chow D, New MI. Progressive adrenal failure in polyglandular autoimmune disease. *Journal of Clinical Endocrinology and Metabolism* 1982;**54**:863–8.

5. Diamond TH, Huddle KRL, Dubb A. Hyperkalaemia secondary to hypoaldosteronism. A report of 2 cases differentiating hyperreninaemic from hyporeninaemic hypo-aldosteronism. *South African Medical Journal* 1987;**71**; 40–2.

6. Silver J, Rosler A, Friedlander M, Popovtzer MM. Unmasking of isolated hypoaldosteronism after renal allotransplantation in familial Mediterranean fever. *Israel Journal of Medical Sciences* 1982;**18**:495–8.

7. Taylor HC, Shah B, Pillay I, Mayes DM. Isolated hyperreninemic hypoaldosteronism due to carcinoma metastatic to the adrenal gland. *American Journal of Medicine* 1988;**85**:441–4.

8. Armanini D, Kuhnle U, Strasser T, Dorr H, Butenandt I, Weber PC, Stockigt JR, Pearce P, Funder JW. Aldosterone-receptor deficiency in pseudohypoaldosteronism. *New England Journal of Medicine* 1985;**313**:1178–81.

9. Stockigt JR, Hewett MJ, Topliss DJ, Higgs EJ, Taft P. Renin and renin substrate in primary adrenal insufficiency. Contrasting effects of glucocorticoid and mineralocorticoid deficiency. *American Journal of Medicine* 1979;**66**:15–22.

10. Rasmussen S, Damkjaer Nielsen M, Giese J. Captopril combined with thiazide lowers renin substrate concentration: Implications for methodology in renin assays. *Clinical Science* 1981;**60**:591–3.

11. Atkinson AB, Cumming AMM, Brown JJ, Fraser R, Leckie B, Lever AF, Morton JJ, Robertson JIS. Captopril treatment: Inter-dose variations in renin, angiotensins I and II, aldosterone and blood pressure. *British Journal of Clinical Pharmacology* 1982;**13**:855–8.

12. Giese J, Rasmussen S, Nielsen MD, Ibsen H. Biochemical monitoring of vasoactive peptides during angiotensin converting enzyme inhibition. *Journal of Hypertension* 1983;**1** (suppl 1):31–6.

13. Stern N, Beck FWJ, Sowers JR, Tuck M, Hsueh WA, Zipser RD. Plasma corticosteroids in hyperreninemic hypoaldosteronism: Evidence for diffuse impairment of the zona glomerulosa. *Journal of Clinical Endocrinolology and Metabolism* 1983;**57**:217–20.

14. Findling JW, Adams AH, Raff H. Selective hypoaldosteronism due to an endogenous impairment in angiotensin II production. *New England Journal of Medicine* 1987;**316**:1632–5.

15. Williams Jr FA, Schambelan M, Biglieri EG, Carey RM. Acquired primary hypoaldosteronism due to an isolated zona glomerulosa defect. *New England Medical Journal* 1983;**309**:1623–7.

16. Braithwaite SS, Barbato AL, Emanuele MA. Acquired partial corticosterone methyl oxidase type II defect in diabetes mellitus. *Diabetes Care* 1990;**13**:790–2.

17. Kokko JP. Primary acquired hypoaldosteronism. *Kidney International* 1985;**27**: 690–702.

18. Muto S, Fujisawa G, Natsume T, Asano Y, Yaginuma T, Hosoda S, Saito T. Hyponatremia and hyperreninemic hypoaldosteronism in a critically ill patient: Combination of insensitivity to angiotensin II and tubular unresponsiveness to mineralocorticoid. *Clinical Nephrology* 1990;**34**:208–13.

19. O'Kelly R, Magee F, McKenna TJ. Routine heparin therapy inhibits adrenal aldosterone production. *Journal of Clinical Endocrinology and Metabolism* 1983;**56**: 108–12.

20. Rebuffat P, Kasprzak A, Andreis PG, Mazzocchi G, Gottardo G, Coi A, Nussdorfer GG. Effects of prolonged cyclosporine-A treatment on the morphology and function of rat adrenal cortex. *Endocrinology* 1989;**125**:1407–13.

21. Carey RM, Thorner MO, Ortt EM. Effects of metoclopramide and bromocriptine on the renin–angiotensin–aldosterone system in man. *Journal of Clinical Investigation* 1979;**63**:727–35.

22. Sequeira SJ, McKenna TJ. Chlorbutol, a new inhibitor of aldosterone biosynthesis identified during examination of heparin effect on aldosterone production. *Journal of Clinical Endocrinology and Metabolism* 1986;**63**:780–4.

23. Biglieri EG, Schambelan M, Slaton Jr PE. Effect of adrenocorticotropin on desoxycorticosterone, corticosterone and aldosterone excretion. *Journal of Clinical Endocrinology and Metabolism* 1969;**29**:1090–101.

24. Kraiem Z, Rosenthal T, Rotzak R, Lunenfeld B. Angiotensin II and K challenge following prolonged ACTH administration in normal subjects. *Acta Endocrinologica* 1979;**91**:657–65.

25. Aguilera G, Fujita K, Catt KJ. Mechanisms of inhibition of aldosterone secretion by adrenocorticotropin. *Endocrinology* 1981;**108**:522–8.

26. McDougall JG, Butkus A, Coghlan JP, Denton DA, Muller J, Oddie CJ, Robinson PM, Scoggins BA. Biosynthetic and morphological evidence for inhibition of aldosterone production following administration of ACTH to sheep. *Acta Endocrinologica* 1980;**94**:559–70.

27. Braley LM, Menachery AI, Conlin PR, Mortensen RM, Hallahan J, Williams GH. Dose effect of ACTH on aldosterone and cortisol biosynthesis in cultured bovine adrenal glomerulosa cells: A possible *in vitro* correlate of hyperreninemic hypoaldosteronism. *Proceedings of the 73rd Annual Meeting*, The Endocrine Society 1991:Abstract **165**.

28. Hermus ARMM, Sweep CGJ. Cytokines and the hypothalamic–pituitary–adrenal axis. *Journal of Steroid Biochemistry and Molecular Biology* 1990;**37**:867–71.

29. Natarajan R, Ploszaj S, Horton R, Nadler J. Tumor necrosis factor and interleukin-1 are potent inhibitors of angiotensin-II-induced aldosterone synthesis. *Endocrinology* 1989;**125**:3084–9.

30. Stern N, Natarajan R, Tuck ML, Laird E, Nadler JL. Selective inhibition of angiotensin-II-mediated aldosterone secretion by 5-hydroxyeicosatetraenoic acid. *Endocrinology* 1989;**125**:3090–5.

31. Vanderhoek JY, Karmin MT, Ekborg SL. Endogenous hydroxyeicosatetraenoic acids stimulate the human polymorphonuclear leukocyte 15-lipoxygenase pathway. *Journal of Biological Chemistry* 1985;**260**:15482–7.

32. Hirai A, Tahara K, Tamura Y, Saito H, Terano T, Yoshida S. Involvement of 5-lipoxygenase metabolites in ACTH-stimulated corticosteroidogenesis in rat adrenal glands. *Prostaglandins* 1985;**30**:749–67.

33. Fourrier F, Leclerc L, Lestavel P, Racadot A, Chambrin M-C, Mangalaboyi J, Chopin C. Decrease of angiotensin-converting enzyme activity after plasma exchange. *Critical Care Medicine* 1988;**16**:105–10.

34. Stalcup SA, Lipset JS, Woan J–M, Leuenberger P, Mellins RB. Inhibition of angiotensin converting enzyme activity in cultured endothelial cells by hypoxia. *Journal of Clinical Investigation* 1979;**63**:966–76.

35. Hollinger MA. Effect of endotoxin on mouse serum angiotensin-converting enzyme. *American Review of Respiratory Diseases* 1983;**127**:756–7.

36. Fourrier F, Chopin C, Wallaert B, Wattre P, Mangalaboyi J, Durocher A, Dubois D, Wattel F. Angiotensin-converting enzyme in human adult respiratory distress syndrome. *Chest* 1983;**83**:593–7.

37. Lan NC, Graham B, Bartter FC, Baxter JD. Binding of steroids to mineralocorticoid receptors:Implications for *in vivo* occupancy by glucocorticoids. *Journal of Clinical Endocrinology and Metabolism* 1982;**54**:332–42.

38. Landier F, Guyene TT, Boutignon H, Nahoul K, Corvol P, Job J–C. Hyporeninemic hypoaldosteronism in infancy: A familial disease. *Journal of Clinical Endocrinology and Metabolism* 1984;**58**:143–8.

39. Anderson JV, Struthers AD, Payne NN, Slater JDH, Bloom SR. Atrial natriuretic peptide inhibits the aldosterone response to angiotensin II in man. *Clinical Science* 1986;**70**:507–12.

70 HYPORENINEMIC HYPOALDOSTERONISM

JAN R STOCKIGT

HISTORY AND INTRODUCTION

Acquired selective hypoaldosteronism was first described in 1957 by Hudson [1], but it was not until 1972 that the frequent association of this syndrome with hyporeninemia was recognized [2,3]. Since then, it has been widely assumed that hypoaldosteronism may be a direct consequence of deficiency of circulating active renin, that is, a classical secondary end-organ deficiency from lack of trophic hormone [2–4]. This view, however, may be an over-simplification because there is evidence of an associated abnormality of aldosterone synthesis in this group of disorders (see later). While it is unsatisfying to evoke two causal mechanisms for one disorder, it has become difficult to identify a single pathogenic

Findings in 81 cases (mean age 65 years, range 32–82 years)	Positive or present (%)
Findings at presentation	
*asymptomatic hyperkalemia	75
muscle weakness	25
cardiac arrhythmia	25
hyperchloremic acidosis	~50
salt wasting	unusual
*normal glucocorticoid function	100
*mild-to-moderate renal insufficiency	70
diabetes mellitus	49
*low or low–normal baseline plasma aldosterone levels with subnormal increase following volume contraction	100
*subnormal baseline and/or stimulated plasma renin levels	82
normal aldosterone response to Ang II infusion	15
normal aldosterone response to adrenocorticotropic hormone	21
* = generally accepted diagnostic criteria	

Fig. 70.1 Clinical and laboratory characteristics in selective hypoaldosteronism. Modified from De Fronzo RA [5].

mechanism in hyporeninemic hypoaldosteronism. The clinical and biochemical features of the syndrome are shown in Fig. 70.1.

Although the condition is frequently referred to as 'hyporeninemic' hypoaldosteronism, it is notable that 18% of the 81 cases reviewed by de Fronzo in 1980 showed normal basal or stimulated plasma renin levels [5]. The hyporeninemic patients reported by Schambelan *et al* in 1972 [2], tended to lose sodium and develop postural hypotension with sodium restriction, but other reports included patients in whom subnormal renin and aldosterone levels were associated with sodium-dependent hypertension [6]. As pointed out by Holland [7], volume retention might be the fundamental abnormality in that situation. Diuretics may then correct hypertension and hyperkalemia; in contrast, 9-α-fluorohydrocortisone (fludrocortisone) was beneficial in the patients reported by Schambelan *et al* [2].

The prevalence of acquired selective hypoaldosteronism is not precisely known, but it has been estimated that up to 50% of patients in hospital with persistent hyperkalemia have this syndrome [8], often aggravated by associated drug therapy (see below). In a study of 31 patients with chronic renal insufficiency and hyperkalemia, including seven with diabetes mellitus, 23 were found to have hypoaldosteronism, associated with subnormal renin levels in 19 [9].

In hyporeninemic hypoaldosteronism, aldosterone and renin values should be interpreted in relation to sodium balance and the prevailing plasma potassium concentration — 'normal' aldosterone levels may be inappropriately low in the presence of hyperkalemia, whereas hyperkalemia *per se* may decrease circulating renin. Since most patients with hyporeninemic hypoaldosteronism are elderly, it is important to consider the normal decline in supine and ambulant renin and ambulant aldosterone, which has been reported with advancing age [10]. Urinary excretion of aldosterone as the acid-labile 18-glucuronide has been shown to correlate closely with plasma aldosterone and with aldosterone secretion rate in patients with renal insufficiency [9], although some suggest that this metabolite may give an underestimate relative to circulating concentrations in the elderly [11].

A classification of hyporeninemic hypoaldosteronism, based on the presence or absence of hypertension, is given in Fig. 70.2. In contrast to the hyperkalemic condition, which is the main focus of this chapter, hyporeninemic hypoaldosteronism in association with hypokalemia and hypertension usually suggests that an alternative mineralocorticoid, endogenous or exogenous, is involved [12,13], or that renal tubular function is abnormal in the absence of a distinct hormonal abnormality. These hypertensive hypokalemic disorders are outside the scope of the present chapter, and have been reviewed in detail elsewhere [12,13] (see *Chapters 55, 63, 65,* and *66*).

In contrast to the acquired form of hyporeninemic hypoaldosteronism associated with renal insufficiency, there is a single report of this association in a salt-wasting syndrome of infancy [14]. Glucocorticoid secretion and the aldosterone response to adrenocorticotropic hormone (ACTH) were normal, but renin activity and angiotensinogen were both subnormal. The disorder was tentatively attributed to a qualitative or quantitative hereditary defect in angiotensinogen [14].

ASSOCIATED DISEASES

The list of diseases associated with hyporeninemic hypoaldosteronism (Fig. 70.3) is so diverse that it is hardly surprising

normotensive (? hypertensive)
hyporeninemic hypoaldosteronism
(see *Fig. 70.3* for associated diseases
and *Fig. 70.8* for drug causes)
anephric state
hypertensive
exogenous mineralocorticoid
pharmaceutical formulations [12]
adrenocorticotropic hormone excess
enzymic defects
17–α–hydroxylase deficiency
11–β–hydroxylase deficiency
hereditary glucocorticoid resistance [55]
ectopic adrenocorticotropic hormone secretion
apparent mineralocorticoid excess
11–β–hydroxysteroid dehydrogenase deficiency [56]
11–β–hydroxysteroid dehydrogenase inhibition [57]
for example, liquorice
excess renal tubular sodium reabsorption
Liddle's syndrome
pseudohypoaldosteronism, type II [58] (*Chapter 65*)

Fig. 70.2 Classification of hyporeninemic hypoaldosteronism.

diabetes mellitus
interstitial nephritis
gout
obstructive uropathy [59]
glomerulonephritis
lead nephropathy [60]
postrenal transplant [61]
analgesic nephropathy
sickle-cell disease [62]
acquired immune deficiency syndrome [63]
*hypopituitarism [64,65]
* = transient, relieved by glucocorticoid

Fig. 70.3 Diseases associated with hyporeninemic hypoaldosteronism.

that no specific renal pathology has been described. In general, the syndrome is recognized when hyperkalemia and metabolic acidosis develop to an extent out of proportion to the degree of renal impairment. Although arrhythmias associated with hyperkalemia were described in some early reports and may be the presenting feature [1,2], most cases are now initially recognized from the biochemical findings. Hormonal findings vary, depending on whether the patients have presented with definite features that suggest hyporeninemic hypoaldosteronism, or whether studies have been done in large groups of patients, usually diabetics, with the aim of seeking this syndrome.

Grande Villoria *et al* [15] compared the frequency of hyporeninemic hypoaldosteronism in nondiabetic and in insulin-dependent diabetic patients with and without renal impairment. They found that a tendency to hyporeninism and impairment of net acid excretion could occur from an early stage of diabetes before renal impairment developed. Diabetes mellitus, independent of changes in renal function, was associated with lower basal and stimulated levels of renin activity and plasma aldosterone. Changes consistent with hyporeninemic hypoaldosteronism were found in the majority of diabetics with renal failure. At the same level of renal impairment, plasma potassium was higher in diabetics (5.0 ± 0.3 versus 4.0 ± 0.5 mmol/l); despite this difference, the ratio of plasma aldosterone to potassium was reduced to approximately half in the presence of diabetes, consistent with subnormal aldosterone responsiveness to Ang II even in the presence of hyperkalemia. Numerous workers have sought to resolve this paradox (*Chapters 65, 75* and *92*).

THE ABNORMALITY OF RENIN SECRETION

Hyporeninemic hypoaldosteronism was initially assumed to be due to selective damage to the juxtaglomerular cells as a result of interstitial renal disease, but direct proof of such a mechanism is lacking. No single pathogenic mechanism that reconciles each of the documented abnormalities has so far been described, but a single cause might emerge if a factor were shown to impair renin release and also to inhibit the final steps in aldosterone biosynthesis.

ABNORMAL RENAL MORPHOLOGY

In diabetic nephropathy, there are descriptions of arteriolar sclerosis with wider than normal separation between macula densa and juxtaglomerular cells [16] and with hyalinization of afferent arterioles [17] (Color Plate 31). These changes have not been directly correlated with a clear abnormality of renin secretion or activation, and there is still a lack of information about the changes in renal morphology that are associated with hyporeninemic hypoaldosteronism in nondiabetics.

IMPAIRED CONVERSION OF PRORENIN TO ACTIVE RENIN

Several studies in diabetic patients have shown impairment of the conversion step from prorenin to active renin [18,19]. DeLeiva *et al* [18] reported that plasma renin concentration (measured after acid activation) was markedly increased in two patients with this disorder, while active renin remained subnormal after sodium restriction; a defect in aldosterone biosynthesis was also present. It is now known, however, that up to 50% of diabetics with microvascular complications have an excess of circulating prorenin of extrarenal origin, usually with normal concentrations of active renin [20], suggesting that the presence of prorenin excess *per se* may not have direct significance in the pathogenesis of hyporeninemic hypoaldosteronism (see *Chapters 6* and *75*).

DEFECTIVE SYMPATHETIC STIMULATION OF RENIN RELEASE

Subnormal renin responses to upright posture and exercise (Fig. 70.4) suggested that renal sympathetic function was impaired in hyperkalemic diabetics with typical hyporeninemic hypoaldosteronism. These diabetics also showed diminished norepinephrine responses to postural change, and a diminished renin response to the β-adrenergic agonist, isoproterenol [21,22]. A possible connection between abnormal sympathetic function and impaired activation of prorenin was suggested by Misbin *et al* [23] who reported that diabetics with autonomic dysfunction (who did not

have hyporeninemic hypoaldosteronism), had elevated levels of trypsin-activatable inactive renin, although active renin was normal. These changes correlated with neuropathy and were not found when microvascular complications were present in the absence of neuropathy. In contrast, Franken *et al* [20] found that microvascular disease, rather than neuropathy *per se*, correlated with increased levels of inactive renin. Hence, it remains uncertain which diabetic complications are directly associated with deficiency of active renin.

SALT AND WATER RETENTION

The fact that sodium retention and volume expansion might be causal factors in hyporeninemic hypoaldosteronism was first suggested by the studies of Oh *et al* [6] who identified a group of hyperkalemic patients with renal insufficiency and hypertension, in whom renin rose significantly after volume depletion. It is notable that aldosterone levels generally remained disproportionately low, consistent with an associated adrenal defect.

Some studies suggest that levels of atrial natriuretic factor (ANF) may be abnormal in diabetic patients. Bell *et al* [24] compared poorly controlled and moderately well-controlled uncomplicated diabetic patients with normal subjects. They found that mean basal ANF levels were higher, and renin activity lower, in the poorly controlled diabetics; ANF did not correlate with plasma potassium or urinary aldosterone. Some studies have shown that diabetics, both normotensive and hypertensive, have higher than normal ANF levels in the basal state, but that their ANF responses to acute sodium loading are attenuated, associated with impaired ability to excrete a sodium load [25]. In contrast, others have not been able to identify any ANF abnormality in diabetic subjects who retain sodium more avidly than normal after acute volume expansion [26]. Although ANF is a substance that could suppress both renin and aldosterone (*Chapter 36*), its role in this syndrome is uncertain.

EFFECT OF POTASSIUM RETENTION

Chronic hyperkalemia can impair renin release [27] but should normally stimulate aldosterone secretion, even in the absence of renal renin [28]. Short-term normokalemia fails to reverse the defect in renin secretion in hyporeninemic hypoaldosteronism [2,29], suggesting that hyperkalemia *per se* is unlikely to be a major causal factor, although it remains possible that long-term correction of hyperkalemia, in the absence of volume changes, might restore renal renin secretion to normal. In diabetic patients, defective insulin secretion with associated hyperglycemia may aggravate hyperkalemia [30] and thus impair renin secretion.

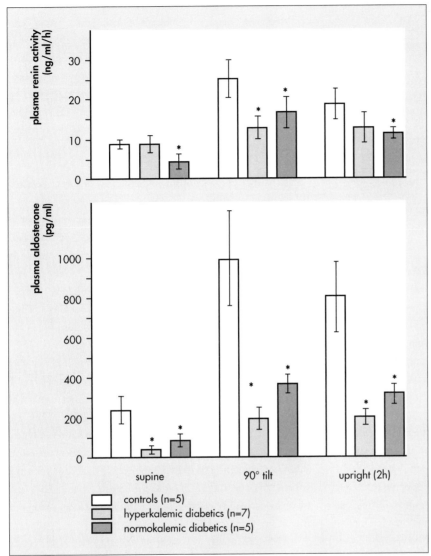

Fig. 70.4 Plasma renin activity and aldosterone responses (mean ± SEM) to upright tilt and walking in control subjects (n=5), hyperkalemic diabetics (n=7), and normokalemic diabetics (n=5). Patients with hyperkalemic diabetes had longer duration of diabetes, with a greater prevalence of renal impairment, hypertension, and neuropathy (*$P<0.05$ to <0.001). Modified from Perez GO *et al* [21].

PROSTAGLANDIN DEFICIENCY

There is evidence that intrarenal prostaglandin deficiency can cause or aggravate hyporeninemia [31] (*Chapter 38*). In patients with renal insufficiency, the nonsteroidal anti-inflammatory drug, indomethacin, can cause transient reversible deficiency of circulating active renin and aldosterone [32]. This drug has also shown to decrease plasma active renin in the absence of renal insufficiency [33]. Nadler *et al* [31] reported that the urinary prostacyclin metabolite, 6-ketoprostacyclin $F_{1\alpha}$, was decreased in hyporeninemic hypoaldosteronism and failed to increase in response to calcium or norepinephrine infusion (Fig. 70.5). A study of patients with rheumatoid arthritis and renal impairment showed that naproxen

decreased urinary 6-keto-prostaglandin $F_{1\alpha}$, renin activity, and urinary aldosterone, associated with increase in serum potassium [34].

OTHER MECHANISMS

It would be of particular interest if a common mechanism were shown to have a dual effect to impair secretion of active renin and to inhibit aldosterone production. There is evidence that peptides of endothelial origin may influence renal renin release by altering the synthesis of prostaglandin derivatives [35] and that endothelin can stimulate aldosterone secretion in mammalian adrenal tissue *in vitro* [36]. Further studies may lead to new insights

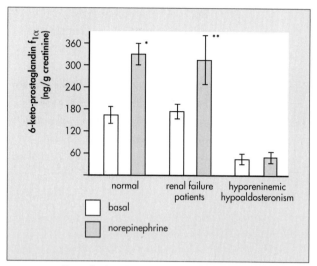

Fig. 70.5 Effect of a four-hour pressor norepinephrine infusion (0.1 µg/kg/min) on four hours' excretion of urinary 6-keto-prostaglandin $F_{1\alpha}$ (mean ± SEM) in normal subjects, in renal failure patients with normal renin, and in hyporeninemic hypoaldosteronism. (*$P<0.02$; **$P<0.05$.) Calcium infusion also failed to stimulate this prostaglandin in hyporeninemic hypoaldosteronism. Modified from Nadler JL et al [31].

into conditions such as diabetes mellitus, where microvascular damage is common and where production of endothelium-derived peptides might be deficient.

The demonstration that the aldosterone response to sodium restriction in rats may be mediated by changes in a distinct self-contained RAS within the adrenal zona glomerulosa [37], raises interesting possibilities. If such a system exists in man, a defect in its activity might reproduce the features of hyporeninemic hypoaldosteronism without concordant changes in the level of circulating renin (see *Chapter 44*).

THE ASSOCIATED ABNORMALITY OF ALDOSTERONE BIOSYNTHESIS

Even when the RAS is markedly suppressed, as in primary aldosteronism or the anephric state, aldosterone normally shows a brisk response to increases in plasma potassium [28,38]. The lack of response to increases in plasma potassium in hyporeninemic hypoaldosteronism is paradoxical if the primary abnormality were simply a defect in renin secretion. There is now accumulating evidence of associated impairment in the final stages of aldosterone formation, although the relationship of this impairment to the abnormality of renal renin secretion remains undefined. The

occurrence of selective hypoaldosteronism with normal renin secretion in some patients [5,39,40] suggests that renin deficiency alone may not account for this syndrome. This view is at variance with that of Kater *et al* [41], who inferred that a defect in aldosterone synthesis could be ruled out in hyporeninemic hypoaldosteronism, on the basis of a normal ratio of 18-hydroxycorticosterone (18OHB) to aldosterone, with normal responses of these steroids to acute high-dose infusion of des-Asp Ang II.

It has not been established whether the apparent defect in aldosterone biosynthesis is related to zona glomerulosa atrophy as a result of renin deficiency, chronic hyperkalemia, or some other factor associated with renal insufficiency. Prolonged renin deficiency may be important as aldosterone production from the remaining adrenal gland may respond poorly to ACTH and Ang II after removal of an aldosterone-producing adenoma [42]. Hyperkalemia *per se* is unlikely to be a factor as prior potassium loading augments the aldosterone responses to acute sodium restriction and to acute potassium infusion [43].

Studies in anephric subjects suggest that chronic lack of renal renin may impair the acute aldosterone responses to Ang II infusion [44]; this response was enhanced, but not restored to normal, by prior dietary sodium restriction [44]. While the hypothesis that a lack of the trophic effect of renal renin on the adrenal zona glomerulosa may explain the apparent defect in aldosterone biosynthesis in hyporeninemic hypoaldosteronism is an attractive one, there is at present no direct proof for this view. Factors that may selectively impair the aldosterone response to Ang II are considered further in *Chapter 69*.

Tuck and Mayes [45] studied four hyperkalemic diabetic patients with hyporeninemic hypoaldosteronism and moderate renal insufficiency and found severely impaired plasma aldosterone responses to Ang II infusion (Fig. 70.6), sodium restriction, and ACTH, associated with normal corticosterone, 18OHB, and cortisol responses to these stimuli. The rates of Ang II infusion were comparable in the controls and the study subjects. These findings suggest an acquired defect of corticosterone methyl-oxidase, type I or II [46]. In contrast to the findings in the classical adrenal enzyme deficiencies, however, there was no associated increase in 18OHB or corticosterone, a difference that may be attributable to the subnormal renin and Ang II levels, or to the fact that 18OHB is not an obligatory aldosterone precursor [46].

Sowers *et al* [47] studied the responses of active and inactive renin, 18OHB, and aldosterone to acute volume depletion by intravenous furosemide in a heterogeneous group of patients with hyporeninemic hypoaldosteronism (Fig. 70.7). Compared with normal subjects, the active renin response was less and was

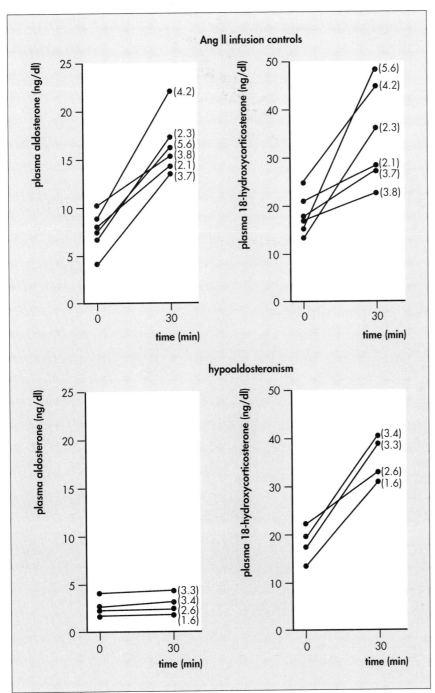

Fig. 70.6 Response of plasma aldosterone and 18-hydroxycorticosterone to Ang II infusion in control subjects (upper; n=6) and hyperkalemic patients with hyporeninemic hypoaldosteronism (lower; n=4). The Ang II infusion rates (ng/kg/min) are shown in parentheses for each subject. Modified from Tuck ML and Mayes DM [45].

associated with subnormal rises in plasma 18OHB and aldosterone, the aldosterone response being much more severely impaired. While these authors concluded that impairment of renin activation was possibly the primary abnormality, their data also showed a markedly diminished aldosterone response to submaximal doses of ACTH, consistent with a late block in biosynthesis.

The findings of Iwasaki et al [40] suggest a possible defect in zona glomerulosa function that is independent of renin deficiency. They studied diabetic patients with marginal renal impairment and subnormal plasma aldosterone levels; renin activity was normal in 9 of 17 patients and low in eight. In response to a graded Ang II infusion, both 18OHB and aldosterone showed subnormal responses. This impairment was more

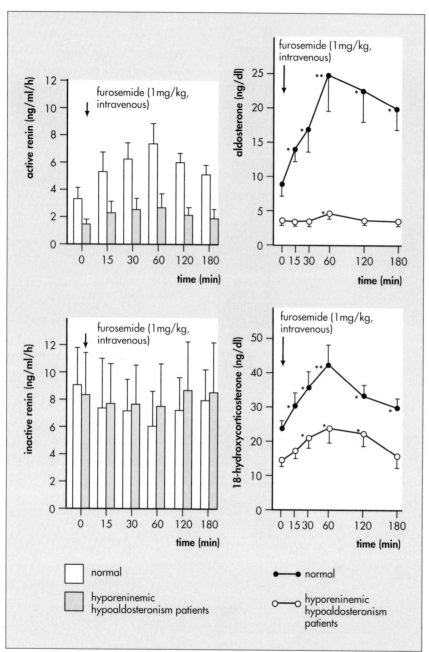

Fig. 70.7 Active and inactive renin, plasma aldosterone, and 18-hydroxycorticosterone (18OHB) responses to furosemide 1mg/kg intravenously in six normal subjects and 10 hyperkalemic patients with hyporeninemic hypoaldosteronism. The acute responses of active renin and aldosterone were severely impaired. It should be noted that low-dose adrenocorticotrophic hormone infusion showed a normal 18OHB response, with severe impairment of the aldosterone response in these subjects with hyporeninemic hypoaldosteronism. (*$P<0.05$; **$P<0.01$.) Modified from Sowers JR *et al* [47].

marked in the group with normal renin levels, a paradox similar to that reported by Schambelan *et al* [9] who found lower aldosterone responses to increasing renin in normoreninemic than in hyporeninemic patients.

There is evidence that the various stimuli to aldosterone secretion continue to show normal interactions in this syndrome. In response to sodium restriction, plasma aldosterone correlated positively with renin activity in both normal subjects and those with hyporeninemic hypoaldosteronism [9]. While the ability of aldosterone to respond to potassium was blunted, plasma aldosterone was higher at equivalent renin levels in the presence of hyperkalemia, and higher at equivalent levels of potassium in response to renin and Ang II [9].

RELATIONSHIPS BETWEEN METABOLIC ACIDOSIS, ALDOSTERONE DEFICIENCY AND HYPERKALEMIA

The hyperchloremic metabolic acidosis of hyporeninemic hypoaldosteronism, which is usually out of keeping with moderate impairment of renal function, has been designated type IV renal tubular acidosis [48]. Mineralocorticoid deficiency may reduce renal hydrogen ion (H^+) excretory capacity by two distinct mechanisms: reduction in direct renal H^+ secretory capacity independent of potassium retention and reduction of renal ammonia production secondary to hyperkalemia [49]. While some have argued that potassium retention *per se* is the major cause of acidosis in hypoaldosteronism [50], others have shown that mineralocorticoids can influence acid–base status independent of potassium balance [51], suggesting that the inability to excrete acid is not simply a consequence of hyperkalemia. In support of this view, recurrence of acidosis after cessation of mineralocorticoid was associated with diminished excretion of titratable acid even when hyperkalemia was prevented [51]. In some studies, supraphysiological doses of fludrocortisone have been required to correct acidosis [48,51], suggesting that the renal tubule is resistant to mineralocorticoid, an effect that may in part be due to impaired renal ammonia excretion as a consequence of hyperkalemia [49].

In hyporeninemic hypoaldosteronism, where aldosterone is not normally responsive to increased plasma potassium, hyperkalemia may worsen acidosis, which may then perpetuate hyperkalemia in a cyclical fashion. In progressive renal failure, there is normally a marked capacity for the remaining nephrons to increase their ability to secrete potassium [52]. Any impairment

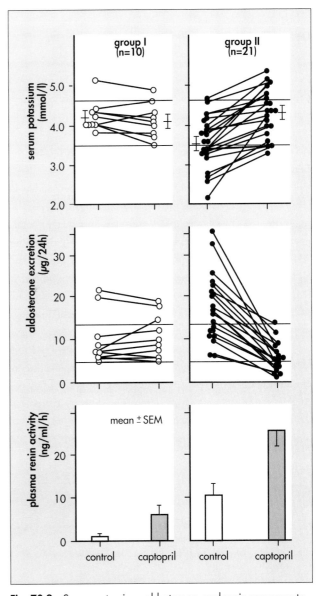

Fig. 70.9 Serum potassium, aldosterone, and renin responses to 4–7 days' treatment with captopril 100–1,000mg/d (mean dose 575mg/d) in 31 hypertensive patients. If aldosterone excretion decreased by >40%, patients were classified into group II. Initial creatinine clearance was 93 ± 9 ml/min in group I and 64 ± 6 ml/min in group II. The hyperkalemic response was greater in the face of normal or high initial renin levels. Normal basal peripheral renin activity was 0.4–2.6ng/ml/h. Modified from Textor SC *et al* [53]. Note that the high doses of captopril used in this early study are now considered excessive, at least in azotemic patients.

---

potassium supplements

potassium-sparing diuretics

nonsteroidal anti-inflammatory agents [32–34]
    ? except sulindac [34]

β-blockers [67]

heparin [68]

cyclosporin A [69]

spironolactone

converting-enzyme inhibitors [53,70]

agents that induce acidosis

agents that induce volume depletion

Fig. 70.8 Drugs that aggravate hyperkalemia in hypoaldosteronism [66].

of this mechanism of potassium adaptation would further pre-dispose to the cycle: potassium retention — impaired ammonia production — acidosis — potassium retention.

TREATMENT

In view of its diversity, there is no single appropriate line of treatment for hyporeninemic hypoaldosteronism, although several general principles apply.

AVOIDANCE OR REMOVAL OF PRECIPITATING FACTORS

Since associated drug therapy can precipitate hyperkalemia in patients with renal insufficiency and hyporeninemic hypoaldo-steronism, it is crucial to review all aspects of drug therapy before instituting specific treatment. The drugs listed in Fig. 70.8 may be contraindicated in patients predisposed to hyperkalemia, and removal of such precipitating factor(s) may be all that is necessary. It is important to note that any degree of volume depletion, for example due to poorly controlled diabetes or abnormal fluid loss, may aggravate hyperkalemia.

Due to the frequent use of ACE inhibitors in diabetic patients who are prone to hyporeninemic hypoaldosteronism, it is impor-tant to establish which patients in this group are at risk of serious ACE inhibitor–induced hyperkalemia. The study by Textor *et al* [53] showed that the tendency to hyperkalemia in response to high-dose captopril was greatest when pretreatment renin and aldosterone levels were normal or increased, that is, when the decrease in aldosterone was greatest (Fig. 70.9). This finding suggests that the risk of hyperkalemia may be small in patients who already have established hypoaldosteronism.

FLUDROCORTISONE AND/OR DIURETICS

Fludrocortisone is clearly beneficial in reversing hyperkalemia, but the dose required may be greater than in generalized adrenocortical insufficiency [48,51], consistent with some degree of diminished sensitivity to mineralocorticoids. Potassium excre-tion is enhanced and metabolic acidosis may be corrected, but hypertension and fluid retention can be worsened.

Diuretics, for example, furosemide, can be used to correct fluid retention, but they must be prescribed with care to avoid intravascular volume depletion which may worsen hyperkalemia and postural hypotension. Furosemide has also been shown to increase net acid excretion and to have a beneficial effect on hyperchloremic metabolic acidosis [54]. Synergism between furosemide and fludrocortisone has not been conclusively demon-strated in hyporeninemic hypoaldosteronism, but might be ex-pected if furosemide increases distal tubular volume and sodium loads in the face of fixed replacement doses of mineralocorticoid. Hence, in some instances, when hyperkalemic metabolic acidosis is associated with a tendency to hypertension and volume overload, the best approach may be judicious use of fludrocortisone and furosemide together. This combination is unusual in any other circumstance.

REFERENCES

1. Hudson JB, Chobanian AV, Relman AS. Hypoaldosteronism: A clinical study of a patient with an isolated adrenal mineralocorticoid deficiency resulting in hyperkalemia and Stokes–Adams attacks. *New England Journal of Medicine* 1957;257:529–36.

2. Schambelan M, Stockigt JR, Biglieri EG. Isolated hypoaldosteronism in adults: A renin-deficiency syndrome. *New England Journal of Medicine* 1972;287:573–8.

3. Perez G, Siegel L, Schreiner GE. Selective hypoaldosteronism with hyperkalemia. *Annals of Internal Medicine* 1972;76:757–63.

4. Brown JJ, Chinn RH, Fraser R, Lever AF, Morton JJ, Robertson JIS, Tree M, Waite MA, Park DM. Recurrent hyperkalemia due to selective aldosterone deficiency: Correction by angiotensin infusion. *British Medical Journal* 1973;1:650–4.

5. DeFronzo RA. Hyperkalemia and hyporeninemic hypoaldosteronism. *Kidney International* 1980;17:118–34.

6. Oh MS, Carroll HJ, Clemmons JE, Vagnucci AH, Levison SP, Whang ESM. A mechanism for hyporeninemic hypoaldosteronism in chronic renal disease. *Metabolism* 1974;23:1157–66.

7. Holland OB. Hypoaldosteronism — disease or normal response? *New England Journal of Medicine* 1991;324:488–9.

8. Tan SY, Burton M. Hyporeninemic hypoaldosteronism: An overlooked cause of hyperkalemia. *Archives of Internal Medicine* 1981;141:30–3.

9. Schambelan M, Sebastian A, Biglieri EG. Prevalence, pathogenesis, and functional significance of aldosterone deficiency in hyperkalemic patients with chronic renal insufficiency. *Kidney International* 1980;17:89–101.

10. Weidmann P, Beretta-Piccoli C, Ziegler WH, Keusc G, Gluck Z, Reubi FC. Age versus urinary sodium for judging renin, aldosterone, and catecholamine levels: Studies in normal subjects and patients with essential hypertension. *Kidney International* 1978;14:619–28.

11. Pratt H, Hawthorne JJ, Debono DJ. Reduced urinary aldosterone excretion rates with normal plasma concentrations of aldosterone in the very elderly. *Steroids* 1988;51:163–71.

12. Mantero F. Exogenous mineralocorticoid-like disorders. *Clinics in Endocrinology and Metabolism* 1981;10:465–78.

13. Biglieri EG. Enzymatic disorders and hypertension. *Clinics in Endocrinology and Metabolism* 1981;10:453–63.

14. Landier F, Guyene TT, Boutignon H, Nahoul K, Corvol P, Job J–C. Hyporeninemic hypoaldosteronism in infancy: A familial disease. *Journal of Clinical Endocrinology and Metabolism* 1984;58:143–8.

15. Grande Villoria J, Macias Nunez JF, Miralles JM, De Castro del Pozo S, Tabernero Romo JM. Hyporeninemic hypoaldosteronism in diabetic patients with chronic renal failure. *American Journal of Nephrology* 1988;8:127–37.

16. Schindler AM, Sommers SC. Diabetic sclerosis of the renal juxtaglomerular apparatus. *Laboratory Investigation* 1966;15:877–84.

17. Sparaganza M. Hyporeninemic hypoaldosteronism with diabetic glomerulosclerosis. *Biochemical Medicine* 1975;14:93–103.

18. DeLeiva A, Christlieb AR, Melby JC, Graham CA, Day RP, Luetscher JA, Zager PG. Big renin and biosynthetic defect of aldosterone in diabetes mellitus. *New England Journal of Medicine* 1976;295:639–43.

19. Tan SY, Antonipillai I, Mulrow PJ. Inactive renin and prostaglandin E_2 production in hyporeninemic hypoaldosteronism. *Journal of Clinical Endocrinology and Metabolism* 1980;51:849–53.

20. Franken AAM, Derkx FHM, Man in't Veld AJ, Hop WCJ, van Rens GH, Peperkamp E, de Jong PTVM, Schalekamp MADH. High plasma prorenin in diabetes mellitus and its correlation with some complications. *Journal of Clinical Endocrinology and Metabolism* 1990;71:1008–15.

21. Perez GO, Lespier L, Jacobi J, Oster JR, Katz FH, Vaamonde CA, Fishman LM. Hyporeninemia and hypoaldosteronism in diabetes mellitus. *Archives of Internal Medicine* 1977;137:852–5.

22. Tuck ML, Sambhi MP, Levin L. Hyporeninemic hypoaldosteronism in diabetes mellitus. *Diabetes* 1979;28:237–41.

23. Misbin RI, Grant MB, Pecker MS, Atlas SA. Elevated levels of plasma prorenin (inactive renin) in diabetic and nondiabetic patients with autonomic dysfunction. *Journal of Clinical Endocrinology and Metabolism* 1987;64:964–8.

24. Bell GM, Bernstein RK, Laragh JH, Atlas SA, James GD, Pecker MS, Sealey JE. Increased plasma atrial natriuretic factor and reduced plasma renin in patients with poorly controlled diabetes mellitus. *Clinical Science* 1989;77:177–82.

25. Opocher G, Mantero F, Rocco S, Trevisan R, Fioretto P, Semplicini A, Morocutti A, Zanette G, Donadon V, Perico N, Giorato C, Carraro A, Remuzzi G, Nosadini R. Atrial natriuretic factor in hypertensive and normotensive insulin-dependent diabetics. *Journal of Hypertension* 1989;7 (suppl 6):S236–7.

26. O'Hare JP, Anderson JV, Millar ND, Dalton N, Tymms DJ, Bloom SR, Corrall RJM. Hormonal response to blood volume expansion in diabetic subjects with and without autonomic neuropathy. *Clinical Endocrinology* 1989;30:571–9.

27. Brunner HR, Baer L, Sealey JE, Ledingham JGG, Laragh JH. The influence of potassium administration and of potassium deprivation on plasma renin in normal and hypertensive subjects. *Journal of Clinical Investigation* 1970;49:2128–38.

28. Cooke CR, Horvath JS, Moore MA, Bledsoe T, Walker WG. Modulation of plasma aldosterone concentration by plasma potassium in anephric man in the absence of a change in potassium balance. *Journal of Clinical Investigation* 1973;52:3028–32.

29. Weidmann P, Reinhart R, Maxwell M, Rowe P, Coburn JW, Massry SG. Syndrome of hyporeninemic hypoaldosteronism and hyperkalemia in renal disease. *Journal of Endocrinology and Metabolism* 1973;36:965–77.

30. DeFronzo RA, Sherwin RS, Felig P, Bia M. Nonuremic diabetic hyperkalemia. *Archives of Internal Medicine* 1977;137:842–3.

31. Nadler JL, Lee FO, Hsueh W, Horton R. Evidence of prostacyclin deficiency in the syndrome of hyporeninemic hypoaldosteronism. *New England Journal of Medicine* 1986;314:1015–20.

32. Tan SY, Shapiro R, Franco R, Stockard H, Mulrow PJ. Indomethacin-induced prostaglandin inhibition with hyperkalemia. *Annals of Internal Medicine* 1979;90:783–5.

33. Franco–Saenz R, Suzuki S, Tan SY. Prostaglandins and renin production: A review. *Prostaglandins* 1980;20:1131–42.

34. Eriksson L–O, Sturfelt G, Thysell H, Wollheim FA. Effects of sulindac and naproxen on prostaglandin excretion in patients with impaired renal function and rheumatoid arthritis. *The American Journal of Medicine* 1990;89:313–21.

35. Campbell WB, Henrich WL. Endothelial factors in the regulation of renin release. *Kidney International* 1990;38:612–7.

36. Cozza EN, Gomez–Sanchez CE, Foecking MF, Chiou S. Endothelin binding to cultured calf adrenal zona glomerulosa cells and stimulation of aldosterone secretion. *Journal of Clinical Investigation* 1989;84:1032–5.

37. Kifor I, Moore TJ, Fallo F, Sperling E, Menachery A, Chiou C–Y, Williams GH. The effect of sodium intake on angiotensin content of the rat adrenal gland. *Journal of Clinical Endocrinology and Metabolism* 1991;128:1277–84.

38. Slaton Jr, PE, Schambelan M, Biglieri EG. Stimulation and suppression of aldosterone secretion in patients with an aldosterone-producing adenoma. *Journal of Clinical Endocrinology* 1969;29:239–50.

39. deChâtel R, Weidmann P, Flammer J, Ziegler WH, Beretta–Piccoli C, Vetter W, Reubi FC. Sodium, renin, aldosterone, catecholamines, and blood pressure in diabetes mellitus. *Kidney International* 1977;12:412–21.

40. Iwasaki R, Kigoshi T, Uchida K, Morimoto S. Plasma 18-hydroxycorticosterone and aldosterone responses to angiotensin II and corticotropin in diabetic patients with hyporeninemic and normoreninemic hypoaldosteronism. *Acta Endocrinologica* 1989;121:83–9.

41. Kater CE, Biglieri EG, Brust N, Chang B, Hirai J, Irony I. Stimulation and suppression of the mineralocorticoid hormones in normal subjects and adrenocortical disorders. *Endocrine Reviews* 1989;10:149–64.

42. Bravo EL, Dustan HP, Tarazi RC. Selective hypoaldosteronism despite prolonged pre- and postoperative hyperreninemia in primary aldosteronism. *Journal of Clinical Endocrinology and Metabolism* 1975;41:611–7.

43. Dluhy RG, Axelrod L, Underwood RH, Williams GH. Studies of the control of plasma aldosterone concentration in normal man: II. Effect of dietary potassium and acute potassium infusion. *Journal of Clinical Investigation* 1972;51:1950–7.

44. Deheneffe J, Cuesta V, Briggs JD, Brown JJ, Fraser R, Lever AF, Morton JJ, Robertson JIS, Tree M. Response of aldosterone and blood pressure to angiotensin II infusion in anephric man. *Circulation Research* 1976;39:183–90.

45. Tuck ML, Mayes DM. Mineralocorticoid biosynthesis in patients with hyporeninemic hypoaldosteronism. *Journal of Clinical Endocrinology and Metabolism* 1980;50:341–7.

46. Veldhuis JD, Melby JC. Isolated aldosterone deficiency in man: Acquired and inborn errors in the biosynthesis or action of aldosterone. *Endocrine Reviews* 1981;2:495–517.

47. Sowers JR, Beck FWJ, Waters BK, Barrett JD, Welch BG. Studies of renin activation and regulation of aldosterone and 18-hydroxycorticosterone biosynthesis in hyporeninemic hypoaldosteronism. *Journal of Clinical Endocrinology and Metabolism* 1985;61:60–7.

48. Sebastian A, Schambelan M, Lindenfeld S, Morris Jr RC. Amelioration of metabolic acidosis with fludrocortisone therapy in hyporeninemic hypoaldosteronism. *New England Journal of Medicine* 1977;297:576–83.

49. Hulter HN, Ilnicki LP, Harbottle JA, Sebastian A. Impaired renal H$^+$ secretion and NH$_3$ production in mineralocorticoid-deficient glucocorticoid-replete dogs. *American Journal of Physiology* 1977;232:F136–46.

50. Szylman P, Better OS, Chaimowitz C, Rosler A. Role of hyperkalemia in the metabolic acidosis of isolated hypoaldosteronism. *New England Journal of Medicine* 1976;294:361–5.

51. Sebastian A, Sutton JM, Hulter HN, Schambelan M, Poler SM. Effect of mineralocorticoid replacement therapy on renal acid–base homeostasis in adrenalectomized patients. *Kidney International* 1980;18:762–73.

52. Silva P, Brown RS, Epstein FH. Adaptation to potassium. *Kidney International* 1977;11:466–75.

53. Textor SC, Bravo EL, Fouad FM, Tarazi RC. Hyperkalemia in azotemic patients during angiotensin-converting enzyme inhibition and aldosterone reduction with captopril. *American Journal of Medicine* 1982;73:719–25.

54. Bosch JP, Godstein MH, Levitt MF, Kahn T. Effect of chronic furosemide administration on hydrogen and sodium excretion in the dog. *American Journal of Physiology* 1977;232:F397–404.

55. Chrousos GP, Vingerhoeds A, Brandon D, Eil C, Pugeat M, DeVroede M, Loriaux DL, Lipsett MB. Primary cortisol resistance in man. A glucocorticoid receptor-mediated disease. *Journal of Clinical Investigation* 1982;69:1261–9.

56. Stewart PM, Corrie JET, Shackleton HL, Edwards CRW. Syndrome of apparent mineralocorticoid excess. A defect in the cortisol–cortisone shuttle. *Journal of Clinical Investigation* 1988;82:340–9.

57. Armanini D, Scali M, Zennaro MC, Karbowiak I, Wallace C, Lewicka S, Vecsei P, Mantero F. The pathogenesis of pseudohyperaldosteronism from carbenoxolone. *Journal of Endocrinological Investigation* 1989;12:337–41.

58. Gordon RD. Syndrome of hypertension and hyperkalemia with normal glomerular filtration rate. *Hypertension* 1986;8:93–102.

59. Battle DC, Arruda JAL, Kurtzman NA. Hyperkalemic distal renal tubular acidosis associated with obstructive uropathy. *New England Journal of Medicine* 1981;304:373–80.

60. Morgan JM. Hyperkalemia and acidosis in lead nephropathy. *Southern Medical Journal* 1976;69:881–6.

61. Roll D, Licht A, Rösler A, Durst AL, Kleeman CR, Czaczkes JR. Transient hypoaldosteronism after renal allotransplantation. *Israel Journal of Medical Sciences* 1979;15:29–34.

62. Battle DC, Itsarayoungyuen K, Arruda JAL, Kurtzman NA. Hyperkalemic hyperchloremic metabolic acidosis in sickle cell hemoglobinopathies. *American Journal of Medicine* 1982;72:188–92.

63. Kalin MF, Poretsky L, Seres DS, Sumoff B. Hyporeninemic hypoaldosteronism associated with acquired immune deficiency syndrome. *American Journal of Medicine* 1987;82:1035–8.

64. Major P, Kuchel O, Boucher R, Nowaczynski W, Genest J. Selective hypopituitarism with severe hyponatremia and secondary hyporeninism. *Journal of Clinical Endocrinology and Metabolism* 1978;46:15–9.

65. Merriam GR, Baer L. Adrenocorticotropin deficiency: Correction of hyponatremia and hypoaldosteronism with chronic glucocorticoid therapy. *Journal of Clinical Endocrinology and Metabolism* 1980;50:10–4.

66. Rimmer JM, Horn JF, Gennari FJ. Hyperkalemia as a complication of drug therapy. *Archives of Internal Medicine* 1987;147:867–9.

67. Waal-Manning HJ. Metabolic effects of ß-adrenergic blockers. *Drugs* 1976;11 (suppl I):121–6.

68. Levesque H, Verdier S, Cailleux N, Elie–Legrand MC, Gancel A, Basuyau JP, Borg JY, Moore N, Courtois H. Low molecular weight heparins and hypoaldosteronism. *British Medical Journal* 1990;300:1437–8.

69. Petersen KC, Silberman H, Berne TV. Hyperkalaemia after cyclosporin therapy. *Lancet* 1984;i:1470.

70. Sakemi T, Ohchi N, Sanai T, Rikitake O, Maeda T. Captopril-induced metabolic acidosis with hyperkalemia. *American Journal of Nephrology* 1988;8:245–8.

71

THE RENIN–ANGIOTENSIN SYSTEM AND THE RESPONSE TO HEMORRHAGE

J IAN S ROBERTSON

EARLY STUDIES

Indications that stimulation of the RAS could be involved in the response of the animal to hemorrhage date from at least half a century ago. Early work showed that after a large acute bleed, dog plasma developed the ability to stimulate smooth muscle *in vitro* [1,2], and to increase blood pressure when injected into nephrectomized dogs [3–5]. Although, as these investigators recognized, their methods were neither specific nor quantitative, it was tentatively suggested that acute hemorrhage stimulated the release of renin from the kidney.

Ziegler and Gross [6], using a more advanced isovolemic cross-circulation technique, demonstrated a 3–4-fold increase in circulating renin-like activity, 10–15 minutes after hemorrhage in the rat.

STUDIES WITH MORE SPECIFIC RENIN ASSAY

Using a more specific assay method for plasma renin concentration (PRC), which assessed together both active and inactive renin, Brown *et al* [7] showed, in pentobarbitone-anesthetized dogs that were bled 26–28ml/kg over some 15 minutes, a marked immediate rise in PRC varying from 50 to 500%. After reinfusing the shed blood, PRC fell again, but did not regain prebleed values (Fig. 71.1a). Hemorrhage of this magnitude was usually, but not in all animals, accompanied by a fall in mean arterial pressure. Control dogs bled only 5ml/kg showed neither a change in systemic arterial pressure nor a rise in PRC (Fig. 71.1b). With bleeding intermediate in extent (12ml/kg over 15 minutes), changes in blood pressure and PRC were small and inconsistent.

In the same paper [7], these workers reported that seven unanesthetized human volunteers bled 400–500 ml (4.8–6.7ml/kg) over 5–11 minutes showed no subsequent change in blood

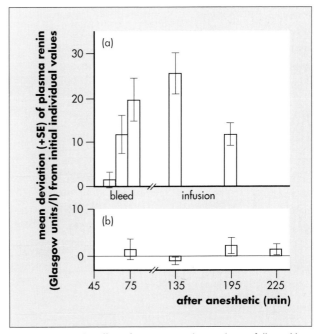

Fig. 71.1 (a) The effect of acute severe hemorrhage, followed by infusion of the shed blood, on plasma renin concentration (PRC) measured in Glasgow units/l, in an experimental group of dogs bled 26–28ml/kg. (b) The variation in PRC in a control group of dogs bled 5ml/kg. The columns refer to the mean deviation for the group from the initial individual levels, and the bars indicate the standard errors. Modified from Brown JJ *et al* [7].

pressure or PRC either immediately in recumbency or after 24–72 hours of normal activity.

Goetz *et al* [8] confirmed that normal adults who were bled an average of 485ml did not show a change in blood pressure, heart rate, plasma renin activity (PRA), or plasma vasopressin.

Hesse *et al* [9] also found that in man, hemorrhage of 400–655ml over 15 minutes did not alter arterial pressure, although right atrial pressure fell. Plasma renin activity was unchanged in seven and slightly increased in two of the nine subjects they studied.

Bleeding to a similar modest extent in man was, in contrast, found by Skillman *et al* (10), to raise PRA; however, unlike Brown *et al* [7] who studied the effects of hemorrhage immediately, and again after 24 or 72 hours, Skillman *et al* [10] examined PRA four hours after the removal of blood.

There is little doubt that massive bleeding in man can elevate circulating renin values. Brown *et al* [7] also reported on a patient who sustained a large hemorrhage from a duodenal ulcer and was found to have a PRC some four times normal; PRC returned to the normal range following transfusion of 3.3 liters of blood over two days (Fig. 71.2).

RANGE OF SPECIES SHOWING THIS PHENOMENON

The response of the RAS to hemorrhage has been demonstrated in a range of mammalian species, including man [7–10], monkey [11], dog [7,12,13], cat [14], rat [15–18], pig [19], sheep [20,21], rabbit [22–24], and guinea pig [25].

By contrast, in the freshwater turtle Pseudemys scripta, Cipolle and Zehr [26] were unable to demonstrate an increase

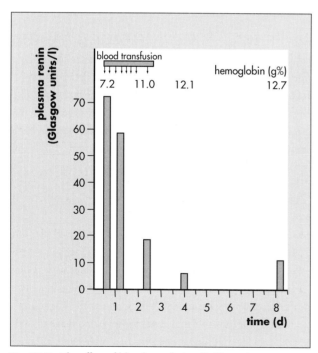

Fig. 71.2 The effect of blood transfusion (3.3l) on plasma renin concentration in a patient after a large hemorrhage from the gut. Renin is measured in Glasgow units/l. Modified from Brown JJ *et al* [7].

in plasma renin even after bleeding up to 60% of estimated blood volume, when arterial pressure had fallen to around 50% of control values. It was concluded that unlike all mammals tested, these turtles do not possess an intrarenal baroreceptor mechanism in the control of renin secretion.

EFFECT OF RATE OF HEMORRHAGE

Claybaugh and Share [27] paid especial attention to the rate of bleeding in anesthetized dogs. Hemorrhage at the rate of 0.42ml/kg/min to a total blood loss of 2.1ml/kg led to significant increases in PRA. By contrast, slower bleeding, at the rate of 0.28ml/kg, but to the same total extent, caused only a transitory rise in PRA.

EFFECT OF FLUID REPLACEMENT

Weber *et al* [28] showed that in the rabbit also, bleeding to a cumulative loss of 6ml/kg (9% of estimated total blood volume) led to a progressive rise in PRA to some three times control values. Replacement of withdrawn plasma by simultaneous infusion of a protein–saline plasma substitute completely prevented the rise in PRA.

STUDIES WITH ASSAY OF ANGIOTENSINS I AND II

Experiments conducted in anesthetized dogs, and employing various assay methods, showed that peripheral blood levels of Ang I and Ang II were increased following hemorrhage [29–33].

CONCURRENT MEASUREMENTS OF RENIN AND ANGIOTENSIN II

In a series of experiments in anesthetized dogs [13], it was demonstrated that with a severe acute hemorrhage there were concurrent increases in arterial PRC, Ang II concentration, and the generation rate of Ang II, with a return towards control values after reinfusion of the shed blood (Figs. 71.3 and 71.4). Inflation of an intra-aortic balloon situated just above the renal arteries so as to reduce renal arterial pressure produced similar concurrent increases in PRC and Ang II (Fig. 71.4).

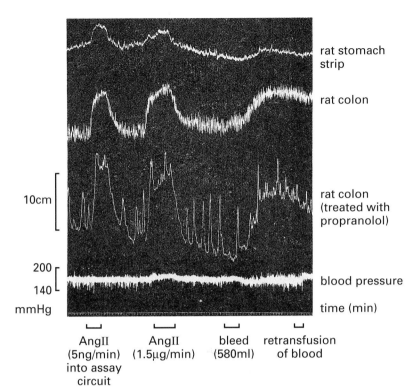

10cm

200
140
mmHg

rat stomach
strip

rat colon

rat colon
(treated with
propranolol)

blood pressure

time (min)

AngII   AngII   bleed   retransfusion
(5ng/min)   (1.5μg/min) (580ml)   of blood
into assay
circuit

Fig. 71.3 The responses of three blood-bathed tissues to Ang II infused at 5ng/min for five minutes into the assay circuit (rate of flow 15ml/min), Ang II intravenously infused at 1.5μg/min for nine minutes into a whole dog (29kg), 580ml bleed from an artery for 5.5 minutes, and retransfusion of shed blood over two minutes. The tissues used were a rat stomach strip and two rat colons (one being treated with propranolol). Arterial blood pressure was also recorded. Modified from Brown JJ *et al* [13].

RENIN SECRETION AND METABOLIC CLEARANCE RATES

As Brown *et al* [7] were at pains to emphasize, while the rise in PRC with bleeding probably indicates an increase in renin secretion rate, this is not necessarily the case; other influences, such as diminished plasma volume, and reduced renin clearance, could contribute (see *Chapter 24*).

Beaty *et al* [34] measured renal blood flow and hence were able to compute renin secretion rate. They showed that the renal secretion rate of renin was increased, accompanying the rise in PRA, during graded hemorrhagic hypotension in the dog.

Johnson *et al* [35] studied the hepatic clearance of renin in conscious dogs before and following hemorrhages of 20ml/kg and 30ml/kg body weight. No significant changes in the hepatic extraction of renin or in the hepatic clearance of renin were observed after a 20ml/kg bleed. Hemorrhage of 30ml/kg, however, resulted in a significant decrease in hepatic plasma flow from mean values of 30 to 17ml/min/kg. At the same time, hepatic extraction of renin increased from 33 to 104ng/min/kg body weight, while the hepatic clearance of renin decreased from 6.5 to 3.4ml/min/kg.

Therefore, the increases of circulating renin with hemorrhage receive contributions both from a rise in the renal secretion rate and a fall in hepatic clearance.

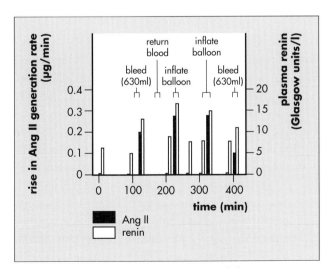

Fig. 71.4 The changes in the concentration of plasma renin measured in Glasgow units/l and the rate of generation of Ang II, associated with arterial bleeds of 630ml, the return of blood, and the inflation of an aortic balloon just above the renal arteries to reduce arterial blood pressure. Modified from Brown JJ *et al* [13].

RESPONSE OF SEVERAL COMPONENTS OF THE RENIN SYSTEM TO HEMORRHAGE

In the anesthetized dog, Michailov et al [33] detected, after acute hemorrhage, 3–4-fold increases in PRC, PRA, Ang I, and Ang II. Concurrently, plasma ACE activity decreased, while circulating Ang II degrading enzymes were unchanged.

Beaty et al [34], also studying anesthetized dogs, confirmed that hemorrhagic hypotension raised PRA, while plasma angiotensinogen (renin substrate) was unchanged. Infusion of the Ang II antagonist saralasin, however, lowered plasma angiotensinogen progressively, while intravenous administration of Ang II restored plasma angiotensinogen concentrations. These experiments were interpreted, inter alia, as confirming the importance of Ang II in stimulating hepatic release of angiotensinogen [34, 36,37].

Barrett et al [38] assayed separately, plasma levels of active, inactive, and total renin in the rat after applying various stimuli, including hemorrhage. Although active renin was increased following hemorrhage plus pentobarbital anesthesia, there was no detectable concomitant change in plasma inactive renin levels.

Richards et al [23] showed by contrast, in the rabbit, that both active and inactive renin increased in plasma in response to hemorrhage, and that this stimulus did not change the relative proportion of the two forms. After ligation of the renal blood vessels, neither form of renin increased in response to bleeding.

EFFECT OF ANESTHESIA

Zimpfer et al [39] examined the effects of graded hemorrhage in dogs either anesthetized with pentobarbital or unanesthetized. Anesthesia did not affect basal hemodynamic measurements appreciably. However, with 30ml/kg blood loss under anesthesia, the reductions of blood pressure and cardiac output were more profound, and the increase in iliac arterial resistance was less than in awake dogs bled to the same extent. The response of the RAS was not affected by anesthesia, but the sympathoadrenal response was depressed.

EFFECT OF PRIOR SALT RESTRICTION

Kopelman et al [12] demonstrated that in conscious dogs, prior salt restriction led to much greater rises in PRA (and catecholamines) after bleeding. The fall in blood pressure and the increase in heart rate were the same in the two states of salt loading.

The studies of Johnson et al [35] referred to above, showed that sodium depletion in the conscious dog caused, as did bleeding, a decrease in hepatic plasma flow, an increase in hepatic extraction of renin, and a fall in hepatic clearance of renin.

EFFECT OF INHIBITORS OF THE RENIN–ANGIOTENSIN SYSTEM

The effect of the Ang II antagonist saralasin on the response to hemorrhage was studied by Cornish et al [11] in chronically instrumented conscious monkeys. Seven animals (four intact and three with renal denervation) were bled so as to lower mean arterial pressure to 50–60mmHg; blood pressure was then allowed to rise spontaneously to values around 80–90mmHg. The infusion of saralasin reduced blood pressure once more to the immediate posthemorrhage levels. By contrast, a vasopressin antagonist had no effect on the blood-pressure recovery.

Freeman et al [40] administered the Ang II antagonist saralasin intravenously to conscious dogs that had more than doubled their PRA and had established a new level of arterial pressure following hemorrhage of 20ml/kg body weight. Infusion of saralasin caused an initial transient rise in arterial pressure which was followed by a substantial further fall. The data were interpreted as strongly supporting the concept of the RAS as an important determinant of arterial pressure during hemorrhage.

Kopelman et al [12] administered the converting enzyme inhibitor teprotide to conscious dogs either on a normal or low salt intake and bled 30ml/kg. As mentioned above, the salt-deprived dogs had bigger rises in PRA and catecholamines following hemorrhage. Teprotide caused substantially greater falls in blood pressure in the salt-deprived bled dogs. Moreover, converting enzyme inhibition blunted the expected rise in catecholamines and heart rate after hemorrhage.

Similarly, following hemorrhage in anesthetized rats, Zerbe et al [17] observed that captopril administration almost completely blocked the spontaneous recovery of blood pressure.

Obika found [18], in the rat, that neither bilateral nephrectomy nor the administration of a converting enzyme inhibitor affected recovery in the first 10 minutes after hemorrhage. Thereafter, recovery was markedly suppressed. Thus, the late recovery requires the presence of the kidneys and depends on the RAS.

In fetal sheep, Iwamoto and Rudolph [41] noted that when bleeding was performed with prior saralasin infusion, blood pressure fell to lower absolute values than in the absence of saralasin.

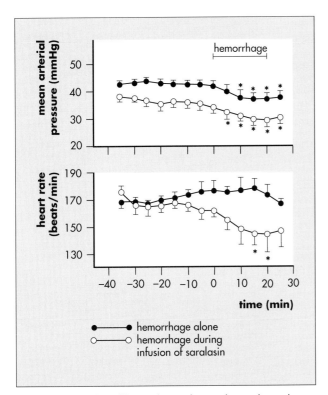

Fig. 71.5 The effect of hemorrhage alone or hemorrhage during infusion of saralasin, on mean arterial pressure and heart rate in fetal sheep. The data are expressed as mean ± SE from 10 experiments on 10 fetal sheep. The time is expressed as minutes relative to the onset of hemorrhage at time zero. *P<0.05, significantly less than all values before hemorrhage. Modified from Iwamoto H and Rudolph AM [41].

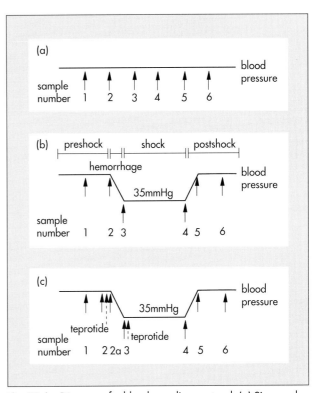

Fig. 71.6 Diagram of a blood sampling protocol. (a) Six samples taken from a control group of dogs (group 1) at hourly intervals, the first taken at least 45 minutes after completion of surgery. (b) Six samples taken from the untreated bled group (group 2): basal (1); prehemorrhage (2); end of hemorrhage, taken within five minutes after blood pressure reached 35mmHg (3); end of shock (4); end of retransfusion (5); and one hour post-transfusion (6). (c) Seven samples taken from the converting enzyme inhibitor-treated and bled group (group 3): basal (1); at five minutes before SQ 20881 (teprotide) injection (2); five minutes postadministration of teprotide and prehemorrhage (2a); end of hemorrhage (3); end of shock (4); end of retransfusion (5); and one hour post-transfusion (6). Modified from Morton JJ et al [32].

However, when saralasin was given, this was due mainly to a reduction of blood pressure before the bleed; the magnitude of the posthemorrhagic drop in pressure was similar with or without saralasin (Fig. 71.5). Heart rate, which was unchanged by bleeding in the absence of saralasin, fell markedly with hemorrhage after saralasin administration (Fig. 71.5).

Morton *et al* [32] studied the hormonal responses in anesthetized dogs subjected to hemorrhagic reduction of mean arterial pressure to the range 35–40mmHg for 30 minutes, followed subsequently by retransfusion of the shed blood so as to restore blood pressure. Experiments were performed both with and without administration of the ACE inhibitor teprotide (Fig. 71.6). Controlled hemorrhagic hypotension led to substantial increases in plasma Ang II concentration (Fig. 71.7). When teprotide was given, the increase in Ang II was prevented, while the circulating concentrations of the precursor peptide Ang I were very high (Fig. 71.8). Of 15 dogs subjected to hemorrhagic

hypotension in the absence of the converting enzyme inhibitor, five died before retransfusion was completed (four of cardiac failure and one of cardiac arrhythmia), whereas none of the 10 dogs in the teprotide-treated group died. Morton *et al* [32] ascribed this protection to abrogation of adverse cardiovascular effects of Ang II, as is discussed further below. It should be emphasized in this connection that blood pressure during hemorrhage was, in these experiments, strictly controlled by regulation of blood loss and by retransfusion.

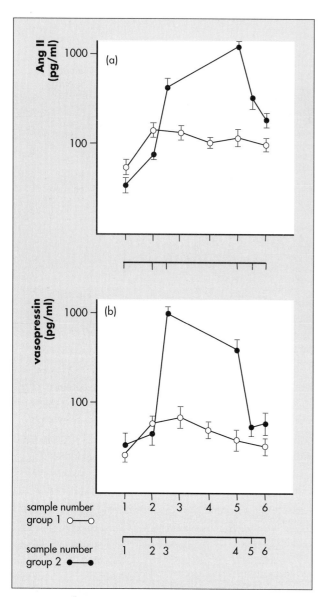

Fig. 71.7 Changes in the plasma concentration of (a) Ang II and (b) vasopressin in the control group of dogs (group 1 discussed in *Fig. 71.6*) and in the untreated bled group of dogs (group 2 discussed in *Fig. 71.6*). The bars indicate ± SEM. Ordinate values are plotted logarithmically. Modified from Morton JJ *et al* [32].

Observations in several respects supportive of those of Morton *et al* [32] were reported by Trachte and Lefer [14], who examined the effects of hemorrhage in pentobarbital-anesthetized cats. Cats that were bled showed a sharp fall in arterial pressure, which rebounded after reinfusion of the shed blood (Fig. 71.9). Blood pressure then declined again in both groups, but this late fall was significantly less in cats given saralasin (Fig. 71.9). Trachte and Lefer concluded [14] that Ang II may in some way

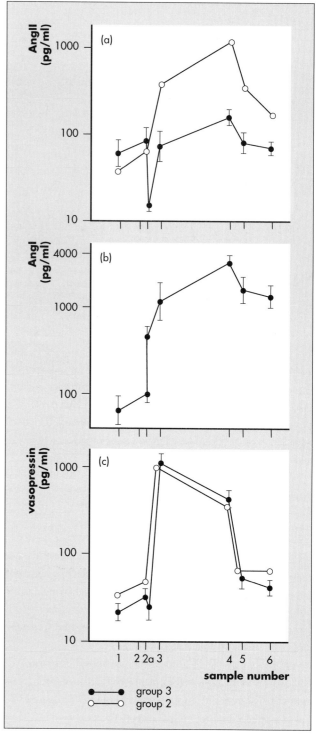

Fig. 71.8 Changes in the plasma concentration of (a) Ang II, (b) Ang I, and (c) vasopressin in the converting enzyme inhibitor-treated group of dogs (group 3 discussed in *Fig. 71.6*). Group 2 (discussed in *Fig. 71.6*) is shown for comparison. The bars indicate ± SEM. Ordinate values are plotted logarithmically. Modified from Morton JJ *et al* [32].

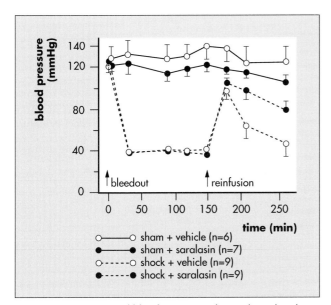

Fig. 71.9 Mean arterial blood pressure in hemorrhaged and sham-shocked cats. Sham-shocked cats exhibited stable pressures over a 4.5-hour experiment. Hemorrhaged cats experienced a sharp decline in pressures after bleedout, which rebounded after reinfusion. Pressures then declined in both shocked groups but this decline was significantly reduced (P<0.05) in the saralasin-treated cats, the final values being 48 and 81mmHg with vehicle and saralasin treatment, respectively. Drug or vehicle infusions were started immediately after time zero. Values are expressed as mean ± SEM. Modified from Trachte GJ and Lefer AM [14].

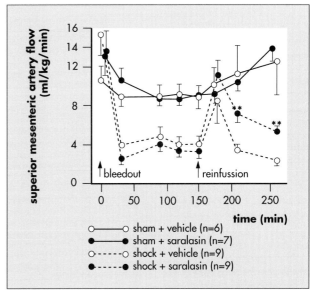

Fig. 71.10 The effect of saralasin on superior mesenteric artery flow. Sham-shocked cats showed minor variations in flow, with no values differing significantly from the initial values. Hemorrhaged animals showed large decreases in superior mesenteric artery flow during oligemia, the values returning to sham-shocked levels after reinfusion. Splanchnic perfusion then decreased again, but saralasin significantly inhibited this reduction of flow (**P<0.005) at 210 and 270 minutes. Modified from Trachte GJ and Lefer AM [14].

impair posthemorrhagic recovery, and that this impairment is corrected by giving saralasin. Superior mesenteric artery blood flow was greater after hemorrhage and reinfusion in the cats given saralasin (Fig. 71.10), while plasma amino-nitrogen concentration was lower.

Averill *et al* [42] demonstrated that baroreceptor-denervated dogs subjected to hypotensive hemorrhage responded with a marked rise in PRA; infusion of the Ang II antagonist saralasin severely lowered blood pressure. These authors concluded that intact baroreceptor reflexes are not essential for the renin response to hemorrhage, but that dogs subjected to baroreceptor denervation are especially dependent on Ang II for the maintenance of arterial pressure after bleeding.

Henrich *et al* [43], studying hemorrhagic hypotension in anesthetized dogs, administered a sarcosine–glycine Ang II analog antagonist into one renal artery. They found that such Ang II antagonism significantly attenuated the posthemorrhagic reductions of both glomerular filtration rate (GFR) and renal blood

flow. This renal protection by the Ang II antagonist was enhanced by concomitant renal denervation.

Katoh *et al* [22] studied the relative importance for the recovery of arterial pressure after acute hemorrhage in the rabbit of four physiological mechanisms: the sinoaortic baroreflex, the vagally mediated baroreflex, vasopressin, and the RAS. Angiotensin II formation was prevented by giving teprotide. They concluded that for the restoration of blood pressure after rapid, mild bleeding, the arterial baroreflex system is far more important than the vagally mediated cardiopulmonary baroreflex, vasopressin, or the RAS.

Schadt and Gaddis [24] evaluated the role of the RAS following hemorrhage in the rabbit using the ACE inhibitor captopril. As in the early studies in dog and man described above [7], the change in PRA in the rabbit after a nonhypotensive bleed was not statistically significant. However, after a more severe hemorrhage, which lowered mean arterial pressure to less than 40mmHg, PRA increased six-fold. In rabbits pretreated with captopril, the blood loss required to decrease mean arterial pressure to below 40mmHg was some 25% less than in untreated animals.

In experiments in the rat, Zerbe et al [17] found that spontaneous recovery of blood pressure after hemorrhage was almost completely blocked by the administration of captopril. This failure of recovery was seen despite increases in plasma catecholamines and vasopressin, which were similar to, or as great as, those that occurred in the absence of captopril. The authors also therefore concluded that increased Ang II generation is not essential for the hemorrhagic stimulation of vasopressin or cathecholamines.

All of these studies are compatible with the concept of the RAS as a critical component of homeostasis following hypotensive hemorrhage. However, the experiments of Morton et al [32] and of Trachte and Lefer [14] also indicate some adverse effects of high plasma Ang II concentrations when blood is reinfused after a large bleed. These latter unwanted actions are discussed further below.

INTERACTION OF THE RENIN SYSTEM WITH OTHER HORMONES FOLLOWING HEMORRHAGE

ALDOSTERONE

Observations that acute hemorrhage was followed by increases in aldosterone secretion in hypophysectomized animals [44–47] were critical in establishing the link between the RAS and aldosterone (see Chapters 1 and 33). Nevertheless, after bilateral nephrectomy, which prevents an increase in PRA, hemorrhage can still cause an increase in plasma aldosterone, emphasizing that in the intact animal, factors other than the RAS, including for example, corticotropin (ACTH), can contribute to the response of aldosterone to hemorrhage [48].

CORTICOTROPHIN AND CORTISOL

Lilly et al [49] studied chronically instrumented conscious dogs, which were bled 10% on two occasions five minutes apart. Plasma renin activity and Ang II were both increased as early as four minutes after each hemorrhage, to a small but definitely greater extent after the second bleed. Corticotropin did not change measurably after the first bleed, but was increased after the second. Cortisol was elevated after each hemorrhage, to a greater extent after the second bleed.

VASOPRESSIN

The detailed experiments of Morton et al [32] conducted in anesthetized dogs, have already been referred to above. Controlled hemorrhagic hypotension led to substantial rises in plasma vasopressin as well as in Ang II. Although the timing of these changes was similar, the patterns of the increase in the two peptides were not strictly parallel (see Fig. 71.7) Moreover, when the increase in Ang II was prevented by the administration of teprotide, the course and pattern of the rise in plasma vasopressin was virtually unaltered (see Fig. 71.8). Thus, an elevation of plasma Ang II was not, in this model, necessary to effect an increase in plasma vasopressin in response to hemorrhage. These considerations do not exclude the possibility that when plasma Ang II is permitted to rise after a bleed, the circulating concentration may sometimes be sufficient to contribute to the enhancement of vasopressin secretion [50]; if this is the case, however, when Ang II is deleted, other mechanisms are recruited so as to achieve the same vasopressin response.

Claybaugh and Share likewise observed [27], in experiments already mentioned earlier, that although rapid bleeding in anesthetized dogs to a total blood loss of 2.1ml/kg caused an increase in PRA, this did not occur with a slower bleed (Fig. 71.11). By contrast, plasma vasopressin increased similarly with both rates of blood loss (Fig. 71.12). Thus, the increase in vasopressin was independent both of the speed of bleeding and of PRA, and was considered to be a consequence of changes in left atrial pressure.

Wang et al, studying conscious dogs [51], found that hemorrhage caused increases in vasopressin which were prevented by prior cardiac denervation. By contrast, there was no evidence that cardiac receptors played a dominant role in mediating increases in renin during hemorrhage; indeed, bleeding to 30ml/kg caused greater increases in PRA in cardiac-denervated dogs than in sham-operated dogs.

The studies of Lilly et al [49], also mentioned above, showed that in conscious dogs bled by 10% on two occasions five minutes apart, plasma vasopressin increased on both occasions but to a greater extent on the second. These authors invoked the rise in vasopressin as possibly mediating the observed increase in ACTH.

In rats of the Brattleboro strain, which have defective vasopressin secretion, vasopressin was undetectable both before and after hemorrhage [52], although both PRA and epinephrine rose to a greater extent than in normal rats bled to the same extent. The recovery of blood pressure after bleeding was subnormal in

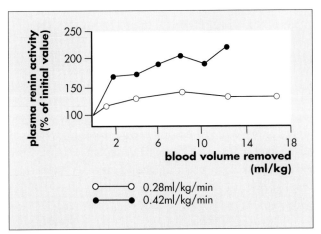

Fig. 71.11 The effect of continual bleeding on plasma renin activity (PRA) in the dog. The 0.42-ml/kg/min rate of blood withdrawal produced a significant elevation in PRA when cumulative hemorrhage was 2.1 (P<0.01). Plasma renin activity remained elevated for the remainder of the experiment (P<0.01). In the group with the slower rate of hemorrhage, PRA was significantly elevated only at a cumulative hemorrhage of 8.4ml/kg (P<0.05). Modified from Claybaugh JR et al [27].

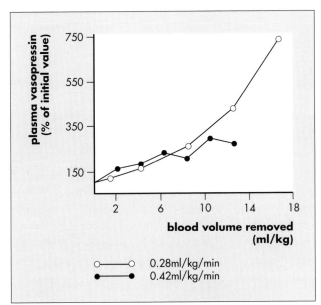

Fig. 71.12 The effect of continuous hemorrhage on plasma vasopressin concentration. Plasma titers of vasopressin were higher than initial values in the group of dogs bled at 0.28ml/kg/min when cumulative hemorrhage was 4.2 (P<0.05), 8.4, 12.6, and 16.8 (P<0.01), and in groups bled at 0.42ml/kg/min when cumulative hemorrhage was 2.1 (P<0.05), 4.2, 6.3, 8.4, 10.5, and 12.6 (P<0.01). Modified from Claybaugh JR et al [27].

the vasopressin-deficient animals, an abnormality attributed directly to their lack of this vasoactive peptide and not to any impairment of the sympathetic or renin systems.

Feuerstein *et al* [53] provided evidence that in the rat, the anterolateral third ventricle is a site responsible for the integration of sympathetic pressor pathways and of vasopressin secretion in response to Ang II. Nevertheless, in rats with experimental lesions of the anterolateral third ventricle, plasma catecholamines, Ang II, and vasopressin responses were unchanged 24 hours after bleeding, although early mortality was higher. It was concluded that the anterolateral third ventricle in the rat is important for recuperation and survival after acute hemorrhage, but via mechanisms unrelated to the sympathetic nervous system, the RAS, or vasopressin.

The balance of evidence indicates that recruitment of vasopressin is a component following hemorrhage which is largely independent of the RAS. Although in some circumstances the RAS may well comprise one stimulus to the secretion of vasopressin, it appears not to be an obligatory one. If the vasopressin response to bleeding is deficient, recovery is accordingly impaired, while other hormonal defences, including the recruitment of catecholamines and the RAS, need to be more active.

CATECHOLAMINES

In the dog, activation of the RAS with hemorrhage was found to be accompanied by a rise in plasma epinephrine and norepinephrine [12,54].

The rise in PRA after hemorrhage in conscious sheep was followed similarly by increases in both plasma epinephrine and norepinephrine [20]. The increase in PRA began earlier than the rise in circulating concentrations of epinephrine and norepinephrine; the maximal elevation in all three occurred near the end of blood withdrawal.

Angiotensin II is necessary for the unimpaired adrenal reflex secretion of catecholamines after hemorrhage in the dog; this is apparently achieved by a central mechanism [54]. The adrenal medullary response to hemorrhage *in vivo* is greatly attenuated by administration of the Ang II antagonist saralasin [54].

Lightman *et al* [15] observed that both PRA and epinephrine were markedly increased in the rat by hemorrhage (5ml/kg). No increase in plasma norepinephrine was seen. Lesions of the dorsal noradrenergic pathway in the midbrain, which had already been shown to attenuate the vasopressin response to hypovolemia [16], were also found to prevent the post-hemorrhagic rise in both PRA and epinephrine.

In rats of the Brattleboro strain, which are deficient in vasopressin, both plasma epinephrine and PRA were found to be higher than in normal rats before hemorrhage, and to increase to a greater extent after bleeding [52]. Thus, as already mentioned, in the absence of vasopressin, the renin and catecholamine responses to hemorrhage appear especially important in defending against hypotension.

ATRIAL NATRIURETIC FACTOR

Experiments in anesthetized dogs [55] have provided evidence that circulating atrial natriuretic factor (ANF) is, as predicted, significantly reduced in hemorrhagic hypotension. Activation of the RAS in this circumstance is independent of the presence or absence of circulating ANF.

VASOACTIVE INTESTINAL PEPTIDE

Vasoactive intestinal peptide (VIP) has been shown to be capable of increasing plasma renin in several species, including dog and man [56,57]. However, following hemorrhage sufficient to cause a rise in PRA, VIP did not measurably increase in the dog. Thus, in this situation, VIP did not appear to be responsible for renin release, at least via a humoral pathway.

PROSTAGLANDINS

Feuerstein et al [58] have shown that the administration of prostacyclin to rats subjected to severe bleeding can aid recuperation and improve survival. The available data suggest that the beneficial effects of prostacyclin may be achieved by a combination of stimulation of the sympathoadrenal axis, and of vasopressin and renin secretion. These workers have, notwithstanding, demonstrated that prostacyclin effected improvement of survival following severe hemorrhage in rats in the absence of overt hemodynamic or sympathetic effects.

Henrich et al [43] concluded that the renal ischemic effects of the RAS during hemorrhagic hypotension are usually modulated by renal prostaglandins.

ENDORPHINS

Injection of naloxone during acute hemorrhagic hypotension in the rabbit did not affect the changes in PRA [24]. It was, however, demonstrated in the guinea pig that β-endorphin inhibits the centrally mediated pressor action of Ang II, and that naloxone prevents this effect [25]. Naloxone indeed reverses hemorrhagic hypotension in the conscious guinea pig [25]. This beneficial effect of naloxone is impeded by the administration of either captopril or saralasin, indicating the involvement of Ang II in the response.

ANGIOTENSIN II-INDUCED LESIONS IN THE HEART, KIDNEY, AND EYE WITH HEMORRHAGE

As discussed earlier, Morton et al [32], with controlled hemorrhagic hypotension in the dog, found that prevention of the rise in circulating Ang II by administering teprotide, protected against cardiac failure and arrhythmia on retransfusion. They speculated that these benefits might have been a result of limitation of Ang II-induced myocardial necrotic lesions [59] (see *Chapter 40*). As emphasized by Kremer et al [59], and discussed further in *Chapter 40*, a maintained or elevated systemic arterial pressure and/or ventricular work load seem to be requisite components of the genesis of these myocardial lesions. Arterial pressure was carefully controlled in the experiments of Morton et al [32], and thus could have remained sufficiently high to permit the development of Ang II-mediated ventricular lesions.

As described in some detail above, Trachte and Lefer [14] found in cats that recovery from posthemorrhagic shock was better when saralasin was given. These authors also speculated that, in part, this might have been due to minimizing the extent of Ang II-induced myocardial lesions [58].

In the face of hemorrhagic hypotension, the renal circulation is diminished at an early stage; renal function is temporarily expendable when more vital organs such as the brain are threatened. In such circumstances of reduced renal blood flow, activation of the RAS can serve for a time to sustain GFR and urea excretion [60] (see *Chapters 21, 26, 55, 76*, and *88*). Excessive activation of the RAS can, however, lead to acute circulatory renal failure (see *Chapters 40* and *56*). Experiments in the dog have shown that local intrarenal administration of an Ang II antagonist can moderate the fall in renal blood flow and glomerular filtration which occur with a large bleed [43]. Thus, with correction of hemorrhagic hypotension, antagonists of the RAS might be expected to minimize the risk of ischemic kidney damage. However, the administration of such agents if the general circulation were still deficient would, although improving the renal blood supply, risk imperilling more immediately, vital organs such as the heart or brain.

Hemorrhagic hypotension in man can be associated with retinal hemorrhages, exudates, and papilledema. Optic atrophy and blindness may follow [61]. Pears and Pickering found that these ocular lesions were not unusual after a major gastrointestinal bleed [61]. They speculated that the rarity of their recognition was a consequence of the unfamiliarity of gastroenterologists with the ophthalmoscope, and they recommended that the deficiency would be remedied if these specialists carried (and regularly used) such instruments. Ophthalmoscopically, the posthemorrhagic lesions are indistinguishable from those of malignant hypertension, and this has suggested a common pathogenesis [61]. One obvious feature often present in both circumstances is elevation of circulating renin and hence Ang II. The possible role of Ang II in causing or exacerbating arterial lesions in the malignant phase of hypertension is discussed in some detail in *Chapters 40* and *60*. While such an aggravating role of Ang II is considered to be a distinct possibility in the malignant phase, if so, it apparently requires to be combined with raised arterial pressure to produce these effects. A raised blood pressure is notably absent after severe hemorrhage. If therefore, Ang II does contribute to the retinal lesions that follow severe hemorrhage, this is achieved without the involvement of systemic hypertension. However, it is possible that in man, as in the dog [32] and cat [14], blood transfusion following hemorrhage may provoke some unwanted effects when the RAS is already stimulated.

ROLE OF RENIN IN THE DEFENCE AGAINST HEMORRHAGE

The evidence summarized in this chapter has pointed to a critical role of the RAS in the defence of the organism against hemorrhagic hypotension. This defence is achieved via multiple actions of Ang II, including most prominently, the direct pressor effect, stimulation of secretion of aldosterone and possibly vasopressin, and facilitation of the sympathetic nervous system and catecholamines. Other routes by which the adverse consequences of hemorrhage are countered by the RAS include an increase in splanchnic arterial resistance [62]; increased jejunal ion and water reabsorption [63]; and renal cortical vasoconstriction [60,64]. Although less well documented, the effects of Ang II in promoting the ingestion of water and salt (see *Chapter 32*), will support this multifaceted reaction. While the secretion of ANF will almost invariably be suppressed in circumstances of threatened or extant hemorrhagic hypotension, the responses of the RAS can be fully mounted even in the presence of ANF [55].

The extreme vulnerability of these defences to administration of antagonists of the RAS [11,12,17,18,24,40,65] re-emphasizes the central importance of the response of the RAS to hemorrhage for the survival of the threatened animal. Even so, there are a few contrary disturbing hints that a hyperactive RAS may cause some adverse effects on the renal and splanchnic circulations, the heart, and the eye when blood is transfused after a large bleed [14,32,43,61], These aspects deserve further critical evaluation.

REFERENCES

1. Sapirstein LA, Ogden E, Southard FD. Renin-like substance in blood after hemorrhage. *Proceedings of the Society for Experimental Biology and Medicine* 1941;48:505–8.

2. Collins DA, Hamilton AS. Changes in the renin–angiotensin system in hemorrhagic shock. *American Journal of Physiology* 1944;140:499–512.

3. Hamilton AS, Collins DA. The homeostatic role of a renal humoral mechanism in hemorrhage and shock. *American Journal of Physiology* 1942;136:275–84.

4. Huidobro F, Braun-Menendez E. The secretion of renin by the intact kidney. *American Journal of Physiology* 1942;137:47–55.

5. Dexter L, Frank HA, Haynes FW, Altschule MD. The effect of hemorrhagic shock on the concentration of renin and hypertensinogen in the plasma of unanesthetized dogs. *Journal of Clinical Investigation* 1943;22:847–52.

6. Ziegler M, Gross F. Effect of blood volume changes on renin-like activity in blood. *Proceedings of the Society for Experimental Biology and Medicine* 1964;116:774–8.

7. Brown JJ, Davies DL, Lever AF, Robertson JIS, Verniory A. The effect of acute haemorrhage in the dog and man on plasma renin concentration. *Journal of Physiology* 1966;182:649–63.

8. Goetz KL, Bond GC, Smith WE. Effect of moderate hemorrhage in humans on plasma ADH and renin. *Proceedings of the Society for Experimental Biology and Medicine* 1974;145:277–80.

9. Hesse B, Nielsen I, Hansen JF. The effect of reduction in blood volume on plasma renin activity in man. *Clinical Science* 1975;49:515–7.

10. Skillman JJ, Lauler DP, Hickler RB, Lyons JH, Olson JE, Ball MR, Moore FD. Hemorrhage in normal man: Effect on renin, cortisol, aldosterone, and urine composition. *Annals of Surgery* 1967;166:865–85.

11. Cornish KG, Barazanji MW, Iaffaldano R. Neural and hormonal control of blood pressure in conscious monkeys. *American Journal of Physiology* 1990;258:H107–12.

12. Kopelman RI, Dzau VJ, Shimabukuro S, Barger AC. Compensatory responses to hemorrhage in conscious dogs on normal and low salt intake. *American Journal of Physiology* 1983;244:H351–6.

13. Brown JJ, Lever AF, Roberson JIS, Hodge RL, Lowe RD, Vane JR. Concurrent measurement of renin and angiotensin in the circulation of the dog. *Nature* 1967;215:853–5.

14. Trachte GJ, Lefer AM. Effect of angiotensin II receptor blockade by [Sar¹–Ala⁸] angiotensin II in hemorrhagic shock. *American Journal of Physiology* 1979;236:H280–5.

15. Lightman SL, Todd K, Everitt BJ, Brown MJ, Causon RC. Ascending brainstem noradrenergic pathways modulate the renin response to haemorrhage. *Clinical Science* 1984;67:269–72.

16. Lightman SL, Everitt BJ, Todd K. Ascending noradrenergic projections from the brainstem: Evidence for a major role in the regulation of blood pressure and vasopressin secretion. *Experimental Brain Research* 1984;224:1–7.

17. Zerbe RL, Feuerstein G, Kopin IJ. Effect of captopril on cardiovascular sympathetic and vasopressin responses to hemorrhage. *European Journal of Pharmacology* 1981;72:391–5.

18. Obika LF. Effect of bilateral nephrectomy on the recovery of blood pressure after acute hemorrhage in rats: Role of renin–angiotensin system. *Experientia* 1986;42:390–2.

19. Broughton Pipkin F, Colenbrander B, MacDonald AA. Changing basal and stimulated activity of the renin–angiotensin system during the second half of gestation in the anaesthetized piglet. *Quarterly Journal of Experimental Physiology* 1986;71:277–84.

20. Starc TJ, Stalcup SA. Time course of changes of plasma renin activity and catecholamines during hemorrhage in conscious sheep. *Circulatory Shock* 1987;21:129–40.

21. Rose JC, Block SM, Flowe K, Morris M, South S, Sundberg DK, Zimmerman C. Responses to converting enzyme inhibition and hemorrhage in newborn lambs and adult sheep. *American Journal of Physiology* 1987;252:R306–13.

22. Katoh N, Sheriff DD, Siu CO, Sagawa K. Relative importance of four pressoregulatory mechanisms after 10% bleeding in rabbits. *American Journal of Physiology* 1989;256:H291–6.

23. Richards HK, Grace SA, Noble AR, Munday KA. Inactive renin in plasma: Effect of haemorrhage. *Clinical Science* 1979;56:105–8.

24. Schadt JC, Gaddis RR. Renin–angiotensin system and opioids during acute hemorrhage in conscious rabbits. *American Journal of Physiology* 1990;258:R543–51.

25. Innanen VT, Jobb E, Korogyi N. Naloxone reversal of hemorrhagic hypotension in the conscious guinea-pig is impeded by inhibition of the renin–angiotensin II system. *Neuroscience* 1987;22:313–5.

26. Cipolle MD, Zehr JE. Renin release in turtles: Effects of volume depletion and furosemide administration. *American Journal of Physiology* 1985;249:R100–5.

27. Claybaugh JR, Share L. Vasopressin, renin, and cardiovascular responses to continuous slow hemorrhage. *American Journal of Physiology* 1973;224:519–23.

28. Weber MA, Thornell IR, Stokes GS. Effect of hemorrhage with and without fluid replacement on plasma renin activity. *American Journal of Physiology* 1973;225:1161–4.

29. Skornik AO, Paladini AC. Angiotensin blood levels in hemorrhagic hypotension and related conditions. *American Journal of Physiology* 1964;206:553–6.

30. Regoli D, Vane JR. The continuous estimation of angiotensin formed in the circulation of the dog. *Journal of Physiology* 1966;183:513–31.

31. Hodge RL, Lowe RD, Vane JR. The effects of alteration of blood volume on the concentration of circulating angiotensin in anaesthetized dogs. *Journal of Physiology* 1966;185:613–26.

32. Morton JJ, Semple PF, Ledingham IA, Stuart B, Tehrani MA, Reyes Garcia A, McGarrity G. Effect of angiotensin-converting enzyme inhibitor (SQ20881) on the plasma concentration of angiotensin I, angiotensin II and arginine vasopressin in the dog during hemorrhagic shock. *Circulation Research* 1977;41:301–8.

33. Michailov ML, Schad H, Dahlheim H, Jacob IC, Brechtelsbauer H. Renin–angiotensin system responses to acute graded hemorrhage in dogs. *Circulatory Shock* 1987;21:217–24.

34. Beaty O, Sloop CH, Schmid HE, Buckelew VM. Renin response and angiotensinogen control during graded hemorrhage and shock in the dog. *American Journal of Physiology* 1976;231:1300–7.

35. Johnson JA, Davis JO, Baumber JS, Schneider EG. Effects of hemorrhage and chronic sodium depletion on hepatic clearance of renin. *American Journal of Physiology* 1971;220:1677–82.

36. Khayyal M, MacGregor J, Brown JJ, Lever AF, Robertson JIS. Increase of plasma renin-substrate concentration after infusion of angiotensin in the rat. *Clinical Science* 1973;44:87–90.

37. Nasjletti A, Masson GMC. Stimulation of angiotensinogen formation by renin and angiotensin. *Proceedings of the Society for Experimental Biology and Medicine* 1973;142:307–10.

38. Barrett JD, Eggena P, Sambhi MP. *In vivo* and *in vitro* alterations of active and inactive plasma renins in the rat. *Hypertension* 1982;4:75–9.

39. Zimpfer M, Manders WT, Barger AC, Vatner SF. Pentobarbital alters compensatory neural and humoral mechanisms in response to hemorrhage. *American Journal of Physiology* 1982;243:H713–21.

40. Freeman RH, Davis JO, Johnson JA, Spielman WS, Zatzman ML. Arterial pressure regulation during hemorrhage: Homeostatic role of angiotensin II. *Proceedings of the Society for Experimental Biology and Medicine* 1975;149:19–22.

41. Iwamoto H, Rudolph AM. Role of renin–angiotensin system in response to hemorrhage in fetal sheep. *American Journal of Physiology* 1981;240:H848–54.

42. Averill DB, Scher AM, Feigl EO. Angiotensin causes vasoconstriction during hemorrhage in baroreceptor denervated dogs. *American Journal of Physiology* 1983;245:H667–73.

43. Henrich WL, Berl T, McDonald KM, Anderson RJ, Schrier RW. Angiotensin II, renal nerves, and prostaglandins in renal hemodynamics during hemorrhage. *American Journal of Physiology* 1978;235:F46–51.

44. Farrell G. Recent contributions to the study of the role of the central nervous system in aldosterone secretion. In: Baulieu EE, Robel P, eds. *Aldosterone*. Oxford: Blackwell Scientific Publications, 1964:243–9.

45. Ganong WF, Mulrow P. Evidence of secretion of an aldosterone-stimulating substance by the kidney. *Nature* 1961;190:1115–6.

46. Davis JO. Mechanisms regulating the secretion and metabolism of aldosterone in experimental secondary hyperaldosteronism. *Recent Progress in Hormone Research* 1961;17:293–331.

47. Bartter FC, Casper AGT, Delea CS, Slater JDH. On the role of the kidney in control of adrenal steroid production. *Metabolism* 1961;10:1006–20.

48. Groza P, Borocs I, Militaru M, Boerescu I, Zagreanu L, Grigoriu M, Nicoara M. Renin and aldosterone reactions after acute hemorrhage. *Physiologie* 1988;25:105–10.

49. Lilly MP, De Maria EJ, Bruhn TO, Gann DS. Potentiated cortisol response to paired hemorrhage: Role of angiotensin and vasopressin. *American Journal of Physiology* 1989;257:R118–26.

50. Padfield PL, Morton JJ. Effects of angiotensin II on arginine-vasopressin in physiological and pathological situations in man. *Journal of Endocrinology* 1977;74:251–9.

51. Wang BC, Sundet WD, Hakumaki MOK, Goetz KL. Vasopressin and renin responses to hemorrhage in conscious, cardiac-denervated dogs. *American Journal of Physiology* 1983;245:H399–405.

52. Zerbe RL, Feuerstein G, Meyer DK, Kopin IJ. Cardiovascular, sympathetic, and renin–angiotensin system responses to hemorrhage in vasopressin-deficient rats. *Endocrinology* 1982;111:608–13.

53. Feuerstein G, Johnson AK, Zerbe RL, Davis-Kramer R, Faden AI. Anteroventral hypothalamus and hemorrhagic shock: Cardiovascular and neuroendocrine responses. *American Journal of Physiology* 1984;246:R551–7.

54. Corwin EJ, Seaton JF, Hamaji M, Harrison TS. Central role for angiotensin in control of adrenal catecholamine secretion. *American Journal of Physiology* 1985;248:R363–70.

55. Edwards BS, Zimmerman RS, Schwab TR, Heublin DM, Burnett JC. Role of atrial peptide system in renal and endocrine adaptation to hypotensive hemorrhage. *American Journal of Physiology* 1988;254:R56–60.

56. Porter JP, Thrasher TN, Said SI, Ganong WF. Vasoactive intestinal peptide in the regulation of renin secretion. *American Journal of Physiology* 1985;249:F84–9.

57. Porter JP, Ganong WF. Vasoactive intestinal peptide and renin secretion. *Annals of the New York Academy of Sciences* 1988;527:465–77.

58. Feuerstein G, Zerbe RL, Meyer DK, Kopin IJ. Alteration of cardiovascular, neurogenic, and humoral responses to acute hypovolemic hypotension by administered prostacyclin. *Journal of Cardiovascular Pharmacology* 1982;4:246–53.

59. Kremer D, Lindop G, Brown WCB, Morton JJ, Robertson JIS. Angiotensin-induced myocardial necrosis and renal failure in the rabbit: Distribution of lesions and severity in relation to plasma angiotensin II concentration and arterial pressure. *Cardiovascular Research* 1981;**15**:43–6.

60. Brown JJ, Davies DL, Johnson VW, Lever AF, Robertson JIS. Renin relationships in congestive cardiac failure, treated and untreated. *American Heart Journal* 1970;**80**:329–42.

61. Pears MA, Pickering GW. Changes in the fundus oculi after haemorrhage. *Quarterly Journal of Medicine* 1960;**29**:153–78.

62. Suvannapura A, Levens NR. Local control of mesenteric blood flow by the renin–angiotensin system. *American Journal of Physiology* 1988;**255**:G267–74.

63. Levens NR. Modulation of jejunal ion and water absorption by endogenous angiotensin after hemorrhage. *American Journal of Physiology* 1984;**246**:G634–43.

64. Hock CE, Passmore JC, Levin JI, Neiberger RE. Angiotensin II and alpha-adrenergic control of the intrarenal circulation in hemorrhage. *Circulatory Shock* 1982;**9**:81–94.

65. Reid IA. The renin–angiotensin system and body function. *Archives of Internal Medicine* 1985;**145**:1475–9.

72

RENIN WITH ANOREXIA NERVOSA, BULIMIA NERVOSA, VOMITING, AND ABUSE OF DIURETICS AND PURGATIVES

J IAN S ROBERTSON

Anorexia nervosa, bulimia nervosa, vomiting, and abuse of diuretics and purgatives are considered together because of their predilection for patients with abnormalities of personality, in whom often more than one of the disturbances may be indulged, frequently in secret. Anorexia nervosa is, for example, often associated with bulimia nervosa, a malady in which a powerful urge to overeat is accompanied by self-induced vomiting and abuse of diuretics and purgatives [1]. Not surprisingly, irrespective of the dominant initial disorder, the resulting clinical and biochemical anomalies in all these syndromes are very similar. The RAS is intimately involved in the pathogenesis of the metabolic disarray.

Wolff *et al* [2] gave a revealing account of nine psychiatrically disturbed women, who were variously suffering from the effects of anorexia nervosa, vomiting, and abuse of diuretics and purgatives (Fig. 72.1). Each of these women had more than one source of electrolyte depletion, and each deliberately concealed at least one of them (Fig. 72.2). All nine were deficient in total body potassium, and all were hypokalemic, in eight cases, markedly so. Sodium depletion was also evident in eight women. Blood pressure was low. Pedal edema was a recurrent feature in at least three of the patients, and proteinuria was prominent in four. During exacerbations, plasma renin concentration (PRC) was raised, sometimes markedly, the secretion rate and plasma concentrations of aldosterone were increased, and the metabolic clearance rate of aldosterone was diminished. In three of the patients, renal biopsies showed hyperplasia and increased granularity of the juxtaglomerular cells, features associated with increased secretion of renin. In another and separate case [3], plasma renin substrate (angiotensinogen) was also elevated, perhaps as a result of stimulation by high levels of Ang II [4].

The complex interrelationships of the multiple pathophysiological disturbances is indicated in Fig. 72.3. It appears that although the initial insult can cause considerable losses of both sodium and potassium, deficiency of potassium is eventually likely to be the more severe. This is because most of the primary anomalies cause greater deficits of potassium than of sodium; potassium loss tends to favor sodium retention, in part, by

reinforcing stimuli to renin secretion; and increased aldosterone secretion, while aiding sodium retention, will promote further elimination of potassium. Hypomagnesemia and hypocalcemia are not unusual accompaniments, and disturbances of cardiac rhythm and heart failure may occur [5]. It is noteworthy that the development of secondary abnormalities, such as constipation and ankle swelling, will often lead to further ingestion of purgatives and diuretics, with worsening potassium depletion, more severe constipation, ingestion of even larger doses of these drugs, and thus, an advancing vicious cycle.

The prevalent proteinuria in this group of conditions is almost certainly a consequence of very high circulating levels of renin and hence Ang II, even though man is a species not particularly susceptible to Ang II-induced proteinuria [6] (see *Chapter 58*). This cause of proteinuria is crucial to recognize. Such patients are notoriously unreliable historians, and the discovery of protein in the urine has more than once suggested incorrectly to an unwary physician that a renal abnormality is the primary cause of the gross electrolyte abnormalities.

The basis of the ankle edema is less clear; it may have multiple origins. Hypoalbuminemia is not unusual, in part perhaps caused by Ang II-induced proteinuria [2], with malnutrition often contributory. Plasma Ang II concentrations can be sufficiently high to stimulate the secretion of vasopressin [7], which could then also be involved, although the kaliopenic kidney is rather insensitive to vasopressin [8]. A direct renal water-conserving action of Ang II might also contribute [9].

In patients in whom vomiting predominates, loss of gastric hydrochloric acid leads to gross alkalosis; a serum bicarbonate concentration in excess of 40mmol/l is strongly suggestive of such abnormality. Trousseau and Chvostek's signs can further be present. Plasma and urinary chloride values will be very low [2,10]. While this route of electrolyte losses is often secret and self-induced [1,10], such is not necessarily the case; the same sequence may be initiated by persistent vomiting as a result for example of duodenal ulceration and pyloric stenosis. Even in patients with organic gastrointestinal disease, however, there is sometimes a surprising reluctance to reveal the extent of the vomiting [10].

The extreme deceptiveness of patients suffering from this group of disorders cannot be overemphasized. As a consequence,

Clinical data	Patient number								
	1	2	3	4	5	6	7	8	9
height (cm)	174	150	168	177	164	168	174	158	155
weight (kg) (theoretical normal in parentheses)	59 (67)	42 (51)	49 (60)	59 (66)	39 (56)	42 (63)	62 (67)	43 (53)	34 (59)
edema	absent	slight	absent	slight	present	slight	present	sometimes severe	sometimes severe
muscular weakness	present	present	present	pronounced	present	pronounced	slight	present	present
constipation	absent	present	present	present	present	present	present	present	present
tendon reflexes	normal	normal	normal	normal	brisk	depressed	depressed	normal	normal
proteinuria	absent	present	present	absent	present	absent	absent	present	absent
blood pressure (mmHg)	100/70	90/60	95/60	80/55	100/80	95/65	85/55	80/50	70/40
gastric acidity	normal	—	normal	normal	diminished	diminished	diminished	—	—
melanosis recti	pronounced	—		present	—	slight	slight	—	—
plasma:									
sodium (mmol/l)	134–138	128–135	126–130	134–142	124–132	119–128	126–138	117–139	121–123
potassium (mmol/l)	2.4–2.8	1.9–2.5	3.0–3.9	2.2	2.0–2.8	1.75–3.1	2.0–2.9	1.7–3.4	2.5–3.1
calcium (mmol/l)	4.6	4.3	5.0	4.9	5.2	5.1	4.6	4.5	5.0
chloride (mmol/l)	98–102	86–92	88–94	94–102	85–88	92–103	80–98	98–101	88–94
bicarbonate (mmol/l)	36	24	25	37	34	32	32	20–26	19–21
urea (mg/100ml)	20	38	32	35	—	52	42	36–150	110–116
creatinine (mg/100ml)	0.77	1.38	1.07	1.14	1.99	2.0	1.5	1.1	2.4
albumin (g/100ml)	3.4	2.7	3.0	4.5	3.2	3.8	3.4	3.4	4.2
pH	7.50	7.42	7.42	7.53	7.47	7.49	7.5	—	7.45
base excess	+ 9.2	+ 0.6	+ 1.7	+ 14	+ 16	+ 12	+ 8.8	—	—
hematocrit (%)	46	41	34	46	42–52	39	48–52	43–51	36
urine/plasma osmolar ratio (after 20 hours' dehydration)	1.2	—	2.2	1.8	2.8	1.9	1.0	3.5	—
inulin clearance (ml/min)	—	95	71	—	23	68	64	43	28
para-amino-hippurate clearance (ml/min)	—	480	338	—	125	394	375	—	—
NH₄ excretion (mmol/l/24h)	26.0	16.4	51.9	8.6	17	11.4	72.0	—	—
Urine titratable acidity (ml 0.1N NaOH)	2.8	5.3	18.3	7.2	3.9	0.04	13.8	—	—
Urine pH	6.60	6.34	5.82	5.6	6.2	7.45	6.01	—	—
Electrocardiogram changes suggestive of hypokalemia	present	present	absent	present	absent	pronounced	present	absent	absent

Fig. 72.1 Summary of clinical and biochemical features in nine psychiatrically disturbed patients, suffering from the effects of anorexia nervosa, vomiting, and abuse of diuretics and purgatives. Data from Wolff HP et al [2].

Causes	Patient number								
	1	2	3	4	5	6	7	8	9
anorexia	+	+	+	+	+	+	+	+	+
vomiting	−	+ (S)	+	+ (S)	+ (S)	+ (S)	+ (S)	+ (S)	−
diuretics	−	−	−	−	+ (S)	−	+	+	−
purgatives	+ (S)	+	+ (S)	+	+	+	+	+ (S)	+ (S)
S = secret									

Fig. 72.2 Various sources of electrolyte losses in nine patients (see *Fig. 72.1*). Data from Wolff HP *et al* [2].

complicated and unnecessary testing, including renal biopsy, metabolic balance studies, and even surgery, have been called upon [10–12]. In some cases, the biochemical features (including renin levels) and microscopic appearances on renal biopsy have led to a provisional diagnosis of Bartter's syndrome [11,12].

One of the most strange instances, at least to come to recognition, was the patient reported by Love *et al* [3]. This was a woman with anorexia nervosa, secret self-induced vomiting, pedal edema, and occult addiction to purgatives and diuretics. In exacerbations, she became markedly depleted of potassium. She also became alkalotic, and had elevation of PRC, angiotensinogen, and aldosterone. During an attempted metabolic balance study, she was discovered to be secretly disposing of uneaten food, vomitus, and stools, which were smuggled from the hospital by her

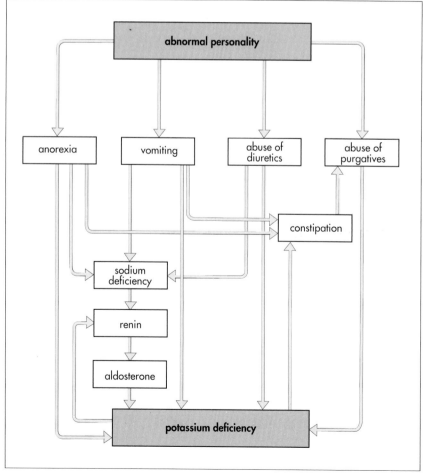

Fig. 72.3 Schema showing the interrelationship of the several disturbances in the group of disorders of anorexia nervosa, bulimia nervosa, vomiting, and abuse of diuretics and purgatives. Modified from Wolff HP *et al* [2].

72.3

sister. Simultaneously, she persuaded her husband to bring his stools into the ward, these then being substituted for her own and offered as part of the metabolic balance material.

This case illustrates, very well, the domineering personalities of many patients of this kind, and the perverse influence they can have over their family, an aspect well recognized by Gull in his original description of anorexia nervosa [13]. Another important epidemiological feature is the overwhelming [1,2], but not exclusive [10], predilection for women, particularly those having a connection with the medical profession (often as nurses or doctor's wives, or both) or with the church.

This account of some of the more bizarre aspects of the RAS may be concluded by returning to the percipient Gull and his 1874 recommendations for therapeutic success in dealing with anorexia nervosa [13]. These comprised firm discipline, the institution of a regular ample diet, exclusion of both the advice and the proximity of relatives and well-wishers, and in particular, the prohibition of medicines. His precepts are even more applicable today, when the ready availability of drugs with profound effects on the bowels, kidneys, and mind can complicate anorexia nervosa to an extent probably not encountered in Victorian times.

REFERENCES

1. Fairburn CG, Cooper PJ. Self-induced vomiting and bulimia nervosa: An undetected problem. *British Medical Journal* 1982;284:1153–5.

2. Wolff HP, Vecsei P, Krück F, Roscher S, Brown JJ, Düsterdieck GO, Lever AF, Robertson JIS. Psychiatric disturbance leading to potassium depletion, sodium depletion, raised plasma-renin concentration, and secondary hyperaldosteronism. *Lancet* 1968;i:257–61.

3. Love DR, Brown JJ, Fraser R, Lever AF, Robertson JIS, Timbury GC, Thomson S, Tree M. An unusual case of self-induced electrolyte depletion. *Gut* 1971;12:284–90.

4. Khayyal M, MacGregor J, Brown JJ, Lever AF, Robertson JIS. Increase of plasma renin-substrate concentration after infusion of angiotensin in the rat. *Clinical Science* 1973;44:87–90.

5. Fonseca V, Havard CWH. Electrolyte disturbances and cardiac failure with hypomagnesaemia in anorexia nervosa. *British Medical Journal* 1985;291:1680–3.

6. Bock KD, Brown JJ, Lever AF, Robertson JIS. Effects of renin and angiotensin on excretion and distribution of water and salts. In: Page IH, McCubbin JW, eds. *Renal Hypertension*. Yearbook Medical Publishers: Chicago, 1968:184–203.

7. Padfield PL, Morton JJ. Effects of angiotensin II on arginine-vasopressin in physiological and pathological situations in man. *Journal of Endocrinology* 1977;74:215–59.

8. Schwartz WB, Relman AS. Metabolic and renal studies in chronic potassium depletion resulting from overuse of laxatives. *Journal of Clinical Investigation* 1953;32:258–71.

9. Brown JJ, Davies DL, Lever AF, Robertson JIS. Renin and angiotensin: A survey of some aspects. *Postgraduate Medical Journal* 1966;42:153–76.

10. Wallace M, Richards P, Chesser E, Wrong O. Persistent alkalosis and hypokalaemia caused by surreptitious vomiting. *Quarterly Journal of Medicine* 1968;37:577–88.

11. Ramos E, Hall–Craggs M, Demers LM. Surreptitious habitual vomiting simulating Bartter's syndrome. *Journal of the American Medical Association* 1980;243:1070–2.

12. Padfield PL, Grekin RJ, Nicholls MG. Clinical syndromes associated with disorders of renal tubular chloride transport: Excess and deficiency of a circulating factor? *Medical Hypotheses* 1984;14:387–400.

13. Gull WW. Anorexia nervosa (apepsia hysterica, anorexia hysterica). *Transactions of the Clinical Society of London* 1874;7:22–8.

73 RENIN, ANGIOTENSIN, AND ANTIDIURESIS IN DIABETES INSIPIDUS

J IAN S ROBERTSON

INTRODUCTION

The possibility that the polyuria of diabetes insipidus (DI) might, in certain circumstances, be inhibited by increases in endogenous renin and hence in Ang II, was first proposed in 1965 [1]. The concept was later developed more fully [2]. These ideas led initially to considerable controversy [3–6]. Subsequent clinical observations, which will be reviewed herein, however, made it clear that such elevation of endogenous Ang II was likely to make, in suitable circumstances, a substantial contribution to the control of polyuria in DI; in some patients, dose–response data suggested that this could provide virtually the full explanation of such antidiuresis [7,8].

Experiments in Brattleboro rats, which have congenital deficiency of vasopressin, and hence DI, have provided more variable information. In these animals, it appears that, as in man, increases in endogenous renin and Ang II contribute to the control of polyuria during dehydration, but that additional mechanisms also participate, perhaps to a greater extent than in patients.

The principal, and in some circumstances the seemingly exclusive, way in which Ang II controls polyuria in DI is by direct actions on the kidney. These are reviewed in detail in *Chapter 26*. Additional, but not obligatory, contributions which can modulate the antidiuretic action of Ang II in several directions are via the stimulant effect of Ang II on the secretion of aldosterone (see *Chapter 33*), on that of vasopressin (see *Chapter 35*), on thirst and sodium appetite (see *Chapter 32*), and on systemic arterial pressure (see *Chapter 28*).

PATHOPHYSIOLOGICAL BASIS

The apparently paradoxical action of diuretics in reducing urine flow in DI was observed in 1905 by Meyer [9] after the administration of theophylline. In 1924, a similar effect was noted after the injection of a mercurial compound [10]. These observations were largely neglected, however, until 1959, when Kennedy and Crawford [11] showed that the administration of benzothiadiazines reduced urine volume in both clinical and experimental DI; later, a similar antidiuresis was found with administration of mercurials [12,13], spirolactones [14–16], ethacrynic acid [17], and furosemide [18]. The effect was seen in both vasopressin-sensitive and in vasopressin-resistant DI [13,19,20]. There were numerous speculations on the possible mechanisms [13–17,21–28].

It was then proposed [1,2] that since the various diuretics found to have an antidiuretic effect in DI had either been observed, or were thought likely to cause increases in renin and Ang II, and since Ang II infusions diminished urine flow in DI, the antidiuresis might be due, at least in part, to increases in circulating and/or renal renin and Ang II. A similar notion was subsequently considered briefly by Orr and Filipich [29]. It was emphasized that a contribution of renin (and hence Ang II) to 'diuretic antidiuresis' does not necessarily exclude other explanations.

ANTIDIURETIC EFFECT OF ANGIOTENSIN II

The intravenous infusion of Ang II in healthy man leads, over a wide dose range, to a fall in urine volume and a reduction in the excretion of sodium, chloride, and potassium [30–37]. Angiotensin II has a similar antidiuretic effect in patients with vasopressin-sensitive DI [31,35,38,39]. The increase in urinary osmolality is, however, modest in comparison with that produced by vasopressin. When the hypothesis was first put forward, the effect of Ang II in vasopressin-resistant ('nephrogenic') DI had not been reported. Since diuretics had been shown to reduce urine flow in this variety of the disease, however, it was pointed out that the viability of the hypothesis required infused Ang II to be antidiuretic here also [1,2]. Subsequently, it was reported that Ang II infusion reduced urine flow and increased urinary osmolality in nephrogenic DI [29,40].

EFFECT OF SODIUM RESTRICTION AND OF DIURETICS ON RENIN AND ANGIOTENSIN

It is now well established that dietary sodium restriction, or the administration of natriuretic drugs, leads, both in animals and man, to an elevation of renin and Ang II in peripheral blood (see *Chapters 1, 24,* and *74*). Similar measures lead to an increase in renal renin [12]. It has been known since 1903 that the polyuria of DI can be diminished by a reduction in the dietary intake of sodium [41], and this has been repeatedly confirmed [42–44]. Furthermore, there is considerable evidence that the beneficial effect of various diuretic drugs is closely related to their natriuretic potency [12,17,23,45]. Thus, the antidiuretic action of theophylline in DI was shown many years ago to follow an initial natriuresis [9,46]. Of the drugs introduced subsequently, benzothiadiazines, ethacrynic acid, furosemide, and the mercurials are, in their usual dosage, generally the most effective [12,17,18,23]. By contrast, spirolactones are much less antidiuretic [14,17], while the weakly natriuretic drugs, triamterene and acetazolamide, are said to be virtually devoid of antidiuretic effect in DI [24,27]. These observations strongly suggested that the antidiuretic effect is related to sodium deprivation or loss, particularly since the beneficial effect of diuretics can be impaired or abolished by salt replacement [13,14,28,44]. It therefore seemed likely that the modes of action of diuretic drugs and of dietary sodium restriction in reducing the polyuria were either closely similar or identical. Since elevation of renin and Ang II is produced by either sodium restriction or the administration of diuretics (see *Chapters 1, 24,* and *74*), the known antidiuretic effect of Ang II suggested this to be the mechanism of the antidiuresis in both situations [1,2].

SODIUM RESTRICTION, DIURETICS, RENIN, AND ANGIOTENSIN II IN CLINICAL VASOPRESSIN-SENSITIVE OR VASOPRESSIN-RESISTANT DIABETES INSIPIDUS

The above-mentioned concepts were pursued experimentally initially in two patients: a 28-year-old woman with typical vasopressin-sensitive DI following a head injury (Case 1) and a 12-year-old boy with congenital vasopressin-insensitive (nephrogenic) DI (Case 2) [2,7]. Both patients were investigated while taking fixed diets of normal, and then of reduced, sodium content. Results were very similar in both patients.

Intravenous infusion of synthetic Ang II (1–4ng/kg/min) for 2–3 hours effectively lowered urine flow and free-water clearance, whether given during periods of normal or reduced sodium intake. Urinary osmolality increased slightly (greatest rise from 52 to 99mosmol/kg). Plasma osmolality was unaffected in Case 1 and fell in Case 2. At all Ang II-infusion rates producing significant reduction in urine flow, the arterial pressure rose at least slightly.

Dietary sodium restriction reduced the pressor sensitivity to

infused Ang II, caused an increase in peripheral venous plasma renin concentration (PRC) and Ang II to abnormally high levels, and diminished urine flow by 43–67%.

Intravenous injections of furosemide caused an initial natriuresis and diuresis and a rise in PRC. Within 90 minutes, this was succeeded by an antidiuretic phase lasting at least 12 hours, in which urine flow fell to 40–60% of control rates. Plasma renin concentration remained elevated throughout this phase, the characteristics of which closely resembled those produced by Ang II infusion. Thus, urine flow and free-water clearance were notably reduced, while osmolality was lowered in plasma and slightly elevated in urine.

Furosemide, bendrofluazide and spironolactone, given orally, all elevated plasma renin and reduced urine flow. The greatest elevation of renin and reduction in polyuria were seen when bendrofluazide and spironolactone were given together.

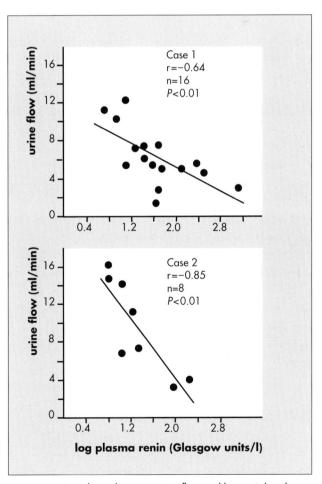

Fig. 73.1 Correlation between urine flow and log peripheral venous plasma renin concentration in two cases of diabetes insipidus. Modified from Brown *et al* [2].

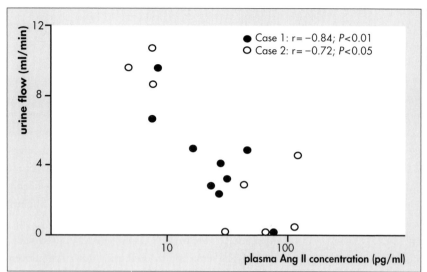

Fig 73.2 Relationship between urine flow and plasma Ang II concentration in two patients with diabetes insipidus. Modified from Chinn RH *et al* [7].

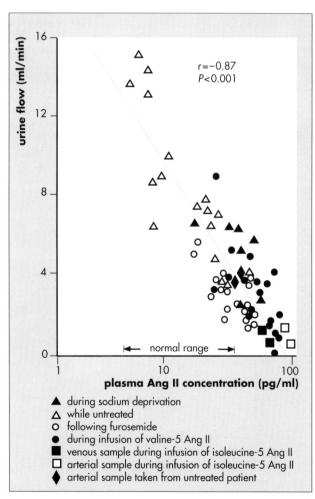

Fig. 73.3 Relationship between plasma Ang II concentration and urine volume in four patients with diabetes insipidus. Modified from MacGregor J *et al* [48].

A comparison was made in each patient between peripheral venous PRC and urine flow rate, on all the occasions on which both were measured concurrently (but excluding samples taken in the phase immediately after intravenous furosemide, where any antidiuretic action of Ang II was overwhelmed by the diuretic, and also during Ang II infusion, for obvious reasons). There was a close inverse correlation between urine flow and log PRC (Fig. 73.1).

In a further report on these patients [7], it was shown that, in each, there was a similar significant inverse correlation between peripheral venous plasma Ang II concentration and urine flow, following furosemide administration and during Ang II infusion (Fig. 73.2).

These relationships were confirmed in observations in four patients with DI (Fig. 73.3) [48]. In man, valine-5 Ang II and isoleucine-5 Ang II were seen to have a similar antidiuretic effect, and the correlation was not disturbed if Ang II was assayed in arterial or venous plasma.

The effects of infused Ang II and of diuretics in DI were clearly similar, but several points of difference were seen. Intravenous furosemide produced a prompt fall in plasma osmolality, whereas this was less consistent with Ang II infusion. This was explained by the initial natriuresis which followed furosemide and which was absent with Ang II infusion. Another point of difference was that while both sodium restriction and diuretics caused an increase in PRC and Ang II and an inhibition of polyuria without a detectable effect on arterial pressure, at effective antidiuretic doses, infused Ang II was usually, at least slightly, pressor, even during periods of sodium restriction. It was noted, however, that sodium depletion attenuated the pressor action of infused Ang II.

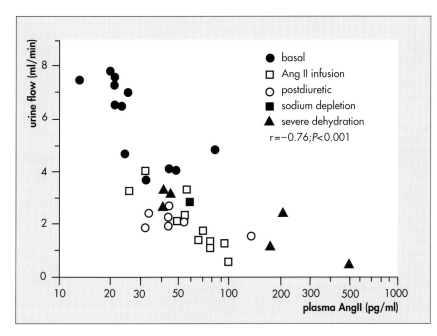

Fig. 73.4 Interrelation of plasma Ang II concentration and urine flow in several situations in a patient with diabetes insipidus. Log abscissa. Modified from Trust PM *et al* [8].

Detailed studies on a further patient enabled the quantitative aspects to be pursued further. Trust *et al* [8] reported on a 20-year-old man with a progressive inoperable hypothalamic tumor, which caused hypopituitarism and DI. He was initially treated with corticosteroid replacement, the polyuria being controlled with a thiazide diuretic, which increased urinary osmolality while lowering plasma osmolality. Dietary sodium restriction was similarly beneficial. Angiotensin II infusion also reduced the urine flow rate, while causing increases in urinary osmolality. Similar peripheral plasma Ang II concentrations, whether endogenous or due to intravenous Ang II infusion, were associated with similar urinary flow rates (Fig. 73.4). Later extension of the tumor led to loss of thirst, whereupon the patient stopped treatment, later being admitted to hospital with severe dehydration, hypernatremia, and oliguria. The oliguria was accompanied by very high plasma Ang II levels (Fig. 73.4), while plasma vasopressin, though detectable, was inappropriately low for the severity of the dehydration. It was concluded that the oliguria with hypertonic urine present during severe dehydration was due to a direct renal action of the very high plasma Ang II concentrations, possibly supplemented by some residual vasopressin secretion, which later might also have been, in part, stimulated by the elevated Ang II [49] (see *Chapter 35*). When all available plasma Ang II data on this patient were assembled, having been obtained variously during uncontrolled DI, postdiuretic administration, during sodium deprivation, when severely dehydrated following loss of thirst, and during Ang II infusion, a highly significant inverse correlation was observed between plasma Ang II and concurrent urine flow (Fig. 73.4).

In this patient, during dehydration, plasma aldosterone appeared disproportionately low for the concurrent plasma Ang II concentrations. As will be described, a similar altered relationship between Ang II and aldosterone has subsequently been reported in rats with DI.

POSSIBLE ANTIDIURETIC MECHANISMS

While the data obtained in patients and presented in the preceding section provided impressive support for the notion that the renal effects were largely controlled directly or indirectly by circulating Ang II, other contributions remain possible, as had been discussed earlier [2,8]. It might be that local release of renin could lead to a rise in Ang II both in renal lymph and renal blood; thus Ang II might reach various renal tissues in sufficient concentration to cause antidiuresis without having a systemic effect.

Among the conceivable mechanisms of Ang II in promoting antidiuresis is that the glomerular filtration rate (GFR) is reduced or that there is a direct effect on the vasa recta or the renal tubules [32,35,50] (*Chapter 26*). Another possibility is that sodium depletion might change the distribution of intrarenal renin, and so divert function from superficial to deep nephrons [51], with consequent changes in water excretion (see *Chapter 21*). Last, it must be emphasized that the renal effects of Ang II might well, if it is raised for a prolonged period, differ from those seen in briefer infusions [34,37] such as were studied in these patients [2,7,8]. This is an important proviso in considering the relevance of renin and Ang II to the long-term actions of diuretics or salt restriction in DI.

DIABETES INSIPIDUS IN OTHER CLINICAL SITUATIONS IN WHICH RENIN IS INCREASED

The data presented thus far suggest further that other clinical circumstances in which renin and Ang II are increased will reduce the polyuria of DI. In several conditions, this seems to be the case. Thus plasma renin and Ang II are high in adrenal insufficiency [52,53] (see *Chapter 68*), in which the polyuria of DI is also diminished [15].

A similar situation prevails in hypopituitarism as touched on in the case of Trust *et al* [8] already described. Both clinically and experimentally, total destruction of the hypophysis does not usually result in chronic polyuria; this only occurs if significant portions of the anterior pituitary remain intact [54–59]. There is no generally agreed explanation of this [54,60], but one possibility, which may occur in some cases and would accord with the concepts advanced here, is that unless corticotropin (adreno-corticotropic hormone; ACTH) is secreted normally, with consequent normal adrenocortical function, renin and Ang II may increase and counter the polyuria which would otherwise follow cessation of posterior pituitary function. In some cases of panhypopituitarism, polyuria and polydipsia have developed only when replacement therapy with glucocorticoids was given [45,58,60,61].

The application of a renal-artery clamp in water-loaded dogs leads to a striking reduction in polyuria [62,63]. Water loading is a situation closely analogous to DI in that the secretion of vasopressin is suppressed throughout, and presumably therefore in these experiments, the inhibition of polyuria is independent of vasopressin. Berliner and Davidson [63] regarded a reduction in GFR as the essential mechanism of the antidiuresis, but renin and Ang II might contribute, since it is probable that after the application of a renal-artery or aortic clamp in the dog, there is a rise in the concentration of renin in renal lymph and renal venous plasma, and in the net secretion rate of renin [64–67] (see *Chapter 55*).

Congestive cardiac failure may also inhibit the polyuria of DI [68], and renin and Ang II might well contribute to this situation, since circulating renin is increased in some (but by no means all)

cases of untreated congestive heart failure [69] (see *Chapter 76*). Treatment with diuretics would obviously modify these effects.

Since plasma renin and Ang II are increased in normal pregnancy [70,71] (see *Chapter 50*), this condition also might be expected to benefit DI. The published evidence on the point seems equivocal, however. Some case reports have indicated improvement during pregnancy [72,73], while others have not [42]. Since the increases in renin and Ang II with pregnancy are variable [70,71], an inconstant response of DI in pregnancy is perhaps not surprising.

DIABETES INSIPIDUS IN VASOPRESSIN-DEFICIENT RATS

Rats of the Brattleboro strain are deficient in vasopressin and consequently have DI. When such rats with DI were deprived of water for 14 hours, they showed, in comparison with normal Long–Evans rats deprived of water for 53 hours, similar reductions in plasma volume [74]. The Brattleboro rats, however, had a greater fall in body weight, in food intake, and in urine volume, while plasma sodium and potassium concentrations and plasma osmolality, were substantially higher. Plasma Ang II also tended to increase to a greater extent in the water-deprived Brattleboro rats, although aldosterone did not [74]. Other workers agree that plasma renin is hyperresponsive to water deprivation in Brattleboro rats [75]. Some investigators have also found that angiotensinogen is elevated in these animals [75], although others have not confirmed this [76]. It has, however, been agreed that the level of plasma aldosterone is less in water-deprived Brattleboro rats than in Long–Evans rats [77]. As noted above [8], in DI in man also, plasma aldosterone can be disproportionately low for the concurrent plasma Ang II concentration. Administration of vasopressin to homozygous Brattleboro rats can decrease plasma renin [76,78,79]. A probably important observation is that water deprivation in Brattleboro rats causes an increase in plasma oxytocin, which appears to cause natriuresis, weak antidiuresis, and maintenance of GFR [80].

Mann *et al* [81] found, in Brattleboro rats, that administration of Ang II or furosemide each decreased urine flow and raised urinary sodium concentration. With furosemide there was a two-fold increase in plasma Ang II. When the formation of Ang II was blocked by giving captopril, plasma Ang II fell 2.5-fold, but furosemide still had an antidiuretic effect. These workers concluded that elevated Ang II could contribute to an antidiuresis. In their opinion, however, the antidiuresis induced by furosemide was not mediated by Ang II. The latter conclusion does not, however, follow from their experiments. Mann *et al* [81] did not measure arterial pressure, but it is known that captopril has a particularly marked hypotensive effect in Brattleboro rats [82]. Such a hypotensive effect would be even more pronounced with concomitant furosemide dosing. Thus, when captopril and furosemide were combined, arterial hypotension, with consequent loss of pressure natriuresis and diuresis, would confound ready interpretation of the data. Mann *et al* [81] further conclude, even more surprisingly, that, in diuretic-induced antidiuresis, an action more important than that of Ang II is the 'intense sodium loss, with a decrease of GFR and renal blood flow [83]'. Their statement exemplifies well the confusion that has persistently afflicted this topic. The intrarenal and circulatory changes in the RAS resulting from 'intense sodium loss' are an inevitable and inextricable consequence of that sodium loss and are largely responsible for the resultant alterations in renal hemodynamics and functions.

CONCLUSIONS

Currently available evidence indicates some differences in physiological emphasis in patients as compared with rats suffering from DI. In man, both in vasopressin-deficient as well as in nephrogenic DI, it appears that increases in renin and Ang II, either in the circulation or in the kidney, or both, make a major contribution to the antidiuresis that follows sodium deprivation or the administration of natriuretic drugs, or in severe dehydration. While similar changes occur in the RAS in water-deprived rats with DI, additional hormonal responses, notably a rise in plasma oxytocin, probably also contribute to the antidiuresis. Studies with combined captopril and furosemide administration in rats are confounded by the presence of arterial hypotension, with loss of pressure diuresis. While the role of the RAS in DI may be further clarified by studies using renin inhibitors (see *Chapter 85*) and newer Ang II antagonists (see *Chapter 86*), caution will again be needed regarding the confounding effect of hypotension.

A curiosity of studies of the RAS in the pathophysiology of DI is the continued antipathy or indifference to, and misunderstanding of, the concepts presented herein [3,5,81]. This is particularly surprising because the dose–response relationships are among those most precisely established for the RAS [7,8,48,84] (*Figs. 73.2–4*). It is for example remarkable that Valtin and Edwards [85] contrived to review the mechanisms of urine concentration in dehydrated Brattleboro rats while avoiding any specific mention of renin or Ang II, although they do concede that 'other peptide hormones' (than vasopressin) may contribute. It is, moreover, sadly inappropriate that many traditional nephrologists have, when considering such issues, often erroneously regarded the kidney as composed of nephrons homogeneous in anatomical structure, biochemistry, and function [3,5,85]. Such evaluations are ill founded [51,86–88] (see *Chapter 21*), and are especially inapt in considering changes in renal hemodynamics and function in relation to the RAS.

REFERENCES

1. Brown JJ, Lever AF, Robertson JIS. Renin in diabetes insipidus. *Lancet* 1965;ii:1349.
2. Brown JJ, Chinn RH, Lever AF, Robertson JIS. Renin and angiotensin as a mechanism of diuretic-induced antidiuresis in diabetes insipidus. *Lancet* 1969;i:237–9.
3. Morgan T, De Wardener HE. Antidiuresis in diabetes insipidus. *Lancet* 1969;i:524–5.
4. Brown JJ, Chinn RH, Lever AF, Robertson JIS. Antidiuresis in diabetes insipidus. *Lancet* 1969;i:729.
5. Del Greco F, Simon NM. Solute load and urine flow in diabetes insipidus. *Lancet* 1969;i:945.
6. Brown JJ, Chinn RH, Lever AF, Robertson JIS. Antidiuresis in diabetes insipidus. *Lancet* 1969;i:1155.
7. Chinn RH, Brown JJ, Düsterdieck GO, Lever AF, Robertson JIS. Plasma angiotensin II concentrations in diabetes insipidus. *Proceedings of the Royal Society of Medicine* 1971;64:1073.
8. Trust PM, Brown JJ, Chinn RH, Lever AF, Morton JJ, Padfield PL, Robertson JIS, Ireland JT, Melville ID, Thomson WST. A case of hypopituitarism with diabetes insipidus and loss of thirst: Role of antidiuretic hormone and angiotensin II in the control of urine flow and osmolality. *Journal of Clinical Endocrinology and Metabolism* 1975;41:346–53.
9. Meyer E. Über Diabetes insipidus und andere Polyurien. *Deutsches Archiv für Klinische Medizin* 1905;83:1–70.
10. Bauer J, Aschner B. Die therapeutische Wirkung des Novasurols bei Diabetes insipidus. *Zentralblatt für Innere Medizin* 1924;34:682–8.
11. Kennedy GC, Crawford JD. Treatment of diabetes insipidus with hydrochlorothiazide. *Lancet* 1959;i:866–7.
12. Blom PS, Rook L, Sonneveldt HA. Sodium economy in the proximal and distal parts of the nephron studied in patients with diabetes insipidus. Their estimation under normal conditions and after salt restriction, chlorothiazide and a mercurial diuretic. *Acta Medica Scandinavica* 1963; 174:201–13.
13. Earley LE, Orloff J. The mechanism of antidiuresis associated with the administration of hydrochlorothiazide to patients with vasopressin-resistant diabetes insipidus. *Journal of Clinical Investigation* 1962;41:1988–97.
14. Havard CWH, Wood PHN. The effect of diuretics on renal water excretion in diabetes insipidus. *Clinical Science* 1961;21:321–32.
15. Kennedy GC, Crawford JD. A comparison of the effects of adrenalectomy and of chlorothiazide in experimental diabetes insipidus. *Journal of Endocrinology* 1961;22:77–86.

16. Kowarski A, Berant M, Grossman MS, Migeon CJ. Antidiuretic properties of aldactone (spironolactone) in diabetes insipidus. Studies on the mechanism of antidiuresis. *Bulletin of Johns Hopkins Hospital* 1966;**119**:413–23.

17. Lant AF. The antidiuretic effect of diuretics in diabetes insipidus. *Journal of the Royal College of Physicians of London* 1968;**2**:298–309.

18. Rado JP, Banos C, Marosi J, Tako J, Szilagyi L. Frusemide antidiuresis. *Lancet* 1967;**ii**:568–9.

19. Crawford JD, Kennedy GC. Chlorothiazid in diabetes insipidus. *Nature* 1959;**183**:891–2.

20. Goodman AD, Carter RD. A study on the mechanism of the antidiuretic action of chlorothiazide in diabetes insipidus. *Metabolism* 1962;**11**:1033–40

21. Robson JS, Lambie AT. The effect of chlorothiazide in diabetes insipidus with particular reference to the osmolality of the serum. *Metabolism* 1962;**11**:1041–53.

22. Kennedy GC, Skadhauge E, Hague P. The effect of hydrochlorothiazide on water intake and plasma osmolality in diabetes insipidus in the rat. *Quarterly Journal of Experimental Physiology* 1964;**49**:417–23.

23. Skadhauge E. Investigations into the thiazide-induced antidiuresis in patients with diabetes insipidus. *Acta Medica Scandinavica* 1963;**174**:739–49.

24. Crawford JD, Kennedy GC, Hill LE. Clinical results of treatment of diabetes insipidus with drugs of the chlorothiazide series. *New England Journal of Medicine* 1960;**262**:737–43.

25. Linke A. Die Behandlung des Diabetes insipidus mit saluretischen Sulfonamiden. *Medizinische Welt* 1960;**218**:968–73.

26. Alexander CS, Gordon GB. Chlorothiazide derivatives for diabetes insipidus? *Archives of Internal Medicine* 1961;**108**:218–25.

27. Rado JP. Mechanism of 'thiazide antidiuresis'. *Lancet* 1965;**ii**:1018.

28. Gillenwater JY. Antidiuretic properties of chlorothiazide in diabetes insipidus dogs. *Metabolism* 1965;**14**:539–58.

29. Orr FR, Filipich RL. Studies with angiotensin in nephrogenic diabetes insipidus. *Canadian Medical Association Journal* 1967;**97**:841–5.

30. Bock KD, Krecke HJ. Die Wirkung von synthetischem hypertensin II auf die PAH und inulin-clearance, die renale Hämodynamik und die Diurese beim Menschen. *Klinische Wochenschrift* 1958;**36**:69–74.

31. Peart WS. Hypertension and the kidney. II. Experimental basis of renal hypertension. *British Medical Journal* 1959;**ii**:1421–9.

32. Brown JJ, Peart WS. The effect of angiotensin on urine flow and electrolyte excretion in hypertensive patients. *Clinical Science* 1962;**22**:1–17.

33. Biron P, Chrétien M, Koiw E, Genest J. Effects of angiotensin infusions on aldosterone and electrolyte excretion in normal subjects and patients with hypertension and adrenocortical disorders. *British Medical Journal* 1962;**i**:1569–75.

34. Brown JJ. Actions of angiotensin on the circulation. *Memoirs of the Society for Endocrinology* 1963;**13**:303–16.

35. de Bono E, Lee G, Mottram FR, Pickering GW, Brown JJ, Keen H, Peart WS, Sanderson PM. The action of angiotensin in man. *Clinical Science* 1963;**25**:123–57.

36. Gantt CL, Carter WJ. Acute effects of angiotensin on calcium, phosphorus, magnesium and potassium excretion. *Canadian Medical Association Journal* 1964;**90**:287–91.

37. Bock KD, Brown JJ, Lever AF, Robertson JIS. Effects of renin and angiotensin on excretion and distribution of water and salts. In: Page IH, McCubbin JW, eds. *Renal hypertension.* Chicago: Year Book Medical Publishers, 1968:184–203.

38. Del Greco F. Comparative effects of valine-5 angiotensin II amide and pitressin on renal excretory function in diabetes insipidus. *Proceedings of the Society for Experimental Biology and Medicine* 1962;**109**:105–10.

39. Gill JR, Barbour BH, Slater JDH, Bartter FC. Effect of angiotensin II on urinary dilution in normal man. *American Journal of Physiology* 1964;**206**:750–4.

40. Brodehl J, Gelissen K. Die antidiuretische Wirkung des Angiotensins beim Diabetes insipidus. *Klinische Wochenschrift* 1966;**44**:101–3.

41. Tallqvist TWZ. Untersuchungen über einen Fall von Diabetes insipidus. *Zeitschrift für Klinische Medizin* 1903;**49**:181–92.

42. Fitz R. A case of diabetes insipidus. *Archives of Internal Medicine* 1914;**14**:706–21.

43. Beaser SB. Renal excretory function and diet in diabetes insipidus. *American Journal of the Medical Sciences* 1947;**213**:441–9.

44. Havard CWH. Thiazide-induced antidiuresis in diabetes insipidus. *Proceedings of the Royal Society of Medicine* 1965;**58**:1005–7.

45. Coggins CH, Leaf A. Diabetes insipidus. *American Journal of Medicine* 1967;**42**:807.

46. Socin CZ. Ueber Diabetes insipidus. *Zeitschrift für Klinische Medizin* 1913;**78**:294–308.

47. Baba WI, Lant AF, Wilson GM. The action of oral diuretics in diabetes insipidus. *Proceedings of the Royal Society of Medicine* 1965;**58**:911–2.

48. MacGregor J, Briggs JD, Brown JJ, Chinn RH, Gavras H, Lever AF, MacAdam RF, Medina A, Morton JJ, Oliver NWJ, Paton A, Powell-Jackson JD, Robertson JIS, Waite MA. Renin and renal function. In: *Modern therapy in the treatment of cardiovascular and renal diseases. International Congress Series No. 268.* Amsterdam: Excerpta Medica, 1972:71–83.

49. Padfield PL, Morton JJ. Effects of angiotensin II on arginine-vasopressin in physiological and pathological situations in man. *Journal of Endocrinology* 1977;**74**:251–9.

50. Lever AF. The vasa recta and countercurrent multiplication. *Acta Medica Scandinavica* 1965;**178** (suppl 434).

51. Horster M, Thurau K. Micropuncture studies on the filtration rate of single superficial and juxtamedullary glomeruli in the rat kidney. *Pflügers Archiv für die gesamte Physiologie des Menschen und der Tiere* 1968;**301**:162–81.

52. Brown JJ, Davies DL, Lever AF, Robertson JIS. Variations in plasma renln concentration in several physiological and pathological states. *Canadian Medical Association Journal* 1964;**90**:201–6.

53. Brown JJ, Fraser R, Lever AF, Robertson JIS, James VHT, McCusker J, Wynn V. Renin, angiotensin, corticosteroids, and electrolyte balance in Addison's disease. *Quarterly Journal of Medicine* 1968;**37**:97–118.

54. Harris GW. *Neural control of the pituitary gland.* London: Edward Arnold, 1955.

55. von Hann F. Über die Bedeutung der Hypophysenveränderungen bei Diabetes insipidus. *Frankfurter Zeitschrift für Pathologie* 1918;**21**:337–65.

56. Sheehan HL, Whitehead R. The neurohypophysis in post-partum hypopituitarism. *Journal of Pathology* 1963;**85**:145–69.

57. Goth A. Sheehan's syndrome in association with diabetes insipidus. *British Medical Journal* 1963;**i**:240.

58. Ahn CS, Kim DS. Sheehan's syndrome associated with diabetes insipidus. *Lancet* 1964;**ii**:1045–6.

59. Carey R, Melby JC. Diabetes insipidus following post-partum shock. *Archives of Internal Medicine* 1966;**118**:9–13.

60. Dingman JF, Despointes RH, Laidlaw JC, Thorn GW. Studies of neurohypophyseal function in man: Effect of adrenal steroids on polyuria in combined anterior and posterior pituitary insufficiency. *Journal of Laboratory and Clinical Medicine* 1958;**51**:690–700.

61. Ikkos D, Luft R, Olivecrona H. Hypophysectomy in man: Effect on water excretion during the first two postoperative months. *Journal of Clinical Endocrinology and Metabolism* 1955;**15**:553–67.

62. Rydin H, Verney EB. The inhibition of water-diuresis by emotional stress and by muscular exercise. *Quarterly Journal of Experimental Physiology* 1937–8;**27**:343–74.

63. Berliner RW, Davidson DG. Production of hypertonic urine in the absence of pituitary antidiuretic hormone. *Journal of Clinical Investigation* 1957;**36**:1416–27.

64. Lever AF, Peart WS. Renin and angiotensin-like activity in renal lymph. *Journal of Physiology (London)* 1962;**160**:548.

65. Skinner SL, McCubbin JW, Page IH. Renal baroceptor control of renin secretion. *Science* 1963;**141**:814–6.

66. Vander AJ, Miller R. Control of renin secretion in the anesthetized dog. *American Journal of Physiology* 1964;**207**:537–46.

67. Hosie KF, Brown JJ, Harper AM, Lever AF, MacAdam RF, MacGregor J, Robertson JIS. The release of renin into the renal circulation of the anaesthetized dog. *Clinical Science* 1970;**38**:157–74.

68. Tuttle EP. Diabetes insipidus. *American Heart Journal* 1965;**69**:577–81.

69. Brown JJ, Davies DL, Johnson VW, Lever AF, Robertson JIS. Renin relationships in congestive cardiac failure, treated and untreated. *American Heart Journal* 1970;**80**:329–42.

70. Weir RJ, Brown JJ, Fraser R, Lever AF, Logan RW, McIlwaine GM, Morton JJ, Robertson JIS, Tree M. Relationship between plasma renin, renin substrate, angiotensin II, aldosterone and electrolytes in normal pregnancy. *Journal of Clinical Endocrinology and Metabolism* 1975;**40**:108–15.

71. Beilin LJ, Deacon J, Michael CA, Vandongen R, Lalor CM, Barden AE, Davidson L, Rouse I. Diurnal rhythms of blood pressure, plasma renin activity, angiotensin II and catecholamines in normotensive and hypertensive pregnancies. *Clinical and Experimental Hypertension* 1983;**B2**:271–93.

72. McKenzie CH, Swain FM. Diabetes insipidus and pregnancy. *Minnesota Medicine* 1955;**38**:809–11.

73. Kaplan NM. Successful pregnancy following hypophysectomy during the twelfth week of gestation. *Journal of Clinical Endocrinology and Metabolism* 1961;**21**:1139–45.

74. Bennett T, Gardiner SM. Water deprivation: Effects of fluid and electrolyte handling and plasma biochemistry in Long–Evans and Brattleboro rats. *Journal of Physiology* 1987;**385**:35–48.

75. Gross F, Dauda G, Kazda S, Kyncl J, Möhring J, Orth H. Increased fluid turnover and the activity of the renin–angiotensin system under various experimental conditions. *Circulation Research* 1972;**30 and 31** (suppl 2):173–81.

76. Gutman Y, Benzakein F. Antidiuretic hormone and renin in rats with diabetes insipidus. *European Journal of Pharmacology* 1974;**28**:114–8.

77. Ezzarani EA, Laulin JP, Brudiex R. Effects of water-deprivation on aldosterone production in Brattleboro male rats congenitally lacking vasopressin. *Hormone and Metabolic Research* 1985;**17**:230–3.

78. Hoffman WE, Ganten U, Schelling P, Phillips PG, Ganten D. The renin and isorenin–angiotensin system in rats with hereditary hypothalamic diabetes insipidus. *Neuropharmacology* 1978;**17**:919–23.

79. Rafaello M, Golin A, Gotoh E, Keil LC, Shackelford RL, Ganong WF. Lack of effect of vasopressin replacement on renin. *American Journal of Physiology* 1989;**257**:R1117–22.

80. Edwards BR, Larochelle FT. Antidiuretic effect of endogenous oxytocin in dehydrated Brattleboro homozygous rats. *American Journal of Physiology* 1984;**247**:F453–65.

81. Mann JFE, Rascher W, Schömig A, Dietz R. Inhibition of the renin–angiotensin-system in Brattleboro rats with hereditary hypothalamic diabetes insipidus. *Klinische Wochenschrift* 1978;**56** (suppl 1):67–70.

82. Gardiner SM, Bennett T. Cardiovascular consequences of water deprivation in female Long Evans and Brattleboro rats. *Journal of the Autonomic Nervous System* 1988;**24**:205–14.

83. Shirley DG, Walter SJ, Laycock JF. The role of sodium depletion in hydrochlorothiazide-induced antidiuresis in Brattleboro rats with diabetes insipidus. *Clinical Science* 1978;**54**:209–15.

84. Brown JJ, Casals-Stenzel J, Cumming AMM, Davies DL, Fraser R, Lever AF, Morton JJ, Semple PF, Tree M, Robertson JIS. Angiotensin II, aldosterone and arterial pressure: A quantitative approach. Arthur C. Corcoran Memorial Lecture. *Hypertension* 1979;**1**:159–79.

85. Valtin H, Edwards BR. GFR and the concentration of urine in the absence of vasopressin: Berliner-Davidson re-explored. *Kidney International* 1987;**31**:634–40.

86. Bankir L, Bouby N, Trinh-Tang-Tan MM. Heterogeneity of nephron anatomy. *Kidney International* 1985;**31** (suppl 20):25–39.

87. Robertson JIS, Richards M. Converting enzyme inhibitors and renal function in cardiac failure. *Kidney International* 1985;**31** (suppl 20):216–9.

88. Gavras H, Brown JJ, Lever AF, Robertson JIS. Changes of renin in individual glomeruli in response to variations of sodium intake in the rabbit. *Clinical Science* 1970;**38**:409–14.

74

CHANGES IN RENIN SECRETION: PHYSIOLOGICAL, PATHOPHYSIOLOGICAL, PHARMACOLOGICAL, AND EPIDEMIOLOGICAL EXPRESSION

M GARY NICHOLLS AND J IAN S ROBERTSON

The several influences on renin secretion have been considered in detail in *Chapter 24*. These are reflected in changes in the RAS in response to a wide array of physiological and pharmacological stimuli and thus present characteristic epidemiological and pathophysiological patterns. While many of these aspects are considered in detail in other chapters, it may be useful to present a summary here.

PHYSIOLOGICAL ROLE OF THE RENIN SYSTEM

In broad terms, the RAS can be considered as protecting the organism against sodium and fluid loss, hemorrhage, and hypotension, and hence as usually running counter to the atrial natriuretic factor (ANF) system (see *Chapter 36*). However, in some pathological circumstances, notably cardiac failure, and some forms of renovascular hypertension, renin and ANF are recruited together (see *Chapters 76* and *55*).

ELECTROLYTE AND WATER INTAKE

SODIUM
A low dietary sodium intake leads to an increase in plasma renin, Ang II, and aldosterone [1–3]. Concurrently, sodium deprivation enhances the stimulant effect of Ang II on aldosterone, while the pressor effect of Ang II is diminished (see *Chapters 33* and *28*) (Fig. 74.1). Conversely, a high sodium intake causes plasma renin to fall [1].

POTASSIUM
Although the situation under highly experimental circumstances and *in vitro* is complex and somewhat controversial [4], in intact animals and man, potassium depletion has a stimulant effect on the RAS while potassium loading has a modest effect in

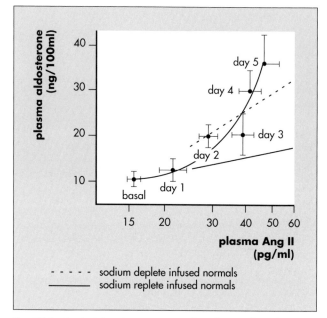

Fig. 74.1 Pooled data (mean ± SEM) from four studies of dietary sodium restriction in normal subjects for up to five days. Compared with the basal mean (on normal intake), mean plasma Ang II was significantly increased by day 1 (*P*<0.02) and on all subsequent days; mean plasma aldosterone was significantly increased by day 2 (*P*<0.02) and on all subsequent days (*t* test). Note the progressive steepening of the relationship of aldosterone to Ang II. The solid straight line indicates part of the regression of plasma Ang II on aldosterone, before and during incremental Ang II infusion in sodium-repleted subjects; the dotted line shows part of the regression similarly found for sodium-depleted subjects. Modified from Brown JJ *et al* [2].

suppressing the renin system [5–7]. The influence of potassium is, however, subordinate to that of sodium intake.

WATER
Dehydration stimulates the RAS (see *Chapter 32*), especially in diabetes insipidus, where the homeostatic influence of vasopressin is lost (see *Chapter 73*). Normally, the influence of water intake on the RAS is also subordinate to that of sodium.

FASTING: NATRIURESIS OF FASTING

Severe dietary salt restriction, as mentioned above, leads to prompt rises in plasma renin concentration (PRC), PRA, Ang II, and aldosterone, and a rapid reduction in urinary sodium output to very low values [1,2].

Both obese and lean subjects, however, excrete more sodium while fasting than when maintained on a low sodium diet [8–11]. Stinebaugh and Schloeder [12] separated the effects produced by salt restriction from those of fasting, by feeding their subjects low sodium diets immediately prior to total fasting. They showed that there was a natriuresis associated with the withdrawal of calories, which began on the second day of fasting, reached a peak on the fourth day, and then subsided. This natriuresis associated with the withdrawal of calories, which occurs at varying levels of sodium intake [13,14], is arrested by refeeding with carbohydrate or protein [13,15]. Indeed some workers have found that fat refeeding temporarily aggravates the natriuresis [14].

Chinn et al studied the relationship of changes in plasma total renin (PRC) and plasma aldosterone concentrations to electrolyte balance during complete fasting and during sodium deprivation followed by fasting [16]. During simple sodium deprivation, obese subjects lost significantly more sodium than did lean subjects, but the rise in PRC was similar in the two groups (Fig. 74.2). During complete fasting, there was a failure of PRC to increase despite a marked negative sodium balance. In the early stages of the fast, PRC decreased in 9 of 11 subjects, while subsequently it increased in all subjects. During sodium deprivation, PRC and plasma aldosterone concentration rose in all subjects studied, but in the first few days of a period of complete fasting immediately following, there was a fall in PRC in 8 of 10 volunteers, while plasma aldosterone continued to rise in five of six subjects in whom it was measured [16].

These investigators concluded that the exaggerated sodium loss in fasted obese people could have three components: exponentially decreasing sodium loss due simply to sodium deprivation; an enhanced sodium loss peculiar to obese subjects; and a secondary natriuresis related to calorie withdrawal. Several possibilities were considered as accounting for the secondary natriuresis. There could be, for example, a net sodium loss from the extracellular compartment with or without a subsequent drain from the intracellular fluid. Alternatively, there might be an influx of sodium into the extracellular fluid from some other sites; in this instance, the extracellular fluid would be expanded and the urinary sodium loss might be a consequence of the expansion. Possible sources of an influx of sodium into the

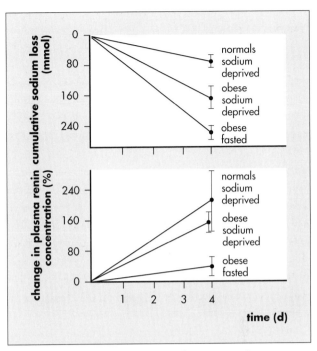

Fig. 74.2 Cumulative sodium loss and percentage change in plasma renin concentration during sodium deprivation in normal and obese subjects and during total fasting in obese subjects. Data are mean ± SEM. Modified from Chinn RH et al [16].

extracellular fluid during fasting, which Chinn et al [16] considered, were bone (thought to be unlikely because any such mobilization of sodium would require to occur early in fasting), gut, and intracellular fluid.

An explanation for the dissociation between PRC and aldosterone was also extensively considered but not resolved [16]. Possibilities included a dissociation of aldosterone from PRC, but not from Ang II; an enhanced stimulant action of Ang II on aldosterone secretion in these circumstances; an alternative to Ang II as a stimulus to aldosterone secretion; and a fall in aldosterone metabolic clearance rate. A further problem was to explain the inability of the elevated plasma aldosterone to prevent the natriuresis. In part, this might have been due to the need for a direct renal antinatriuretic effect of Ang II (see *Chapters 26* and *27*), as well as of aldosterone, a need that was not supplied in the absence of a rise in Ang II.

While this early study was invaluable in defining the phenomenon and in posing the problems to be solved, as Chinn et al conceded [16], it did not succeed in resolving the issue; indeed, it raised more questions than it answered.

Nocenti et al [17] showed that the natriuresis of fasting in the rabbit was accompanied by a significant reduction in PRC, unchanged plasma renin activity (PRA), markedly increased plasma angiotensinogen, a fall in plasma Ang I, and a significant increase in Ang II.

Boulter et al [18] demonstrated in man, that during the natriuretic phase of starvation, aldosterone secretion rose while PRA fell. Renal tubular mineralocorticoid sensitivity was diminished. Kolanowski et al [19] showed that on day four of a fast in man, infused aldosterone had a 60% diminished mineralocorticoid effect. North et al [20], noting that the natriuresis of fasting can be virtually abolished by giving ammonium chloride beforehand, reported that a major factor responsible for the increased excretion of sodium on fasting (and for the excessive retention of sodium on refeeding) was a failure of ammonium excretion to keep pace with the changing output of organic acid.

Spark et al [21] noted that during fasting, peak natriuresis and loss of renal tubular sensitivity to both endogenous and exogenous mineralocorticoids were accompanied by a rise in plasma levels of immunoactive glucagon. Conversely, during carbohydrate refeeding, with augmented renal tubular sensitivity to mineralocorticoid, glucagon levels become very low or undetectable. In fed subjects, infusion of glucagon to produce levels calculated to mimic those during fasting caused natriuresis. Spark et al proposed that the inability of the elevated plasma aldosterone to control natriuresis during fasting might be in part explained by an antimineralocorticoid action of elevated plasma glucagon values [21].

Cooke et al [22] proposed that the magnitude and persistence of the exaggerated sodium retention on refeeding was consistent with 'resetting' of sodium homeostatic mechanisms.

FEEDING

The ingestion of a meal can stimulate the RAS (see *Chapter 15*).

CAFFEINE

In a controlled experiment, Robertson et al [23] showed that a single dose of oral caffeine increased PRA by 57%, plasma norepinephrine by 75%, and plasma epinephrine by 207%.

Brown et al [24] reported that caffeine, in a dose selected to cause adenosine receptor blockade, augmented the PRA response to diazoxide in healthy volunteers.

However, a subsequent study by Robertson et al [25] showed more minor and less consistent effects, with an insignificant rise in mean PRA and unchanged plasma Ang II, 60 minutes after caffeine administration. Likewise, Passmore and

colleagues [26] showed no effect of caffeine in doses up to 360mg on PRA in healthy volunteers.

TILTING

Circulating total PRC [27], plasma active renin concentration [28], and plasma Ang II [28] are increased by upright tilting on a tilt table. This effect can be lost or diminished in patients with orthostatic hypotension and autonomic nervous lesions of the efferent component of the reflex arc [29]. However, the renin response to tilting is preserved if an autonomic lesion is restricted to the afferent component of the arc [29]. Prolonged upright tilting can in part overcome the renin-suppressing effect of massive β-adrenergic blockade [28].

A rise in PRA on tilting has been found in tetraplegic patients [30] (see below).

TETRAPLEGIA

As mentioned above, PRA increases on tilting in patients who are tetraplegic. In tetraplegic subjects, PRA has been found not to be affected by bladder stimulation or the infusion of norepinephrine, but to respond to isoproterenol and to insulin-induced hypoglycemia to the same extent as in normal subjects [31]. Thus, renin-release mechanisms in tetraplegic patients do not seem to be hypersensitive to catecholamines.

STANDING AND WALKING

Both renin and Ang II are increased on ambulation. The rise in renin on standing can be minimized by applying positive pressure to the lower extremities [32].

EXERCISE

Exercise, either acute or when continued over some days, induces increments in PRA [33–36].

EXERCISE PROTEINURIA

It has been proposed that the proteinuria that can accompany severe exercise can be a result of increases in renin, and hence of a renal action of Ang II [37]. The effects of Ang II in causing proteinuria are discussed in more detail in *Chapters 26, 55, 58,* and *72*.

STRESS

RESTRAINT

The stress accompanying restraint has been shown to enhance PRA in spontaneously hypertensive rats (SHR) but not in Wistar–Kyoto animals [38].

HEAT STRESS

Increased PRA, Ang II, and aldosterone levels were noted during and after heat stress in a sauna bath [39,40] (Fig. 74.3). Brandenberger *et al* [40] observed that after propranolol administration, although PRA was depressed, the aldosterone response to heat exposure increased. Concurrently, propranolol reduced heat tolerance, leading to increased release of adrenocorticotropic hormone and cortisol in three of the six subjects studied. Thus, the aldosterone response to heat exposure appears not to be primarily or necessarily mediated via the RAS.

AIR STRESS

Directing a jet of air to the face stimulated an increase in PRA in young, restrained SHR; this effect was diminished by propranolol treatment [38].

MENTAL ARITHMETIC

The performance of mental arithmetic has been shown to increase PRA and Ang II in control subjects [41].

AGGRESSION

Aggressive behaviour in mice can result in a 600-fold increase in PRC [42,43] (see *Chapter 43*). This increase is due mainly to release of submaxillary renin, although there is also significant renal renin release. The extent of renin release is influenced by the duration of aggression and by previous exposure to other mice, both of which diminish renin output.

NOISE

Intensities of noise below the human pain threshold can acutely increase PRA in conscious rats, an effect which is enhanced by sodium deprivation [44].

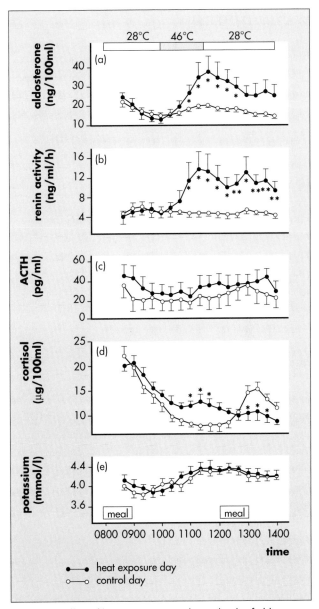

Fig. 74.3 Effect of heat exposure on plasma levels of aldosterone (a), renin activity (b), adrenocorticotropic hormone (c), cortisol (d), and potassium (e) in six sodium-restricted subjects (mean ± SEM). The asterisks indicate significant differences (*P*<0.05) in the corresponding levels between the two experimental days. Modified from Brandenberger G *et al* [40].

WATER IMMERSION

Water immersion to the neck causes a profound suppression of plasma renin and aldosterone (Fig. 74.4) [45]. The mechanisms effecting this include increased release of ANF, with ANF-mediated inhibition of renin secretion (see *Chapter 36*), and decreased renal sympathetic nerve traffic [45].

DIURNAL CHANGE

There is a distinct, albeit modest, variation of PRC through 24 hours in ambulant subjects, with a zenith at about time 1000 and a nadir around time 2200 [46–48]. This normal diurnal cycle is influenced by posture; in recumbent subjects, plasma active renin concentration, PRA, and Ang II are either unchanged or fall slightly between time 0900 and 1200 [49,50].

SLEEP

In man, during sleep, a strong ultradian rhythm in PRA has been observed, closely linked to the rapid eye movement (REM) and non-REM sleep cycles. Increasing PRA values mark the transition from REM to non-REM sleep, while declining levels coincide with the transition from deep to lighter sleep [46,48]. Plasma renin activity curves thus reflect the pattern of sleep stages.

Pretreatment with furosemide or the administration of a sodium-deficient diet enhance both the nocturnal upward trend of PRA and the superimposed oscillations corresponding to the stages of sleep [48] (Fig. 74.5). Conversely, the β-blocker atenolol lowers the underlying PRA and flattens the increase associated with non-REM sleep.

Thus, the normal nocturnal secretion of renin during sleep remains intermittent, corresponding to the stages of sleep, even when renin release is enhanced or depressed by other influences.

MENSTRUAL CYCLE

Plasma renin and Ang II are generally higher in the luteal phase of the menstrual cycle [49–51]. These aspects are considered in detail in *Chapter 50*.

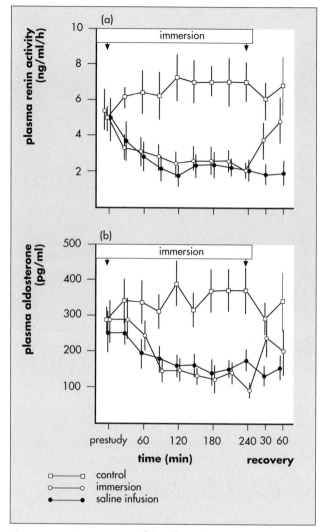

Fig. 74.4 (a) Comparison of the effects of control, water immersion, and acute saline infusion (2l/120min), in the seated posture, on plasma renin activity (PRA) in nine normal subjects in balance on a 10-mmol sodium diet. Immersion resulted in a progressive decrement in PRA beginning as early as 30 min, with maximal suppression during the final 2h of immersion. The saline-induced suppression of PRA was indistinguishable from that observed during immersion. Results are the mean ± SEM. (b) Comparison of the effects of control, water immersion, and acute saline infusion (2l/120min), in the seated posture, on plasma aldosterone in nine normal subjects in balance on a 10-mmol sodium diet. Immersion resulted in a progressive decrement in plasma aldosterone beginning as early as 60 min of immersion. Saline-induced suppression of plasma aldosterone was indistinguishable from that observed during immersion. Modified from Epstein M *et al* [45].

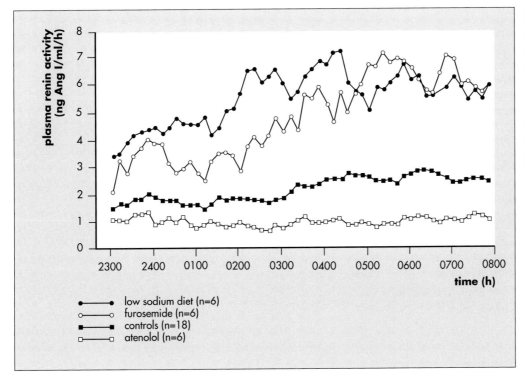

Fig. 74.5 Mean plasma renin activity profiles from three groups of six subjects who received either furosemide or atenolol or who were on a low sodium diet for three days, together with mean profiles observed during control nights. Modified from Brandenberger G *et al* [48].

PREGNANCY

Very marked, and rather variable, increases in active and inactive renin, angiotensinogen, and Ang II occur in normal human pregnancy. A detailed account of these changes is presented in *Chapter 50*.

THYROID DEFICIENCY

Plasma renin is low in patients with hypothyroidism, possibly because of diminished β-adrenergic activity [114]. Renin returns to normal when the euthyroid state is restored.

HEMORRHAGE

Bleeding is a marked stimulus to renin secretion, a topic considered in detail in *Chapter 71*.

HEMOGLOBIN

Hemoglobin blood level is positively correlated with PRA in man [52,53]. Plasma renin activity is elevated with polycythemia [54].

LEUKOCYTE COUNT

Leukocyte count is positively correlated with PRA in man [52,54].

FACTOR VIII

Clotting factor VIII in man has been found to be positively correlated with PRA [52].

CHOLESTEROL

In man, blood cholesterol is positively correlated with PRA [52,55].

AGE

Numerous studies have shown a progressive fall in PRC, PRA, and Ang II with age in man [52,56–58]. This fall is exponential, being very rapid in early childhood, and continuing into old age (see *Chapter 83, Fig. 83.1*).

ARTERIAL PRESSURE

Studies in man, both ostensibly normal and with essential hypertension, have usually shown either no relationship, or an inverse correlation, between blood pressure and PRC, PRA, or Ang II [52,56,59–62]. The inverse relationship is more marked in men than in women [52]. In one report, there was a weak, and probably a chance, positive correlation between systolic pressure and Ang II in essential hypertension [63]. These findings contrast with the positive corrrelation between Ang II and blood pressure consistently observed in both clinical and experimental renovascular hypertension (see *Chapter 55*). Importantly, with progressive lowering of renin and Ang II in essential hypertension, the adrenocortical aldosterone response to Ang II is enhanced [2,64–66] (see *Fig. 74.1*) (see *Chapters 33* and *62*).

Most investigators consider that this inverse correlation between blood pressure and the RAS reflects diminished neural stimulation of renin release and/or afferent renal glomerular arteriolar sclerosis with higher blood pressures [55,59,67]. However, Gordon [68] has proposed, rather differently, that the RAS lowers, rather than elevates, arterial pressure; this latter view has not found general acceptance.

In essential hypertension, total peripheral resistance is negatively correlated with plasma renin, indicating that 'high-renin' essential hypertension is not necessarily associated with arteriolar constriction [59].

GENDER

Plasma renin activity is lower in women than in age-matched men [52].

RACE

Both in the USA and Britain, blacks have been found to have consistently lower PRA than have whites [52,69–71].

CIGARETTE SMOKING

Mean PRA has been found in smokers and ex-smokers to be approximately 20% higher than in nonsmokers [52].

EFFECTS OF THERAPEUTIC DRUGS

DIURETICS
A full account of diuretics is given in *Chapter 80*. Diuretic agents, including thiazides and related drugs, loop-acting agents, and potassium-conserving drugs such as spironolactone and amiloride, stimulate an increase in plasma renin and Ang II. In large measure, this reflects their varied natriuretic potency (see *Chapter 73*), and, to a less extent, their differing capacity also to cause potassium loss [72]. However, loop-acting diuretics can stimulate renin release directly: for example, with intravenous furosemide, marked and rapid increases in plasma active renin concentration and Ang II are seen, with peak levels 15–30 minutes after injection; values then subside despite continuing natriuresis [28].

MINERALOCORTICOIDS
Drugs with mineralocorticoid activity, such as fludrocortisone, deoxycorticosterone (DOC), and carbenoxolone, and also licorice-containing compounds, suppress the RAS in proportion to the extent of induced sodium retention. In the cases of aldosterone and DOC at least, there is no direct feedback on renin secretion but rather, suppression of renin secondary to sodium retention [73–75]. These matters are dealt with in detail in *Chapter 63*.

SYMPATHOLYTIC AGENTS
Guanethidine and bethanidine have been reported to have inconsistent effects on the RAS [76].

BETA-ADRENERGIC BLOCKERS
Beta-blockers, including labetalol which has also an α-blocking component, nearly always induce a fall in PRA, PRC, and Ang II. Nevertheless, this suppressant effect can be partly overcome by the administration of furosemide or by upright tilting [28]. Moreover, β-blockers with marked agonist activity, such as pindolol, can stimulate an increase in PRA [77].

A detailed account of effects of β-blockers on the renin system is given in *Chapter 84*.

ALPHA-ADRENERGIC BLOCKERS

Early studies, as discussed in *Chapter 24*, indicated that the postsynaptic α-blocker prazosin was either neutral in its effect on renin release or actually inhibitory. However, more recent studies in man show that the acute effect of prazosin is to stimulate a rise in plasma active renin concentration and Ang II [78]. This stimulant effect on renin release is blunted or lost with continued prazosin therapy [79]. Further details are given in *Chapter 80*.

CENTRALLY ACTING ANTIHYPERTENSIVE DRUGS

Reserpine, methyldopa, and clonidine all tend to inhibit renin release and to blunt the increases in PRA following stimuli such as hemorrhage or furosemide administration [76]. This topic is considered also in *Chapters 37 and 80*.

KETANSERIN

The serotonergic S$_2$ antagonist ketanserin, which also possesses some α-blocking effects, has been reported variously to cause in man, a small transient increase in PRA [80] or to leave both plasma active renin concentration and Ang II unchanged [81] (see *Chapter 80*).

ANGIOTENSIN II ANTAGONISTS

Antagonists of Ang II, whether peptide analogs of Ang II such as saralasin, or nonpeptide Ang II antagonists, cause increases in PRC, PRA, and Ang II [82,83] (see *Chapter 86*).

ANGIOTENSIN-CONVERTING ENZYME INHIBITORS

Angiotensin-converting enzyme inhibitors are discussed extensively in *Chapters 87–99*. They cause a fall in plasma Ang II, with converse increases in circulating renin and Ang I. With long-term therapy in man [84], the rise in Ang I is proportionately less than the rise in active renin concentration. This has been considered by some investigators (see *Chapters 8, 86, and 88*) possibly to reflect the fall in plasma angiotensinogen seen with long-term ACE inhibition [85], which in turn is largely due to loss of the stimulant effect of Ang II on angiotensinogen release [86]. However, others (see *Chapter 23*) have opposed this concept.

RENIN INHIBITORS

Administration of a renin inhibitor in man causes a fall in circulating Ang I and Ang II, with concomitant increases in circulating concentrations of active and inactive renin [87,88].

However, renin concentration measured by enzymic methods, and PRA, are low. Renin inhibitors are described in detail in *Chapter 85*.

CALCIUM ANTAGONISTS

Calcium antagonists are considered in detail in *Chapter 80*, and therefore receive only brief mention here.

There is remarkable inconsistency concerning descriptions of the effects of dihydropyridine calcium antagonists on the RAS in man. In part, the very varied reports reflect the conflicting views on whether or not these agents, when used to treat hypertension, do or do not cause sodium retention [89–92].

Marone *et al* [89] found that nifedipine lowered blood pressure in essential hypertension while causing an average 27% expansion in total exchangeable sodium and also weight gain; concurrently, PRA was slightly, but insignificantly, increased. Lederballe-Pedersen *et al* [93] found nifedipine in essential hypertension to cause a significant increase in PRA. Pevahouse *et al* [90], on withdrawing long-term therapy with nifedipine in hypertension, saw sodium rentention and a fall in PRA.

Aoki and Sato [94] found that niludipine lowered blood pressure in essential hypertension without affecting PRA.

With amlodipine, Cappuccio *et al* [95] found blood-pressure reduction and no measurable change in sodium balance, but a significant rise in PRA.

Waeber *et al* [96] found that administration of the phenylalkylamine calcium antagonist verapamil to rats with 1-clip, 1-kidney hypertension (see *Chapter 55*) lowered blood pressure while markedly stimulating renin release. They found no evidence that the blood-pressure reduction was influenced by the state of sodium balance or PRA.

VASODILATORS

The vasodilating antihypertensive agents diazoxide, minoxidil, hydralazine, nitroprusside, and guancidine all consistently stimulate the RAS [76] as discussed fully in *Chapter 80*.

CARDIAC GLYCOSIDES

Ouabain has been demonstrated to inhibit the secretion of renin from rat kidney slices [97]. In man, Cody *et al* [98] showed a modest lowering of PRA with the acute administration of digoxin. As discussed in *Chapter 76*, cardiac glycosides can, in the short term, suppress plasma renin in patients with cardiac failure, but long-term therapy has little or no effect.

CALCITONIN

The intravenous infusion of salmon calcitonin in man has been observed to cause significant increases in PRA, aldosterone, and serum ACE [99]. These effects were considered to be, at least in part, consequences of renal losses of sodium and calcium.

PROSTAGLANDINS

As discussed above, and also extensively in *Chapter 38*, the ability of prostaglandins to enhance renin secretion has been reported [100–102], but also remains a matter of some controversy [103].

INDOMETHACIN

Indomethacin administration in dogs with caval constriction had very modest effects in lowering PRA, although causing marked decreases in both creatinine clearance and renal plasma flow [102]. Moreover, indomethacin failed to suppress the rise in PRA on administration of saralasin to sodium-depleted dogs, despite a 58% fall in the rate of excretion of PGE_2 [104]. A detailed account is given in *Chapter 80*.

INSULIN

Insulin has been shown to produce a dose-dependent reduction in renin release in the isolated perfused rat kidney [105]. This inhibitory effect of insulin on renin release was abrogated by perfusion with a calcium-free solution or by the addition of verapamil. In healthy volunteers, however, insulin-induced hypoglycemia induces a brisk rise in PRA, which can be blocked by propranolol [106].

Several related aspects are discussed in *Chapters 75* and *92*.

VITAMIN D₃

No evidence was found that 1,25 dihydroxyvitamin D_3 influenced renin output [107].

COLCHICINE

Colchicine was found to be without effect on the basal level of renin release from isolated rat glomeruli [108].

VINCA ALKALOIDS

Vincristine and vinblastine caused a progressive increase in basal renin release from isolated rat glomeruli [108].

CYCLOSPORIN

Siegl and Ryffel [109] reported an increase in PRA in dogs and rats given cyclosporin. A similar effect was seen in rats by Baxter *et al* [110]. In man and marmoset, however, most reports suggest that cyclosporin alters renin little or has a suppressive effect [111–113].

ERYTHROPOIETIN

The interrelationships between erythropoietin and the RAS are discussed in detail in *Chapter 39*.

SUMMARY

In summary, renal renin secretion is modified by a host of physiological and pharmacological stimuli acting through known input signals to the juxtaglomerular apparatus (see *Chapters 24* and *38*). While our knowledge of these modulating factors and the mechanisms by which they alter renal renin secretion and release is considerable, there are still large areas of uncertainty and ignorance. Interpretation of circulating levels of renin and Ang II (see *Chapter 83*) in health and disease requires nevertheless an understanding of these modulating influences.

REFERENCES

1. Brown JJ, Davies DL, Lever AF, Robertson JIS. Influence of sodium deprivation and loading on the plasma-renin in man. *Journal of Physiology* 1964;173:408–19.
2. Brown JJ, Casals-Stenzel J, Cumming AMM, Davies DL, Fraser R, Lever AF, Morton JJ, Semple PF, Tree M, Robertson JIS. Angiotensin II, aldosterone and arterial pressure: A quantitative approach. Arthur C Corcoran Memorial Lecture. *Hypertension* 1979;1:159–79.
3. Fraser R, James VHT, Brown JJ, Davies DL, Lever AF, Robertson JIS. Changes in plasma aldosterone, cortisol, corticosterone, and renin concentration in a patient with sodium-losing renal disease. *Journal of Endocrinology* 1966;35:311–20.
4. Churchill MC, Churchill PC, McDonald FD. Comparison of the effects of rubidium and potassium on renin secretion from rat kidney slices. *Endocrinology* 1983;112:777–82.
5. Sealey JE, Clark I, Bull MB, Laragh JH. Potassium balance and the control of renin secretion. *Journal of Clinical Investigation* 1970;49:2119–27.
6. Dluhy RG, Underwood RH, Williams GH. Influence of dietary potassium on plasma renin activity in normal man. *Journal of Applied Physiology* 1970;28:299–302.
7. Linas SL, Dickmann D, Arnold P. Mechanism of hyperreninemia in the potassium-depleted rat. *Journal of Clinical Investigation* 1981;68:347–55.
8. Gamble JL, Ross GS, Tisdall FF. Metabolism of fixed base during fasting. *Journal of Biological Chemistry* 1923;57:633–95.
9. Hervey GR, McCance RA. Effects of carbohydrate and seawater on metabolism of men without food or sufficient water. *Proceedings of the Royal Society of London. Series B: Biological Sciences* 1952;139:527–545.

10. Bloom WL, Mitchell W. Salt excretion of fasting patients. *Archives of Internal Medicine* 1960;**106**:312–26.

11. Rapaport A, From GLA, Husdan H. Metabolic studies in prolonged fasting. I. Inorganic metabolism and kidney function. *Metabolism* 1965;**14**:31–46.

12. Stinebaugh BJ, Schloeder FX. Studies on the natriuresis of fasting. I. Effect of prefast intake. *Metabolism* 1966;**15**:828–37.

13. Bloom WL. Inhibition of salt excretion by carbohydrate. *Archives of Internal Medicine* 1962;**109**:80–6.

14. Veverbrants E, Arky RA. Effects of fasting and refeeding. I. Studies on sodium potassium and water excretion on a constant electrolyte and fluid intake. *Journal of Clinical Endocrinology and Metabolism* 1969;**29**:55–62.

15. Katz AI, Hollingsworth DR, Epstein FH. Influence of carbohydrate and protein on sodium excretion during fasting and refeeding. *Journal of Laboratory and Clinical Medicine* 1969;**72**:93–104.

16. Chinn RH, Brown JJ, Fraser R, Heron SM, Lever AF, Murchison L, Robertson JIS. The natriuresis of fasting: Relationship to changes in plasma renin and plasma aldosterone concentrations. *Clinical Science* 1970;**39**:436–55.

17. Nocenti MR, Simchon S, Cizek LJ. Analysis of the renin–angiotensin system during fasting in adult male rabbits. *Proceedings of the Society for Experimental Biology and Medicine* 1975;**150**:142–7.

18. Boulter PR, Spark RF, Arky RA. Dissociation of the renin–aldosterone system and refractoriness to the sodium-retaining action of mineralocorticoid during starvation in man. *Journal of Clinical Endocrinology and Metabolism* 1974;**38**:248–54.

19. Kolanowski J, Desmecht P, Crabbé J. Sodium balance and renal tubular sensitivity to aldosterone during total fast and carbohydrate refeeding in the obese. *European Journal of Clinical Investigation* 1976;**6**:75–8.

20. North KAK, Lascelles D, Coates P. The mechanisms by which sodium excretion is increased during a fast but reduced on subsequent carbohydrate refeeding. *Clinical Science* 1974;**46**:423–32.

21. Spark RF, Arky RA, Boulter PR, Saudek CK, O'Brien JT. Renin, aldosterone and glucagon in the natriuresis of fasting. *New England Journal of Medicine* 1975;**292**:1335–9.

22. Cooke CR, Turin MD, Whelton A, Walker WG. Studies of marked and persistent sodium retention in previously fasted and sodium-deprived obese subjects. *Metabolism* 1987;**36**:609–15.

23. Robertson D, Frölich JC, Carr RK, Watson JT, Hollifield JW, Shand DG, Oates JA. Effects of caffeine on plasma renin activity, catecholamines and blood pressure. *New England Journal of Medicine* 1978;**298**:181–6.

24. Brown NJ, Porter J, Ryder D, Branch RA. Caffeine potentiates the renin response to diazoxide in man. Evidence of a regulatory role of endogenous adenosine. *Journal of Pharmacology and Experimental Therapeutics* 1991;**256**:56–61.

25. Robertson D, Hollister AS, Kincaid D, Workman R, Goldberg MR, Tung CS, Smith B. Caffeine and hypertension. *American Journal of Medicine* 1984;**77**:54–60.

26. Passmore AP, Kondowe GB, Johnston GD. Renal and cardiovascular effects of caffeine: A dose–response study. *Clinical Science* 1987;**72**:749–56.

27. Brown JJ, Davies DL, Lever AF, McPherson D, Robertson JIS. Plasma renin concentration in relation to changes in posture. *Clinical Science* 1966;**30**:279–84.

28. Sonkodi S, Agabati-Rosei E, Fraser R, Leckie BJ, Morton JJ, Cumming AMM, Sood VP, Robertson JIS. Response of the renin–angiotensin–aldosterone system to upright tilting and to intravenous frusemide: Effect of prior metoprolol and propranolol. *British Journal of Clinical Pharmacology* 1982;**13**:341–50.

29. Love DR, Brown JJ, Chinn RH, Johnson RH, Lever AF, Park DM, Robertson JIS. Plasma renin in idiopathic orthostatic hypotension: Differential response in subjects with probable afferent and efferent autonomic failure. *Clinical Science* 1971;**41**:289–99.

30. Mathias CJ, Christiansen NJ, Corbett JL, Frankel HL, Goodwin TJ, Peart WS. Plasma catecholamines, plasma renin activity and plasma aldosterone in tetraplegic man, horizontal and tilted. *Clinical Science* 1975;**49**:291–9.

31. Mathias CJ, Frankel HL, Davies IB, James VHT, Peart WS. Renin and aldosterone release during sympathetic stimulation in tetraplegia. *Clinical Science* 1981;**60**:399–404.

32. McGivern D, Hardcastle A, Millar JGB, Warren DJ. Modification of the normal postural changes in plasma renin activity by the application of positive pressure to the legs. *Clinical Endocrinology* 1979;**11**:105–9.

33. Kotchen TA, Hartley LH, Rice TW, Mougey EH, Jones LG, Mason JW. Renin, norepinephrine, and epinephrine responses to graded exercise. *Journal of Applied Physiology* 1971;**31**:178–84.

34. Kosunen JK, Pakarinen AJ. Plasma renin, angiotensin II and plasma and urinary aldosterone in running exercise. *Journal of Applied Physiology* 1976;**41**:26–9.

35. Milledge JS, Bryson EI, Catley DM, Hesp R, Luff N, Minty BD, Older MWJ, Payne NN, Ward MP, Withey WR. Sodium balance, fluid homeostasis and the renin–aldosterone system during the prolonged exercise of hill walking. *Clinical Science* 1982;**62**:595–604.

36. Convertino VA, Keil LC, Greenleaf JE. Plasma volume, renin, and vasopressin responses to graded exercise after training. *Journal of Applied Physiology* 1983;**54**:508–14.

37. Castenfors J. Exercise and renal function. *Acta Physiologica Scandinavica* 1967;**70** (suppl 293):1–44.

38. Porter JP. Effect of stress on the control of renin release in spontaneously hypertensive rats. *Hypertension* 1990;**15**:310–7.

39. Kosunen KJ, Pakarinen AJ, Kuoppasalmi K, Adlercreutz H. Plasma renin activity, angiotensin II, and aldosterone during intense heat stress. *Journal of Applied Physiology* 1976;**41**:323–7.

40. Brandenberger G, Follenius M, Oyono S, Reinhardt B, Simeone M. Effect of propranolol on aldosterone response to heat exposure in sodium-restricted men. *Journal of Endocrinological Investigation* 1980;**4**:395–400.

41. Kosunen KJ. Plasma renin activity, angiotensin II, and aldosterone after mental arithmetic. *Scandinavian Journal of Clinical and Laboratory Investigation* 1977;**37**:425–9.

42. Bing JB, Poulsen K. In mice aggressive behaviour provokes vast increase in plasma renin concentration, causing only slight, if any increase in blood pressure. *Acta Physiologica Scandinavica* 1979;**105**:64–72.

43. Bing J, Poulsen K. Aggression-provoked renin release from extrarenal and extrasubmaxillary sources in mice. *Acta Physiologica Scandinavica* 1979;**107**:251–6.

44. Vander AJ, Kay LL, Dugan E, Mouw DR. Effects of noise on plasma renin activity in rats. *Proceedings of the Society for Experimental Biology and Medicine* 1977;**156**:24–6.

45. Epstein M, Richard RE, Preston S, Haber E. Comparison of the suppressive effects of water immersion and saline administration of renin–aldosterone in normal man. *Journal of Clinical Endocrinology and Metabolism* 1979;**49**:358–63.

46. Mullen PE, James VHT, Lightman SL, Linsell C, Peart WS. A relationship between plasma renin activity and the rapid eye movement phase of sleep in man. *Journal of Clinical Endocrinology and Metabolism* 1980;**50**:466–9.

47. Brandenberger G, Follenius M, Muzet A, Ehrhat J, Schieber JP. Ultradian oscillations in plasma renin activity: Their relationships to meals and sleep stages. *Journal of Clinical Endocrinology and Metabolism* 1985;**61**:280–4.

48. Brandenberger G, Krauth MO, Ehrhart J, Libert JP, Simon Ch, Follenius M. Modulation of episodic renin release during sleep in humans. *Hypertension* 1990;**15**:370–5.

49. Brown JJ, Davies DL, Lever AF, Robertson JIS. Variations in plasma renin during the menstrual cycle. *British Medical Journal* 1964;**ii**:1114–5.

50. Lightman A, Tarlatzis BC, Rzasa PJ, Culler MD, Caride VJ, Negro-Vilar AF, Lennard D, DeCherney AF, Naftolin F. The ovarian renin–angiotensin system: Renin-like activity and angiotensin II/III immunoreactivity in gonadotrophin-stimulated and unstimulated human follicular fluid. *American Journal of Obstetrics and Gynecology* 1987;**156**:808–14.

51. Cedard L, Mignot ThM, Giuchard A, Boyer P, Zorn JR. Immunoreactive renin variations during fertile and infertile hyperstimulated cycles with *in-vitro* fertilisation and embryo transfer or gamete intra-Fallopian transfer. *Human Reproduction* 1989;**4**:403–7.

52. Meade TW, Imeson JD, Gordon D, Peart WS. The epidemiology of plasma renin. *Clinical Science* 1983;**64**:273–80.

53. Meyer P, Ménard J, Alexandre J-M, Weil B. Correlations between plasma renin, hematocrit and natriuresis. *Revue Canadienne de Biologie* 1966;**25**:111–3.

54. Wallis PJW, Cunningham J, Few JD, Newland AC, Empey DW. Effects of packed cell volume reduction on renal haemodynamics and the renin–angiotensin–aldosterone system in patients with secondary polycythaemia and hypoxic cor pulmonale. *Clinical Science* 1986;**70**:81–90.

55. Russell GI, Bing RF, Thurston H, Swales JD. Plasma renin in hypertensive patients: Significance in relation to clinical and other biochemical features. *Quarterly Journal of Medicine* 1980;**49**:385–94.

56. Karlberg BE, Tolagen K. Relationships between blood pressure, age, plasma renin activity and electrolyte excretion in normotensive subjects. *Scandinavian Journal of Clinical and Laboratory Investigation* 1977;**37**:521–8.

57. Van Acker KJ, Scharpe SL, Deprettere AJR, Neels HM. Renin–angiotensin–aldosterone system in the healthy infant and child. *Kidney International* 1979;**16**:196–203.

58. Weidmann P, Beretta-Piccoli C, Ziegler WH, Keusch G, Gluck Z, Reubi FC. Age versus urinary sodium for judging renin, aldosterone, and catecholamines levels. Studies in normal subjects and patients with essential hypertension. *Kidney International* 1978;**14**:619–28.

59. Fagard R, Amery A, Reybrouck T, Lijnen P, Billiet L, Joossens JV. Plasma renin levels and systemic haemodynamics in essential hypertension. *Clinical Science* 1977;**52**:591–7.

60. Beevers DG, Morton JJ, Nelson CS, Padfield PL, Titterington N, Tree M. Angiotensin II in essential hypertension. *British Medical Journal* 1977;**1**:415.

61. Thomas GW, Ledingham JGG, Beilin LJ, Stott AN, Yeates KM. Reduced renin activity in essential hypertension: A reappraisal. *Kidney International* 1978;**13**:513–8.

62. James GD, Pickering TG, Laragh JH. Ambulatory blood pressure variation is related to plasma renin activity in borderline hypertensive men. *American Journal of Hypertension* 1991;**4**:525–8.

63. Beretta-Piccoli C, Davies DL, Boddy K, Brown JJ, Cumming AMM, East K, Fraser R, Lever AF, Padfield PL, Semple PF, Robertson JIS, Weidmann P, Williams ED. Relation of arterial pressure with body sodium, body potassium and plasma potassium in essential hypertension. *Clinical Science* 1982;**63**:257–70.

64. Kisch ES, Dluhy RG, Williams GH. Enhanced aldosterone response to angiotensin II in human hypertension. *Circulation Research* 1976;**38**:502–5.

65. Wisgerhof M, Brown RD. Increased adrenal sensitivity to angiotensin II in low-renin essential hypertension. *Journal of Clinical Investigation* 1978;**61**:1456–62.

66. Fraser R, Beretta-Piccoli C, Brown JJ, Cumming AMM, Lefer AF, Mason PA, Morton JJ, Robertson JIS. Response of aldosterone and 18-hydroxycorticosterone to angiotensin II in normal subjects and patients with essential hypertension. Conn's syndrome, and non-tumorous hyperaldosteronism. *Hypertension* 1981; **3** (suppl 1):87–92.

67. Swales JD. Low-renin hypertension: Nephrosclerosis? *Lancet* 1975;**i**:75–7.

68. Gordon DB. Hypothesis: Renin lowers blood pressure. *Lancet* 1978;**ii**:970–2.

69. Channick BJ, Adlin EV, Marks AD. Suppressed plasma renin activity in hypertension. *Archives of Internal Medicine* 1969;**123**:131–40.

70. Mroczek WJ, Finnerty FA, Catt KJ. Lack of association between plasma-renin and history of heart-attack or stroke in patients with essential hypertension. *Lancet* 1973;**ii**:464–9.

71. Creditor MC, Loschky UK. Plasma renin activity in hypertension. *American Journal of Medicine* 1967;**43**:371–82.

72. Singh BN, Hollenberg NK, Poole-Wilson PA, Robertson JIS. Diuretic-induced potassium and magnesium deficiency: Relation to drug-induced QT prolongation, cardiac arrhythmias and sudden death. *Journal of Hypertension* 1992;**10**:301–6.

73. Geelhoed GW, Vander AJ. The role of aldosterone in renin secretion. *Life Sciences* 1967;**6**:525–35.

74. Goodwin FJ, Knowlton AI, Laragh JH. Absence of renin suppression by deoxycorticosterone acetate in rats. *American Journal of Physiology* 1969;**216**:1476–80.

75. de Champlain J, Genest J, Veyrat R, Boucher R. Factors controlling renin in man. *Archives of Internal Medicine* 1966;**117**:355–63.

76. Guthrie GP, Genest J, Kuchel O. Renin and the therapy of hypertension. *Annual Review of Pharmacology and Toxicology* 1976;**16**:287–308.

77. Weber MA, Stokes GS, Gain JM. Comparison of the effects on renin release of beta adrenergic antagonists with differing properties. *Journal of Clinical Investigation* 1974;**54**:1413–9.

78. McAreavey D, Cumming AMM, Sood VP, Leckie BJ, Morton JJ, Murray GD, Robertson JIS. The effect of oral prazosin on blood pressure and plasma concentrations of renin and angiotensin II in man. *Clinical Science* 1981; **61** (suppl):457–60.

79. Webb DJ, Fulton JD, Leckie BJ, Malatino LS, McAreavey D, Morton JJ, Murray GD, Robertson JIS. The effect of chronic prazosin therapy on the responses of the renin–angiotensin system in patients with essential hypertension. *Journal of Human Hypertension* 1987;**1**:195–200.

80. Wenting GJ, Man in't Veld AJ, Woittiez AJJ, Boomsma F, Schalekamp MA. Treatment of hypertension with ketanserin, a new selective 5HT$_2$ receptor antagonist. *British Medical Journal* 1982;**284**:537–9.

81. Vanhoutte PM, Amery A, Birkenhäger WH, Breckenridge A, Bühler F, Distler A, Dormandy J, Doyle AE, Frohlich E, Hansson L, Hedner T, Hollenberg NK, Jensen H-E, Lund-Johansen P, Meyer P, Opie L, Robertson JIS, Safar M, Schalekamp MA, Trap-Jensen J, Zanchetti A. Serotonergic mechanisms in hypertension: Focus on the effects of ketanserin. *Hypertension* 1988;**11**:111–33.

82. Pettinger WA, Mitchell HC. Angiotensin antagonists as diagnostic and pharmacologic tools. *Progress in Biochemical Pharmacology* 1976;**12**:203–13.

83. Brown JJ, Brown WCB, Fraser R, Lever AF, Morton JJ, Robertson JIS, Rosei EA, Trust PM. The effect of the angiotensin II antagonist saralasin on blood pressure and plasma aldosterone in man in relation to the prevailing plasma angiotensin II concentration. *Progress in Biochemical Pharmacology* 1976;**12**:230–41.

84. Hodsman GP, Brown JJ, Cumming AMM, Davies DL, East BW, Lever AF, Morton JJ, Murray GD, Robertson JIS. Enalapril in treatment of hypertension with renal artery stenosis: Changes in blood pressure, renin, angiotensin I and II, renal function, and body composition. *American Journal of Medicine* 1984; **77** (2A):52–60.

85. Rasmussen S, Nielsen MD, Giese J. Captopril combined with thiazide lowers renin substrate concentration: Implications for methodology in renin assays. *Clinical Science* 1981;**60**:591–3.

86. Khayyall M, MacGregor J, Brown JJ, Lever AF, Robertson JIS. Increase of plasma renin-substrate concentration after infusion of angiotensin in the rat. *Clinical Science* 1973;**44**:87–90.

87. Webb DJ, Manhem PJO, Ball SG, Inglis G, Leckie BJ, Lever AF, Morton JJ, Robertson JIS, Murray GD, Ménard J, Jones DM, Szelke M. A study of the renin inhibitor H142 in man. *Journal of Hypertension* 1985;**3**:653–8.

88. Haber E. Renin inhibitors. *New England Journal of Medicine* 1984;**311**: 1631–3.

89. Marone C, Luisoli S, Bomio F, Beretta-Piccoli C, Bianchetti MG, Weidmann. Body sodium-blood volume state, aldosterone, and cardiovascular responsiveness after calcium entry blockade with nifedipine. *Kidney International* 1985;**28**: 658–65.

90. Pevahouse JB, Markandu ND, Cappuccio FP, Buckley MG, Sagnella GA, MacGregor GA. Long term reduction in sodium balance: Possible additional mechanism whereby nifedipine lowers blood pressure. *British Medical Journal* 1990;**301**:580–4.

91. Robertson JIS. Long-term reduction in sodium balance. *British Medical Journal* 1990;**301**:1159–60.

92. Cappuccio FP, Markandu ND, Sagnella GA, Singer DRJ, Buckley MG, Miller A, MacGregor GA. Acute and sustained changes in sodium balance during nifedipine treatment in essential hypertension. *American Journal of Medicine* 1991;**91**:233–8.

93. Lederballe-Pederson O, Mikkelsen E, Christensen NJ, Kornerup HJ, Pedersen EB. Effects of nifedipine on plasma renin, aldosterone, and catecholamines in hypertension. *European Journal of Clinical Pharmacology* 1979;**15**:235–40.

94. Aoki K, Sato K. Acute hypotensive, hemodynamic effects of long-term treatment with niludipine, a Ca^{2+}-antagonist, in patients with essential hypertension. *Drug Research* 1982;9:1141–5.

95. Cappuccio FP, Markandu ND, Sagnella GA, SInger DRJ, Buckley MG, Miller A, MacGregor GA. Effects of amlodipine on urinary sodium excretion, renin–angiotensin–aldosterone system, atrial natriuretic peptide and blood pressure in essential hypertension. *Journal of Human Hypertension* 1991;5:115–9.

96. Waeber B, Nussberger J, Brunner HR. Does renin determine the blood pressure response to calcium entry blockers? *Hypertension* 1985;7:223–7.

97. Churchill PC. Possible mechanism of the inhibitory effect of ouabain on renin secretion from rat renal cortical slices. *Journal of Physiology* 1979;294:123–34.

98. Covit AB, Schaer GL, Sealey JE, Laragh JH, Cody RJ. Suppression of the renin–angiotensin system by intravenous digoxin in chronic congestive heart failure. *American Journal of Medicine* 1983;75:445–7.

99. Malatino LS, Fiore CE, Fotti R, Tamburino FGG. Acute effects of salmon calcitonin in man include stimulation of the renin–angiotensin–aldosterone system. *Mineral and Electrolyte Metabolism* 1987;13:316–22.

100. Seymour AA, Davis JO, Freeman RH, DeForrest JM, Rowe BP, Williams GM. Renin release from filtering and nonfiltering kidneys stimulated by PGI_2 and PGD_2. *American Journal of Physiology* 1979;237:F285–90.

101. Osborn JL, Kopp UC, Thames MD, DiBona GF. Interactions among renal nerves, prostaglandins, and renal arterial pressure in the regulation of renin release. *American Journal of Physiology* 1984;247:F706–13.

102. Echtenkamp SF, Davis JO, DeForest JM, Rowe BP, Freeman RH, Seymour AA, Dietz JR. Effects of indomethacin, renal denervation, and propranolol on plasma renin activity in conscious dogs with chronic thoracic caval constriction. *Circulation Research* 1981;49:492–500.

103. Henrich WL. Role of prostaglandins in renin secretion. *Kidney International* 1981;19:822–30.

104. Dietz JR, Davis JO, Freeman RH, Echtenkamp SF, Villarreal D. Failure of indomethacin to inhibit saralasin-stimulated plasma renin activity in conscious dogs with mild sodium depletion. *Proceedings of the Society for Experimental Biology and Medicine* 1981;167:567–71.

105. Cohen AJ, Laurens P, Fray JCS. Suppression of renin secretion by insulin: Dependence on extracellular calcium. *American Journal of Physiology* 1983;245:E531–4.

106. Lowder SC, Frazer MG, Liddle GW. Effect of insulin-induced hypoglycemia upon plasma renin activity in man. *Journal of Clinical Endocrinology and Metabolism* 1975;41:97–102.

107. Mayfield RK, Bell NK. No evidence of regulation of plasma renin by 1,25-dihydroxyvitamin D_3. *New England Journal of Medicine* 1985;312:1195–6.

108. Baumbach L. Renin release from isolated rat glomeruli: Effects of colchicine, vinca alkaloids, dimethylsulphoxide, and cytochalasins. *Journal of Physiology* 1980;299:145–55.

109. Siegl H, Ryffel B. Effect of cyclosporin on renin–angiotensin–aldosterone system. *Lancet* 1982;ii:1274.

110. Baxter CR, Duggin GG, Willis NS. Cyclosporin A-induced increases in renin storage and release. *Research Communications in Chemical Pathology and Pharmacology* 1982;37:305–11.

111. Bantle CR, Duggin GG, Willis NS. Cyclosporin A-induced increases in renin storage and release. *American Journal of Medicine* 1987;83:59–64.

112. Editorial. Cyclosporin hypertension. *Lancet* 1988;ii:1234.

113. Clozel J-P, Fischli W. Cyclosporin-induced hypertension in marmosets: A new model of hypertension sensitive to angiotensin-converting enzyme inhibition. *Journal of Cardiovascular Pharmacology* 1989;14:77–81.

114. Bing RF. Thyroid disease and hypertension. In: Robertson JIS, ed. *Handbook of hypertension, volume 15. Clinical hypertension.* Amsterdam: Elsevier, 1992: chapter 18.

75

RENIN IN DIABETES MELLITUS

PETER WEIDMANN, PAOLO FERRARI, AND
SIDNEY G SHAW

Diabetes mellitus is a metabolic disease involving many tissues, organs, and functions. The RAS and its actions are among the various regulatory mechanisms that may be affected.

POSSIBLE EFFECTS OF DIABETES MELLITUS ON THE REGULATION OF THE RENIN–ANGIOTENSIN SYSTEM

SYNTHESIS AND SECRETION OF PRORENIN AND RENIN

Renin production and secretion by the juxtaglomerular cells of the kidney is often disturbed in diabetes mellitus (Figs. 75.1 and 75.2). The secretory rate and plasma levels of prorenin are often increased in absolute terms and relative to levels of active renin [1–14]. This alteration develops at the clinically latent stage of diabetic renal involvement in some cases and becomes more prominent as the duration of diabetes increases and nephropathy progresses [6,10,12,14]. The underlying mechanisms are unclear.

The processing of prorenin to renin is probably less efficient [14,15], and glycosylation of prorenin-processing enzyme(s) could theoretically be involved; for example, cathepsin B, a kidney protease that can convert prorenin to active renin, becomes inactive after incubation with glucose in high concentrations [15,16]. Furthermore, a contributory role of autonomic neuropathy has been suggested [7,8].

Renin production and/or secretion could be altered in diabetes because of disturbances in neuroendocrine and other regulatory control mechanisms. Decreased sympathetic nervous activity [17,18], impaired β-receptor mediated responsiveness of renin release [18,19], renal prostaglandin deficiency [20,21], sodium retention [22,23], and hypertension [17,24] are diabetic complications that tend to lower renin secretion. Increased levels of plasma atrial natriuretic factor (ANF) [25–27] may also contribute. Ultimately the renin production capacity of the kidneys may become impaired due to replacement of juxtaglomerular cells by hyalinosis of the afferent (and efferent) glomerular arterioles [28].

Situations where renin is stimulated in diabetes mellitus are much less common but occur occasionally in the form of sodium depletion, hypovolemia, and sympathetic activation (for instance, during diabetic ketoacidosis) [29–32] and perhaps also as a

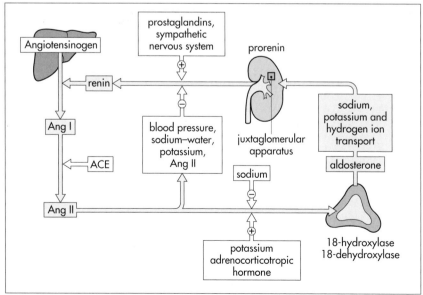

Fig. 75.1 Regulation of the RAS. Diabetes mellitus may cause disturbances at various regulatory levels (see Color Plate 31).

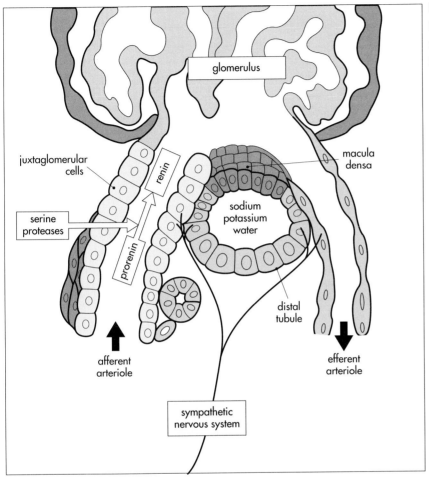

Fig. 75.2 The juxtaglomerular apparatus, illustrating sites of possible disturbance of renin release in diabetes mellitus (see Color Plate 31).

consequence of alterations in renal hemodynamics [33]. Finally, treatment with various drugs may either inhibit or enhance prorenin and renin release.

Changes in plasma glucose concentrations *per se* probably have no direct influence on renal renin release. Hyperglycemia, however, and concomitant alterations in acid–base balance, can modulate renin-regulating factors such as blood volume, renal sodium handling, and potassium metabolism. Insulin was reported to inhibit renin secretion from isolated perfused kidneys [34], but the physiological and pathophysiological relevance of this observation is uncertain. Hyperinsulinemia could also modify renin release indirectly by promoting renal sodium retention [35] and stimulating sympathetic nervous activity [36]. In normal man, acute increases in plasma glucose and insulin in response to glucose loading are accompanied by a mild rise in plasma renin [37] (Fig. 75.3); the latter may well result from a concomitant decrease in plasma potassium and/or activation of the sympathetic nervous system.

PLASMA RENIN IN EXPERIMENTAL DIABETES MELLITUS

Considering the numerous and complex interactions between renin-regulating factors, observations on circulating renin in rats with experimental diabetes of varying severity and studied under different protocols [20,38–40] are particularly difficult to interpret. In rats with streptozotocin- or alloxan-induced diabetes, plasma renin levels range from low to elevated [20,38,41–44]. In some experiments, plasma Ang II and/or renin levels were high in the early stages of diabetes and decreased into the lower range a few weeks after streptozotocin administration [38,40,42,43]. Low renin levels were noted in severely hyperglycemic animals [20,38,40,42,44], and insulin treatment restored circulating renin to the normal or supranormal range [35,36,38,40,44].

Streptozotocin-diabetic rats differ from diabetic man not only in species and the pathogenesis of diabetes mellitus, but also in the evolution of complications that may contribute to the regulation of renin levels. In animals, the induced diabetes starts as

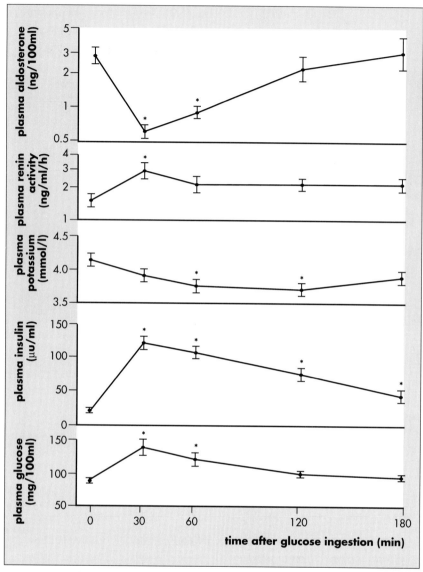

Fig. 75.3 Effects of a standard oral glucose load on fasting supine plasma glucose, insulin, potassium, renin, and aldosterone levels in normal subjects (mean ± SEM). Asterisks denote a significant (*P*<0.02) difference from the control (preglucose load) value. Modified from Beretta–Piccoli C *et al* [37].

an abrupt, severe, and widespread metabolic decompensation. Streptozotocin-diabetic rats also tend to develop hypertension rapidly in association with hypervolemia [41,45,46]. In contrast, patients with insulin-dependent (type 1) diabetes mellitus remain normotensive until the development of incipient diabetic nephropathy (see later), and metabolically stable diabetes mellitus type 1 or 2 (noninsulin-dependent) is not accompanied by hypervolemia [22,47–49]. Sodium intake deserves consideration here, since diabetic rats ingest more sodium than control animals as a consequence of catabolism and hyperphagia [38,42]. It follows that experimental diabetes in rats, and human diabetes, are likely to affect the RAS quite differently, and indiscriminate extrapolation from animal studies to the human condition is unwarranted.

PLASMA ANGIOTENSINOGEN, ANGIOTENSINS, AND ANGIOTENSIN-CONVERTING ENZYME

Circulating angiotensinogen (renin substrate) concentrations seem to be unaltered both in metabolically stable [1,8,13,49,50] and uncontrolled diabetes mellitus [31]. Nevertheless, most of the available information relates specifically to type 1 diabetes mellitus [1,13,49,50].

Plasma Ang I levels have been reported to be slightly low in some patients with diabetes mellitus [49,50], but an analysis of its relationship with angiotensinogen levels was not provided.

Circulating Ang II paralleled Ang I levels at least in type 1 diabetes mellitus [49–55]; observations relating to patients with type 2 diabetes mellitus are scarce [52]. In a group of patients, most of whom had type 2 diabetes mellitus, the plasma clearance rate of infused Ang II was, on average, normal [56].

Serum ACE activity has been variously reported to be mildly increased [57–63], normal [57,62,64–67], or low [68] in patients with either type 1 or type 2 diabetes mellitus. Discrepant findings may reflect differences between the patient groups studied or in methodological aspects. It seems reasonable to conclude that serum ACE activity is raised in a minority (approximately 10–25%) of unselected diabetic patients with stable metabolic control. In approximately half of these patients, the increase in ACE activity is intermittent, while in the other half, it is persistent. Serum ACE activity tends to rise with increasing severity of diabetes mellitus [60,61,63], although values are often still normal even when there is frank diabetic retinopathy or nephropathy [57,62,64,67] (see later).

It is not clear why ACE activity is increased in some patients. In that vascular endothelial cells are major sites of ACE synthesis, diffuse vascular damage, including diabetic microangiopathy, may promote the release of ACE into the bloodstream [57,60,63]. The poor correlation between serum ACE activity and diabetic microvascular complications does not necessarily mitigate against this possibility, since reported findings relate to peripheral (usually antecubital) venous blood rather than to the immediate effluent from major organs, particularly those prone to diabetic microangiopathy; the state of the lung vasculature, a major source of ACE, cannot be judged from these clinical studies; and concomitant abnormalities in endothelial ACE production and/or ACE degradation in diabetes have not been excluded.

Long-term metabolic control of carbohydryate metabolism seems to be at most, a minor determinant of serum ACE activity. Reports of a weak inverse relationship of ACE activity with plasma or urinary glucose or HbA1c levels [58,64] were not confirmed in several other studies [60,61,63]. Moreover, diabetic ketoacidosis is accompanied by a decline in serum ACE activity [58]. On the other hand, insulin can inhibit ACE activity *in vitro* [69] or *in vivo* [70], but the relevance of this potential interaction in human diabetes is uncertain. Finally, since ACE is normally present in excess, a further rise has no known or postulated biological consequence.

CONCLUSION

The diabetic state in man can induce numerous functional and morphological alterations which can, in turn, modify the juxtaglomerular production and/or secretion of prorenin and active renin. Active renin seems to remain the governing determinant of plasma Ang II levels, although the kinetics of Ang I and Ang II generation and metabolism in diabetes of different types and severity deserve further study. The available data neither show, nor entirely exclude fundamental differences in the impact of type 1 diabetes mellitus as compared with type 2 on the circulating components of the RAS. Nevertheless, patients with type 2 diabetes mellitus are on average considerably older than those with type1, and aging is accompanied by a progressive decrease in the basal activity and responsiveness of the RAS [71,72]. This, and the effect of age on other biological processes, must be considered when evaluating the different types of diabetes mellitus. Finally, important aspects of the physiological and pathogenetic role of Ang II, such as the function of local tissue renin–angiotensin systems and of Ang II receptors particularly in cardiovascular tissue, the kidneys, and brain, have so far been inaccessible to study and are, therefore, of unknown pathophysiological relevance in human diabetes mellitus.

THE RENIN–ANGIOTENSIN SYSTEM IN THE DIFFERENT STAGES OF DIABETES MELLITUS

DIABETIC KETOACIDOSIS

Plasma renin, Ang II, and aldosterone usually rise acutely during diabetic ketoacidosis [29–32,73,74] while ACE activity tends to decline [58]. Plasma catecholamines, arginine vasopressin, and cortisol also increase, and ANF levels decrease [32]. Activation of the RAS (Fig. 75.4) probably results from the combined effects of sodium, fluid, and potassium depletion, raised adrenergic activity, ANF suppression [32], and perhaps additional factors. In diabetics with long-term complications such as nephropathy, retinopathy, and/or neuropathy, impaired renin production and/or secretion may preclude an appropriate compensatory rise in plasma renin, Ang II, and aldosterone (Fig. 75.4). Nevertheless, aldosterone levels may be raised because of stimulation by high levels of adrenocorticotropic hormone (ACTH) and hyponatremia, despite the fact that potassium depletion tends to antagonize these effects. With dehydration and shock, hepatic blood flow and the clearance of aldosterone by the liver may be reduced, thereby contributing to high circulating levels of aldosterone. Activation of the RAS, aldosterone, catecholamines, vasopressin, and the ACTH–cortisol axis, and inhibition of ANF, seem to be orchestrated to counteract sodium and fluid depletion and the resulting risk of hypotension and shock.

These homeostatic hormonal reactions contribute importantly to the rapid restoration of sodium and water balance upon institution of treatment with insulin, fluid, and electrolytes. On the other hand, hyperaldosteronism promotes renal potassium

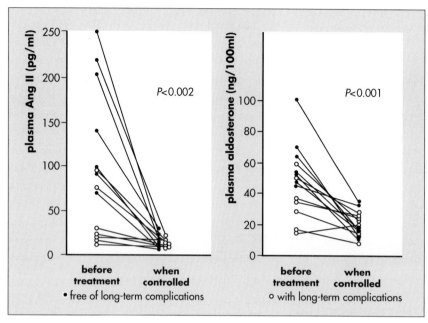

Fig. 75.4 Plasma Ang II and aldosterone concentrations in 14 diabetic patients with ketoacidosis before treatment and when metabolic control was restored (mean interval nine days). Mean blood glucose (± SEM) before treatment was 33.3 ± 4.2mmol/l, and when control was restored, the mean fasting blood glucose was 11.5 ± 1.7mmol/l ($P<0.001$). The shaded areas represent the respective normal ranges in supine subjects. Modified from Ferriss JB *et al* [31].

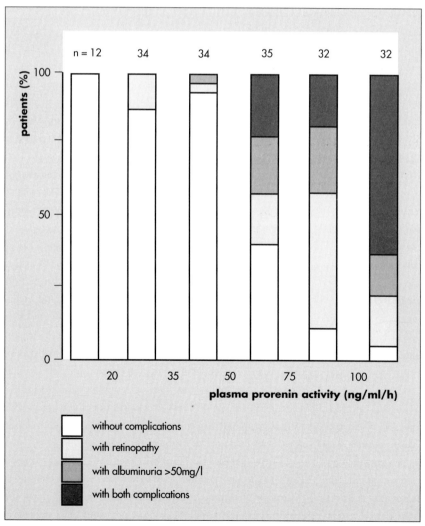

Fig. 75.5 Levels of plasma prorenin in relation to frequency of complications of type 1 or 2 diabetes. On the abscissa, the first bar includes all plasma prorenin values below 20ng/ml/h, and the last bar, all values above 100ng/ml/h; n shows the number of observations indicated by each bar. Modified from Luetscher JA *et al* [6].

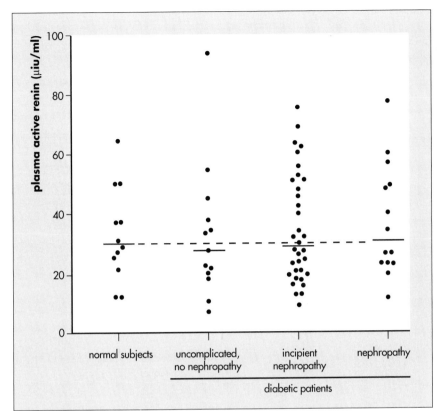

Fig. 75.6 Plasma active renin concentrations in type 1 diabetic patients with different levels of urinary albumin excretion. Incipient nephropathy = microalbuminuria, 30–300mg/24h, and clinical nephropathy = proteinuria >300mg/24h. Modified from Feldt–Rasmussen B *et al* [49].

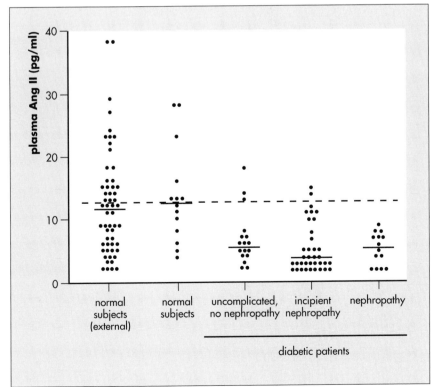

Fig. 75.7 Plasma Ang II concentrations in type 1 diabetic patients with different levels of urinary albumin excretion. Incipient nephropathy = microalbuminuria, 30–300mg/24h, and clinical nephropathy = proteinuria >300mg/24h. Difference between normal control subjects and diabetic patients groups: *P*<0.001. Modified from Feldt–Rasmussen B *et al* [49].

loss, and the lipolytic and ketogenic action of catecholamines can further accentuate established ketoacidosis. Correction of keto-acidosis restores plasma renin, Ang II, aldosterone (Fig. 75.4), and ACE activity, as well as the other 'stress' hormones to pre-ketoacidosis levels.

UNCOMPLICATED DIABETES MELLITUS

During the early uncomplicated stages (initial 3–5 years, of type 1 diabetes mellitus), plasma prorenin and active renin levels, measured under stable metabolic conditions, are generally normal relative to the patients age and sodium intake [14].

In uncomplicated type 1 diabetes mellitus of more than 3–5 years' duration and in uncomplicated type 2 diabetes mellitus, values of plasma prorenin range from normal to high [4–7] (Fig.

75.5) and are on average significantly higher than in age-matched normal subjects [5,6]. Plasma active renin levels are often normal [49,50,55,73–78] but are occasionally low [4,48] or high [37,79–81] (Fig. 75.6). Plasma renin responsiveness to assumption of the upright posture or to administration of furosemide tends to be slightly impaired [11,23,24,77]. Nevertheless, the feedback control of active renin is still largely intact, as evidenced by decreases in plasma active renin levels during Ang II infusion [24,56] or sodium loading [2]. Plasma Ang II concentrations are, at least in uncomplicated type 1 diabetes mellitus, often normal and occasionally low or high [49–55] (Fig. 75.7), thus resembling the pattern of active renin levels. Plasma ACE activity varies from normal to slightly elevated values [57,58,60, 61,64,66] (Fig. 75.8).

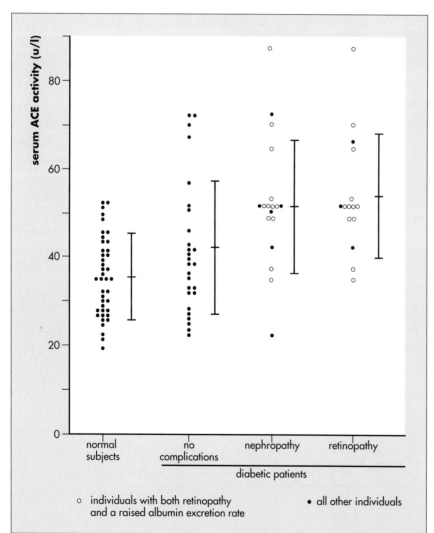

Fig. 75.8 Serum ACE activity (u/l) in normal subjects and in insulin-dependent (type 1) diabetic patients with no complications, raised urinary albumin excretion rate (nephropathy), and/or retinopathy. The bars represent the mean ± SD. Modified from Toop MJ *et al* [61].

o individuals with both retinopathy and a raised albumin excretion rate

• all other individuals

DIABETES MELLITUS COMPLICATED BY NEPHROPATHY

Plasma prorenin is often increased in patients with diabetic nephropathy (see *Fig. 75.3*). Considering the different stages of diabetic renal involvement [82], plasma prorenin activity is, on average, progressively higher in the presence of intermittent albuminuria, incipient nephropathy as defined by continuous microalbuminuria (≥20–200mg/g creatinine or ≥20 or 30– 300 mg/d) and, finally, overt clinical nephropathy (proteinuria >200mg/g creatinine or >300mg/d) [1,6,8,10,12,14,83). Thus, maximal plasma prorenin activity (that is, the highest of several values measured consecutively) was shown to correlate positively with the urinary albumin/creatinine ratio [83]. On follow-up of diabetics with microalbuminuria or clinical proteinuria, plasma prorenin activity tended to rise further in patients continuing to receive their conventional antidiabetic therapy, but decreased in some patients whose metabolic control was improved by intensified treatment [14].

In diabetics with microalbuminuria or clinical proteinuria, plasma levels of active renin and Ang II range from normal to low (see *Figs. 75.6* and *75.7*), and tend to be low in the phase of clinical nephropathy [17,18,51,76,78,80,84,85]. In the later stages of nephropathy, there is unresponsiveness of plasma active renin although prorenin responds to the acute administration of furosemide, which points to impaired feedback control of active renin [2,11]. On the other hand, a tendency for high circulating renin levels was reported in type 1 diabetic patients with early renal involvement, a high glomerular filtration rate (GFR), and without evidence of clinical nephropathy [33,86], and also in teenage type 1 diabetic subjects going on to develop microalbuminuria [81].

Levels of serum ACE activity are often normal or sometimes high in diabetic patients with nephropathy [6,59,61,67] (Fig. 75.8) and do not correlate with the severity of renal involvement. Urinary ACE excretion, however, has recently been reported to be normal in type 2 diabetics with or without incipient nephropathy and elevated in those with overt clinical nephropathy [87,88]. Urinary ACE correlated positively with proteinuria of tubular origin, suggesting that increased ACE excretion may reflect renal tubular damage [87,88].

Renal responses to Ang II may be altered in diabetes mellitus. In rats with experimental diabetes, the number of glomerular Ang II receptors was found to be decreased after a few weeks of the disease and with severe hyperglycemia [42]. Insulin treatment rendering severely hyperglycemic animals only moderately hyperglycemic, normalized the number of Ang II receptors [42]. Angiotensin II-receptor numbers were also restored [40] or even

increased [89] with longer duration of diabetes mellitus when plasma Ang II levels fell [89]. In regard to renal hemodynamics, decreases in glomerular filtration and renal blood flow, which normally occur in response to Ang II, may be blunted in diabetic rats [90], although effects of higher doses of Ang II were unremarkable [91]. The contractile response of glomeruli to Ang II has been variously described as normal [92] or reduced [89,93], the latter suggesting altered functioning of mesangial cells. On the other hand, diabetes mellitus may be associated with an enhanced effect of Ang II on filtration fraction [94]. Based on these experimental observations, it appears possible that dysregulation of Ang II-mediated renal hemodynamic control may be one of the mechanisms facilitating the development of increased glomerular flow, pressure, and filtration [80,94,95] which characterize the early stage of diabetic renal involvement.

DIABETES COMPLICATED BY RETINOPATHY OR NEUROPATHY

Plasma prorenin activity is usually elevated in patients with retinopathy or neuropathy (see *Fig 75.5*) and, as in clinical nephropathy, is significantly higher on average than in uncomplicated diabetes mellitus [2,3,6,8,13,14]. In addition, diabetics with proliferative retinopathy have increased concentrations of prorenin in their ocular vitreous fluid [13]. Based on the latter observation, it has been postulated that an increased intraocular production of prorenin and thence possibly also of renin and Ang II could perhaps promote the development of diabetic retinal vasculopathy [13].

Plasma levels of active renin in diabetics with retinopathy or neuropathy range from normal to low [2,3,6–8,11,13,14,56], although type 1 diabetic patients with proliferative retinopathy were reported by Drury *et al* to have elevated renin values [51]. Serum ACE activity ranges from normal to high [57,60, 61,63,64,67] and, therefore lacks the sensitivity and specificity for use as a marker for diabetic microangiopathy (Fig. 75.8).

In diabetics with retinopathy, retinal vascular reactivity to Ang II or norepinephrine was reported to be blunted [96], whereas systemic pressor responsiveness was described as exaggerated [97].

CONCLUSION

The regulation and activity of the RAS seem to be largely normal in the early stages of diabetes mellitus. The prevalence and magnitude of renin dysregulation increase with the duration of diabetes mellitus and the development of microvascular and neural complications. The presence of microvascular and neurologic complications is associated with increased plasma prorenin, independent of age or duration of diabetes [3,5,10,12,14].

VALUE OF PRORENIN IN PREDICTING MICROVASCULAR COMPLICATIONS

In type 1 diabetes mellitus, a rise in plasma prorenin level and the presence of microalbuminuria seem to be markers of early diabetic renal disease. Prorenin levels tend to increase 1–2 years before the appearance of incipient nephropathy, diabetic retinopathy, or neuropathy [12,14]. Among children and adults with currently uncomplicated type 1 diabetes mellitus and normal blood pressure, those with raised plasma prorenin levels were much more likely to develop subsequently microvascular complications than patients with normal prorenin values [12,14] (Fig. 75.9). Nevertheless, intraindividual variations in plasma prorenin were considerable, and the highest value among several consecutive determinations was used for prognostic appraisal. On this basis, the sensitivity and specificity of high prorenin values in predicting the subsequent development of retinopathy and/or nephropathy in children and adolescents were noted to be approximately 90% and 80%, respectively [14], suggesting that the test could be clinically useful. It follows that in patients with uncomplicated type 1 diabetes mellitus, repetitive measurements of plasma prorenin may help to identify a high-risk subgroup, in which special therapeutic efforts might be desirable to achieve optimal glycemic control. Additional predictors of an increased risk of nephropathy are said to be a positive family history of hypertension [98] and enhanced Na^+/Li^+ countertransport in red blood cells [99,100].

In type 2 diabetes mellitus, a prognostic value for plasma prorenin seems to be limited to a minority of patients who are normotensive and not receiving drugs that modify prorenin levels

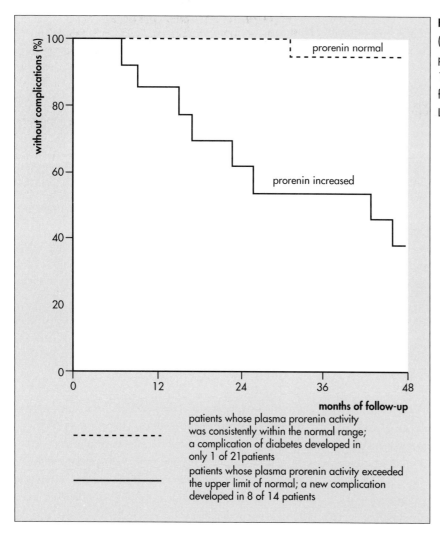

Fig. 75.9 Incidence of complications (retinopathy or overt albuminuria) in 34 patients with previously uncomplicated type 1 diabetes mellitus during 12–54 months of follow-up. Modified from Wilson DM and Luetscher JA [14].

patients whose plasma prorenin activity was consistently within the normal range; a complication of diabetes developed in only 1 of 21 patients

patients whose plasma prorenin activity exceeded the upper limit of normal; a new complication developed in 8 of 14 patients

[6,10]. Plasma prorenin is not a reliable marker of microvascular complications in hypertensive patients (at least 50% of the type 2 diabetic population) and in those treated with prorenin-modifying drugs. As blood pressure rises, plasma prorenin and renin levels tend to decline, whereas the prevalence of microalbuminuria and clinical nephropathy increases. Various antihypertensive drugs can increase (that is, diuretics, converting-enzyme inhibitors, direct arteriolar vasodilators) or decrease (β-blockers) plasma prorenin levels (see *Chapters* 6 and 7). Circulating prorenin concentrations may also be lowered by glipizide [6] and perhaps by other oral antidiabetic agents. It appears therefore that in the majority of type 2 diabetics, the level of arterial pressure and urinary albumin excretion may be more reliable predictors of diabetic complications than are plasma prorenin values.

RENIN, ANGIOTENSIN, AND OTHER FACTORS IN HYPERTENSION ACCOMPANYING DIABETES MELLITUS

The prevalence of hypertension in patients with type 1 or type 2 diabetes mellitus is approximately double that in persons of similar age in the general population [101]. In type 1 diabetes mellitus, the blood pressure is usually normal in the absence of nephropathy, tends to rise slightly with the appearance of incipient nephropathy as indicated by microalbuminuria, and increases further during the stage of clinical nephropathy [82,102–104]. In type 2 diabetes, hypertension may either precede or follow the development of diabetes mellitus or nephropathy [105]. The frequent, although often temporally dissociated development of both hypertension and type 2 diabetes mellitus in a given individual probably involves a strong hereditary contribution. Thus, a familial trait for essential hypertension seems often to be accompanied by a concomitant propensity to decreased insulin sensitivity and reactive hyperinsulinemia, which can be detected in numerous normotensive, young lean offspring of nondiabetic essential hypertensive parents [106] as well as in some nonobese, nondiabetic essential hypertensive patients [107,108]. Obesity and other acquired factors undoubtedly contribute also to the clustering of type 2 diabetes mellitus and hypertension.

BODY SODIUM–FLUID VOLUME STATUS

The pathogenesis of hypertension accompanying diabetes mellitus involves various mechanisms. Sodium retention and a functional and/or morphological vasculopathy seem to play major roles, while a genetic predisposition and nephropathy are probably also important contributory factors [109,110] (Fig. 75.10).

In metabolically stable nonazotemic type 1 or 2 diabetes, exchangeable body sodium is increased by 10% on average, regardless of age, body habitus, or the presence or absence of diabetic retinopathy or clinical nephropathy [22,47,111,112] (Fig. 75.11). Mean plasma and blood volumes are normal in normotensive and low in hypertensive diabetics [22,111,112]. This result points to accumulation of sodium and probably also fluid volume within the extravascular (interstitial and/or intracellular) space, and a tendency for blood-volume contraction in diabetic patients who are also hypertensive. In type 1 diabetes, exchangeable sodium and extracellular fluid volume tend to increase even before the development of incipient diabetic nephropathy, and both changes become more pronounced at the stage of clinical nephropathy [49,113].

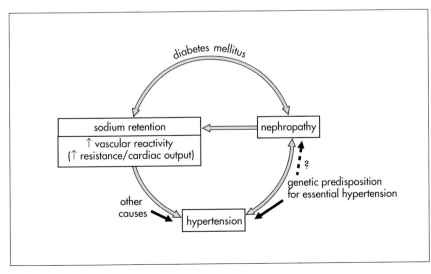

Fig. 75.10 A schematic diagram of some factors involved in the pathogenesis of hypertension accompanying diabetes mellitus.

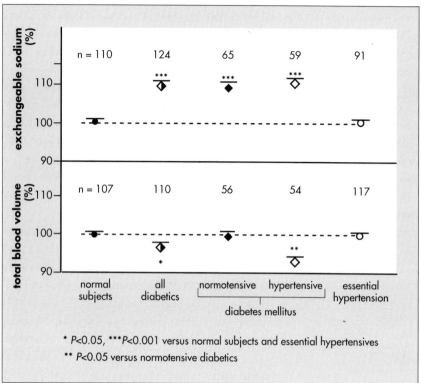

Fig. 75.11 Exchangeable sodium and blood volume in normal subjects and patients with diabetes mellitus or essential hypertension. Results are expressed as per cent of mean in normal subjects according to sex (mean ± SEM). Modified from Weidmann P *et al* [112].

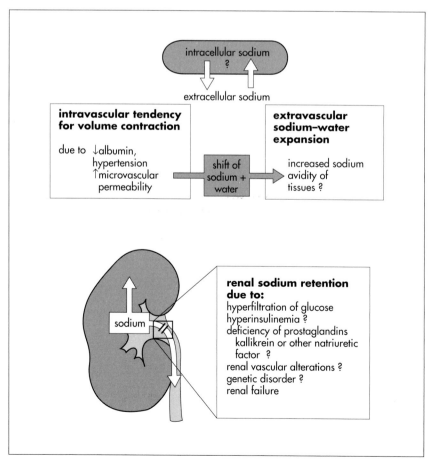

Fig. 75.12 Possible mechanisms of sodium retention in diabetes mellitus. Modified from Weidmann P and Ferrari P [110].

The natriuretic response to acute sodium loading or volume expansion induced by water immersion was found to be impaired even at the uncomplicated stage of type 1 diabetes mellitus [114,115]. Moreover, when changing from a low to a high sodium diet, patients with type 2 diabetes mellitus retained more sodium than did nondiabetic control subjects [116].

A role for sodium retention in the pathogenesis of diabetes-associated hypertension is supported by some additional observations. In nonazotemic hypertensive diabetics, systolic blood pressure correlated with exchangeable body sodium [111], and diuretic treatment removed the excess sodium, further reduced blood volume, and restored blood pressure towards normal [47]. In type 1 diabetics with incipient nephropathy, mean arterial pressure correlated with exchangeable sodium [49]. The lack of such a relationship (that is, normal blood-pressure values in the presence of sodium retention) in some normotensive diabetics [111] suggests differences in cardiovascular sensitivity to perturbations in body sodium balance. In fact, changing from a low to a high salt intake increased arterial pressure in hypertensive but not in normotensive type 2 diabetics or nondiabetic control subjects [116]. The excess in body sodium content is thus characteristic of diabetics but not of uncomplicated essential hypertension [117–120] (see *Fig 75.10*).

Mechanisms that may contribute to renal sodium retention in diabetes mellitus include increased glomerular filtration of glucose leading to enhanced proximal-tubular sodium–glucose cotransport [110], and increased distal tubular sodium reabsorption due to hyperinsulinemia [35] resulting from excessive endogenous insulin release in type 2 diabetes mellitus and from systemic insulin administration with inadequate suppression of hepatic glucose output in type 1 diabetes mellitus (Fig. 75.12). A shift of sodium and fluid from the vascular compartment into the extravascular space [22,112] and renal failure, are additional factors promoting sodium retention. Plasma ANF levels tend to be increased in diabetics with nephropathy and/or hypertension, possibly as a response to concomitant sodium retention and/or raised systemic blood pressure [25–27]. The natriuretic response to ANF, however, appears to be impaired, at least in some diabetics [121,122].

RENIN, ANGIOTENSIN, AND ALDOSTERONE

Plasma active renin, Ang II, and aldosterone levels in relation to age and/or urinary sodium excretion are usually normal or low in hypertensive patients with type 1 or 2 diabetes mellitus [23,24,47,48,49,50,56,76,78] (Fig. 75.13). Hypertension accompanying diabetes mellitus cannot therefore be easily attributed to activation of the RAS. Nevertheless, even normal levels of plasma renin and Ang II could be inappropriately high in the presence of an excessive body sodium content [112]. Some findings are indeed consistent with this notion. In a group of 100 diabetic patients whose renin levels are depicted in Fig. 75.13, plasma renin activity (PRA) correlated positively, although not closely, with both systolic and diastolic blood pressures (r=0.30 and 0.34, respectively, $P<0.05$) [23]. An interaction in the opposite direction, namely a regulatory effect of blood pressure and possible associated factors such as sodium retention and aging on renin release [23], would promote an inverse rather than a positive relationship. In this regard, patients with type 1 diabetes mellitus and clinical nephropathy had minimally lower plasma Ang II levels than patients with a normal urinary albumin excretion or with incipient nephropathy, although their exchangeable sodium was distinctly higher [49].

It may be surmised that the tendency for a hypoactive and/or hyporesponsive RAS with advancing duration and severity of diabetes mellitus may help to protect such patients from the development of malignant hypertension [123].

CATECHOLAMINES

Total plasma catecholamines, norepinephrine and epinephrine concentrations, and urinary catcholamine excretion rates, are also usually normal or sometimes low [22,23,49,124] relative to the age and/or urinary sodium excretion in hypertensive diabetics [72,125]. An acute, high-dose infusion of insulin increased sympathetic outflow in experimental animals and normal man [126–128]. Whether this effect persists under chronic conditions and contributes to the genesis of hypertension in hyperinsulinemic states [129] is presently unknown. Of course, any initial tonic influence of hyperinsulinemia on sympathetic function might be negated once autonomic neuropathy develops.

CARDIOVASCULAR REACTIVITY

Variations in cardiovascular reactivity modulate the responses to vasoactive stimuli and are, therefore, very important in blood-pressure regulation. Under normal conditions, blood-pressure responses to norepinephrine or Ang II are inversely related to basal blood levels of norepinephrine and renin–Ang II, respectively [130,131]. In human diabetes, pressor responsiveness to these hormones is often exaggerated. In patients with metabolically stable, nonazotemic type 1 or 2 diabetes mellitus, the dose of infused norepinephrine required to elevate mean blood pressure by 20mmHg was less than 50% of that needed in normal subjects, despite the absence of any significant difference in pre-infusion plasma norepinephrine levels. The relationship between increases in plasma norepinephrine and concomitant changes in

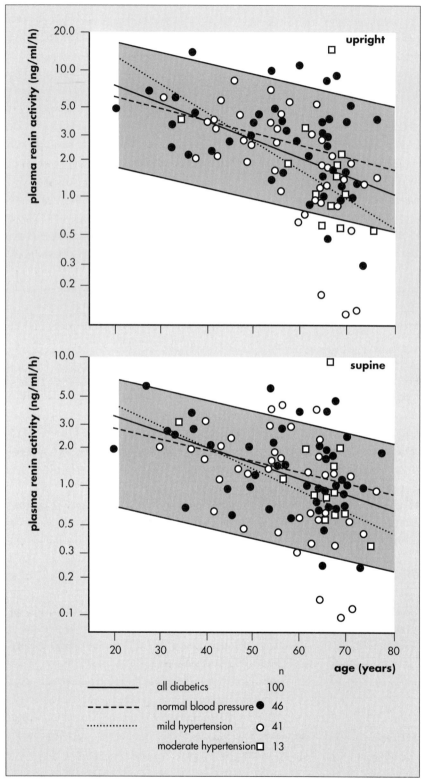

Fig. 75.13 Plasma renin activity related to age in 100 nonazotemic diabetic patients with a normal or high blood pressure. The shaded areas represent the 95% confidence ranges obtained from healthy subjects. The regression lines indicate statistically significant correlations (r = −0.36 to −0.58, P<0.01 to <0.001). Modified from Beretta–Piccoli C *et al* [23].

arterial pressure was significantly displaced to the left in the diabetic group [56,112].

The dose of infused Ang II required to increase diastolic pressure by 20mmHg was also significantly reduced in these diabetics, despite the fact that basal (pre-infusion) PRA was not low [47,56,112,116] (Fig. 75.14]. More recent studies in which plasma Ang II levels were measured suggest that even normotensive patients with uncomplicated type 1 diabetes mellitus have an exaggerated blood-pressure responsiveness to Ang II [132] and an inappropriate increase in Ang II binding sites on platelets [55]. It seems therefore, that vascular hyperreactivity tends to develop early in the course of diabetes mellitus, and may precede the onset of hypertension and other complications such as retinopathy and neuropathy [47,56].

Pressor responsiveness to Ang II was reported to be normal in moderately diabetic rats and reduced in severely diabetic animals,

and to correlate inversely with basal plasma renin levels [38]. Other workers have noted a reduced contractile response in aortic rings from diabetic rats [133] or rabbits [39]. The relevance of these animal and *in vitro* experiments to human diabetes and its complications is, again, uncertain.

Mechanisms contributing to vascular hyperreactivity in human diabetes mellitus may include sodium retention and functional and morphological alterations of resistance vessels. In nonazotemic diabetic patients with mild hypertension, treatment with a thiazide diuretic restored the pressor responsiveness to norepinephrine and Ang II to normal and produced a concomitant increase in PRA [47] (Fig. 75.15). Thiazide diuretics, apart from removing extracellular sodium and water, may also modify the intracellular content of sodium and/or calcium which triggers contraction of vascular smooth muscle [134]. In contrast to diuretic treatment, short-term dietary sodium restriction, which reduces blood pressure responsiveness in normal subjects, failed to alter the pressor hyperreactivity to Ang II in type 2 diabetic patients [116]. Observations before and after treatment with the calcium-channel blocker, nitrendipine, in 10 patients with type 2 diabetes mellitus and mild hypertension suggested that vascular hyperreactivity is, at least in part, calcium dependent [135]. Calcium-channel blockade reduced arterial pressure and diminished pressor responsiveness to both norepinephrine and Ang II, although the total exchangeable body sodium and blood volume were unchanged [135].

Functional and morphological vascular changes occur in diabetes. Alterations in resistance vessels develop quite early in the course of diabetes mellitus [109]. Hyperinsulinemia may stimulate the proliferation of vascular smooth-muscle cells and accelerate atherosclerosis which, in turn, results in luminal narrowing, increased arterial stiffness, and heightened resistance to blood flow [136]. Whether hyperinsulinemia *per se* can modulate vascular tone and arterial pressure through influences on transmembrane electrolyte pumps is still unclear.

When administered acutely, insulin increased myocardial contractility *in vitro* [137,138] and produced *in vivo* net vasoconstriction in diabetic patients [139]. Hyperinsulinemia may possibly also upregulate Ang II receptors in renal efferent glomerular arterioles [93]. Information regarding Ang II receptors on platelets, however, is controversial. One report described a reduced number of Ang II receptors on platelets from patients with uncomplicated type 1 diabetes [54], whereas others have observed increased Ang II binding to platelets [55].

The relationship between Ang II, norepinephrine, or other vasculotrophic hormones and vasculopathy in diabetes mellitus is unknown. Once hypertension (whatever its pathogenesis) has

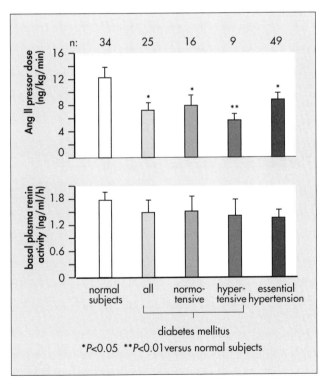

Fig. 75.14 Angiotensin II pressor doses and basal (preinfusion) plasma renin levels in healthy subjects, nonazotemic diabetics with normal blood pressure or mild to moderate hypertension, and patients with mild to moderate essential hypertension.
The Ang II pressor dose is defined as the infusion rate required to increase diastolic arterial pressure by 20mmHg (mean ± SEM). Modified from Weidmann P *et al* [112].

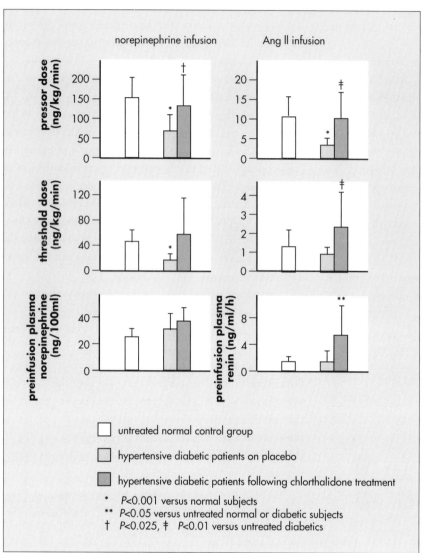

Fig. 75.15 Norepinephrine and Ang II pressor doses, and basal (preinfusion) plasma norepinephrine and renin levels in an untreated normal control group and in hypertensive diabetic patients on placebo and following chlorthalidone treatment (100mg/day for six weeks) (data are means ± SEM). The pressor dose is defined as the infusion rate required to increase diastolic arterial pressure by 20mmHg. Modified from Weidmann P *et al* [47].

developed, secondary hypertrophy of the vascular wall occurs [140]. Finally, dysfunction of the autonomic reflex arch may complicate long-term diabetes and is yet another factor that promotes exaggerated pressor responses [56,124].

ANTIHYPERTENSIVE THERAPY INVOLVING RENIN–ANGIOTENSIN INHIBITION IN DIABETES

This topic is discussed in detail in *Chapter 86*.

It might be surmised that diuretics, by decreasing total-body sodium content [47], may be particularly effective in controlling the hypertension in diabetes. Diuretics, however, particularly in

high dosages, are no longer recommended as first-line antihypertensive agents in diabetes mellitus because of their metabolic and other side effects [141,142]. Beta-blockers have also been used widely in hypertensive diabetic patients. Some of these agents reduce plasma renin levels while others do not, but no difference in their antihypertensive potency has been apparent. Beta-blockers can decrease awareness of hypoglycemia, interfere with autonomic cardiovascular homeostasis, and adversely affect carbohydrate and lipoprotein metabolism and, therefore, are no longer considered ideal antihypertensive agents in diabetes [141,142].

Angiotensin-converting enzyme inhibitors are said to have no adverse 'metabolic' effects [143–146] and seem to be equally effective in lowering arterial pressure in hypertensive patients with either type 1 or type 2 diabetes mellitus [141,147] (Figs. 75.16 and 75.17). The relative importance of reduced Ang II production *per se* in the antihypertensive mechanism of ACE inhibitors in diabetes mellitus is unknown but the recent availability of specific renin inhibitors may help to clarify this question. The usually normal or low levels of circulating renin and Ang II in hypertensive diabetics do not preclude a satisfactory antihypertensive response to ACE inhibitors. The latter could theoretically improve the relationship between plasma levels of, and vascular reactivity to, Ang II, but this appears not to be the case, at least in nondiabetic essential hypertensive patients [148,149]. Nevertheless, tissue Ang II concentrations in diabetic blood vessels, and their possible modification by ACE inhibition, remain to be examined. Moreover, other potential interactions, such as reduced vascular norepinephrine reactivity relative to prevailing sympathetic activity [149–151] and/or increased tissue or circulating levels of vasodilator kinins or prostaglandins (see

Chapters 38, 87, and *98*), deserve particular consideration with regard to clarification of the mechanisms whereby ACE inhibitors reduce arterial pressure in diabetic patients.

Proteinuria is an index of renal prognosis [82,102–104] and kidney function is a critical co-determinant of wellbeing and life expectancy in diabetic patients. In type 1 diabetes mellitus, antihypertensive drug treatment was noted to decrease protein excretion in patients with incipient or nonazotemic clinical nephropathy [152,153], and in some [154], but not all [155], patients with azotemia and clinical nephropathy. Likewise, antihypertensive therapy slowed the rate of decline in GFR in patients with nonazotemic [152,153] or mildly azotemic [154, 155] clinical nephropathy. Data in type 2 diabetes mellitus are still too scarce for interpretation. Whether a renal protective influence results from specific pharmacological properties of individual antihypertensive agents as well as from the reduction in arterial pressure *per se*, awaits clarification.

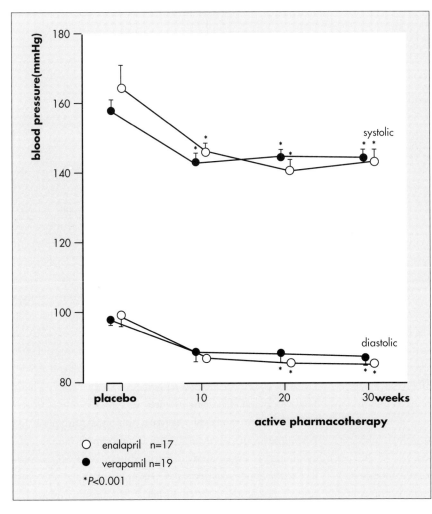

Fig. 75.16 Antihypertensive therapy with the ACE inhibitor, enalapril, or the calcium-channel blocker, verapamil, in the 36 patients responding satisfactorily to monotherapy. A satisfactory response was defined as a decrease in diastolic blood pressure to less than 85mmHg if pretreatment values on placebo ranged from 90 to 95mmHg, or to less than 90mmHg if pretreatment values ranged from 96 to 115mmHg. Data are means ± SEM. Modified from Ferrier C *et al* [147].

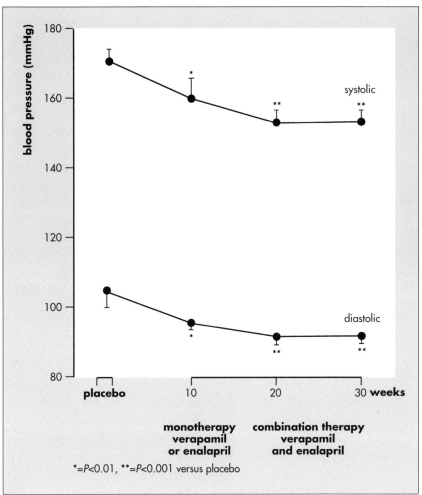

Fig. 75.17 Antihypertensive therapy with the ACE inhibitor, enalapril, and the calcium-channel blocker, verapamil, in hypertensive diabetic patients: blood pressure in the 18 patients with insufficient control after 10 weeks of monotherapy and who, thereafter, received both drugs. A satisfactory response was defined as a decrease in diastolic blood pressure to less than 85mmHg if pretreatment values on placebo ranged from 90 to 95mmHg, or to less than 90mmHg if pretreatment values ranged from 96 to 115mmHg. Data are means ± SEM.

With regard to their effect on glomerular arterioles, ACE inhibitors preferentially dilate the efferent vessels by reducing levels of Ang II [45,156]. The net effect of ACE inhibition on glomerular hemodynamics is a decrease in glomerular capillary pressure and flow [45,157]. The latter are elevated in diabetic kidney disease, thereby promoting proteinuria, and probably also the evolution of chronic progressive kidney failure [158]. Since efferent arteriolar Ang II receptors are said to be up-regulated in diabetes mellitus [95], these vessels may be especially responsive to ACE inhibition. Therefore, patients with diabetic nephropathy could theoretically be at an increased risk from excessive falls in glomerular filtration pressure and rate with ACE inhibition. Although this is not a frequent complication, it necessitates monitoring of serum creatinine after initiation of ACE inhibitor therapy in nephropathic patients.

On the other hand, administration of an ACE inhibitor to diabetic or nondiabetic rats subjected to subtotal nephrectomy slowed further renal functional deterioration and reduced proteinuria. These studies were performed in diabetic and nondiabetic rats. The beneficial effects were, at least in nondiabetic rats, more marked than those obtained with conventional antihypertensive therapy [45,156,157]. In a very small study of patients with type 1 diabetes mellitus, microproteinuria decreased in those receiving the ACE inhibitor, captopril, but increased in patients taking the calcium antagonist, nifedipine [159]. A similar, although statistically insignificant, trend was noted in hypertensive type 2 diabetics after 30 weeks of treatment with enalapril as compared with verapamil [147]. Other workers have, however, found that some calcium antagonists (diltiazem and nifedipine) are as effective as ACE inhibitors (lisinopril and perindopril) in decreasing clinical proteinuria and micro-albuminuria in hypertensive diabetic subjects [160,161]. Regardless of the exact renal protective potential of various antihypertensive agents, the early initiation of treatment is important.

Control of both blood pressure and metabolic indices is vital in the prevention of cardiovascular and renal disease in diabetic patients.

RENIN IN DIABETIC PATIENTS WITH ORTHOSTATIC HYPOTENSION

Diabetic patients with orthostatic hypotension often have supine hypertension. Such patients typically exhibit both a decrease in sympatho-adrenergic activity and a tendency to a low plasma volume [162] although the body sodium content is increased [22]. Efferent parasympathetic function is usually disturbed, but not necessarily more so in orthostatic hypotensive than in age-matched, nonhypotensive diabetics [162–164]. Functional and morphologic diabetic vasculopathy, markedly exaggerated reactivity to norepinephrine, and less-pronounced pressor hyper-responsiveness to Ang II may promote supine hypertension, but are insufficient to prevent orthostatic falls in blood pressure.

In diabetics with orthostatic hypotension, PRA is normal or low [18,165]. Postural increases in plasma renin are often blunted [22–24,76–78,81) and even 'normal' renin responses to upright body posture [22,47,51,75–78,81,84] may be inappropriately low relative to the concomitant fall in blood pressure. In nonazotemic patients with type 1 or 2 diabetes mellitus, orthostatic changes in mean arterial pressure were found to correlate positively with basal supine PRA, but not with concomitant postural changes in PRA [22] (Fig. 75.18). In this situation, it is not clear whether supine plasma renin levels merely reflect the degree of sympatho-adrenergic dysregulation, or whether a low activity of the RAS contributes to the development of orthostatic hypotension.

HYPORENINEMIC (HYPOANGIOTENSINEMIC) HYPOALDOSTERONISM

After an early case report [166], several groups in the early 1970s reported cases of selective hypoaldosteronism due to a deficiency in circulating renin [19,167–171]. We termed this syndrome hyporeninemic hypoaldosteronism [19] (Figs. 75.19 and 75.20). Subsequent series have confirmed that decreased activity of the

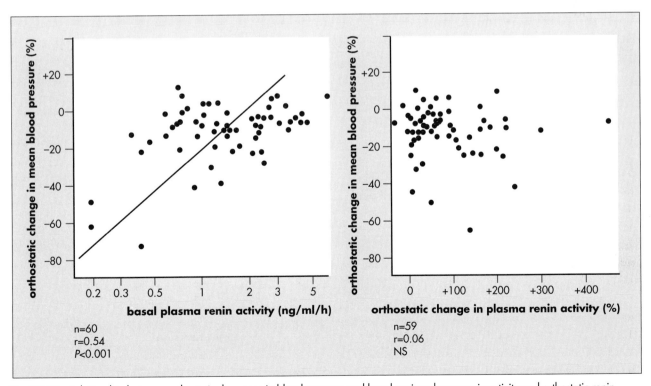

Fig. 75.18 Relationship between orthostatic decreases in blood pressure and basal supine plasma renin activity and orthostatic renin changes in nonazotemic diabetic patients. Modified from de Châtel R *et al* [22].

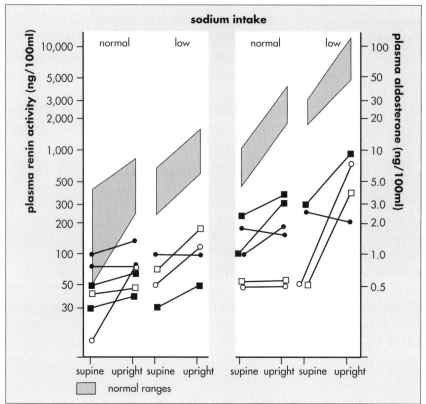

Fig. 75.19 Plasma renin activity and aldosterone levels in hyperkalemic patients with hyporeninemic hypoaldosteronism. Five patients were diabetic and all patients had nephropathy with serum creatinine ranging from 1.8 to 5.4mg/dl. Data from Weidmann P *et al* [19,171].

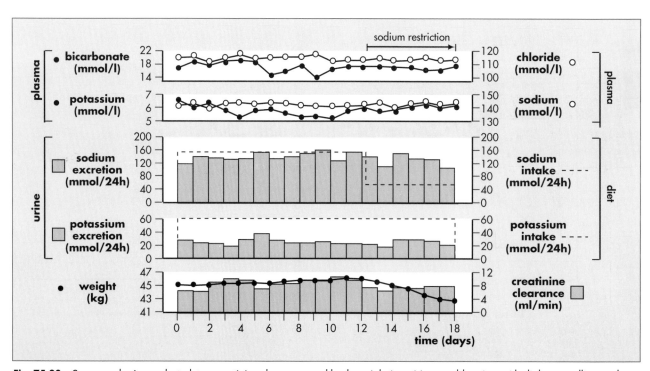

Fig. 75.20 Serum and urinary electrolytes, creatinine clearance, and body weight in a 66-year-old patient with diabetes mellitus and hyporeninemic hypoaldosteronism during dietary sodium intakes of 120–140mmol and 40mmol daily. Modified from Weidmann P *et al* [19].

RAS, caused either by a number of disorders or by drugs, is the most common cause of selective hypoaldosteronism in adults [172–178]. Additional causes of selective hypoaldosteronism include defects in adrenocortical 18-hydroxylase or 18-hydroxydehydrogenase, which are sometimes associated with low active plasma renin and/or high prorenin [167,179–181], Liddles syndrome, and the syndrome of apparent mineralocorticoid excess, the latter two being characterized by low levels of renin (see *Chapter 66*).

Diabetic patients are particularly prone to develop hyporeninemic hypoaldosteronism [2,19,171–174,177,179,180]. Other causes include various types of nephropathy and renin-lowering drugs such as cyclo-oxygenase inhibitors or, to a lesser extent, β-blockers [172–178]. ACE inhibitors can promote hypoaldosteronism by lowering plasma levels of Ang II [176]. Aging *per se* is associated with a fall in activity of the RAS [71,72] and most adults with symptomatic selective hypoaldosteronism are older than 50 years of age. Since Ang II rather than renin is the proximate regulator of aldosterone production, it would seem

logical to change the term 'hyporeninemic hypoaldosteronism' to 'hypoangiotensinemic hypoaldosteronism'.

Hypoaldosteronism promotes the development of hyperkalemia and, through diminished renal excretion of hydrogen and ammonium ions, the development of hyperchloremic acidosis ('renal tubular acidosis type 4') [182,183] (Fig. 75.21). Apart from the severity of aldosterone deficiency, the expression of these metabolic alterations, hyperkalemia in particular, depends on the functional reserve of renal and extrarenal compensatory mechanisms [19,171–178]. In adult patients with normal kidney function and an intact extrarenal potassium disposal capacity, selective hypoaldosteronism rarely, if ever, leads to a clinically relevant increase in serum potassium [184] (Fig. 75.22). Nevertheless, hyperkalemia may occur with hypoaldosteronism when normal kidney function is compromised by volume depletion, heart failure, or hypotension, or in diabetic patients with acute generalized cellular potassium leakage due to severe hyperglycemia resulting from insulin deficiency [185]. The large majority of patients with hyperkalemia and type 4 renal-tubular

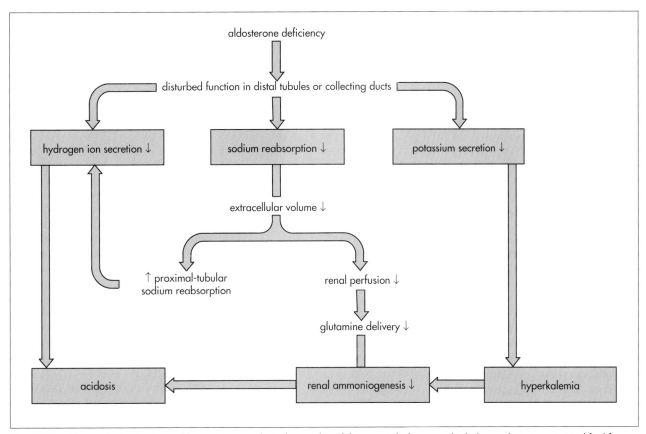

Fig. 75.21 Effects of selective hypoaldosteronism on electrolyte and acid–base metabolism: renal-tubular acidosis type 4. Modified from Weidmann P *et al* [174].

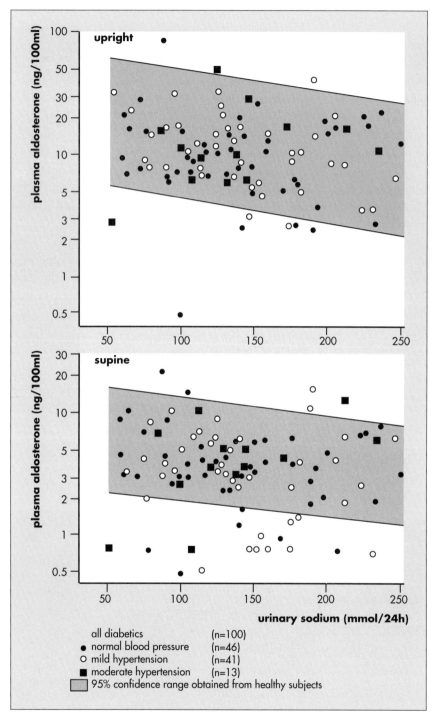

Fig. 75.22 Plasma aldosterone as related to age in 100 diabetic patients with normal serum creatinine levels. This is the same study population as in *Fig. 75.13*. Of the patients with low plasma aldosterone, none had hyperkalemia. Data from Weidmann P *et al* [184].

acidosis due to hyporeninemic hypoaldosteronism have mild to marked chronic renal functional impairment, and renal failure is usually also accompanied by reduced extrarenal potassium disposal [186].

For further details on the pathogenesis, differential diagnosis, and therapeutic management of hypoaldosteronism, the reader is referred to Chapters 65, 66, and 68–70 of this book.

75.21

REFERENCES

1. Day RP, Luetscher JA, Gonzales CM. Occurrence of big renin in human plasma, amniotic fluid and kidney extracts. *Journal of Clinical Endocrinology and Metabolism* 1975;**40**:1078–84.

2. Hsueh WA, Carlson EJ, Luetscher JA, Grislis G. Activation and characterization of inactive big renin in plasma of patients with diabetic nephropathy and unusual active renin. *Journal of Clinical Endocrinology and Metabolism* 1980;**51**:535–43.

3. Fujii S, Shimojo N, Wada M, Funae Y. Plasma active and inactive renin in patients with diabetes mellitus. *Endocrinologia Japonica* 1980;**27**:65–8.

4. Antonipillai I, Tan SY, Suzuki S, Franco-Saenz R, Mulrow PJ. Active and inactive renin in low renin states: Studies in human plasma. *Journal of Clinical Endocrinology and Metabolism* 1981;**53**:694–7.

5. Bryer–Ash M, Ammon RA, Luetscher JA. Increased inactive renin in diabetes mellitus without evidence of nephropathy. *Journal of Clinical Endocrinology and Metabolism* 1983;**56**:557–61.

6. Luetscher JA, Kraemer FB, Wilson DM, Schwartz HC, Bryer-Ash M. Increased plasma inactive renin in diabetes mellitus. *New England Journal of Medicine* 1985;**312**:1412–7.

7. Chimori K, Miyazaki S, Kosaka J, Sakanaka A, Yasuda K, Miura K. The significance of autonomic neuropathy in the elevation of inactive renin in diabetes mellitus. *Clinical and Experimental Hypertension. Part A, Theory and Practice* 1987;**A9**:1–18.

8. Misbin RI, Grant MB, Pecker MS, Atlas SA. Elevated levels of plasma prorenin (inactive renin) in diabetic and nondiabetic patients with autonomic dysfunction. *Journal of Clinical Endocrinology and Metabolism* 1987;**64**:964–8.

9. Derkx FHM, Schalekamp MADH. Human prorenin, pathophysiology and clinical implications. *Clinical and Experimental Hypertension. Part A, Theory and Practice* 1988;**A10**:1213–25.

10. Mossetti G, Megna SA, Maddaloni D, Motti C, Gravina E. La prorenina plasmatica quale indice di valutazione prognostica nella malattia diabetica. *Minerva Medica* 1988;**79**:931–6.

11. Bryer-Ash M, Fraze EB, Luetscher JA. Plasma renin and prorenin (inactive renin) in diabetes mellitus, effects of intravenous furosemide. *Journal of Clinical Endocrinology and Metabolism* 1988;**66**:454–8.

12. Luetscher JA, Kraemer FB, Wilson DM. Prorenin and vascular complications of diabetes. *American Journal of Hypertension* 1989;**2**:382–6.

13. Danser AHJ, van den Dorpel MA, Deinum J, Derkx FHM, Franken AAM, Peperkamp E, de Jong PTVM, Schalekamp MADH. Renin, prorenin, and immunoreactive renin in vitreous fluid from eyes with and without diabetic retinopathy. *Journal of Clinical Endocrinology and Metabolism* 1989;**68**:160–7.

14. Wilson DM, Luetscher JA. Plasma prorenin activity and complications in children with insulin-dependent diabetes mellitus. *New England Journal of Medicine* 1990;**323**:1101–6.

15. Dzau VJ, Burt DW, Pratt RE. Molecular biology of the renin–angiotensin system. *American Journal of Physiology* 1988;**255**:F563–73.

16. Coradello H, Pollak A, Pagano M, Leban J, Lubec G. Non-enzymatic glycosylation of cathepsin B, possible influence on conversion of proinsulin to insulin. *IRCS Journal of Medical Science* 1981;**9**:766–9.

17. Christlieb AR. Diabetes and hypertensive vascular disease. *American Journal of Cardiology* 1973;**32**:592–606.

18. Tuck ML, Sambhi MP, Levin L. Hyperreninemic hypoaldosteronism in diabetes mellitus, studies of the autonomic nervous system's control of renin release. *Diabetes* 1972;**28**:237–41.

19. Weidmann P, Reinhart R, Maxwell MH, Massry SC, Lupu AN, Coburn JW, Kleeman CR. Syndrome of hyporeninemic hypoaldosteronism and hyperkalemia in renal disease. *Journal of Clinical Endocrinology and Metabolism* 1973;**36**:965–77.

20. Katayama S, Lee JB. Hypertension in experimental diabetes mellitus. Renin–prostaglandin interaction. *Hypertension* 1985;**7**:554–61.

21. Nadler JL, Lee FO, Hsueh W, Horton R. Evidence of prostacyclin deficiency in the syndrome of hyporeninemic hypoaldosteronism. *New England Journal of Medicine* 1986;**314**:1015–20.

22. de Châtel R, Weidmann P, Flammer J, Ziegler WH, Beretta-Piccoli C, Vetter W, Reubi FC. Sodium, renin, aldosterone, catecholamines and blood pressure in diabetes mellitus. *Kidney International* 1977;**12**:412–21.

23. Beretta-Piccoli C, Weidmann P, de Châtel R, Ziegler W, Glück Z, Keusch G. Plasma catecholamines and renin in diabetes mellitus, relationships with age, posture, sodium and blood pressure. *Klinische Wochenschrift* 1979;**57**:681–91.

24. Beretta-Piccoli C, Weidmann P, Keusch G. Responsiveness of plasma renin and aldosterone in diabetes mellitus. *Kidney International* 1981;**20**:259–66.

25. Sawicki PT, Heinemann L, Rave K, Hohmann A, Berger M. Atrial natriuretic factor in various stages of diabetic nephropathy. *Journal of Diabetic Complications* 1988;**2**:207–9.

26. Jungmann E, Höll E, Konzok C, Fassbinder W, Schöffling K. Welchen pathophysiologischen Stellenwert haben erhöhte Plasmaspiegel des humanen atrialen natriuretischen Peptids bei Patienten mit Diabetes mellitus? *Zeitschrift für Kardiologie* 1988;**77** (suppl 2):114–8.

27. Weidmann P, Saxenhofer H, Ferrier C, Shaw SG. Atrial natriuretic peptide in man. *American Journal of Nephrology* 1988;**8**:1–14.

28. Schindler AM, Sheldon CS. Diabetic sclerosis of the juxtaglomerular apparatus. *Laboratory Investigation* 1966;**15**:877–84.

29. Scott RS, Espiner EA, Donald RA, Livesey JH. Hormonal responses during treatment of acute diabetic ketoacidosis and constant insulin infusions. *Clinical Endocrinology* 1978;**9**:463–74.

30. Waldhäusl W, Kleinberger G, Korn A, Dudczak R, Bratusch–Marrain P, Nowotny P. Severe hyperglycemia, effects of rehydration on endocrine derangements and blood glucose concentration. *Diabetes* 1979;**28**:577–84.

31. Ferriss JB, O'Hare JA, Kelleher CCM, Sullivan PA, Cole MM, Ross HF, O'Sullivan DJ. Diabetic control and the renin–angiotensin system, catecholamines, and blood pressure. *Hypertension* 1985;**7** (suppl II):58–63.

32. Tulassay T, Rascher W, Körner A, Miltényi M. Atrial natriuretic peptide and other vasoactive hormones during treatment of severe diabetic ketoacidosis in children. *Journal of Pediatrics* 1987;**III**:329–34.

33. Wiseman MJ, Drury PL, Keen H, Viberti GC. Plasma renin activity in insulin-dependent diabetics with raised glomerular filtration rate. *Clinical Endocrinology* 1984;**21**:409–14.

34. Cohen AJ, Laurens P, Fray JCS. Suppression of renin secretion by insulin: Dependence on extracellular calcium. *American Journal of Physiology* 1983;**245**:E531–4.

35. De Fronzo RA. The effect of insulin on renal sodium metabolism. *Diabetologia* 1981;**21**:165–71.

36. Rowe JW, Young JB, Minaker KL, Stevens AL, Pallotta J, Landsberg L. Effect of insulin and glucose infusions on sympathetic nervous system activity in normal man. *Diabetes* 1981;**20**:219–25.

37. Beretta–Piccoli C, Weidmann P, Flammer J, Glück Z, Bachmann C. Effects of standard oral glucose loading on the renin–angiotensin–aldosterone system and its relationship to circulating insulin. *Klinische Wochenschrift* 1980;**58**:467–74.

38. Christlieb AR. Renin, angiotensin, and norepinephrine in alloxan diabetes. *Diabetes* 1974;**23**:962–70.

39. Head RJ, Longhurst PA, Panek RL, Stitzel RE. A contrasting effect of the diabetic state upon the contractile responses of aortic preparations from the rat and rabbit. *British Journal of Pharmacology* 1987;**91**:275–86.

40. Wilkes B. Reduced glomerular angiotensin II receptor density in diabetes mellitus in the rat. Time course and mechanism. *Endocrinology* 1987;**120**:1291–8.

41. Kohler L, Boillat N, Lüthi P, Atkinson J, Peters-Haefeli L. Influence of streptozotocin-induced diabetes on blood pressure and on renin formation and release. *Archives of Pharmacology* 1980;**313**:257–61.

42. Ballermann B, Skorecki KL, Brenner BM. Reduced glomerular angiotensin II receptor density in early untreated diabetes mellitus in the rat. *American Journal of Physiology* 1984;247:F110–6.

43. Kikkawa R, Kitamura E, Fujiwara Y, Haneda M, Shigeta Y. Biphasic alteration of renin–angiotensin–aldosterone system in streptozotocin-diabetic rats. *Renal Physiology* 1986;9:187–92.

44. Pratt JH, Parkinson CA, Weinberger MH, Duckworth WC. Decreases in renin and aldosterone secretion in alloxan diabetes, an effect of insulin deficiency. *Endocrinology* 1985;116:1712–6.

45. Zatz R, Dunn BR, Meyer TW, Anderson S, Rennke HG, Brenner BM. Prevention of diabetic glomerulosclerosis by pharmacological amelioration of glomerular capillary hypertension. *Journal of Clinical Investigation* 1986;77:1925–30.

46. Jackson CV, Carrier GO. Influence of short-term experimental diabetes on blood pressure and heart rate in response to norepinephrine and angiotensin II in the conscious rat. *Journal of Cardiovascular Pharmacology* 1983;5:260–5.

47. Weidmann P, Beretta-Piccoli C, Keusch G, Glück Z, Mujagic M, Grimm M, Meier A, Ziegler WH. Sodium-volume factor, cardiovascular reactivity and hypotensive mechanisms of diuretic therapy in hypertension associated with diabetes mellitus. *American Journal of Medicine* 1979;67:779–84.

48. O'Hare JA, Ferriss JB, Brady D, Twomey B, O'Sullivan DJ. Exchangeable sodium and renin in hypertensive diabetic patients with and without nephropathy. *Hypertension* 1985;7 (suppl II):43–8.

49. Feldt-Rasmussen B, Mathisen ER, Deckert T, Giese J, Christensen NJ, Bent-Hansen L, Nielsen MD. Central role for sodium in the pathogenesis of blood pressure changes independent of angiotensin, aldosterone and catecholamines in type 1 (insulin-dependent) diabetes mellitus. *Diabetologia* 1987;30:610–7.

50. Hommel E, Mathiesen ER, Giese J, Nielsen MD, Schütten HJ, Parving HH. On the pathogenesis of arterial blood pressure elevation early in the course of diabetic nephropathy. *Scandinavian Journal of Clinical and Laboratory Investigation* 1989;49:537–44.

51. Drury PL, Bodansky HJ, Oddie CJ, Cudworth AG, Edwards CRW. Increased plasma renin activity in type I diabetes with microvascular disease. *Clinical Endocrinology* 1982;16:453–61.

52. Ferriss JB, Sullivan PA, Gongrijp H, Cole M, O'Sullivan DJ. Plasma angiotensin II and aldosterone in unselected diabetic patients. *Clinical Endocrinology* 1982;17:261–9.

53. Björck S, Delin K, Herlitz H, Larsson O, Aurell M. Renin secretion in advanced diabetic nephropathy. *Scandinavian Journal of Urology and Nephrology* 1984;79 (suppl):53–7.

54. Connell JMC, Ding YA, Fisher BM, Frier BM, Semple PF. Reduced number of angiotensin II receptors on platelets in insulin-dependent diabetes. *Clinical Science* 1986;71:217–20.

55. Mann JFE, Mürtz H, Sis J, Usadel K, Hasslacher Ch, Ritz E. Specific binding of angiotensin II and atrial natriuretic factor in non-nephrotic type I diabetes mellitus. *Nephrology, Dialysis, Transplantation* 1989;4:530–4.

56. Beretta-Piccoli C, Weidmann P. Exaggerated pressor responsiveness to norepinephrine in nonazotemic diabetes mellitus. *American Journal of Medicine* 1981;71:829–35.

57. Lieberman J, Sastre A. Serum angiotensin-converting enzyme, elevations in diabetes mellitus. *Annals of Internal Medicine* 1980;93:825–6.

58. Schmitz O, Rømer FK, Alberti KGMM, Hreidarsson AB, Orskov H. Angiotensin-converting enzyme in diabetes mellitus dependence on metabolic aberration. *Diabetes/Metabolism Reviews* 1983;9:179–82.

59. Miura H, Nakayama M, Sato T. Serum angiotensin converting enzyme (S-ACE) activity in patients with chronic renal failure on regular hemodialysis. *Japanese Heart Journal* 1984;25:87–92.

60. Schernthaner G, Schwarzer Ch, Kuzmits R, Müller MM, Klemen U, Freyler H. Increased angiotensin-converting enzyme activities in diabetes mellitus, analysis of diabetes type, state of metabolic control and occurrence of diabetic vascular disease. *Journal of Clinical Pathology* 1984;37:307–12.

61. Toop MJ, Dallinger KJC, Jennings PE, Barnett AH. Angiotensin-converting enzyme (ACE): Relationship to insulin-dependent diabetes and microangiopathy. *Diabetic Medicine* 1986;3:455–7.

62. Ninomiya Y, Arakawa M. Serum angiotensin converting enzyme activity in type 2 (non-insulin-dependent) diabetic patients with chronic glomerulonephritis. *Diabetes Research* 1989;11:121–4.

63. Migdalis IN, Iliopoulou V, Kalogeropoulou K, Koutoulidis K, Samartzis M. Elevated serum levels of angiotensin-converting enzyme in patients with diabetic retinopathy. *Southern Medical Journal* 1990;83:425–7.

64. Canivet B, Squara P, Raybaud M, Iordache A, Dujardin P, Freychet P. Enzyme de conversion de l'angiotensine et diabète sucré. *Revue de Médicine Interne* 1983;IV:115–8.

65. Schweisfurth H, Heinrich J, Brugger E, Steinl C, Maiwald L. The value of angiotensin-I-converting enzyme determinations in malignant and other diseases. *Clinical Physiology and Biochemistry* 1985;3:184–92.

66. Giampietro O, Lenzi S, Sampietro T, Miccoli R, Navalesi R. Serum angiotensin-converting enzyme in diabetes mellitus, a negative report. *Enzyme* 1986;35:102–5.

67. Porta M, Passera P, Bertagna A, La Selva M, Ricchetti I, Molinatti GM. Levels of serum angiotensin-converting enzyme before and after forearm venous stasis in diabetic microangiopathy. *Diabetes Research* 1987;4:117–20.

68. Aoyagi T, Wada T, Kojima F, Nagai M, Akanuma Y, Akanuma H, Umezawa H. Relation of blood glucose levels to the changes in plasma levels of various hydrolytic enzymes in diabetes patients. *Biochemistry International* 1985;10:821–7.

69. Bing J, Poulsen K, Markussen J. The ability of various insulins and insulin fragments to inhibit the angiotensin I converting enzyme. *Acta Pathologica et Microbiologica Scandinavica {A}* 1974;82:777–82.

70. Igic R, Erdös EG, Yeh HSJ, Serrels K, Nakajima T. Angiotensin I converting enzyme of the lung. *Circulation Research* 1972;31 (suppl II):51–61.

71. Weidmann P, De Myttenaere-Bursztein S, Maxwell MH, De Lima J. Effect of aging on plasma renin and aldosterone levels in normal man. *Kidney International* 1975;8:325–33.

72. Weidmann P, de Châtel R, Schiffmann A, Bachmann E, Beretta-Piccoli C, Ziegler WH, Vetter W, Reubi FC. Interrelations among age and plasma renin, aldosterone and cortisol, urinary catecholamines and the body sodium/volume state in normal man. *Klinische Wochenschrift* 1977;55:725–33.

73. Christlieb AR, Assal JP, Katsilambros N, Williams GH, Kozak GP, Suzuki T. Plasma renin activity and blood volume in uncontrolled diabetes. Ketoacidosis, a state of secondary aldosteronism. *Diabetes* 1975;24:190–3.

74. Sullivan PA, Gonggrijp H, Crowley MJ, Ferriss JB, O'Sullivan DJ. Plasma angiotensin II and the control of diabetes mellitus. *Clinical Endocrinology* 1980;13:387–92.

75. Christlieb AR. Renin–angiotensin system in diabetes mellitus. *Diabetes* 1976;25:820–5.

76. Christlieb AR, Kaldany A, D'Elia JA. Plasma renin activity and hypertension in diabetes mellitus. *Diabetes* 1976;25:969–74.

77. Campbell IW, Ewing DJ, Anderton JL, Thompson JH, Horn DB, Clarke BF. Plasma renin activity in diabetes autonomic neuropathy. *European Journal of Clinical Investigation* 1976;6:381–5.

78. Christlieb AR, Kaldany A, D'Elia JA, Williams GH. Aldosterone responsiveness in patients with diabetes mellitus. *Diabetes* 1978;27:732–7.

79. Gossain VV, Werk EE, Sholiton LJ, Srivastava L, Knowles HC. Plasma renin activity in juvenile diabetes mellitus and effect of diazoxide. *Diabetes* 1975;24:833–5.

80. Manchandia MR, Gossain VV, Michelakis AM, Rovner DR. Plasma cryoactivated renin and active renin in diabetes mellitus. *Journal of Clinical Endocrinology and Metabolism* 1981;53:1025–9.

81. Paulsen EP, Seip RL, Ayers CR, Croft BY, Kaiser DL. Plasma renin activity and albumin excretion in teenage type I diabetic subjects. A prospective study. *Hypertension* 1989;13:781–8.

82. Mogensen CE. Microalbuminuria as a predictor of clinical diabetic nephropathy. *Kidney International* 1987;31:673–89.

83. Luetscher JA, Kraemer FB. Microalbuminuria and increased plasma prorenin. Prevalence in diabetics followed up for fours years. *Archives of Internal Medicine* 1988;148:937–41.

84. Tomita K, Matsuda O, Ideura T, Shiigai T, Takeuchi J. Renin–angiotensin–aldosterone system in mild diabetic nephropathy. *Nephron* 1982;31:361–7.

85. Fernandez-Cruz A, Noth RH, Lassman MN, Hollis JB, Mulrow PJ. Low plasma renin activity in normotensive patients with diabetes mellitus. Relationship to neuropathy. *Hypertension* 1981;3:87–92.

86. Solerte SB, Fioravanti M, Petraglia F, Facchinetti F, Aprile C, Genazzani AR, Ferrari E. Circulating opioids and plasma renin activity in insulin-dependent diabetics with renal hemodynamic alterations. *Nephron* 1987;46:194–8.

87. Baggio B, Briani G, Cicerello E, Gambaro G, Bruttomesso D, Tiengo A, Borsatti A, Crepaldi G. Urinary glycosaminoglycans, sialic acid and lysosomal enzymes increase in nonalbuminuric diabetic patients. *Nephron* 1986;43:187–90.

88. Hosojima H, Miyauchi E, Morimoto S. Urinary excretion of angiotensin-converting enzyme in NIDDM patients with nephropathy. *Diabetes Care* 1989;12:580–2.

89. Kikkawa R, Kitamura E, Fujiwara Y, Arimura T, Haneda M, Shigeta Y. Impaired contractile responsiveness of diabetic glomeruli to angiotension II. A posssible indication of mesangial dysfunction in diabetes mellitus. *Biochemical and Biophysical Research Communications* 1986;136:1185–90.

90. Reineck HJ, Kreisberg JL. Renal vascular response to angiotensin II in rats with streptozotocin-induced diabetes mellitus [Abstract]. *Kidney International* 1983;24:247.

91. McCormack AJ, Finn WF. Effect of indomethacin on angiotensin II induced natriuresis and diuresis in normal and diabetic rats. *Proceedings of the Xth International Congress of Nephrology, London* 1987:32.

92. Barnett R, Scharschmidt L, Ko YH, Schlondorff D. Comparison of glomerular and mesangial prostaglandin synthesis and glomerular contraction in two rat models of diabetes mellitus. *Diabetes* 1987;36:1468–75.

93. Kreisberg JI. Insulin requirements for contraction of cultured mesangial cells in response to angiotensin II, possible role for insulin in modulating glomerular hemodynamics. *Proceedings of the National Academy of Sciences of the USA* 1982;79:4190–2.

94. Bank N, Lahorra MAG, Aynedjin HS, Schlondorff D. Vasoregulatory hormones and the hyperfiltration of diabetes. *American Journal of Physiology* 1988;254:F202–9.

95. Zatz R, Brenner BM. Pathogenesis of diabetic microangiopathy, the hemodynamic view. *American Journal of Medicine* 1986;80:443–53.

96. Rhie FH, Christlieb AR, Sandor T, Gleason RE, Rand LI, Shah ST, Soeldner JS. Retinal vascular reactivity to norepinephrine and angiotensin II in normals and diabetics. *Diabetes* 1982;31:1056–60.

97. Christlieb AR, Janka HU, Kraus B, Gleason RE, Icasas-Cabral EA, Aiello LM, Cabral BV, Solano A. Vascular reactivity to angiotensin II and to norepinephrine in diabetic subjects. *Diabetes* 1976;25:268–74.

98. Krolewsky AS, Canessa M, Rand LI, Warram JH, Christlieb AR, Knowler WC, Kahn CR. Genetic predisposition to hypertension as a major determinant of development of diabetic nephropathy. *Kidney International* 1987;31:388.

99. Krolewsky AS, Canessa M, Warram JH. Laffel LMB, Christlieb R, Knowler WC, Rand LI. Predisposition to hypertension and susceptibility to renal disease in insulin-dependent diabetes mellitus. *New England Journal of Medicine* 1988;318:140–5.

100. Mangili R, Bending JJ, Scott G, Li LK, Gupta A, Viberti GC. Increased sodium–lithium countertransport activity in red cells of patients with insulin-dependent diabetes mellitus and nephropathy. *New England Journal of Medicine* 1988;318:146–50.

101. Christlieb AR, Warram JH, Krolewski AS, Busick EJ, Ganda OP, Asmal AC, Soeldner JS, Bradley RF. Hypertension: The major risk factor in juvenile-onset insulin-dependent diabetics. *Diabetes* 1981;31 (suppl 2):90–6.

102. Parving HH, Anderssen AR, Smidt UM, Oxenbøll B, Edsberg B, Sandahl Christiansen J. Diabetic nephropathy and arterial hypertension. *Diabetologia* 1983;24:10–2.

103. Feldt-Rasmussen B, Borch–Johnsen K, Mathiesen ER. Hypertension in diabetes as related to nephropathy. *Hypertension* 1985;7 (suppl II):18–20.

104. Mogensen CE, Christensen CK. Blood pressure changes and renal function in incipient and overt diabetic nephropathy. *Hypertension* 1985;7 (suppl II):64–73.

105. Hasslacher Ch. Nephropathie bei Typ-II-Diabetes. *GIT Labor-Medizin* 1988;5:278–80.

106. Ferrari P, Weidmann P, Shaw S, Giachino D, Riesen W, Allemann Y, Heynen G. Altered insulin sensitivity, hyperinsulinemia and dyslipidemia in hypertension-prone humans. *Clinical Research* 1991;39:351A.

107. Ferrannini E, Buzzigoli G, Giorico MA, Oleggini M, Graziadei L, Pedrinelli R, Brandi L, Bevilacqua S. Insulin resistance in essential hypertension. *New England Journal of Medicine* 1987;317:350–7.

108. Pollare T, Lithell H, Berne C. Insulin resistance is a characteristic feature of primary hypertension independent of obesity. *Metabolism* 1990;39:167–74.

109. Blumenthal HT, Goldenberg S, Berns AW. Pathology and pathogenesis of the disseminated angiopathy of diabetes mellitus. On the nature and treatment of diabetes. In: Liebel BS, Wrenshall GA, eds. *International Congress Series nr 84* Amsterdam: Excerpta Medica, 1965:397–408.

110. Weidmann P, Ferrari P. Hypertension in the diabetic: Central role of sodium. *Diabetes Care* 1991;14:220–32.

111. Beretta-Piccoli C, Weidmann P. Body sodium-blood volume state in nonazotemic diabetes mellitus. *Mineral and Electrolyte Metabolism* 1982;7:36–47.

112. Weidmann P, Beretta-Piccoli C, Trost BN. Pressor factors and responsiveness in hypertension accompanying diabetes mellitus. *Hypertension* 1985;7 (suppl II):33–42.

113. Mathiesen ER, Rønn B, Jensen T, Storm B, Deckert T. Relationship between blood pressure and urinary albumin excretion in development of microalbuminuria. *Diabetes* 1990;39:245–9.

114. Roland JM, O'Hare JP, Walters C, Corrall RJM. Sodium retention in response to saline infusion in uncomplicated diabetes mellitus. *Diabetes Research* 1986;3:213–5.

115. O'Hare JP, Roland JM, Walters G, Corrall RJM. Impaired sodium excretion in response to volume expansion induced by water immersion in insulin dependent diabetes mellitus. *Clinical Science* 1986;71:403–9.

116. Tuck M, Corry D, Trujillo A. Salt-sensitive blood pressure and exaggerated vascular reactivity in the hypertension of diabetes mellitus. *American Journal of Medicine* 1990;68:210–6.

117. Lebel M, Schalekamp MA, Beevers DG, Brown JJ, Davies DL, Fraser R, Kremer D, Lever AF, Morton JJ, Robertson JIS, Tree M, Wilson A. Sodium and the renin–angiotensin system in essential hypertension and mineralocorticoid excess. *Lancet* 1974;ii:308–10.

118. Schalekamp MA, Lebel M, Beevers DG, Fraser R, Klosters G, Birkenhäger WH. Body-fluid volume in low-renin hypertension. *Lancet* 1974;ii:310–1.

119. Weidmann P, Hirsch D, Beretta-Piccoli C, Ziegler WH, Reubi FC. Interrelations among blood pressure, blood volume, plasma renin activity and urinary catecholamines in benign essential hypertension. *American Journal of Medicine* 1977;62:209–18.

120. Beretta-Piccoli C, Weidmann P. Circulatory volume in essential hypertension. Relationship with age, blood pressure, exchangeable sodium, renin, aldosterone and catecholamines. *Mineral Electrolyte Metabolism* 1984;10:292–300.

121. de Châtel R, Toth M, Barna I. Exchangeable body sodium: Its relationship with blood pressure and atrial natriuretic factor for patients with diabetes mellitus. *Journal of Hypertension* 1986;4 (suppl 6):526–8.

122. Haak T, Jungmann E, Rosak C, Schwab N, Fassbinder W, Althoff PH, Schöffling K. Evidence for a decreased natriuretic efficacy of human atrial natriuretic peptide in patients with type 1 diabetes mellitus. *Diabetologia* 1986;29:544–5.

123. Christlieb AR. Nephropathy, the renin angiotensin system, and hypertensive vascular disease in diabetes mellitus. *Cardiovascular Medicine* 1978;3:417–32.

124. Christensen NJ. Catecholamines and diabetes mellitus. *Diabetologia* 1979;16:211–24.

125. Weidmann P, Beretta-Piccoli C, Ziegler WH, Keusch G, Glück Z. Age versus urinary sodium for judging renin, aldosterone and catecholamine levels. Studies in normal subjects and patients with essential hypertension. *Kidney International* 1978;14:619–28.

126. Christensen NJ, Gundersen, HJG, Hegedüs L, Jacobsen F, Mogensen CE, Osterby R, Vittinghus E. Acute effects of insulin on plasma noradrenaline and the cardiovascular system. *Metabolism* 1980;29:1138–45.

127. Landsberg L, Young JB. Insulin-mediated glucose metabolism in the relationship between dietary intake and sympathetic nervous system activity. *International Journal of Obesity* 1985;9:63–8.

128. Berne C, Fagius J. Sympathetic response to oral carbohydrate administration. Evidence from microelectrode nerve recordings. *Journal of Clinical Investigation* 1989;84:1403–9.

129. Reaven GM. Role of insulin resistance in human disease. *Diabetes* 1988;37:1595–1607.

130. Chinn RH, Düsterdieck G. The response of blood pressure to infusion of angiotensin II. Relation to plasma concentrations of renin and angiotensin II. *Clinical Science* 1972;42:489–504.

131. Philipp T, Distler A, Cordes U. Sympathetic nervous system and blood pressure control in essential hypertension. *Lancet* 1978;ii:959–63.

132. Drury PL, Smith GM, Ferriss JB. Increased vasopressor responsiveness to angiotensin II in type I (insulin dependent) diabetic patients without complications. *Diabetologia* 1984;27:174–9.

133. Turlapaty PDMV, Lum G, Altura BM. Vascular responsiveness and biochemical parameters in alloxan diabetes mellitus. *American Journal of Physiology* 1980;239:E412–21.

134. Erne P, Bolli P, Burgisser E, Bühler F. Correlation of platelet calcium with blood pressure. Effect of antihypertensive therapy. *New England Journal of Medicine* 1984;310:1084–8.

135. Trost BN, Weidmann P, Beretta–Piccoli C. Antihypertensive therapy in diabetic patients. *Hypertension* 1985;7 (suppl II):II-102–8.

136. Ferrari P, Weidmann P. Insulin, insulin sensitivity and hypertension. *Journal of Hypertension* 1990;8:491–500.

137. Snow TR. Study of the characteristics of the inotropic effect of insulin in rabbit papillary muscle. *Experientia* 1976;32:1550–1.

138. Imanaga I. Effects of insulin on mammalian cardiac muscle. In: Kobayashi T, Sano T, Dhalla NS, eds. *Recent advances in studies on cardiac structure and metabolism, volume 11.* Baltimore: University Park Press, 1978:441–50.

139. Gundersen HJG, Christensen NJ. Intravenous insulin causing loss of intravascular water and albumin and increased adrenergic nervous activity in diabetics. *Diabetes* 1977;26:551–7.

140. Folkow B. The hemodynamic consequences of adaptive structural changes of the resistance vessels in hypertension. *Clinical Science* 1971;41:1–12.

141. Weidmann P, Trost BN, Ferrari P. Treatment of the hypertensive diabetic: Focus on calcium channel blockade. In: Omae T, Zanchetti A, eds. *How should elderly hypertensive patients be treated?* Heidelberg: Springer, 1989:85–99.

142. Ferrari P, Rosman J, Weidmann P. Antihypertensive agents, serum lipoprotein and glucose metabolism. *American Journal of Cardiology* 1991;67:26–35B.

143. Veterans Administration Cooperative Study Group on Antihypertensive Agents. Low dose captopril for the treatment of mild to moderate hypertension. *Hypertension* 1983;5 (suppl III):139–44.

144. Perani G, Muggia C, Martignoni A, Bongarzoni A, Radaelli A, Testa F, Finardi G. Increase in plasma HDL-cholesterol in hypertensive patients treated with enalapril. *Clinical Therapy* 1987;9:635–9.

145. Costa FV, Borghi C, Mussi A, Ambrosioni E. Hypolipidemic effects of long-term antihypertensive treatment with captopril. *American Journal of Medicine* 1988;84 (3A):159–61.

146. Pollare T, Lithell H, Berne C. A comparison of the effects of hydrochlorothiazide and captopril on glucose and lipid metabolism in patients with hypertension. *New England Journal of Medicine* 1989;321:868–73.

147. Ferrier C, Ferrari P, Weidmann P, Keller U, Riesen W. Antihypertensive therapy with the calcium channel blocker verapamil and/or the ACE inhibitor enalapril in non-insulin dependent diabetic patients. *Diabetes Care* 1991;14:911–4.

148. Koletsky RJ, Gordon MB, LeBoff MS, Moore TJ, Dluhy RG, Hollenberg NK, Williams GH. Captopril enhances vascular and adrenal responsiveness to angiotensin II in essential hypertension. *Clinical Science* 1984;66:299–305.

149. Uehlinger DE, Ferrier CP, Matthieu R, Reuter K, Gnädinger MP, Saxenhofer H, Shaw S, Weidmann P. Antihypertensive contribution of sodium depletion and the sympathetic axis during chronic angiotensin II converting enzyme inhibition. *Journal of Hypertension* 1989;7:901–7.

150. Fruncillo RJ, Rotmensch HH, Vlasses PH, Koplin JR, Swanson BN, Ferguson RK. Effect of captopril and hydrochlorothiazide on the response to pressor agents in hypertensives. *European Journal of Clinical Pharmacology* 1985;28:5–9.

151. Weidmann P. Pathogenetic and therapeutic relevance of cardiovascular pressor reactivity to norepinephrine in human hypertension. *Clinical and Experimental Hypertension* 1989;A11 (suppl 1):257–73.

152. Christensen CK, Mogensen CE. Effect of antihypertensive treatment on progression of incipient diabetic nephropathy. *Hypertension* 1985;7 (suppl II):109–13.

153. Parving HH, Hommel E, Smidt UM. Protection of kidney function and decrease in albuminuria by captopril in insulin-dependent diabetics with nephropathy. *British Medical Journal* 1988;297:1086–91.

154. Parving HH, Andersen AR, Smidt UM, Hommel E, Mathiesen ER, Svendsen PA. Effect of antihypertensive treatment on kidney function in diabetic nephropathy. *British Medical Journal* 1987;294:1443–7.

155. Björk S, Nyberg G, Mulec H, Granerus G, Herlitz H, Aurell M. Beneficial effects of angiotensin converting enzyme inhibition on renal function in patients with diabetic nephropathy. *British Medical Journal* 1986;293:471–4.

156. Anderson S, Meyer TW, Rennke HG, Brenner BM. Control of glomerular hypertension limits glomerular injury in rats with reduced renal mass. *Journal of Clinical Investigation* 1985;76:612–9.

157. Anderson S, Rennke HG, Brenner BM. Therapeutic advantage of converting enzyme inhibitors in arresting progressive renal disease associated with hypertension in the rat. *Journal of Clinical Investigation* 1986:77:1993–2000.

158. Anderson S, Brenner BM. Role of intraglomerular hypertension in the initiation and progression of renal disease. In: Kaplan N, Brenner BM, Laragh JH, eds. *The kidney in hypertension. Perspectives in hypertension, volume 1.* New York: Raven Press, 1987:67–76.

159. Mimran A, Insua A, Ribstein J, Monnier L, Bringer J, Mirouze J. Contrasting effects of captopril and nifedipine in normotensive patients with incipient diabetic nephropathy. *Journal of Hypertension* 1988;6:919–23.

160. Bakris GL. Effects of diltiazem or lisinopril on massive proteinuria associated with diabetes mellitus. *Annals of Internal Medicine* 1990;112:707–8.

161. Melbourne Diabetic Nephropathy Study Group. Comparison between perindopril and nifedipine in hypertensive and normotensive diabetic patients with microalbuminuria. *British Medical Journal* 1991;302:210–6.

162. Savopol MAV. Orthostatic hypotension in diabetes mellitus or certain other disorders with autonomic deficiency: Pathogenic and therapeutic studies. [Thesis supervised by P Weidmann]. Berne, Switzerland: University of Berne, 1986:1–45.

163. Low PA, Walsh JC, Huang CY, McLeod JG. The sympathetic nervous system in diabetic neuropathy. A clinical and pathological study. *Brain* 1975;98:341–56.

164. Ewing DJ, Campbell IW, Clarke BF. The natural history of diabetic autonomic neuropathy. *Quarterly Journal of Medicine* 1980;49:95–108.

165. Christlieb AR, Munichoodappa C, Braaten JT. Decreased response of plasma renin activity to orthostasis in diabetic patients with orthostatic hypotension. *Diabetes* 1974;23:835–40.

166. Hudson JB, Chobanian AB, Relman AS. Hypoaldosteronism. A clinical study of a patient with an isolated adrenal mineralocorticoid deficiency, resulting in hyperkalemia and Stokes–Adams attacks. *New England Journal of Medicine* 1957;257:529–36.

167. Perez G, Siegel L, Schreier GE. Selective hypoaldosteronism with hyperkalemia. *Annals of Internal Medicine* 1972;76:757–63.

168. Schambelan M, Stockigt J, Biglieri EG. Isolated hypoaldosteronism in adults: A renin deficiency syndrome. *New England Journal of Medicine* 1972;**287**:573–8.

169. Weidmann P, Reinhart R, Massry SG, Coburn JW, Lupu A, Maxwell MH, Kleeman CR. Failure of renin–angiotensin system and selective hypoaldosteronism causing hyperkalemia in chronic renal disease. *Clinical Research* 1972;**20**:249.

170. Brown JJ, Chinn RH, Fraser R, Lever AF, Morton JJ, Robertson JIS, Tree M, Waite MA, Park DM. Recurrent hyperkalaemia due to selective aldosterone deficiency: Correction by angiotensin infusion. *British Medical Journal* 1973;**1**:650–4.

171. Weidmann P, Maxwell MH, Rowe P, Winer R, Massry SG. Role of the renin–angiotensin–aldosterone system in the regulation of plasma potassium in chronic renal disease. *Nephron* 1975;**15**:35–49.

172. Schambelan M, Sebastian A. Hyporeninemic hypoaldosteronism. *Advances in Internal Medicine* 1979;**24**:385–405.

173. De Fronzo RA. Hyperkalemia and hyporeninemic hypoaldosteronism. *Kidney International* 1980;**17**:118–34.

174. Weidmann P. Hyporeninämischer Hypoaldosteronismus und Differential-diagnose der Hyperkalämie. *Schweizerische Medizinische Wochenschrift* 1982;**112**:1764–74.

175. Tan SY, Shapiro R, Franco R, Stockard H, Mulrow PJ. Indomethacin-induced prostaglandin inhibition with hyperkalemia: A reversible cause of hyporeninemic hypoaldosteronism. *Annals of Internal Medicine* 1979;**90**:783–5.

176. Textor SC, Bravo EL, Fouad FM, Tarazi RC. Hyperkalemia in azotemic patients during angiotensin-converting enzyme inhibition and aldosterone reduction with captopril. *American Journal of Medicine* 1982;**73**:719–25.

177. Large DM, Laing I, Carr PH, Davies M. Hyperkalaemia in diabetes mellitus — potential hazards of coexisting hyporeninaemic hypoaldosteronism. *Postgraduate Medical Journal* 1984;**60**:370–3.

178. Ruilope LM, Robles RG, Paya C, Alcazar JM, Miravalles E, Sancho-Rof J, Rodicio J, Knox FG, Romero JC. Effects of long-term treatment with indomethacin on renal function. *Hypertension* 1986;**8**:677–84.

179. DeLeiva A, Christlieb AR, Melby JC, Graham CA, Day RP, Luetscher JA, Zager PG. Big renin and biosynthetic defect of aldosterone in diabetes mellitus. *New England Journal of Medicine* 1976;**295**:639–43.

180. Tuck ML, Sambhi MP, Levin L. Hyporeninemic hypoaldosteronism in diabetes mellitus. Studies of the autonomic nervous system's control of renin release. *Diabetes* 1979;**28**:237–41.

181. Iwasaki R, Kigoshi T, Uchida K, Morimoto S. Plasma 18-hydroxycorticosterone and aldosterone responses to angiotensin II and corticotropin in diabetic patients with hyporeninemic and normoreninemic hypoaldosteronism. *Acta Endocrinologica* 1989;**121**:83–9.

182. Morris RC Jr, Sebastian A. Disorders of the renal tubule that cause disorders of fluid, acid–base, and electrolyte metabolism. In: Maxwell MH, Kleeman CR, eds. *Clinical disorders of fluid and electrolyte metabolism.* New York: McGraw-Hill, 1980:883.

183. Sebastian A, Schambelan M, Lindfeld S, Morris RC Jr. Amelioration of metabolic acidosis with fludrocortisone therapy in hyporeninemic hypoaldosteronism. *New England Journal of Medicine* 1977;**297**:576–83.

184. Weidmann P, Beretta-Piccoli C, Glück Z, Keusch G, Reubi FC, de Châtel R, Cottier C. Hypoaldosteronism without hyperkalemia. *Klinische Wochenschrift* 1980;**58**:185–94.

185. Cox M, Sterns RH, Singer I. The defense against hyperkalemia: The roles of insulin and aldosterone. *New England Journal of Medicine* 1978;**299**:525–32.

186. Van Ypersele de Strihou C. Potassium homeostasis in renal failure. *Kidney International* 1977;**11**:491–504.

76 RENIN IN CARDIAC FAILURE

M GARY NICHOLLS AND AJ GÜNTER RIEGGER

Few studies have documented activity of the RAS in untreated patients, and for obvious reasons there is comparatively little information on changes in renin and Ang II levels as heart failure evolves. In contrast, there are numerous reports on the RAS in various animal models of heart failure. This chapter briefly summarizes animal data before discussing the RAS in human heart failure prior to and during treatment. Finally, the control of renin secretion and its importance in the pathophysiology of heart failure and relevance to treatment are addressed.

RENIN IN EXPERIMENTAL HEART FAILURE

Early studies in high- and low-output models of heart failure reported increased circulating renin levels in most instances [1–4]. Since renal renin content, and hyperplasia and hypergranulation of juxtaglomerular cells were frequently present [5,6] (Fig. 76.1), increased renin production was suspected and later confirmed by formal measurements of renal renin-secretion rates in dogs with aortic-caval fistulae [3]. Nevertheless, a reduced hepatic-clearance rate contributes to the raised renin levels in high-output cardiac failure in dogs, but not apparently in low-output failure [2].

Not all animals with heart failure have high plasma renin levels [1,7–12], but studies where sequential measurements have been performed suggest there is a pattern. The initial response is a rise in circulating renin, often to extremely high values, whether cardiac failure is induced by constriction of the aorta [13], constriction of the pulmonary artery and/or the thoracic inferior vena cava [14–17], rapid cardiac pacing [18–20], tricuspid incompetence [21], administration of adriamycin [22], or by construction of an arteriovenous fistula [23] (Fig. 76.2). This early rise in renin is usually accompanied by a parallel increase in circulating aldosterone levels (Fig. 76.2) and avid renal sodium retention. Renin levels remain high as long as the circulatory status deteriorates, the arterial pressure is low, and the kidneys retain sodium. When, however, a new steady state is achieved, plasma renin plateaus or declines — sometimes to preheart failure values [12,14,16]. The usual, initial rise in renin in the early or acute phase of heart failure is not always seen, perhaps because of the inhibitory action of high circulating levels of atrial natriuretic factor (ANF) [10,11,24]. Of course, species differences and variations of experimental methodology may contribute to discrepant patterns of renin release [11,25].

RENIN IN HUMAN HEART FAILURE

IN THE ABSENCE OF TREATMENT

Single measurements of plasma renin in untreated but symptomatic patients have given widely differing results. This is so from early studies involving small numbers of patients and using relatively insensitive assays [26–30] and from later studies with more refined assays; for example, of 21 untreated patients with congestive heart failure, studied by Brown and colleagues, plasma renin concentration (PRC) was subnormal in three, normal in 12, and high in six [31]. A wide range in levels of PRA was reported also by Vandongen et al [32], Nicholls et al [33], and Anand et al [34]. Patients with left ventricular dysfunction but no symptoms, who were receiving no treatment, were found to have normal levels of PRA [35].

Variable study conditions and small patient numbers make interpretation of available information difficult. Furthermore, assay techniques vary between different laboratories, and measurements of PRA can underestimate active renin concentration and Ang II levels in patients with severe heart failure which causes liver dysfunction [230]. Nevertheless, it appears that renin levels are often low or normal in mild or stable heart failure [35,36] or when there is a 'spontaneous' diuresis [33]. On the other hand, high renin levels are seen when there is acute or severe cardiac failure with renal sodium retention [33,37,38]. This apparent pattern of renin release in man is similar to that described above in animal models of heart failure. As discussed in *Chapter 77*, there is also activation of the RAS after acute myocardial infarction, particularly if left ventricular failure supervenes.

Whether the etiology of heart failure has a bearing on renin release is unclear, although Ikram et al [39] noted that activation

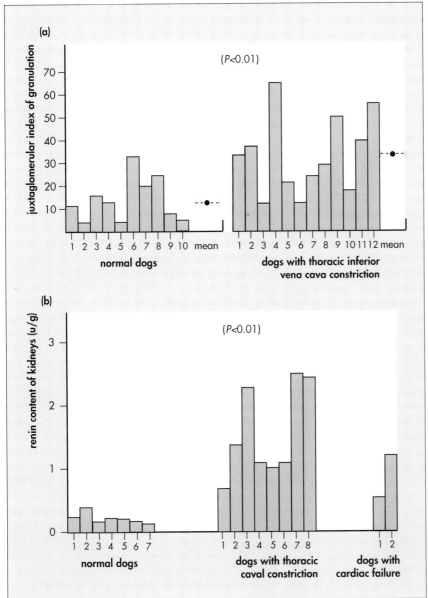

Fig. 76.1 (a) Degree of granulation of juxtaglomerular cells and (b) renin content in kidneys of normal dogs and dogs with thoracic caval constriction. Results from individual animals are shown and differences between the two groups of animals were statistically significant (P<0.01). Modified from Davis JO *et al* [5].

of the RAS in high-output cardiac failure due to beri-beri was less than that in patients with low-output failure. Bayliss and colleagues noted similar levels of PRA and aldosterone whether heart failure was due to coronary disease or to idiopathic dilated cardiomyopathy [36]. Plasma renin concentration was high in a patient with cardiac tamponade, rising as the condition worsened, and falling with treatment [31]. In peripartum heart failure in Nigeria, PRA and aldosterone levels were lower than in age-matched women post partum, but rose with treatment [231].

RENIN RESPONSES

Nonpharmacologic maneuvers

Sodium restriction increased PRA in patients with valvular heart disease and a cardiac index of >2.5l/min/m², but uniformly reduced PRA in those whose cardiac index was <2.5l/min/m² [40]. Genest and colleagues reported a paradoxical decline in renin levels during sodium depletion in cardiac failure [41]. Withdrawal of maintenance diuretic therapy and institution of a

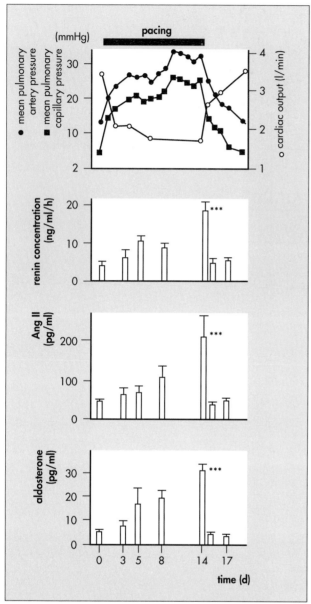

Fig. 76.2 Hemodynamic and plasma hormone indices before, during, and after right ventricular pacing at 240–280 beats/min for 14 days in six dogs (mean ± SEM). Modified from Riegger AJG *et al* (18). ***P<0.001 compared with pre-pacing values.

high sodium diet (300mmol/d for five days) suppressed PRA in four patients whose baseline renin values were low; high PRA values, however, persisted in four other patients [42] (Fig. 76.3). An earlier study noted a paradoxical rise in aldosterone secretion during sodium loading in two patients with advanced heart failure, but renin levels were not recorded [43].

Although definitive data do not exist for obvious reasons, it appears that sodium loading and sodium restriction evoke 'normal' directional responses of renin in patients with mild, stable cardiac failure, whereas those subjects with more severe myocardial dysfunction often exhibit a rise in renin during sodium loading and a fall with sodium restriction. The explanation, one assumes, is that any added burden of sodium causes a deterioration in cardiac function in severe heart failure and hence further renin release through mechanisms discussed later in this chapter. Sodium restriction, by contrast, may improve cardiac function through a reduction in the excessive preload, thereby inducing a fall in renin release. In the case of mild, stable heart failure, cardiac responses to changes in sodium intake are directionally normal, and changes in renin release are also likely to be normal.

Mannitol infusion, but not lower-body positive pressure, suppressed PRA in patients with severe, treated heart failure [44,45]. Neither lower-body negative pressure nor head-up tilt elicited a clear response of PRA in patients with severe heart failure and high renin levels [46–48]. In contrast, patients with less-severe failure showed a clear rise in PRA with head-up tilt [47] and their PRA values doubled during strenuous exercise [49], although interpretation of the latter study is hampered by treatment with digitalis and furosemide. Isometric exercise did not affect PRA in patients with severe heart failure or in healthy volunteers [50].

Overall, it appears that patients with severe cardiac failure and high baseline levels of renin have little or no response to stimuli such as lower-body negative pressure, and little suppression of renin during sodium loading. When cardiac dysfunction is less severe, renin secretion can be inhibited by a high sodium intake and stimulated by exercise or tilt. Interpretation of the above studies requires caution, however, since in many instances, drugs capable of altering renin release were being prescribed.

Drugs

A summary of drug effects on plasma renin levels is given in Fig. 76.4.

Diuretics

Renin responses to diuretic administration are extremely variable [28,29,31–33,36,40,41,51–53], but scrutiny of the literature suggests there are patterns of response depending on the presence or absence of edema, the severity of cardiac failure and, of course, timing of blood sampling in relation to diuretic administration. For edematous patients with raised or 'normal' renin levels, the institution of diuretic therapy induces a fall in renin often to very low values during the natriuretic phase

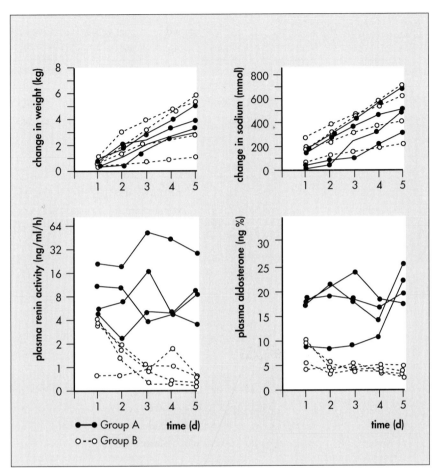

Fig. 76.3 Weight gain, cumulative sodium retention, plasma renin activity (PRA), and plasma aldosterone over five days of high sodium intake (300mmol/d) in eight patients with congestive heart failure. Some patients showed suppression of plasma aldosterone and PRA (Group B) whereas others did not (Group A). Modified from Chonko AM et al [42].

(Fig. 76.5). Continued treatment, particularly with high doses of diuretic, however, elicits a steep rise in renin as the natriuretic effect diminishes [31–33,52] (Fig. 76.5). This so-called triphasic pattern is biphasic in patients whose baseline renin levels are low, because a 'spontaneous' natriuresis has developed or the heart failure is mild or stable [33,36,40,52,54], or even monophasic in terminal cases when diuretic administration serves only to stimulate further already high renin levels.

Intravenous loop diuretics elicited minor short-term responses in plasma renin, Ang II, and aldosterone in edematous patients who showed a brisk natriuresis [52,55]. In contrast, nonedematous patients exhibited a doubling of PRA within 10 minutes of intravenous furosemide [56,57]. Few studies have compared different diuretics, but Peltola et al [58] reported that hydrochlorothiazide had a greater and more prolonged stimulatory effect on renin than did furosemide.

Once diuretic therapy has been established and stabilized, there is a positive relationship between the maintenance dose of diuretic and plasma levels of renin, Ang II, and aldosterone [59,60] (Fig. 76.6) and a gradual, progressive rise in both PRA and norepinephrine with time [61]. Interestingly, the daily maintenance dose of an oral loop diuretic in stable heart failure has only a modest short-term stimulatory effect on renin and aldosterone levels [60] although this varies according to the severity of cardiac dysfunction, the dose of the diuretic, and body posture [55]. The addition of either amiloride or spironolactone for two months to chronic furosemide therapy has been shown to elicit a vigorous rise in renin, Ang II, and aldosterone levels [62].

Digoxin

Digoxin given intravenously in a dose of 0.5mg was associated with a 50% fall in PRA over three hours in patients with severe chronic cardiac failure [63]. This observation is consistent with reports in essential hypertension that a single 0.5-mg oral dose of digoxin can inhibit the renin response to furosemide [64]. The same dose given intravenously reduced PRA by more than 90%

Drug	Duration of treatment	Renin response	References	Comments
diuretic loop	short term	variable: triphasic	28,29,31–33,36, 40,41,51–57	
	long term	increase	59,60	
spironolactone amiloride		increase	62	
digoxin	short term	decrease	63	
	long term	little effect	66,67	
β₁-partial agonists dopaminergic agents	short term	increase	69–76	dopamine has little effect
	long term	little effect		xamoterol may suppress renin
phosphodiesterase inhibitors	short term	increase	74,77–79	some reports indicate no change or even a fall
	long term	little effect		
nitrates	short term	increase	80–83	usually modest effect
	long term	little effect		information sparse
	transdermal	no effect	84–86	
prazosin	short term	increase	88–97	modest effect
	long term	transient increase		no effect in some reports
calcium-channel antagonists	acute			
	nifedipine	increase	98–100	
	nisoldipine	little effect	101	
	nitrendipine	little effect	102	
hydralazine	acute	increase	100,103	no effect in one report
minoxidil	acute	increase	104	
nitroprusside		little effect	99,106	
prostaglandin I₂ and E₂		increase or little effect	106,107	
atrial natriuretic factor	acute	little effect	108–116	

Fig. 76.4 Effects of drugs on plasma renin in human heart failure.

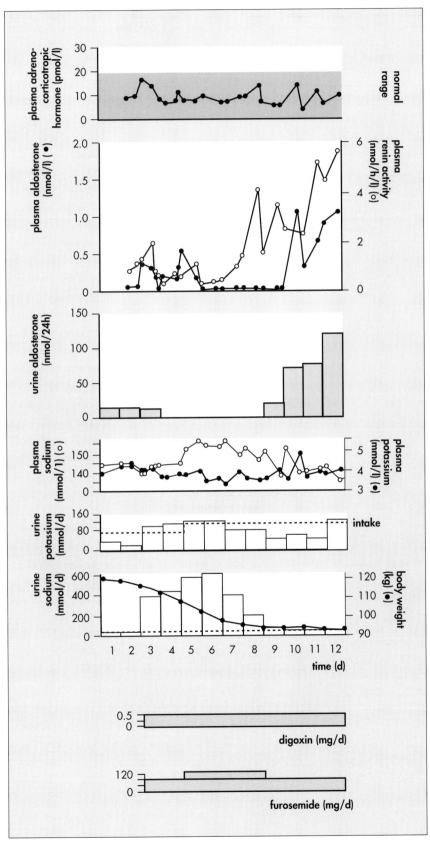

Fig. 76.5 Electrolyte, hormone, plasma renin activity, and body weight changes before and during treatment with furosemide and digoxin in a previously untreated 45-year-old patient with heart failure. Modified from Nicholls MG *et al* [33].

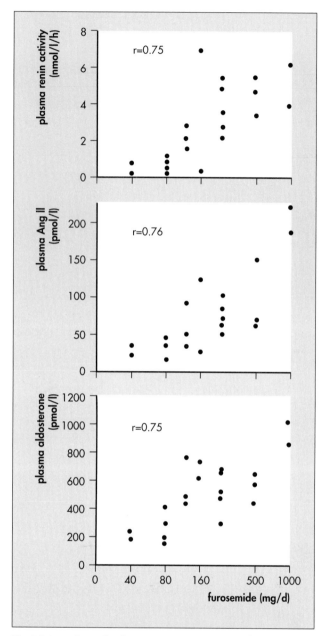

Fig. 76.6 Relationship between maintenance daily furosemide dose (log scale) and hormone levels in 21 patients (20 for Ang II) with heart failure. Each point represents a mean of two values (drawn at 0830 and 1500 hours) in each patient. Modified from Fitzpatrick MA *et al* [60].

over three hours in hypertensive subjects [65]. In contrast, digoxin given for six weeks in a placebo-controlled study did not alter PRA or aldosterone levels in 19 patients with mild cardiac failure who were on maintenance hydrochlorothiazide therapy [66]. Furthermore, Alicandri and colleagues [67] reported no change in PRA

after four weeks of digoxin treatment in 16 patients with mild to moderate heart failure. It appears therefore, that digoxin can suppress renin in the short term but has little or no effect with chronic treatment in heart failure. Whether the vascular (pressor) response to Ang II is enhanced by digoxin as it is in normal volunteers [68], is not known.

Beta-agonists, partial agonists, and dopaminergic agents
Beta-agonists, partial agonists, and dopaminergic agents can stimulate renin levels in the short term but there is little information from prolonged studies. A three-day incremental infusion of prenalterol doubled PRA, Ang II, and aldosterone levels in patients with moderate, stable cardiac failure who were receiving maintenance furosemide and digoxin [69]. The same drug given orally in an incremental fashion (20, 30, and 50mg every two hours) stimulated PRA two-fold although the change did not achieve statistical significance [70]. By contrast, prenalterol 20–100mg twice daily for one month had no effect on PRA in a placebo-controlled study [70] while another β_1-adrenoceptor partial agonist, xamoterol, blunted the PRA response to a diuretic in patients with impaired left ventricular function after acute myocardial infarction [71]. Intravenous dobutamine (5–15µg/kg/min) increased PRC and PRA by 32–58% in patients with severe heart failure [72–74]. Dopamine infusion at 5µg/kg/min for 20 minutes, however, did not alter PRC in six patients with low cardiac output after acute myocardial infarction [72]. Likewise, an incremental dopamine infusion in severe chronic heart failure failed to affect PRA [75]. A single 100-mg oral dose of the dopamine$_1$-agonist, fenoldapam, induced a two-fold rise of PRA in patients with chronic cardiac failure [76]. When given for three days (100mg four times daily) to the same patients, PRA and aldosterone levels rose slightly but not statistically significantly, although the final dose of fenoldapam increased PRA by 81% at two hours [76].

Phosphodiesterase inhibitors
Phosphodiesterase inhibitors tend to increase plasma renin in short-term studies but the response can be variable. Uretsky [77] reported a minor rise in PRA after a single oral or intravenous dose of enoximone, while a bolus of amrinone on top of dobutamine infusion elicited a vigorous increase in PRA [74]. Likewise, Petein *et al* [78] observed a sizeable (65%) rise in PRA after bolus injections of piroximone. In contrast, a brief intravenous infusion of the phosphodiesterase inhibitor, ICI 153110, suppressed PRA by nearly 50% in 10 patients with chronic heart failure [79].

Vasodilator drugs

Vasodilator drugs either increase circulating renin levels in cardiac failure or have little effect. Nitroglycerin given continuously by intravenous infusion for 48 hours elicited a 70% rise in PRA whereas intermittent (12-hour) infusions had little effect in patients with severe heart failure [80]. More recent information from short-term (4–72-hour) infusions of nitroglycerin, in moderate or severe cardiac failure revealed a modest and probably transient stimulatory action on PRA [81–83]. Transdermal nitroglycerin, however, has no clear effect on PRA in heart failure [84–86]. The possibility that hemodynamic tolerance to nitroglycerin is contributed to by stimulation of the RAS seems unlikely since ACE inhibition with captopril failed to modify the development of tolerance [87].This topic is discussed in greater depth in *Chapter 98*.

The postsynaptic α_1-adrenoceptor blocker, prazosin, increases circulating renin slightly according to some workers, especially with single-dose or short-term treatment [88–93], although diuretic doses were sometimes adjusted, which complicates interpretation. Other studies noted a transient stimulation of renin [94] or no effect [95–97].

The calcium-channel blocker, nifedipine, has been reported to stimulate renin levels in cardiac failure [98–100] without a concomitant rise in aldosterone concentration [98,100]. Acute studies with nisoldipine [101] and nitrendipine [102] by contrast, failed to show any effect on PRA.

Acute administration of hydralazine [103] and minoxidil [104] increased PRA in cardiac failure, although Elkayam and colleagues [100] noted no change in PRC after intravenous hydralazine (5–30mg) in severe cardiac failure. Flosequinan, a direct-acting venous and arteriolar dilator, suppressed renin slightly but not significantly in a four-week, double-blind, placebo-controlled crossover study in 11 patients with chronic ischemic heart failure [105]. Intravenous infusion of viprostol, a prostaglandin E_2 analog, stimulated PRA five-fold in nine patients with chronic cardiac failure [106], but PGI_2 had little or no stimulatory effect on PRA in patients with severe heart failure [107]. Nitroprusside infusion failed to alter PRA in cardiac failure [99,106].

Since ANF, or at least drugs that limit its breakdown, may have therapeutic potential in heart failure, it is of interest to note that brief infusion of the 28 amino-acid peptide in high dose had little or no effect on plasma renin or Ang II levels, despite often sizeable falls in arterial pressure [108–116]. Likewise, a rise in levels of endogenous ANF induced by inhibition of its degradation by endopeptidase 24:11 did not alter plasma active renin concentration [117].

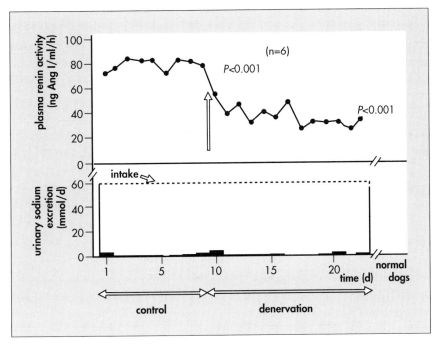

Fig. 76.7 Effect of bilateral denervation of the kidneys on plasma renin activity and urine sodium in dogs with thoracic caval constriction. Modified from Witty RT *et al* [119].

REGULATION OF RENIN
IN HEART FAILURE

Many input signals to the juxtaglomerular apparatus, both stimulatory and inhibitory, are activated in heart failure [118]. Of these, the sympathetic system, the intrarenal afferent arteriolar baroreceptor, and the macula densa appear particularly important.

ANIMAL STUDIES

Detailed studies in dogs with thoracic caval constriction indicate that the sympathetic nervous system contributes to high circulating renin levels since renal denervation reduced PRA by 50% (Fig. 76.7) and intrarenal propranolol inhibited renin secretion from kidneys whether with or without a functional macula densa [119,120]. Since renal denervation and propranolol together failed to prevent a rise in PRA [120], however, it appears that activation of the sympathetic system is not a prerequisite for stimulation of renin in this animal model.

Armstrong and colleagues observed a close correlation (r=0.83) between concurrent norepinephrine and PRA in dogs with pacing-induced heart failure [121] but this need not necessarily reflect sympathetic stimulation of the juxtaglomerular apparatus. Elsner et al noted a two-fold rise in PRA with blockade of the vagi in dogs with pacing-induced heart failure despite a 20-fold increase in vasopressin, and in the absence of hemodynamic change [122]. These data suggest that afferent traffic in the vagi, presumably from stimulation of cardiopulmonary stretch receptors, exerts a tonic inhibitory action on the juxtaglomerular apparatus via renal sympathetic innervation. These observations pertain to the early phases of cardiac failure, and the authors are cautious in extrapolating to the chronic state where atrial distension and blunting of atrial receptor sensitivity may decrease vagal tone, thereby increasing sympathetic traffic to the juxtaglomerular apparatus.

The fact that the intrarenal baroreceptor contributes, whether or not the macula densa is functional, was shown by a 50% fall in renin secretion during intrarenal papaverine infusion in caval dogs [119]. It is probable that the macula densa is also involved since the renin secretory rate was considerably higher in dogs with filtering kidneys than in those with nonfiltering kidneys although other explanations (for example, loss of juxtaglomerular cells in nonfiltering kidneys) cannot be ruled out [119].

There will be, inevitably, complex interrelationships between the above-mentioned three stimuli [123]; for example, Kirchheim and colleagues suggest that activation of renal sympathetic nerves in cardiac failure lowers the threshold of the renal artery baroreceptor for renin release [124].

Other likely contributors to control of renin secretion in cardiac failure are renal prostaglandins, plasma electrolyte levels, circulating Ang II, vasopressin, ANF, and endothelin. The relative importance of these, however, is impossible to gauge from available information.

The fact that prostaglandins contribute to renin secretion is suggested by the 43% inhibition of PRA by intravenous indomethacin in dogs with thoracic caval constriction [120], and by the exaggerated rise in PRC in response to the prostacyclin derivative, iloprost, in dogs with pacing-induced heart failure [125]. Dogs with high-output heart failure, however, failed to show an inhibitory effect of indomethacin [126].

Infusion of hypertonic sodium chloride [127] or sodium lactate [128] into the renal artery of intact kidneys in caval dogs reduced renin secretion, suggesting that plasma sodium concentration (or at least the sodium ion) may modulate renin release in this model [118]. Since the intrarenal infusion of potassium chloride into intact or nonfiltering kidneys reduced renin secretion in the same animal model [127], it seems possible that a rise in circulating potassium concentration might inhibit renin or, more importantly, any decline in plasma potassium might contribute to high levels of renin.

Both Ang II and vasopressin can inhibit renin release under many circumstances (see Chapter 24), and although little attention has been directed to this question in cardiac failure, one would expect that a high circulating level of either peptide could exert a restraining effect on the juxtaglomerular apparatus. Evidence that blockade of Ang II by a competitive antagonist [129] or by an ACE inhibitor [130,131] stimulates renin release in experimental cardiac failure is consistent with this premise, although other factors (especially a major fall in renal perfusion pressure) complicate interpretation. Confirmation of any renin-suppressant action of vasopressin in heart failure is needed. Blockade of the vascular vasopressin type I (V_1) receptor failed to elicit a change in PRA in chronic caval dogs [132] and, an unexpected fall in PRA occurred in rabbits with adriamycin-induced cardiac failure [133]. Either the antagonist failed to block juxtaglomerular actions of vasopressin, or circulating vasopressin was not contributing in any major way to the regulation of renin under these circumstances.

In experimental heart failure, infusion of ANF in high doses can suppress renin [10,21,134–137] although no change in PRC or Ang II levels was noted in two studies [138,139], and Langton and colleagues reported a rise in PRA in rabbits with

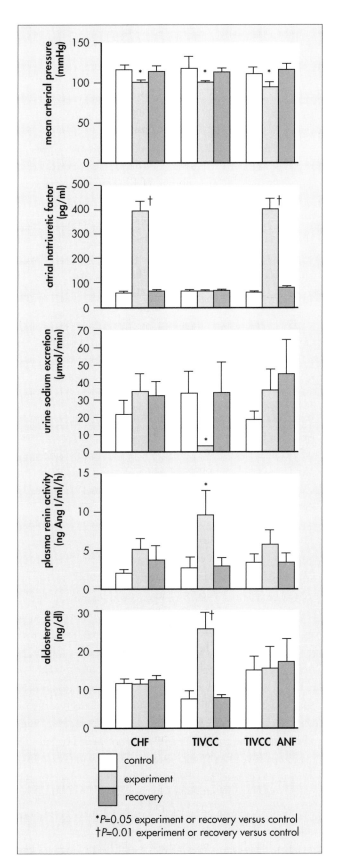

Fig. 76.8 Effect of rapid right ventricular pacing (CHF), thoracic inferior vena caval constriction (TIVCC), and TIVCC plus exogenous atrial natriuretic factor (ANF) on mean arterial pressure, plasma ANF, urine sodium excretion, plasma renin activity, and plasma aldosterone (mean ± SEM). Modified from Lee ME *et al* [10].

adriamycin-induced heart failure [140]. The study by Lee *et al* [10] suggests that endogenous ANF serves as an inhibitor of renin (and aldosterone) in dogs with congestive heart failure due to rapid right ventricular pacing. (Fig. 76.8).

Since circulating levels of endothelin are elevated in pacing-induced heart failure [141] and the peptide has been shown to suppress PRA [141], it is possible that endothelin serves to restrain renin release; further information, however, is awaited.

HUMAN STUDIES

The obvious difficulty of performing detailed studies in man leaves many unanswered questions regarding control of renin. Most information comes from statistical associations between plasma renin levels and putative input signs, and from renin responses to administration of known stimuli to renin or to agents that block endogenous secretagogues.

Inverse relations between arterial pressure and renin levels [37,60,142] and between urinary (or fractional) excretion of sodium and renin levels [143,144] (Fig. 76.9) are consistent with an important role of the renal afferent arteriolar baroreceptor and the macula densa in regulating renin production. Since many workers, though by no means all, have found positive correlations between renin and concomitant plasma norepinephrine levels [145–147], and in view of the observation that renal sympathetic activity is increased in heart failure [148], it is likely that sympathetic stimulation of the juxtaglomerular apparatus contributes to renin secretion in cardiac failure. Heightened sympathetic activity may result from cardiac and arterial baroreceptor dysfunction, which leads to a reduction in inhibitory input stimuli to the central nervous system. The failure of upright tilt and lower-body negative pressure to raise renin levels in heart failure [46–48] is consistent with this premise. An abnormality within the central nervous system has also been claimed to contribute to supranormal sympathetic activity [149].

Positive associations between levels of renin and metabolites of PGI_2 and PGE_2 [150] suggest a role for prostaglandins in the regulation of renin in cardiac failure. The possibility is strengthened by reports that a PGE_2 analog stimulates renin levels [106] while inhibitors of prostaglandin synthesis reduce renin in heart failure.

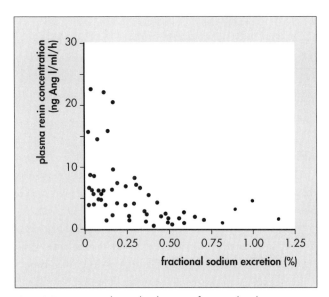

Fig. 76.9 Inverse relationship between fractional sodium excretion and plasma renin concentration in 40 patients with chronic congestive heart failure. The patients were taking a low or normal sodium diet and digoxin. Diuretics were withdrawn seven days prior to the study. Measurements were made twice in some patients. Modified from Riegger AJG, unpublished data.

Renal ischemia in heart failure might increase local formation of adenosine, which could enhance renin secretion, although the interrelationship is complex [225].

Inverse correlations between plasma sodium and renin levels have often been noted in cardiac failure [31,37,151–153]. The correlation is especially close in untreated patients [31]. Although this might indicate that hyponatremia augments renin release, it more likely reflects the multiple effects of Ang II to lower plasma sodium concentration [31] (see *Chapter 21*).

High circulating levels of Ang II are presumed to restrain renin release. Indeed, infusion of the octapeptide inhibits plasma renin levels in patients whether or not they are taking an ACE inhibitor [154,155] and, blockade of the Ang II receptor [142, 156] or of Ang II production [157,158] elicits a vigorous rise in renin levels.

As pointed out by Richards and colleagues [159] and confirmed by others [160,161], there is a positive relationship between plasma levels of ANF and renin in cardiac failure which contrasts with the inverse association in healthy volunteers. This altered relationship in heart failure presumably reflects both the abnormal atrial distension (a plausible mechanism for ANF

release) [226] and decreased renal perfusion (the basis for raised renin secretion in heart failure) [227]. Although proof is lacking, it is likely that the high ANF concentrations restrain renin release and indeed, high-dose short-term infusions of the peptide either suppress renin or have little effect in the face of often vigorous falls in arterial pressure [108–116].

To summarize, available data suggest that the intrarenal baroreceptor, the macula densa, and sympathetic innervation of the juxtaglomerular apparatus are important regulators of renal renin production in cardiac failure. Additional contributions are likely to come from renal prostaglandins and adenosine, plasma sodium and potassium concentrations, circulating Ang II and vasopressin, ANF, and endothelin. A final point is that a contribution to plasma renin levels from extrarenal sources is entirely possible in heart failure, but data are lacking.

PATHOPHYSIOLOGICAL IMPORTANCE OF THE RENIN–ANGIOTENSIN SYSTEM IN HEART FAILURE

The role of the RAS can be assessed, albeit imperfectly, by relating plasma levels of its components to the severity of organ or tissue dysfunction, or by blocking the system at various sites. Imperfections in measurement techniques (particularly for Ang II), incomplete blockade of Ang II formation or action, and alterations in other vasoactive systems (especially with ACE inhibition) necessitate that conclusions reached must be less than definitive.

ANIMAL STUDIES
Early suggestions that the RAS may play a pathophysiological role [162] were confirmed when competitive inhibitors of Ang II [129], the ACE inhibitors [14,130,163–166], and renin inhibitors [166,167] were shown to have definite hemodynamic, hormonal, and renal effects in various models of cardiac failure. In brief, these reports suggest that the RAS contributes to control of arterial pressure, to aldosterone and cortisol secretion, and to regulation of renal function (Fig. 76.10). One contrary report, that increased vascular resistance in hindquarters of guinea pigs with constriction of the pulmonary artery was not altered by infusion of a competitive Ang II antagonist [168], does not exclude a longer-term effect of Ang II. Of particular note is that a renin inhibitor and an ACE inhibitor produced similar effects on systemic hemodynamics and left ventricular function in dogs with acute heart failure [166], suggesting that the main hemodynamic consequences of ACE inhibition in this particular animal model resulted from a fall in Ang II production.

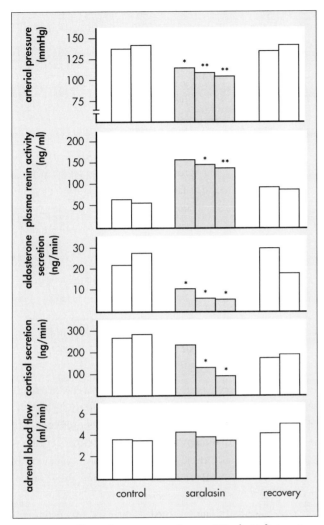

Fig. 76.10 Effects of intravenous infusion of [Sar^1, Ala^8] Ang II (saralasin), a competitive inhibitor of Ang II, on arterial pressure, plasma renin activity, aldosterone and cortisol secretion, and on adrenal blood flow in five dogs with thoracic caval constriction (mean). Modified from Johnson JA and Davis JO [129]. *$P<0.05$, **$P<0.01$, compared with control.

HUMAN STUDIES

Statistically significant associations have been reported in heart failure between plasma renin and hemodynamic indices such as systemic vascular resistance, right heart and wedge pressures, and cardiac output, and with clinical status [60,161,169–171], although such observations are by no means universal [143]. The initial hemodynamic response to a competitive Ang II-receptor blocker [142,156,172] or an ACE inhibitor relates, in many studies, to pretreatment activity of the RAS [96,173–177]. Likewise, positive correlations have been reported between central

hemodynamic indices and plasma Ang II levels over the first few days of treatment with ACE inhibitors [158,176,178].

The fact that the RAS contributes to the set point of vascular resistance in the heart, kidneys, and brain is suggested by the increase in blood flow to these organs with competitive Ang II blockers and ACE inhibitors [179] (see *Chapter 93*). Since hepatic blood flow falls with ACE inhibition [180,181], factors other than Ang II must dictate flow to the liver.

Some authors have noted that whereas limb vascular resistance is reduced and blood flow is increased by long-term ACE inhibition, these indices are altered little by ACE inhibitors in the short term [179,182–186]. This observation raised the possibility that perturbations in vasoactive systems other than the RAS dictate vascular resistance in skeletal muscle, that a component of the vasoconstrictor action of Ang II has a long half-life, or that a vascular RAS is pathophysiologically important but is not blocked immediately by some ACE inhibitors.

The response to infusion of an ACE inhibitor, directly into both coronary arteries of patients with idiopathic dilated cardiomyopathy, suggests that the RAS contributes not only to coronary artery constriction but also has a positive inotropic action [187]. The relative contribution of circulating and tissue renin systems, however, remains to be determined. It is also likely that activation of renin systems hastens hemodynamic deterioration through direct effects on myocytes, for example, via impairment of relaxation, promotion of hypertrophy, and direct toxic actions. Stimulation of fibroblast function may contribute to excessive wall stiffness. Finally, cardiac work will ultimately be increased through the many additional actions of Ang II, which lead to an increase in preload and afterload.

In patients with heart failure, positive statistical associations between various measurements of renin on one hand and crude indices of renal function (such as plasma urea and creatinine concentrations) on the other have been observed [31,37,60,171]. These, together with the fact that blockade of the RAS increases renal blood flow while decreasing filtration fraction, support a prominent role for the RAS in regulating renal function in cardiac failure [188]. It is suggested that Ang II serves to maintain glomerular filtration rate (GFR) in cardiac failure [31,189,190]. While this is certainly so, Brown *et al* [31] found that plasma renin and blood urea were positively correlated in clinical cardiac failure. By contrast, Cody and colleagues reported insignificant statistical associations between PRA and GFR in 34 patients [191]. Responses in GFR to ACE inhibition are extremely variable depending on a number of factors, including the magnitude of fall in arterial pressure and the duration of treatment [192].When plasma renin and Ang II are modestly elevated in heart failure, ACE inhibition often causes a deterioration in GFR and a rise in blood urea and creatinine [205,206,226]. However, with very severe hyponatremia and renal failure in cardiac impairment, ACE inhibitors can improve renal function [228]. Another possible role of Ang II in heart failure may be regulation of vasa recta blood flow and hence facilitation of urea excretion [31,193]. Whether redistribution of the intrarenal circulation in heart failure [194] relates to alterations in activity and distribution of renin within the kidney [193,227], remains to be seen.

The often observed inverse relationship between plasma sodium and renin levels [31,37,151–153,195] (Fig. 76.11) supports a water-retaining action of high plasma Ang II concentrations, presumably through stimulation of thirst and secretion of vasopressin [196,197] and through direct renal effects of the octapeptide [31]. Consistent with this thesis is the fact that ACE inhibitors correct hyponatremia [157,198,199] whereas alternative vasodilator drugs fail to do so [199]. As noted earlier, the inverse renin/sodium relationship may reflect, in part, a renin-stimulating action of hyponatremia.

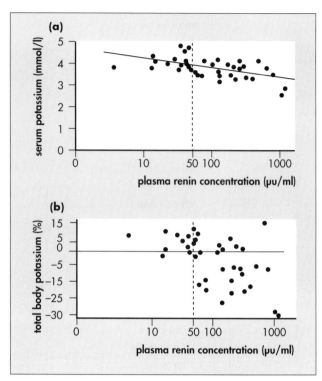

Fig. 76.12 Relations between plasma active renin concentration (log scale) and serum potassium (a) and total body potassium (expressed as percentage of predicted normal, b) in patients with heart failure. Modified from Cleland JGF et al [203].

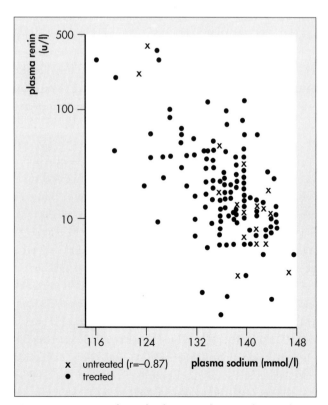

Fig. 76.11 Inverse relationship between plasma sodium and renin concentrations (log scale) in patients with congestive heart failure. All patients, r=−0.55. Modified from Brown JJ et al [31]

Many factors probably contribute to control of aldosterone secretion in heart failure but the RAS is dominant. Most reports document positive associations between concomitant levels of renin (or Ang II) and aldosterone [33,37,40,42,52,60,62,157, 158,170]. Infusion of Ang II stimulates aldosterone levels in the presence [154] or absence [155] of an ACE inhibitor. Finally, Ang II and aldosterone levels fall in parallel during the initiation of ACE inhibitor therapy [157,158] despite the fact that cumulative potassium balance is positive and plasma potassium levels rise [200].

Angiotensin II, through direct actions on the kidney and via aldosterone secretion, is, no doubt, one factor of importance in the excessive sodium retention of heart failure. It is not clear whether renal responses to Ang II are altered in cardiac failure, but inability of the kidney to 'escape' from the sodium-retaining action of aldosterone [201] and evidence from animals for heightened renal responsiveness to aldosterone [202] support a major role of the renin–angiotensin–aldosterone system in renal sodium retention. The ACE inhibitors have variable effects on urine sodium excretion [192] as discussed in *Chapter 93*.

Plasma renin and potassium concentrations have been found to be significantly and positively correlated in untreated cardiac failure in man [31]. One assumes that the inverse relationship between plasma renin and both serum and total body potassium levels in treated heart failure [203,204] (Fig. 76.12) is largely accounted for by Ang II-related aldosterone secretion, to which diuretic therapy no doubt contributes. Consistent with this premise is the rise in serum and total body potassium during ACE inhibition [205,206]. An effect of hypokalemia to stimulate renin release (see *Chapter 74*) may contribute to the potassium–renin relationship in diuretic-treated cases.

As with animal studies, there is some suggestive evidence for an association, not necessarily causative, between activity of the RAS and cortisol secretion. A fall in cortisol excretion has been noted during introduction of an ACE inhibitor in severe cardiac failure [207] and a brisk rise occurred when the ACE inhibitor was stopped [208]. Infusion of Ang II in the presence [154] or absence [155] of an ACE inhibitor, however, failed to elicit a change in plasma cortisol. Overall, the evidence is not strong for Ang II being an important secretagog either directly or via stimulation of corticotropin secreting factor or adrenocorticotropic hormone, for cortisol secretion in cardiac failure. It must be said, however, that little attention has been directed to this question.

Whether the phylogenetically ancient action of Ang II to stimulate the sympathetic system is important in human cardiac failure, is disputed. Some authors report statistically significant correlations between plasma norepinephrine and renin levels [145–147] and a decline in norepinephrine during ACE inhibition [205,206,209]. Although this might reflect, in part, stimulation of global sympathetic activity by high circulating levels of Ang II, it may equally suggest parallel but separate activation of both systems, or stimulation of the juxtaglomerular apparatus by heightened sympathetic activity. Finally, some authors have failed to find either a relationship between renin and norepinephrine levels or a decline in norepinephrine concentrations during ACE inhibition [209]. Overall, evidence for activation of sympathetic activity by circulating Ang II in cardiac failure is unconvincing.

Angiotensin-converting enzyme inhibition sensitizes the parasympathetic baroreceptor heart-rate reflex in cardiac failure [210,211]. It is possible that high circulating Ang II levels contribute to the inhibition of parasympathetic activity, which is a characteristic of the disorder, particularly during treatment with cardiac glycosides [229].

Positive associations between activity of the RAS and vasodilator PGE_2 and PGI_2 (or their metabolites) have been noted [150]. Whereas this might be taken to indicate a stimulatory action of Ang II on prostaglandin synthesis, it is more likely there is a common stimulus to both systems and, as mentioned earlier, prostaglandins may contribute to renin secretion in cardiac failure. Since two groups have noted a rise in PGE_2 metabolite levels during captopril treatment [178,212], it is difficult to sustain a dominant role for Ang II in regulating prostaglandin synthesis in cardiac failure.

Erythropoietin levels are high in cardiac failure and decline with ACE inhibitor treatment [213], but whether or not this reflects a direct effect of the RAS to stimulate erythropoietin secretion, is unclear (see *Chapter 39*).

The RAS may directly or indirectly contribute to the generation of cardiac arrhythmias as witnessed by a positive (though weak) relationship between PRA and ventricular ectopy [204]. Furthermore, ACE inhibitors reduce ectopic frequency in cardiac failure according to some but not all authors (see *Chapter 93*). It is likely that the RAS is one amongst many contributors to arrhythmogenesis in heart failure.

The possibility that the degree of activation of the RAS is one determinant of longevity in cardiac failure has been discussed [214–216]. It is noteworthy, however, that quite a number of neurohormonal and electrolyte indices, apart from the RAS, have been related statistically to longevity [214,215,217]. Nevertheless, the fact that ACE inhibitors increase longevity in patients with moderate [218,232] or severe heart failure [219], whereas alternative vasodilators have little or no effect [214,220], supports the concept that high circulating Ang II levels hasten hemodynamic deteroriation and shorten the lifespan.

A contribution of tissue renin systems to the pathophysiology of cardiac failure is possible and has been discussed [221–224]. At present, however, there is little understanding of the role of such tissue systems in human heart failure.

In summary, evidence from studies in animals and man, point to the RAS being an important contributor to the pathophysiology of cardiac failure. It plays a major role in central and peripheral hemodynamics, in the regulation of renal and cardiac function, in the control of aldosterone secretion, and in water and electrolyte balance. It may also contribute to the secretion of cortisol and erythropoietin, and to activation of the sympathetic system. Finally, the RAS is likely to be one determinant of arrhythmogenesis and the rapidity of hemodynamic deterioration and hence longevity. The relative importance of the kidney-based circulating RAS and various tissue systems to the pathophysiology of cardiac failure remains to be defined.

REFERENCES

1. Johnston CI, Davis JO, Robb CA, Mackenzie JW. Plasma renin in chronic experimental heart failure and during renal sodium 'escape' from mineralocorticoids. *Circulation Research* 1968;**22**:113–25.

2. Schneider EG, Davis JO, Robb CA, Baumber JS. Hepatic clearance of renin in canine experimental models for low- and high-output heart failure. *Circulation Research* 1969;**24**:213–9.

3. Spielman WS, Davis JO, Gotshall RW. Hypersecretion of renin in dogs with a chronic aortic-caval fistula and high-output heart failure. *Proceedings of the Society for Experimental Biology and Medicine* 1973;**143**:479–82.

4. Galla JH, Schneider G, Kotchen TA, Hayslett JP. Renin and aldosterone in the cardiomyopathic hamster in congestive heart failure. *Endocrinology* 1977;**101**:389–95.

5. Davis JO, Hartroft PM, Titus EO, Carpenter CCJ, Ayers CR, Spiegel HE. The role of the renin–angiotensin system in the control of aldosterone secretion. *Journal of Clinical Investigation* 1962;**41**:378–89.

6. Davis JO, Urquhart J, Higgins JT, Rubin EC, Hartroft PM. Hypersecretion of aldosterone in dogs with a chronic aortic-caval fistula and high output heart failure. *Circulation Research* 1964;**14**:471–85.

7. Belleau L, Mion H, Simard S, Granger P, Bertranou E, Nowaczynski W, Boucher R, Genest J. Studies on the mechanism of experimental congestive heart failure in dogs. *Canadian Journal of Physiology and Pharmacology* 1970;**48**:450–6.

8. Hodsman GP, Kohzuki M, Howes LG, Sumithran E, Tsunoda K, Johnston CI. Neurohumoral responses to chronic myocardial infarction in rats. *Circulation* 1988;**78**:376–81.

9. Wilson JR, Lanoce V, Frey MJ, Ferraro N. Effect on peripheral arterioles of chronic fluid and sodium retention in heart failure. *Journal of the American College of Cardiology* 1988;**12**:202–8.

10. Lee ME, Miller WL, Edwards BS, Burnett JC. Role of endogenous atrial natriuretic factor in acute congestive heart failure. *Journal of Clinical Investigation* 1989;**84**:1962–6.

11. Riegger AJG, Elsner D, Kromer EP. Circulatory and renal control by prostaglandins and renin in low cardiac output in dogs. *American Journal of Physiology* 1989;**256**:H1079–86.

12. Villarreal D, Freeman RH, Brands MW. ANF and postprandial control of sodium excretion in dogs with compensated heart failure. *American Journal of Physiology* 1990;**258**:R232–9.

13. Morris BJ, Davis JO, Zatzman ML, Williams GM. The renin–angiotensin–aldosterone system in rabbits with congestive heart failure produced by aortic constriction. *Circulation Research* 1977;**40**:275–82.

14. Watkins L, Burton JA, Haber E, Cant JR, Smith FW, Barger AC. The renin–angiotensin–aldosterone system in congestive failure in conscious dogs. *Journal of Clinical Investigation* 1976;**57**:1606–17.

15. Scriven TA, Burnett JC. Effects of synthetic atrial natriuretic peptide on renal function and renin release in acute experimental heart failure. *Circulation* 1985;**72**:892–7.

16. Freeman RH, Villarreal D, Vari RC, Verburg KM. Endogenous atrial natriuretic factor in dogs with caval constriction. *Circulation Research* 1987;**61** (suppl I):I-96–9.

17. Paganelli WC, Cant JR, Pintal RR, Kifor I, Barger AC, Dzau VJ. Plasma atrial natriuretic factor during chronic thoracic inferior vena caval constriction. *Circulation Research* 1988;**62**:279–85.

18. Riegger AJG, Liebau G. The renin–angiotensin–aldosterone system, antidiuretic hormone and sympathetic nerve activity in an experimental model of congestive heart failure in the dog. *Clinical Science* 1982;**62**:465–9.

19. Fitzpatrick MA, Nicholls MG, Espiner EA, Ikram H, Bagshaw P, Yandle TG. Neurohumoral changes during onset and offset of ovine heart failure: Role of ANP. *American Journal of Physiology* 1989;**256**:H1052–9.

20. Moe GW, Stopps TP, Angus C, Forster C, De Bold AJ, Armstrong PW. Alterations in serum sodium in relation to atrial natriuretic factor and other neuroendocrine variables in experimental pacing-induced heart failure. *Journal of the American College of Cardiology* 1989;**13**:173–9.

21. Koepke JP, DiBona GF. Blunted natriuresis to atrial natriuretic peptide in chronic sodium-retaining disorders. *American Journal of Physiology* 1987;**252**:F865–71.

22. Arnolda L, McGrath B, Cocks M, Sumithran E, Johnston C. Adriamycin cardiomyopathy in the rabbit: An animal model of low output cardiac failure with activation of vasoconstrictor mechanisms. *Cardiovascular Research* 1985;**19**:378–82.

23. Villarreal D, Freeman RH, Davis JO, Verburg KM, Vari RC. Atrial natriuretic factor secretion in dogs with experimental high-output heart failure. *American Journal of Physiology* 1987;**252**:H692–6.

24. Holmer SR, Riegger AJG, Notheis WF, Kromer EP, Kochsiek K. Hemodynamic changes and renal plasma flow in early heart failure: Implications for renin, aldosterone, norepinephrine, atrial natriuretic peptide and prostacyclin. *Basic Research in Cardiology* 1987;**82**:101–8.

25. Turini GA, Brunner HR. The role of hormones in congestive heart failure: New frontiers in therapy? *Clinical Science* 1982;**63**:333–8.

26. Merrill AJ, Morrison JL, Brannon ES. Concentration of renin in renal venous blood in patients with chronic heart failure. *American Journal of Medicine* 1946;**1**:468–72.

27. Fasciolo JC, De Vito E, Romero JC, Cucchi JN. The renin content of the blood of humans and dogs under several conditions. *Canadian Medical Association Journal* 1964;**90**:206–9.

28. Genest J, Boucher R, De Champlain J, Veyrat R, Chretien M, Biron P, Tremblay G, Roy P, Cartier P. Studies on the renin–angiotensin system in hypertensive patients. *Canadian Medical Association Journal* 1964;**90**:263–8.

29. Veyrat R, De Champlain J, Boucher R, Genest J. Measurement of human arterial renin activity in some physiological and pathological states. *Canadian Medical Association Journal* 1964;**90**:215–20.

30. Ripa R, Alvisi R, Salzano S, Baggioni GF, Alvisi V, Pipani A. La renina plasmatica nei soggetti con scompenso cardiaco congestizio. *Giornale di Clinica Medica* 1970;**51**:580–90.

31. Brown JJ, Davies DL, Johnson VW, Lever AF, Robertson JIS. Renin relationships in congestive cardiac failure, treated and untreated. *American Heart Journal* 1970;**80**:329–42.

32. Vandongen R, Gordon RD. Plasma renin in congestive heart failure in man. *Medical Journal of Australia* 1970;**1**:215–7.

33. Nicholls MG, Espiner EA, Donald RA, Hughes H. Aldosterone and its regulation during diuresis in patients with gross congestive heart failure. *Clinical Science and Molecular Medicine* 1974;**47**:301–15.

34. Anand IS, Ferrari R, Kalra GS, Wahi PL, Poole–Wilson PA, Harris PC. Edema of cardiac origin. Studies of body water and sodium, renal function, hemodynamic indexes, and plasma hormones in untreated congestive cardiac failure. *Circulation* 1989;**80**:299–305.

35. Francis GS, Benedict C, Johnstone DE, Kirlin PC, Nicklas J, Liang C, Kubo SH, Rudin–Toretsky E, Yusuf S. Comparison of neuroendocrine activation in patients with left ventricular dysfunction with and without congestive heart failure. A substudy of the studies of left ventricular dysfunction (SOLVD). *Circulation* 1990;**82**:1724–9.

36. Bayliss J, Norell M, Canepa–Anson R, Sutton G, Poole–Wilson P. Untreated heart failure: Clinical and neuroendocrine effects of introducing diuretics. *British Heart Journal* 1987;**57**:17–22.

37. Dzau VJ, Colucci WS, Hollenberg NK, Williams GH. Relation of the renin–angiotensin–aldosterone system to clinical state in congestive heart failure. *Circulation* 1981;**63**:645–51.

38. Fyhrquist F, Tikkanen I. Atrial natriuretic peptide in congestive heart failure. *American Journal of Cardiology* 1988;**62**:20–4A.

39. Ikram H, Maslowski AH, Smith BL, Nicholls MG. The haemodynamic, histopathological and hormonal features of alcoholic cardiac beriberi. *Quarterly Journal of Medicine* 1981;**50**:359–75.

40. Judson WE, Helmer OM. Relationship of cardiorenal function to renin–aldosterone system in patients with valvular heart disease. *Circulation* 1971;**44**:245–53.

41. Genest J, Granger P, De Champlain J, Boucher R. Endocrine factors in congestive heart failure. *American Journal of Cardiology* 1968;**22**:35–42.

42. Chonko AM, Bay WH, Stein JH, Ferris TF. The role of renin and aldosterone in the salt retention of edema. *American Journal of Medicine* 1977;**63**:881–9.

43. Laragh JH. Hormones and the pathogenesis of congestive heart failure: Vasopressin, aldosterone, and angiotension II. *Circulation* 1962;**25**:1015–23.

44. Uretsky BF, Verbalis JG, Murali S, Betschart AR, Kolesar JA, Reddy PS. Control of atrial natriuretic peptide secretion in patients with severe congestive heart failure. *Journal of Clinical Endocrinology and Metabolism* 1990;**71**:146–51.

45. Creager MA, Hirsch AT, Nabel EG, Cutler SS, Colucci WS, Dzau VJ. Responsiveness of atrial natriuretic factor to reduction in right atrial pressure in patients with chronic congestive heart failure. *Journal of the American College of Cardiology* 1988;**11**:1191–8.

46. Levine TB, Francis GS, Goldsmith SR, Cohn JN. The neurohumoral and hemodynamic response to orthostatic tilt in patients with congestive heart failure. *Circulation* 1983;**67**:1070–5.

47. Kubo SH, Cody RJ. Circulatory autoregulation in chronic congestive heart failure: Responses to head-up tilt in 41 patients. *American Journal of Cardiology* 1983;**52**:512–8.

48. Mohanty PK, Arrowood JA, Ellenbogen KA, Thames MD. Neurohumoral and hemodynamic effects of lower body negative pressure in patients with congestive heart failure. *American Heart Journal* 1989;**118**:78–85.

49. Kirlin PC, Grekin R, Das S, Ballor E, Johnson T, Pitt B. Neurohumoral activation during exercise in congestive heart failure. *American Journal of Medicine* 1986;**81**:623–9.

50. Elkayam U, Roth A, Weber L, Hsueh W, Nanna M, Freidenberger L, Chandraratna AN, Rahimtoola SH. Isometric exercise in patients with chronic advanced heart failure: Hemodynamic and neurohumoral evaluation. *Circulation* 1985;**72**:975–81.

51. Meurer KA, Rosskamp E, Krause DK, Kaufmann W. Stimulatory action of various drugs on plasma renin activity and angiotensin II concentration in normals, patients with arterial hypertension and congestive heart failure. In: Genest J, Koiw J, eds. *Hypertension '72.* Berlin: Springer–Verlag, 1972: 140–8.

52. Ikram H, Chan W, Espiner EA, Nicholls MG. Haemodynamic and hormone responses to acute and chronic frusemide therapy in congestive heart failure. *Clinical Science* 1980;**59**:443–9.

53. Sinoway L, Minotti J, Musch T, Goldner D, Davis D, Leaman D, Zelis R. Enhanced metabolic vasodilation secondary to diuretic therapy in decompensated congestive heart failure secondary to coronary artery disease. *American Journal of Cardiology* 1987;**60**:107–11.

54. Kubo SH, Clark M, Laragh JH, Borer JS, Cody RJ. Identification of normal neurohormonal activity in mild congestive heart failure and stimulating effect of upright posture and diuretics. *American Journal of Cardiology* 1987;**60**:1322–8.

55. Ring–Larsen H, Henriksen JH, Wilken C, Clausen J, Pals H, Christensen NJ. Diuretic treatment in decompensated cirrhosis and congestive heart failure: Effect of posture. *British Medical Journal* 1986;**292**:1351–3.

56. Francis GS, Siegel RM, Goldsmith SR, Olivari MT, Levine TB, Cohn JN. Acute vasoconstrictor response to intravenous furosemide in patients with chronic congestive heart failure. *Annals of Internal Medicine* 1985;**103**:1–6.

57. Goldsmith SR, Francis G, Cohn JN. Attenuation of the pressor response to intravenous furosemide by angiotensin converting enzyme inhibition in congestive heart failure. *American Journal of Cardiology* 1989;**64**:1382–5.

58. Peltola P, Lahovaara S, Paasonen MK. Effect of furosemide and hydrochlorothiazide on plasma renin activity in man. *Annales Medicinae Experimentalis et Biologiae Fenniae* 1970;**48**:122–4.

59. Knight RK, Miall PA, Hawkins LA, Dacombe J, Edwards CRW, Hamer J. Relation of plasma aldosterone concentration to diuretic treatment in patients with severe heart disease. *British Heart Journal* 1979;**42**:316–25.

60. Fitzpatrick MA, Nicholls MG, Ikram H, Espiner EA. Stability and inter-relationships of hormone, haemodynamic and electrolyte levels in heart failure in man. *Clinical and Experimental Pharmacology and Physiology* 1985;**12**:145–54.

61. Francis GS, Rector TS, Cohn JN. Sequential neurohumoral measurements in patients with congestive heart failure. *American Heart Journal* 1988;**116**:1464–8.

62. Nicholls MG, Espiner EA, Hughes H, Rogers T. Effect of potassium-sparing diuretics on the renin–angiotensin–aldosterone system and potassium retention in heart failure. *British Heart Journal* 1976;**38**:1025–30.

63. Covit AB, Schaer GL, Sealey JE, Laragh JH, Cody RJ. Suppression of the renin–angiotensin system by intravenous digoxin in chronic congestive heart failure. *American Journal of Medicine* 1983;**75**:445–7.

64. Montanaro D, Antonello A, Baggio B, Finotti P, Melacini P, Ferrari M. Effects of digoxin on plasma renin activity in hypertensive patients. *International Journal of Clinical Pharmacology, Therapy, and Toxicology* 1980;**18**:322–3.

65. Antonello A, Cargnielli G, Ferrari M, Melacini P, Montanaro D. Effect of digoxin on plasma-renin-activity in man. *Lancet* 1976;**ii**:850.

66. Kromer EP, Elsner D, Riegger AJG. Digoxin, converting-enzyme inhibition (Quinapril), and the combination in patients with congestive heart failure functional class II and sinus rhythm. *Journal of Cardiovascular Pharmacology* 1990;**16**:9–14.

67. Alicandri C, Fariello R, Boni E, Zaninelli A, Castellano M, Beschi M, Rosei EA, Muiesan G. Captopril versus digoxin in mild–moderate chronic heart failure: A crossover study. *Journal of Cardiovascular Pharmacology* 1987;**9** (suppl 2): S61–7.

68. Guthrie GP. Effect of digoxin on responsiveness to the pressor actions of angiotensin and norepinephrine in man. *Journal of Clinical Endocrinology and Metabolism* 1984;**58**:76–80.

69. Fitzpatrick D, Ikram H, Nicholls MG, Espiner EA. Hemodynamic, hormonal and electrolyte responses to prenalterol infusion in heart failure. *Circulation* 1983;**67**:613–9.

70. Wathen CG, Mackay IG, Glover DR, Roulston JE. Effect of the partial beta-agonist prenalterol on plasma renin activity in patients with left ventricular failure. *Clinica Chimica Acta* 1987;**162**:97–100.

71. McMurray JJ, Lang CC, MacLean D, McDevitt DG, Struthers AD. Neuroendocrine changes post myocardial infarction: Effects of xamoterol. *American Heart Journal* 1990;**120**:56–62.

72. Kho TL, Henquet JW, Punt R, Birkenhager WH, Rahn KH. Influence of dobutamine and dopamine on hemodynamics and plasma concentrations of noradrenaline and renin in patients with low cardiac output following acute myocardial infarction. *European Journal of Clinical Pharmacology* 1980;**18**: 213–7.

73. Uretsky BF, Generalovich T, Verbalis JG, Valdes AM, Reddy PS. Comparative hemodynamic and hormonal response of enoximone and dobutamine in severe congestive heart failure. *American Journal of Cardiology* 1986;**58**:110–6.

74. Uretsky BF, Lawless CE, Verbalis JG, Valdes AM, Kolesar JA, Reddy PS. Combined therapy with dobutamine and amrinone in severe heart failure. *Chest* 1987;**92**:657–62.

75. Maskin CS, Ocken S, Chadwick B, LeJemtel TH. Comparative systemic and renal effects of dopamine and angiotensin-converting enzyme inhibition with enalaprilat in patients with heart failure. *Circulation* 1985;**72**:846–52.

76. Francis GS, Wilson BC, Rector TS. Hemodynamic, renal, and neurohumoral effects of a selective oral DA$_1$ receptor agonist (Fenoldapam) in patients with congestive heart failure. *American Heart Journal* 1988;**116**:473–9.

77. Uretsky BF, Generalovich T, Verbalis JG, Valdes AM, Reddy PS. MDL 17,043 therapy in severe congestive heart failure: Characterization of the early and late hemodynamic, pharmacokinetic, hormonal and clinical response. *Journal of the American College of Cardiology* 1985;**5**:1414–21.

78. Petein M, Levine TB, Cohn JN. Hemodynamic effects of a new inotropic agent, piroximone (MDL 19205), in patients with chronic heart failure. *Journal of the American College of Cardiology* 1984;4:364–71.

79. Jafri SM, Reddy BR, Budzinski D, Goldberg AD, Pilla A, Levine TB. Acute neurohormonal and hemodynamic response to a new peak III phosphodiesterase inhibitor (ICI 153, 110) in patients with chronic heart failure. *Journal of Cardiovascular Pharmacology* 1990;16:360–6.

80. Packer M, Lee WH, Kessler PD, Gottlieb SS, Medina N, Yushak M. Prevention and reversal of nitrate tolerance in patients with congestive heart failure. *New England Journal of Medicine* 1987;317:799–804.

81. Webster MWI, Sharpe DN, Coxon R, Murphy J, Hannan S, Nicholls MG, Espiner EA. Effect of reducing atrial pressure on atrial natriuretic factor and vasoactive hormones in congestive heart failure secondary to ischemic and nonischemic dilated cardiomyopathy. *American Journal of Cardiology* 1989;63:217–21.

82. Dupuis J, Lalonde G, Lebeau R, Bichet D, Rouleau JL. Sustained beneficial effect of a seventy-two hour intravenous infusion of nitroglycerin in patients with severe chronic congestive heart failure. *American Heart Journal* 1990;120:625–37.

83. Dupuis J, Lalonde G, Lemieux R, Rouleau JL. Tolerance to intravenous nitroglycerin in patients with congestive heart failure: Role of increased intravascular volume, neurohumoral activation and lack of prevention with N-acetylcysteine. *Journal of the American College of Cardiology* 1990;16:923–31.

84. Ogasawara B, Ogawa K, Sassa H. Effects of nitroglycerin ointment on plasma norepinephrine and cyclic nucleotides in congestive heart failure. *Journal of Cardiovascular Pharmacology* 1981;3:867–75.

85. Olivari MT, Carlyle PF, Levine TB, Cohn JN. Hemodynamic and hormonal response to transdermal nitroglycerin in normal subjects and in patients with congestive heart failure. *Journal of the American College of Cardiology* 1983;2:872–8.

86. Elkayam U, Roth A, Henriquez B, Weber L, Tonnemacher D, Rahimtoola SH. Hemodynamic and hormonal effects of high-dose transdermal nitroglycerin in patients with chronic congestive heart failure. *American Journal of Cardiology* 1985;56:555–9.

87. Dakak N, Makhoul N, Flugelman MY, Merdler A, Shehadeh H, Schneeweiss A, Halon DA, Lewis BS. Failure of captopril to prevent nitrate tolerance in congestive heart failure secondary to coronary artery disease. *American Journal of Cardiology* 1990;66:608–13.

88. Colucci WS, Wynne J, Holman BL, Braunwald E. Long-term therapy of heart failure with prazosin: A randomized double blind trial. *American Journal of Cardiology* 1980;45:337–44.

89. Pierpoint GL, Franciosa JA, Cohn JN. Effect of prazosin on renal function in congestive heart failure. *Clinical Pharmacology and Therapeutics* 1980;28:335–9.

90. Ogasawara B, Ogawa K, Hayashi H, Sassa H. Plasma renin activity and plasma concentrations of norepinephrine and cyclic nucleotides in heart failure after prazosin. *Clinical Pharmacology and Therapeutics* 1981;29:464–71.

91. Bayliss J, Norell MS, Canepa-Anson R, Reid C, Poole-Wilson P, Sutton G. Clinical importance of the renin–angiotensin system in chronic heart failure: Double blind comparison of captopril and prazosin. *British Medical Journal* 1985;290:1861–5.

92. Packer M, Medina N, Yushak M. Role of the renin–angiotensin system in the development of hemodynamic and clinical tolerance to long-term prazosin therapy in patients with severe chronic heart failure. *Journal of the American College of Cardiology* 1986;7:671–80.

93. Packer M, Medina N, Yushak M. Comparative hemodynamic and clinical effects of long-term treatment with prazosin and captopril for severe chronic congestive heart failure secondary to coronary artery disease or idiopathic dilated cardiomyopathy. *American Journal of Cardiology* 1986;57:1323–7.

94. Riegger AJG, Haeske W, Kraus C, Kromer EP, Kochsiek K. Contribution of the renin–angiotensin–aldosterone system to development of tolerance and fluid retention in chronic congestive heart failure during prazosin treatment. *American Journal of Cardiology* 1987;59:906–10.

95. Stein L, Henry DP, Weinberger MH. Increase in plasma norepinephrine during prazosin therapy for chronic congestive heart failure. *American Journal of Medicine* 1981;70:825–32.

96. Kluger J, Cody RJ, Laragh JH. The contributions of sympathetic tone and the renin–angiotensin system to severe chronic congestive heart failure: Response to specific inhibitors (prazosin and captopril). *American Journal of Cardiology* 1982;49:1667–74.

97. Markham RV, Corbett JR, Gilmore A, Pettinger WA, Firth BG. Efficacy of prazosin in the management of chronic congestive heart failure: A 6-month randomized, double-blind, placebo-controlled study. *American Journal of Cardiology* 1983;51:1346–52.

98. Prida XE, Kubo SH, Laragh JH, Cody RJ. Evaluation of calcium-mediated vasoconstriction in chronic congestive heart failure. *American Journal of Medicine* 1983;75:795–800.

99. Fifer MA, Colucci WS, Lorell BH, Jaski BE, Barry WH. Inotropic, vascular and neuroendocrine effects of sublingual nifedipine in heart failure: Comparison with nitroprusside. *Journal of the American College of Cardiology* 1985;5:731–7.

100. Elkayam U, Roth A, Hsueh W, Weber L, Freidenberger L, Rahimtoola SH. Neurohumoral consequences of vasodilator therapy with hydralazine and nifedipine in severe congestive heart failure. *American Heart Journal* 1986;111:1130–8.

101. Moe GW, Karlinsky SJ, Frankel D, Armstrong PW. Intravenous nisoldipine in severe congestive heart failure. *Journal of Cardiovascular Pharmacology* 1988;12:160–6.

102. Cohn JN. Calcium antagonists and left ventricular function: Effects of nitrendipine in congestive heart failure. *American Journal of Cardiology* 1986;58:27–30D.

103. Schofer J, Mathey DG, Polster J, Bode V, Dietlein G. Hemodynamic and neurohumoral response to hydralazine versus captopril: A controlled study in idiopathic dilated cardiomyopathy. *Journal of Cardiovascular Pharmacology* 1987;9 (suppl 2):S46–9.

104. Franciosa JA, Cohn JN. Effects of minoxidil on hemodynamics in patients with congestive heart failure. *Circulation* 1981;63:652–7.

105. Cowley AJ, Wynne RD, Stainer K, Fullwood L, Rowley JM, Hampton JR. Flosequinan in heart failure: Acute haemodynamic and longer term symptomatic effects. *British Medical Journal* 1988;297:169–73.

106. Olivari MT, Levine TB, Cohn JN. Evidence for direct renal stimulating effect of prostaglandin E$_2$ on renin release in patients with congestive heart failure. *Circulation* 1986;74:1203–7.

107. Yui Y, Nakajima H, Kawai C, Murakami T. Prostacyclin therapy in patients with congestive heart failure. *American Journal of Cardiology* 1982;50:320–4.

108. Riegger AJG, Kromer EP, Kochsiek K. Der natriuretische Vorhoffaktor bei schwerer kongestiver Herzinsuffizienz. *Deutsche Medizinische Wochenschrift* 1985;110:1607–10.

109. Cody RJ, Atlas SA, Laragh JH, Kubo SH, Covit AB, Ryman KS, Shaknovich A, Pondolfino K, Clark M, Camargo MJF, Scarborough RM, Lewicki JA. Atrial natriuretic factor in normal subjects and heart failure patients – plasma levels and renal, hormonal, and hemodynamic responses to peptide infusion. *Journal of Clinical Investigation* 1986;78:1362–74.

110. Crozier IG, Nicholls MG, Ikram H, Espiner EA, Gomez HJ, Warner NJ. Haemodynamic effects of atrial peptide infusion in heart failure. *Lancet* 1986;ii:1242–5.

111. Riegger AJG, Kromer EP, Kochsiek K. Human atrial natriuretic peptide: Plasma levels, hemodynamic, hormonal, and renal effects in patients with severe congestive heart failure. *Journal of Cardiovascular Pharmacology* 1986;8:1107–12.

112. Saito Y, Nakao K, Nishimura K, Sugawara A, Okumura K, Obata K, Sonoda R, Ban T, Yasue H, Imura H. Clinical application of atrial natriuretic polypeptide in patients with congestive heart failure: Beneficial effects on left ventricular function. *Circulation* 1987;76:115–24.

113. Goy JJ, Waeber B, Nussberger J, Bidiville J, Biollaz J, Nicod P, Mooser V, Kappenberger L, Brunner HR. Infusion of atrial natriuretic peptide to patients with congestive heart failure. *Journal of Cardiovascular Pharmacology* 1988;12:562–70.

114. Molina CR, Fowler MB, McCrory S, Peterson C, Myers BD, Schroeder JS, Murad F. Hemodynamic, renal and endocrine effects of atrial natriuretic peptide infusion in severe heart failure. *Journal of the American College of Cardiology* 1988;12:175–86.

115. Anand IS, Kalra GS, Ferrari R, Harris P, Poole–Wilson PA. Hemodynamic, hormonal, and renal effects of atrial natriuretic peptide in untreated congestive cardiac failure. *American Heart Journal* 1989;118:500–5.

116. Fifer MA, Molina CR, Quiroz AC, Giles TD, Herrman HC, De Scheerder IR, Clement DL, Kubo S, Cody RJ, Cohn JN, Fowler MB. Hemodynamic and renal effects of atrial natriuretic peptide in congestive heart failure. *American Journal of Cardiology* 1990;65:211–5.

117. Northridge DB, Jardine AG, Findlay IN, Archibald M, Dilly SG, Dargie HJ. Inhibition of the metabolism of atrial natriuretic factor causes diuresis and natriuresis in chronic heart failure. *American Journal of Hypertension* 1990;3: 682–7.

118. Davis JO, Freeman RH. Renin release mechanisms in congestive heart failure. *Journal of Hypertension* 1984;2 (suppl 1):89–94.

119. Witty RT, Davis JO, Shade RE, Johnson JA, Prewitt RL. Mechanisms regulating renin release in dogs with thoracic caval constriction. *Circulation* 1972;31:339–47.

120. Echtenkamp SF, Davis JO, DeForrest JM, Rowe BP, Freeman RH, Seymour AA, Dietz JR. Effects of indomethacin, renal denervation, and propranolol on plasma renin activity in conscious dogs with chronic thoracic caval constriction. *Circulation Research* 1981;49:492–500.

121. Armstrong PW, Stopps TP, Ford SE, De Bold AJ. Rapid ventricular pacing in the dog: Pathophysiologic studies of heart failure. *Circulation* 1986;74:1075–84.

122. Elsner D, Kromer EP, Riegger AJG. Effects of vagal blockade on neurohumoral systems in conscious dogs with heart failure. *Journal of Cardiovascular Pharmacology* 1990;15:586–91.

123. Gibbons GH, Dzau VJ, Farhi ER, Barger AC. Interaction of signals influencing renin release. *Annual Review of Physiology* 1984;46:291–308.

124. Kirchheim H, Ehmke H, Persson P. Physiology of the renal baroreceptor mechanism of renin release and its role in congestive heart failure. *American Journal of Cardiology* 1988;62:68–71E.

125. Elsner D, Kromer EP, Riegger AJG. Hemodynamic, hormonal, and renal effects of the prostacyclin analogue iloprost in conscious dogs with and without heart failure. *Journal of Cardiovascular Pharmacology* 1990;16:601–8.

126. Villarreal D, Davis JO, Freeman RH, Dietz JR, Echtenkamp SF. Effects of indomethacin in conscious dogs with experimental high-output heart failure. *American Journal of Physiology* 1983;245:H942–6.

127. Shade RE, Davis JO, Johnson JA, Witty RT. Effects of renal arterial infusion of sodium and potassium on renin secretion in the dog. *Circulation Research* 1972;31:719–27.

128. Stephens GA, Davis JO, Freeman RH, Watkins BE. Effects of sodium and potassium salts with anions other than chloride on renin secretion in the dog. *American Journal of Physiology* 1978;234:F10–5.

129. Johnson JA, Davis JO. Angiotensin II: important role in the maintenance of arterial blood pressure. *Science* 1973;179:906–7.

130. Riegger AJG, Liebau G, Holzschuh M, Witkowski D, Steilner H, Kochsiek K. Role of the renin–angiotensin system in the development of congestive heart failure in the dog as assessed by chronic converting-enzyme blockade. *American Journal of Cardiology* 1984;53:614–8.

131. Fitzpatrick MA, Rademaker MT, Frampton CM, Espiner EA, Yandle TG, A'Court G, Ikram H. Renal effects of ACE inhibition in ovine heart failure: A comparison of intermittent and continuous ACE inhibition. *Journal of Cardiovascular Pharmacology* 1990;16:629–35.

132. Vari RC, Freeman RH, Davis JO, Sweet WD. Systemic and renal hemodynamic responses to vascular blockade of vasopressin in conscious dogs with ascites. *Proceedings of the Society for Experimental Biology and Medicine* 1985;179:192–6.

133. Arnolda L, McGrath BP, Cocks M, Johnston CI. Vasoconstrictor role for vasopressin in experimental heart failure in the rabbit. *Journal of Clinical Investigation* 1986;78:674–9.

134. Freeman RH, Davis JO, Vari RC. Renal response to atrial natriuretic factor in conscious dogs with caval constriction. *American Journal of Physiology* 1985; 248:R495–500.

135. Scriven TA, Burnett JC. Effects of synthetic atrial natriuretic peptide on renal function and renin release in acute experimental heart failure. *Circulation* 1985;72:892–7.

136. Carson P, Carlyle P, Rector TS, Cohn JN. Cardiovascular and neurohormonal effects of atrial natriuretic peptide in conscious dogs with and without chronic left ventricular dysfunction. *Journal of Cardiovascular Pharmacology* 1990;16: 305–11.

137. Levy M. Comparative effects of diuretics and atrial peptide in chronic caval dogs. *American Journal of Physiology* 1990;258:F768–74.

138. Riegger AJG, Elsner D, Kromer EP, Daffner C, Forssman WG, Muders F, Pascher EW, Kochsiek K. Atrial natriuretic peptide in congestive heart failure in the dog: Plasma levels, cyclic guanosine monophosphate, ultrastructure of atrial myoendocrine cells, and hemodynamic, hormonal, and renal effects. *Circulation* 1988;77:398–406.

139. Sweet CS, Ludden CT, Frederick CM, Ribeiro LGT, Nussberger J, Slater EE, Blaine EH. Hemodynamic effects of synthetic atrial natriuretic factor (ANF) in dogs with acute left ventricular failure. *European Journal of Pharmacology* 1985;115:267–76.

140. Langton D, Jover BF, Trigg L, Fullerton M, Blake DW, McGrath BP. Regional distribution of the cardiac output and renal responses to atrial natriuretic peptide infusion in rabbits with congestive heart failure. *Clinical and Experimental Pharmacology and Physiology* 1989;16:939–51.

141. Cavero PG, Miller WL, Heublein DM, Margulies KB, Burnett JC. Endothelin in experimental congestive heart failure in the anesthetized dog. *American Journal of Physiology* 1990;259:F312–7.

142. Turini GA, Brunner HR, Ferguson RK, Rivier JL, Gavras H. Congestive heart failure in normotensive man. Haemodynamics, renin and angiotensin II blockade. *British Heart Journal* 1978;40:1134–42.

143. Cohn JN, Levine TB. Angiotensin-converting enzyme inhibition in congestive heart failure: The concept. *American Journal of Cardiology* 1982;49:1480–3.

144. Cody RJ, Covit AB, Schaer GL, Laragh JH, Sealey JE, Feldschuh J. Sodium and water balance in chronic congestive heart failure. *Journal of Clinical Investigation* 1986;77:1441–52.

145. Levine TB, Francis GS, Goldsmith SR, Simon AB, Cohn JN. Activity of the sympathetic nervous system and renin–angiotensin system assessed by plasma hormone levels and their relation to hemodynamic abnormalities in congestive heart failure. *American Journal of Cardiology* 1982;49:1659–66.

146. Staroukine M, Devriendt J, Decoodt P, Verniory A. Relationships between plasma epinephrine, norepinephrine, dopamine and angiotensin II concentrations, renin activity, hemodynamic state and prognosis in acute heart failure. *Acta Cardiologica* 1984;39:131–8.

147. Rouleau J–L, Kortas C, Bichet D, de Champlain J. Neurohumoral and hemodynamic changes in congestive heart failure: Lack of correlation and evidence of compensatory mechanisms. *American Heart Journal* 1988;116: 746–57.

148. Hasking GJ, Esler MD, Jennings GL, Burton D, Korner PI. Norepinephrine spillover to plasma in patients with congestive heart failure: Evidence of increased overall and cardiorenal sympathetic nervous activity. *Circulation* 1986;73:615–21.

149. Porter TR, Eckberg DL, Fritsch JM, Rea RF, Beightol LA, Schmedtje JF, Monhanty PK. Autonomic pathophysiology in heart failure patients: Sympathetic–cholinergic interrelations. *Journal of Clinical Investigation* 1990;85:1362–71.

150. Dzau VJ, Packer M, Lilly LS, Swartz SL, Hollenberg NK, Williams GH. Prostaglandins in severe congestive heart failure: Relation to activation of the renin–angiotensin system and hyponatremia. *New England Journal of Medicine* 1984;310:347–52.

151. Levine TB, Franciosa JA, Vrobel T, Cohn JN. Hyponatraemia as a marker for high renin heart failure. *British Heart Journal* 1982;47:161–6.

152. Schaer GL, Covit AB, Laragh JH, Cody RJ. Association of hyponatremia with increased renin activity in chronic congestive heart failure: Impact of diuretic therapy. *American Journal of Cardiology* 1983;51:1635–8.

153. Lilly LS, Dzau VJ, Williams GH, Rydstedt L, Hollenberg NK. Hyponatremia in congestive heart failure: Implications for neurohumoral activation and response to orthostasis. *Journal of Clinical Endocrinology and Metabolism* 1984;59:924–30.

154. Chambers S, Nicholls MG, Espiner EA, Ikram H, Livesey JH. Hormone and haemodynamic effects of angiotensin II infusion during captopril treatment for heart failure. *Hormone and Metabolic Research* 1984;17:159–62.

155. Nicholls MG, Espiner EA, Donald RA. Aldosterone and renin–angiotensin responses to stimuli in patients with treated congestive heart failure. *Journal of Laboratory and Clinical Medicine* 1976;87:1005–15.

156. Gavras H, Flessas A, Ryan TJ, Brunner HR, Faxon DP, Gavras I. Angiotensin II inhibition. Treatment of congestive cardiac failure in a high-renin hypertension. *Journal of the American Medical Association* 1977;238:880–2.

157. Dzau VJ, Colucci WS, Williams GH, Curfman G, Meggs L, Hollenberg NK. Sustained effectiveness of converting-enzyme inhibition in patients with severe congestive heart failure. *New England Journal of Medicine* 1980;302:1373–9.

158. Maslowski AH, Ikram H, Nicholls MG, Espiner EA. Haemodynamic, hormonal, and electrolyte responses to captopril in resistant heart failure. *Lancet* 1981;i:71–4.

159. Richards AM, Tonolo G, Tree M, Robertson JIS, Montorsi P, Leckie BA, Polonia J. Atrial natriuretic peptides and renin release. *American Journal of Medicine* 1988;84 (suppl 3A):112–8.

160. Carlone S, Palange P, Mannix ET, Salatto MP, Serra P, Weinberger MH, Aronoff GR, Cockerill EM, Manfredi F, Farber MO. Atrial natriuretic peptide, renin and aldosterone in obstructive lung disease and heart failure. *American Journal of The Medical Sciences* 1989;298:243–8.

161. Fyhrquist F, Tikkanen I. Atrial natriuretic peptide in congestive heart failure. *American Journal of Cardiology* 1988;62:20–24A.

162. Urquhart J, Davis JO. Role of the kidney and the adrenal cortex in congestive heart failure (II). *Modern Concepts of Cardiovascular Disease* 1963;32:787–92.

163. Freeman RH, Davis JO, Williams GM, DeForrest JM, Seymour AA, Rowe BP. Effects of the oral converting enzyme inhibitor, SQ 14225, in a model of low cardiac output in dogs. *Circulation Research* 1979;45:540–5.

164. Williams GM, Davis JO, Freeman RH, DeForrest JM, Seymour AA, Rowe BP. Effect of the oral converting enzyme inhibitor SQ 14225 in experimental high output failure. *American Journal of Physiology* 1979;236:541–5.

165. Ichikawa I, Pfeffer JM, Pfeffer MA, Hostetter TH, Brenner BM. Role of angiotensin II in the altered renal function of congestive heart failure. *Circulation Research* 1984;55:669–75.

166. Sweet CS, Ludden CT, Frederick CM, Bush LR, Ribeiro LGT. Comparative hemodynamic effects of MK-422, a converting enzyme inhibitor, and a renin inhibitor in dogs with acute left ventricular failure. *Journal of Cardiovascular Pharmacology* 1984;6:1067–75.

167. Fitzpatrick MA, Rademaker MT, Frampton CM, Charles CJ, Yandle TG, Espiner EA, Ikram H. Hemodynamic and hormonal effects of renin inhibition in ovine heart failure. *American Journal of Physiology* 1990;258:H1625–31.

168. McNamara RF, Schmid PG, Schmidt JA, Lund DD, Bhatnagar RK. Humoral regulation of vascular resistance after 30 days of pulmonary artery constriction. *American Journal of Physiology* 1979;236:H866–72.

169. Hayduk K, Riegger G, Hepp A. Electrolyte and water balance in cardiac insufficiency. Recent clinical and experimental data. *Basic Research in Cardiology* 1980;75:289–93.

170. Kubo S, Nishioka A, Nishimura H, Sonotani N, Takatsu T. The renin–angiotensin–aldosterone system and catecholamines in chronic congestive heart failure. Effect of angiotensin I converting enzyme inhibitor SQ 14225 (captopril). *Japanese Circulation Journal* 1980;44:427–38.

171. Creager MA, Faxon DP, Cutler SS, Kohlmann O, Ryan TJ, Gavras H. Contribution of vasopressin to vasoconstriction in patients with congestive heart failure: Comparison with the renin–angiotensin system and the sympathetic nervous system. *Journal of the American College of Cardiology* 1986;7:758–65.

172. Cody RJ, Covit AB, Schaer GL, Laragh JH. Estimation of angiotensin II receptor activity in chronic congestive heart failure. *American Heart Journal* 1984;108:81–9.

173. Curtiss C, Cohn JN, Vrobel T, Franciosa JA. Role of the renin–angiotensin system inthe systemic vasoconstriction of chronic congestive heart failure. *Circulation* 1978;58:763–800.

174. Cohn JN, Mashiro I, Levine TB, Mehta J. Role of vasoconstrictor mechanisms in the control of left ventricular performance of the normal and damaged heart. *American Journal of Cardiology* 1979;44:1019–22.

175. Creager MA, Halperin JL, Bernard DB, Faxon DP, Melidossian CD, Gavras H, Ryan TJ. Acute regional circulatory and renal hemodynamic effects of converting-enzyme inhibition in patients with congestive heart failure. *Circulation* 1981;64:483–9.

176. Fitzpatrick D, Nicholls MG, Ikram H, Espiner EA. Haemodynamic, hormonal, and electrolyte effects of enalapril in heart failure. *British Heart Journal* 1983;50:163–9.

177. Packer M, Medina N, Yushak M, Lee WH. Usefulness of plasma renin activity in predicting haemodynamic and clinical responses and survival during long term converting enzyme inhibition in severe chronic heart failure. Experience in 100 consecutive patients. *British Heart Journal* 1985;54:298–304.

178. Silberbauer K, Punzengruber C, Sinzinger H. Endogenous prostaglandin E$_2$ metabolite levels, renin–angiotensin system and catecholamines versus acute hemodynamic response to captopril in chronic congestive heart failure. *Cardiology* 1983;70:297–307.

179. Crozier IG, Ikram H, Nicholls MG, Jans S. Global and regional hemodynamic effects of ramipril in congestive heart failure. *Journal of Cardiovascular Pharmacology* 1989;14:688–93.

180. Creager MA, Halperin JL, Bernard DB, Faxon DP, Melidossian CD, Gavras H, Ryan TJ. Acute regional circulatory and renal hemodynamic effects of converting-enzyme inhibition in patients with congestive heart failure. *Circulation* 1981;64:483–9.

181. Crossley IR, Bihari D, Gimson AES, Westaby D, Richardson PJ, Williams R. Effects of converting enzyme inhibition on hepatic blood flow in man. *American Journal of Medicine* 1984;76 [5B]:62–70.

182. Faxon DP, Halperin JL, Creager MA, Gavras H, Schick EC, Ryan TJ. Angiotensin inhibition in severe heart failure: Acute central and limb hemodynamic effects of captopril with observations on sustained oral therapy. *American Heart Journal* 1981;101:548–56.

183. Cowley AJ, Rowley JM, Stainer KL, Hampton JR. Captopril therapy for heart failure: A placebo controlled study. *Lancet* 1982;ii:730–2.

184. Creager MA, Faxon DP, Rockwell SM, Gavras H, Coffman JD. The contribution of the renin–angiotensin system to limb vasoregulation in patients with heart failure: Observations during orthostasis and α-adrenergic blockade. *Clinical Science* 1985;68:659–67.

185. Wilson JR, Ferraro N. Effect of the renin–angiotensin system on limb circulation and metabolism during exercise in patients with heart failure. *Journal of the American College of Cardiology* 1985;6:556–63.

186. Drexler H, Hiroi M, Riede U, Banhardt U, Meinertz T, Just H. Skeletal muscle blood flow, metabolism and morphology in chronic congestive heart failure and effects of short- and long-term angiotensin-converting enzyme inhibition. *American Journal of Cardiology* 1988;62:82–5E.

187. Foult J–M, Tavolaro O, Antony I, Nitenberg A. Direct myocardial and coronary effects of enalaprilat in patients with dilated cardiomyopathy: Assessment by a bilateral intracoronary infusion technique. *Circulation* 1988;77:337–44.

188. Kubo S, Nishioka A, Nishimura H, Kawamura K, Takatsu T. Effects of converting-enzyme inhibition on cardiorenal hemodynamics in patients with chronic congestive heart failure. *Journal of Cardiovascular Pharmacology* 1985;7:753–9.

189. Packer M. Is the renin–angiotensin system really unnecessary in patients with severe chronic heart failure: The price we pay for interfering with evolution. *Journal of the American College of Cardiology* 1985;6:171–3.

190. Packer M, Lee WH, Kessler PD. Preservation of glomerular filtration rate in human heart failure by activation of the renin–angiotensin system. *Circulation* 1986;74:766–74.

191. Cody RJ, Ljungman S, Covit AB, Kubo SH, Sealey JE, Pondolfino K, Clark M, James G, Laragh JH. Regulation of glomerular filtration rate in chronic congestive heart failure patients. *Kidney International* 1988;34: 361–7.

192. Nicholls MG. Overview: Angiotensin, angiotensin converting enzyme inhibition, and the kidney — congestive heart failure. *Kidney International* 1987;31 (suppl 20):S200–2.

193. Robertson JIS, Richards AM. Converting enzyme inhibitors and renal function in cardiac failure. *Kidney International* 1987;31 (suppl 20):S-216–9.

194. Kilcoyne MM, Schmidt DH, Cannon PJ. Intrarenal blood flow in congestive heart failure. *Circulation* 1973;47:786–97.

195. Packer M, Medina N, Yushak M. Relation between serum sodium concentration and the hemodynamic and clinical responses to converting enzyme inhibition with captopril in severe heart failure. *Journal of the American College of Cardiology* 1984;3:1035–43.

196. Goldsmith SR, Francis GS, Cowley AW, Levine TB, Cohn JN. Increased plasma arginine vasopressin levels in patients with congestive heart failure. *Journal of the American College of Cardiology* 1983;1:1385–90.

197. Stanek B, Bruckner U, Silberbauer K. Plasma vasopressin as influenced by acute and chronic blockade of the renin–angiotensin system. *Journal of Hypertension* 1985;3 (suppl 2):S129–31.

198. Dzau VJ, Hollenberg NK. Renal response to captopril in severe heart failure: Role of furosemide in natriuresis and reversal of hyponatremia. *Annals of Internal Medicine* 1984;100:777–82.

199. Packer M, Medina N, Yushak M. Correction of dilutional hyponatremia in severe chronic heart failure by converting-enzyme inhibition. *Annals of Internal Medicine* 1984;100:782–9.

200. Nicholls MG, Espiner EA, Ikram H, Maslowski AH, Lun S, Scandrett MS. Angiotensin II is more potent than potassium in regulating aldosterone in cardiac failure: Evidence during captopril therapy. *Journal of Clinical Endocrinology and Metabolism* 1981;52:1253–6.

201. Nelson DH, August JT. Abnormal response of oedematous patients to aldosterone or deoxycortone. *Lancet* 1959;i:883–6.

202. Barger AC, Muldowney FP, Liebowitz MR. Role of the kidney in the pathogenesis of congestive heart failure. *Circulation* 1959;20:273–85.

203. Cleland JGF, Dargie HJ, Robertson I, Robertson JIS, East BW. Total body electrolyte composition in patients with heart failure: A comparison with normal subjects and patients with untreated hypertension. *British Heart Journal* 1987;58:230–8.

204. Dargie HJ, Cleland JGF, Leckie BJ, Inglis CG, East BW, Ford I. Relation of arrhythmias and electrolyte abnormalities to survival in patients with severe chronic heart failure. *Circulation* 1987;75 (suppl IV):IV98–107.

205. Cleland JGF, Dargie HJ, Hodsman GP, Ball SG, Robertson JIS, Morton JJ, East BW, Robertson I, Murray GD, Gillen G. Captopril in heart failure. A double blind controlled trial. *British Heart Journal* 1984;52:530–5.

206. Cleland JGF, Dargie HJ, Ball SG, Gillen G, Hodsman GP, Morton JJ, East BW, Robertson I, Ford I, Robertson JIS. Effects of enalapril in heart failure: A double blind study of effects on exercise performance, renal function, hormones, and metabolic state. *British Heart Journal* 1985;54:305–12.

207. Nicholls MG, Ikram H, Espiner EA, Maslowski AH, Scandrett MA, Penman T. Hemodynamic and hormonal responses during captopril therapy for heart failure: Acute, chronic and withdrawal studies. *American Journal of Cardiology* 1982;49:1497–501.

208. Maslowski AH, Nicholls MG, Ikram H, Espiner EA, Turner JG. Haemodynamic, hormonal, and electrolyte responses to withdrawal of long-term captopril treatment for heart failure. *Lancet* 1981;ii:959–61.

209. Crozier IG, Teoh R, Kay R, Nicholls MG. Sympathetic nervous system during converting enzyme inhibition. *American Journal of Medicine* 1989;87 (suppl 6B):29–32S.

210. Vogt A, Unterberg C, Kreuzer H. Acute effects of the new angiotensin converting enzyme inhibitor ramipril on hemodynamics and carotid sinus baroreflex activity in congestive heart failure. *American Journal of Cardiology* 1987;59:149–54D.

211. Osterziel KJ, Dietz R, Schmid W, Mikulaschek K, Manthey J, Kübler W. ACE inhibition improves vagal reactivity in patients with heart failure. *American Heart Journal* 1990;120:1120–9.

212. Dzau VJ, Swartz SL. Dissociation of the prostaglandin and renin angiotensin systems during captopril therapy for chronic congestive heart failure secondary to coronary artery disease. *American Journal of Cardiology* 1987;60:1101–5.

213. Fyhrquist F, Karppinen K, Honkanen T, Saijonmaa O, Rosenlöf K. High serum erythropoietin levels are normalized during treatment of congestive heart failure with enalapril. *Journal of Internal Medicine* 1989;226:257–60.

214. Lee WH, Packer M. Prognostic importance of serum sodium concentration and its modification by converting-enzyme inhibition in patients with severe chronic heart failure. *Circulation* 1986;73:257–67.

215. Packer M, Lee WH, Kessler PD, Gottlieb SS, Bernstein JL, Kukin ML. Role of neurohormonal mechanisms in determining survival in patients with severe chronic heart failure. *Circulation* 1987;75 (suppl IV):IV80–92.

216. Rockman HA, Juneau C, Chatterjee K, Rouleau J–L. Long-term predictors of sudden and low output death in chronic congestive heart failure secondary to coronary artery disease. *American Journal of Cardiology* 1989;64:1344–8.

217. Swedberg K, Eneroth P, Kjekshus J, Wilhelmsen L. Hormones regulating cardiovascular function in patients with severe congestive heart failure and their relation to mortality. *Circulation* 1990;82:1730–6.

218. Newman TJ, Maskin CS, Dennick LG, Meyer JH, Hallows BG, Cooper WH. Effects of captopril on survival in patients with heart failure. *American Journal of Medicine* 1988;84 (suppl 3A):140–4.

219. The Consensus Trial Study Group. Effects of enalapril on mortality in severe congestive heart failure. Results of the cooperative North Scandinavian Enalapril Survival Study (Consensus). *New England Journal of Medicine* 1987;316: 1429–35.

220. Cohn JN, Archibald DG, Ziesche S, Franciosa JA, Harston WE, Tristani FE, Dunkman WB, Jacobs W, Francis GS, Flohr KH, Goldman S, Cobb FR, Shah PM, Saunders R, Fletcher RD, Loeb HS, Hughes VC, Baker B. Effects of vasodilator therapy on mortality in chronic congestive heart failure. Results of a Veterans Administration Cooperative Study. *New England Journal of Medicine* 1986;314:1547–52.

221. Dzau VJ. Contributions of neuroendocrine and local autocrine–paracrine mechanisms to the pathophysiology and pharmacology of congestive heart failure. *American Journal of Cardiology* 1982;62:76–81E.

222. Lindpaintner K, Jin M, Wilhelm MJ, Suzuki F, Linz W, Schoelkens BA, Ganten D. Intracardiac generation of angiotensin and its physiologic role. *Circulation* 1988;77 (suppl I):I-18–23.

223. Fabris B, Jackson B, Kohzuki M, Perich R, Johnston CI. Increased cardiac angiotensin-converting enzyme in rats with chronic heart failure. *Clinical and Experimental Pharmaceology and Physiology* 1990;17:309–14.

224. Urata H, Healy B, Stewart RW, Bumpus FM, Husain A. Angiotensin II-forming pathways in normal and failing human hearts. *Circulation Research* 1990;66:883–90.

225. Spielman WS, Arend LJ. Adenosine receptors and signaling in the kidney. *Hypertension* 1991;17:117–30.

226. Richards AM, Cleland JGF, Tonolo G, Ball SG, Dargie HJ, Robertson JIS. Plasma alpha natriuretic peptide in cardiac impairment. *British Medical Journal* 1986;293:409–12.

227. Robertson JIS, Richards AM. Cardiac failure, the kidney, renin and atrial peptides. *European Heart Journal* 1988;9 (suppl H):11–4.

228. Montgomery AJ, Shepherd AN, Elmslie–Smith B. Severe hyponatraemia and cardiac failure successfully treated with captopril. *British Medical Journal* 1982;284:1085–6.

229. Scroop GC, Lowe RD. Efferent pathways of the cardiovascular response to vertebral artery infusions of angiotensin II in the dog. *Clinical Science* 1969;37:605–19.

230. Arnal J–F, Cudek P, Plouin P–F, Guyenne T–T, Michel J–B, Corvol P. Low angiotensinogen levels are related to the severity and liver dysfunction of congestive heart failure: implications for renin measurements. *American Journal of Medicine* 1991;**90**:17–22.

231. Adesanya CO, Anjorin FI, Sada IA, Parry EHO, Sagnella GA, MacGregor GA. Atrial natriuretic peptide, aldosterone, and plasma renin activity in peripartum heart failure. *British Heart Journal* 1991;**65**:152–4.

232. The SOLVD Investigators. Effect of enalapril on survival in patients with reduced left ventricular ejection fractions and congestive heart faiure. *New England Journal of Medicine* 1991;**325**:293–302.

77

RENIN IN MYOCARDIAL INFARCTION

PASCAL NICOD, BERNARD WAEBER AND
HANS R BRUNNER

INTRODUCTION

Numerous investigations are currently underway to determine the role of the RAS in myocardial infarction, and to evaluate the potentially beneficial effect of ACE inhibition to treat patients with myocardial infarction. This enthusiasm can be explained by the convergence of several findings pointing to the increased risk of developing a myocardial infarction associated with a stimulated RAS in hypertensive patients, the detrimental physiopathological effects of enhanced Ang II production [1–3] (see *Chapter 40*), and the well-documented efficacy of ACE inhibitors in prolonging life and improving symptoms in patients with congestive heart failure [4,5] (see *Chapter 93*).

In this chapter, the neurohormonal consequences of myocardial infarction are described initially, and the potential harmful effect of activation of the RAS on the cardiovascular system during myocardial infarction is subsequently discussed. In addition, the known experimental and clinical results on the use of ACE inhibitors in the acute and subacute phases of myocardial infarction are reviewed. The preliminary data available to date suggest that ACE inhibition might indeed be beneficial in such conditions, but the long-term clinical efficacy of this therapeutic approach remains to be confirmed in large-scale clinical studies.

NEUROHORMONAL ACTIVATION DURING MYOCARDIAL INFARCTION

Myocardial infarction causes an acute disturbance of hemodynamic balance which triggers wide fluctuations in the neurohormonal control of the circulation. Factors other than changes in hemodynamics, such as pain, fear, and medications, can also contribute to such neurohormonal activation. Neurohormonal stimulation therefore may facilitate cardiovascular homeostasis and maintain adequate blood pressure and perfusion of vital organs in the presence of pump failure. Sometimes, however, the intense neurohormonal responses may also have detrimental effects by increasing peripheral resistance and afterload, by inducing metabolic disturbances, and by promoting potentially deleterious cardiac ventricular changes such as expansion, dilation, or compensatory hypertrophy.

THE SYMPATHETIC NERVOUS SYSTEM

Intense stimulation of the sympathetic nervous system has been well documented in man in the initial 24–48 hours following myocardial infarction [6-11]. Both plasma catecholamine levels and urinary catecholamine excretion are increased in the acute phase of myocardial infarction. There is a correlation between the magnitude of this increase and the occurrence of complications such as left ventricular failure, cardiogenic shock, and ventricular fibrillation [6–11]. Patients with large infarcts, as assessed by a depressed left ventricular ejection fraction and high plasma creatine kinase levels, are particularly prone to activation of their sympathetic nervous system. This activation seems maximal on admission, particularly in the group of patients with heart failure (Fig 77.1). The adrenergic response may be to some extent beneficial by maintaining systemic arterial pressure at an adequate level and by preserving perfusion of vital organs in the presence of a failing heart. On one hand, catecholamines appear to have a protective role since they can prevent the development of hypotension by inducing vasoconstriction and since they may increase cardiac output by improving myocardial contractility, accelerating heart rate, and facilitating venous return. On the other hand, however, the compensatory activation of the sympathetic nervous system also has potentially harmful effects. It increases myocardial oxygen demand due to the positive chronotropic and inotropic effects of β-adrenergic stimulation, it causes coronary vasoconstriction, it increases cardiac load because of peripheral vasoconstriction, it may have direct toxic effects on myocardium, and finally, it seems to promote arrhythmias in part via β_2-mediated hypokalemia.

THE RENIN–ANGIOTENSIN SYSTEM

The first evidence of an activated renin–angiotensin–aldosterone system following myocardial infarction was indirect, via the finding of abnormally high urinary and plasma aldosterone levels.

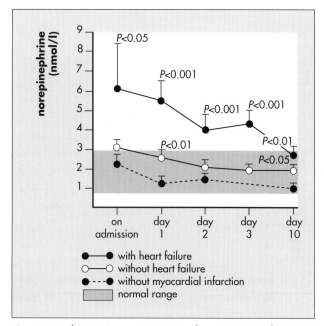

Fig. 77.1 Changes (means ± SEM) in plasma norepinephrine concentration over 10 days in patients with heart failure or without heart failure, following acute myocardial infarction, and in those without myocardial infarction. Modified from McAlpine HM *et al* [9].

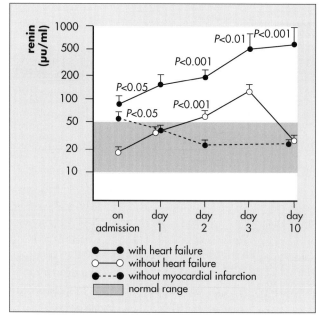

Fig. 77.2 Changes (means ± SEM) in plasma active renin concentration over 10 days in patients with heart failure or without heart failure, following acute myocardial infarction, and in those without myocardial infarction. Modified from McAlpine HM *et al* [9].

This was true particularly in patients who developed heart failure [12–13]. Elevated plasma renin levels following myocardial infarction were described in an early study by Kedra *et al* who reported peak values of PRA on the third postinfarction day [14]. The increase of renin correlated with complications such as left ventricular failure, cardiogenic shock, and ventricular fibrillation [15–18]. These findings were confirmed by sequential measures of plasma renin and Ang II following myocardial infarction. McAlpine *et al* followed 78 patients admitted for myocardial infarction within six hours of the onset of symptoms [9]. Venous blood samples were drawn on admission. The presence of left ventricular failure was assessed by standard criteria. Sixteen patients had confirmed myocardial infarction; in 18 other patients, myocardial infarction was ruled out. Plasma active renin (Fig 77.2) and Ang II concentrations were slightly elevated on admission only in patients with evidence of left ventricular failure. Renin and Ang II rose in the days following myocardial infarction whether or not the patients had left ventricular failure. This increase was particularly prominent in patients with heart failure. Although medications such as diuretics and nitrates may have played a role in the elevation of renin and Ang II, five patients with heart failure on admission, who received no such

medication, were also found to increase their plasma renin and Ang II levels. Thus, substantial evidence shows that the RAS is activated during the course of myocardial infarction, mainly in patients with heart failure. This activation is generally moderate on admission and peaks between the 3rd and the 10th day after the infarction. This is of note since activation of the sympathetic nervous system seems maximal on admission.

Several factors may trigger the release of renin following myocardial infarction [19–21]. Beta-adrenoceptor stimulation at the level of juxtaglomerular cells is one likely mechanism. The correlation between plasma catecholamines and plasma renin would support such a view [9–16]. The slower elevation of plasma renin than that of catecholamines following myocardial infarction, however, suggests that other factors play a role. Changes in intrarenal hemodynamics may result in stimulation of the renal baroreceptor and a decreased sodium delivery at the level of the macula densa and thereby cause renin release. Furthermore, drugs such as vasodilators and diuretics may also lead to activation of the RAS.

Stimulation of renin release following myocardial infarction may be regarded primarily as a mechanism aimed to maintain an adequate blood pressure in the presence of pump failure.

Angiotensin II is indeed a potent vasoconstrictor hormone. This peptide can even reinforce the sympathetic nervous system, for instance, by enhancing norepinephrine release at the presynaptic level [22]. Angiotensin II itself is a powerful antinatriuretic hormone (see *Chapters 26* and *27*) and is a well-established stimulus of aldosterone secretion (see *Chapter 33*), and can thus cause sodium retention and an increase in cardiac preload. Finally, Ang II might have a positive inotropic effect, as suggested by *in vitro* experiments.

As was the case for the sympathetic nervous system, activation of the RAS is also likely to have some detrimental effects. Angiotensin II is a powerful vasoconstrictor of coronary arteries, while at the same time, it increases afterload [23–26]. This could increase myocardial oxygen demand in the face of a decreased oxygen supply and therefore aggravate the ischemia and possibly increase the size of the myocardial infarct. Administration of large doses of Ang II to rabbits can cause multifocal myocardial necrosis [23,24]. Similar lesions can be found at postmortem examination of patients known to have had high renin levels before death [24]. The Ang II- and aldosterone-induced increase in preload and afterload may contribute adversely to the development of heart failure. Moreover, arrhythmias can be precipitated by electrolytic disturbances (hypokalemia secondary to the hyperaldosteronism or by the Ang II-mediated facilitation of norepinephrine release).

VASOPRESSIN

A significant retention of free water, with an average of 774ml in the first 24 hours according to one study [27], has been described following myocardial infarction. This retention during the acute phase of myocardial infarction could well be, in part, a consequence of increased Ang II, as discussed in the preceding paragraph. It could, however, also be partly due to an enhanced secretion of vasopressin involving a nonosmotic mechanism. As for other vasopressor systems, the increase is mostly seen in patients with left ventricular failure or those dying following myocardial infarction, and is maximal on admission [9–11].

Besides water retention, vasopressin might theoretically have a vasoconstrictor effect on peripheral and coronary arteries. Whether this peptide participates actively in the regulation of vascular tone in patients suffering from a myocardial infarction is unknown. Current evidence in patients with congestive heart failure suggests a significant vasoconstrictor effect only in patients with severely compromised hemodynamics and very elevated plasma Ang II and vasopressin levels [28]. Other studies suggest that moderate elevations of plasma vasopressin concentrations, such as seen in congestive heart failure [29] or following cigarette smoking [30], have a limited physiologic effect with regard to blood-pressure control.

INFARCT EXPANSION AND LEFT VENTRICULAR REMODELING FOLLOWING MYOCARDIAL INFARCTION

Infarct size and residual left ventricular function have been shown by many authors to determine prognosis following myocardial infarction [31,32]. Cardiac size has also been shown to correlate with the outcome after myocardial infarction [33]. Kostuk *et al* demonstrated the prognostic significance of an enlarged cardiac silhouette on chest X-ray in patients with a myocardial infarction [34]. Subsequently, other investigators have documented left ventricular dilation following myocardial infarction using echocardiography [35], radionuclide studies [36,37], and contrast ventriculography [38–39]. These papers have shown that infarct expansion occurs in the first few days following myocardial infarction. This expansion is seen in approximately one-third of infarcts. It occurs mostly in patients with large anterior Q-waves as shown in the electrocardiogram. Factors such as increased afterload, the use of anti-inflammatory drugs, and non-reperfusion of the artery responsible for the infarct may play a role in this process. Infarct expansion can occur in the absence of new myocardial necrosis. It may be explained by cell slippage, by damaged collagen connections, and less likely by cell stretch [40].

Left ventricular dilation following myocardial infarction can be attributed only in part to early infarct expansion. Left ventricular remodeling in noninfarcted areas also appears to be involved. Thus, McKay *et al* [38] showed that endocardial length increased by 13% in the infarcted segment and by 19% in the noninfarcted segment in a group of patients with large infarcts. These observations were made two weeks following myocardial infarction using left ventriculography on admission. Left ventricular dilation has also been shown to occur late following myocardial infarction. Warren *et al* studied left ventricular end-diastolic volume by radionuclide left ventriculography performed 11 days and again 10 months following myocardial infarction [37]. They showed a substantial left ventricular dilation occurring between the two evaluations, mostly in the noninfarct-related segment. Pfeffer *et al* reported similar findings using contrast left ventriculography. In the latter experience, late dilation occurred mostly in patients with large myocardial infarction and areas of left ventricular akinesis or dyskinesis [39].

In addition to cardiac dilation, myocardial hypertrophy of noninfarcted areas may occur early after myocardial infarction [41,42]. In a rat model, such myocardial hypertrophy can be seen as early as three days following an experimental infarct. Hypertrophy is more marked in rats with large infarcts and is characterized by an increase in myocyte diameter and length. Hypertrophy appears therefore to be a compensatory mechanism following a loss of myocardium. In man, hypertrophy is difficult to assess given the inaccuracy of noninvasive methods. Left ventricular hypertrophy, however, was documented by echocardiography in patients nine months following myocardial infarction [43]. It was associated with an improvement of left ventricular wall motion as compared with data in patients with no left ventricular hypertrophy. Ventricular hypertrophy may conceivably also be detrimental, by rendering myocardium more vulnerable to ischemia, by decreasing diastolic compliance, and by inducing further diastolic enlargment. Whether left ventricular hypertrophy occurring following myocardial infarction is a desirable response tending to restore a normal wall stress is still debated [44,45].

The RAS may have a pivotal role in all the remodeling of the cardiac structure described above (see *Chapter 94*). The early activation of the RAS may cause an increase in afterload. In animal models, an increase in afterload early following myocardial infarction causes infarct expansion [46]. In man, the activated RAS possibly contributes to infarct expansion through increased afterload, increased wall stress, and systolic bulging in the infarcted region. The RAS is, however, also likely to play a role in the process of left ventricular dilation in noninfarcted areas, particularly in patients with poor left ventricular function and long-standing cardiac failure, in whom the RAS remains stimulated beyond the first few days following infarction [9]. It is precisely in this group with left ventricular failure that dilation is most often observed, as discussed earlier. The concomitant increasing preload and afterload resulting from the activation of the RAS may contribute to left ventricular dilation and worsening failure. Animal and clinical studies showing a beneficial effect of captopril in preventing left ventricular dilation, as will be discussed later in the chapter, tend to support the notion of implication of the RAS in the left ventricular remodeling. The RAS might also be involved in producing left ventricular hypertrophy, for instance by raising systolic wall stress. In addition, there is good evidence that Ang II *per se* promotes myocardial hypertrophy [47] (see *Chapter 42*). Thus, protein synthesis is increased by incubating cultured myocytes with Ang II. Even more convincing, in a rat model of pressure overload using aortic banding, left ventricular hypertrophy could be prevented by

inhibiting the generation of Ang II using ACE inhibitors [48]. This effect was seen despite the fact that blood pressure remained elevated.

Altogether, there is ample evidence to support the concept that the RAS is involved in both the early and late changes in cardiac geometry, as well as in the processes of cardiac hypertrophy which occur following myocardial infarction. Since these changes are major determinants of residual left ventricular function and therefore of the prognosis after myocardial infarction, there is considerable hope that blocking the RAS may prevent some of the cardiac remodeling and, in this way, improve the outcome of patients who have suffered a myocardial infarction.

ACUTE AND DELAYED EFFECTS OF ANGIOTENSIN-CONVERTING ENZYME INHIBITION FOLLOWING MYOCARDIAL INFARCTION

Infarct expansion occurring very early following myocardial infarction is directly proportional to infarct size and represents a major determinant of left ventricular dilation [35,38,49]. An enormous effort has been made towards limiting infarct size by early thrombolysis and recanalization. Preservation of subepicardial layers of myocardium through reperfusion should limit infarct expansion, although this has been difficult to demonstrate in patients, because of the inaccuracy of, and the difficulty in obtaining, serial noninvasive measurements of left ventricular function following myocardial infarction.

There is experimental evidence that ACE inhibition in the acute stage of myocardial infarction may have a cardioprotective effect [3]. Acute afterload reduction is expected to improve the balance of myocardial oxygen demand and supply. Angiotensin-converting enzyme inhibitors may prevent the coronary vasoconstrictor effect of Ang II [50] and impair the degradation of bradykinin, a vasodilator peptide [51]. The accumulation of bradykinin could in turn trigger the synthesis of vasodilating prostaglandins [52–55]. This has, however, been difficult to substantiate in clinical studies; for instance, in angina, there is no consistent evidence that ACE inhibition has a significant therapeutic effect in improving coronary flow [56]. Angiotensin-converting enzyme inhibition may alternatively have a cardioprotective effect by reducing reperfusion injury [57–64]. This could be due to the oxygen-scavenging effect of sulfhydryl-containing ACE inhibitors [57,58], or to the antioxidant properties of ACE inhibitors via a reduction in the concentration of cytochrome C [62], by stimulating the production of prostacyclin [52], or through a reduced sympathetic nerve activity [61, 63,64]. Despite all these potentially favorable effects of ACE inhibition, however, human studies do not show a consistent effect of these agents in reducing infarct size [65].

In contrast, ACE inhibition during the subacute phase of experimental myocardial infarction in rats seems to prevent some of the cardiac remodeling [66]. Thus, Pfeffer et al [66] showed a reduction of left ventricular mass and left ventricular end-diastolic pressure and volume, and a prolongation of survival in rats given captopril from the 3rd week to the 12th month following myocardial infarction. In clinical studies, the effect of late ACE inhibition (starting 1–2 weeks after myocardial infarction) on cardiac geometry is well documented and is comparable with that found in animal experiments. The effect of early ACE inhibition on infarct expansion, remodeling, and clinical outcome is less clear. In many studies, it is difficult to document whether early administration of ACE inhibitors (within 24 hours) is advantageous compared with later treatment. Indeed, some of the side effects such as hypotension may be more common following early ACE inhibition and may offset any beneficial effect. No study to date has, to our knowledge, compared early and late administration of ACE inhibitors following myocardial infarction.

The Survival and Ventricular Englargement (SAVE) trial is a large multicenter study involving over 2,300 patients following acute Q-wave myocardial infarction. Patients were randomized to receive captopril or placebo 3–16 days following onset of symptoms. Preliminary data, presented at the 41st Annual Scientific Session of the American College of Cardiology in Dallas, United States of America, in April 1992, indicate that after a median follow-up period of 3.6 years, those receiving captopril had a statistically significant improvement in overall survival and reduction in cardiovascular morality and morbidity. Divergence between the treatment groups for a number of end-points was not apparent until approximately 10 months. Full details from this important trial are awaited.

ANGIOTENSIN-CONVERTING ENZYME INHIBITORS IN THE ACUTE PHASE OF MYOCARDIAL INFARCTION

Nabel et al [67] randomized 38 patients with acute myocardial infarction to receive either captopril or placebo within three hours following the onset of symptoms. Only one patient had to discontinue therapy because of symptomatic hypotension. At day seven, there was a significant trend towards smaller left ventricular end-diastolic volumes in patients treated with captopril compared with those on placebo.

Similarly, Kingma et al [68] showed the safety of the early administration of captopril (within six hours of onset) in patients undergoing thrombolysis with streptokinase for acute myocardial infarction. They showed, in the treated group, a significant reduction in norepinephrine levels and a trend towards increased left ventricular ejection fraction at three months.

In the ISIS 4 pilot study [69], 81 patients with acute myocardial infarction undergoing thrombolysis were randomized to receive captopril, isosorbide dinitrate, or placebo within 13 hours from the onset of infarction. The authors showed an increased cardiac output, and a decreased systemic peripheral resistance without an increased heart rate. These potential advantages persisted for six weeks in the group treated with captopril. The ISIS 4 definitive study is expected to include some 50,000 patients.

Pye et al [70] reported in a group of 99 patients with acute myocardial infarction, that early treatment with captopril (within 24 hours of infarction) resulted in a decreased left ventricular endsystolic index and prevented left ventricular expansion, compared with a placebo group, mostly in patients with anterior infarcts. In a double-blind, placebo–controlled study of 100 patients with acute myocardial infarction, Sharpe et al [71] also found a significant decrease in left ventricular endsystolic volume index, and an increase in ejection fraction and stroke volume index in those receiving early captopril (within 24–48 hours) compared with those receiving placebo (Fig. 77.3).

In the pilot Chinese study (CEI AMI trial), 1,519 patients with acute myocardial infarction were randomized to captopril or placebo within 36 hours following the onset of symptoms. Captopril did not cause significant side effects. Furthermore, there was a nonsignificant trend toward decreased mortality and morbidity in the treated group. The definitive trial is expected to recruit a total of 10,000 patients.

Several other studies are under way. The CATS study by Kingma et al is expected to enroll 280 patients with acute myocardial infarction undergoing thrombolysis with streptokinase. Patients will be randomized to captopril or placebo with six hours following onset of symptoms. The CAPTIN study by Sonnenblick et al will enroll 280 patients with acute myocardial infarction undergoing thrombolysis with tissue plasminogen activator, who will be randomized to receive either captopril or placebo within six hours of infarction. The Gissi III trial will randomize 20,000 patients with acute myocardial infarction to a treatment with lisinopril, mononitrate, or placebo. Results are expected in 1993. The Consensus II study which enrolled 9,000 patients to receive enalapril or placebo within 24 hours of onset of symptoms has been stopped, and full results are pending.

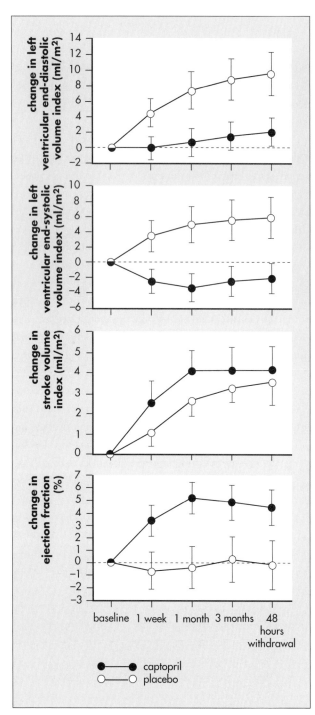

Fig. 77.3 Mean differences from baseline (with 95% confidence limits) for left ventricular volume and function in patients treated with captopril or placebo after myocardial infarction. Modified from Sharpe N *et al* [71].

In summary, early cautious administration of ACE inhibitors following myocardial infarction appears safe and may improve hemodynamics and have a favorable effect on left ventricular geometry. Whether these encouraging changes will translate into long-term benefits with regard to mortality and morbidity seems likely from SAVE data. It is not known, however, whether early administration of ACE inhibitors is better than delayed administration.

ANGIOTENSIN-CONVERTING ENZYME INHIBITORS IN THE SUBACUTE PHASE OF MYOCARDIAL INFARCTION

Pfeffer *et al* [39] randomized 59 patients with acute electrocardiographic Q-wave anterior myocardial infarction to receive either captopril or placebo, on average 20 days following the onset of symptoms. They showed that after one year of treatment, left ventricular end-diastolic volume or area was lower in patients receiving captopril than in those receiving placebo (Fig 77.4). This was particularly prominent in the subgroup of patients with persistent occlusion of their left anterior descending artery. Exercise testing in a subgroup of 36 patients suggested improved exercise tolerance in those treated with captopril compared with those given placebo.

Similar observations were made by Sharpe *et al* [72] on a group of 60 patients with electrocardiographic Q-wave myocardial infarction and left ventricular ejection fraction of less than 0.45. Patients were randomized to receive captopril or placebo within seven days of onset of symptoms. The captopril group showed a significant reduction in end-systolic volume index and significant increases in stroke volume index and left ventricular ejection fraction. Sharpe *et al* confirmed these findings in a subsequent study including 90 patients [73].

As noted earlier, the SAVE study has shown that captopril, starting 3–16 days after acute myocardial infarction in patients with an ejection fraction of 40% or less, improves the outcome for both mortality and cardiovascular morbidity over a median period of follow up of 3.6 years.

CONCLUSIONS

Activation of the RAS has been clearly shown to occur in patients with acute myocardial infarction. Although the RAS in this condition may be useful to maintain an adequate blood pressure and tissue perfusion in the face of a failing heart, it may be, in other respects, detrimental, for example, by increasing both cardiac pre- and afterload. There are therefore theoretical reasons

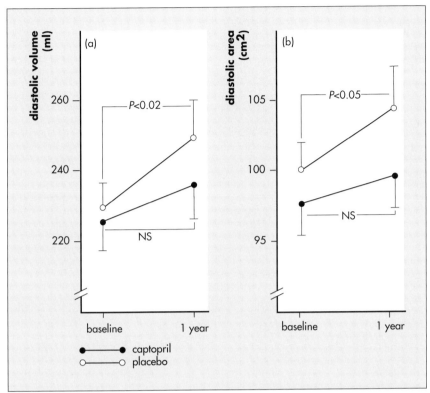

Fig. 77.4 Increase in ventricular end-diastolic volume (a) and area (b) in patients treated with captopril or placebo after myocardial infarction (mean ± SEM). Modified from Pfeffer MA *et al* [39].

to block the RAS after myocardial infarction. In some animal models, this approach can limit infarct size and prevent left ventricular remodeling. In patients, acute and subacute administration of ACE inhibitors following myocardial infarction can be done safely. Blockade of Ang II generation seems to have a favorable effect in limiting remodeling following infarction. Whether ACE inhibition, early (within 24 hours) or delayed (between 24 hours and 10 days), is safer or has more impact on left ventricular geometry and function remains to be shown in comparative studies. Most importantly, the influence of blocking the RAS on morbidity and mortality following myocardial infarction needs to be confirmed by ongoing large multicenter studies.

Until the results of these trials are known, it will remain unclear whether the influence of ACE inhibition on cardiac geometry following infarction translates into better clinical outcome.

ACKNOWLEDGMENTS

We thank MA Blanc for her expert secretarial assistance in preparing the manuscript. This work was supported by grants of the Swiss National Science Foundation and the Cardiovascular Research Foundation.

REFERENCES

1. Brunner HR, Laragh JH, Baer L, Newton MA, Goodwin FT, Krakoff LR, Bard RH, Bühler FR. Essential hypotension: Renin and aldosterone, heart attack and stroke. *New England Journal of Medicine* 1972;286:441–9.

2. Alderman MH, Madhaven S, Ooi WL, Cohen H, Sealey JE, Laragh JH. Association of the renin–sodium profile with the risk of myocardial infarction in patients with hypertension. *New England Journal of Medicine* 1991;324:1098–104.

3. Gavras H, Gavras I. Cardioprotective potential of angiotensin converting enzyme inhibitors. *Journal of Hypertension* 1991;9:385–92.

4. The CONSENSUS Trial Study Group. Effects of enalapril on mortality in severe congestive heart failure: Results of the Cooperative North Scandinavian Enalapril Survival Study (CONSENSUS). *New England Journal of Medicine* 1987;316:1429–35.

5. The SOLVD Investigators. Effect of enalapril on survival in patients with reduced left ventricular ejection fractions and congestive heart failure. *New England Journal of Medicine* 1991;325:293–302.

6. Jewitt DE, Mercer CJ, Reid D, Valori C, Thomas M, Shillingford JP. Free noradrenaline and adrenaline excretion in relation to the development of cardiac arrhythmias and heart-failure in patients with acute myocardial infarction. *Lancet* 1969;i:635–41.

7. Prakash R, Parmley WW, Horvat M, Swan JHC. Serum cortisol, plasma free fatty acids, and urinary catecholamines as indicators of complications in acute myocardial infarction. *Circulation* 1972;45:736–45.

8. Karlsberg RP, Cryer PE, Roberts R. Serial plasma catecholamine response early in the course of clinical acute myocardial infarction: Relationship to infarct extent and mortality. *American Heart Journal* 1981;102:24–9.

9. McAlpine HM, Morton JJ, Leckie B, Rumley A, Gillen G, Dargie HJ. Neuroendocrine activation after acute myocardial infarction. *British Heart Journal* 1988;60:117–24.

10. Cohn JN. Neuroendocrine activation after acute myocardial infarction. *American Journal of Cardiology* 1990;65:28–31I.

11. Schaller MD, Nussberger J, Feihl F, Waeber B, Brunner HR, Perret C, Nicod P. Clinical and hemodynamic correlates of elevated plasma arginine vasopressin after acute myocardial infarction. *American Journal of Cardiology* 1987;60:1178–80.

12. Wolff HP, Koczorek KHR, Buchborn E, Kuehler M. Ueber die Aldosteronaktivitaet und Natriumretention bei Herzkranken und ihre Pathophysiologische Bedeutung. *Klinische Wochenschrift* 1956;34:1105–14.

13. Wedler B, Voss W, Osten B, Kalweit UH. Das Verhalten des Aldosteronserumspiegels in der akuten Phase des Myokardinfarktes. *Deutsche Gesundheit wesen (Berlin)* 1979;34:348–51.

14. Kedra M, Kedrowa S, Rzesniowiecta G, Plasma renin activity in myocardial infarction. *Cor et Vasa* 1972;14:16–21.

15. Michorowski B, Ceremuzynski L. The renin–angiotensin system and the clinical course of acute myocardial infarction. *European Heart Journal* 1983;4:259–64.

16. Vaney C, Waeber B, Turini G, Margalith D, Brunner HR, Perret C. Renin and the complications of myocardial infarction. *Chest* 1984;86:40–3.

17. Wenting GJ, Man In't Veld AJ, Woittiez AJ, Boomsma F, Laird-Meeter K, Simoons ML, Hugenholtz PG, Schalekamp MADH. Effects of captopril in acute and chronic heart failure. Correlation with plasma levels of noradrenaline, renin and aldosterone. *British Heart Journal* 1983;49:65–76.

18. Dzau V, Colucci WS, Hollenberg NK,Williams GH. Relation of the renin–angiotensin–aldosterone system to clinical state in congestive heart failure. *Circulation* 1981;63:645–51.

19. McAlpine HM, Cobbe SM. Neuroendocrine changes in acute myocardial infarction. *American Journal of Medicine* 1988;84 (suppl 3A):61–6.

20. Ertl G, Meesmann M, Kochsiek K. On the mechanism of renin release during experimental myocardial ischemia. *European Journal of Clinical Investigation* 1985;15:375–81.

21. Davis JO, Freeman RH. Mechanisms regulating renin release. *Physiological Reviews* 1976;56:1–56.

22. Zimmerman BG, Sybertz EJ, Wong PC. Interaction between sympathetic and renin–angiotensin system. *Journal of Hypertension* 1984;2:581–8.

23. Gavras H, Brown JJ, Lever AF, MacAdam RF, Robertson JIS. Acute renal failure, tubular necrosis and myocardial infarction induced in the rabbit by intravenous angiotensin II. *Lancet* 1971;ii:19–22.

24. Gavras H, Kremer D, Brown JJ, Gray B, Lever AF, MacAdam RF, Medina A, Morton JJ, Robertson JIS. Angiotensin- and norepinephrine-induced myocardial lesions: Experimental and clinical studies in rabbits and man. *American Heart Journal* 1975;89:321–32.

25. Liang CS, Gavras H, Hood WB. Renin–angiotensin system inhibition in conscious sodium-depleted dogs: Effects on systemic and coronary hemodynamics. *Journal of Clinical Investigation* 1978;61:874–83.

26. Gavras H, Liang CS, Brunner HR. Redistribution of regional blood flow after inhibition of the angiotensin converting enzyme. *Circulation Research* 1978;43 (suppl I):59–63.

27. Col J, Petein M, Van Eyll C, Cheron P, Charlier AA, Pouleur H. Early changes in sodium and water balances in patients with acute myocardial infarction; relationship to haemodynamics and creatine kinase. *European Journal of Clinical Investigation* 1984;14:247–54.

28. Nicod P, Biollaz J, Waeber B, Goy JJ, Polikar R, Schlapfer J, Schaller MD, Turini GA, Nussberger J, Hofbauer KG, Brunner HR. Hormonal, global, and regional haemodynamic responses to a vascular antagonist of vasopressin in patients with congestive heart failure with and without hyponatraemia. *British Heart Journal* 1986;56:433–9.

29. Goldsmith SR, Francis GS, Cowley AW, Goldenberg IF, Cohn JN. Hemodynamic effects of infused arginine vasopressin in congestive heart failure. *Journal of the American College of Cardiology* 1986;8:779–83.

30. Waeber B, Schaller MD, Nussberger J, Bussien JP, Hofbauer KG, Brunner HR. Skin blood flow reduction induced by cigarette smoking: The role of vasopressin. *American Journal of Physiology* 1984;247:H895–901.

31. Killip T, Kimball JT. Treatment of myocardial infarction in a coronary care unit. *American Journal of Cardiology* 1967;20:457–64.

32. Nicod P, Gilpin E, Dittrich H, Chappuis F, Ahnve S, Engler R, Henning H, Ross J Jr. Influence on prognosis and morbidity of left ventricular ejection fraction with and without signs of left ventricular failure after acute myocardial infarction. *American Journal of Cardiology* 1988;61:1165–71.

33. White HD, Norris RM, Brown MA, Brandt PWT, Whitlock RML, Wild CJ. Left ventricular end-systolic volume as the major determinant of survival after recovery from myocardial infarction. *Circulation* 1987;76:44–51.

34. Kostuk W, Barr JW, Simon AL, Ross J Jr. Correlations between the chest film and hemodynamics in acute myocardial infarction. *Circulation* 1973;48:624–32.

35. Eaton LW, Weiss JL, Bulkley BH, Garrison JB, Weisfeldt ML. Regional cardiac dilation after acute myocardial infarction. Recognition by two-dimensional echocardiography. *New England Journal of Medicine* 1979;300:57–62.

36. Jeremy RW, Hackworthy RA, Bautovich G, Hutton BF, Harris PJ. Infarct artery perfusion and changes in left ventricular volume in the month after acute myocardial infarction. *Journal of the American College of Cardiology* 1987;9:989–95.

37. Warren SE, Royal HD, Markis JE, Grossman W, McKay RG. Time course of left ventricular dilation during acute myocardial infarction: Influence of infarct-related artery and success of coronary thrombolysis. *Journal of the American College of Cardiology* 1988;11:12–9.

38. McKay RG, Pfeffer MA, Pasternak RC, Markis JE, Come PC, Nakao S, Alderman JD, Ferguson JJ, Safian RD, Grossman W. Left ventricular remodeling following myocardial infarction: A corollary to infarct expansion. *Circulation* 1986;74:693–711.

39. Pfeffer MA, Lamas GA, Vaughan DE, Parisi AF, Braunwald E. Effect of captopril on progressive ventricular dilatation after anterior myocardial infarction. *New England Journal of Medicine* 1988;319:80–6.

40. Anversa P, Beghi C, Kikkawa Y, Olivetti G. Myocardial infarction in rats. Infarct size, myocyte hypertrophy, and capillary growth. *Circulation Research* 1986;58:26–37.

41. Fletcher PJ, Pfeffer JM, Pfeffer MA, Braunwald E. Left ventricular diastolic pressure–volume relations in rats with healed myocardial infarction. Effects on systolic function. *Circulation Research* 1981;49:618–26.

42. Rubin SA, Fishbein M, Swan HJC, Rabines A. Compensatory hypertrophy in the heart after myocardial infarction in the rat. *Journal of the American College of Cardiology* 1983;1:1435–41.

43. Ginzton LE, Conant R, Rodrigues DM, Laks MM. Functional significance of hypertrophy of the noninfarcted myocardium after myocardial infarction in humans. *Circulation* 1989;80:816–22.

44. Pfeffer MA, Pfeffer JM, Steinberg C, Finn P. Survival after an experimental myocardial infarction: Beneficial effects of long-term therapy with captopril. *Circulation* 1985;72:406–12.

45. Michel JB, Lattion AL, Salzmann JL, Cerol ML, Philippe M, Camilleri JP, Corvol P. Hormonal and cardiac effects of converting enzyme inhibition in rat myocardial infarction. *Circulation Research* 1988;62:641–50.

46. Hammerman H, Kloner RA, Alker KJ, Schoen FJ, Braunwald E. Effects of transient increased afterload during experimentally induced acute myocardial infarction in dogs. *American Journal of Cardiology* 1985;55:566–70.

47. Aceto JF, Baker KM. [Sar^1] angiotensin II receptor-mediated stimulation of protein synthesis in chick heart cells. *American Journal of Physiology* 1990;258:H806–13.

48. Baker KM, Chernin MI, Wixson SK, Aceto JF. Renin–angiotensin system involvement in pressure-overload cardiac hypertrophy in rats. *American Journal of Physiology* 1990;259:H324–32.

49. Pirolo JS, Hutchins GM, Moore W. Infarct expansion: Pathologic analysis of 204 patients with a single myocardial infarct. *Journal of the American College of Cardiology* 1986;**7**:349–54.

50. Magrini F, Shimizu M, Roberts N, Fouad F, Tarazi RC, Zanchetti A. Converting enzyme inhibition and coronary blood flow. *Circulation* 1987;**75** (suppl I): 168–74.

51. Erdös EG. Angiotensin I converting enzyme. *Circulation Research* 1975;**36**: 247–55.

52. Chen X, Pi XJ, Li DY, Li YJ, Deng HW. Prostacyclin-mediated cardioprotection of captopril and ramiprilat against lipid peroxidation in rat. *Progress in Clinical and Biological Research* 1989;**301**:167–73.

53. Scholkens BA, Linz W. Local inhibition of angiotensin II formation and bradykinin degradation in isolated hearts. *Clinical and Experimental Hypertension. Part A, Theory and Practice* 1988;**10**:1259–70.

54. Woodman OL, Dusting GJ, Nolan RD. Pericardial release of prostacyclin induced by bradykinin and angiotensin II: Effects on coronary blood flow in the dog. *Journal of Cardiovascular Pharmacology* 1983;**5**:954–60.

55. McGiff JC, Terragno N, Malik KU, Lonigro AJ. Release of a prostaglandin-like substance from canine kidney by bradykinin. *Circulation Research* 1972;**31**: 36–43.

56. Klein WW, Khurmi NS, Eber B, Dusleag J. Effects of benazepril and metoprolol OROS alone and in combination on myocardial ischaemia in patients with chronic stable angina. *Journal of the American College of Cardiology* 1990;**16**:948–56.

57. Przyklenk K, Kloner RA. Relationship between structure and effects of ACE inhibitors: Comparative effects in myocardial ischaemic/reperfusion injury. *British Journal of Clinical Pharmacology* 1989;**28** (suppl 2):167–75S.

58. De Graeff PA, De Langen CD, VanGilst WH, Bel K, Scholtens E, Kingma JH, Wesseling H. Protective effects of captopril against ischemia/reperfusion-induced ventricular arrhythmias *in vitro* and *in vivo*. *American Journal of Medicine* 1988;**84** (suppl 3A):67–74.

59. Hock CE, Ribeiro LGT, Lefer AM. Preservation of ischemic myocardium by a new converting enzyme inhibitor, enalaprilic acid, in acute myocardial infarction. *American Heart Journal* 1985;**109**:222–8.

60. Li K, Chen X. Protective effects of captopril and enalaprilat on myocardial ischemia and reperfusion damage of rat. *Journal of Molecular and Cellular Cardiology* 1987;**19**:909–15.

61. de Langen CDJ, De Graeff PA, van Gilst WH, Bel KJ, Kingma JH, Wesseling H. Effects of angiotensin II and captopril on inducible sustained ventricular tachycardia two weeks after myocardial infarction in the pig. *Journal of Cardiovascular Pharmacology* 1989;**13**:186–91.

62. Sweet CS. Issues surrounding a local cardiac renin system and the beneficial actions of angiotensin-converting enzyme inhibitors in ischemic myocardium. *American Journal of Cardiology* 1990;**65**:111–31.

63. Tio RA, de Langen CDJ, de Graeff PA, van Gilst WH, Bel KJ, Wolters KGTP, Mook PH, van Wijngaarden J, Wesseling H. The effects of oral pretreatment with zofenopril, an angiotensin converting enzyme inhibitor, on early reperfusion and subsequent electrophysiologic stability in the pig. *Cardiovascular Drugs and Therapy* 1990;**4**:695–704.

64. Fleetwood G, Boutinet S, Meier M, Wood JM. Involvement of the renin–angiotensin system in ischemic damage and reperfusion arrhythmias in the isolated perfused rat heart. *Journal of Cardiovascular Pharmacology* 1991;**17**:351–6.

65. McMurray J, MacLenachan J, Dargie HJ. Unique cardioprotective potential of angiotensin converting enzyme inhibitors: A hypothesis still to be tested on humans. *Journal of Hypertension* 1991;**9**:393–7.

66. Pfeffer JM, Pfeffer MA, Braunwald E. Influence of chronic captopril therapy on the infarcted left ventricle of the rat. *Circulation Research* 1985;**57**:84–95.

67. Nabel EG, Topol EJ, Galeana A, Ellis SG, Bates ER, Werns SW, Walton JA, Muller SW, Schwaiger M, Pitt B. A randomized placebo-controlled trial of combined early intravenous captopril and recombinant tissue-type plasminogen activator therapy in acute myocardial infarction. *Journal of the American College of Cardiology* 1991;**17**:467–73.

68. Kingma JH, Van Gilst WH, Peels CH, Jaarsma W, Verheugt FW. Converting enzyme inhibition during thrombolytic therapy in acute myocardial infarction. *Circulation* 1990;**82** (suppl III):666.

69. Pipilis A, Flather M, Collins R, Conway M, Sleight P, ISIS-4 pilot study: Serial hemodynamic changes with oral captopril and oral isosorbide mononitrate in a randomized double-blind trial in acute myocardial infarction. *Journal of the American College of Cardiology* 1991;**17** (suppl A):115A.

70. Pye M, Oldroyd KG, Ray SG, Christie J, Ford I, Cobbe SM, Dargie HJ. Effects of early captopril administration on left ventricular dilatation and function after acute myocardial infarction. *Circulation* 1990;**82** (suppl III):674.

71. Sharpe N, Smith H, Murphy J, Greaves S, Hart H, Gamble G. Early prevention of left ventricular dysfunction after myocardial infarction with angiotensin-converting-enzyme inhibition. *Lancet* 1991;**337**:872–6.

72. Sharpe N, Murphy J, Smith H, Hannan S. Treatment of patients with symptomless left ventricular dysfunction after myocardial infarction. *Lancet* 1988;**331**:255–9.

73. Sharpe N, Murphy J, Smith H, Hannan S. Preventive treatment of asymptomatic left ventricular dysfunction following myocardial infarction. *European Heart Journal* 1990;**11** (Suppl B):147–56.

78 THE RENIN SYSTEM IN LIVER DISEASE

NANCY WY LEUNG AND M GARY NICHOLLS

INTRODUCTION

Laennec (1781–1826) was unaware of the existence of the RAS when he described the clinical picture of end-stage hepatic cirrhosis. Such patients had central cyanosis, arterial hypotension, a hyperdynamic circulation with cutaneous vasodilation, abdominal distension from ascites, and anasarca.

Sodium and water retention is well documented in patients with cirrhosis but investigations to elicit the underlying mechanisms have failed to define clearly the time-related sequence of changes in, and importance of, the various humoral, hemodynamic, renal, and neural factors. Likewise, the pathogenic basis for the hemodynamic alterations in cirrhosis is far from clear, as are the mechanisms underlying the alterations in renal function which are most striking in the hepatorenal syndrome.

In this chapter, available information on the RAS and its level of activity and likely pathophysiological role in liver disease are reviewed. The emphasis is on data from man but some studies in animals are mentioned.

MEASUREMENTS OF RENIN AND CONVERTING ENZYME

The most commonly used index of activity of the RAS in patients with disorders of the liver has been plasma renin activity (PRA). There are, as detailed in *Chapters 8, 13*, and *14*, theoretical limitations inherent in PRA assays, especially under circumstances when angiotensinogen (renin substrate) levels are low. Angiotensinogen is synthesized in the liver (see *Chapter 8*). Numerous studies have, indeed, reported low circulating levels of renin substrate in patients with disordered hepatic function [1–9] with some authors noting an inverse relationship between substrate concentrations and the severity of liver dysfunction [7,8]. For patients with severe impairment of liver function and hence of renin substrate production, PRA may underestimate the level of circulating active renin concentration [8]. This is especially so in cirrhotics with gross ascites and in the hepatorenal syndrome when extremely high levels of active renin are the rule (see below) and further deplete circulating renin substrate levels. Nevertheless, the few studies that have reported both PRA and plasma renin concentration (PRC) in patients with disorders of the liver have noted close correlations between the two indices [10–12]. In addition, Kondo *et al* [13] and Wernze *et al* [14] observed that PRA and/or PRC accurately reflected circulating Ang II levels in cirrhotic patients.

Since the metabolism of circulating renin is determined predominantly by the liver (see *Chapter 23*), hepatic dysfunction results in a decrease in the plasma clearance rate of renin. This has been shown in animal studies of severe hemorrhage (see *Chapter 71*), sodium depletion (see *Chapter 23*), and high-output heart failure [15]; it has also been shown in man [16,17]. As a consequence, plasma levels of renin are likely to reflect the rate of renin secretion less accurately in patients with hepatic dysfunction than under circumstances when liver function is normal.

An additional effect of disordered liver function on the RAS is to increase plasma ACE activity [18–22]; for example, Borowsky *et al* reported that 30% of 151 patients with alcoholic liver disease had elevated ACE levels [18]. Some authors found ACE activity to be high in patients with intrahepatic disorders, but normal or low in others with extrahepatic biliary obstruction [19,20], although overlap between groups was considerable. It seems unlikely that the minor and variable increase in ACE activity in some patients with disordered liver function would significantly alter the rate of Ang II production from Ang I. The report by Loyke [3] that the plasma of cirrhotic patients contains an inhibitor of ACE, requires confirmation.

ACTIVITY OF THE CIRCULATING RENIN–ANGIOTENSIN SYSTEM

Numerous studies have been designed to document activity of the RAS in patients with liver disease, most commonly by measuring PRA but also by reporting on the histological appearance of the juxtaglomerular apparatus, on PRC levels and on circulating concentrations of Ang II. Conditions of study have varied with regard to factors known to alter activity of the RAS (age of patients, body posture and time of day for venous sampling, dietary sodium intake, and drug treatment); thus, comparisons of results between studies are not always possible.

Reeves and colleagues, in an autopsy study in 45 patients with cirrhosis and ascites, reported in 1963 that whereas the total renal juxtaglomerular cell counts were similar to those in control (noncirrhotic) patients, type II and III juxtaglomerular cells (moderately granulated) were more numerous in the cirrhotics [23]. This suggested to the authors that the rate of renal renin secretion in these patients increased prior to their demise.

Subsequent studies indicated that activity of the circulating RAS is normal or low in patients with cirrhosis who have no ascites or peripheral edema, and is normal or high in those with ascites, compared with healthy control subjects. This appears to be true whether the measurements are of PRC [2,4,11,13,24], Ang II [13,25–27] or, as in most instances, PRA [13,28–47]. Levels of renin are almost invariably high in patients, most of whom have ascites, who are actively retaining sodium. By contrast, renin levels are often low in those undergoing a natriuresis [26] as is the case also in patients with cardiac failure (see *Chapter 76*). Activation of the circulating RAS is most striking in patients with the hepatorenal syndrome (see later). As noted by Wernz *et al* [14], diuretic treatment stimulates the RAS in patients with cirrhosis, as was reported also by Wilkinson *et al* [48] and Jespersen and colleagues [27].

Patients with activation of the RAS differ from those with normal or near-normal renin levels in excreting less of a water load [36,40], or of a high sodium intake [31]. They also exhibit a lesser natriuretic response to head-out water immersion [45]

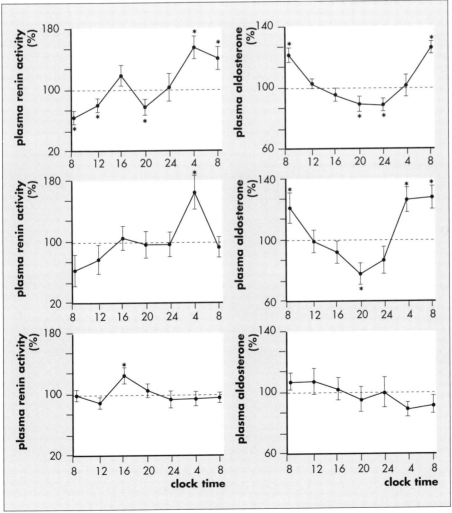

Fig. 78.1 Circadian patterns of plasma renin activity and plasma aldosterone, expressed as percentage of mesor values (=100) in: upper, healthy subjects (controls, n=7); centre, seven patients with cirrhosis but no ascites; and lower, nine patients with cirrhosis and ascites. Data are mean ± SEM. *$P<0.05$ compared with mesor value. Modified from Bernardi M *et al* [43].

and to loop diuretics [34,39]. Patients with ascites were reported by Bernardi *et al* [43] and Colantonio *et al* [49] to have raised PRA and to lose their normal diurnal pattern of fluctuations in PRA (Fig. 78.1). The former group also showed an exaggerated rise in PRA upon changing from the supine to the sitting position [41].

CONTROL OF RENIN SECRETION

As noted already, the clearance rate of renin is impaired when liver function is deranged, thus, extrapolation from circulating PRC to renal renin secretion rates should be made with more caution than when liver function is normal. Nevertheless, Arroyo *et al* reported a close correlation (r=0.93) between the logarithm of the rate of renal renin secretion and arterial PRC in 12 patients with nonazotemic cirrhosis and ascites [37]. The extrapolation is hampered more in the case of PRA, which is dependent not only on the concentration of active renin in the plasma sample being assayed, but also upon the level of renin substrate, which is frequently below normal in patients with disordered liver function (see *Chapter 5*) (see above).

Of the factors known to modulate renal renin release (see *Chapter 24*), there is evidence from studies in man to support a role for sympathetic innervation of kidneys, the delivery of sodium and chloride to the distal portions of the nephron, prostaglandins, the level of arterial pressure, and changes in regional blood flow within the kidney. Less clear are the roles, if any, of atrial natriuretic factor (ANF) and vasopressin.

Strong circumstantial evidence supports a role for sympathetic innervation of the kidneys, presumably to the juxtaglomerular apparatus, in contributing to the rate of renal renin secretion in patients with liver disease. A number of authors have observed positive associations between peripheral circulating levels of norepinephrine and PRA in these patients [36,37,41]. This evidence alone is frail, but Esler and colleagues have shown that renal norepinephrine 'spillover' (which is an index of the rate at which norepinephrine is released from the kidney and thus presumably of the sympathetic nerve firing rate) is increased in patients with decompensated cirrhosis as part of a generalized activation of the sympathetic nervous system [50].

Heightened sympathetic outflow to the kidneys might be expected to stimulate renin release, and under these circumstances, blockade of β_1-adrenoceptors should suppress plasma renin levels. This, in fact, is the case [32,48,51–53]. Furthermore, muscle sympathetic activity in the peroneal nerve is increased in patients with cirrhosis and ascites, and relates directly

to both plasma norepinephrine and PRA levels [46] (Fig. 78.2). It seems, therefore, that the level of sympathetic 'tone' to the kidneys is increased in the late stages of cirrhosis and contributes to the raised levels of renin in the circulation. Why the sympathetic system in general, and to the kidneys in particular, should be stimulated is beyond the scope of this chapter and is discussed in detail elsewhere [54–56]. It is worthy of note here, however, that some authors [11,55], though not all [17,57], have observed a positive relationship between the level of portal venous pressure (or hepatic venous wedge pressure) and circulating levels of renin in patients with cirrhosis (Fig. 78.3). Furthermore, Anderson and colleagues demonstrated in anesthetized dogs that acute portal hypertension induced an increase in the renin secretion rate, along with a decline in glomerular filtration rate (GFR) and renal plasma flow, in innervated kidneys, but a decrease of renin production and no change in GFR or renal plasma flow in denervated kidneys [58]. Subsequent studies by Levy *et al* in conscious dogs with cirrhosis and ascites, likewise showed that portal hypertension activates the RAS [59]. Earlier data from the same group suggested that a rise in portal pressure might be a prerequisite for heightened renin secretion in dogs with cirrhosis [60]. These data suggest that one afferent limb in the reflex activation of sympathetic tone to the kidneys, and thus presumably to the juxtaglomerular apparatus, involves a hepatorenal reflex [54–56].

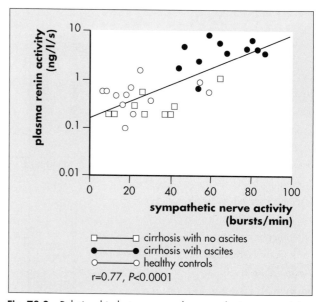

Fig. 78.2 Relationship between muscle sympathetic nerve activity and plasma renin activity in patients with cirrhosis but no ascites, in patients with cirrhosis and ascites, and in healthy controls. Modified from Floras JS *et al* [46].

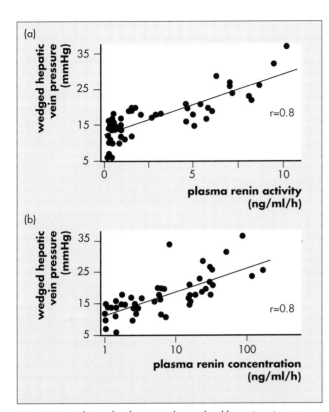

Fig. 78.3 Relationship between the wedged hepatic vein pressure and plasma renin activity (a) or concentration (b) in 44 patients with alcoholic cirrhosis, 36 of whom had ascites. Modified from Bosch J *et al* [11].

The rate of delivery of sodium and chloride to the distal portions of the renal tubule and hence the macula densa, is likely to contribute to the level of renin secretion in patients with disordered hepatic function, but data from studies in man are suggestive rather than definitive. Although it is not a universal finding, numerous authors have reported an inverse relationship between plasma levels of renin and the rate of urine sodium excretion [4,11,41,44,53,61]. Furthermore, Nicholls and colleagues observed an inverse relationship between urine sodium excretion and PRA during water immersion (with and without norepinephrine infusion) in patients with cirrhosis and ascites [62]. Conversely, head-out water immersion can lower elevated plasma renin levels in patients who have little or no natriuretic response [45] (see also *Chapter 74*). On balance, it seems that delivery of sodium and chloride to the distal renal tubules can modulate renal renin secretion in patients with liver disease, but it is one amongst a number of stimuli, and its effect can be overcome by other regulatory factors.

Available evidence strongly suggests that the RAS and prostaglandins, especially PGI_2 and PGE_2, are closely and functionally linked in patients and in experimental animals with disordered liver function. The action of Ang II to stimulate prostaglandin production and thereby preserve renal function and contribute to pressor hyporeponsiveness to Ang II, is of major pathophysiological significance [53,59]. Here it should be noted that some [40], although not all, authors have reported a positive association between activity of the RAS and urinary PGE_2 [37]. In rats with cirrhosis induced by carbon tetrachloride, Sola *et al* reported a close temporal relationship between activation of the RAS, the renal production of prostacyclin, and urinary retention of sodium [63], although which of these is stimulus and which the response is open to debate. The fact that prostaglandins do at least contribute to renin secretion is indicated by the fact that cyclo-oxygenase inhibitors (indomethacin, ibuprofen) reduce high levels of PRA in cirrhotic patients with ascites [53,64] (see also *Chapter 38*).

The renal artery perfusion pressure and distribution of blood flow within the kidney may be determinants of renin secretion in patients with cirrhosis. Systemic arterial pressure was noted by Bernardi *et al* [38] to relate inversely to PRA in patients with ascites but not in those without ascites. The same authors found statistically significant inverse correlations between renal plasma flow and GFR on one hand, and PRA on the other hand, but again, only in patients with ascites [38]. Although there are exceptions [10,17], other authors concur that PRA or PRC relate in a reciprocal fashion to renal plasma flow [30] and/or the GFR [4,30,37]. Pre-dating the above studies, Reeves *et al* documented a positive, if statistically weak, relationship between antemortem serum creatinine concentrations and the number of moderately granulated juxtaglomerular cells on microscopy (r=0.44, $P<0.05$) at postmortem in 45 patients with cirrhosis, ascites, and edema [23].

Schroeder and colleagues in 1967 concluded from studies in 22 patients with cirrhosis, ascites, and a wide range of levels of renal function, that there was a redistribution of blood flow within the kidneys as a result of renal cortical vasoconstriction, and a relative increase in medullary blood flow [65]. Subsequent and more detailed investigation using the [133]xenon washout technique and renal arteriography [66] showed that cirrhotic patients with renal impairment have a marked reduction in renal cortical perfusion and extreme hemodynamic instability (characterized by variability and irregularity of xenon washout). The authors considered that active vasoconstriction accounted for these changes, but increased sympathetic activity was deemed an unlikely mechanism since phentolamine, injected into the renal artery, failed to alter intrarenal hemodynamics [66]. Later studies by Wilkinson and colleagues [32,67] in patients with cirrhosis, ascites in most, and normal (or near normal) total renal perfusion, revealed a redistribution of plasma flow from outer cortical to juxtamedullary nephrons. They further noted an inverse correlation between effective plasma flow to outer cortical nephrons and logarithm PRA [67]. The authors speculated that outer cortical ischemia, of uncertain cause, might be the stimulus to activation of the RAS, although the alternative possibility that outer cortical ischemia was the result (rather than the cause) of high Ang II levels could not be ruled out [67]. These issues are considered from another aspect in *Chapter 21*.

As described in *Chapter 36*, ANF can inhibit renin release under many circumstances although studies where ANF infusion reduces arterial pressure often show activation of the RAS. In patients with cirrhosis and ascites, intravenous injection or infusion of ANF, sufficient to lower arterial pressure, had little effect on [68,69], or stimulated a rise in, PRA [61]. Petrillo *et al* demonstrated a fall in PRA with ANF infusion at 0.015μg/kg/min, which did not alter arterial pressure, but a rise in PRA in association with a decline in blood pressure at higher rates of ANF infusion in patients with cirrhosis and ascites [70]. These data are consistent with the premise that ANF, whether secreted endogenously or infused, might serve to restrain renin release in patients with cirrhosis except if the achieved plasma levels of ANF were sufficient to reduce blood pressure, when the opposite effect, stimulation of the RAS, can occur. If, indeed, endogenous ANF has a powerful restraining influence on the juxtaglomerular release of renin, an inverse relationship between renin and ANF might be expected. Such an association of weak statistic magnitude has been noted by Lai and colleagues in patients with cirrhosis and gross ascites [47]. Furthermore, reciprocal changes in ANF and renin levels have been observed with head-out water immersion [45,71] and peritoneovenous shunting [72] in patients with ascites. Somewhat against a potent restraining action of ANF on renin release in such patients is the observation that renin levels can be high in patients whose ANF levels are normal [47]. In summary, the role of ANF, if any, in modulating renin release in patients with disordered liver function is uncertain. Studies using specific inhibitors of ANF secretion or of its action, are needed to clarify this issue.

Since vasopressin can suppress renin secretion (see *Chapters 24* and *35*), it is pertinent to enquire whether the former is an important regulator of the latter in patients with cirrhosis. Evidence one way or the other in man is sparse, and definitive studies using specific blockers of vasopressin receptors are lacking. In conscious dogs with ascites due to chronic constriction of the inferior vena cava, infusion of the vascular receptor V_1 antagonist of vasopressin had no effect on PRA [73]. Gentile and colleagues [44] reported a positive and statistically significant association between PRA and vasopressin levels in 26 patients with cirrhosis and ascites (r=0.69, $P<0.001$) as did Burmeister *et al* [42], and the trend appears to be that activity of the RAS and vasopressin levels are often increased in the same patient [40,74] or that they are both normal. Such data do not support a major regulatory role for vasopressin on the juxtaglomerular apparatus, but a restraining effect cannot be ruled out with current information. More likely, it seems the RAS when stimulated, may contribute to vasopressin secretion.

An inhibitory action of Ang II on the juxtaglomerular apparatus is to be expected in this condition (see *Chapter 24*). Administration of a competitive Ang II-receptor blocker [5] or an ACE inhibitor stimulates renin release in patients with cirrhosis and ascites [75,76], but this most likely reflects changes in a number of input signals to the juxtaglomerular apparatus of which withdrawal (or antagonism) of Ang II and a fall in renal artery perfusion pressure, are presumably the most important.

A fall in plasma sodium concentration can stimulate renin under experimental circumstances, and cirrhotic patients with ascites not infrequently have hyponatremia and evidence of activation of the RAS. Since a number of workers, though not all, have reported an inverse relationship between plasma sodium and renin levels (see below), it is possible that hyponatremia contributes to hypersecretion of renin. More likely is the possibility that high circulating levels of Ang II, along with vasopressin, induce water retention, thereby resulting in hyponatremia (see below).

In summary, the factors that regulate renin and their relative importance in patients with liver disease are not well understood, but sympathetic innervation of the kidneys, delivery of sodium and chloride to the distal tubules, prostaglandins, renal artery perfusion pressure, redistribution of blood flow from outer cortical regions to the renal medulla, and Ang II, all appear to contribute. The role of ANF and vasopressin is less certain.

PATHOPHYSIOLOGICAL ROLE OF THE RENIN–ANGIOTENSIN SYSTEM

There is no doubt that the RAS is of major pathophysiological importance in cirrhotic patients with gross ascites, and especially in those with the hepatorenal syndrome (see below). Less clear is its place in the early stages of hepatic dysfunction and, specifically, whether or not it contributes directly or indirectly to excessive urinary sodium retention.

ALDOSTERONE

Liver dysfunction slows the plasma clearance rate of aldosterone [77,78] and alters the profile of aldosterone metabolites excreted in the urine [79]. Despite the latter observation, Wilkinson *et al* reported a close relationship between the renal excretion of aldosterone 18-glucuronide and aldosterone secretion rates (r=0.94, P< 0.001) in eight patients with cirrhosis [80].

Early studies documented high aldosterone secretion or excretion rates in cirrhotic patients with ascites [81–83]. Subsequent observations, mostly using plasma measurements, have been that aldosterone levels are in the normal or low-normal range in cirrhotic patients with little or no fluid retention, but are above the normal range in those with ascites and especially in the hepatorenal syndrome. This pattern is the same as that for plasma levels of renin. Within studies, there have generally been close positive statistical associations between concurrent levels of plasma renin (or Ang II) and plasma aldosterone [10–12,17,38,42,43,52] especially in patients with evidence of fluid retention. The directional change in the two indices is the same, for example, with head-out water immersion, peritoneovenous shunting, or β-blockade (6,32,52,84]. These reports point to the primacy of the RAS in regulating aldosterone secretion in such patients, although dissociations between renin and aldosterone have been reported [40,51] and might be explained under some circumstances by an inhibitory effect of ANF on the zona glomerulosa [69].

Studies of the effects of competitive Ang II-receptor antagonists and of ACE inhibitors support the central role of the RAS in controlling aldosterone secretion in patients with cirrhosis; for example, Schroeder *et al* [5] showed a fall in plasma aldosterone levels in four of five patients with cirrhosis and ascites during an intravenous infusion of saralasin. Saito and colleagues reported a clear decline in plasma aldosterone in only one of seven patients with ascites during Sar[1] Ile[8] Ang II infusion, but this was the only patient who had raised baseline levels of PRA and aldosterone [85]. The ACE inhibitors, captopril and enalapril, reduce plasma aldosterone levels in the short term in most patients with cirrhosis, with or without the presence of ascites [57,75,76,86] (Fig. 78.4) and even when baseline aldosterone values are not elevated [57]. The effect on aldosterone of long-term ACE inhibitors in these patients is not known.

Responsiveness of the adrenal glomerulosa to Ang II in patients with impaired liver function is disputed. Ames *et al* [82] observed a lesser rise in the aldosterone secretion rate, from a

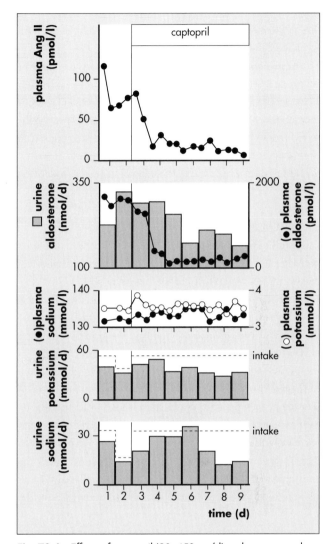

Fig. 78.4 Effects of captopril (30–450mg/d) on hormone and electrolyte indices in one patient with cirrhosis and gross ascites and peripheral edema. Modified from Espiner EA and Nicholls MG [86].

high baseline, during high-dose Ang II infusions (2.4–20.7μg/min) over 2–6 days, in patients with cirrhosis and ascites, compared with healthy volunteers. Epstein and colleagues [6] reported that slopes of regression lines relating PRA and plasma aldosterone during head-out water immersion in 16 cirrhotic patients were similar to those in normal subjects under the same experimental circumstances. In a study of diurnal patterns, Bernardi *et al* made note that slopes of regression lines for logarithm PRA versus logarithm plasma aldosterone were steeper in cirrhotic patients than in volunteers with normal hepatic function [43]. Henley's interpretation of Wong's data [33] from infusions of saline or albumin in cirrhotic patients with ascites is that aldosterone responsiveness to changes in activity of the RAS is enhanced compared to normal subjects [87].

An overview is that the RAS is the primary regulator of aldosterone secretion in patients with liver disease, although other factors (for example, ANF, plasma potassium and sodium concentrations, adrenocorticotropic hormone) may play a modulating role. Whether aldosterone responsiveness to Ang II is altered in cirrhotic patients is uncertain and requires construction of full dose–response (Ang II/aldosterone) curves for clarification.

ARTERIAL PRESSURE

Early studies by Laragh [81] and Ames et al [82] demonstrated a striking and specific impairment in arterial pressor responsiveness to infused Ang II in cirrhotic patients with ascites. The phenomenon, which has been confirmed repeatedly [5,53,88] may relate to downregulation of Ang II receptors on vascular smooth muscle (see Chapter 12) and Ang II-induced stimulation of vasodilator substances including prostaglandins [53] and nitric oxide (see Chapter 29). Whereas these data might be taken to suggest that the RAS plays little role in maintaining blood pressure in such patients, results from studies utilizing Ang II-receptor antagonists or ACE inhibitors point clearly to a pivotal role for circulating Ang II in patients with activation of the RAS, that is, those with ascites and, in particular, patients with the hepatorenal syndrome; for example, saralasin reduced arterial pressure in all of five patients with cirrhosis and ascites in the study of Schroeder et al [4] but, in contrast, raised blood pressure in cirrhotic patients without ascites. Arroyo and colleagues [89] made similar observations and documented a significant relationship between the pre-infusion level of PRA and the magnitude of fall in blood pressure in response to saralasin. As might be predicted, the hypotensive response to saralasin infusion is marked in the hepatorenal syndrome where activation of the RAS is, in most patients, equally striking [9]. The ACE inhibitors cause an acute fall in blood pressure in most cirrhotic patients with or without ascites [57,75,76,86,90,91] and again a relationship between baseline renin levels and the fall in blood pressure has been reported [75].

Overall, the above results suggest that the RAS plays only a minor role in maintaining arterial pressure in cirrhotic patients who have normal or low levels of plasma renin and who do not have fluid retention. One caveat here is that a slow pressor action of Ang II (see Chapter 28) may not be apparent from the available short-term studies with agents that block activity of the RAS. In patients with definite evidence for activation of the

RAS, it is clear that this pressor system is an important contributor to the maintenance of arterial pressure.

SODIUM BALANCE

A perplexing and widely debated issue is the pathophysiology of sodium and water retention in hepatic cirrhosis [92–98]. Three hypotheses have dominated center stage. The 'underfilling' theory proposes that the formation of ascites is an early, and perhaps primary, event which leads to circulatory hypovolemia. This, in turn, induces renal sodium retention through stimulation of the sympathetic nervous system, the RAS, vasopressin, and no doubt other mechanisms. The 'overflow' hypothesis suggests that renal sodium retention precedes and results in the development of ascites and edema. The third, and more recent 'peripheral arterial vasodilation' theory proposes that widespread dilatation of arterioles, which is an early phenomenon in cirrhotic patients, initiates the renal retention of sodium and water through stimulation of neurohormonal systems (Fig. 78.5). The role of the RAS in sodium retention in cirrhosis, whichever of these three hypotheses is more correct, is far from clear.

As noted earlier, a number of workers have reported an inverse relationship between plasma levels of renin and the rate of urinary sodium excretion in patients with cirrhosis [4,11,41,44,53,61]. This might suggest that retention of sodium by the kidneys is a response, at least in part, to activation of the RAS. Equally, and as discussed previously, it may reflect the importance of the rate of delivery of sodium and chloride to the area of the macula densa in the regulation of renal renin secretion (see Chapter 24).

The antinatriuretic effect of Ang II has been emphasized in Chapter 26 [98]. However, the renal tubular action of Ang II to promote sodium reabsorption may be overcome by its pressor action which can induce 'escape' [98] (see Chapter 63). Few studies have concentrated on the renal effects of administered Ang II in patients with disordered liver function, and most have used short-term pressor doses of the peptide. Laragh [81], Ames et al [82] and Schroeder et al [65] reported a variable but often striking natriuretic effect of intravenous Ang II in cirrhotic patients with ascites. The occurrence and magnitude of the natriuresis, however, was related to the pressor response and the dose of Ang II infused [82]. Gutman and colleagues reported that a 120-minute pressor infusion of Ang II induced a vigorous natriuresis in four cirrhotic patients with ascites, but had little or no effect in four others [88]. In all these patients, preinfusion rates of urinary sodium excretion were low but, as in other studies, there was no assessment of the urinary response to subpressor doses of

Ang II. The possibility remains, therefore, that a potent tubular action of Ang II is an important contributor to the renal retention of sodium and water in patients with cirrhosis [98]. Administration of partial agonist, Ang II-receptor blocking agents, or of ACE inhibitors has not proved especially helpful in this regard. A substantial decline in systemic arterial pressure from low baseline values results, not unexpectedly, in urinary sodium retention [86,90,91] despite ACE inhibitor-induced falls in

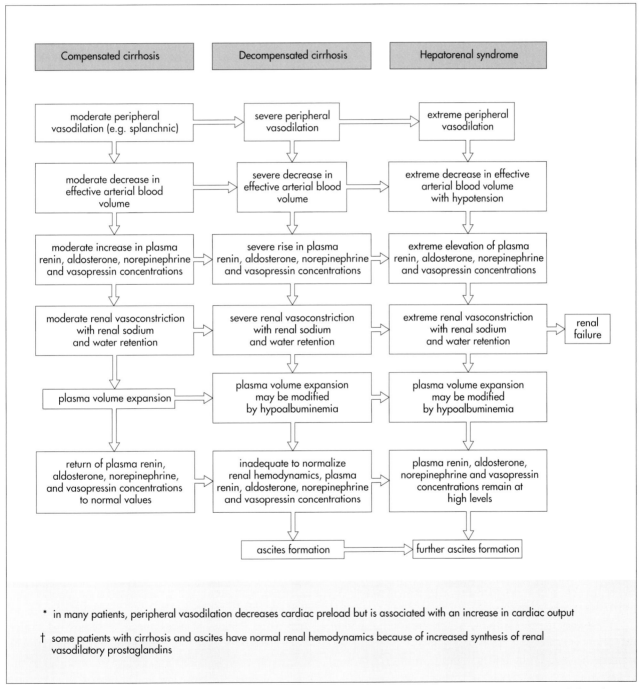

Fig. 78.5   The peripheral arterial vasodilation hypothesis has been taken to explain the hemodynamic, renal, hormone, and electrolyte changes in patients with cirrhosis. Modified from Schrier RW *et al* [96].

circulating Ang II (see *Fig. 78.4*). Under these conditions, any natriuretic response to a decline in plasma and/or renal Ang II concentrations is likely to be countered, completely or in part, by a dramatic fall in renal arterial perfusion pressure (see *Chapter 26*). Ohnishi and colleagues reported a natriuretic response to captopril or enalapril in cirrhotic patients, but time-matched control data were not given [76].

To summarize, pressor doses of exogenous Ang II often, but not always, induce a natriuretic response in cirrhotic patients with ascites. It seems entirely possible that the much lower endogenous circulating levels of Ang II seen in such patients have a renal tubular action in the reabsorption of sodium, thereby contributing significantly to abnormal sodium and water retention, but this is unproven. Infusions of nonagonist Ang II-receptor antagonists (see *Chapter 86*) into the renal artery of experimental animals or patients with cirrhosis and ascites should clarify this issue.

Apart from a direct action on renal tubular cells, Ang II appears to contribute to excessive sodium retention through stimulation of aldosterone secretion. The observation that aldosterone levels relate inversely to the rate of urine sodium excretion has been made on numerous occasions [6,11,12,38,53,99] (Fig. 78.6). Sola and colleagues noted a temporal relationship between a rise in urinary aldosterone excretion and decline in sodium excretion in rats with cirrhosis [63]. An additional observation in man is that there is a shift in the relationship between the two indices such that for any level of aldosterone, urinary sodium excretion is lower than in noncirrhotic subjects [38,99]. This has been taken, along with data from dogs with chronic caval obstruction [100], to indicate that the kidney is hyperresponsive to the sodium-retaining action of aldosterone [92,101]. Of further possible relevance is that the kidney, in at least some patients and animals with cirrhosis, in contrast to the normal situation [102], fails to 'escape' from the antinatriuretic action of long-term mineralocorticoid administration [103–106] (*Chapter 63*). The doses of mineralocorticoid used in these studies, however, were very high and the relevance to the clinical situation is unclear. A final point is that aldosterone levels are not suppressed by sodium or volume-loading to the same extent in many cirrhotic patients, especially those with ascites, compared with healthy subjects [31,107].

These data, together with the fact that drugs that inhibit aldosterone secretion or its action on the kidney, frequently (if not always) induce a natriuresis in cirrhotic patients with ascites and/or edema [12,39,83,92], point firmly to involvement of the RAS, through aldosterone secretion, in the excessive renal sodium retention in patients with cirrhosis.

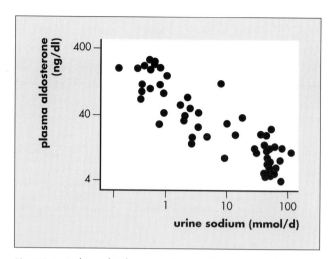

Fig. 78.6 Relationship between plasma aldosterone and urinary sodium excretion in 56 nonazotemic cirrhotic patients with ascites ($r=-0.87$, $P<0.001$). Modified from Arroya V *et al* [10].

WATER BALANCE

Angiotensin II can influence water balance through a number of mechanisms including stimulation of vasopressin secretion (see *Chapter 35*) and thirst (see *Chapter 32*), and by direct actions on the kidney (see *Chapters 21, 26,* and *27*). An inverse relationship between renin or juxtaglomerular granularity and plasma sodium levels has been noted in cirrhotic patients, especially those with ascites, by some authors [7,14,23,38,43,67,75] and might point to an action of Ang II to retain water, in excess of sodium, through the mechanisms noted above. In this regard, Ames *et al* [82] reported the development of hyponatremia in some cirrhotic patients during long-term, high-dose infusions of Ang II. An alternative explanation of this relationship, as mentioned earlier, is that hyponatremia serves to stimulate renin release. The former of these two hypotheses might be tested by sustained blockade of the RAS which, in patients with cardiac failure, does correct hyponatremia (see *Chapter 93*). No comparable information is available in cirrhotic patients, but Stanek *et al* noted that acute captopril administration failed to alter vasopressin levels [75]. Currently, therefore, a role of the RAS in the development of hyponatremia in patients with cirrhosis is likely, but unproven.

PORTAL HYPERTENSION

Angiotensin II infusion increased hepatic venous and wedged hepatic venous pressures in cirrhotic patients [108]. This observation, together with the positive relationship noted between activity of the RAS and portal venous (or hepatic venous wedge) pressure [11,55] in some studies, suggests that the RAS might contribute to the degree of portal venous hypertension in cirrhosis. Furthermore, Arroyo and colleagues documented a fall in wedged hepatic venous pressure (a measure of portal pressure) during infusion of the competitive Ang II antagonist, saralasin, in 14 patients with cirrhosis and ascites, the magnitude of which related to the preinfusion level of PRA [89]. Conversely, Eriksson et al reported little change in hepatic venous wedge pressures over a time period of 90 minutes after captopril administration (12.5mg or 25mg) in seven cirrhotic patients [57]. Pariente et al [90] likewise found that 25mg captopril in six nonazotemic patients with cirrhosis and ascites did not affect the hepatic venous pressure gradient either after 30 minutes or two hours.

Overall, it seems likely that the RAS is one contributory factor in determining the level of portal venous pressure, although its importance relative to other determinants remains to be defined. In two reviews of the topic, Lebrec [109,110] does not regard ACE inhibitors as useful drugs for the treatment of portal hypertension.

Indeed, Jørgensen et al [111] have reported that the combination of captopril with diuretic in alcoholic cirrhosis with ascites can provoke confusion, independently of hypotension, electrolyte disturbance, or hepatic or renal failure.

THE PITUITARY–ADRENAL AXIS IN CIRRHOSIS

Relationships between the RAS and the pituitary–adrenal axis have been reported under a variety of circumstances (see *Chapter 34*). It is of interest in this regard that prolonged infusions of pressor doses of Ang II stimulated a vigorous rise in the rate of cortisol secretion in cirrhotic patients with ascites [82]. Further information is needed to determine at what level in the hypothalamic–pituitary–adrenal axis Ang II was acting, and whether such an effect is seen from the levels of plasma Ang II commonly measured in patients with cirrhosis.

PROGNOSIS AND THE RENIN–ANGIOTENSIN SYSTEM

Long-term survival in patients with cirrhosis and ascites has been related, statistically, to a number of variables including arterial pressure, plasma norepinephrine, urinary sodium excretion, and the combination of hyponatremia and impaired renal function [112–115]. Three reports found plasma levels of renin to be of prognostic value [113–115]. Less obvious are the implications of these observations. As is the case in cardiac failure (see *Chapter 76*), it is conceivable that severe activation of the RAS hastens the demise of cirrhotic patients through its

pathophysiological actions noted above, and particularly by its likely role in the hepatorenal syndrome.

THE RENIN–ANGIOTENSIN SYSTEM IN HEPATORENAL SYNDROME

Severe liver disease in cirrhosis and fulminant hepatic failure is often complicated by renal impairment. An oliguric, azotemic clinical picture is accompanied by avid urinary sodium retention. The term 'hepatorenal syndrome', introduced in the 1930s, has raised much controversy over its exact definition. In recent years, a general agreement has been developed limiting the definition of hepatorenal syndrome to the unexplained progressive renal impairment (that is, decreased renal blood flow and GFR) that develops during the course of severe liver failure. The clinical picture is very similar to prerenal failure due to hypovolemia and it is indeed very important to differentiate the two clinical entities. Hepatorenal syndrome should be diagnosed only if renal failure cannot be explained by other known clinical disorders or diseases causing histological lesions of the kidney.

The mechanisms underlying the hepatorenal syndrome are many and complex [116]. The reduction in cortical renal perfusion is striking [66], but the cause of this intense cortical vasoconstriction is unknown [116]. In that circulating renin levels are very high [116,117], and despite low renin substrate concentrations [117–119], it is tempting to ascribe a role for activation of the RAS in the renal cortical vasoconstriction. Interactions between the RAS, sympathetic innervation of the kidney (including the juxtaglomerular apparatus), prostaglandins, the kallikrein system, and various dilators and constrictors produced by endothelial cells (see *Chapter 29*) are likely participants in the syndrome. The availability of selective nonagonist Ang II-receptor blocking agents (see *Chapter 86*) should help clarify the present uncertain role of the RAS in this obscure disorder. From a therapeutic standpoint, ACE inhibitors cannot, on current evidence, be recommended [119].

PANCREATIC RENIN SYSTEM

On a more peripheral issue, the presence of angiotensinogen mRNA, angiotensinogen protein, Ang II, and Ang II binding sites has been reported in dog pancreas [120]. The significance of these observations in relation to pancreatic exocrine and/or endocrine functions remains to be determined.

CONCLUSION

Activity of the RAS is normal or reduced in most patients with cirrhosis in the absence of edema or ascites, but is activated in the majority of those with clinical evidence of excessive fluid retention. Extremely high plasma levels of renin are the rule in the hepatorenal syndrome. Renin substrate concentrations in plasma relate inversely to the severity of liver dysfunction, and ACE activity is increased in some patients with hepatic disease. Control of renin secretion is complex in such patients, but a contribution from sympathetic innervation of the kidneys, delivery of sodium and chloride to the distal tubule, prostaglandins, and changes in regional blood flow within the kidney is likely. Once there is activation of the RAS, it contributes importantly to control of aldosterone secretion, the level of arterial pressure, and to renal sodium retention, although the contribution of a direct tubular action of Ang II to reabsorb sodium, remains to be defined. Possible additional effects of high circulating levels of Ang II include retention of body water, an increase in portal venous pressure, and less certainly, the regulation of cortisol secretion.

A possible role for renin systems in various tissues in patients with hepatic dysfunction has not been investigated.

REFERENCES

1. Ayers CR. Plasma renin activity and renin-substrate concentration in patients with liver disease. *Circulation Research* 1967;20:594–8.

2. Imai M, Sokabe H. Plasma renin and angiotensinogen levels in pathological states associated with oedema. *Archives of Diseases in Childhood* 1968;43:475–9.

3. Loyke HF. Liver enzymes in hypertension. *American Journal of Gastroenterology* 1970;53:339–51.

4. Schroeder ET, Eich RH, Smulyan H, Gould AB, Gabuzda GJ. Plasma renin level in hepatic cirrhosis. *American Journal of Medicine* 1970;49:186–91.

5. Schroeder ET, Anderson GH, Goldman SH, Streeten DHP. Effect of blockade of angiotensin II on blood pressure, renin and aldosterone in cirrhosis. *Kidney International* 1976;9:511–9.

6. Epstein M, Levinson R, Sancho J, Haber E. Re R. Characterization of the renin–aldosterone system in decompensated cirrhosis. *Circulation Research* 1977;41:818–29.

7. Wilkinson SP, Smith IK, Williams R. Changes in plasma renin activity in cirrhosis: A reappraisal based on studies in 67 patients and 'low-renin' cirrhosis. *Hypertension* 1979;1:125–9.

8. Arnal JF, Cudek P, Plouin PF, Guyenne TT, Michel JB, Corvol P. Low angiotensinogen levels are related to the severity and liver dysfunction of congestive heart failure: Implications for renin measurements. *American Journal of Medicine* 1991;90:17–22.

9. Schroeder ET, Anderson GH, Smulyan H. Effects of a portacaval or peritoneovenous shunt on renin in the hepatorenal syndrome. *Kidney International* 1979;15:54–61.

10. Arroya V, Bosch J, Mauri M, Viver J, Mas A, Rivera F, Rodes J. Renin, aldosterone and renal haemodynamics in cirrhosis with ascites. *European Journal of Clinical Investigation* 1979;9:69–73.

11. Bosch J, Arroyo V, Betriu A, Mas A, Carrilho F, Rivera F, Navarro-Lopez F, Rodes J. Hepatic hemodynamics and the renin–angiotensin–aldosterone system in cirrhosis. *Gastroenterology* 1980;78:92–9.

12. Sellars L, Shore AC, Mott V, Wilkinson R. The renin–angiotensin–aldosterone system in decompensated cirrhosis: Its activity in relation to sodium balance. *Quarterly Journal of Medicine* 1985;56:485–96.

13. Kondo K, Nakamura R, Saito I. Saruta T, Matsuki S. Renin, angiotensin II and juxtaglomerular apparatus in liver cirrhosis. *Japanese Circulation Journal* 1974;38:913–21.

14. Wernze H, Spech HJ, Muller G. Studies on the activity of the renin–angiotensin–aldosterone system (RAAS) in patients with cirrhosis of the liver. *Klinische Wochenschrift* 1978;56:389–97.

15. Schneider EG, Davis JO, Robb CA, Baumber JS. Hepatic clearance of renin in canine experimental models for low- and high-output heart failure. *Circulation Research* 1969;24:213–9.

16. Barnardo DE, Strong CG, Baldus WP. Failure of the cirrhotic liver to inactivate renin: Evidence for a splanchnic source of renin-like activity. *Journal of Laboratory and Clinical Medicine* 1969;74:495–506.

17. Mitch WE, Whelton PK, Cooke CR, Walker WG, Maddrey WC. Plasma levels and hepatic extraction of renin and aldosterone in alcoholic liver disease. *American Journal of Medicine* 1979;66:804–10.

18. Borowsky SA, Lieberman J, Strome S, Sastre A. Elevation of serum angiotensin-converting enzyme level. Occurrence in alcoholic liver disease. *Archives of Internal Medicine* 1982;142:893–5.

19. Matsuki K, Sakata T. Angiotensin-converting enzyme in diseases of the liver. *American Journal of Medicine* 1982;73:549–51.

20. Johnson DA, Diehl AM, Sjogren MH, Lazar J, Cattau EL, Smallridge RC. Serum angiotensin converting enzyme activity in evaluation of patients with liver disease. *American Journal of Medicine* 1987;83:256–60.

21. Ohnishi A, Tsuboi Y, Ishizaki T, Kubota K, Ohno T, Yoshida H, Kanezaki A, Tanaka T. Kinetics and dynamics of enalapril in patients with liver cirrhosis. *Clinical Pharmacology and Therapeutics* 1989;45:657–65.

22. Yamada Y, Ishizaki M, Kido T, Honda R, Tsuritani I, Ikai E, Yamaya H. Elevations of serum angiotensin-converting enzyme and gamma-glutamyl transpeptidase activities in hypertensive drinkers. *Journal of Human Hypertension* 1991;5:183–8.

23. Reeves G, Lowenstein LM, Sommers SC. The macula densa and juxtaglomerular body in cirrhosis. *Archives of Internal Medicine* 1963;112:708–15.

24. Brown JJ, Davies DL, Lever AF, Robertson JIS. Variations in plasma renin concentration in several physiological and pathological states. *Canadian Medical Association Journal* 1964;90:201–6.

25. Genest J, Boucher R, de Champlain J, Veyrat R, Chretien M, Biron P, Tremblay G, Roy P, Cartier P. Studies on the renin–angiotensin system in hypertensive patients. *Canadian Medical Association Journal* 1964;90:263–8.

26. Madsen M, Pedersen EB, Danielsen H, Jensen LS, Sorensen SS. Imparied renal water excretion in early hepatic cirrhosis. *Scandinavian Journal of Gastroenterology* 1986;21:749–55.

27. Jespersen B, Jensen L, Sorensen SS, Pedersen EB. Atrial natriuretic factor, cyclic 3',5'-guanosine monophosphate and prostaglandin E_2 in liver cirrhosis: Relation to blood volume and changes in blood volume after furosemide. *European Journal of Clinical Investigation* 1990;20:632–41.

28. Fasciolo JC, De Vito E, Romero JC, Cucchi JN. The renin content of the blood of humans and dogs under several conditions. *Canadian Medical Association Journal* 1964;90:206–9.

29. Veyrat R, de Champlain J, Boucher R, Genest J. Measurement of human arterial renin activity in some physiological and pathological states. *Canadian Medical Association Journal* 1964;90:215–20.

30. Barnardo DE, Summerskill WHJ, Strong CG, Baldus WP. Renal function, renin activity and endogenous vasoactive substances in cirrhosis. *Digestive Diseases* 1970;**15**:419–25.

31. Chonko AM, Bay WH, Stein JH, Ferris TF. The role of renin and aldosterone in the salt retention of edema. *American Journal of Medicine* 1977;**63**:881–9.

32. Wilkinson SP, Bernardi M, Smith IK, Jowett TP, Slater JDH, Williams R. Effect of beta-adrenergic blocking drugs on the renin–aldosterone system, sodium excretion, and renal hemodynamics in cirrhosis with ascites. *Gastroenterology* 1977;**73**:659–63.

33. Wong PY, Carroll RE, Lipinski TL, Capone RR. Studies on the renin–angiotensin–aldosterone system in patients with cirrhosis and ascites: Effect of saline and albumin infusion. *Gastroenterology* 1979;**77**:1171–6.

34. Arroyo V, Bosch J, Casamitjana R, Cabrera J, Rivera F, Rodes J. Use of piretanide, a new loop diuretic, in cirrhosis with ascites. Relationship between the diuretic response and the plasma aldosterone level. *Gut* 1980;**21**:855–9.

35. Sellars L, Shore AC, Wilkinson R, James OFW, Robson V. Sodium status and the renin–angiotensin–aldosterone system in compensated liver disease. *European Journal of Clinical Investigation* 1981;**11**:299–304.

36. Bichet DG, Van Putten VJ, Schrier RW. Potential role of increased sympathetic activity in impaired sodium and water excretion in cirrhosis. *New England Journal of Medicine* 1982;**307**:1552–7.

37. Arroyo V, Planas R, Gaya J, Deulofeu R, Rimola A, Perez-Ayuso RM, Rivera F, Rodes J. Sympathetic nervous activity, renin–angiotensin system and renal excretion of prostaglandin E_2 in cirrhosis. Relationship to functional renal failure and sodium and water excretion. *European Journal of Clinical Investigation* 1983;**13**:271–8.

38. Bernardi M, Trevisani F, Santini C, De Palma R, Gasbarrini G. Aldosterone related blood volume expansion in cirrhosis before and during the early phase of ascites formation. *Gut* 1983;**24**:761–6.

39. Perez-Ayuso RM, Arroyo V, Planas R, Gaya J, Bory F, Rimola A, Rivera F, Rodes J. Randomized comparative study of efficacy of furosemide versus spironolactone in nonazotemic cirrhosis with ascites. *Gastroenterology* 1983;**84**:961–8.

40. Perez-Ayuso RM, Arroyo V, Camps J, Rimola A, Gaya J, Costa J, Rivera F, Rodes J. Evidence that renal prostaglandins are involved in renal water metabolism in cirrhosis. *Kidney International* 1984;**26**:72–80.

41. Bernardi M, Santini C, Trevisani F, Baraldini M, Ligabue A, Gasbarrini G. Renal function impairment induced by change in posture in patients with cirrhosis and ascites. *Gut* 1985;**26**:629–35.

42. Burmeister P, Scholmerich J, Diener W, Gerok W. Renin, aldosterone and arginine vasopressin in patients with liver cirrhosis: The influence of ascites retransfusion. *European Journal of Clinical Investigation* 1986;**16**:117–23.

43. Bernardi M, De Palma R, Trevisani F, Santini C, Capani F, Baraldini M, Gasbarrini G. Chronobiological study of factors affecting plasma aldosterone concentration in cirrhosis. *Gastroenterology* 1986;**91**:683–91.

44. Gentile S, Angelico M, Chiappini MG, Peruzzi G, Vulterini S. Clinical and hormonal conditions associated with sodium retention in cirrhotic patients with ascites. *Digestive Diseases and Sciences* 1987;**32**:569–76.

45. Skorecki KL, Leung WM, Campbell P, Warner LC, Wong PY, Bull S, Logan AG, Blendis LM. Role of atrial natriuretic peptide in the natriuretic response to central volume expansion induced by head-out water immersion in sodium-retaining cirrhotic subjects. *American Journal of Medicine* 1988;**85**:375–82.

46. Floras JS, Legault L, Morali GA, Hara K, Blendis LM. Increased sympathetic outflow in cirrhosis and ascites: Direct evidence from intraneural recordings. *Annals of Internal Medicine* 1991;**114**:373–80.

47. Lai KN, Li PKT, Law E, Swaminathan R, Nicholls MG. Large-volume paracentesis versus dialytic ultrafiltration in the treatment of cirrhotic ascites. *Quarterly Journal of Medicine* 1991;**78**:33–41.

48. Wilkinson SP, Wheeler PG, Bernardi M, Smith IK, Williams R. Diuretic-induced renal impairment without volume depletion in cirrhosis: Changes in the renin–angiotensin system and the effect of beta-adrenergic blockade. *Postgraduate Medical Journal* 1979;**55**:862–7.

49. Colantonio D, Pasqualetti P, Casale R, Desiati P, Giandomenico G, Natali G. Atrial natriuretic peptide–renin–aldosterone system in cirrhosis of the liver: Circadian study. *Life Sciences* 1988;**45**:631–5.

50. Esler MD, Hasking GJ, Willett IR, Leonard PW, Jennings GL. Noradrenaline release and sympathetic nervous system activity. *Journal of Hypertension* 1985;**3**:117–29.

51. Gatta A, Sacerdoti D, Merkel C, Caregaro L, Borsato M, Bolognesi M, Ruol A. Renal effects of nadolol in cirrhosis. *European Journal of Clinical Pharmacology* 1987;**33**:473–7.

52. Bernardi M, De Palma R, Trevisani F, Tame MR, Ciancaglini GC, Pesa O, Ligabue A, Baraldini M, Gasbarrini G. Renal function and effective beta-blockade in cirrhosis with ascites. Relationship with baseline sympathoadrenergic tone. *Journal of Hepatology* 1989;**8**:279–86.

53. Zipser RD, Hoefs CJ, Speckart PF, Zia PK, Horton R. Prostaglandins: Modulators of renal function and pressor resistance in chronic liver disease. *Journal of Clinical Endocrinology and Metabolism* 1979;**48**:895–900.

54. Rocco VK, Ware AJ. Cirrhotic ascites. Pathophysiology, diagnosis, and management. *Annals of Internal Medicine* 1986;**105**:573–85.

55. Seifter JL, Skorecki LK, Stivelman JC, Haupert G, Brenner BM. Control of extracellular fluid volume and pathophysiology of edema formation. In: Brenner BM, Rector FC, eds. *The kidney*. Philadelphia: WB Saunders, 1986;343–84.

56. DiBona GF. Renal neural activity in hepatorenal syndrome. *Kidney International* 1984;**25**:841–53.

57. Eriksson LSIW, Kagedal B, Wahren J. Effects of captopril on hepatic venous pressure and blood flow in patients with liver cirrhosis. *American Journal of Medicine* 1984;**76** [5B]:66–70.

58. Anderson RJ, Cronin RE, McDonald KM, Schrier RW. Mechanisms of portal hypertension-induced alterations in renal hemodynamics, renal water excretion, and renin secretion. *Journal of Clinical Investigation* 1976;**58**:964–70.

59. Levy M, Wexler MJ, Fechner C. Renal perfusion in dogs with experimental hepatic cirrhosis: Role of prostaglandins. *American Journal of Physiology* 1983;**245**:F521–9.

60. Levy M, Wexler MJ. Renal sodium retention and ascites formation in dogs with experimental cirrhosis but without portal hypertension or increased splanchnic vascular capacity. *Journal of Laboratory and Clinical Medicine* 1978;**91**:520–36

61. Laffi G, Pinzani M, Meacci E, La Villa G, Renzi D, Baldi E, Cominelli F, Marra F, Gentilini P. Renal hemodynamic and natriuretic effects of human atrial natriuretic factor infusion in cirrhosis with ascites. *Gastroenterology* 1989;**96**:167–77.

62. Nicholls KM, Shapiro MD, Kluge R, Chung HM, Bichet DG, Schrier RW. Sodium excretion in advanced cirrhosis: Effect of expansion of central blood volume and suppression of plasma aldosterone. *Hepatology* 1986;**6**:235–8.

63. Sola J, Camps J, Arroyo V, Guarner F, Gaya J, Rivera F, Rodes J. Longitudinal study of renal prostaglandin excretion in cirrhotic rats: Relationship with the renin–aldosterone system. *Clinical Science* 1988:**75**:263–9.

64. Boyer TD, Zia P, Reynolds TB. Effect of indomethacin and prostaglandin A_1 on renal function and plasma renin activity in alcoholic liver disease. *Gastroenterology* 1979;**77**:215–22.

65. Schroeder ET, Shear L, Sancetta SM, Gabuzda GJ. Renal failure in patients with cirrhosis of the liver. *American Journal of Medicine* 1967;**43**:887–96.

66. Epstein M, Berk DP, Hollenberg NK, Adams DF, Chalmers TC, Abrams HL, Merrill JP. Renal failure in the patient with cirrhosis. *American Journal of Medicine* 1970;**49**:175–85.

67. Wilkinson SP, Smith IK, Clarke M, Arroyo V, Richardson J, Moodie H, Williams R. Intrarenal distribution of plasma flow in cirrhosis as measured by transit renography: Relationship with plasma renin activity, and sodium and water excretion. *Clinical Science and Molecular Medicine* 1977;**52**:469–75.

68. Laffi G, Marra F, Pinzani M, Meacci E, Tosti-Guerra C, De Feo ML, Gentilini P. Effects of repeated atrial natriuretic peptide bolus injections in cirrhotic patients with refractory ascites. *Liver* 1989;**9**:315–21.

69. Fyhrquist F, Totterman KJ, Tikkanen I. Infusion of atrial natriuretic peptide in liver cirrhosis with ascites. *Lancet* 1985;**ii**:1439.

70. Petrillo A, Scherrer U, Gonvers JJ, Nussberger J, Marder H, de Vane Ph, Waeber B, Hofstetter JR, Brunner HR. Atrial natriuretic peptide administered as intravenous infusion or bolus injection to patients with liver cirrhosis and ascites. *Journal of Cardiovascular Pharmacology* 1988;12:279–85.

71. Fernandez-Cruz A, Marco J, Cuadrado LM, Gutkowska J, Rodriguez-Puyol D, Caramelo C, Lopez-Novoa JM. Plasma levels of atrial natriuretic peptide in cirrhotic patients. *Lancet* 1985;ii:1439–40.

72. Campbell PJ, Skorecki KL, Logan AG, Wong PY, Leung WM, Greig P, Blendis LM. Acute effects of peritoneovenous shunting on plasma atrial natriuretic peptide in cirrhotic patients with massive refractory ascites. *American Journal of Medicine* 1988;84:112–9.

73. Vari RC, Freeman RH, Davis JO, Sweet WD. Systemic and renal hemodynamic responses to vascular blockade of vasopressin in conscious dogs with ascites. *Proceedings of the Society for Experimental Biology and Medicine* 1985;179:192–6.

74. Nicholls KM, Shapiro MD, Groves BS, Schrier RW. Factors determining renal response to water immersion in non-excretor cirrhotic patients. *Kidney International* 1986;30:417–21.

75. Stanek B, Renner F, Sedlmayer A, Silberbauer K. Effect of captopril on renin and blood pressure in cirrhosis. *European Journal of Clinical Pharmacology* 1987;33:249–54.

76. Ohnishi A, Ishizaki T, Murakami S, Tanaka T. Intrapatient comparison of acute hemodynamic, hormonal and natriuretic responses to captopril versus enalapril in liver cirrhosis. *Clinical Pharmacology and Therapeutics* 1990;48:67–75.

77. Coppage WS, Island DP, Cooner AE, Liddle GW. The metabolism of aldosterone in normal subjects and in patients with hepatic cirrhosis. *Journal of Clinical Investigation* 1962;41:1672–80.

78. Vecsei P, Düsterdieck G, Jahnecke J, Lommer D, Wolff HP. Secretion and turnover of aldosterone in various pathological states. *Clinical Science* 1969;36:241–56.

79. Hurter R, Nabarro JDN. Aldosterone metabolism in liver disease. *Acta Endocrinologica* 1960;33:168–74.

80. Wilkinson SP, Wheeler PG, Jowett TP, Smith IK, Keenan J, Slater JDH, Williams R. Factors relating to aldosterone secretion rate, the excretion of aldosterone 18-glucuronide, and the plasma aldosterone concentration in cirrhosis. *Clinical Endocrinology* 1981;14:355–62.

81. Laragh JH. Hormones and the pathogenesis of congestive heart failure: Vasopressin, aldosterone and angiotensin II. *Circulation* 1962;25:1015–23.

82. Ames RP, Borkowski AJ, Sicinski AM, Laragh JH. Prolonged infusions of angiotensin II and norepinephrine and blood pressure, electrolyte balance, and aldosterone and cortisol secretion in normal man and in cirrhosis with ascites. *Journal of Clinical Investigation* 1965;44:1171–86.

83. Kuchel O, Horky K, Gregorova I. The treatment of secondary hyperaldosteronism with oedema by amino-glutethimide. *Pharmacologia Clinica* 1970;2:138–42.

84. Greig PD, Blendis LM, Langer B, Ruse J, Taylor BR. The acute effects of sustained volume expansion on the renin–aldosterone system and renal function in human hepatic ascites. *Journal of Laboratory and Clinical Medicine* 1981;98:127–34.

85. Saito I, Saruta T, Eguchi T, Nakamura R, Kondo K, Iyori S, Kato E. Role of renin–angiotensin system in the control of blood pressure and aldosterone in patients with cirrhosis and ascites. *Japanese Heart Journal* 1978;19:741–47.

86. Espiner EA, Nicholls MG. Hormones and fluid retention in cirrhosis. *Lancet* 1982;ii:501–2.

87. Henley KS. Hormones and fluid retention in cirrhosis. *Lancet* 1982;ii:328.

88. Gutman RA, Forrey SW, Fleet WP, Cutler RE. Vasopressor-induced natriuresis and altered intrarenal haemodynamics in cirrhotic man. *Clinical Science and Molecular Medicine* 1973;45:19–34.

89. Arroyo V, Bosch J, Mauri M, Ribera F, Navarro-Lopez F, Rodes J. Effect of angiotensin II blockade on systemic and hepatic haemodynamics and on the renin–angiotensin–aldosterone system in cirrhosis with ascites. *European Journal of Clinical Investigation* 1981;11:221–9.

90. Pariente EA, Bataille C, Bercoff E, Lebrec D. Acute effects of captopril on systemic and renal hemodynamics and on renal function in cirrhotic patients with ascites. *Gastroenterology* 1985;88:1255–9.

91. Wood LJ, Goergen S, Stockigt JR, Powell LW, Dudley FJ. Adverse effects of captopril in treatment of resistant ascites, a state of functional bilateral renal artery stenosis. *Lancet* 1985;ii:1008–9.

92. Wilkinson SP, Williams R. Renin–angiotensin–aldosterone system in cirrhosis. *Gut* 1980;21:545–54.

93. Henriksen JH. The 'overflow' theory of ascites formation: A fading concept? *Scandinavian Journal of Gastroenterology* 1983;18:833–7.

94. Sewell RB, Poston L, Wilkinson SP. Sodium and fluid retention in hepatic cirrhosis: A role for circulating hormones? *Australian and New Zealand Journal of Medicine* 1984;14:297–304.

95. Epstein M. The kidney in liver disease. In: Arias IM, Jakoby WB, Popper H, Schachter D, Shafritz DA, eds. *The liver: Biology and Pathobiology, 2nd edition.* New York: Raven Press, 1988;1043–62.

96. Schrier RW. Pathogenesis of sodium and water retention in high-output and low-output cardiac failure, nephrotic syndrome, cirrhosis, and pregnancy. *New England Journal of Medicine* 1988;319:1127–34.

97. Schrier RW, Arroyo V, Bernardi M, Epstein M, Henriksen JH, Rodes J. Peripheral arterial vasodilation hypothesis: A proposal for the initiation of renal sodium and water retention in cirrhosis. *Hepatology* 1988;8:1151–7.

98. Hall JE, Guyton AC, Mizelle HL. Role of the renin–angiotensin system in control of sodium excretion and arterial pressure. *Acta Physiologica Scandanavica* 1990;139 (suppl 591):48–62.

99. Wilkinson SP, Jowett TP, Slater JDH, Arroyo V, Moodie H, Williams R. Renal sodium retention in cirrhosis: Relation to aldosterone and nephron site. *Clinical Science* 1979;56:169–77.

100. Davis JO, Holman JE, Carpenter CCJ, Urquhart J, Higgins JT. An extra-adrenal factor essential for chronic renal sodium retention in presence of increased sodium-retaining hormone. *Circulation Research* 1964;14:17–31.

101. Bernardi M, Gasbarrini G. The renin–angiotensin–aldosterone system in human hepatic cirrhosis. *Israel Journal of Medical Sciences* 1986;22:70–7.

102. August JT, Nelson DH, Thorn GW. Response of normal subjects to large amounts of aldosterone. *Journal of Clinical Investigation* 1958;37:1549–55.

103. Nelson DH, August JT. Abnormal response of oedematous patients to aldosterone or deoxycortone. *Lancet* 1959;ii:883–6.

104. Denison EK, Lieberman FL, Reynolds TB. 9-alpha-fluorohydrocortisone induced ascites in alcoholic liver disease. *Gastroenterology* 1971;61:497–503.

105. Wilkinson SP, Smith IK, Moodie H, Poston L, Williams R. Studies on mineralocorticoid 'escape' in cirrhosis. *Clinical Science* 1979;56:401–6.

106. Chaimovitz C, Alon U, Better OS. Pathogenesis of salt retention in dogs with chronic bile-duct ligation. *Clinical Science* 1982;62:65–70.

107. Duncan LE, Liddle GW, Bartter FC. The effect of changes in body sodium on extracellular fluid volume and aldosterone and sodium excretion by normal and edematous men. *Journal of Clinical Investigation* 1956;35:1299–305.

108. Segel N, Bayley TJ, Paton A, Dykes PW, Bishop JM. The effects of synthetic vasopressin and angiotensin on the circulation in cirrhosis of the liver. *Clinical Science* 1963;25:43–5.

109. Lebrec D. Drugs for portal hypertension. *Journal of Gastroenterology and Hepatology* 1987;2:361–74.

110. Lebrec D. Current status and future goals of the pharmacologic reduction of portal hypertension. *American Journal of Surgery* 1990;160:19–25.

111. Jørgensen F, Badskjaer J, Nordin H. Captopril and resistant ascites. *Lancet* 1983;ii:405.

112. Arroyo V, Rodes J, Gutierrez-Lizarraga MA, Revert L. Prognostic value of spontaneous hyponatremia in cirrhosis with ascites. *Digestive Diseases* 1976;21:249–56.

113. Arroya V, Bosch J, Gaya-Beltran J, Kravetz D, Estrada L, Rivera F, Rodes J. Plasma renin activity and urinary sodium excretion as prognostic indicators in nonazotemic cirrhosis with ascites. *Annals of Internal Medicine* 1981;94:198–201.

114. Llach J, Gines P, Arroyo V, Rimola A, Tito L, Badalamenti S, Jimenez W, Gaya J, Rivera F, Rodes J. Prognostic value of arterial pressure, endogenous vasoactive systems and renal function in cirrhotic patients admitted to the hospital for the treatment of ascites. *Gastroenterology* 1988;94:482–7.

115. Genoud E, Gonvers J-J, Schaller M-D, Essinger A, Haller E, Brunner H-R. Valeur pronostique du systeme renine–angiotensine dans la reponse a la restriction sodee et le pronostic de l'ascite cirrhotique d'origine alcoolique. *Schweizerische Medizinische Wochenschrift* 1986;116:463–9.

116. Pinzani M, Zipser RD. The hepatorenal syndrome. *Intensive Care Medicine* 1987;13:148–53.

117. Iwatsuki S, Popovtzer MM, Corman JL, Ishikawa M, Putman CW, Katz FH, Starzl TE. Recovery from 'hepatorenal syndrome' after orthotopic liver transplantation. *New England Journal of Medicine* 1973;289:1155–9.

118. Ziegler TW. Hepatorenal syndrome: A disease mediated by the intrarenal action of renin. *Medical Hypotheses* 1976;2:15–21.

119. Cobden I, Shore A, Wilkinson R, Record CO. Captopril in hepatorenal syndrome. *Journal of Clinical Gastroenterology* 1985;7:354–60.

120. Chappell MC, Millsted A, Diz DI, Brosnihan KB, Ferrario CM. Evidence for an intrinsic angiotensin system in the canine pancreas. *Journal of Hypertension* 1991;9:751–9.

79 THE RENIN–ANGIOTENSIN SYSTEM IN CONNECTIVE TISSUE DISORDERS

STEVEN L STRONGWATER AND JEFFREY S STOFF

The role of the RAS has been investigated in systemic sclerosis, rheumatoid arthritis, systemic lupus erythematosus (SLE), and in other disorders associated with joint effusions. These diverse disorders have in common activation of the inflammatory cascade and modulation of the immune system with resulting tissue injury. The exact function of the RAS in these disorders is unknown, but various investigations have focused on systemic and/or local renin systems as potential immunomodulators; markers of endothelial or vascular injury; active participants in vascular damage; modulators of hypertension leading to renal failure; and stimulators of the release and/or production of other vasoactive substances.

The RAS is comprised of a complex of proenzymes, enzymes, and other proteins synthesized and metabolized at a number of sites, the details of which are reviewed elsewhere in this book. This chapter discusses the possible role of prorenin, renin, and isorenins (locally produced renins), angiotensins, and ACE as they relate to the connective tissue disorders. The use of ACE inhibitors will also be reviewed in the context of the etiology, pathogenesis, and therapy of these diseases. Figure 79.1 provides an overview of the RAS in the connective tissue disorders.

Disease	Plasma renin	Plasma Ang II	ACE activity in vivo (serum)	ACE activity in vitro (monocyte culture)
rheumatoid arthritis	normal	not available	decreased, normal, increased*	increased
Sjögren's syndrome	not available	not available	normal	not available
scleroderma	normal, increased	normal, increased	normal, increased	not available
systemic lupus erythematosus	not available	not available	normal, increased	not available
osteoarthritis	not available	not available	normal	normal
ankylosing spondylitis	not available	not available	normal	not available
psoriatic arthritis	not available	not available	normal	not available
Behçet's syndrome	not available	not available	normal	not available

*joint fluid activity — normal, increased

Fig. 79.1 The RAS in connective tissue diseases. Modified from Lowe JR *et al* [42], Machin ND *et al* [43], Aoyagi T *et al* [44], Sheikh IA and Kaplan AP [45], Goto M *et al* [46], Specks U *et al* [47], and Boers M *et al* [50].

SYSTEMIC SCLEROSIS

Systemic sclerosis or scleroderma is a disorder of unknown etiology characterized by a generalized increase in skin thickening due to fibrosis and increased collagen production [1,2]. There is variable and unpredictable involvement of visceral structures such as the heart, lungs, kidneys, gastrointestinal tract, and the vasculature. Five clinical subsets of the disease are recognized, the most progressive being diffuse scleroderma (Fig. 79.2) [1].

Almost all patients with scleroderma have Raynaud's phenomenon which is a consequence of vascular constriction leading to a three-phase color response in the digits: pallor, cyanosis, and erythema [1–4] (see *Chapter 97*). Cold exposure, emotional stress, and a number of drugs (for example, ergotamines, β-blockers, and phenyl-propanolamine) may precipitate this phenomenon [4]. Typically, vasospasm involves arterioles but occasionally larger vessels are affected. Pathologically, there can be intimal hyperplasia with narrowing and obliteration of the arteriolar lumen [4,5] leading to digital ischemia, cutaneous ulceration, abnormalities of the nail capillary bed (capillary dilatation, branching, and dropout), and perhaps telangiectasias (1–4). The latter are present in many patients with scleroderma but tend not to occur in idiopathic Raynaud's disease [3–5].

The development of nailfold capillary abnormalities and telangiectasias may be due, in part, to a circulating humoral substance such as Ang II. A circulating stimulator of angiogenesis has been postulated in the development of new collateral

```
(1) systemic sclerosis
      diffuse — systemic sclerosis
      limited (for example, CREST syndrome — calcinosis,
        Raynaud's phenomenon, esophageal abnormalities,
        sclerodactyly, and telangiectasia)
(2) overlap syndromes
(3) undifferentiated and mixed connective tissue diseases
(4) diffuse fasciitis with eosinophilia
(5) localized scleroderma (cutaneous, morphea)
```

Fig. 79.2 Classification of scleroderma. There are also scleroderma-like illnesses due to drugs (for example, tryptophan, vinyl chloride, pentazocine, rape-seed oil-associated toxic oil syndrome, etc) and in association with juvenile diabetes mellitus. Look-alike disorders include scleroderma adultorum of Buschke, scleromyxedema, lichen sclerosis et atrophicus, and porphyria cutanea tarda. Modified from Rocco VK and Hurd ER [1].

vessels under ischemic conditions. In this regard, Fernandez *et al* reported that Ang II induced neovascularization in the rabbit cornea [6]. As discussed in detail below, some patients with scleroderma have sustained and significant increases in plasma renin activity (PRA), which in turn may cause a rise in circulating and local tissue Ang II, which might account for or contribute to these changes.

In addition to acral ischemia, varying degrees of visceral ischemia occur in scleroderma [1–4,7,8]. Perhaps Raynaud's phenomenon, which is an early event in scleroderma, causes or contributes to alterations in activity of the local vascular RAS, which then leads to more advanced abnormalities such as nailfold capillary changes, telangiectasias, and progressive skin, renal, and other organ dysfunction (Fig. 79.3). Surprisingly however, in other diseases, *de novo* Raynaud's phenomenon has been precipitated by ACE inhibitor therapy [9,10]. It is not likely that this is a common side effect. The scenario in Fig. 79.3 receives some support from a report that the powerful vasoconstrictor cocaine appeared to influence the development of scleroderma [11]. Indeed, reduced blood flow to the renal and pulmonary circulations is probably important in the development of scleroderma lung (interstitial fibrosis) and renal disease [1,7,8].

The role of the RAS in scleroderma-associated pulmonary hypertension has been partially explored. It is postulated that pulmonary hypertension in scleroderma develops as a result of vasoconstriction, intravascular obstruction secondary to endothelial swelling and intimal hyperplasia, or due to a reduction in the functional pulmonary vasculature secondary to interstitial fibrosis [7,8]. Infusions of cold saline, cause increases in intrapulmonary vascular resistance, a rise in pulmonary artery pressure, and functional abnormalities of gas exchange. This response is postulated to be mediated, in part, by renin release [7,8,62]. Hypoxia-induced pulmonary vasoconstriction is also believed to be influenced by the RAS [63]. In animals as well as in man, Ang II may contribute to increases in pulmonary arterial pressure, independent of its effects on the systemic blood pressure [63].

The therapeutic role of ACE inhibition in scleroderma-associated pulmonary hypertension is unclear. Sfikakis *et al* reported no effect on measured pulmonary vascular resistance or blood pressure with a single dose of captopril [64]. Other investigators have described varying results, depending on the duration of observation and treatment. Ikram *et al* treated patients with primary pulmonary hypertension for four days with captopril and noted a reduction in mean arterial pulmonary pressure [63]. Long-term definitive studies with ACE inhibitors have not been undertaken in scleroderma.

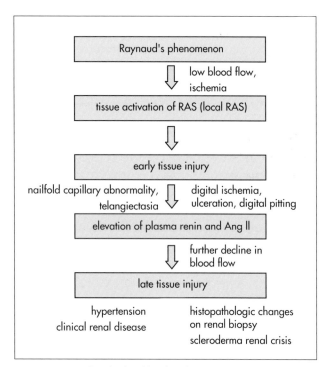

Fig. 79.3 Postulated role of local and systemic renin systems in progressive tissue injury in scleroderma.

Renal disease and hypertension are responsible for considerable morbidity and mortality in scleroderma [1]. Approximately 20% of patients die as a consequence of renal disease [12–15]. Cannon *et al* reported, in a study of 210 patients with 20 years of follow-up, that 45% had renal involvement as defined by the presence of hypertension (24%, with progression to the malignant phase in 7%), proteinuria (24%), or azotemia (19%) [14]. Other studies have found that 20% of patients with scleroderma develop renal failure and malignant hypertension [13] (*Chapter 56*). Renal involvement is noted typically 2–3 years after the diagnosis of scleroderma [1,12–15], and three patterns have been described. First, there may be rapidly progressive renal failure in association with malignant hypertension, central nervous system abnormalities, congestive heart failure, and microangiopathic hemolytic anemia. This syndrome is scleroderma renal crisis. The second is characterized by normal blood pressure or stable hypertension with rapidly progressive renal failure. The third is isolated proteinuria and azotemia [16–18]. There is very limited information regarding involvement of the RAS in the last of these three categories, but its role in the two former conditions is suggested from a review of the histopathology.

Generally, renal pathology in scleroderma is confined to the microcirculation of the cortex [1,12–18] where interlobular and arcuate vessels are most often affected. The presence of perivascular adventitial fibrosis helps to distinguish scleroderma from other causes of malignant hypertension [14]. Concentric proliferation of intimal cells between intact endothelium and internal elastic membranes and the deposition of a mucoid substance, leads to vascular occlusion and ischemia. Careful morphometric studies have confirmed the significance of these intimal changes, which typically appear in association with fibrinoid necrosis of small- and medium-sized vessels [18]. With the exception of adventitial fibrosis, the presence of concentric intimal prolifer-ation, vasospasm, smooth-muscle hyalinization, and ischemic necrosis (fibrinoid necrosis) are similar to the changes in malignant hypertension [19]. Damage to the vascular endothelium, fibrin deposition, and a microangiopathy are critical components in this syndrome, and deposition of complement and immunoglobulin have been reported [12,15]. Arteriography and xenon washout studies have confirmed a reduction in renal cortical blood flow [14].

Cannon *et al* [14] postulated that two factors act alone or in combination to reduce renal cortical blood flow and precipitate scleroderma renal crisis. They are vasoconstriction of renal cortical vessels, and mucoid intimal proliferation of the interlobular arteries [14]. The exact initiating events, however, have yet to be elucidated. Irrespective of the primary event(s), a series of changes occurs leading to increased renin release, high circulating and perhaps also high intrarenal levels of Ang II, exaggerated renal vasoconstriction, further reductions in renal cortical blood flow, and ultimately, acute renal failure [1]. Predictably, Ang II also increases total peripheral vascular resistance and blood pressure.

Several sites within the kidney are important targets for Ang II, including the afferent and efferent arterioles and the mesangial cells. The initial response of the intrarenal circulation to Ang II is to maintain the glomerular filtration rate by preferential constriction of the efferent arterioles as renal blood flow declines [20]. A progressive rise of Ang II concentration will then subsequently compromise both glomerular filtration and renal blood flow as the afferent arterioles constrict, inducing renal insufficiency and ischemia. Angiotensin II or similar substances have been implicated in the development of fixed structural lesions such as myointimal cell hypertrophy or hyperplasia, hyalinization of vessel-wall media, and fibrinoid necrosis, all of which are commonly seen in scleroderma renal crisis and malignant hypertension [20,21]. The RAS has also been implicated in proliferative responses in sites other than blood vessels, including the myocardium [22]. In this regard, patients with rapidly increasing skin involvement, anemia, pericarditis, or congestive heart failure appear to be at particular risk of developing scleroderma crisis [13].

Several factors are believed to contribute to the development of severe hypertension and/or renal failure in scleroderma. These include activation of the RAS and perhaps other circulating humoral substances which may damage the endothelium of renal vessels or affect intrarenal hemodynamics; alterations in intravascular volume (as a result of treatment with diuretics or calcium-channel blockers or as a consequence of a 'pressure natriuresis'); a decline in renal cortical perfusion (see earlier); and structural or functional changes in interlobular arteries including endothelial-cell proliferation, swelling, and collagen deposition, which may lead to vascular occlusion and ischemia [1,14,15].

Details of the interactions of these factors and the role of hypertension *per se* in the precipitation of acute renal failure are unclear. While hypertension may accelerate the progression of renal disease, Helfrich *et al* reported that accelerated renal failure may also occur in the absence of significant hypertension [16]. Indeed, 15 of 131 (11%) patients whose blood pressures were recorded at the University of Pittsburgh were normotensive during the course of rapidly progressive renal failure. Renin levels were measured in five of these normotensive patients and were high in every case [16]. Normotensive patients more often had microangiopathic hemolytic anemia and thrombocytopenia, and had received high doses of corticosteroids (prednisone, 30mg/d or greater) in the two months preceding scleroderma renal crisis. One-year survival in this group was significantly reduced, even when compared to patients with scleroderma renal crisis who had hypertension (13% versus 35% [16]). Nonsteroidal anti-inflammatory agents or other nephrotoxic drugs could not be implicated in this process. A minor increase in blood pressure to levels not expected to cause renal crisis or malignant hypertension has been implicated, but in Helfrich's series, the mean increase in diastolic blood pressure in 14 of 15 normotensive patients was only 7.5mmHg, and in only two patients was there an increase of 20mmHg [16].

Trostle has pointed out that the prevalence of hypertension in the 'normal' adult population is estimated at 20% and that a similar frequency exists in scleroderma [18]. Conversely, pre-existing hypertension in scleroderma does not predict evolution to scleroderma renal crisis [1,16]. Bennet *et al* described five patients with scleroderma and blood pressure in excess of 180/100mmHg who did not develop renal crisis [23].

These data support the view that although hypertension is an important contributor to the morbidity of scleroderma renal crisis, other factors such as changes in the RAS, endothelial-derived relaxing factors, cytokines, and endothelin, may play a more critical role in the evolution of this disorder.

A number of locally functioning renin systems, identified in several organs, and in vascular tissue, are postulated to function as autocrine, paracrine, or intracrine systems [24]. Angiotensinogen mRNA has been detected in many extrahepatic tissues [24], and it has been possible to demonstrate, by *in situ* hybridization, altered mRNA expression of renin and angiotensinogen at various sites in response to sodium depletion, experimental heart failure, and hypertension in the spontaneously hypertensive rat [25,26]. Abnormalities in these local tissue renin systems may be important in the pathogenesis of scleroderma kidney disease even in the absence of high circulating levels of renin and Ang II. These tissue renin systems might be responsible for the trophic and/or mitogenic abnormalities seen in the vasculature and kidneys which lead to progressive scleroderma and renal crisis, and may explain the progression of disease in the absence of systemic hypertension.

The importance of the RAS in scleroderma has been evaluated clinically by measurements of PRA. Gavras reported that high levels of PRA just preceded or coincided with the development of accelerated renal failure in 23 patients [27]. Renin levels, therefore, were suggested as predictive markers for renal crisis [27]. Other investigators, however, have found no correlation between PRA and the development of hypertension in scleroderma [12,28]. Indeed, Kovalchik *et al* reported prominent vascular abnormalities on renal biopsy in four patients who were normotensive and had normal renal function but who manifested an exaggerated renin response on cold pressor testing [12]. Steen and colleagues [13] described three patients with renal involvement and elevated PRA six months prior to the development of scleroderma renal crisis, but noted a similar number of patients with high PRA without clinical evidenc of renal disease or progression to renal crisis. These latter patients were normotensive, had normal renal function, and were not on diuretics [13].

In contrast marked hyperreninemia has been described in virtually all patients during scleroderma renal crisis. These data suggest that moderate elevations in PRA are not predictive of imminent renal involvement but that the RAS is important in the pathophysiology of scleroderma renal crisis. The role, if any, of local renin systems remains unexplored.

Scleroderma is to a large extent a microvascular endothelial disorder characterized by arterial thrombosis, occlusion, and tissue injury. Indices of endothelial injury have therefore been sought as markers of disease activity. In 17 patients with scleroderma and in nine with Raynaud's phenomenon, von Willebrand factor activity and von Willebrand factor antigen were significantly increased, suggesting the presence of endothelial injury [29]. These findings are not specific for scleroderma, however, since similar abnormalities have been described in diabetes mellitus, severe atherosclerosis, myocardial infarction, thromboembolic disease, and chronic renal failure. Diminished ACE activity was found in 26 patients with scleroderma (mean duration of disease 9.6 years) as compared with values in age- and sex-matched controls [30]. Patients receiving corticosteroids were excluded from the study since it is known that these drugs decrease high ACE levels in patients with sarcoidosis. The significance of these results is unclear but the investigators speculated that decreased endothelial ACE production may result from endothelial injury or interference by unknown circulating factors. Abnormalities of ACE activity have also been described in a number of other immune-mediated disorders including chronic active hepatitis, rheumatoid arthritis (see later), and granulomatous disorders such as leprosy and tuberculosis [31].

Claman has proposed a pathophysiologic scheme for scleroderma which incorporates vascular changes, immune dysfunction, and increased collagen synthesis (Fig. 79.4). In this model, elements of the vascular system (especially the endothelial cell), the immune system (via multiple cytokines and growth factors, the mast cell, and heparin-binding growth factors), and the

fibroblast (producing collagen) combine to cause scleroderma [32] although the precipitating event(s) is not specified. Heparin, a potent angiogenic factor, is released from mast cells, and bound and internalized by endothelial cells and which then release endothelial cell-derived growth factor. Other heparin-binding growth factors (which are produced by endothelium, macrophages, and fibroblasts) are released, including acidic and basic fibroblast growth factors (which in addition to being mitogenic for endothelial cells, stimulate fibroblasts). Platelet-derived growth factor and transforming growth factor-β stimulate fibroblasts and may be generated by platelets that are injured as a result of the vascular abnormalities described above. Multiple cytokines figure prominently in this proposed schema, with interleukins 3 and 4 being capable of activating mast cells. There is accumulating support for several elements of this model from both clinical investigation and laboratory studies. Goronzy and Weyand reported clinical improvement in scleroderma in two patients treated with a monoclonal antibody directed against T-cells bearing CD3+, CD4+ antigens [33].

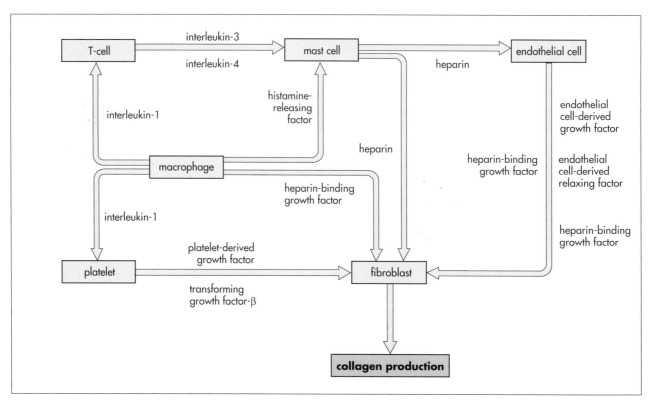

Fig. 79.4 The immune system in scleroderma. The interaction of cellular and humoral elements contributes to the formation of collagen and to the development of systemic sclerosis. The principal elements are the endothelial cell, the fibroblast, and other immunologically active cells including the mast cell, macrophage, and T-lymphocyte. Renin systems may be important in endothelial physiology and in growth factor production. Modified from Claman HN [32].

79.5

Does the RAS play a role in immune regulation? Several lines of evidence suggest that it may. High levels of components of the RAS system have been detected in a murine system of hepatic granulomata induced by schistosoma eggs. Angiotensin I, Ang II, and ACE were detected in the supernatants of cultured macrophages [34]. In this murine-induced granuloma system, pretreatment with captopril reduced granuloma size as well as ACE activity and Ang II levels [35]. Similarly, captopril has been reported to reduce the size of bacille Calmette–Guerin murine-induced granulomata [36]. Angiotensin II receptors have been expressed on human mononuclear leukocytes derived from schistosoma egg-induced granuloma [37]. A chemotactic role has also been ascribed to Ang II for human macrophages and T-lymphocytes from schistosoma-infected mice [37,38]. Furthermore, Ang II has a concentration-dependent effect on migration and phagocytosis by murine and rat peritoneal macrophages, respectively. Finally, in tissue culture experiments employing human aorta and pulmonary arterial endothelium, Ang II induced the production of a neutrophil chemoattractant, independent of the presence of bradykinin [39].

Although circulating ACE activity is sometimes reduced in scleroderma, plasma renin and Ang II levels are usually increased at least in renal crisis. There is accumulating evidence that renal failure which develops as a consequence of scleroderma renal crisis can be reversed by chemically distinct ACE inhibitors such as captopril and enalapril [40]. Improvement in renal function often occurs several months after ACE inhibitor-induced normalization of the blood pressure, which indirectly raises the possibility that nonvascular actions of the RAS are involved in the pathophysiology. It is important to recognize also that improvements in hemodynamic and renal function with ACE inhibitor therapy may result in part, from alterations in bradykinin and prostaglandin metabolism (see later). The extent to which the RAS influences growth factors other than Ang II, and cellular, immunologic, and endothelial function in scleroderma, awaits further investigation.

RHEUMATOID ARTHRITIS, SYSTEMIC LUPUS ERYTHEMATOSUS, AND OTHER CONNECTIVE TISSUE DISORDERS

The role of the RAS in rheumatoid arthritis, SLE, and other connective tissue disorders is just beginning to be explored. Studies have focused on monocyte production of ACE, as well as circulating levels of prorenin, renin, and ACE. The etiology of rheumatoid arthritis is unknown but class II gene products

(HLA-DR, DQ, DP) of the major histocompatibility complex appear important in its pathogenesis. In patients with rheumatoid factor activity (seropositive), HLA-DR4 confers a several-fold risk for developing rheumatoid arthritis. The earliest pathology within the joints includes microvascular injury, edema of the subsynovial tissues, and synovial lining proliferation. Over time, the synovial tissue hypertrophies and there are progressive vascular abnormalities including venous distention, capillary obstruction, thrombosis, and perivascular hemorrhage. The subsynovial stroma becomes filled with immunologically activated cells including T-lymphocytes (both CD4$^+$ and CD8$^+$ cells), plasma cells, and macrophages (antigen-presenting cells). The interplay between these cellular elements, antibodies (rheumatoid factors), and ingress of humoral agents results in a local inflammatory reaction that ultimately leads to pannus formation, joint effusions, and cartilage destruction [41].

Angiotensin-converting enzyme activity in serum and synovial fluid, and production of ACE by isolated monocytes have been evaluated in rheumatoid arthritis. Serum ACE activity was found to be normal in 48 patients by Lowe and colleagues [42]. Synovial fluid levels were higher in rheumatoid arthritis than in osteoarthritis, but when corrected for protein levels, were considered to be similar. Normal serum ACE activity was also reported in patients with osteoarthritis (11 patients), ankylosing spondylitis (24 patients), psoriatic arthritis (12 patients), and

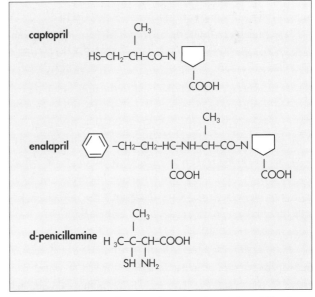

Fig. 79.5 Structures of captopril, enalapril, and d-penicillamine. The shared thiol group may be responsible for some common toxic effects.

Behçet's syndrome (20 patients). Very limited clinical information, however, was provided in this study. There was, for example, no comment regarding disease duration, drug therapy (specifically with corticosteroids), or seropositivity [42].

Machin *et al* found no significant changes in ACE activity in 21 patients with Sjögren's syndrome, 12 of whom had rheumatoid arthritis [43]. Decreased levels of ACE activity were described by Aoyagi *et al* in rheumatoid arthritis [44] whereas increased levels were described in five patients with rheumatoid arthritis and five with SLE by Sheikh and Kaplan [45]. These authors likewise provided little clinical information, making it difficult to reach firm conclusions.

Goto *et al* assayed ACE activity and interleukin-1 production by peripheral blood mononuclear cells in 32 patients with rheumatoid arthritis and 11 patients with osteoarthritis [46]. Serum ACE activity was normal in all groups, but mononuclear production of ACE was elevated in 29 of the 32 patients with rheumatoid arthritis. Interleukin-1 activity was increased in 11 of 32 patients. Most of the increase was in interleukin-1β. Monocytes from patients who had the disease for less than three years released more ACE and interleukin-1. These authors also reported (data not provided) that cells other than monocytes, including those from rheumatoid synovial membranes and nodules, produced increased amounts of ACE and interleukin-1. They suggested that this provides a rationale for the early use of monocyte inhibitors in the treatment of rheumatoid arthritis.

Angiotensin-converting enzyme levels, measured in bronchoalveolar lavage specimens from patients with interstitial fibrosis and rheumatoid arthritis, were not elevated [47].

It is interesting to note that captopril has been reported as an effective therapy for rheumatoid arthritis [48]. Due to its structural similarity to d-penicillamine, there has been debate as to whether its therapeutic properties rest in the thiol group that is present in both d-penicillamine and captopril (Fig. 79.5), or in its ability to inhibit ACE. Although this issue has yet to be resolved, Bird *et al* evaluated the effect of a nonthiol-containing ACE inhibitor and found no clinical or biochemical improvement in disease activity [49]. These authors argued therefore that ACE inhibition alone has little, if any therapeutic role in rheumatoid arthritis although no data regarding disease duration were provided in this study [49].

Plasma renin and prorenin levels were measured by Boers *et al* in 34 patients with rheumatoid arthritis, seven of whom had vasculitis before and five days after discontinuing nonsteroidal anti-inflammatory drugs [50]. As expected, renin and prorenin levels increased after stopping the anti-inflammatory drug. Median levels of prorenin and renin tended to be higher than in controls but most patients had levels within the normal range. Those with vasculitis, however, did have slightly elevated values for both renin and prorenin. These data continue to raise questions as to the role of the RAS in rheumatoid arthritis and in other immunologically mediated connective tissue disorders.

ANGIOTENSIN-CONVERTING ENZYME INHIBITOR THERAPY IN SCLERODERMA AND UNDIFFERENTIATED CONNECTIVE TISSUE DISEASE

At least three components of scleroderma and/or undifferentiated connective tissue disease may be influenced by the RAS and therefore by blockade of the RAS: the peripheral microvascular bed (Raynaud's phenomenon), sclerodermatous skin changes, and scleroderma renal crisis. This section focuses mainly on the effects of ACE inhibition on renal function in scleroderma renal crisis where there is the most compelling evidence for therapeutic benefit.

There are major problems in determining the efficacy of treatment in many connective tissue disorders since the natural history is variable with individuals showing unpredictable progression or spontaneous recovery. Nevertheless, it is clear that the onset and progression of scleroderma renal disease is heralded by stimulation of renin release and the subsequent generation of high circulating levels of Ang II (see *Fig. 79.3*) [1,2,12–17]. The primary stimulus to renin release is most likely at the level of the renal afferent arteriolar baroreceptor in response to diminished blood flow caused by intimal hyperplasia and/or superimposed Raynaud's phenomenon (see earlier) [12–17]. Despite modest success with the institution of dialysis, blood-pressure control with a number of agents, and bilateral nephrectomy, little change in the overall mortality of 75% [13] was achieved in scleroderma renal crisis until the advent of ACE inhibitors. There are now numerous reports that document the remarkable efficacy of ACE inhibitors in controlling blood pressure and slowing or reversing the progression of renal failure [13,40]. The effectiveness of these agents is most dramatic in the setting of dialysis-dependent renal failure where several reports confirm recovery of renal function in approximately 50% of patients even after several months of dialysis support [12,13,40]. This point is highlighted by a study from Pittsbrough which reported that 20 patients (55%) with scleroderma renal crisis who survived dialysis more than three months and continued ACE inhibitors were able to discontinue dialysis after 3–15 months compared with none of 15 patients who did not receive ACE inhibitors [65]. These authors also documented the dramatic improvement in one-year survival with ACE inhibitors (76%) compared to other forms of therapy (15%) in patients with scleroderma renal crisis.

It proved nearly impossible to predict which patients would recover renal function in scleroderma renal crisis prior to the widespread use of ACE inhibitors, although several risk factors for a poor outcome were identified, including the presence of advanced renal failure, inability to control hypertension, thrombocytopenia, and the presence of microangiopathic hemolytic anemia [13]. In the absence of these risk factors, the long-term outcome of patients with scleroderma and undifferentiated connective tissue disorders who recovered renal function, was excellent. Nevertheless, most investigators nowadays maintain such patients on ACE inhibitor therapy indefinitely despite the absence of long-term studies to support this practice.

The initial reports on the efficacy of ACE inhibition in scleroderma renal crisis were with captopril [51–54]. Similar efficacy seems likely with other ACE inhibitors [12,13,15,40] but there are no controlled trials that have formally compared individual ACE inhibitors in this disorder. Some reports have suggested that the sulfhydryl group in captopril (in common with d-penicillamine) may provide additional benefit from an anti-inflammatory action independent of effects on the RAS. (see Fig. 79.5) [55].

It is possible that recovery of renal function in scleroderma renal crisis with ACE inhibitors results not only from blockade of the circulating RAS, but also from inhibition of Ang II formation within the kidney and renal vessels, and increased levels of the potent vasodilator bradykinin. Indeed, it has been postulated that altered bradykinin metabolism may be important not only in scleroderma but also in the regulation of disease activity in rheumatoid arthritis [45,49], but there is no good evidence that this is so.

ACE inhibitors, especially captopril in excessive doses, have been reported to cause a variety of side effects including interstitial nephritis [56], vasculitis [57], proteinuria [58], and immunologic or bone marrow toxicity such as leukopenia, thrombocytopenia, and an SLE-like illness (see Chapter 99). Patients with diminished renal perfusion can develop a decline in glomerular filtration when ACE inhibitors are administered. This is particularly important in scleroderma where there is both a functional and pathologic compromise in renal blood flow. The RAS may initially preserve the glomerular filtration rate through relatively selective constriction of the renal efferent arterioles. If the RAS is blocked under these circumstances an acute fall in glomerular filtration may, at least in theory, ensue [59]. This could further accelerate the progression to renal failure. In addition, hyperkalemia may develop during ACE inhibition in patients with advanced and progressive renal disease [60].

Several reports have suggested that ACE inhibitors may be efficacious in the management of the cutaneous manifestations of scleroderma [13–15,51,53] and Raynaud's phenomenon (see Chapter 97). If this is so, one could postulate that circulating or tissue Ang II in scleroderma contributes to the pathogenesis through immune modulation, direct vasculotoxic and trophic effects, and a reduction in regional blood flow. Presently, however, there are no carefully controlled clincial trials to assess the efficacy of ACE inhibitors with regard to skin manifestations and especially Raynaud's phenomenon in scleroderma. It should also perhaps be pointed out that in other conditions, Raynaud's phenomenon has been reported as a side effect of therapy with both captopril [9] and enalapril [10].

Finally, Kahan and colleagues stated that captopril significantly decreased the number of segments with thallium 201 myocardial perfusion defects in 12 patients with scleroderma whereas no such effect was observed in eight other patients who did not receive an ACE inhibitor [61]. Further studies of larger number of patients with documentation of vascular and tissue effects of ACE inhibition versus other forms of treatment, are awaited.

REFERENCES

1. Rocco VK, Hurd EF. Scleroderma and scleroderma-like disorders. *Seminars in Arthritis and Rheumatism* 1986;16:22–69.

2. Lally EV, Jimenez SA, Kaplan SR. Progressive systemic sclerosis: Mode of presentation, rapidly progressive disease course, and mortality based on an analysis of 91 patients. *Seminars in Arthritis and Rheumatism* 1988;18:1–13.

3. Spencer–Green G. Raynaud phenomenon. *Bulletin on the Rheumatic Diseases* 1983;33:1–8.

4. Campbell PM, LeRoy C. Raynaud phenomenon. *Seminars in Arthritis and Rheumatism* 1986;16:92–103.

5. Belch JJF. Raynaud's phenomenon. *Current Opinion in Rheumatology* 1989;1:490–8.

6. Fernandez LA, Twickler J, Mead A. Neovascularization produced by angiotensin II. *Journal of Laboratory and Clinical Medicine* 1985;105:141–5.

7. Fahey PJ, Utell MJ, Condemi JJ, Green R, Hyde RW. Raynaud's phenomenon of the lung. *American Journal of Medicine* 1984;76:263–9.

8. Ohar JM, Robichaud AM, Fowler AA, Glauser FL. Increased pulmonary artery pressure in association with Raynaud's phenomenon. *American Journal of Medicine* 1986;81:361–2.

9. Havelka J, Vetter H, Studer A, Greminger P, Lüscher T, Wollnik S, Siegenthaler W, Vetter W. Acute and chronic effects of the angiotensin converting enzyme inhibitor captopril in severe hypertension. *American Journal of Cardiology* 1982;49:1467–74.

10. Hodsman GP, Brown JJ, Cumming AMM, Davies DL, East BW, Lever AF, Morton JJ, Murray GD, Robertson JIS. Enalapril in the treatment of hypertension with renal artery stenosis. *Journal of Hypertension* 1983;1 (suppl 1): 109–17.

11. Kerr HD. Cocaine and scleroderma. *Southern Medical Journal* 1989;82:1275–6.

12. Kovalchik MT, Guggenheim SJ, Silverman MH, Robertson JS, Steigerwald JC. The kidney in systemic sclerosis. A prospective study. *Annals of Internal Medicine* 1978;89:881–7.

13. Steen VD, Medsger TA, Osial TA, Ziegler GL, Shapiro AP, Rodnan GP. Factors predicting development of renal involvement in progressive systemic sclerosis. *American Journal of Medicine* 1984;76:779–86.

14. Cannon PJ, Hassar M, Case DB, Casarella WJ, Sommers SC, LeRoy C. The relationship of hypertension and renal failure in scleroderma (progressive systemic sclerosis) to structural and functional abnormalities of the renal cortical circulation. *Medicine* 1974;53:1–46.

15. Traub YM, Shapiro AP, Rodnan GP, Medsger TA, McDonald RH, Steen VD, Osial TA, Tolchin SF. Hypertension and renal failure (scleroderma renal crisis) in progressive systemic sclerosis. Review of a 25 year experience with 68 cases. *Medicine* 1983;62:335–52.

16. Helfrich DJ, Banner B, Steen VD, Medsger TA. Normotensive renal failure in systemic sclerosis. *Arthritis and Rheumatism* 1989;32:1128–34.

17. Heptinstall RH. Hemolytic uremic syndrome, thrombotic thrombocytopenic purpura and scleroderma (progressive systemic sclerosis). In: Heptinstall RH, ed. *Pathology of the Kidney*. Boston: Little, Brown and Company, 1983:938–61.

18. Trostle DC, Bedetti CD, Steen VD, Al-Sabbagh MR, Zee B, Medsger TA. Renal vascular histology and morphometry in systemic sclerosis. A case control autopsy study. *Arthritis and Rheumatism* 1988;31:393–400.

19. Kashgarian M. Pathology of small blood vessel disease in hypertension. *American Journal of Kidney Disease* 1985;5(4):A104–10.

20. Skorecki KL, Ballerman BJ, Rennke HG, Brenner BM. Angiotensin II receptor regulation in isolated renal glomeruli. *Federation Proceedings* 1983;41:3064–70.

21. Chapman PJ, Van Zyl-Smit P, Van Zyl-Smit R. Successful use of captopril in the treatment of 'scleroderma renal crisis.' *Clinical Nephrology* 1986;26:106–8.

22. Sweet CS. Issues surrounding a local cardiac renin system and the beneficial actions of angiotensin-converting enzyme inhibitors in ischemic myocardium. *American Journal of Cardiology* 1990;65:11–13I.

23. Bennet R, Bluestone R, Holt PJL, Bywaters EGL. Survival in scleroderma. *Annals of Rheumatic Diseases* 1971;30:581–8.

24. Frohlich ED, Iwata T, Sasaki O. Clinical and physiologic significance of local tissue renin–angiotensin systems. *American Journal of Medicine* 1989;87: 6B-19–23S.

25. Dzau VJ, Ingelfinger JR. Molecular biology and pathophysiology of the intrarenal renin–angiotensin system. *Journal of Hypertension* 1989;7 (Suppl):3–8.

26. Unger T, Gohlke P. Tissue renin–angiotensin system in the heart and vasculature: Possible involvement in the cardiovascular actions of converting enzyme inhibitors. *American Journal of Cardiology* 1990;65:3–10I.

27. Gavras H, Gavras I, Cannon PJ, Brunner HR, Laragh JH. Is elevated plasma renin activity of prognostic importance in progressive systemic sclerosis? *Archives of Internal Medicine* 1977;137:1554–8.

28. Fleischmajer R, Gould AB. Serum and renin substrate levels in scleroderma. *Proceedings of the Society for Experimental Biology and Medicine* 1975;150:374–9.

29. Kahaleh MB, Osborn I, LeRoy EC. Increased factor VIII/von Willebrand factor activity in scleroderma and in Raynaud's phenomenon. *Annals of Internal Medicine* 1981;94:482–4.

30. Matucci-Cerinic M, Pignone A, Lotti T, Spillantini G, Curradi C, Leoncini G, Iannone F, Falcini F, Cagnoni M. Reduced angiotensin converting enzyme plasma activity in scleroderma. A marker of endothelial injury? *Journal of Rheumatology* 1990;17:328–30.

31. Studdy P, Bird R, James GD, Sherlock S. Serum angiotensin converting enzyme in sarcoidosis and other granulomatous disorders. *Lancet* 1978;ii:1331–4.

32. Claman HN. On scleroderma. Mast cells, endothelial cells, and fibroblasts. *Journal of the American Medical Association* 1989;262:1206–9.

33. Goronzy JJ, Weyand CM. Long term immunomodulatory effects of T lymphocyte depletion in patients with systemic sclerosis. *Arthritis and Rheumatism* 1990;33:511–9.

34. Weinstock JV, Blum AM. Synthesis of angiotensin by cultured granuloma macrophages in murine schistosomiasis mansoni. *Cellular Immunology* 1987;107:273–80.

35. Weinstock JV, Ehrinpreis MN, Boros DL, Gee JB. Effect of SQ 14225, an inhibitor of angiotensin of angiotensin I-converting enzyme, on the granulomatous response to shistosoma mansoni eggs in mice. *Journal of Clinical Investigation* 1981;67:931–6.

36. Schrier DJ, Ripani LM, Katzenstein A, Moore VL. Role of angiotensin converting enzyme in bacille Calmette-Guerin-induced granulomatous inflammation. *Journal of Clinical Investigation* 1982;69:651–7.

37. Shimada K, Yazaki Y. Binding sites of angiotensin II in human mononuclear leukocytes. *Journal of Biochemistry* 1978;84:1013–5.

38. Weinstock JV, Kassab JT. Functional angiotensin II receptors on macrophages from isolated liver granulomas of murine schistosoma mansoni. *Journal of Immunology* 1984;132:2598–602.

39. Farber HW, Center DM, Rounds S, Danilov SM. Components of the angiotensin system cause release of a neutrophil chemoattractant from cultured bovine and human endothelial cells. *European Heart Journal* 1990;11 (suppl B):100–7.

40. Strongwater SL, Galvanek EG, Stoff JS. Control of hypertension and reversal of renal failure in undifferentiated connective tissue disease by enalapril. *Archives of Internal Medicine* 1989;149:582–5.

41. Zvaifler NJ. Rheumatoid arthritis. Epidemiology, etiology, rheumatoid factor, pathology, pathogenesis. In: Schumacher HR Jr, Klippel JH, Robinson DR, eds. *Primer on the rheumatic diseases*. Atlanta GA: Arthritis Foundation, 1988:83–7.

42. Lowe JR, Dixon JS, Guthrie JA, McWhinney P. Serum and synovial fluid levels of angiotensin converting enzyme in polyarthritis. *Annals of the Rheumatic Diseases* 1986;45:921–4.

43. Machin ND, Chard MD, Paice EW. Serum angiotensin converting enzyme in Sjogren's syndrome — a case report and study of 21 further cases. *Postgraduate Medical Journal* 1984;60:270–1.

44. Aoyagi T, Wada T, Kojima F, Nagai M, Akanuma Y, Akanuma H. Decreased serum levels of various hydrolytic enzymes in patients with rheumatoid arthritis. *Biochemistry International* 1985;8:529–35.

45. Sheikh IA, Kaplan AP. Assessment of kininases in rheumatic diseases and the effect of therapeutic agents. *Arthritis and Rheumatism* 1987;30:138–45.

46. Goto M, Fujisawa F, Yamada A, Okabe T, Takaku F, Sassano M, Nishioka K. Spontaneous release of angiotensin converting enzyme and interleukin 1 beta from peripheral blood monocytes from patients with rheumatoid arthritis under a serum free condition. *Annals of the Rheumatic Diseases* 1990;49:172–6.

47. Specks U, Martin II WJ, Rohrbach MS. Bronchoalveolar lavage fluid angiotensin-converting enzyme in interstitial lung disease. *American Review of Respiratory Diseases* 1990;141:117–23.

48. Martin MFR, McKenna F, Bird HA, Surrall KE, Dixon JS, Wright V. Captopril: A new treatment for rheumatoid arthritis? *Lancet* 1984;i:1325–8.

49. Bird HA, LeGallez P, Dixon JS, Catalano MA, Traficante A, Liauw L, Sussman H, Rotman H, Wright V. A clinical and biochemical assessment of a nonthiol ACE inhibitor (pentopril; CGS-12945) in active rheumatoid arthritis. *Journal of Rheumatology* 1990;17:603–8.

50. Boers M, Breedveld FC, Dijkmans BAC, Chang PC, van Brummelen P, Derkx FHM, Cats A. Raised plasma renin and prorenin in rheumatoid vasculitis. *Annals of the Rheumatic Diseases* 1990;49:517–20.

51. Lopez–Ovejero JA, Saal SD, D'Angelo WA, Cheigh JS, Stenzel KH, Laragh JH. Reversal of vascular and renal crises of scleroderma by oral angiotensin converting enzyme blockade. *New England Journal of Medicine* 1979;300: 1417–9.

52. Zawada ET Jr, Clements PJ, Furst DA, Bloomer HA, Paulus HE, Maxwell MH. Clinical course of patients with scleroderma renal crisis treated with captopril. *Nephron* 1981;27:74–8.

53. Sorenson LB, Paunicka K, Harris M. Reversal of scleroderma renal crisis for more than two years in a patient treated with captopril. *Arthritis and Rheumatism* 1983;26:797–801.

54. Thurm RH, Alexander JC. Captopril in the treatment of scleroderma renal crisis. *Archives of Internal Medicine* 1984;144:733–5.

55. Igic RP, Gafford JT, Erdos EG. Effect of captopril on proteins and peptide hormones. *Biochemical Pharmacology* 1981;30:683–5.

56. Smith WR, Neill J, Cushman WC, Butkus DE. Captopril-associated acute interstitial nephritis. *American Journal of Nephrology* 1989;9:230–5.

57. Barlow RJ, Schulz EJ. Lisinopril-induced vasculitis. *Clinical and Experimental Dermatology* 1988;13:117–20.

58. Case DB, Atlas SA, Mouradian JA, Fishman RA, Sherman RL, Laragh JH. Proteinuria during long-term captopril therapy. *Journal of the American Medical Association* 1980;244:346–9.

59. Navar IG, Rosivall L. Contribution of the renin angiotensin system to the control of intrarenal hemodynamics. *Kidney International* 1984;25:857–68.

60. Atlas SA, Case DB, Sealey JE, Laragh JH, McKinney DN. Interruption of the renin–angiotensin system in hypertensive patients by captopril induces sustained reduction in aldosterone secretion, potassium retention and natriuresis. *Hypertension* 1979;1:274–80.

61. Kahan A, Devaux JY, Amor B, Menkes CJ, Weber S, Venot A, Strauch G. The effect of captopril in thallium 201 myocardial perfusion in systemic sclerosis. *Clinical Pharmacology and Therapeutics* 1990;47:483–9.

62. Ohar J, Polatty C, Robichaud A, Fowler A, Vetrovec G, Glauser F. The role of vasodilators in patients with systemic sclerosis. Interstitial lung disease and pulmonary hypertension. *Chest* 1985;88:263–5S.

63. Ikram H, Maslowski AH, Nicholls MG, Espiner EA, Hull FT. Haemodynamic and hormonal effects of captopril in primary pulmonary hypertension. *British Heart Journal* 1982;48:541–5.

64. Sfikakis PP, Kyriakidis MK, Vergos CG, Vyssoulis GP, Psarros TK, Kyriakidis CA, Mavrikakis ME, Sfikakis PP, Toutouzas PK. Cardiopulmonary hemodynamics in systemic sclerosis and response to nifedipine and captopril. *American Journal of Medicine* 1991;90:541–6.

65. Steen VD, Costantino JP, Shapiro AP, Medsger TA. Outcome of renal crisis in systemic sclerosis: Relation to availability of angiotensin converting enzyme (ACE) inhibitors. *Annals of Internal Medicine* 1990;113:352–7.

80

THE EFFECT OF DRUGS ON THE RENIN–ANGIOTENSIN SYSTEM IN MAN

JOHN K DOIG, KENNEDY R LEES, AND JOHN L REID

INTRODUCTION

Renin is released from the renal juxtaglomerular apparatus by four mechanisms (see *Chapter 24*):

- *Intrarenal receptors*, including baroreceptors which respond to stretch of the afferent arterial wall and are therefore sensitive to changes in plasma volume or renal hemodynamics, and the macula densa which is sensitive to the amount of sodium chloride delivered to the distal nephron. These mechanisms themselves may be dependent on synthesis and release of prostaglandins which act in a local autocrine manner in stimulating the juxtaglomerular apparatus.

- *Sympathetic mechanisms*, where β-adrenoceptor activation, as a result of stimulation of the renal sympathetic nerves or circulating catecholamines, has a direct stimulatory effect on juxtaglomerular renin release.

- *Humoral factors*, including those which either stimulate (for example, prostaglandins and catecholamines) or inhibit (for example, Ang II, potassium, aldosterone, and atrial natriuretic factor — ANF) renin release.

- *Intracellular second messenger mechanisms*, within the juxtaglomerular cell, with cAMP being important in stimulating of renin release and calcium ions inhibiting renin release.

These mechanisms are interrelated. Drugs may therefore influence the RAS by either direct or indirect interaction with one of the controlling mechanisms of renin release (Fig. 80.1).

The drugs that are considered in this chapter are those that have a direct interaction with the above mechanisms. Angiotensin-converting enzyme inhibitors and inhibitors of renin and Ang II are covered more fully in *Chapters 85–87*: these latter drugs will be discussed only with reference to their interaction with other agents. Beta-adrenoceptor antagonists are also considered in detail in *Chapter 84* and are therefore only briefly included in this review.

It is emphasized that while some experimenters have assessed renin secretion as such [1–3], more often, and especially in intact animals and man, the effect of drugs in either stimulating or inhibiting renin release is inferred from changes in plasma renin levels. Although such inferences are generally true, plasma renin values are subject to other influences (such as clearance rate). Nevertheless, in many of the papers discussed herein, the term 'renin release' is used in this inferential sense.

DRUGS AFFECTING THE SYMPATHETIC AND ADRENERGIC MECHANISMS

Stimulation of the sympathetic nervous system results in renin release and therefore drugs interacting with the sympathetic nervous system will modulate renin release. Agonists and antagonists of α- and β-receptors are also associated with systemic and renovascular hemodynamic responses which could independently affect renin release by activation of renal baroreceptors, altering sodium delivery to the macula densa, or via secondary sympathetic activation (Fig. 80.2).

ALPHA AGONISTS AND ANTAGONISTS

De Leeuw *et al* [1–3] have studied hypertensive patients undergoing diagnostic renal angiography with regard to the role of α-adrenergic receptors in renin release. Intrarenal arterial infusions of the selective α_1-antagonist, doxazosin, did not increase basal or exercise-induced renin secretion [1,2]. However, infusions of the nonselective α-antagonist, phentolamine, and the selective α_2-antagonist, yohimbine, significantly increased both basal and exercise-induced renin secretion, in association with an increase in renal perfusion and norepinephrine secretion [2,3]. Pretreatment with atenolol blocked the renin response to yohimbine but not the increase in norepinephrine release [3]. It appears that α_2-adrenoceptors are important in inhibition of renin release, probably at a prejunctional site.

There have also been many noninvasive studies investigating the effects of α-antagonists on the RAS. Systemic α-adrenergic antagonism, however, causes systemic hemodynamic effects with secondary activation of the sympathetic nervous system which alone could stimulate renin release.

Phentolamine activates the RAS with a fall in blood pressure and an increase in heart rate [4,5]. At low rates of intravenous infusion (0.5μg/min), however, a two-fold increase in plasma renin activity (PRA) is observed, with little effect on mean arterial blood pressure or heart rate, though this is blocked by pretreatment with the β-blocker, oxprenolol [5]. Phentolamine [6] and prazosin [7] also enhance insulin-induced activation of the RAS during hypoglycemia.

Although early reports suggested that the α_1-adrenoceptor antagonist, prazosin, may reduce blood pressure without an increase in PRA [8,9], there are now several acute studies demonstrating an increase in PRA [10,11], active renin concentration, and Ang II [12] in association with a fall in blood pressure and increased plasma norepinephrine levels. Furthermore, there is a strong inverse relationship between the first-dose acute fall in erect blood pressure and basal PRA. The absolute increase in PRA is greater in hypertensive patients who have a high basal PRA, these patients tending not to develop significant postural hypotension [11]. This suggests that activation of the RAS is an important homeostatic mechanism in prevention or limitation of first-dose hypotension with α_1-antagonists.

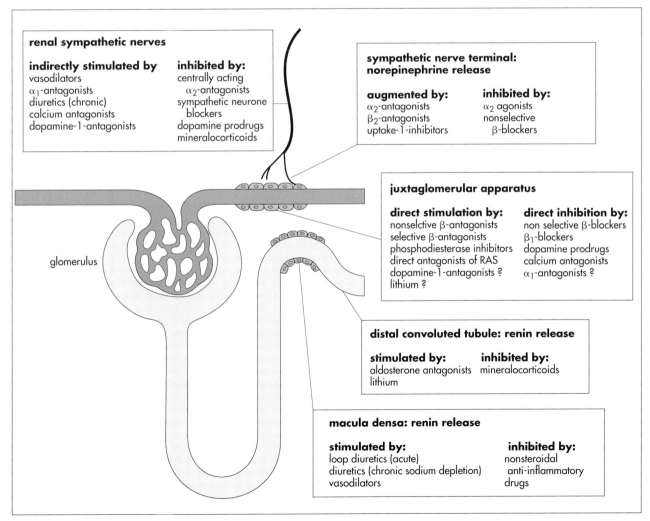

Fig. 80.1 Mode of interaction of drugs with renal renin release.

Doxazosin, which has a longer half-life than prazosin, also results in significant first-dose blood-pressure reduction with associated secondary activation of the sympathetic nervous system. There is, however, no associated activation of the RAS in patients with essential hypertension [13,14]. This may reflect doxazosin's more gradual onset of hypotensive effect: there may be no direct antagonistic effect of α_1-antagonists on renin release, only activation in response to a reduction in blood pressure. This would be in keeping with the observations of De Leeuw *et al* [1,2] using intrarenal arterial infusions.

Type	Drug	Mechanisms affecting renin release	References
nonselective α-antagonists	phentolamine	reflex sympathetic activation	2–6
		presynaptic augmentation of norepinephrine release	
selective α_1-antagonists	prazosin	reflex activation of sympathetic nervous system	7,10,11, 12
		possible direct antagonism of α-adrenergic inhibitory receptors	
selective α_2-antagonists	yohimbine RX 781094	augment presynaptic norepinephrine release	2,3,19
nonselective β-agonists	isoproterenol	predictable direct stimulation of renin release	29–33
selective β_2-agonists	prenalterol	variable direct stimulation of renin release	37–41
	dobutamine	?inhibition via systemic baroreflexes	
selective β_2-agonists	salbutamol	variable stimulation of renin release	29,33,36, 37
	fenoterol	presynaptic augmentation of norepinephrine release and induction of hypokalemia	

Fig. 80.2 Sympathetic and adrenergic drugs that stimulate renin release.

Prazosin also potentiates the PRA response to isoproterenol infusion [15]. While enhancement of a direct renal hemodynamic effect can not be excluded to explain this, α_1- as well as α_2- adrenoceptors may inhibit renin release.

There is no evidence that α_1-antagonists significantly activate the RAS following chronic treatment of volunteers [16], patients with essential hypertension [12–14,17], or patients with congestive cardiac failure [18].

The α_2-antagonist, yohimbine, significantly stimulates basal renin release when infused into the renal artery [2,3]. Intravenous infusion of the α_2-antagonist, RX 781094, in normal volunteers increases PRA by 200% after 20 minutes. The increase in PRA is associated with a 60% increase in plasma norepinephrine levels and a small but significant pressor response [19]. This is consistent with α_2-adrenergic inhibition of renin release in man.

The centrally acting α_2-adrenoceptor agonist, clonidine, has been reported either to suppress PRA [20–23] or to have little effect [23–25], despite significant blood-pressure reductions which alone should stimulate renin release.

Clonidine exerts its antihypertensive effect mainly by central inhibition of sympathetic tone [26]. Its inhibitory effect on PRA may be secondary to the reduction in sympathetic tone. Experimentally, clonidine has a direct inhibitory effect on renin release at the level of renal adrenoceptors [27]. In man, however, intrarenal infusion of the α_2-agonist, B-HT933, does not alter renin release [2]. In view of the significantly enhanced renin release following renal infusion of α_2-antagonists [2,3] and the lack of response to renal infusion of an α_2-agonist, it appears that α_2-adrenoceptors tonically suppress renin release. Any effect observed on PRA following parenteral administration of clonidine is likely to be secondary to a central effect.

In patients with essential hypertension, clonidine significantly reduces PRA, in association with a fall in blood pressure and decreased plasma norepinephrine levels, both acutely and chronically [20–22]. There is a significant correlation between the fall in blood pressure and decrease in PRA following a single day's therapy [20] but not after chronic treatment [21].

Suppression of the RAS may therefore contribute to the acute fall in blood pressure following administration of clonidine, but effects on the RAS do not appear to influence the chronic response to clonidine.

In hypertensive patients with renal parenchymal disease, single doses of clonidine also reduce blood pressure, PRA (64%), and plasma norepinephrine levels (50%) [25], though the reduction in PRA is not observed after chronic treatment [28]. No reduction in PRA is observed in patients with renovascular hypertension, however, despite reduced plasma norepinephrine levels [23,26]. In renovascular hypertension, the increased PRA is probably not driven by sympathetic stimulation.

In conclusion, stimulation of α-adrenoceptors inhibits renin release in man. This is primarily mediated by the α_2 subtype, both peripherally at the presynaptic sympathetic nerve terminal and in the central nervous system. Although α_1-adrenoceptors may also inhibit renin release, antagonists may stimulate renin secretion by producing systemic vasodilation, resulting in hypotension and secondary activation of the sympathetic nervous system.

BETA-AGONISTS AND ANTAGONISTS

Beta-adrenoceptor activation of the juxtaglomerular cells is one of the major stimulatory pathways for renin release. The non-selective β-agonist, isoproterenol, invariably increases PRA in man [29–33]. During intravenous infusion of isoproterenol, there is a dose-related increase in PRA [29,30] of up to 500% [29]. The peak response occurs rapidly, within 10 minutes of intravenous administration to volunteers [30].

Sympathetic-induced renin release is probably mediated mainly via the β_1-adrenoceptor. Pretreatment of volunteers with the cardioselective β_1-blockers, atenolol, acebutolol, metoprolol, or betaxolol, all block the PRA response to an isoproterenol infusion almost as efficiently as propranolol [29,31].

The cardioselective β-blockers also inhibit both resting and exercise-induced renin release [34,35]. However, the selective β_2-receptor antagonist, ICI 118151, which has 200 times greater affinity for β_2- than for β_1-adrenoceptors, does not suppress resting or exercise-induced increase in plasma renin activity [35].

Evidence for β_1-mediated renin release in man is less conclusive when studies using selective β-agonists are used. There have been reports that the selective β_2-agonists, salbutamol and fenoterol, stimulate renin release [36,37] as well as fail to stimulate renin release [29,30,32,33]. Beta$_2$-agonists also induce a significant reduction in serum potassium and increase plasma norepinephrine levels [36,37] and therefore the increase in PRA may not be a result of direct interaction with juxtaglomerular β_2-adrenoceptors.

Similarly, there are conflicting results on renin release with the selective β_1-agonist prenalterol [37–40] and with dobutamine [29,41] which also has β_2-agonistic activity as well as a high affinity for α-adrenoceptors.

Overall, β_1-adrenoceptors are probably the main adrenergic receptors involved in stimulation of renin release. The reason for failure of selective β-agonists to stimulate renin release predictably, and with potency equivalent to isoproterenol, is not clear, though it could be a result of activation of mechanisms that inhibit renin release. Beta$_1$-agonists produce inotropic, chronotropic, and pressor effects which may in turn, inhibit sympathetic stimulation of the juxtaglomerular cells. Other possibilities include alterations in renal hemodynamics or electrolyte excretion, or partial agonist effects, or it might be that the β-adrenoceptor involved in renin release may not fit the normal classification of β-adrenoceptors.

Effects of β-adrenergic blockade on renin release are discussed in detail in *Chapter 84*.

DOPAMINERGIC AGONISTS AND ANTAGONISTS

In 1969, Barbeau *et al* [42] demonstrated that patients with Parkinson's disease treated with levodopa had significantly reduced PRA when compared with a control group of untreated patients. The PRA of the control patients fell to unrecordable levels after commencing treatment. It was inferred that dopamine inhibits renin secretion.

The effect of dopamine on the RAS appears to depend on the dose, probably as a result of varying effects on dopamine DA$_1$ and DA$_2$ receptors and on α- and β-adrenergic receptors.

When given by intravenous infusion in low doses, $3\mu g/kg/min$, dopamine does not produce systemic hemodynamic effects or a change in PRA, but does increase renal blood flow, and produces a natriuresis and increased renal prostaglandin production [43,44].

At a higher dose of $4\mu g/kg/min$, significant pressor effects have been observed, with slight, but not significant, increases in PRA [45]. At a yet higher dose level of $9\mu g/kg/min$, dopamine produces pressor effects with significant elevation of PRA [46]. At concentrations achieved with this dose, dopamine would produce adrenergic effects and therefore the increase in PRA may not be a direct and specific dopaminergic receptor effect.

Studies with the prodrugs levodopa and gludopa have produced results more in keeping with the observation of Barbeau *et al* [42]. Levodopa, unlike dopamine, crosses the blood–brain barrier and is decarboxylated to dopamine both peripherally and in the central nervous system.

In normal volunteers, levodopa induces a natriuresis, with increased effective renal plasma flow, but little, if any, pressor effect. However, PRA is reduced by 50% after an intravenous infusion ($7\mu g/kg/min$) [47] or with oral levodopa 500mg [48]. The PRA response to an erect posture is inhibited [45] and there is also a significant suppression of plasma aldosterone levels which precedes the fall in PRA. This suggests that dopamine directly inhibits aldosterone secretion [48].

Gludopa, another dopamine prodrug, is transformed to dopamine by gamma-glutamyl transferase, and by L-dopa decarboxylase. When given to volunteers by intravenous infusion at 12.5μg/kg/min or above, gludopa also produces significant reductions in PRA without a pressor effect. However, there is a dose-related natriuresis, an increase in effective renal plasma flow, and an increase in urinary dopamine excretion [49,50].

The activity of gamma-glutamyl transferase in the kidney is 200 times higher than in the central nervous system. It is therefore likely that the major site of dopamine production from gludopa is in the periphery and that the suppression of PRA by dopamine is a peripheral effect. Certainly, the suppression of PRA, but not the natriuretic effect of gludopa, is blocked by pretreatment with domperidone, a DA_2 antagonist that does not cross the blood–brain barrier [51].

Similarly, Lightman et al [45] demonstrated that concurrent use of carbidopa (an inhibitor of peripheral dopa-decarboxylase) antagonizes the levodopa-induced decrease in PRA, although others have not confirmed this [48].

In keeping with dopamine exerting an inhibitory effect on renin secretion, metoclopramide, a drug which has predominantly DA_2 antagonistic activity, may either enhance PRA [52–54] or have no effect [55–57]. The dopaminergic system assumes greater importance in salt-depleted states, when metoclopramide induces greater increments in PRA, Ang II, and aldosterone than in salt-replete subjects [53]. All of these studies, however, have demonstrated a significant increase in plasma aldosterone [52–57] within 15 minutes of metoclopramide administration. This effect is not blocked by previous ACE inhibition, and therefore appears to be independent of changes in the RAS.

Chlorpromazine also produces a dose-related increase in PRA, peaking at 60 minutes after administration. The rise in aldosterone after chlorpromazine, however, seems to be more closely related to the RAS than that associated with metoclopramide [58].

Dopaminergic receptors may be directly involved in stimulating renin release. The DA_1-receptor agonist, fenoldopam, which is a potent vasodilator, significantly enhances PRA [59–61]. This is associated with increases in effective renal plasma flow and glomerular filtration rate (GFR), and a fall in blood pressure with a reflex tachycardia. The rise in PRA is not observed in hypertensive patients who are taking β-blockers, despite a large fall in blood pressure and increased heart rate [62,63]. This suggests that the stimulation of PRA may be mediated via secondary activation of renal sympathetic nerves. There is, however, in vitro and in vivo evidence in animals which suggests a direct DA_1 mechanism in renin release that is independent of sympathetic or macula densa mechanisms [64,65].

In conclusion, it appears that renin secretion in man is inhibited via a peripheral dopamine receptor most probably of the DA_2 subtype. The role of the DA_1 receptor is less clear. This receptor may be involved in direct stimulation of renin release but sympathetic activation secondary to hypotension also occurs. Central suppression of the sympathetic nervous system may contribute to diminution of renin release following levodopa.

OTHER SYMPATHOLYTIC AND VASODILATOR DRUGS

Sympathetic blocking drugs such as the ganglion-blocking agents [106], reserpine [107], and methyldopa [107,108] reduce blood pressure without an associated renin response in hypertensive patients; indeed PRA may fall [107,108]. The inhibitory effect on renin release is unlikely to contribute significantly to the hypotensive effect of these drugs as any change in renin is usually modest.

Conversely, guanethidine, which inhibits postganglionic adrenergic transmission, reportedly stimulates PRA in patients with low-renin hypertension [109], an effect which could be explained by reductions in renal blood flow and GFR which are not observed following treatment with methyldopa. Despite depleting catecholamines at sympathetic nerve terminals, guanethidine also possesses uptake inhibitory effects and does not inhibit adrenal medullary catecholamines which may contribute to stimulation of renin release.

Unlike the direct-acting vasodilators, ketanserin, a type 2 5-hydroxytryptamine antagonist with also some a_1-adrenoceptor blocking activity, inconsistently and only transiently activates the RAS in volunteers [110,111] or hypertensive patients [112].

CALCIUM ANTAGONISTS

Intracellular calcium is reported to inhibit renin release and to augment Ang II-induced aldosterone production and vasoconstriction [66]. One would therefore expect calcium antagonists to stimulate renin release via a direct action of reduced calcium transport into juxtaglomerular cells.

Most calcium antagonists are vasodilators, reducing peripheral vascular resistance and systemic blood pressure, which reflexly activates the sympathetic nervous system. Several also have an initial diuretic and natriuretic action [67–69]. These effects should cause indirect activation of the RAS.

In man, there is, however, great variability in reports of activation of the RAS by calcium antagonists, depending on the type of drug, the dose used, the duration of treatment, the timing of investigation after drug administration [70], the age of the subject, and the type of population studied, that is, hypertensive or normotensive.

After single-dose administration of the dihydropyridine derivatives, acute activation of the RAS usually occurs in normotensive and hypertensive subjects, reflected by increased PRA and Ang II. This activation is associated with a reduction in blood pressure and stimulation of the sympathetic nervous system, as indicated by a tachycardia and increased plasma norepinephrine levels [71–73]. No associated rise in plasma aldosterone concentration has, however, been observed. There are also other reports that each of these drugs fails to activate the RAS [67,74,75], and after long-term treatment, there is little evidence that any calcium antagonist activates the RAS to a significant degree [76–78].

Age has an important effect on the ability of nifedipine to activate the RAS. Volunteers with a mean age of 28 and young patients with essential hypertension (mean age 24), showed significant activation of the RAS with increments of PRA of 80% and 65%, respectively, and increases in Ang II of 35% and 30%, respectively. However, older volunteers (mean age 56), and older hypertensive patients (mean age 58), showed no significant activation of the RAS with the same single oral dose of nifedipine (10mg), despite greater reductions in blood pressure and similar increases in heart rate [79].

Following prolonged treatment from 6 to 16 weeks, there is no evidence that nifedipine results in any significant activation of the RAS despite sustained reduction in blood pressure and evidence of sustained increase in sympathetic activity as reflected by increased plasma norepinephrine levels [76,77]. Failure of activation of the RAS in these circumstances may be explained by substantial retention of total body sodium during chronic treatment with nifedipine [80].

Pretreatment of hypertensive patients with either atenolol or metoprolol blocks the renin response to felodipine [81,82], and in situations where dihydropyridine calcium antagonists have not lowered blood pressure or increased plasma norepinephrine levels, there has been no rise in PRA or plasma renin concentration (PRC) [67,75,83].

The homoveratrylamine derivatives, verapamil and triapamil, and the benzazepine derivative, diltiazem, have consistently shown no activation of the RAS in normal volunteers or patients with essential hypertension following either single doses [67,84] or long-term treatment [85–87]. Why these calcium antagonists do not activate the RAS is not clear. It may reflect a reduced

peripheral vasodilator effect and less stimulation of the sympathetic nervous system than is achieved by the dihydropyridine derivatives. In keeping with this, these calcium antagonists do not increase plasma norepinephrine levels [84,86,87].

Overall, these results suggest that activation of the sympathetic nervous system is, in part, responsible for the stimulation of renin release following calcium antagonist administration. The degree of activation of the sympathetic nervous system with nitrendipine [88,89], however, as reflected by increased heart rate and serum catecholamines, appears to be less than that produced by nifedipine, despite greater increases in PRA. This indicates that other mechanisms such as a direct juxtaglomerular action, natriuretic effect, or alteration in renal hemodynamics, may be involved.

The main mechanism by which calcium antagonists appear to interact with the RAS is by reducing the pressor effect of Ang II. Evidence for this is provided by studies in volunteers which show that all types of calcium antagonists produce a shift to the right in the Ang II pressor dose–response curve [75,85,90,91]. This is nonspecific, since the pressor dose–response curve of norepinephrine is similarly shifted to the right [84].

Acute administration of nifedipine [91] and felodipine [69] attenuates the aldosterone response to administration of Ang II. After prolonged treatment [92,93], the effect on the aldosterone response is not observed although attenuation of the pressor response to Ang II persists [92].

No attenuation of aldosterone's response to Ang II was observed after administration of verapamil [94], nicardipine [75], or isradipine [95].

In conclusion, stimulation of the RAS by dihydropyridine calcium antagonists is transient and occurs mainly as a result of secondary activation of the sympathetic nervous system. In hypertensive patients, the increase in Ang II levels is of little significance in the homeostatic blood-pressure response, particularly as the pressor response of Ang II is attenuated.

DIRECT VASODILATORS

Vasodilating agents that have a direct action on vascular smooth muscle include hydralazine, minoxidil, and diazoxide. They have all been used in the treatment of hypertension or congestive cardiac failure. Their use, however, is now limited due to symptomatic side effects. They usually have to be given with diuretics and β-blockers. They have been largely superseded by ACE inhibitors and calcium antagonists.

Vasodilating drugs have been reported to activate the RAS [96–99]. This is associated with significant reductions in blood pressure, with tachycardia, and with increased plasma norepinephrine concentrations, indicating secondary generalized sympathetic nervous activation.

The increase in PRA correlates positively with the increase in plasma norepinephrine concentration and negatively with the change in mean arterial pressure following oral hydralazine [96]. Pretreatment with β-blockers significantly attenuates the renin response to hydralazine [97], minoxidil [98], or diazoxide [100], thus indicating the importance of sympathetic activation stimulating renin release following administration of vasodilators.

Other mechanisms that could be involved in renin release following administration of vasodilators include reduced renal perfusion and/or an antinatriuretic effect [101] which may result in activation of renal baroreceptors or macula densa mechanisms.

In patients with congestive cardiac failure, the effect of vasodilators on the RAS is less profound, with some reports demonstrating activation with significant increments in PRA [102,103] and others showing no overall effect [104,105]. In these patients, small depressor responses have been observed; however, there is a marked increase in cardiac output secondary to reduced vascular resistance [104,105] which may suppress secondary activation of the sympathetic nervous system and therefore activation of the RAS.

NONSTEROIDAL ANTI-INFLAMMATORY DRUGS

Prostaglandins are important mediators of renin release in man and animals. In particular, stimulation of renin release via the macula densa and renal baroreceptors appears to be prostaglandin dependent, with prostaglandin PGI_2 (prostacyclin) being the most attractive direct mediator [113–115]. Prostaglandins are also involved in the control of electrolyte excretion and of renal and systemic hemodynamics (see *Chapter 38*). Inhibitors of prostaglandin synthetase may therefore inhibit renin release directly, particularly in situations where the macula densa or baroreceptor mechanisms have been activated, and also indirectly by salt and water retention, pressor effects, and alterations in renal blood flow [116].

Indomethacin reduces PRA in normal recumbent salt-replete volunteers by over 50% after single or multiple dosing [117–120], with continued suppression of PRA for over 12 hours following a single dose [117]. This is associated with moderate or significant reduction in sodium excretion [118,119,121].

The reduction in PRA is associated with equal reductions in total renin and prorenin as measured by acid activation [122] and by direct immunological techniques [123], that is, there is no significant alteration in the active:total renin ratio after one week's treatment; 24-hour aldosterone excretion is reduced after one week's treatment with indomethacin.

When sodium intake in volunteers is moderately restricted (60mmol/d), indomethacin again causes significant suppression of basal PRA by 60% after three days [118]. Under conditions of severe sodium-restriction (10mmol/d) in normal volunteers, however, indomethacin did not reduce basal PRA or posturally stimulated PRA. In contrast, in a group of hypertensive patients on the same sodium-restricted diet, and pretreated with β-blockers, indomethacin inhibited both basal and posturally stimulated PRA. Under conditions of severe sodium restriction, both prostaglandins and sympathetic stimulation appear important in stimulation of renin release [124]. These findings, however, should be interpreted cautiously since the two groups of subjects were not entirely comparable, and a crossover volunteer study would have been more appropriate.

In volunteers, the reduction in PRA and renin concentration is associated with reduced excretion of urinary prostaglandins [120–122]. There is, however, no effect on basal GFR as measured by creatinine or inulin clearance, or on basal renal plasma flow as measured by p-aminohippurate clearance [118,121].

In patients with essential hypertension, indomethacin significantly suppresses PRA by 70–90% in association with reduced urinary excretion of PGE_2 and 6-keto-$PGF_{1\alpha}$ (the stable metabolic product of prostacyclin) [125,126]. A mild pressor effect occurs which antagonizes the antihypertensive action of β-blockers, diuretics, and converting-enzyme inhibitors. This may result from reduced concentrations of vasodilator prostaglandins, rather than by interaction with the RAS. Other nonsteroidal anti-inflammatory drugs, including piroxicam and ibuprofen, antagonize antihypertensive agents but there is less evidence that this occurs with sulindac or aspirin [127].

Short-term treatment (three days) with the prostaglandin synthetase inhibitor, oxindac, inhibits basal PRA by 50% in normal volunteers on a controlled daily sodium intake of 120mmol [128]. However, short-term treatment with ibuprofen (400mg or 800mg three times daily for three days) does not significantly affect basal PRA in either sodium-replete or moderately sodium-restricted volunteers [118,129]. Similarly, short-term treatment with low-dose aspirin [130], sulindac [131], or naproxen [129] does not significantly affect basal PRA.

After six days' treatment with ibuprofen or sulindac, however, volunteers have shown significant reductions in basal renin activity of 55% and 30%, respectively [132]. Likewise, seven days' treatment with naproxen or sulindac resulted in reductions of PRA by 38% and 22%, respectively, this time in patients with rheumatoid arthritis [133].

The lack of suppression of basal PRA after short-term treatment with most nonsteroidal anti-inflammatory drugs, other than indomethacin, probably reflects their lower potency. Relative sparing of renal prostaglandins is another possible factor in the case of sulindac.

Renal prostaglandins may not become a significant regulatory influence in renal hemodynamics or in renin release until renal baroreceptors or the macula densa are activated. Inhibitors of prostaglandin synthetase have little influence on basal unstimulated PRA. In situations where these mechanisms are activated, such as with loop diuretics, salt depletion, or renal artery stenosis, prostaglandin inhibitors exhibit greater inhibitory effects on PRA [118,129,132,134]. Indeed, there is some evidence that the pressor response to indomethacin may be countered by its effects on renin release, with reversible depressor effects being noted in patients with renovascular hypertension [124].

Further indications that this may be the case are provided by the report that intravenous aspirin significantly reduced mean arterial pressure by 10mmHg in patients with confirmed untreated renovascular hypertension [135]. This fall in blood pressure correlated with the reduction in PRA in the aorta and also PGE_2 concentration in the renal vein on the stenotic side. Conversely, in patients with essential hypertension, intravenous aspirin produced a small but significant increase in mean arterial pressure, consistent with previous reports on the pressor effects of nonsteroidal anti-inflammatory drugs in essential hypertension [135].

This suggests that renal prostaglandins play an important role in the pathogenesis of hyperreninemic hypertension in renal artery stenosis, and the effects of nonsteroidal anti-inflammatory drugs in this situation merit further investigation.

CORTICOSTEROIDS

MINERALOCORTICOIDS

It has been realized for many years that corticosteroids have the ability to alter renin release, and that aldosterone is one of the principal physiological regulators of renin secretion. In adrenocortical insufficiency, where sodium depletion may be severe, activation of the RAS is almost invariable and appears to be an important homeostatic mechanism for maintenance of supine blood pressure [136] (see Chapter 68). Steroid replacement therapy with dexamethasone and fludrocortisone results in normalization of the activated RAS. Indeed, monitoring of PRA may allow

mineralocorticoid replacement therapy to be optimized [137]. It is therefore clear that mineralocorticoids have an inhibitory effect on the RAS (see Chapter 63).

The administration of fludrocortisone (0.6 mg/d) for four days to salt-replete volunteers results in an increase in blood pressure, sodium and water retention, and hypokalemia. Plasma renin activity is also suppressed by between 50 and 90% with associated significant reductions in plasma and urinary aldosterone [138–140]. The inhibitory effect of mineralocorticoids on the RAS is probably secondary to sodium retention and expansion of extracellular fluid volume. Fludrocortisone also suppresses sympathetic nervous activity, reflected by decreased plasma norepinephrine levels [139], and increases ANF levels [140,141] which in themselves have been demonstrated to have an inhibitory effect on renin release [142]. However, changes in sympathetic nervous activity and ANF are unlikely to contribute substantially to the suppression of PRA since glucocorticoids induce identical changes without suppression of PRA [140].

Conversely, low-dose fludrocortisone (0.15mg/d) produces significant metabolic effects including suppression of PRA without a pressor response [143].

Fludrocortisone enhances the pressor response to Ang II but not to norepinephrine [140]. In view of the reduction in PRA, however, it is unlikely that the RAS makes any contribution to the pressor effects of mineralocorticoids.

Glycyrrhetinic acid, the active component in liquorice, and its derivative carbenoxolone, previously used in the treatment of peptic ulcer disease, have mineralocorticoid activity. Metabolic effects following long-term ingestion of liquorice, and the side effects of carbenoxolone, are similar to those of mineralocorticoid excess: hypertension, sodium retention, and hypokalemia [144,145]. Liquorice and carbenoxolone also suppress PRA [146–149]. As with fludrocortisone, there is a significant increase in ANF, but unlike fludrocortisone, there is also an increase in urinary-free cortisol [146–148].

Initially, the mineralocorticoid effects of these drugs were believed to be achieved by direct interaction with aldosterone receptors. The affinity of glycyrrhetinic acid and carbenoxolone for the aldosterone receptor is, however, poor (1×10^{-4} and 6×10^{-4} compared with aldosterone, respectively) although greater than that of dexamethasone [150]. More recent evidence suggests that the main mineralocorticoid effect of liquorice and carbenoxolone is through inhibition of 11β-dehydrogenase, as measured by an increased half-life of tritiated 11β cortisol. The resulting increased plasma cortisol concentration allows overspill into the urine, and therefore increased urinary-free cortisol and activation of type I mineralocorticoid receptors [147–149].

GLUCOCORTICOIDS

The effects of glucocorticoids on the RAS are much less pronounced than those of mineralocorticoids.

Prednisolone, when given in pharmacological doses (50mg/d) to salt-replete volunteers, has no effect on PRA, sodium retention, or blood pressure. It is, however, associated with an increase in ANF and suppression of plasma norepinephrine levels almost equivalent to those produced by fludrocortisone in doses of 0.6mg/d. There is no modulation of the pressor response to Ang II or norepinephrine [140]. This absence of PRA suppression is consistent with earlier studies with dexamethasone and prednisolone [151,152].

Cortisol possesses both mineralocorticoid and glucocorticoid effects. It produces glucose intolerance, sodium retention, kaliuresis, and suppression of PRA and of active renin concentration. It also increases renin substrate (angiotensinogen) levels, which is believed to be a glucocorticoid effect [153,154]. The increased renin substrate levels following glucocorticoid administration may cause elevated PRA in the absence of a change in renin concentration. Measurement of immunologically active renin is necessary for an accurate assessment of effects on renin release.

Since the carbohydrate intolerance produced by hydrocortisone is selectively blocked by the glucocorticoid antagonist RU486, and since the mineralocorticoid effects, including PRA suppression, are attenuated by the mineralocorticoid antagonist spironolactone, the effects on PRA are probably mediated by the mineralocorticoid receptor [154].

LITHIUM

Lithium is widely used for research purposes as well as being employed therapeutically in the treatment of manic-depressive illness. It is reabsorbed in the proximal renal tubules in similar proportions to sodium, but unlike sodium, is neither reabsorbed nor secreted to any great extent in the distal nephron. As lithium's renal handling is so similar to that of sodium, it is not surprising that it also affects renin release.

In 1969, Murphy *et al* [155] demonstrated that when patients are first given lithium, there is an initial natriuresis, followed by a rise in aldosterone secretion. There are now many reports of lithium stimulating the RAS; however, the exact mechanism remains unclear and there are few data on the dose– and time–response relationships.

In single small doses, lithium carbonate 300mg (8.1mmol lithium) has little effect on PRA, and at most, a moderate [60,156]

natriuretic effect. In higher doses, lithium carbonate 750mg (20.4mmol lithium) is natriuretic, and significantly increases PRA by 50%–70%, 12 hours after dosing [44,50,157].

In psychiatric patients, lithium has been shown to cause a significant four- to six- fold increase in PRA within 24 hours of starting treatment, an effect that persists over one week's treatment [158].

There is, however, some variation in the reports following long-term therapy. Whilst some report a return to basal levels of PRA [158,159], others suggest a sustained increase in PRC [160] or PRA and in aldosterone concentration when compared to a control group [161].

The exact mechanism for the stimulation of the RAS by lithium in man remains unclear. Experimentally, lithium has a direct effect on the juxtaglomerular apparatus which is not attenuated by blockade of the sympathetic nervous system, macula densa, or baroreceptors, although it is attenuated by nonsteroidal anti-inflammatory drugs [162]. Lithium inhibits inositol phosphate recycling to phosphoinositides. How interaction with this intracellular second messenger system contributes to lithium's effects on renin release is not known [163]. In man only, there is evidence that lithium may interact with aldosterone at the distal nephron and induce a state of resistance to mineralocorticoids [160,161,164,165].

Further evidence for the antagonistic effect of lithium on mineralocorticoids is the observation of significantly increased aldosterone levels (greater than 100%) in psychiatric patients treated with lithium when compared with normal controls [160,161], with a positive correlation between plasma aldosterone and serum lithium levels [161,165]. The absence of hypokalemia or signs of hypovolemia [161] suggests that this observation is not simply a result of secondary hyperaldosteronism following sodium depletion. This may lead to compensatory activation of the renin–angiotensin–aldosterone axis to maintain blood pressure and electrolyte homeostasis. Further investigation is needed to confirm this hypothesis.

DIURETICS

There have been reports since 1965 [166] that diuretics stimulate the RAS. The mechanisms are complex and involve the activation of the macula densa, renal baroreceptors, renal sympathetic nerves, and prostaglandins [167]. Loop diuretics, thiazides, and potassium- sparing diuretics are considered separately.

LOOP DIURETICS

Loop diuretics, particularly furosemide and bumetanide, are widely used in clinical practice. Intravenous administration induces an acute activation of the RAS in normal volunteers, hypertensive patients, and patients with chronic cardiac failure.

The mechanisms by which loop diuretics stimulate the RAS vary in importance depending on the time after administration (Fig. 80.3). Factors such as the diuretic dose [168,169], sodium intake, age of subjects, and route of administration also affect the degree of activation.

In salt-deplete and replete volunteers, intravenous furosemide caused a significant increase in PRA; in volunteers maintained on a high sodium diet (250mmol/d), intravenous furosemide (80mg) failed to stimulate the RAS acutely [170].

In volunteers aged between 18 and 29, an intravenous bolus of furosemide 0.5mg/kg induced an acute increase in PRA of above 100% which was sustained for over four hours; the same dose of furosemide failed to stimulate the RAS in volunteers over the age of 50 [171].

Plasma renin activity rises within five minutes of intravenous loop-diuretic administration, and peak increments of between 95 and 200% occur between 10 and 15 minutes [118,134,172,173] and are sustained for up to eight hours in hypertensive patients [174] and for over four hours in volunteers

[171,175]. Plasma Ang II concentrations increase by up to 100% [169,173] lagging behind the rise in PRA by 20–40 minutes in moderately salt-depleted volunteers [169].

Associated with the acute increase in PRA, there is a brisk natriuresis with increased urinary flow, increased urinary prostaglandin excretion, increased urinary excretion of dopamine, and increased renal plasma flow and GFR. There is, however, no evidence of acute sympathetic activation as assessed by plasma catecholamines, although there is a report of significantly increased plasma norepinephrine and epinephrine levels 60 minutes after administration [176].

Loop diuretic-induced activation of the RAS could thus result from one or more of these mechanisms.

RENAL HEMODYNAMICS AND ACUTE RENIN RESPONSE

Acute increases in renal plasma flow of up to 30% and in GFR of up to 70% have been reported to occur after intravenous furosemide, but these increases are very dependent on the salt status of the subjects, becoming more significant in salt-depleted subjects [118,173,177] as does the activation of the RAS.

Although Passmore *et al* [169] demonstrated that the furosemide-induced acute rise in PRA was accompanied by a significant increase in effective renal plasma flow, bumetanide,

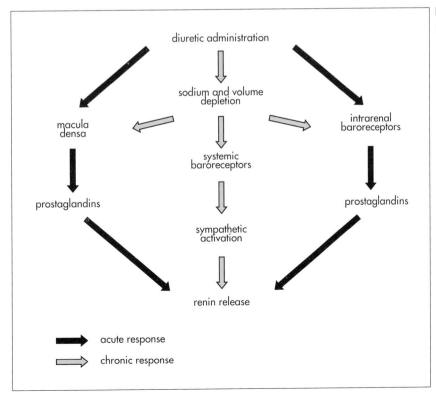

Fig. 80.3 Mechanisms of loop diuretic-induced renin release.

which produced an equivalent natriuresis, failed to stimulate PRA or increase renal plasma flow. Larger doses of both diuretics resulted in equivalent increments in PRA and renal plasma flow. Changes in renal plasma flow may, therefore, play a role in the activation of the RAS following the administration of loop diuretics.

NATRIURESIS AND ACUTE RENIN RESPONSE
The acute rise in PRA following furosemide intravenously, is probably unrelated to natriuresis: following intravenous furosemide, there is a poor correlation between cumulative urinary sodium excretion and acute increase in PRA, or between reduction in plasma volume and increase in PRA [178].

PROSTAGLANDINS AND ACUTE RENIN RESPONSE
Intravenous furosemide increases synthesis and urinary excretion of PGE_2, $PGF_{2\alpha}$, prostacyclin, and thromboxane B_2 (the inactive product of thromboxane A_2, a potent vasoconstrictor) [115,169,175,179]. Pretreatment of subjects with indomethacin or ibuprofen invariably attenuates the acute PRA response to furosemide [118,134,180] and reduces prostaglandin excretion [180], which in itself, is evidence that prostaglandins play a major role in renin release.

Experimentally PGI_2, but not PGE_2, stimulates renin release from renal cortical slices [181] suggesting that prostacyclin is the main direct mediator of renin release. In man, PGI_2 infusions produced a dose-related increase in PRA which was unaffected by combined pretreatment with propranolol and indomethacin [115]. This indicates that prostacyclin induces renin release independently of sympathetic or prostaglandin synthetase mechanisms. There was, however, a marked fall in blood pressure which may have contributed to the PRA response.

Excretion of both PGE_2 and 6-keto-$PGF_{1\alpha}$ (the stable metabolic product of prostacyclin) correlates with the acute rise in PRA following furosemide [115,179,180,182]. The increase in urinary excretion of PGE_2 is, however, blocked by pretreatment with the ACE inhibitors captopril [183] or cilazapril [173], despite augmentation of the furosemide-induced PRA response. This argues against PGE_2 having a direct stimulatory effect on renin release following furosemide. It suggests that the increased PGE_2 excretion may be secondary to an increase in plasma Ang II. Unfortunately, in these studies, urinary 6-keto-$PGF_{1\alpha}$ was not measured; therefore one cannot infer that the renin response is a result of increased renal prostacyclin. In another study, however, the ACE inhibitor ramipril had no significant effect on the furosemide-induced excretion of PGE_2 or 6-keto-$PGF_{1\alpha}$, though it did significantly enhance the PRA response [182].

Further evidence against PGE_2 having a direct effect on acute renin release is implied by the observation that a low dose of bumetanide (0.25mg) significantly increased urinary PGE_2 equivalent to furosemide 10mg [169]; however, unlike furosemide, it fails to increase PRA [169,184].

It therefore appears that furosemide-induced acute renin release is mediated through prostaglandins, probably as a result of activation of either the macula densa or renal baroreceptors [113], with prostacyclin probably having a direct effect on the juxtaglomerular cells. Renal prostaglandins are also important in renal hemodynamics and electrolyte excretion, however, particularly during salt depletion, and therefore may also affect renin release indirectly.

DOPAMINERGIC AND SYMPATHETIC ACTIVATION AND THE RENIN RESPONSE
Furosemide causes an acute increase in urinary dopamine excretion which closely follows the rise in PRA [182,185]. Dopamine, however, is not important in the acute renin increase as carbidopa blocks the urinary dopamine response but not the PRA response [185].

The acute renin response is also independent of reflex sympathetic activation, being unaffected by replacing voided urine loss with intravenous saline [186] and at most, is moderately attenuated by β-blockers [186,187].

Increased plasma catecholamine concentrations have, however, been observed from one to eight hours following furosemide given intravenously to hypertensive patients [174,176], and propranolol blocks the furosemide-induced PRA response in volunteers who are salt depleted (60mmol/d) having received furosemide 80mg/d orally for three days prior to testing [188]. Sympathetic mechanisms may therefore become more important late in the response and during salt depletion.

ORAL ADMINISTRATION OF LOOP DIURETICS
As described earlier, intravenous administration of furosemide results in an acute increase in PRA which correlates poorly with net sodium loss and plasma-volume reduction. Following oral administration of furosemide, the response differs in that there is a progressive increase in PRA over two hours which correlates closely with urinary sodium excretion [178]. This may simply reflect differences in the pharmacokinetics of the two routes of administration.

Acute but not chronic oral dosing with loop diuretics results in increased urinary excretion of prostaglandins [120,128,189, 190]. Pretreatment with nonsteroidal anti-inflammatory drugs, however, significantly reduces urinary prostaglandin excretion and attenuates the acute and chronic diuretic-induced increase in PRA and sodium excretion [128,189,190].

Following oral administration of loop diuretics, net sodium excretion may therefore play a role in the degree of activation of the RAS. As with intravenous administration, prostaglandins also play a major role in the stimulation of renin release following oral administration. However, in view of the incomplete blockade of the increase in PRA following chronic treatment, other mechanisms such as sympathetic activation may also be involved.

NEGATIVE FEEDBACK AND PHYSIOLOGICAL CONSEQUENCES OF LOOP-DIURETIC ADMINISTRATION

Although intravenous loop diuretics induce an acute increase in PRA and Ang II, there is evidence that this acute activation of the RAS is limited by negative feedback mechanisms through Ang II. In several studies, pretreatment with the ACE inhibitors, captopril, cilazapril, or ramipril, significantly augmented the absolute and percentage increase in PRA [173,182,183,191].

Activation of the RAS also has physiological consequences. Following intravenous administration of furosemide to volunteers, frequently a small increase in mean arterial pressure is observed from 5 up to 30 minutes postinjection [134,168,184]. The increase in blood pressure is dose dependent and correlates with the increase in PRA [168]. The pressor effect is not observed following low doses (0.25mg) of intravenous bumetanide [184] where there is no activation of the RAS.

There is also, with loop-diuretic administration, an associated increase in venous capacitance as a result of increased prostaglandin production [168,184,191]. These pressor and venous capacitance effects are blocked by nonsteroidal anti-inflammatory drugs [134,185] and ACE inhibitors [191].

The pressor effect of intravenous furosemide has also been observed in hypertensive patients [174] and in patients with chronic congestive cardiac failure [192]. In patients with congestive cardiac failure, the rise in PRA is associated with an acute increase in systemic vascular resistance and reduced stroke volume. This may account for the occasional acute deterioration in symptoms following intravenous furosemide. Following the acute response, however, there is a fall in left ventricular filling pressure probably as a result of reduced preload secondary to increased venous capacitance.

In summary, loop diuretics, when given intravenously, induce an acute activation of the RAS in man. The most important factors involved in this stimulation appear to be increased renal prostaglandins, with prostacyclin probably interacting directly with the juxtaglomerular cells to release renin. The main origin of prostaglandins following loop diuretics is probably the macula densa following blockade of chloride transport. Intrarenal baroreceptors, however, may also be a source following alterations in renal hemodynamics. Changes in renal hemodynamics are themselves influenced by renal prostaglandins and increased Ang II levels. Volume contraction, net sodium loss, and activation of renal sympathetic nerves may be important in the late renin response to intravenous furosemide and during oral treatment.

THIAZIDE DIURETICS

As with loop diuretics, thiazides activate the RAS. There have been few studies, however, to investigate the dose- or time response and mechanism of activation of the RAS by these agents.

The thiazide diuretics increase PRA in normal volunteers and hypertensive patients. In volunteers commenced on hydrochlorothiazide 50mg/d, supine and erect PRA progressively increase. The increase reaches significance by day two and peaks with a two- to four-fold increase by day three [120,193]. Thereafter, PRA tends to decline, leveling out at lower values but remaining significantly elevated during chronic treatment. There is also a significant increase in plasma aldosterone levels over the first week of treatment, and increased urinary aldosterone excretion which persists throughout treatment. The initial increase in PRA is associated with a net sodium deficit, a decrease in weight, and an increased hematocrit. After seven days' treatment, however, these tend to normalize, probably as a result of secondary hyperaldosteronism [194,195]. The observed kaliuresis, as plasma aldosterone levels rise, would be in keeping with this.

In hypertensive patients, chlorthiazide [195], hydrochlorthiazide [196–198], polythiazide [199], and bendrofluazide [200,201] all increase PRA two- to four-fold and increase Ang II two-fold following chronic treatment. There is also an increase in plasma norepinephrine levels, but no change in epinephrine or dopamine levels, body weight, or hematocrit.

The rise in PRA occurs to a comparable extent in hypertensive patients whether or not there is a hypotensive effect, although there is a greater increase in norepinephrine in patients who do so respond [197].

Thiazide diuretics do not appear to stimulate urinary prostaglandin excretion either in the first few days of administration or during chronic treatment [120,201]. The nonsteroidal anti-inflammatory drugs indomethacin and ibuprofen, however, attenuate the increase in PRA in association with decreased renal excretion of prostaglandins [120,194,196,202]. These drugs antagonize the hypotensive effect of hydrochlorthiazide and attenuate the hydrochlorthiazide-induced decrease in body weight.

Sulindac also reduces urinary excretion of prostaglandins during thiazide diuretic treatment but does not inhibit the diuretic-induced increase in PRA or the fall in body weight [202].

Prostaglandins may therefore play a role in renin release following thiazide treatment. Another explanation, however, could be that prostaglandin-synthetase inhibitors, particularly the more potent ones, simply antagonize the diuretic and hypotensive action of thiazides, thereby reducing subsequent renal sympathetic stimulation.

In keeping with sympathetic-induced activation of renin release following thazides is the observation that β-blockers attenuate the increase in PRA [203–205]. In addition, patients with longstanding tetraplegia due to cord transections have a diminished PRA response to thiazides [206].

In 50–75% of patients with essential hypertension, blood pressure does not normalize on diuretic therapy alone. Activation of the RAS may limit the therapeutic response. Consistent with this is the observation that treatment with thiazides and ACE inhibitors together has an additive hypotensive effect [198]. Furthermore, the Ang II antagonist, saralasin, enhances the hypotensive effect of thiazide diuretics, particularly in those patients who have had a greater increase in PRA as a result of commencing diuretic therapy [199]. These increased hypotensive effects occur despite enhanced PRA resulting from removal of negative feedback by Ang II.

In conclusion, thiazide diuretics stimulate an increase in PRA during long-term treatment, probably as a result of volume depletion with resulting sympathetic stimulation. However, a prostaglandin-mediated process through activation of the macula densa, as a result of sodium and volume depletion, is possible.

The extent to which the RAS is activated appears to be limited by negative feedback mechanisms through Ang II, and by secondary hyperaldosteronism.

POTASSIUM-SPARING DIURETICS

The potassium-sparing diuretics — amiloride, spironolactone, and triamterene — all increase PRA, induce a natriuresis, and increase plasma potassium concentration in both volunteers and hypertensive patients.

Amiloride and spironolactone induce a dose-related increase in PRA, renin concentration, plasma Ang II, and plasma and urinary aldosterone [120,207,208]. The peak increase in PRC occurs between 10 and 12 days following initiation of treatment with high doses (amiloride 75mg, spironolactone 300mg).

The correlation between aldosterone increase and rising Ang II levels is less with spironolactone than amiloride. This is consistent with spironolactone partially blocking aldosterone synthesis [208].

Neither spironolactone nor amiloride increases urinary prostaglandin excretion. Indomethacin, however, completely blocks the plasma renin response to spironolactone 300mg/d [120,209].

Unlike spironolactone and amiloride, triamterene induces a four-fold increase in urinary PGE_2 and $PGF_{2\alpha}$ in association with increased PRA, these changes being blocked by indomethacin. Indeed, the increase in renal prostaglandin synthesis following triamterene may be a necessary renal hemodynamic homeostatic mechanism, and if blocked by nonsteroidal anti-inflammatory drugs, results in acute renal failure [120,210].

Type	Drug	Other possible effects that influence renin release	References
direct vasodilators	hydralazine diazoxide minoxidil	may alter renal hemodynamics and reduce sodium delivery to macula densa	96–100
calcium antagonists	dihydropyridine derivatives only	have possible direct stimulatory effect by reducing intracellular calcium; no observed stimulation of RAS after chronic usage	see text
nonselective α- and selective α_1-antagonists	phentolamine prazosin	possible direct effect on α-adrenergic inhibitory receptors	4–7,10,11
diuretics	loop diuretics thiazides potassium sparing	have direct renal effects including activation of macula densa and renal baroreceptors; stimulation of renal prostaglandins and altered renal blood flow	see text
dopamine-1-agonists	fenoldopam	direct stimulatory effect	59–61

Fig. 80.4 Drugs that stimulate renin release via reflex activation of the sympathetic nervous system.

There is a report [211] of the PRA response following spironolactone being blocked by propranolol. No similar data on amiloride or triamterene are available.

The mechanisms by which amiloride and spironolactone activate the RAS in man are therefore unclear. As with loop diuretics and thiazides, intrarenal prostaglandins may be involved. Evidence that this is an important mechanism is limited in that neither drug enhances renal excretion of prostaglandins.

Potassium-sparing diuretics do, however, produce a significant sodium deficit, though little weight reduction [120, 207, 208]. This may, in turn, result in activation of the macula densa mechanisms and therefore explain the inhibitory effect of indomethacin on the stimulation of the RAS. The evidence for prostaglandin-induced renin release by triamterene is stronger and is supported by the marked induction of urinary prostaglandin excretion and inhibition of the stimulatory effects on renin release by indomethacin.

Activation of the sympathetic nervous system secondary to volume depletion may also act as a mediator of renin release by potassium-sparing diuretics. Further studies with β-blockers would be needed to confirm this.

SUMMARY

In summary, β-agonists stimulate renin release by a direct effect on juxtaglomerular β_1-adrenoceptors and presynaptic β_2 augmentation of norepinephrine release. Diuretics, dopamine-1 agonists, and calcium antagonists stimulate renin release by a direct effect on the juxtaglomerular cells or macula densa/renal baroreceptor mechanisms. These drugs, however, as well as α_1-antagonists and vasodilators which have a direct action on vascular smooth muscle, induce secondary sympathetic nervous activation which indirectly stimulates renin release (Fig. 80.4). The observed stimulation of the RAS is limited by negative feedback mechanisms through Ang II, and is therefore augmented by direct inhibitors of the RAS.

Similarly, β-blockers, α_2-agonists, dopamine agonists (levodopa), nonsteroidal anti-inflammatory drugs, and mineralocorticoids have a direct inhibitory effect on renal mechanisms of renin release and an indirect effect via suppression of sympathetic nervous activity and via sodium and fluid retention.

REFERENCES

1. De Leeuw PW, De Bos R, Van Es PN, Birkenhäger WH. Effect of sympathetic stimulation and intrarenal alpha-blockade on the secretion of renin by the human kidney. *European Journal of Clinical Investigation* 1985;15:166–70.

2. De Leeuw PW, Van Es PM, De Bos R, Tchang PT, Birkenhäger WH. Tonic suppression of renin by alpha 2-adrenoceptors in hypertension. *Journal of Hypertension* 1987;5 (suppl 5):S15–7.

3. De Leeuw PW, Van Es PN, Tchang PT, De Bos R, Birkenhäger WH. Stimulation of renin by blockade of α2-adrenoceptors in man: Role of the β1-adrenoceptor. *Journal of Hypertension* 1988;6 (suppl 4):S416–7.

4. Drayer JIM, Weber MA, Atlas SA, Laragh JH. Phentolamine testing for alpha-adrenergic participation in hypertensive patients. Independence from renin profiles. *Clinical Pharmacology and Therapeutics* 1977;22:286–92.

5. Pedrinelli R, Sassano P, Arzilli F, Magagna A, Salvetti A. Mediation of renin release in essential hypertension by α-adrenoceptors. *Journal of Cardiovascular Pharmacology* 1981;3:1153–61.

6. Travoti M, Massucco P, Cavalot F, Anfossi G, Mularoni E, Busca G, Orecchia C, Emanuelli G. Alpha-adrenergic blockade with phentolamine increases the response of the renin–angiotensin–aldosterone system to insulin-induced hypoglycaemia in man. *Hormone and Metabolic Research* 1989;21:290–1.

7. Cuneo RC, Livesey JH, Nicholls MG, Espiner ER, Donald RA. Effects of alpha-1-adrenergic blockade on the hormonal response to hypoglycaemic stress in normal man. *Clinical Endocrinology* 1987;26:1–8.

8. Bolli P, Wood AJ, Pharm M, Simpson FO. Effects of prazosin in patients with hypertension. *Clinical Pharmacology and Therapeutics* 1976;20:138–41.

9. Hayes JM, Graham RM, O'Connell BP, Speers E, Humphry TS. Effect of prazosin on plasma renin activity. *Australian and New Zealand Journal of Medicine* 1976;6:90.

10. Rubin PC, Blaschke TF. Studies on the clinical pharmacology of prazosin 1: Cardiovascular, catecholamine and endocrine changes following a single dose. *British Journal of Clinical Pharmacology* 1980;10:23–32.

11. Nicholson JP, Resnick LM, Pickering TG, Marion R, Sullivan P, Laragh JH. Relationship of blood pressure response and the renin–angiotensin system to first-dose prazosin. *American Journal of Medicine* 1985;78:241–4.

12. McAreavey D, Cumming AMM, Sood VP, Leckie BJ, Morton JJ, Murray GD, Robertson JIS. The effect of oral prazosin on blood pressure and plasma concentrations of renin and angiotensin II in man. *Clinical Science* 1981;61: 457–60S.

13. Shionoiri H, Yasuda G, Yoshimura H, Umemura S, Miyajima E, Miyakawa T, Takagi N, Kaneko Y. Antihypertensive effects and pharmacokinetics of single and consecutive administration of doxazosin in patients with mild to moderate essential hypertension. *Journal of Cardiovascular Pharmacology* 1987;10:90–5.

14. Donnelly R, Elliott HL, Meredith PA, Reid JL. Concentration–effect relationships and individual responses to doxazosin in essential hypertension. *British Journal of Clinical Pharmacology* 1989;28:517–26.

15. Morganti A, Sala C, Palermo A, Turolo C, Zanchetti A, Laragh J. Dissociation of the effects of α1 adrenergic blockade on blood pressure and renin release in patients with essential hypertension. *Journal of Cardiovascular Pharmacology* 1982;4 (suppl 1):S158–61.

16. Bianchetti L, Ferrier C, Beretta–Piccoli C, Fraser R, Morton JJ, Ziegler WH. Adrenergic activity and aldosterone regulation: No evidence for an alpha-1 adrenoceptor-mediated influence in normal subjects. *Clinical Endocrinology* 1986;25:87–95.

17. Beretta–Piccoli C, Ferrier C, Weidmann P. Alpha-1-adrenergic blockade and cardiovascular pressor responses in essential hypertension. *Hypertension* 1986;8: 407–14.

18. Riegger GA, Haeske W, Kraus C, Kromer EP, Kochsiek K. Contribution of the renin–angiotensin–aldosterone system to development of tolerance and fluid retention in chronic congestive heart failure during prazosin treatment. *American Journal of Cardiology* 1987;59:906–10.

19. Elliott HL, Jones CR, Reid JL. Peripheral pre and post junctional α2-adrenoceptors in man: Studies with RX 781094, a selective α2-antagonist. *Journal of Hypertension* 1983;**1** (suppl 2):109–11.

20. Weber MA, Drayer JIM, Hubbell FA. Effects on the renin–angiotensin system of agents acting at central and peripheral adrenergic receptors. *Chest* 1983;**83** (suppl l):374–7.

21. Manhem P, Paalzow L, Hökfelt B. Plasma clonidine in relation to blood pressure, catecholamines, and renin activity during long-term treatment of hypertension. *Clinical Pharmacology and Therapeutics* 1982;**31**:445–51.

22. Hui TP, Krakoff LR, Felton K, Yeager K. Diuretic treatment alters clonidine suppression of plasma norepinephrine. *Hypertension* 1986;**8**:272–6.

23. Mathias CJ, Wilkinson AH, Pike FA, Sever PS, Peart WS. Clonidine in unilateral renal artery stenosis and unilateral renal parenchymal disease. Similar antihypertensive but different renin suppressive effects. *Journal of Hypertension* 1983;**1** (suppl 2):123–5.

24. Golub MS, Thananopavarn C, Eggena P, Barrett JD, Sambhi MP. Humoral and hemodynamic effects of short- and long-term clonidine therapy in patients with mild-to-moderate hypertension. *Chest* 1983;**83** (suppl 1):377–9.

25. Mathias CJ, Wilkinson A, Lewis PS, Peart WS, Sever PS, Snell ME. Clonidine lowers blood pressure independently of renin suppression in patients with unilateral renal artery stenosis. *Chest* 1983;**83** (suppl 1):357–9.

26. Reid JL, Wing LMH, Mathias CJ, Frankel HL, Neill E. The central hypotensive effect of clonidine: Studies in tetraplegic subjects. *Clinical Pharmacology and Therapeutics* 1977;**21**:375–81.

27. Pettinger WA, Keeton TK, Campbell WB, Harper DC. Evidence for a renal alpha-adrenergic receptor inhibiting renin release. *Circulation Research* 1976;**38**:338–46.

28. Morgan TB. The use of centrally acting antihypertensive drugs in patients with renal disease. *Chest* 1983;**83** (suppl 1):383–6.

29. Weber F, Brodde OE, Anlauf M, Bock KD. Subclassification of human beta-adrenergic receptors mediating renin release. *Clinical and Experimental Hypertension* 1983;**A5**:225–38.

30. Davies R, Slater JDH, Rudolf M, Geddes DM. The effect of isoprenaline on plasma renin activity in man: A dose–response curve. *Clinical Endocrinology* 1977;**6**:395–9.

31. Pringle TH, Riddell JG, Shanks RG. A comparison of the cardioselectivity of five β-adrenoceptor blocking drugs. *Journal of Cardiovascular Pharmacology* 1987;**10**:228–37.

32. Johnson BF, Smith IK, La Brooy J, Bye C. The nature of the beta-adrenoceptor controlling plasma renin activity in man. *Clinical Science and Molecular Medicine* 1976;**51**:113–8S.

33. Wiggins R, Davies R, Basar I, Slater JDH. The inhibition of adrenergically provoked renin release by salbutamol in man. *British Journal of Clinical Pharmacology* 1978;**5**:213–15.

34. Bühler FR, Burkhart F, Lütold BE, Kung M, Marbet G, Pfisterer M. Antihypertensive beta-blocking action as related to renin and age. A pharmacological tool to identify pathogenetic mechanisms in essential hypertension. *American Journal of Cardiology* 1975;**36**:653–69.

35. Vanhees L, Fagard R, Hespel P, Lijnen P, Amery A. Renin release: β1- or β2-receptor mediated? (Letter) *New England Journal of Medicine* 1985;**312**:123–4.

36. Scheinin M, Koulu M, Laurikainen E, Allonen H. Hypokalaemia and other non-bronchial effects of inhaled fenoterol and salbutamol: A placebo-controlled dose-response study in healthy volunteers. *British Journal of Clinical Pharmacology* 1987;**24**:645–53.

37. Tantucci C, Santeusanio F, Beschi M, Castellano M, Sorbini C, Grassi V. Metabolic and hormonal effects of preferential beta-1 and beta-2 adrenoceptor stimulation in man. *Journal of Endocrinological Investigation* 1988;**11**:279–87.

38. Staessen J, Cattaert A, De Schaepdryver A, Fagard R, Lijnen P, Moerman E, Amery A. Effects of β1-adrenoceptor agonism on plasma renin activity in normal man. *British Journal of Clinical Pharmacology* 1983;**16**:553–6.

39. Meurer KA, Lang R, Homback V, Helber A. Effects of a β1 selective adrenergic agonist in normal human volunteers. *Klinische Wochenschrift* 1980;**58**:425–7.

40. Fitzpatrick D, Ikram H, Nicholls MG, Espiner EA. Haemodynamic, hormonal and electrolyte responses to prenalterol infusion in heart failure. *Circulation* 1983;**67**:613–9.

41. Uretsky BF, Lawless CE, Verbalis JG, Valdes AM, Kolesar JA, Reddy PS. Combined therapy with dobutamine and amrinone in severe heart failure. Improved haemodynamics and increased activation of the renin–angiotensin system with combined intravenous therapy. *Chest* 1987;**92**:657–62.

42. Barbeau A, Gillo–Joffroy L, Boucher R, Nowaczynski W, Genest J. Renin–aldosterone system in Parkinson's disease. *Science* 1969;**165**:291–2.

43. Horton R, Bughi S, Jost-Vu E, Antonipillai I, Nadler J. Effect of dopamine on renal blood flow, prostaglandins, renin and electrolyte excretion in normal and hypertensive humans. *American Journal of Hypertension* 1990;**3**:108–11S.

44. Schoors DF, Dupont AG. Lithium does not reduce the natriuretic response to dopamine in man. *British Journal of Clinical Pharmacology* 1990;**29**:581–2.

45. Lightman SL. Studies on the response of plasma renin activity and aldosterone and cortisol levels to dopaminergic and opiate stimuli in man. *Clinical Endocrinology* 1981;**15**:45–52.

46. Wilcox CS, Aminoff MJ, Kurtz AB, Slater JDH. Comparison of the renin response to dopamine and noradrenaline in normal subjects and patients with autonomic insufficiency. *Clinical Science and Molecular Medicine* 1974;**46**:481–8.

47. Worth D, Harvey J, Brown J, Lee M. The effects of intravenous L-dopa on plasma renin activity, renal function and blood pressure in man. *European Journal of Clinical Pharmacology* 1988;**35**:137–41.

48. Barbieri C, Caldara R, Ferrari C, Crossignani RM, Recchia M. Inhibition of the renin–angiotensin–aldosterone system by L-dopa with and without inhibition of extracerebral dopa decarboxylase in man. *Clinical Science* 1981;**61**:187–90.

49. Worth DP, Harvey JN, Brown J, Lee MR. Gamma-L-glutamyl-L-dopa is a dopamine prodrug relatively specific for the kidney in normal subjects. *Clinical Science* 1985;**69**:207–14.

50. Jeffrey RF, Macdonald TM, Brown J, Rae PW, Lee MR. The effect of lithium on the renal response to the dopamine prodrug gludopa in normal man. *British Journal of Clinical Pharmacology* 1988;**25**:725–32.

51. Worth DP, Harvey JN, Brown J, Worral A, Lee MR. Domperidone treatment in man inhibits the fall in plasma renin activity induced by intravenous gamma-L-glutamyl-L-dopa. *British Journal of Clinical Pharmacology* 1986;**21**:497–502.

52. Sowers JR, Brickman AS, Sowers DK, Berg G. Dopaminergic modulation of aldosterone secretion in man is unaffected by glucocorticoids and angiotensin blockade. *Journal of Clinical Endocrinology and Metabolism* 1981;**52**:1078–84.

53. Gordon MB, Moore TJ, Dluhy RG, Williams GH. Dopaminergic blockade of the renin–angiotensin–aldosterone system: Effect of high and low sodium intakes. *Clinical Endocrinology* 1983;**19**:415–25.

54. Gilchrist NL, Espiner EA, Nicholls MG, Donald RA. Effect of metoclopramide on aldosterone and regulatory factors in man. *Clinical Endocrinology* 1984;**21**:1–7.

55. Noth RH, McCallum RW, Contino C, Havelick J. Tonic dopaminergic suppression of plasma aldosterone. *Journal of Clinical Endocrinology and Metabolism* 1980;**51**:64–9.

56. Carey RM, Thorner MO, Ortt EM. Effects of metoclopramide and bromocriptine on the renin–angiotensin–aldosterone system in man. *Journal of Clinical Investigation* 1979;**63**:727–35.

57. Dupont AG, Vanderniepen P, Smitz JJ, Six RO. Stimulation of aldosterone secretion by metoclopramide is not affected by chronic converting enzyme inhibition. *European Journal of Clinical Pharmacology* 1985;**29**:207–10.

58. Robertson D, Michelakis AM. The effect of chlorpromazine on plasma renin activity and aldosterone in man. *Journal of Clinical Endocrinology and Metabolism* 1975;**41**:1166–8.

59. Harvey JN, Worth DP, Brown J, Lee MR. The effect of oral fenoldopam (SKF 82526), a peripheral dopamine receptor agonist, on blood pressure and renal function in normal man. *British Journal of Clinical Pharmacology* 1985;**19**:21–7.

60. Girbes ARJ, Smit AJ, Meijer S, Reitsma WD. Lack of effect of lithium on the renal response to DA1 dopamine receptor stimulation by fenoldopam in normal man. *British Journal of Clinical Pharmacology* 1990;**29**:413–5.

61. Carey RM, Stote RM, Dubb JW, Townsend LH, Rose CE, Kaiser DL. Selective peripheral dopamine-1-receptor stimulation with fenoldopam in human essential hypertension. *Journal of Clinical Investigation* 1984;74:2198–207.

62. Ruilope LM, Robles RG, Miranda B, Tovar J, Alcazar JM, Sancho J, Rodicio JC, Martinez A, Astorga A, Beck T. Renal effects of fenoldopam in refractory hypertension. *Journal of Hypertension* 1988;6:665–9.

63. White WB, Halley SE. Comparative renal effects of intravenous administration of fenoldopam mesylate and sodium nitroprusside in patients with severe hypertension. *Archives of Internal Medicine* 1989;149:870–4.

64. Antonipillai I, Broers DMI, Lang D. Evidence that specific dopamine-I receptor activation is involved in dopamine induced renin release. *Hypertension* 1989;13:463–8.

65. Montier F, Katchadourian P, Pratz L, Cavero I. Increase in plasma renin activity evoked by fenoldopam in dogs is directly mediated by DA_1 receptor stimulation. *Journal of Cardiovascular Pharmacology* 1989;13:739–47.

66. Kotchen TA, Guthrie GP. Effects of calcium on renin and aldosterone. *American Journal of Cardiology* 1988;62:41–6G.

67. Chellingsworth MC, Kendall MJ. Effects of nifedipine, verapamil and diltiazem on renal function. *British Journal of Clinical Pharmacology* 1988;25:599–602.

68. Young MA, Watson RDS, Stallard TJ, Littler WA. Calcium channel blockers — are they diuretics? *British Journal of Clinical Pharmacology* 1985;20:95–8S.

69. Sluiter HE, Wetzels JFM, Huysmans FTM, Koene R. The natriuretic effect of the dihydropyridine calcium antagonist felodipine: A placebo-controlled study involving intravenous angiotensin II in normotensive volunteers. *Journal of Cardiovascular Pharmacology* 1987;10 (suppl 10):S154–61.

70. Katzman PL, Hulthén UL, Hökfelt B. Effects of the calcium antagonist felodipine on the sympathetic and renin–angiotensin–aldosterone system in essential hypertension. *Acta Medica Scandinavica* 1988;223:125–31.

71. Saito I, Takeshita E, Saruta T, Nagano S, Sekihara T. Effect of a calcium entry blocker on blood pressure, plasma renin activity, aldosterone and catecholamines in normotensive subjects. *Clinical Endocrinology* 1986;24:565–70.

72. Resnick LM, Nicholson JP, Laragh JH. Calcium, the renin–aldosterone system, and the hypotensive response to nifedipine. *Hypertension* 1987;10:254–8.

73. Glorioso N, Manunta P, Troffa C, Pazzola A, Soro A, Pala F, Melis MG, Madeddu P, Tonolo G. Effects of nitrendipine on blood pressure, renin–angiotensin system, and kidney function in essential hypertension. *Journal of Cardiovascular Pharmacology* 1988;12 (suppl 4):S142–5.

74. Ventura HO, Messerli FH, Oigman W, Dunn FG, Reisin E, Frolich ED. Immediate hemodynamic effects of a new calcium-channel blocking agent (nitrendipine) in essential hypertension. *American Journal of Cardiology* 1983;51:783–6.

75. Elliott HL, Pasanisi F, Reid JL. Effects of nicardipine on aldosterone release and pressor mechanisms. *British Journal of Clinical Pharmacology* 1985;20:99–102s.

76. Ferrara LA, Pasanisi F, Marotta T, Rubba P, Mancini M. Calcium antagonists and thiazide diuretics in the treatment of hypertension. *Journal of Cardiovascular Pharmacology* 1987;10 (suppl 10):S136–7.

77. McLeay RAB, Stallard TJ, Watson RDS, Littler WA. The effect of nifedipine on arterial pressure and reflex cardiac control. *Circulation* 1983;67:1084–90.

78. Weber MA. Prolonged calcium channel blocker therapy of hypertension. *Journal of Cardiovascular Pharmacology* 1988;12 (suppl 4):S16–21.

79. Hiramatsu K, Yamagishi F, Kubota T, Yamada T. Acute effects of the calcium antagonist nifedipine, on blood pressure, pulse rate, and the renin–angiotensin–aldosterone system in patients with essential hypertension. *American Heart Journal* 1982;104:1346–9.

80. Marone C, Luisoli S, Bomio F, Beretta–Piccoli C, Bianchetti MG, Weidmann P. Body sodium-blood volume state, aldosterone, and cardiovascular responsiveness after calcium entry blockade with nifedipine. *Kidney International* 1985;28:658–65.

81. Andersson OK, Granérus G, Hedner T. Felodipine: A calcium inhibiting vasodilator in refractory hypertension. *Drugs* 1985;29 (suppl 2):102–8.

82. Fagard R, Lijnen P, Amery A. The acute haemodynamic and humoral responses to felodipine and metoprolol in mild hypertension. *European Journal of Pharmacology* 1987;32:71–5.

83. Cluzel P, Chatellier G, Rivalan J, Bellet M, Corvol P, Ménard J. Predictive factors of the blood pressure fall induced by intravenous nicardipine. *Journal of Cardiovascular Pharmacology* 1989;13:370–5.

84. Laederach K, Weidmann P, Lauener F, Gerber A, Ziegler WH. Comparative acute effects of the calcium channel blockers triapamil, nisoldipine and nifedipine on blood pressure and some regulatory factors in normal and hypertensive subjects. *Journal of Cardiovascular Pharmacology* 1986;8:294–302.

85. Magometschnigg D, Hortnagl H, Rameis H. Diltiazem and verapamil: Functional antagonism of exogenous noradrenaline and angiotensin II in man. *European Journal of Clinical Pharmacology* 1984;26:303–7.

86. De Leeuw PW, Birkenhäger WH. Effects of verapamil in hypertensive patients. *Acta Medica Scandinavica* 1984;681 (suppl):125–8.

87. Stadler P, Leonardi L, Riesen W, Ziegler W, Marone C, Beretta–Piccoli C. Cardiovascular effects of verapamil in essential hypertension. *Clinical Pharmacology and Therapeutics* 1987;42:485–92.

88. Luft FC, Aronoff GR, Sloan RS, Fineberg NS, Weinberger MH. Calcium channel blockade with nitrendipine: Effects on sodium homeostasis, the renin–angiotensin system, and the sympathetic nervous system in humans. *Hypertension* 1985;7:438–42.

89. Simon G, Snyder DK. Altered pressor responses in long-term nitrendipine treatment. *Clinical Pharmacology and Therapeutics* 1984;36:315–9.

90. Mohanty PK, Sowers JR, McNamara C, Welch B, Beck F, Thames MD. Effects of diltiazem on hormonal and hemodynamic responses to lower body negative pressure and tilt in patients with mild to moderate systemic hypertension. *American Journal of Cardiology* 1985;56:28–33H.

91. Millar JA, Struthers AD, Beastall GH, Reid JL. Effect of nifedipine on blood pressure and adrenocortical responses to trophic stimuli in humans. *Journal of Cardiovascular Pharmacology* 1982;4 (suppl 3):S330–4.

92. Millar JA, McLean KA, Sumner DJ, Reid JL. The effect of the calcium antagonist nifedipine on pressor and aldosterone responses to angiotensin II in normal man. *European Journal of Clinical Pharmacology* 1983;24:315–21.

93. Bianchetti MG, Beretta–Piccoli C, Wiedmann P, Boehringer K, Link L, Morton JJ. Studies on aldosterone responsiveness to angiotensin II during clinical variations in calcium metabolism in normal man. *Clinical Science* 1982;63:325–8.

94. Guthrie GP, McAllister RG, Kotchen TA. Effects of intravenous and oral verapamil upon pressor and adrenal steroidogenic responses in normal man. *Journal of Clinical Endocrinology and Metabolism* 1983;57:339–43.

95. Staessen J, Fagard R, Hespel P, Lijnen P, Moerman E, Amery A. Acute calcium entry blockade inhibits the blood pressure but not the hormonal response to angiotensin II. *European Journal of Clinical Pharmacology* 1989;36:567–73.

96. Velasco M, McNay JL. Physiologic mechanisms of bupicomide- and hydralazine-induced increase in plasma renin activity in hypertensive patients. *Mayo Clinic Proceedings* 1977;52:430–2.

97. Reeves RA, Smith DL, Leenen FHH. Hemodynamic interaction of non-selective vs beta-1-selective beta-blockade with hydralazine in normal humans. *Clinical Pharmacology and Therapeutics* 1987;41:326–35.

98. O'Malley K, Velasco M, Wells J, McNay JL. Mechanism of the interaction of propranolol and a potent vasodilator anti-hypertensive agent — minoxidil. *European Journal of Clinical Pharmacology* 1976;9:355–60.

99. Brown NJ, Porter J, Ryder D, Branch RA. Caffeine potentiates the renin response to diazoxide in man. Evidence for a regulatory role of endogenous adenosine. *Journal of Pharmacology and Experimental Therapeutics* 1991;256:56–61.

100. Winer N, Chokshi DS, Yoon MS, Freedman AD. Adrenergic receptor mediation of renin secretion. *Journal of Clinical Endocrinology and Metabolism* 1969;29:1168–75.

101. Koch–Weser J. Vasodilator drugs in the treatment of hypertension. *Archives of Internal Medicine* 1974;133:1017–27.

102. Schofer J, Mathey DG, Polster J, Bode V, Dietlein G. Hemodynamic and neurohormonal response to hydralazine versus captopril: A controlled study in idiopathic dilated cardiomyopathy. *Journal of Cardiovascular Pharmacology* 1987; 9 (suppl 2):S46–9.

103. Levine TB, Olivari MT, Cohn JN. Dissociation of the responses of the renin–angiotensin system and sympathetic nervous system to a vasodilator stimulus in congestive heart failure. *International Journal of Cardiology* 1986;12:165–73.

104. Markham RV Jr, Gilmore A, Pettinger WA, Brater DC, Corbett JR, Firth BG. Central and regional hemodynamic effects and neurohormonal consequences of minoxidil in severe congestive cardiac failure and comparison to hydralazine and nitroprusside. *American Journal of Cardiology* 1988;52:774–81.

105. Elkayam U, Roth A, Hsueh W, Weber C, Freidenberger L, Rahimtoola SH. Neurohumoral consequences of vasodilator therapy with hydralazine and nifedipine in severe congestive heart failure. *American Heart Journal* 1986;111: 1130–8.

106. Kenko Y, Takeda T, Ikeda T, Tagawa H, Ishi M, Takadatake Y, Ueda H. Effect of ganglion-blocking agents on renin release in hypertensive patients. *Circulation Research* 1970;27:97–103.

107. Safar ME, Weiss YA, Corvol PL, Menard JE, London GM, Milliez PL. Anti-hypertensive adrenergic-blocking agents: Effects on sodium balance, the renin–angiotensin system and haemodynamics. *Clinical Science and Molecular Medicine* 1975;49 (suppl 2):93–5.

108. Halushka PV, Keiser HR. Effects of alpha-methyldopa on blood pressure and plasma renin activity. *Circulation Research* 1974;35:458–63.

109. Lowder SC, Liddle MD. Effects of guanethidine and methyldopa on a standardized test for renin responsiveness. *Annals of Internal Medicine* 1975;82:757–60.

110. Zoccali C, Zabludowski JR, Isles CG, Murray GD, Inglis GC, Robertson JIS, Fraser R, Ball SG. The effect of a 5-HT$_2$ antagonist, ketanserin, on blood pressure, the renin–angiotensin system and sympathoadrenal function in normal man. *British Journal of Clinical Pharmacology* 1983;16:305–11.

111. Reimann IW, Ratge D, Wisser H, Klotz U. Effect of intravenous ketanserin on plasma catecholamines and renin activity in normal volunteers. *European Journal of Clinical Pharmacology* 1985;28:273–7.

112. Donnelly R, Elliott HL, Meredith PA, Reid JL. Acute and chronic ketanserin in essential hypertension: Antihypertensive mechanisms and pharmacokinetics. *British Journal of Clinical Pharmacology* 1987;24:599–606.

113. Gerber JG, Olson RD, Nies AS. Inter-relationship between prostaglandins and renin release. *Kidney International* 1981;19:818–21.

114. Henrich WL. Role of prostaglandins in renin secretion. *Kidney International* 1981;19:822–30.

115. Patrono C, Pugliese F, Ciabattoni G, Patrignani P, Maseri A, Chierchia S, Peskar BA, Cinotti GA, Simonetti BM, Pierucci A. Evidence for a direct stimulatory effect of prostacyclin on renin release in man. *Journal of Clinical Investigation* 1982;69:231–9.

116. Brater DC. Effect of indomethacin on salt and water homeostasis in man. *Clinical Pharmacology and Therapeutics* 1979;25:322–30.

117. Rumpf KW, Frenzel S, Lowitz HD, Scheler F. The effect of indomethacin on plasma renin activity in man under normal conditions and after stimulation of the renin angiotensin system. *Prostaglandins* 1975;10:641–8.

118. Passmore AP, Copeland S, Johnston GD. A comparison of the effects of ibuprofen and indomethacin upon renal haemodynamics and electrolyte excretion in the presence and absence of frusemide. *British Journal of Clinical Pharmacology* 1989;27:483–90.

119. Frölich JC, Hollifield JW, Dormois JC, Frölich BL, Seyberth H, Michelakis AM, Oates JA. Suppression of plasma renin activity by indomethacin in man. *Circulation Research* 1976;39:447–52.

120. Favre L, Glasson PH, Riondel A, Vallotton MB. Interaction of diuretics and non-steroidal anti-inflammatory drugs in man. *Clinical Science* 1983;64: 407–15.

121. Prescott LF, Mattison P, Menzies DG, Manson LM. The comparative effects of paracetamol and indomethacin on renal function in healthy female volunteers. *British Journal of Clinical Pharmacology* 1990;29:403–12.

122. Lijnen P, Staessen J, Fagard R, Groeseneken D, M'Buyamba–Kabungu JR, Grauwels R, Amery A. Active and acid-activable inactive renin during inhibition by indomethacin of prostaglandin synthesis in sodium-replete man. *European Journal of Clinical Investigation* 1985;15:141–5.

123. Toffelmire EB, Slater K, Corvol P, Menard J, Schambelan M. Responses of plasma prorenin and active renin to chronic and acute alterations of renin secretion in normal humans: Studies using a direct immunoradiometric assay. *Journal of Clinical Investigation* 1989;83:679–87.

124. Frölich JC, Hollifield JW, Michelakis AM, Vesper BS, Wilson JP, Shand DG, Seyberth HJ, Frölich WH, Oates JA. Reduction of plasma renin activity by inhibition of the fatty acid cyclo-oxygenase in human subjects: Independence of sodium retention. *Circulation Research* 1979;44:781–7.

125. Ylitalo P, Pitkajarvi T, Pyykonen ML, Nurmi AK, Seppala E, Vappaatalo H. Inhibition of prostaglandin synthesis by indomethacin interacts with the anti-hypertensive effect of atenolol. *Clinical Pharmacology and Therapeutics* 1985;38:443–9.

126. Puddey IB, Beilin LJ, Vandongen R, Banks R, Rouse I. Differential effects of sulindac and indomethacin on blood pressure in treated essential hypertensive subjects. *Clinical Science* 1985;69:327–36.

127. Oates JA. Antagonism of anti-hypertensive drug therapy by non-steroidal anti-inflammatory drugs. *Hypertension* 1988;11 (suppl II):II4–6.

128. Tamm C, Favre L, Spence S, Pfister S, Vallotton MB. Interaction of oxindac and frusemide in man. *European Journal of Clinical Pharmacology* 1989;37: 17–21.

129. Brater DC, Anderson S, Baird B, Campbell WB. Effects of ibuprofen, naproxen and sulindac on prostaglandins in man. *Kidney International* 1985;27:66–73.

130. Wilson TW, McCauley FA, Wells HD. Effects of low dose aspirin on responses to frusemide. *Journal of Clinical Pharmacology* 1986;26:100–5.

131. Waslen TA, McCauley FA, Wilson TW. Sulindac does not spare renal prostaglandins. *Clinical and Investigative Medicine* 1989;12:77–81.

132. Riley LJ Jr, Vlasses PH, Rotmensch HH, Swanson BN, Chremos AN, Johnson CL, Ferguson RK. Sulindac and ibuprofen inhibit frusemide-stimulated renin release but not natriuresis in men on a normal sodium diet. *Nephron* 1985;41:283–8.

133. Eriksson LO, Sturfelt G, Thysell H, Wollheim FA. Effects of sulindac and naproxen on prostaglandin excretion in patients with impaired renal function and rheumatoid arthritis. *American Journal of Medicine* 1990;89:313–21.

134. Passmore AP, Copeland S, Johnston GD. The effects of ibuprofen and indomethacin on renal function in the presence and absence of frusemide in healthy volunteers on a restricted sodium diet. *British Journal of Clinical Pharmacology* 1990;29:311–9.

135. Imanishi M, Kawamura M, Akabane S, Matsushima Y, Kuramochi M, Ito K, Ohta M, Kimura K, Tahamiya M, Omae T. Aspirin lowers blood pressure in patients with renovascular hypertension. *Hypertension* 1989;14: 461–8.

136. Stockigt JR, Hewett MJ, Topliss DJ, Higgs EJ, Taft P. Renin and renin substrate in primary adrenal insufficiency: Contrasting effects of glucocorticoid and mineralocorticoid deficiency. *American Journal of Medicine* 1979;66:915–22.

137. Smith SJ, MacGregor GA, Markandu N, Bayliss J, Banks RA, Prentice MG, Dorrington–Ward P, Wise P. Evidence that patients with Addison's disease are under-treated with fludrocortisone. *Lancet* 1984;i:11–4.

138. Martin K, Zipser R, Horton R. Effect of prostaglandin inhibition on the hypertensive action of sodium retaining steroids. *Hypertension* 1981;3:622–8.

139. Izzo JL Jr, Horwitz D, Lawton WJ, Keiser HR. Fludrocortisone suppression of sympathetic nervous activity. *Clinical Pharmacology and Therapeutics* 1983;33: 102–6.

140. Weidmann P, Matter DR, Matter EE, Gnädinger MP, Uehlinger DE, Shaw S, Hess C. Glucocorticoid and mineralocorticoid stimulation of atrial natriuretic peptide release in man. *Journal of Clinical Endocrinology and Metabolism* 1988;66: 1233–9.

141. Kelly TM, Nelson DH. Sodium excretion and atrial natriuretic peptide levels during mineralocorticoid administration: A mechanism for the escape from hyperaldosteronism. *Endocrine Research* 1987;13:363–83.

142. Richards AM, Tonolo G, Tree M, Robertson JIS, Montorsi P, Leckie BJ, Polonia J. Atrial natriuretic peptides and renin release. *American Journal of Medicine* 1988;**84** (suppl 3A):112–8.

143. Whitworth JA, Saines D, Thatcher R. Differential blood pressure and metabolic effects of 9 alpha-fludrocortisol in man. *Clinical and Experimental Pharmacology and Physiology* 1983;**10**:351–4.

144. Conn JW, Rovner DR, Cohen EL. Liquorice-induced pseudoaldosteronism: Hypertension, hypokalaemia, aldosteronopaenia and suppressed plasma renin activity. *Journal of the American Medical Association* 1968;**205**:492–6.

145. Turpie AGG, Thomson TJ. Carbenoxolone sodium in the treatment of gastric ulcers with special reference to side-effects. *Gut* 1965;**6**:591–4.

146. Forslund T, Fyhrquist F, Froseth B, Tikkanen I. Effects of liquorice on plasma natriuretic peptide in healthy volunteers. *Journal of Internal Medicine* 1989;**225**:95–9.

147. Stewart PM, Wallace AM, Valentino R, Burt D, Shackleton CHL, Edwards CRW. Mineralocorticoid activity of liquorice: 11 beta-hydroxysteroid dehydrogenase deficiency comes of age. *Lancet* 1987;**ii**:821–4.

148. Mackenzie MA, Hoefnagels WH, Jansen RW, Benraad TJ, Kloppenborg PW. The influence of glycyrrhetinic acid on plasma cortisol and cortisone in healthy young volunteers. *Journal of Clinical Endocrinology and Metabolism* 1990;**70**:1637–43.

149. Stewart PM, Wallace AM, Atherden SM, Shearing CH, Edwards CRW. Mineralocorticoid activity of carbenoxolone: Contrasting effects of carbenoxolone and liquorice on 11 β-hydroxysteroid dehydrogenase activity in man. *Clinical Science* 1990;**78**:49–54.

150. Armanini D, Karbowiak I, Funder JW. Affinity of liquorice derivatives for mineralocorticoid and glucocorticoid receptors. *Clinical Endocrinology* 1983;**19**:609–12.

151. Newton MA, Laragh JH. Effects of glucocorticoid administration on aldosterone excretion and plasma renin in normal subjects in essential hypertension and in primary aldosteronism. *Journal of Clinical Endocrinology and Metabolism* 1968;**28**:1014–27.

152. Kelsch RC, Light GS, Luciano JR, Oliver WJ. The effect of prednisolone on plasma norepinephrine concentration and renin activity in salt depleted man. *Journal of Laboratory and Clinical Medicine* 1971;**77**:267–77.

153. Whitworth JA, Saines D, Scoggins BA. Blood pressure and metabolic effects of cortisol and deoxycorticosterone in man. *Clinical and Experimental Hypertension* 1984;**A6**:795–809.

154. Clore JN, Estep H, Ross–Clunis H, Watlington CO. Adrenocorticotrophic and cortisol-induced changes in urinary sodium and potassium excretion in man: Effects of spironolactone and RU486. *Journal of Clinical Endocrinology and Metabolism* 1988;**67**:824–31.

155. Murphy DL, Goodwin FK, Bunney WE. Aldosterone and sodium response to lithium administration in man. *Lancet* 1969;**ii**:458–61.

156. Strazzullo P, Iacoviello L, Iacone R, Giorgione N. Use of fractional lithium clearance in clinical and epidemiological investigation: A methodological assessment. *Clinical Science* 1988;**74**:651–7.

157. Freestone S, Jeffrey RF, Bonner CV, Lee MR. Effect of lithium on the renal actions of α-human atrial natriuretic peptide in normal man. *Clinical Science* 1990;**78**:371–5.

158. Shopsin B, Sathananthan G, Gershon S. Plasma renin response to lithium in psychiatric patients. *Clinical Pharmacology and Therapeutics* 1973;**14**:561–4.

159. Miller PD, Dubovsky SL, McDonald KM, Katz FH, Robertson GL, Schrier RW. Central, renal and adrenal effects of lithium in man. *American Journal of Medicine* 1979;**66**:797–803.

160. Transbol I, Christiansen C, Baastrup PC, Nilsen MD, Giese J. Endocrine effects of lithium. *Acta Endocrinologica* 1978;**88**:619–24.

161. Stewart PM, Atherden SM, Stewart SE, Whalley L, Edwards CRW, Padfield PL. Lithium carbonate — a competitive aldosterone antagonist? *British Journal of Psychology* 1988;**153**:205–7.

162. Nally JV, Rutecki GW, Ferris TF. The acute effect of lithium on renal renin and prostaglandin E synthesis in the dog. *Circulation Research* 1980;**46**:739–44.

163. Berridge MJ. Inositol trisphosphate, calcium, lithium, and cell signaling. *Journal of the American Medical Association* 1989;**262**:1834–41.

164. Stewart PM, Grieve J, Nairn IM, Padfield PL, Edwards CRW. Lithium inhibits the action of fludrocortisone on the kidney. *Clinical Endocrinology* 1987;**27**:63–8.

165. Pedersen EB, Darling S, Hansen AK, Amdisen A. Plasma aldosterone during lithium treatment. *Neurophysiology* 1977;**3**:153–9.

166. Fraser R, James VHT, Brown JJ, Isaac P, Lever AF, Robertson JIS. Effect of angiotensin and of frusemide on plasma aldosterone, corticosterone, cortisol and renin in man. *Lancet* 1965;**ii**:989–91.

167. Keeton TK, Campbell WB. The pharmacologic alteration of renin release. *Pharmacological Reviews* 1980;**32**:81–226.

168. Johnston GD, Nicholls DP, Leahey WJ. The dose–response characteristics of the acute non-diuretic peripheral vascular effects of frusemide in normal subjects. *British Journal of Clinical Pharmacology* 1984;**18**:75–81.

169. Passmore AP, Whitehead EM, Johnston GD. Comparison of the acute renal and peripheral vascular response to frusemide and bumetanide at low and high dose. *British Journal of Clinical Pharmacology* 1989;**27**:305–12.

170. Johnston GD, Hiatt WR, Nies AS, Payne NA, Murphy RC, Gerber JG. Factors modifying the early nondiuretic vascular effects of frusemide in man: The possible role of renal prostaglandins. *Circulation Research* 1983;**53**:630–5.

171. Wilson TW, McCauley FA, Waslen TA. Effects of ageing on responses to frusemide. *Prostaglandins* 1989;**38**:675–87.

172. McKay IG, Nath K, Cumming AD, Muir AL, Watson ML. Haemodynamic and endocrine responses of the kidney to frusemide in mild hypertension. *Clinical Science* 1985;**68**:159–64.

173. Johnston GD, Passmore AP. The effects of cilazapril alone and in combination with frusemide in healthy subjects. *British Journal of Clinical Pharmacology* 1989;**27**:235–42S.

174. Van Hooff MEJ, Does RJMM, Rahn KH, Van Baak MA. Time course of blood pressure changes after intravenous administration of propranolol or frusemide in hypertensive patients. *Journal of Cardiovascular Pharmacology* 1983;**5**:773–7.

175. Ciabattoni G, Pugliese F, Cinotti GA, Stirati G, Ronci R, Castrucci G, Pierucci A, Patrono C. Characterisation of frusemide-induced activation of the renal prostaglandin system. *European Journal of Pharmacology* 1979;**60**:181–7.

176. Cannella G, Galva MD, Campanini M, Cesura AM, De Marinis S, Picotti GB. Sequential changes in plasma renin activity and plasma catecholamines in mildly hypertensive patients during acute frusemide-induced body-fluid loss. *European Journal of Clinical Pharmacology* 1983;**23**:299–302.

177. Gerber JG. Role of prostaglandins in the hemodynamic and tubular effects of frusemide. *Federation Proceedings* 1983;**42**:1707–10.

178. Noda Y, Fukiyama K, Kumamoto K, Takishita S, Eto T, Kawasaki T, Omae T. Renin response to frusemide differs with the routes of administration in healthy man. *Japanese Circulation Journal* 1982;**46**:552–8.

179. Wilson TW, Loadholt CB, Privitera PJ, Halushka PV. Frusemide increases urinary 6-keto-prostaglandin-$F_{1\alpha}$: Relation to natriuresis, vasodilation and renin release. *Hypertension* 1982;**4**:634–41.

180. Mackay IG, Muir AL, Watson ML. Contribution of prostaglandins to the systemic and renal vascular response to frusemide in normal man. *British Journal of Clinical Pharmacology* 1984;**17**:513–9.

181. Whorton AR, Misono K, Hollfield J, Frölich JC, Inagami T, Oates JA. Prostaglandins and renin release. Stimulation of renin release from rabbit renal cortical slices by PGI_2. *Prostaglandins* 1977;**14**:1095–104.

182. MacDonald TM, Craig K, Watson ML. Frusemide: Ace inhibition, renal dopamine and prostaglandins: Acute interactions in normal man. *British Journal of Clinical Pharmacology* 1989;**28**:683–94.

183. Fujimura A, Ebihara A. Role of angiotensin II in renal prostaglandin E_2 production after frusemide administration. *Hypertension* 1988;**11**:491–4.

184. Johnston GD, Nicholls DP, Kondowe GB, Finch MB. Comparison of the acute vascular effects of frusemide and bumetanide. *British Journal of Clinical Pharmacology* 1986;**21**:359–64.

80.18

185. Jeffrey RF, MacDonald TM, Ruttier M, Freestone S, Brown J, Samson RR, Lee MR. The effect of intravenous frusemide on urine dopamine in normal volunteers: Studies with indomethacin and carbidopa. *Clinical Science* 1987;73: 151–7.

186. Elmgreen J, Hesse B, Christensen NJ. Lack of adrenergic influence on renin release after frusemide in normal man. *European Journal of Clinical Pharmacology* 1981;20:339–42.

187. Hummerich W, Konrads A, Krause DK, Fischer JH, Kaufmann W. Renin release after frusemide and ethacrynic acid in man: Evidence for neural reflex mechanisms. *Klinische Wochenschrift* 1981;59:791–5.

188. Johnston GD, O'Connor PC, Nicholls DP, Leahey WJ, Finch MB. The effects of propranolol and digoxin on the acute vascular responses to frusemide in normal man. *British Journal of Clinical Pharmacology* 1985;19:417–21.

189. Herchuelz A, Derenne F, Deger F, Juvent M, Van Ganse E, Staroukine M, Verniory A, Voeynaens JM, Douchamps J. Interaction between non-steroidal anti-inflammatory drugs and loop diuretics: Modulation by sodium balance. *Journal of Pharmacology and Experimental Therapeutics* 1989;248:1175–81.

190. Pedrinelli R, Magagna A, Arzilli F, Sassano P, Salvetti A. Influence of indomethacin on the natriuretic and renin-stimulating effect of bumetanide in essential hypertension. *Clinical Pharmacology and Therapeutics* 1980;28:722–31.

191. Johnston GD, Nicholls DP, Leahey WJ, Finch MB. The effects of captopril on the acute vascular response to frusemide in man. *Clinical Science* 1983;65: 359–63.

192. Francis GS, Siegel RM, Goldsmith SR, Olivari MT, Levine TB, Cohn JN. Acute vasoconstrictor response to intravenous furosemide in patients with chronic congestive heart failure: Activation of the neurohumoral axis. *Annals of Internal Medicine* 1985;103:1–6.

193. Griffing GT, Sindler BH, Aurecchia SA, Melby JC. The effects of hydrochlorothiazide on the renin–aldosterone system. *Metabolism* 1983;32: 197–201.

194. Koopmans PP, Kateman WGPM, Tan Y, Van Ginnetken CAM, Gribnau FWJ. The effects of indomethacin and sulindac on hydrochlorothiazide kinetics. *Clinical Pharmacology and Therapeutics* 1985;37:625–8.

195. Saito I, Misumi J, Kondo K, Saruta T, Matsuki S. Effects of frusemide and chlorthiazide on blood pressure and plasma renin activity. *Cardiovascular Research* 1976;10:149–52.

196. Koopmans PP, Thien TH, Gribnau FWJ. The influence of ibuprofen, diclofenac and sulindac on the blood pressure lowering effect of hydrochlorthiazide. *European Journal of Clinical Pharmacology* 1987;31:553–7.

197. Fernandez PG, Snedden W, Nath C, Vasdev S, Lee C, Darke A. Hemodynamic and neurohormonal factors in the response of hypertensives to hydrochlorthiazide therapy. *Clinical and Investigative Medicine* 1987;10:513–9.

198. Chalmers JP, Wing LM, West MJ, Bune AJ, Elliot JM, Morris MJ, Chain MD, Graham JR, Southgate DO. Effects of enalapril and hydrochlorthiazide on blood pressure, renin–angiotensin system and atrial natriuretic factor in essential hypertension: A double blind factorial crossover study. *Australian and New Zealand Journal of Medicine* 1986;16:475–80.

199. Vaughan ED, Carey RM, Peach MJ, Ackerly JA, Ayers CR. The renin response to diuretic therapy: A limitation of anti-hypertensive potential. *Circulation Research* 1978;42:376–81.

200. Swales JD, Thurston H. Plasma renin and angiotensin II measurement in hypertensive and normal subjects: Correlation in basal and stimulated states. *Journal of Clinical Endocrinology and Metabolism* 1977;45:159–63.

201. Lijnen P, Staessen J, Fagard R, Amery A. Effect of bendrofluazide on the renin–angiotensin–aldosterone system and prostaglandins in captopril-resistant hypertensive patients. *Clinical and Experimental Hypertension* 1983;A5:285–95.

202. Koopmans PP, Thien T, Thomas CM, Van Den Berg RJ, Gribnau FW. The effects of sulindac and indomethacin on the anti-hypertensive and diuretic action of hydrochlorthiazide in patients with mild to moderate essential hypertension. *British Journal of Clinical Pharmacology* 1986;21:417–23.

203. Fernandez PG, Snedden W, Vasdev S, Bolli P. Bevantolol attenuates thiazide stimulated renin secretion and catecholamine release in diuretic resistant hypertensives. *Canadian Journal of Cardiology* 1989;5:93–7.

204. Johnson BF, Weiner B, Marwahu R, Johnson J. The influence of pindolol and hydrochlorthiazide on blood pressure and plasma renin and plasma lipid levels. *Journal of Clinical Pharmacology* 1986;26:258–63.

205. Lancaster R, Goodwin TJ, Peart WS. The effect of pindolol on plasma renin activity and blood pressure in hypertensive patients. *British Journal of Clinical Pharmacology* 1976;3:453–60.

206. Claus–Walker J, Cardus D, Griffith D, Hastead LS. Metabolic effects of sodium restriction and thiazides in tetraplegic patients. *Paraplegia* 1978;15:3–10.

207. Ramsay LE, Hettiarachchi J, Fraser R, Morton JJ. Amiloride, spironolactone and potassium chloride in thiazide-treated hypertensive patients. *Clinical Pharmacology and Therapeutics* 1980;27:533–43.

208. Millar JA, Fraser R, Mason P, Leckie B, Cumming AMM, Robertson JIS. Metabolic effects of high dose amiloride and spironolactone: A comparative study in normal subjects. *British Journal of Clinical Pharmacology* 1987;18: 369–75.

209. Favre L, Vallotton MB. Relationship of renal prostaglandins to three diuretics. *Prostaglandins Leukotrienes and Medicine* 1984;14:313–9.

210. Favre L, Glasson P, Vallotton MB. Reversible acute renal failure from combined triamterine and indomethacin. *Annals of Internal Medicine* 1982;96:317–20.

211. Karlberg BE, Kågedal B, Tegler L, Tolagen K, Bergman B. Controlled treatment of primary hypertension with propranolol and spironolactone: A crossover study with special reference to initial plasma renin activity. *American Journal of Cardiology* 1976;37:642–9.

81 RENIN WITH ANESTHESIA AND SURGERY

EDWARD D MILLER

INTRODUCTION

The role of the RAS during anesthesia and surgery has only recently been investigated in detail. Many of the factors that control renin release are activated during the perioperative period. Anesthesia may, however, modify the renin response, and the stress hormones that increase with surgery may not exert their usual effects during anesthesia.

It must be recognized that 'anesthesia' is a specific term. Some of the confusion concerning the influence of anesthetics on the RAS, however, derives from the fact that steady-state conditions have not existed at the time of renin measurements; for example, volatile anesthetics have equal potency at a specific end-tidal concentration.

Anesthetics may be compared at equal minimum alveolar concentration (MAC), at which 50% of patients do not move in response to a painful stimulus. Unfortunately, intravenous anesthetics, in particular, narcotics, do not demonstrate a similar narrow range of potency. It also must be noted that whereas a variety of chemical agents can produce a state of unconsciousness, not all are analgesic. A true anesthetic induces both loss of consciousness and analgesia, and prevents reflex responses to noxious stimuli. Some anesthetics also produce muscle relaxation. This chapter examines the RAS during anesthesia and surgery. Inhibition of the RAS has allowed for a better appreciation of its importance in the perioperative period.

GENERAL ANESTHESIA

The first systematic study in experimental animals which examined the influence of anesthetic agents *per se* on the RAS was performed by Miller and colleagues [1]. In rats, halothane, fluroxene, or ketamine were administered at equipotent anesthetic doses, and blood pressure, heart rate, and plasma renin activity (PRA) were measured. No surgery was performed. Control measurements were taken in the awake state prior to anesthesia. The important finding was that despite a significant decrease in mean arterial pressure during anesthesia, there was no significant rise in PRA. When the competitive Ang II-receptor antagonist, saralasin, however, was infused, a 20-mm decrease in blood pressure occurred in animals anesthetized with halothane but not in those given ketamine or fluroxene (Fig. 81.1). These data clearly demonstrated that during anesthesia, PRA was not an accurate predictor of the blood-pressure response to inhibitors of the RAS. Robertson and Michelakis subsequently reported that patients anesthetized with halothane had no increase in PRA, but that a three-fold rise in PRA occurred midway through the surgical procedure [2]. Ketamine given to healthy volunteers increased blood pressure and heart rate but PRA was unaltered [3]. No inhibitors of the RAS were used in these studies but the importance of the RAS to the support of blood pressure during anesthesia has been demonstrated in patients anesthetized with halothane or isoflurane [4].

Not only does surgical stimulation confound studies of the RAS during the perioperative period, but the volume status and sodium intake are also relevant to interpretation of results. In rats on a low-sodium diet, the average decrease in blood pressure during anesthesia was almost two-fold greater than in animals given a normal sodium diet. Furthermore, anesthesia for one hour with halothane, enflurane, or ketamine stimulated PRA in sodium-depleted rats, and saralasin reduced blood pressure by 30mmHg in each case [5]. It is not surprising then that patients who are either volume depleted or salt restricted prior to surgical procedures have an exaggerated response in PRA [6].

Regional anesthesia (spinal or epidural) does not stimulate an increase in PRA despite relative hypotension.

CONVERTING-ENZYME ACTIVITY

I am aware of only two studies that have directly examined the effect of anesthetic agents on ACE activity. Miller and co-workers examined the influence of anesthetic agents on ACE activity *in vitro* and *in vivo* [7]. In one set of experiments, isolated pulmonary converting enzyme was exposed to air, halothane, or fluroxene. The results demonstrated minimal effect of the anesthetic agents

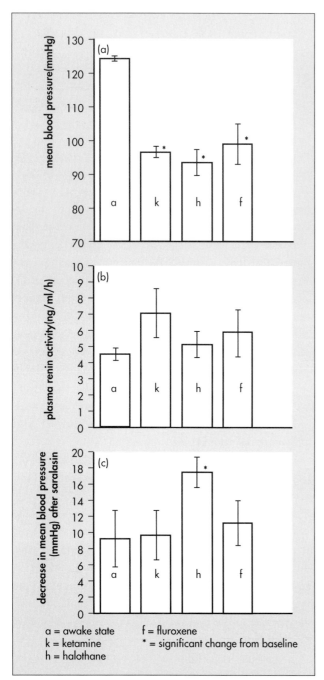

Fig. 81.1 (a) Decrease in mean arterial pressure after one hour of stable anesthesia with ketamine, halothane, or fluroxene as compared to the awake state in rats. (b) Plasma renin activity (PRA) in rats when awake or during stable anesthesia. No significant increase in PRA occurred despite significant decreases in blood pressure. (c) Blood-pressure response to the Ang II-receptor antagonist, saralasin. A significant decrease in blood pressure was seen only in animals anesthetized with halothane. This response was not predicted by the measurement of PRA. Results are given as mean ± SEM. Modified from Miller ED *et al* [1].

on this *in vitro* system. Perhaps more important were the *in vivo* experiments in which animals, either awake or anesthetized, were given Ang I and Ang II and the blood-pressure responses recorded [7]. Angiotensin I and Ang II induced similar blood-pressure responses in awake and anesthetized rats (Fig. 81.2). In man, Knight and co-workers measured PRA and Ang II in anesthetized patients and saw a close correlation between the two indices over a wide range of values [8].

DELIBERATE HYPOTENSION

One of the commonly used methods to limit blood loss during surgical procedures is the introduction of deliberate or controlled hypotension. The mean arterial pressure is lowered to 50–60 mmHg through the use of a variety of drugs, the most common being sodium nitroprusside. Activation of the RAS during the infusion of sodium nitroprusside has been known for some time [9]. Toxicity and even death have, however, occurred with nitroprusside infusion [10], thus a careful study of a possible role of the RAS was undertaken.

Sodium nitroprusside was infused in awake rats in order to lower the mean blood pressure from 120 to 80mmHg. The PRA increased four-fold, and subsequent saralasin induced a dramatic further decrease in blood pressure. Similar observations were made during enflurane anesthesia [11].

It was at this time that the rebound hypertension associated with discontinuation of sodium nitroprusside was recognized clinically [12]. Delany and Miller demonstrated that inhibition of the RAS could prevent this rebound hypertension and allow a more stable hypotensive period [13] (Fig. 81.3).

The measurement of blood pressure alone, however, does not adequately describe the importance of the RAS during deliberate hypotension. What is more important is the distribution of blood flow. Using the microsphere technique, the importance of the RAS was quantified. Blood pressure was reduced to a similar degree with either sodium nitroprusside or saralasin in rats anesthetized with halothane [14]. Blood flow to various organ beds was then determined. At similar levels of arterial pressure, renal blood flow was markedly reduced by nitroprusside but not by saralasin. The decrease in renal blood flow induced by nitroprusside was reversed by the addition of saralasin. This finding clearly showed that distribution of blood flow to the kidney under these circumstances was under the control of the RAS system (Fig. 81.4).

The knowledge that deliberate hypotension could be more readily and smoothly accomplished in animals if the RAS was

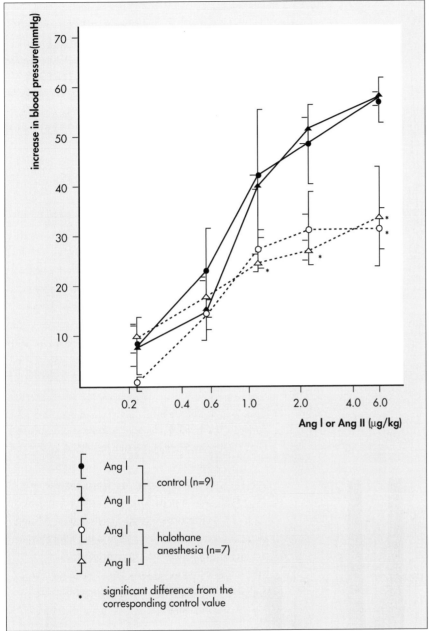

Fig. 81.2 Dose–response curves to Ang I and II in awake or anesthetized rats. The increase in blood pressure was significantly less in animals anesthetized with halothane as compared to the awake state but the two peptides induced similar increments in blood pressure under either circumstance. Results are shown as mean ± SEM. Modified from Miller ED *et al* [7].

inhibited led to studies in man. Woodside and co-workers pretreated patients with captopril prior to major orthopedic surgery [15]. These authors were able to show that for similar degrees of hypotension, significantly less sodium nitroprusside was necessary if captopril was also used — as documented by plasma levels of cyanide in the two groups (Fig. 81.5). Judicious use of β-blocking agents also reduces both the nitroprusside dose requirement and the likelihood of developing cyanide toxicity [16]. Subsequently, the similar use of an intravenous ACE inhibitor, enalaprilat, was investigated [17].

HYPERTENSION

Two experimental forms of hypertension have been studied with commonly used anesthetic agents. Halothane and enflurane anesthesia was administered in rats made hypertensive by clipping of one renal artery (1-clip, 2-kidney model) [18]. Clipping increased the mean arterial pressure to approximately 200mmHg. Both halothane and enflurane anesthesia induced marked decreases in pressure, which was further lowered by the infusion of saralasin.

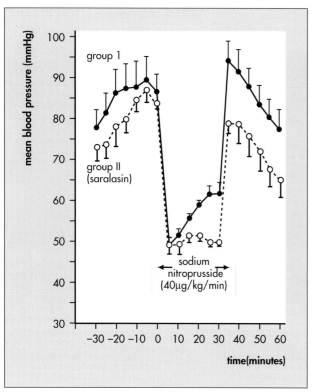

Fig. 81.3 Blood-pressure (mean ± SEM) response to sodium nitroprusside in rats treated with saralasin and in control animals. It should be noted that the period of hypotension was well controlled in animals treated with saralasin and there was no rebound hypertension once the nitroprusside infusion was discontinued. Group I animals (controls) did not receive saralasin. Modified from Delaney TJ and Miller ED [13].

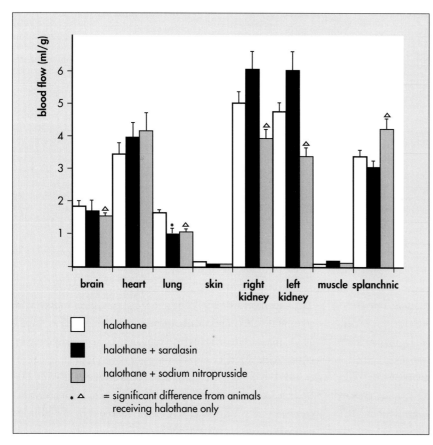

Fig. 81.4 Blood flow to various organs in rats anesthetized with halothane, or receiving halothane and then saralasin or sodium nitroprusside. Blood pressure was similar in both the saralasin- and sodium-nitroprusside-treated animals. A significant decrease in blood flow to the kidneys is seen in animals treated with sodium nitroprusside only. Results are shown as mean ± SEM. Modified from Miller ED, Delaney TJ [14].

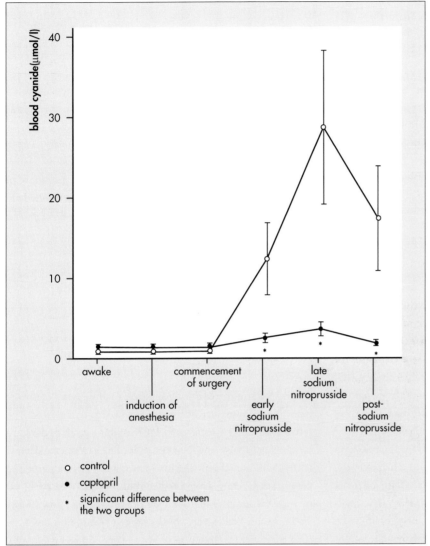

Fig. 81.5 Blood cyanide levels in patients (n=12) receiving sodium nitroprusside. The group that did not receive captopril (control, n=6) required eight times as much sodium nitroprusside to reduce blood pressure to a similar degree. Results are shown as mean ± SEM. Modified from Woodside J *et al* [15].

In spontaneously hypertensive rats (SHR), halothane and enflurane anesthesia acted in a manner different from that seen in normotensive rats or in rats with renovascular hypertension [19]. The major differences were that in the SHR, a 25% reduction in mean arterial pressure with anesthesia did not result in an increase in PRA, whereas in control Wistar – Kyoto (WKY) animals, a five-fold rise in PRA did occur. Only in animals treated with halothane did saralasin induce a further decline in blood pressure in SHR. These data clearly demonstrated not only that the hypertensive and normotensive animals responded differently to anesthesia, but also that normotensive animals (WKY and the Wistar normotensive rat) had discrepant responses. Appropriate controls must therefore be used for proper interpretation of data.

Hypertension in the perioperative period in man has received

limited study. Cardiac surgery has been most closely examined because hypertension at this time may have deleterious effects [20–22]. An increased incidence of bleeding, cerebrovascular accidents, and/or myocardial ischemia are the major concerns. Involvement of the RAS in perioperative hypertension and its complications remains controversial and it is likely that many factors such as the depth of anesthesia, volume status of the patient, and the degree of sympathetic stimulation, play key roles [23].

Several clinical studies suggest that the hypertension associated with intubation may be partially blunted by ACE inhibitors [24–27]. Most studies show that whereas the blood-pressure response to this noxious stimulus is attenuated by ACE inhibitors, the heart rate response is not. Since diastolic filling time is the prime determinant of coronary artery flow, agents that decrease heart rate at intubation are more important than those that decrease pressure. It is unlikely therefore that ACE inhibitors will find a place in routine practice under these circumstances.

Postoperative hypertension has been treated with ACE inhibitors [28,29]. In these studies, patients with the highest PRA showed the greatest fall in arterial pressure. Other factors, however, also seem to be important in cardiovascular control in the postoperative period. One reason why ACE inhibitors have not found universal favor in the treatment of perioperative hypertension is the delayed hypotension seen in some patients when these drugs are given [30].

SURGERY ON THE AORTA

Procedures that require either infrarenal or suprarenal aortic clamping have been extensively studied. The characteristic systemic hemodynamic consequences are well known [31–33]. Renal blood flow and specifically renal cortical blood flow are decreased and remain low for some time after release of the clamp. Renal failure in this setting is associated with a high mortality rate. Visceral blood flow also declines and vasculitis of the mesenteric arterial vessels may develop. It has been proposed that these hemodynamic responses may relate to activation of the RAS.

Experimental data demonstrate that when the thoracic aorta is clamped in dogs, PRA is elevated both during and after the clamp is released. After 60 minutes of aortic cross-clamping, renal cortical blood flow had returned to baseline values in animals treated with enalaprilat but not in control dogs or in those receiving saralasin [34]. It appears from this study that the level of blood pressure is not as important as is the distribution of the blood flow with a particular arterial pressure.

In patients undergoing infrarenal aortic cross-clamping, a single oral dose of 25mg of captopril was given prior to induction of anesthesia [35]. When compared with control patients, the urine output was almost twice as high in the captopril-treated group and remained high for the first 24 hours postoperatively. Whether the improved urine output was due to a renoprotective effect of captopril or to the additional volume replacement that was required to maintain cardiovascular stability in captopril-treated patients, is unclear from this trial. The use of enalaprilat in this context is currently being studied [36].

Activation of the RAS during cardiopulmonary bypass stimulated a study of captopril administration in patients undergoing coronary artery bypass surgery [37]. Compared with placebo (n=10 patients), captopril given as 100mg twice daily prior to surgery (n=8 patients) maintained effective renal plasma flow and glomerular filtration rates at higher levels. Blood pressure was similar in the two groups but urine sodium excretion was greater in those receiving captopril. Whether ACE inhibitors are renoprotective under these conditions seems possible but requires further study.

SUMMARY

The RAS is stimulated during anesthesia and surgery. Its importance in cardiovascular homeostasis, however, is not clear. The recent availability of intravenous ACE inhibitors and the development of nonagonist Ang II-receptor blocking agents should allow better definition of how the RAS controls the circulation in the perioperative period. Unfortunately, our ability to measure blood pressure far surpasses our ability to measure blood flow in different organs. Preliminary studies suggest that inhibition of the RAS may offer protection to the viscera and kidneys. Certainly, the common use of ACE inhibitors in patients who undergo surgery has not been associated with severe complications; thus these drugs do not usually need to be discontinued prior to surgical procedures.

REFERENCES

1. Miller ED, Longnecker DE, Peach MJ. The regulatory function of the renin–angiotensin system during general anesthesia. *Anesthesiology* 1978;48: 399–403.

2. Robertson D, Michelakis AM. Effect of anesthesia and surgery on plasma renin activity in man. *Journal of Clinical Endocrinology* 1972;34:831–6.

3. Miller ED, Bailey DR, Kaplan JA, Rogers PW. The effect of ketamine on the renin–angiotensin system. *Anesthesiology* 1975;42:503–5.

4. Kataja J, Viinamaki O, Punnonen R, Kaukinen S. Renin–angiotensin–aldosterone system and plasma vasopressin in surgical patients anesthetized with halothane or isoflurane. *European Journal of Anaesthesia* 1988;5:121–9.

5. Miller ED, Ackerly JA, Peach MJ. Blood pressure support during general anesthesia in a renin-dependent state in the rat. *Anesthesiology* 1978;48:404–8.

6. Bailey DR, Miller ED, Kaplan JA, Rogers PW. The renin–angiotensin–aldosterone system during cardiac surgery with morphine-nitrous oxide anesthesia. *Anesthesiology* 1975;42:538–44.

7. Miller ED, Gianfagna W, Ackerly JA, Peach MJ. Converting enzyme activity and pressor responses to angiotensin I and II in the rat awake and during anesthesia. *Anesthesiology* 1979;50:88–92.

8. Knight PR, Lane GA, Hensinger RN, Bolles RS, Bjoraker DG. Catecholamine and renin–angiotensin response during hypotensive anesthesia induced by sodium nitroprusside or trimethaphan camsylate. *Anesthesiology* 1983;**59**:248–53.

9. Kaneko Y, Ikeda T, Ueda H. Renin release during acute reduction of arterial pressure in normotensive subjects and patients with renovascular hypertension. *Journal of Clinical Investigation* 1967;**46**:705–16.

10. Davies DW, Kadar D, Stewart DJ. A sudden death associated with the use of sodium nitroprusside for induction of hypotension during anesthesia. *Canadian Anaesthetists Society Journal* 1975;**22**:547–52.

11. Miller ED, Ackerly JA, Vaughan ED, Peach MJ, Epstein RM. The renin–angiotensin system during controlled hypotension with sodium nitroprusside. *Anesthesiology* 1977;**47**:257–62.

12. Khambatta HJ, Stone JG, Khan E. Hypertension during anesthesia on discontinuation of sodium nitroprusside-induced hypotension. *Anesthesiology* 1979;**51**:127–30.

13. Delaney TJ, Miller ED. Rebound hypertension after sodium nitroprusside prevented by saralasin in rats. *Anesthesiology* 1980;**52**:154–6.

14. Miller ED, Delaney TJ. Blood flow alteration induced by saralasin or sodium nitroprusside in rats. *Anesthesiology* 1981;**54**:199–203.

15. Woodside J, Garner L, Bedford RF, Sussman MD, Miller ED, Longnecker DE, Epstein RM. Captopril reduces the dose requirements for sodium nitroprusside induced hypotension. *Anesthesiology* 1984;**60**:413–7.

16. Bedford RF, Berry FA, Longnecker DE. Impact of propranolol on hemodynamic responses and blood cyanide levels during nitroprusside infusion: A prospective study in anesthetized man. *Anesthesia and Analgesia* 1979;**58**:466–9.

17. Murphy JD, Vaughan RS, Rosen M. Intravenous enalaprilat and autonomic reflexes. *Anaesthesia* 1989;**44**:816–21.

18. Woodside JR, Beckman JJ, Althaus JS, Peach MJ, Longnecker DE, Miller ED. Renovascular hypertension: Effect of halothane and enflurane. *Anesthesiology* 1984;**60**:440–7.

19. Miller ED, Beckman JJ, Althaus JS. Hormonal and hemodynamic responses to halothane and enflurane in spontaneously hypertensive rats. *Anesthesia and Analgesia* 1985;**64**:136–42.

20. Taylor KM, Morton JJ, Brown JJ, Bain WH, Caves PK, Shumway N. Hypertension and renin–angiotensin system following open heart surgery. *Journal of Thoracic and Cardiovascular Surgery* 1977;**74**:840–5.

21. Landymore RW, Murphy DA, Kinley E, Parrott J, Sai O, Quirbi AA. Suppression of renin production in patients undergoing coronary artery bypass. *Annals of Thoracic Surgery* 1980;**30**:558–63.

22. Roberts AJ, Niarchos AP, Subramanian VA, Abel RM, Steven D, Herman SD, Sealey JE, Case DB, White RP, Johnson GA, Laragh JH, Gay WA Jr, Okinaka AJ. Systemic hypertension associated with coronary artery bypass surgery. *Journal of Thoracic and Cardiovascular Surgery* 1977;**74**:846–57.

23. Miller ED, Longnecker DE, Peach MJ. Renin response to hemorrhage in awake and anesthetized rats. *Shock* 1979;**6**:271–6.

24. Cashman JN, Jones RM, Thompson MA. Renin–angiotensin activation is not primarily responsible for the changes in mean arterial pressure during sternotomy in patients undergoing cardiac surgery. *European Journal of Anaesthesia* 1984;**1**:299–303.

25. Yates AP, Hunter DN. Anaesthesia and angiotensin-converting enzyme inhibitors. The effect of enalapril on peri-operative cardiovascular stability. *Anaesthesia* 1988;**43**:935–8.

26. McCarthy GJ, Hainsworth M, Lindsay K, Wright JM, Brown TA. Pressor responses to tracheal intubation after sublingual captopril. A pilot study. *Anaesthesia* 1990;**45**:243–5.

27. Murphy JD, Vaughan RS, Rosen M. Intravenous enalaprilat and autonomic reflexes. *Anaesthesia* 1989;**44**:816–21.

28. Niarchos AP, Roberts AJ, Case DB, Gay WA, Laragh JH. Hemodynamic characteristics of hypertension after coronary bypass surgery and effects of the converting enzyme inhibitor. *American Journal of Cardiology* 1979;**43**:586–93.

29. Roberts AJ, Niarchos AP, Subramanian VA, Abel RM, Hoover EL, McCabe JC, Case DB, Laragh JH, Gay WA. Hypertension following coronary artery bypass graft surgery. Comparison of hemodynamic responses to nitroprusside, phentolamine, and converting enzyme inhibitor. *Circulation* 1978;**58** (suppl 1):I43–9.

30. Selby DG, Richards JD, Marshman JM. ACE inhibitors [Letter]. *Anaesthesia Intensive Care* 1989;**17**:110–1.

31. Meloche R, Pottecher T, Audet J, Dufresne O, LePage C. Haemodynamic changes due to clamping of the abdominal aorta. *Canadian Anaesthetists Society Journal* 1977;**24**:20–34.

32. Lunn JK, Dannemiller FJ, Stanley TH. Cardiovascular responses to clamping of the aorta during epidural and general anesthesia. *Anaesthesia and Analgesia* 1979;**58**:372–6.

33. Silverstein PR, Caldera DL, Culler DJ, Davison JK, Darling RC, Emerson CW. Avoiding the hemodynamic consequences of aortic cross-clamping and unclamping. *Anesthesiology* 1979;**50**:462–6.

34. Joob AW, Harman PK, Kaiser DL, Kron IL. The effect of renin–angiotensin system blockade of visceral blood flow during and after thoracic aortic cross-clamping. *Journal of Thoracic and Cardiovascular Surgery* 1986;**91**:411–8.

35. Kataja JH, Kaukenin S, Viinamaki OV, Metsa-Keleta TJ, Vapaalata H. Hemodynamic and hormonal changes in patients pretreated with captopril for surgery of the abdominal aorta. *Journal of Cardiothoracic Anesthesia* 1989;**3**:425–32.

36. Mirenda JV, Grissom TE. Anesthetic implications of the renin–angiotensin system and angiotensin-converting enzyme inhibitors. *Anesthesia and Analgesia* 1991;**72**:667–83.

37. Colson P, Ribstein J, Mimran A, Grolleau D, Chaptal PA, Roquefeuil B. Effect of angiotensin converting enzyme inhibition in blood pressure and renal function during open heart surgery. *Anesthesiology* 1990;**72**:23–7.

82

THE RENIN–ANGIOTENSIN–ALDOSTERONE SYSTEM, ALTITUDE, AND SPACE TRAVEL

JAMES S MILLEDGE

THE RENIN–ANGIOTENSIN–ALDOSTERONE SYSTEM AT ALTITUDE

The renin–angiotensin–aldosterone system has been extensively studied in subjects at high altitude. This is not only because of a general interest in the effects of hypoxia on any physiological system, but also because of the belief that acute mountain sickness (AMS) is due, at least in part, to a disturbance of fluid and sodium balance. Acute mountain sickness is a condition affecting previously healthy subjects who go rapidly to altitude. The symptoms include headache, nausea, vomiting, sleep disturbance, and general malaise. There is a delay of 6–24 hours after arrival at altitude before symptoms arise. They usually disappear in 3–5 days at altitude without treatment or on descent. In a few cases, however, the condition progresses to a potentially fatal outcome as acute pulmonary edema or cerebral edema of high altitude. The incidence of the condition depends on the rate of ascent; in a typical trek in the great mountain ranges, half of a party may be at least mildly affected. When large numbers of trekkers going above 4,000m are studied, 1–2% are found to progress to one of the malignant forms of AMS.

In considering the effect of altitude on the RAS therefore, it is necessary to consider the situation in subjects who are free of AMS compared with those who develop the condition, that is, the physiological response compared with the pathological response. Exercise has a profound effect on the RAS (see *Chapters 24* and *74*), especially the day-long type of exercise involved in mountaineering. It is therefore necessary to consider the effects on the RAS in subjects in whom exercise is excluded and in whom altitude hypoxia has been imposed. Finally, there is the distinction to be made between acute hypoxia lasting for a few hours up to a few days, that is, before acclimatization to altitude, and the chronic hypoxia of a few weeks' duration when acclimatization has taken place.

The RAS is intimately related to a number of other hormones and neural–humoral systems, including the sympathetic (see *Chapter 37*), pituitary–adrenal (see *Chapters 33* and *34*), atrial natriuretic factor (ANF) (see *Chapter 36*), and vasopressin (see *Chapter 35*) systems. The effect of hypoxia on these systems will have secondary effects on the RAS.

THE PHYSIOLOGICAL RESPONSE TO ALTITUDE HYPOXIA

Aldosterone

Within a few years of the discovery of aldosterone in 1952, Williams (then a medical student at the Middlesex Hospital) carried out a study of salivary electrolytes in subjects at altitude in the Karakoram. He inferred that there was a reduction in aldosterone levels [1]. This observation was later confirmed by measurements of aldosterone in urine or blood [2–7] (Fig. 82.1). Slater *et al* [2] showed that this was due to reduced secretion of aldosterone at altitude rather than increased elimination. These studies were on subjects at rest and who were presumably healthy, although their condition as regards AMS was often not stated.

This depression of aldosterone secretion lasts for approximately two weeks after arrival at altitude; by three weeks, aldosterone has returned to sea level values [8].

Exercise results in stimulation of the RAS and a consequent rise in plasma aldosterone levels (see *Chapters 33* and *74*). If exercise is continued for some hours, and especially if repeated for a number of days as in hill walking, there is a significant retention of sodium and also some water retention. There is expansion of the extracellular fluid compartment at the expense of the intracellular compartment. Both plasma volume and interstitial fluid volume are increased, with a reduction in hematocrit and a tendency to the development of dependent edema [9,10]. If subjects exercise in getting to altitude, as is usually the case in the mountains, then the effect of exercise in increasing plasma aldosterone concentration overrides the decrease due to altitude and results in levels similar to those found with comparable exercise at sea level, and there is sodium and fluid retention [11]. Exercise also stimulates release of ANF, as does hypoxia, so it is not surprising that ANF levels are elevated modestly in subjects climbing to high altitudes [12,13]. However, the effect of this

Reference	Altitude above sea level (m)	Exercise	Method of study of aldosterone	Aldosterone	Renin activity
1	4,570+	uncontrolled	salivary sodium/potassium	decreased	not measured
30	4,350+	eliminated	urine	decreased	not measured
2	3,500	eliminated	circulating and secretion	decreased	increased
15	4,279 (equivalent)	eliminated	urine sodium/potassium	decreased	increased
31	4,300	uncontrolled	urine sodium/potassium	decreased	not measured
3	3,660 (equivalent)	eliminated	urine	decreased	decreased
16	5,330	uncontrolled	circulating	increased	increased
4	4,300	eliminated mandatory	circulating circulating	decreased increased	decreased increased
5	4,760 (equivalent)	eliminated	circulating and urine	decreased	no change
6	6,600+	uncontrolled	urine	decreased	not measured
7	4,350	eliminated	circulating and urine	decreased	decreased
11	3,100	mandatory	circulating	increased	increased

Fig. 82.1 The effect of hypoxia on aldosterone secretion and plasma renin activity in man. Modified from Milledge JS *et al* [10].

rise in ANF is overriden by that of aldosterone at both high and low altitude [14].

Renin

While all studies in which exercise has been excluded have reported reduced values of aldosterone on going to altitude, the renin levels have been variously reported as increased [2,15,16] unchanged [5], or decreased [3,4,7] (Fig. 82.1). The differing results may be due to differing amounts of light exercise taken by the subjects, the different timing of sampling in relation to ascent, the different rates of ascent, and the altitude attained. Where even the modest exercise of walking around the base camp is allowed, or where ascent is rapid enough to cause stress and sympathetic stimulation, plasma renin will be increased.

The aldosterone response to renin at altitude

At sea level, when renin secretion is stimulated by exercise, the consequent increase in plasma Ang II stimulates the release of aldosterone from the adrenals (see *Chapter 33*). At altitude,

however, the aldosterone response to a rise in renin is blunted or absent [4,11,17,18]. The different relationships between plasma aldosterone and plasma renin at sea level and at 3,100 and 6,300m, are shown in Fig. 82.2.

The cause of this hypoxic blunting of the response is not clear. The possibility that it might be due to reduced ACE activity was once considered, but is now believed to be unlikely. Raff *et al* [19] found evidence that adrenal cortical cells, *in vitro*, were less responsive to Ang II under hypoxic conditions. Colice and Ramirez, however, had previously found no difference in aldosterone response to infused Ang II between normoxic and hypoxic human subjects [20]. The same group later showed that adrenocorticotropic hormone-stimulated secretion of aldosterone was inhibited by hypoxia whereas cortisol secretion was unaffected [21]. Another possible explanation for this reduced aldosterone response at altitude is that ANF, which is increased at altitude [12], inhibits the secretion of aldosterone [22] (see *Chapter 36*), as well as opposing its effect on sodium retention by the kidney. The rise in ANF levels with altitude in

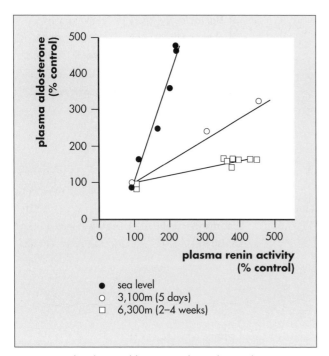

Fig. 82.2 The plasma aldosterone relationship to plasma renin at sea level and two altitudes. Data are from three studies [10,11,32]. At 6,300 meters, each point represents the result for one subject either at rest (left) or after exercise (right). At sea level and at 3,100 meters, each point is the mean of five and six subjects, respectively. Modified from Milledge JS *et al* [32].

resting subjects is rather variable and is at most, quite modest [12,23]. On exercise, however, there is a rise in ANF which is greater under acute hypoxia than with normoxia and this may contribute to the blunted aldosterone response [18].

THE PATHOLOGICAL RESPONSE TO ALTITUDE HYPOXIA

Acute mountain sickness can be considered as a pathological response to altitude hypoxia. Individuals tend to be either susceptible or resistant to AMS. To date, no risk indicators have been identified apart from a history of AMS and possibly obesity. Fitness, age, gender, or race appear not to be predictive. The evidence that some disturbance of salt or water balance may be involved in the genesis of AMS is circumstantial. In subjects taken rapidly to altitude, there is a delay of some hours before the onset of symptoms. Perhaps during this time, sodium and water are retained or redistributed. Subjects destined to develop AMS tend to have an antidiuresis on arrival at altitude, whereas subjects who remain free of symptoms have a diuresis [13,24,25]. Trekkers who gained weight (presumably due to

fluid retention) were found to have more prevalent AMS than those who lost weight [26]. In two studies on groups of climbers, there was an inverse correlation between sodium excretion on the day of ascent to altitude and AMS symptom scores, that is, those who later developed AMS appeared to retain more sodium on the day of ascent than those who remained symptom free [12,13].

The relation of aldosterone and AMS has been considered in a few studies. In a low-pressure chamber experiment, Hogan *et al* [3] reported that subjects who developed AMS had lower aldosterone levels than fit subjects. In two field studies [12,13], however, aldosterone, together with renin and Ang II levels, were higher in AMS sufferers, probably accounting for their greater sodium retention. Bartsch *et al* [13] also found higher levels of norepinephrine and epinephrine in subjects with AMS, suggesting that the exercise of climbing caused greater sympathetic stimulation in these individuals.

Clearly, there is more to the genesis of AMS than an overactive RAS. Hypoxia is an essential ingredient; the symptoms of AMS are not found at sea level in any syndrome of salt or water disturbance. It would seem, however, that given acute hypoxia and possibly a failure to respond by an adequate degree of hyperventilation [26], the RAS, stimulated by exercise, may cause sodium retention and thus contribute to the condition.

SUMMARY

The known response of the RAS to altitude is shown in *Figs. 82.1* and *82.3*. The physiological response in subjects at rest is for there to be a fall in aldosterone levels. This is probably due to a blunting of the aldosterone response to renin (via Ang II), the mechanism of which is unclear. Subjects who later go on to develop AMS have a pathological response to the hypoxic stress of altitude and possibly have a greater depression of aldosterone secretion. However, this evidence is from only one small chamber study [3]. If exercise is taken in reaching high altitude, there is activation of the RAS as with exercise at sea level, with consequent elevation of plasma aldosterone levels. In subjects who later develop AMS, the rise in aldosterone is higher; data for renin are lacking.

THE RENIN–ANGIOTENSIN– ALDOSTERONE SYSTEM IN SPACE TRAVEL

The major physiological factor associated with space travel is weightlessness or microgravity. This has effects on the circulatory system because of the redistribution of blood from the lower

	No exercise		With exercise	
	Physiological	Pathological	Physiological	Pathological
aldosterone	↓	? ↓↓	↑	↑↑
renin	↑ or ↓	↑ or ↓	↑	?

Fig. 82.3 Summary of the changes in plasma aldosterone and renin on ascent to altitude. There may be either a physiological or pathological response. Subjects having a pathological response go on to have acute mountain sickness.

body towards the heart and head. The RAS is involved in the adaptation of the body to this situation. In order to get into space, travelers have to go through the stress of liftoff involving high gravitational forces for a short time, and the stresses of re-entry and splashdown on landing. If things go wrong, they may be exposed to extreme heat, hypoxia, and decompression; however, this chapter only considers the 'normal' stresses of liftoff and microgravity. There is no hypoxic stress because the atmosphere provided to the space traveler has an oxygen content at least that of sea level on Earth. Indeed, the hazard of hyperoxia is more likely, since it is easier in engineering terms, to provide an atmosphere of virtually 100% oxygen at a reduced pressure than one containing nitrogen at a higher total pressure. The earlier spacecraft used the former method until the disastrous fire in Apollo on the ground. For space walks, the suits are still provided with 100% oxygen at a reduced pressure. Finally, the traveler has to return to Earth's gravity and, having adapted to the microgravity of space, there is a danger of syncope because of a reduced blood volume now pooling in the lower body in the upright position. The RAS plays a part in the adaptation to life on Earth again.

CIRCULATORY AND HORMONAL CHANGES ON ENTERING MICROGRAVITY

A general scheme of changes in the distribution and composition of the blood and relevant hormone levels on entering microgravity has been proposed and is shown in Fig. 82.4. This is based on work in which microgravity has been simulated by bed rest, head-down tilt, or water immersion. None of these simulations is perfect. There have been more limited studies of astronauts in real space and, in general, these have supported the proposed scheme, though results in this less-controlled environment are more variable.

With the removal of gravity, there is a shift of blood from the legs and lower body towards the upper body and head. There is a sensation of 'fullness' in the head, and the face feels rounded and may become puffy [27]. The right atrial pressure is increased and release of ANF is stimulated. Plasma renin activity, Ang I, Ang II, aldosterone, and vasopressin levels are reduced. These

changes result in a diuresis and natriuresis and a loss of plasma volume in the first few hours of weightlessness. The reduction in plasma volume increases the hematocrit which then leads to a suppression of bone marrow function, so that over a few weeks, there is a reduction also in red cell mass. Once the blood volume

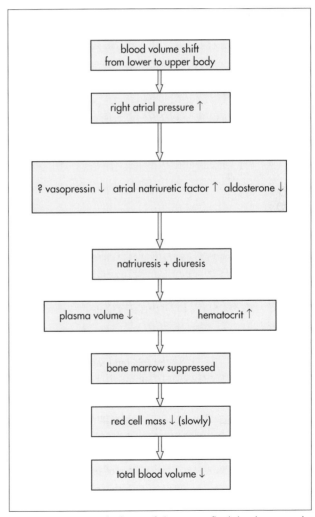

Fig. 82.4 Suggested scheme of changes in fluid distribution and hormones with the imposition of microgravity, derived mainly from work on bed rest, head-down tilt, or water immersion.

82.4

Factor	Changes observed	Mission
total body fluid	reduced	all
total body sodium and potassium	reduced	all
plasma renin activity	variable possibly increased then decreased possibly decreased then increased	Skylab Shuttle
aldosterone	decreased or no change at first increased later in mission	
vasopressin	suppressed unless stimulated by motion sickness	
atrial natriuretic factor	increased then decreased	

Fig. 82.5 Changes observed in astronauts in the Skylab, Shuttle, and Salute-7 missions. Modified from Leach-Huntoon *et al* [29].

Hormone	Changes observed
plasma renin activity	increased
aldosterone	increased
vasopressin	no change
atrial natriuretic factor	increased at first then decreased

Fig. 82.6 Hormone changes measured after space missions and compared with levels at the end of the missions.

is reduced, the various hormone levels return to baseline values and the space traveler can be considered to have adapted to the new environment.

This scheme represents the likely course of changes in an ideal experiment where microgravity would be imposed in controlled conditions on a relaxed, seated subject. In the reality of a space mission, this is not the case: there will be a number of confounding factors, as now discussed.

The stress, psychological and physiological, of the liftoff stimulates the sympathetic system and hence the RAS to a variable degree in different individuals, such as occurs even in ordinary military flight [28]. The preflight procedures require astronauts to spend some hours recumbent before liftoff. This position initiates many of the above changes and so further changes due to weightlessness will be reduced if baseline measures are taken to be those just before liftoff. Fluid intake is important in the whole scheme. In controlled experiments, intake

is kept constant, but in a space mission, fluid intake is usually limited both before and after liftoff. This is partly deliberate for obvious practical reasons and partly because the sensation of thirst seems to be blunted [29]. Many astronauts suffer from a form of motion sickness (space adaptation syndrome) during the first few days of the flight. This will have the effect of stimulating vasopressin release, and the drugs taken to combat the condition may have an effect on fluid balance.

The actual changes observed in astronauts in the Skylab, Shuttle, and Salute-7 missions have been summarized by Leach-Huntoon *et al* [29] in Fig. 82.5.

CHANGES ON RE-ENTRY INTO EARTH GRAVITY

The reduced blood volume resulting from adaptation to life in microgravity causes a tenency to syncope if the astronaut stands up after landing. Re-adaptation to normal gravity is rapid, with retention of electrolytes and fluid, so that the plasma volume is expanded. Hemodilution causes a mild anemia which stimulates the erythropoietic system. Over a few weeks, the red cell mass is increased to normal values, with restoration of normal hematocrit.

Hormone changes measured after space missions and compared with levels at the end of the missions are as shown in Fig. 82.6 [29]. With restoration of the blood volume in 1–2 days, the risk of syncope is removed and hormone levels return to normal.

REFERENCES

1. Williams ES. Salivary electrolyte composition at high altitude. *Clinical Science* 1961;21:37–42.
2. Slater JDH, Tuffley RE, Williams ES, Beresford CH, Sonksen PH, Edwards RHT, Ekins RP, McLaughlin M. Control of aldosterone secretion during acclimatization to hypoxia in man. *Clinical Science* 1969;37:327–41.
3. Hogan RP, Kotchen TA, Boyd AE, Hartley LH. Effect of altitude on renin–aldosterone system and metabolism of water and electrolytes. *Journal of Applied Physiology* 1973;35:385–90.
4. Maher JT, Leeroy G, Jones L, Hartley H, Williams GH, Rose LI. Aldosterone dynamics during graded exercise at sea level and high altitude. *Journal of Applied Physiology* 1975;39:18–22.

5. Sutton JR, Viol GW, Gray GW, McFadden M, Keanem PM. Renin, aldosterone, electrolyte, and cortisol responses to hypoxic decompression. *Journal of Applied Physiology* 1977;43:421–4.

6. Pines A, Slater JDH, Jowett TP. The kidney and aldosterone in acclimatization at altitude. *British Journal of Diseases of the Chest* 1977;71:203–7.

7. Kaynes RJ, Smith GW, Slater JDH, Brown MM, Brown SE, Payne NN, Jowett TP, Monge CC. Renin and aldosterone at high altitude in man. *Journal of Endocrinology* 1982;92:131–40.

8. Milledge JS, Catley DM, Ward MP, Williams ES, Clarke CRA. Renin–aldosterone and angiotensin-converting enzyme during prolonged altitude exposure. *Journal of Applied Physiology* 1983;55:699–702.

9. Williams ES, Ward MP, Milledge JS, Withey WR, Older MWJ, Forsling ML. Effect of the exercise of seven consecutive days hill-walking on fluid homeostasis. *Clinical Science* 1979;56:305–16.

10. Milledge JS, Bryson EI, Catley DM, Hesp R, Luff N, Minty BD, Older MWJ, Payne NN, Ward MP, Withey WR. Sodium balance, fluid homeostasis and the renin–aldosterone system during the prolonged exercise of hill walking. *Clinical Science* 1982;62:595–604.

11. Milledge JS, Catley DM, Williams ES, Withey WR, Minty BD. Effect of prolonged exercise at altitude on the renin–aldosterone system. *Journal of Applied Physiology* 1983;55:413–8.

12. Milledge JS, Beeley JM, McArthur S, Morice AH. Atrial natriuretic peptide, altitude and acute mountain sickness. *Clinical Science* 1989;77:509–14.

13. Bartsch P, Shaw S, Franciolli M, Gnadinger MP, Weidmann P. Atrial natriuretic peptide in acute mountain sickness. *Journal of Applied Physiology* 1988;65:1929–37.

14. Milledge JS, McArthur S, Morice A, Luff N, Abrahams R, Thomas PS. Atrial natriuretic peptide and exercise-induced fluid retention in man. *Journal of Wilderness Medicine* 1991;2:94–101.

15. Tuffley RE, Rubenstein D, Slater JDH, Williams ES. Serum renin activity during exposure to hypoxia. *Journal of Endocrinology* 1970;48:497–510.

16. Frayser R, Rennie ID, Gray GW, Houston CS. Hormonal and electrolyte response to exposure to 17,500 ft. *Journal of Applied Physiology* 1975;38:636–42.

17. Shigeoka JW, Colice GL, Ramirez G. Effect of normoxemic and hypoxemic exercise on renin and aldosterone. *Journal of Applied Physiology* 1985;59:142–8.

18. Lawrence DL, Shenker Y. Effect of hypoxic exercise on atrial natriuretic factor and aldosterone regulation. *American Journal of Hypertension* 1991;4:341–7.

19. Raff H, Kohandarvish S, Jankowski B. The effect of oxygen on aldosterone release from bovine adrenocortical cells *in vitro*. *Journal of Endocrinology* 1990;127:682–7.

20. Colice GL, Ramirez G. Aldosterone response to angiotensin II during hypoxemia. *Journal of Applied Physiology* 1986;61:150–4.

21. Ramirez G, Bittle PA, Hammond M, Ayers CW, Dietz JR, Colice GL. Regulation of aldosterone secretion during hypoxemia at sea level and moderately high altitude. *Journal of Clinical Endocrinology and Metabolism* 1988;67:1162–5.

22. Anderson JV, Struthers AD, Payne NN, Slater JDH, Bloom SR. Atrial natriuretic peptide inhibits the aldosterone response to angiotensin II in man. *Clinical Science* 1986;70:507–12.

23. Lawrence DL, Skatrud JB, Shenker Y. Effect of hypoxia on atrial natriuretic factor and aldosterone regulation in humans. *American Journal of Physiology* 1990;258:E243–8.

24. Singh I, Malhotra MS, Khanna PK, Nanda RB, Purshottam T, Upadhyoy TD, Radakrichnan U, Brahamachan HD. Changes in plasma cortisol, blood antidiuretic hormone and urinary catecholamines in high-altitude pulmonary oedema. *Indian Journal of Biometrology* 1974;18:211–21.

25. Bartsch P, Pfluger N, Audetat MS, Shaw S, Weidmann P, Vock P, Vetter W, Rennie D, Olez O. Effects of slow ascent to 4559m on fluid homeostasis. *Aviation, Space, and Environmental Medicine* 1991;62:105–10.

26. Hackett PH, Rennie D, Hofmeister SE, Grover RF, Grover EB, Reeves JT. Fluid retention and relative hypoventilation in acute mountain sickness. *Respiration* 1982;43:321–9.

27. Berry CA. Medical legacy of Apollo. *Aerospace Medicine* 1974;45:1049–57.

28. Wang YM, Sheng DY. Flight influence on the plasma level of renin–angiotensin–aldosterone system and atrial natriuretic peptide. *Aviation, Space and Environmental Medicine* 1990;61:999–1001.

29. Leach-Huntoon C, Johnson PC, Cintron NM. Hematology, immunology, endocrinology and biochemistry In: Nicogoss AE, Huntoon CL, Pool SL, eds. *Space physiology and medicine. 2nd edition.* Philadelphia: Lea & Febiger, 1989:227–39.

30. Williams ES, Electrolyte regulation during adaptation of humans to life at high altitude. *Proceedings of the Royal Society of London. Series B: Biological Sciences* 1966;165:266–80.

31. Janowski AH, Whitten BK, Shields JL, Hannon JP. Electrolyte patterns and regulation in man during acute exposure to high altitude. *Federation Proceedings* 1969;28:1185–9.

32. Milledge JS, Catley DM, Blume FD, West JB. Renin, angiotensin-converting enzyme, and aldosterone in humans on Mount Everest. *Journal of Applied Physiology* 1983;55:1109–12.

83

CLINICAL VALUE OF MEASUREMENTS OF THE RENIN–ANGIOTENSIN SYSTEM

M GARY NICHOLLS AND J IAN S ROBERTSON

Although methods are established for measuring individual components of the RAS (see *Chapters 13–16*), these are used predominantly for research purposes. Nevertheless, activity of the RAS as measured in peripheral blood or in blood draining a specific organ can be useful in clinical diagnosis and in the management of patients with certain disorders.

For clinical purposes, by far the most common measurement is plasma renin activity (PRA). As noted in *Chapter 13*, the plasma sample to be assayed for PRA is incubated for some hours at 37°C and the amount of Ang I formed is measured, usually by radioimmunoassay. The PRA value reflects the mass concentration of the active enzyme renin, but it also depends on the level of plasma angiotensinogen (renin substrate). Under most circumstances, PRA can be taken as reflecting also plasma active renin concentration (PRC), but this is less so when angiotensinogen levels are either very high — as during pregnancy (see *Chapter 50*), with estrogen treatment (see *Chapter 53*), and in Addison's disease (see *Chapter 68*) — or low as is seen with severe liver disease (see *Chapter 78*) [1]. As discussed in *Chapters 13* and *17* and *Appendix II*, measurements of PRA are not usually expressed in terms of a recognized renin standard. Thus, the 'normal' range for PRA in one laboratory may differ markedly from that established elsewhere, since the final result is dependent upon incubation conditions (for example, the pH, molarity, and duration of incubation). The practical point, therefore, is that the PRA value for a patient must be interpreted in relation to the established 'normal' range for that particular laboratory. Use of the 'normal' range from other laboratories, or from the literature, can lead to erroneous conclusions.

Interpretation of plasma renin levels is also importantly dependent upon the age of the patient, on dietary sodium intake and on body posture prior to blood sampling, on current or recent drug treatment and, to a lesser extent, on the recent ingestion of food, the phase of the menstrual cycle, and the time of day when the sample was drawn (see *Chapter 74*) (Fig. 83.1). To elaborate, PRA values in healthy subjects are highest in early childhood, falling steeply until early teenage years (Fig. 83.2) and more gradually thereafter [2–5]. There is an inverse relationship between dietary sodium (as mirrored by 24-hour urinary

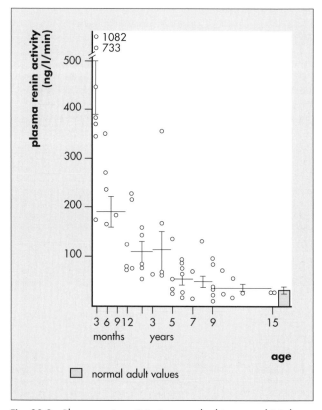

Fig. 83.2 Plasma renin activity in normal subjects aged 15 days to 15 years. Individual levels together with the mean ± SEM are shown. Modified from Sassard J *et al* [2].

| Patient age |
| Dietary sodium intake |
| Body posture |
| Medications |
| Time of day |
| Relation to last meal |
| Other, e.g. phase of menstrual cycle |

Fig. 83.1 Factors affecting interpretation of plasma renin levels.

sodium excretion) and levels of renin and Ang II, the relationship being rectilinear when logarithmic plots are used (Fig. 83.3) [6]. Values of renin increase with upright body posture and fall when the supine position is assumed [7–9]. Numerous drugs alter PRA as discussed in detail in *Chapters 74* and *80*. In addition, renin-inhibiting drugs may give misleading results when a conventional PRA assay is used [10,11] (see *Chapter 85*). A diurnal rhythm in PRA values, of moderate amplitude, is described, with higher levels occurring in the early morning and the nadir late in the evening [12,13]. These factors, and especially also some forms of drug treatment (β-blockers, diuretics, and ACE inhibitors, for example) (see *Chapters 74* and *80*), can so alter renin values that their diagnostic usefulness may be lost. Where antihypertensive therapy is deemed essential, the calcium-channel antagonists nifedipine or nicardipine [14,15] and post-synaptic α-adrenergic blocking agents [16] are useful as they have little effect on renin levels.

If attention is paid, however, to the above influences, and assays are performed in a laboratory with expertise, experience, and attention to quality control, clinically useful information can be obtained from measurements of plasma renin in a number of clinical circumstances (Fig. 83.4).

HYPERTENSIVE DISORDERS

HYPERTENSION AND HYPOKALEMIA

Measurements of renin and aldosterone together are vital to the proper diagnosis of disorders causing the combination of hypertension and hypokalemia. The classic disease is primary hyperaldosteronism (Conn's syndrome; aldosterone-secreting adrenocortical adenoma) which is characterized by suppressed plasma renin and by levels of aldosterone that are inappropriately high considering the inhibitory effects of hypokalemia on aldosterone secretion (see *Chapter 63*). Related disorders, which are discussed in detail in *Chapter 63*, include Ang II-responsive adrenocortical adenoma, aldosterone-secreting carcinoma, and dexamethasone-suppressible aldosterone excess. All of these conditions show low plasma levels of potassium and renin, while aldosterone is elevated. These same biochemical trends are seen but are less marked in idiopathic ('nontumorous', 'pseudo-primary') aldosterone excess. This is now considered to be a part of the spectrum of essential hypertension (see *Chapters 62* and *63*).

A diagnosis of primary hyperaldosteronism should not be made in the absence of clear evidence that renin is suppressed. This rule generally applies also to some patients with the rare

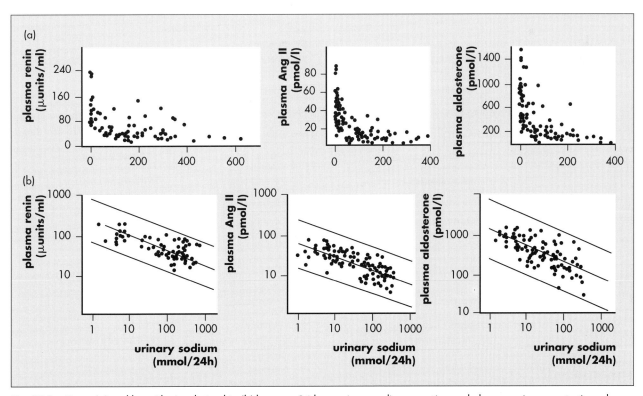

Fig. 83.3 Linear (a) and logarithmic relationship (b) between 24-hour urinary sodium excretion and plasma renin concentration, plasma Ang II, and plasma aldosterone in 64 healthy volunteers. The regression line ± 2 SD is shown in (b). Modified from Agabiti Rosei E *et al* [6].

Essential for diagnosis

hypertension	primary hyperaldosteronism and its variants and related disorders
	DOC-secreting tumor
	corticosterone secreting tumor
	surreptitious licorice intake
	renin-secreting tumor
	Liddle's syndrome
	syndrome of apparent mineralocorticoid excess
	Gordon's syndrome
hypotension	hyperreninemic selective hypoaldosteronism
	Bartter's syndrome
other:	hyporeninemic hypoaldosteronism

Useful in diagnosis (but not essential)

hypertension	renovascular hypertension
	scleroderma renal crisis
	17α-hydroxylase deficiency
	11β-hydroxylase deficiency
hypotension	Addison's disease
	21-hydroxylase deficiency
	surreptitious vomiting, anorexia, and abuse of diuretics and purgatives

Useful in monitoring therapy

hypertension	17α-hydroxylase deficiency
	Liddle's syndrome
	syndrome of apparent mineralocorticoid excess
	Gordon's syndrome
hypotension:	Addison's disease
	21-hydroxylase deficiency

Fig. 83.4 The clinical value of renin measurements.

combination of primary hyperaldosteronism in pregnancy, in whom renin levels are low whether the measurement is of PRC [17] or PRA [18]; the situation can be more complicated in other pregnant patients, however, where renin secretion may become unsuppressed and the hypokalemia and hypertension are corrected [19].

There are other circumstances where plasma renin levels are not necessarily suppressed in primary hyperaldosteronism.

The first is in patients who are taking antihypertensive drugs that stimulate renin release, and especially potassium-retaining diuretics [20,21]. As described above, drugs that activate the RAS (see *Chapter 80*) should always be avoided prior to sampling for measurements of renin and aldosterone. Second, severe sodium restriction can stimulate renin secretion in primary hyperaldosteronism, occasionally to levels that call the diagnosis into doubt [22]. Third, the occasional patient with primary hyperaldosteronism develops malignant hypertension (see *Chapter 60*), in which case renin levels can sometimes rise into or above the normal range [23,24]. Fourth, concomitant renovascular or renal disorders are not uncommon in primary hyperaldosteronism [25] and could stimulate renin release.

Last, there is a single case report of a patient presenting with hypertension, hypokalemia, and virilism whose adrenal adenoma produced not only aldosterone in excess, but also renin and sex steroids [26].

Primary hyperaldosteronism must be differentiated from other causes of hypertension and hypokalemia as detailed below. A careful clinical history and physical examination, together with determination of routine biochemical indices, will often point to the correct diagnosis, but measurements of renin are essential in many cases.

Diuretic intake

Diuretic intake in essential hypertension will usually be obvious as a cause of hypokalemia. Surreptitious self-medication must be suspected where renin levels are high and no underlying cause for secondary aldosterone excess is detected. Purgative abuse and persistent vomiting, both of which can be indulged in secret, should also be considered in this context (see *Chapter 72*).

Licorice or carbenoxolone ingestion

Regular licorice or carbenoxolone ingestion as a cause of hypertension and hypokalemia (see *Chapter 63*) is normally diagnosed readily by careful questioning and can be confirmed by the finding of low renin and aldosterone levels [27]. This unusual combination of suppressed renin and aldosterone should raise the possibility of surreptitious licorice intake.

Adrenal tumor secreting deoxycorticosterone or corticosterone

Cases of an adrenal tumor secreting deoxycorticosterone or corticosterone are rare (see *Chapter 63*), but these diagnoses should be entertained in the hypertensive hypokalemic patient in whom plasma renin and aldosterone levels are low and an adrenal tumor is visualized radiologically [28].

17α- and 11β-hydroxylase deficiency

The same conjunction of low renin and low aldosterone should also bring to mind the possibility of 17α-hydroxylase deficiency (see *Chapter 63*). In this disease, renin levels are low as a result of mineralocorticoid-induced renal sodium retention, and aldosterone secretion is suppressed because of reduced activity of the RAS, hypokalemia, sustained hypersecretion of adrenocorticotropic hormone (ACTH), and probably high circulating concentrations of atrial natriuretic factor [29,30]. Here again, careful clinical assessment of the hypertensive hypokalemic patient, and particularly the abnormal sexual status [31], should direct attention to appropriate specialist investigations that include the documentation of diminished secretion of glucocorticoid and sex hormones and excessive production of 17-hydroxycorticosteroids.

Even rarer is 11β-hydroxylase deficiency, which also presents with hypokalemia, low plasma aldosterone, and suppression of the RAS (see *Chapter 63*).

Malignant hypertension

Malignant hypertension is a clinical (or pathological) complication of very high blood pressure. Plasma renin is very often, but not always, high. Many such patients have hypokalemia as a result of high aldosterone levels [32–34] secondary to activation of the RAS [35–37] (see *Chapter 60*). Some patients have, in addition, hyponatremia (the hyponatremic–hypertensive syndrome) (see *Chapters 55* and *88*) in which case circulating levels of renin are very high [38–41], there is both sodium and potassium depletion, volume depletion can be extreme [39], ACE inhibitors can reduce arterial pressure precipitously [39,41], and judicious salt and volume repletion may be indicated [40–42]. A similar syndrome is well described in experimental animals [43–46]. Here again, the clinician does not require measurements of renin to diagnose the hyponatremic–hypertensive syndrome or to initiate appropriate emergency treatment. Nevertheless, a case can be made for obtaining a blood sample before and after control of arterial pressure for determining renin levels when an underlying secondary form of hypertension (renovascular or renal disease, or Conn's syndrome, for example) is suspected. Certainly, this would be routine in units with a special or research interest in hypertension.

Renin-secreting tumors

Measurements of peripheral plasma renin are central to the diagnosis of renin-secreting tumors (see *Chapter 54*) whether the lesion is of renal [47–49] or of extrarenal origin [50]. Where hyperreninemia in a hypertensive patient is associated with an abnormally high percentage of circulating inactive renin [49,50], a renin-secreting tumor, which in these circumstances can be malignant and extrarenal, must be suspected. Selective regional venous sampling for renin or Ang II measurements has been successful in localizing the tumor in some cases [47,48,51,52] but this is not always so [49,53,54].

Liddle's syndrome and apparent mineralocorticoid excess

As described in *Chapter 66*, peripheral plasma renin levels are low or very low in Liddle's syndrome as a consequence of excessive renal sodium retention and perhaps other factors. Measurements of renin and aldosterone are vital for the diagnosis of this hypertensive–hypokalemic syndrome. Similarly, low renin (and aldosterone) levels are integral features of the syndrome of apparent mineralocorticoid excess (see *Chapters 63* and *66*).

RENAL AND RENOVASCULAR HYPERTENSION

Despite early enthusiasm [55], peripheral plasma renin or Ang II assays have not proved useful in screening for renovascular hypertension (see *Chapters 55* and *88*). Although some workers have found elevated peripheral venous levels of renin to predict curability of renovascular hypertension [56,57] few, if any, clinicians would rely upon this index alone. A number of groups make use of renal venous renin ratios (ischemic:nonischemic kidney ratio of 1.5:1 or greater, for example) with or without evidence of suppression of renin secretion from the nonischemic kidney, together with raised peripheral venous renin levels, to predict the blood-pressure response to balloon angioplasty, renovascular surgery, or nephrectomy [58–63] (see *Chapter 55*). Additional predictive value has been gained in some reports by documenting an exaggerated peripheral renin response or a rise in the ratio of renin in the involved to uninvolved renal vein, with the short-term stimulation of renin secretion by administration of an ACE inhibitor [64–72]. Alternative maneuvers to augment activity of the RAS include dietary sodium restriction or administration of a diuretic or a vasodilating agent (see *Chapters 55* and *88*). Whatever protocol is used, the 'normal range' for renin in healthy volunteers or preferably essential hypertensives should ideally be documented under the same conditions, and attention to details of quality control in the renal assay are necessary. Final decisions regarding the choice of treatment (surgery, balloon angioplasty, or antihypertensive drugs) always take into account vital clinical information such as the patient's age, the underlying renovascular pathology (atheroma, fibromuscular dysplasia, Takayasu's disease, and so on), the presence or absence of concomitant disorders and, of course, the level of surgical expertise — with or without renin measurements. It is noteworthy that there are well-documented cases of surgical cure of renovascular hypertension when clinical predictors were favorable although renin or Ang II estimations were not [73–79,123]. At best, therefore, renin measurements may be viewed as useful predictors of the blood-pressure response to therapeutic intervention when used in conjunction with full clinical information, and in clinical centers that have a wide experience in renin measurements under standardized conditions, and when the available therapeutic experience and expertise is considerable.

The usefulness of renin measurements in detecting bilateral renal ischemia as a cause of hypertension, or in predicting its response to treatment, is much less clear than for unilateral renovascular hypertension.

Measurements of renin have also been used to predict the blood-pressure response to uninephrectomy in hypertensive patients with unilateral renal disease due to a variety of underlying disorders (including pyelonephritis, reflux nephropathy (*Color Plates 26–28*), renal cyst, tuberculosis, or renal carcinoma — see Color Plate 47). Some authors have found that renin values (usually high levels of renin in renal venous blood draining the diseased kidney compared with that from the normal kidney, or raised peripheral renin levels) have provided a useful index of the subsequent blood-pressure response to surgery [80–88]. Many of these studies, however, are of single cases and are carried out in uncontrolled circumstances. Other worker's experience is less satisfactory [89]. As with unilateral renovascular disease, renin assays should be used in conjunction with full clinical information when deciding on the advisability of surgery.

For patients with bilateral renal disease and hypertension, information on peripheral renin levels can be clinically helpful, and can, for example, suggest but not confirm definitively, scleroderma renal crisis (see *Chapter 79*). For patients with other causes of renal impairment, data on circulating renin levels may provide some assistance to the clinician when blood pressure proves resistant to dialysis or to conventional antihypertensive drugs (see *Chapter 56*). Under these circumstances, and along with routine clinical and biochemical information, very low renin values point to excessive extracellular fluid volume, whereas high plasma renin suggests that the hypertension may be dependent on the RAS and is possibly responsive to its blockade with or without expansion of extracellular fluid volume.

MISCELLANEOUS SECONDARY FORMS OF HYPERTENSION

Peripheral levels of renin are not infrequently elevated at least in some circumstances in hypertensive patients with polycystic kidney disease, aortic coarctation, and pheochromocytoma (see *Chapters 57, 59,* and *67*). In none of these disorders, however, is the role of the RAS in the pathogenesis of the hypertension

clearly established, nor is the measurement of renin central to either the diagnosis or the treatment.

In contrast, the hypertensive–hyperkalemic syndrome of Gordon is characterized by low levels of renin, without which the diagnosis cannot be made with confidence (see *Chapter 65*).

The use of renin measurements in hypertensive patients with hypokalemia, and with malignant, renovascular, or renal hypertension, has been discussed. A practical problem is that the results of renin assays take some hours, or even days or weeks, to be reported, depending on the local circumstances. In the interim, an index of peripheral renin levels, albeit an imperfect one, is the plasma (or serum) sodium concentration. An inverse relationship between plasma sodium and the level of renin secretion was suspected in 1958 from the correlation between antemortem plasma sodium concentrations and the postmortem juxtaglomerular index in 24 patients (details of whose clinical status are not available [90]). This negative association of plasma sodium with plasma renin was later documented in cardiac failure (see *Chapter 76*) and in patients with hypertension of diverse etiologies [38] (Fig. 83.5). Although there is considerable scatter of renin values for any level of plasma sodium, and some authors have been unimpressed with the association [91], high renin levels should be suspected in the hyponatremic patient. This is of clinical importance if use of an ACE inhibitor is contemplated since the first dose, especially if large, can induce a precipitous fall in arterial pressure in those with severe hypertension, hyponatremia, and high plasma renin [39]. At the other end of the spectrum, a mineralocorticoid-type of hypertension should be suspected in the hypokalemic patient who has a high or high–normal level of plasma sodium and in whom plasma renin is likely to be low. Of course, a definitive diagnosis demands proper renin measurements.

ESSENTIAL HYPERTENSION

Peripheral plasma renin assays are not useful in the routine management of patients with essential hypertension [92]. As discussed in *Chapters 62* and *63*, many patients with essential hypertension have low plasma renin values. For reasons given in detail in those chapters, low-renin essential hypertension is now considered to be part of a continuum with idiopathic ('nontumorous', or 'pseudo-primary') hyperaldosteronism. Plasma renin assay can be of assistance where the blood pressure proves resistant to various antihypertensive regimens or where reconsideration of the possibility of an underlying secondary type of hypertension (see earlier) is necessary. These instances, however, represent a small percentage of the total hypertensive population.

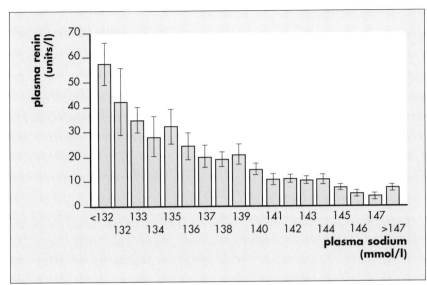

Fig. 83.5 Relation between plasma renin concentration and plasma sodium in 253 patients with essential hypertension or various forms of secondary hypertension. Some patients were receiving antihypertensive medication (ganglion-blocking and sympatholytic drugs, methyldopa, reserpine, thiazide diuretics, or spironolactone). Data are presented as mean ± SEM. Modified from Brown JJ *et al* [38].

For the patient who is asymptomatic, who has no abnormal findings on careful physical examination, and who has normal urine testing, blood count, renal function, and plasma potassium and sodium levels, measurements of renin are not indicated either for diagnosis or to direct clinical management.

Questions have arisen from time to time regarding the prognostic value of plasma renin levels in essential hypertension (see *Chapters 40* and *62*). Whereas there is enthusiasm in some quarters for the concept that a high renin value is a marker of increased risk from various cardiovascular consequences of essential hypertension, others are unconvinced. There is similar controversy and uncertainty as to whether renin assays are helpful in the choice of drug for therapy (see *Chapters 40, 62* and *84*). Until further information is available, good medical care for patients with essential hypertension need not involve the performance of renin assays.

HYPOTENSIVE DISORDERS

HYPERRENINEMIC SELECTIVE HYPOALDOSTERONISM

A diagnosis of hyperreninemic selective hypoaldosteronism cannot be made with confidence in the absence of renin measurements (see *Chapter 69*). In these critically ill patients with hypotension and hyperkalemia, the assay technique for renin (that is, whether of PRA or PRC) should be taken into account when interpreting the result (see *Chapter 69*).

ADDISON'S DISEASE

A diagnosis of Addison's disease did not traditionally require documentation of elevated levels of peripheral renin. Furthermore, the technique of measuring renin may have a bearing on the result since glucocorticoids (and Ang II) are important regulators of angiotensinogen production which, in turn, contributes to PRA but not to PRC (see *Chapter 68*). Nevertheless, many centers make diagnostic use of high renin levels in conjunction with appropriate measurements of cortisol, its reserve, and its metabolites, and of ACTH and aldosterone. In the rare case where loss of function of the zona glomerulosa appears to precede that of the zona fasciculata [93], determination of plasma renin and aldosterone levels is crucial to the diagnosis.

Renin assays have been used to monitor replacement therapy in Addison's disease (see *Chapter 68*). Again, interpretation of the renin results is dependent in part on whether PRA (which utilizes endogenous renin substrate) or PRC (for which an excess of exogenous substrate is added to the assay) is used. Such data can indeed be clinically useful in deciding the level of maintenance therapy and especially whether or not mineralocorticoid replacement with 9α-fludrocortisone is indicated. Clinical information including change in body weight, the energy level, posture-related alterations in blood pressure, 24-hour urinary sodium excretion, and routine plasma biochemical indices must be taken into account, along with renin levels, in deciding on the type and extent of replacement hormone treatment in Addison's disease [94–96].

21-HYDROXYLASE DEFICIENCY

Congenital adrenal hyperplasia is most commonly the result of 21-hydroxylase deficiency. The diagnosis may be suspected on clinical grounds as a result of a sodium-losing state or abnormal sexual features, and is confirmed by measurements of high levels of 17-hydroxyprogesterone, androstenedione, and testosterone, and of low concentrations of cortisol and aldosterone. Renin levels are much higher than in age-matched healthy controls [97]. As in Addison's disease, replacement hormone therapy is assisted by serial measurements of renin but again, such data do not stand alone. Rather, renin values must be used in conjunction with full clinical information and with measurements of plasma electrolytes, 17-hydroxyprogesterone, androstenedione, and testosterone [97–99].

BARTTER'S SYNDROME

A diagnosis of Bartter's syndrome requires documentation of hyperreninemia (see *Chapter 64*). Of course, high renin levels in a hypotensive or normotensive patient with hypokalemia, and even with documented juxtaglomerular hyperplasia (see Color Plate 29), are only consistent with, rather than diagnostic of, Bartter's syndrome. As noted in *Chapters 64* and *72*, the plasma electrolyte, renin, and aldosterone features of Bartter's syndrome are shared with diuretic abuse and, to some extent, also with purgative abuse, vomiting, and anorexia nervosa.

OTHER DISORDERS AND INDICES

As mentioned, PRA or PRC are the most common measurements made to assess activity of the RAS in clinical diagnosis and management. These along with determination of ACE activity, are of some use in assessing compliance with ACE inhibitor therapy in hypertension and, to a lesser extent, in cardiac failure. Diagnosis of hyporeninemic hypoaldosteronism requires documentation of low levels of renin and aldosterone (*Chapter 70*).

PRORENIN

Prorenin (inactive renin) measurements are rarely performed outside research studies. Nevertheless, very high prorenin values that are disproportionate to the level of active renin raise the possibility of a renin-secreting tumor in the hypertensive–hypokalemic patient. Some patients harbor tumors that secrete predominantly or solely prorenin, and these could pass undetected in the absence of prorenin assay (see *Chapter 54*). Additionally, as noted in *Chapter 75*, prorenin is often increased in diabetic patients who have nephropathy. Indeed, elevated plasma prorenin may be an early predictor of nephropathy and microangiopathy and can appear before other biochemical or clinical features are evident. With more experience, measurements of prorenin might be advisable soon after type I diabetes is diagnosed in order to ensure that preventive steps are taken in those patients predisposed to microangiopathy.

Use of prorenin or total renin assay in these and obstetric circumstances is also discussed in *Chapter 7*.

ANGIOTENSIN–CONVERTING ENZYME ACTIVITY

Measurements of plasma ACE activity have found clinical use in confirming a diagnosis of sarcoidosis (where values are elevated), in distinguishing these patients from those with other pulmonary diseases, and in monitoring the therapeutic response to glucocorticoids [100–105], especially when hypercalcemia is present [106–108]. It must be appreciated, however, that there is considerable overlap in values between healthy subjects and patients with sarcoidosis. Furthermore, a number of other disorders are sometimes associated with increased plasma ACE activity including diabetes mellitus [109], liver diseases [110,111], hyperthyroidism [112], Addison's disease [113], peptic ulceration [114], Gaucher's disease, leprosy [115], pneumonia due to *Pneumocystis carinii* [116], and malignant histiocytosis [117]. Low plasma ACE activity has been reported in association with hypoxic states [118,119], especially the adult respiratory-distress syndrome [120,121], and with acute inflammation [122], but clinical usefulness under these circumstances is limited.

CONCLUSION

Determination of plasma renin is central to the diagnosis of a number of disorders and is valuable in several others (see Fig. 83.4). It also finds use in assessing the adequacy of treatment in a few diseases (see Fig. 83.4). Depending on the results of further studies, renin assays might prove helpful in identifying patients with essential hypertension, who are at particular risk of cerebrovascular and coronary artery events. Elevated prorenin levels in hypertensive–hypokalemic patients raise the possibility of an underlying renin-secreting tumor, and in type I diabetics might find a place in determining the risk of developing microvascular complications or nephropathy. Measurements of ACE activity can assist in the differential diagnosis of a number of disorders and in assessing drug compliance with ACE inhibitor treatment.

Whatever the disorder under investigation, attention to details of the renin assay and its quality control, and to factors that are known to alter renin levels (see Fig. 83.1) are essential for the correct interpretation of results.

REFERENCES

1. Arnal JF, Cudek P, Plouin PF, Guyenne TT, Michel JB, Corvol P. Low angiotensinogen levels are related to the severity and liver dysfunction of congestive heart failure: Implications for renin measurements. *American Journal of Medicine* 1991;**90**:17–22.

2. Sassard J, Sann L, Vincent M, Francois R, Cier JF. Plasma renin activity in normal subjects from infancy to puberty. *Journal of Clinical Endocrinology and Metabolism* 1975;**40**:524–5.

3. Dillon MJ, Ryness JM. Plasma renin activity and aldosterone concentration in children. *British Medical Journal* 1975;**4**:316–9.

4. Weidmann P, De Myttenaere-Bursztein S, Maxwell MH, de Lima J. Effect of aging on plasma renin and aldosterone in normal man. *Kidney International* 1975;**8**:325–33.

5. Tsunoda K, Abe K, Goto T, Yasujima M, Sato M, Omata K, Seino M, Yoshinaga K. Effect of age on the renin–angiotensin–aldosterone system in normal subjects: Simultaneous measurement of active and inactive renin, renin substrate and aldosterone in plasma. *Journal of Clinical Endocrinology and Metabolism* 1986;**62**:384–9.

6. Agabiti Rosei E, Brown JJ, Cumming AMM, Fraser R, Semple PF, Lever AF, Morton JJ, Robertson AS, Robertson JIS, Tree M. Is the 'sodium index' a useful way of expressing clinical plasma renin, angiotensin and aldosterone values? *Clinical Endocrinology* 1978;**8**:141–7.

7. Brown JJ, Davies DL, Lever AF, McPherson D, Robertson JIS. Plasma renin concentration in relation to changes in posture. *Clinical Science* 1966;**30**:279–84.

8. Cohen EL, Conn JW, Rovner DR. Postural augmentation of plasma renin activity and aldosterone excretion in normal people. *Journal of Clinical Investigation* 1967;**46**:418–28.

9. Tuck ML, Dluhy RG, Williams GH. Sequential responses of the renin–angiotensin–aldosterone axis to acute postural change: Effect of dietary sodium. *Journal of Laboratory and Clinical Medicine* 1975;**86**:754–63.

10. Cordero P, Fisher ND, Moore TJ, Gleason R, Williams GH, Hollenberg NK. Renal and endocrine responses to a renin inhibitor, enalkiren, in normal humans. *Hypertension* 1991;**17**:510–6.

11. Derkx FHM, van den Meiracker AH, Fischli W, Admiraal PJJ, Man in't Veld AJ, van Brummelen P, Schalekamp MADH. Nonparallel effects of renin inhibitor treatment on plasma renin activity and angiotensin I and II in hypertensive subjects. An assay-related artifact. *American Journal of Hypertension* 1991;**4**:602–9.

12. Gordon RD, Wolfe LK, Island DP, Liddle GW. A diurnal rhythm in plasma renin activity in man. *Journal of Clinical Investigation* 1966;**45**:1587–92.

13. Kawaski T, Uezono K, Ueno M, Omae T, Matsuoka M, Haus E, Halberg F. Comparison of circadian rhythms of the renin–angiotensin–aldosterone system and electrolytes in clinically healthy young women in Fukuoka (Japan) and Minnesota (USA). *Acta Endocrinologica* 1983;**102**:246–51.

14. Nadler JL, Hsueh W, Horton R. Therapeutic effect of calcium channel blockade in primary aldosteronism. *Journal of Clinical Endocrinology and Metabolism* 1985;**60**:896–9.

15. Veglio F, Pinna G, Bisbocci D, Rabbia F, Piras D, Chiandussi L. Efficacy of nicardipine slow release (SR) on hypertension, potassium balance and plasma aldosterone in idiopathic aldosteronism. *Journal of Human Hypertension* 1990;**4**:579–82.

16. McAreavey D, Cumming AMM, Sood VP, Leckie BJ, Morton JJ, Murray GD, Robertson JIS. The effect of oral prazosin on blood pressure and plasma concentrations of renin and angiotensin II in man. *Clinical Science* 1981;**61** (suppl):457–60s.

17. Hammond TG, Buchanan JD, Scoggins BA, Thatcher R, Whitworth JA. Primary aldosteronism in pregnancy. *Australian and New Zealand Journal of Medicine* 1982;**12**:537–9.

18. Gordon RD, Fishman LM, Liddle GW. Plasma renin activity and aldosterone secretion in a pregnant woman with primary aldosteronism. *Journal of Clinical Endocrinology* 1967;**27**:385–8.

19. Gordon RD, Tunny TJ. Aldosterone-producing-adenoma (A-P-A): Effect of pregnancy. *Clinical and Experimental Hypertension. Part A, Theory and Practice* 1982;**A4** (9&10):1685–93.

20. Ferriss JB, Beevers DG, Boddy K, Brown JJ, Davies DL, Fraser R, Kremer D, Lever AF, Robertson JIS. The treatment of low-renin ('primary') hyperaldosteronism. *American Heart Journal* 1978;**96**:97–109.

21. Kater CE, Biglieri EG, Schambelan M, Arteaga E. Studies of impaired aldosterone response to spironolactone-induced renin and potassium elevations in adenomatous but not hyperplastic primary aldosteronism. *Hypertension* 1983;**5** (suppl V):V-115–21.

22. Brown JJ, Chinn RH, Davies DL, Dusterdieck G, Fraser R, Lever AF, Robertson JIS, Tree M, Wiseman A. Plasma electrolytes, renin and aldosterone in the diagnosis of primary hyperaldosteronism. *Lancet* 1968;**ii**:55–9.

23. Murphy BF, Whitworth JA, Kincaid-Smith P. Malignant hypertension due to an aldosterone producing adrenal adenoma. *Clinical and Experimental Hypertension. Part A, Theory and Practice* 1985;**A7**:939–50.

24. Ideishi M, Kishikawa K, Kinoshita A, Sasaguri M, Ikeda M, Takebayashi S, Arakawa K. High-renin malignant hypertension secondary to an aldosterone-producing adenoma. *Nephron* 1990;**54**:259–63.

25. Beevers DG, Brown JJ, Ferriss JB, Fraser R, Lever AF, Robertson JIS, Tree M. Renal abnormalities and vascular complications in primary hyperaldosteronism. Evidence on tertiary hyperaldosteronism. *Quarterly Journal of Medicine* 1976;**45**:401–10.

26. Iimura O, Shimamoto K, Hotta D, Nakata T, Mito T, Kumamoto Y, Dempo K, Ogihara T, Naruse K. A case of adrenal tumor producing renin, aldosterone and sex steroid hormones. *Hypertension* 1986;**8**:951–6.

27. Nicholls MG, Espiner EA. Liquorice, carbenoxolone and hypertension. In: Robertson JIS, ed. *Handbook of hypertension, volume 2: Clinical aspects of secondary hypertension.* Amsterdam: Elsevier 1983:189–95.

28. Brown JJ, Ferriss JB, Fraser R, Lever AF, Love DR, Robertson JIS, Wilson A. Apparent isolated excess deoxycorticosterone in hypertension: A variant of the mineralocorticoid excess syndrome. *Lancet* 1972;**ii**:243–7.

29. Biglieri EG. Mechanisms establishing the mineralocorticoid hormone patterns in the 17-alpha-hydroxylase deficiency syndrome. *Journal of Steroid Biochemistry* 1979;**11**:653–7.

30. Rovner DR, Conn JW, Cohen EL, Berlinger FG, Kem DC, Gordon DL. 17-alpha-hydroxylase deficiency. A combination of hydroxylation defect and reversible blockade in aldosterone biosynthesis. *Acta Endocrinologica* 1979;**90**:490–504.

31. Yanase T, Simpson ER, Waterman MR. 17-alpha-hydroxylase/17,20-lyase deficiency: From clinical investigation to molecular definition. *Endocrine Reviews* 1991;**12**:91–108.

32. Holten C, Petersen VP. Malignant hypertension with increased secretion of aldosterone and depletion of potassium. *Lancet* 1956;**ii**:918–22.

33. Laragh JH, Ulick S, Januszewicz V, Deming QB, Kelly WG, Lieberman S. Aldosterone secretion and primary and malignant hypertension. *Journal of Clinical Investigation* 1960;**39**:1091–106.

34. Barraclough MA. Sodium and water depletion with acute malignant hypertension. *American Journal of Medicine* 1966;**40**:265–71.

35. Kahn JR, Skeggs LT, Shumway NP, Wisenbaugh PE. The assay of hypertensin from the arterial blood of normotensive and hypertensive human beings. *Journal of Experimental Medicine* 1952;**95**:523–9.

36. Brown JJ, Davies DL, Lever AF, Robertson JIS. Plasma renin concentration in human hypertension III: Renin in relation to complications of hypertension. *British Medical Journal* 1966;**1**:505–8.

37. Fyhrquist F, Kala R, Standertskiold-Nordenstam CG, Eisalo A. Angiotensin II plasma levels in hypertensive patients. *Acta Medica Scandinavica* 1972;**192**:507–11.

38. Brown JJ, Davies DL, Lever AF, Robertson JIS. Plasma renin concentration in human hypertension. 1: Relationship between renin, sodium, and potassium. *British Medical Journal* 1965;**2**:144–8.

39. Atkinson AB, Brown JJ, Davies DL, Fraser R, Leckie B, Lever AF, Morton JJ, Robertson JIS. Hyponatraemic hypertensive syndrome with renal-artery occlusion corrected by captopril. *Lancet* 1979;**ii**:606–9.

40. Kaneda H, Yamauchi T, Murata T, Matsumoto J, Haruyama T. Treatment of malignant hypertension with infusion of sodium chloride; a case report and a review. *Tohoku Journal of Experimental Medicine* 1980;**132**:179–86.

41. Heslop H, Richards AM, Nicholls MG, Espiner EA, Ikram H, Maslowski AH. Hyponatraemic–hypertensive syndrome due to unilateral renal ischaemia in women who smoke heavily. *New Zealand Medical Journal* 1985;**98**:739–42.

42. Hilden T. Hypertensive encephalopathy associated with hypochloremia. *Acta Medica Scandinavica* 1950;**76**:199–202.

43. Möhring J. Pathogenesis of malignant hypertension: Experimental evidence from the renal hypertensive rat. *Clinical Nephrology* 1975;**5**:167–74.

44. Shibota M, Nagaoka A, Shino A, Fujita T. Renin–angiotensin system in stroke-prone spontaneously hypertensive rats. *American Journal of Physiology* 1979;**236**:H409–16.

45. Lohmeier TE, Tillman LJ, Carroll RG, Brown AJ, Guyton AC. Malignant hypertensive crisis induced by chronic intrarenal norepinephrine infusion. *Hypertension* 1984;**6** (suppl I):I-177–82.

46. Möhring J, Petri M, Szokol M, Haack D, Mohring B. Effects of saline drinking on malignant course of renal hypertension in rats. *American Journal of Physiology* 1976;**230**:849–57.

47. Conn JW, Cohen EL, Lucas CP, McDonald WJ, Mayor GH, Blough WM, Eveland WC, Bookstein JJ, Lapides J. Primary reninism. Hypertension, hyperreninemia, and secondary aldosteronism due to renin-producing juxtaglomerular cell tumors. *Archives of Internal Medicine* 1972;**130**:682–96.

48. Brown JJ, Fraser R, Lever AF, Morton JJ, Robertson JIS, Tree M, Bell PRF, Davidson JK, Ruthven IS. Hypertension and secondary hyperaldosteronism associated with a renin-secreting renal juxtaglomerular-cell tumour. *Lancet* 1973;**ii**:1228–32.

49. Baruch D, Corvol P, Alhenc-Gelas F, Dufloux MA, Guyenne TT, Gaux JC, Raynaud A, Brisset JM, Duclos JM, Menard J. Diagnosis and treatment of renin-secreting tumors. *Hypertension* 1984;**6**:760–6.

50. Anderson PW, Macaulay L, Do YS, Sherrod A, D'Ablaing G, Koss M, Shinagawa T, Tran B, Montz FJ, Hsueh WA. Extrarenal renin-secreting tumors: Insights into hypertension and ovarian renin production. *Medicine* 1989;**68**:257–68.

51. Bonnin JM, Cain MD, Jose JS, Mukherjee TM, Perrett LV, Scroop GC, Seymour AE. Hypertension due to a renin-secreting tumour localised by segmental renal vein sampling. *Australian and New Zealand Journal of Medicine* 1977;**7**:630–5.

52. Schambelan M, Howes EL Stockigt JR, Noakes CA, Biglieri, EG. Role of renin and aldosterone in hypertension due to a renin-secreting tumor. *American Journal of Medicine* 1973;**55**:86–92.

53. Brand G, Beilin LJ, Vandongen R, Matz L. Juxtaglomerular tumour: Diagnostic renal vein measurements obscured by chronic captopril therapy. *Australian and New Zealand Journal of Medicine* 1985;**15**:755–7.

54. Handa N, Fukunaga R, Yoneda S, Kimura K, Kamada T, Ichikawa Y, Takaha M, Sonoda T, Tokunaga K, Kuroda C, Onishi S. State of systemic hemodynamics in a case of juxtaglomerular cell tumor. *Clinical and Experimental Hypertension. Part A, Theory and Practice* 1986;**A8**:1–19.

55. Cohen EL, Rovner DR, Conn JW. Postural augmentation of plasma renin activity. Importance in diagnosis of renovascular hypertension. *JAMA* 1966;**197**:143–8.

56. Swales JD. The hunt for renal hypertension. *Lancet* 1976;**i**:577–9.

57. Hansson B-G, Bergentz S-E, Dymling J-F, Hedeland H, Hokfelt B. Pre- and postoperative studies in 72 hypertensive patients with renal artery stenosis, with special reference to renin activity and aldosterone. *Acta Medica Scandinavica* 1981;**210**:249–55.

58. Strong CG, Hunt JC, Sheps SG, Tucker RM, Bernatz PE. Renal venous renin activity. *American Journal of Cardiology* 1971;**27**:620–11.

59. Ernst CB, Bookstein JJ, Montie J, Baumgartel E, Hoobler SW, Fry WJ. Renal vein renin ratios and collateral vessels in renovascular hypertension. *Archives of Surgery* 1972;**104**:496–502.

60. Vaughan ED, Buhler FR, Laragh JH, Sealey JE, Baer L, Bard RH. Renovascular hypertension: Renin measurements to indicate hypersecretion and contralateral suppression, estimate renal plasma flow, and score for surgical curability. *American Journal of Medicine* 1973;**55**:402–14.

61. Messerli FH, Genest J, Nowaczynski W, Kuchel O, Cartier P, Rojo-Ortega JM, Schurch W, Honda M, Boucher R. Hypertension with renal arterial stenosis: Humoral, hemodynamic and histopathologic factors. *American Journal of Cardiology* 1975;**36**:702–6.

62. Stanley JC, Gewertz BL, Fry WJ. Renal: Systemic renin indices and renal vein renin ratios as prognostic indicators in remedial renovascular hypertension. *Journal of Surgical Research* 1976;**20**:149–55.

63. Staessen J, Wilms G, Baert A, Fagard R, Lijnen P, Suy R, Amery A. The prediction of blood pressure after percutaneous transluminal renal angioplasty. *Journal of Hypertension* 1987;**5** (suppl 5):S385–7.

64. Lyons DF, Streck WF, Kem DC, Brown RD, Galloway DC, Williams GR, Chrysant SG, Danisa K, Carollo M. Captopril stimulation of differential renins in renovascular hypertension. *Hypertension* 1983;**5**:615–22.

65. Thibonnier M, Joseph A, Sassano P, Guyenne IT, Corvol P, Raynaud A, Seurot M, Gaux JC. Improved diagnosis of unilateral renal artery lesions after captopril administration. *JAMA* 1984;**251**:56–60.

66. Muller FB, Sealey JE, Case DB, Atlas SA, Pickering TG, Pecker MS, Preibisz JJ, Laragh JH. The captopril test for identifying renovascular disease in hypertensive patients. *American Journal of Medicine* 1986;**80**:633–44.

67. Pedersen EB, Danielsen H, Fjeldborg O, Kornerup HJ, Madsen B. Renovascular hypertension. Ability of renal vein ratio to predict the blood pressure level 18–24 months after surgery. *Nephron* 1986;**44** (suppl 1):29–31.

68. Wilcox CS, Williams CM, Smith TB, Frederickson ED, Wingo C, Bucci CM. Diagnostic uses of antiotensin-converting enzyme inhibitors in renovascular hypertension. *American Journal of Hypertension* 1988;**1**:344–9S.

69. Grosse P, Dupas JY, Reynaud P, Jullien E, Dallocchio M. Captopril test in the detection of renovascular hypertension in a population with low prevalence of the disease. A prospective study. *American Journal of Hypertension* 1989;**2**:191–3.

70. Pedersen EB, Jensen FT, Eiskjaer H, Hansen HH, Jensen JD, Jespersen B, Madsen B, Nielsen HK, Sorensen SS. Differentiation between renovascular and essential hypertension by means of changes in single kidney 99mTc-DTPA clearance induced by angiotensin-converting enzyme inhibition. *American Journal of Hypertension* 1989;**2**:323–34.

71. Svetkey LP, Himmelstein SI, Dunnick NR, Wilkinson RH, Bollinger RR, McCann RL, Beytas EM, Klotman PE. Prospective analysis of strategies for diagnosing renovascular hypertension. *Hypertension* 1989;**14**:247–57

72. Tomoda F, Takata M, Ohashi S, Ueno H, Ikeda K, Yasumoto K, Iida H, Sasayama S. Captopril-stimulated renal vein renin in hypertensive patients with or without renal artery stenosis. *American Journal of Hypertension* 1990;**3**:918–26.

73. Marks LS, Maxwell MH, Kaufman JJ. Non-renin-mediated renovascular hypertension: A new syndrome? *Lancet* 1977;**i**:615–7.

74. Maxwell MH, Marks LS, Lupu AN, Cahill PJ, Franklin SS, Kaufman JJ. Predictive value of renin determinations in renal artery stenosis. *JAMA* 1977;**238**:2617–20.

75. Kreft C, Menard J, Corvol P. Value of renin measurements, saralasin test, and acebutolol treatment in hypertension. *Kidney International* 1979;**15**:176–83.

76. Fouad FM, Gifford RW, Fighali S, Mujais SK, Novick AC, Bravo EL, Tarazi RC. Predictive value of angiotensin II antagonists in renovascular hypertension. *JAMA* 1983;**249**:368–73.

77. Sellars L, Shore AC, Wilkinson R. Renal vein studies in renovascular hypertension — do they really help? *Journal of Hypertension* 1985;**3**:177–81.

78. Carmichael DJS, Mathias CJ, Snell ME, Peart WS. Detection and investigation of renal artery stenosis. *Lancet* 1986;**i**:667–70.

79. Luscher TF, Greminger P, Kuhlmann U, Siegenthaler W, Largiader F, Vetter W. Renal venous renin determinations in renovascular hypertension. *Nephron* 1986;**44** (suppl 1):17–24.

80. Kala R, Fyhrquist F, Halttunen P, Rauste J. Solitary renal cyst, hypertension and renin. *Journal of Urology* 1976;**116**:710–1.

81. Rose HJ, Pruitt AW. Hypertension, hyperreninemia and a solitary renal cyst in an adolescent. *American Journal of Medicine* 1976;**61**:579–82.

82. Stockigt JR, Challis DR, Mirams JA. Hypertension due to renal tuberculosis: Assessment by renal vein renin sampling. *Australian and New Zealand Journal of Medicine* 1976;**6**:229–33.

83. Delin K, Aurell M, Granerus G. Renin-dependent hypertension in patients with unilateral kidney disease not caused by renal artery stenosis. *Acta Medica Scandinavica* 1977;**201**:345–51.

84. Weidmann P, Beretta-Piccoli C, Hirsch D, Reubi FC, Massry SG. Curable hypertension with unilateral hydronephrosis. Studies on the role of circulating renin. *Annals of Internal Medicine* 1977;**87**:437–40.

85. Dahl T, Eide I, Fryjordet A. Hypernephroma and hypertension. *Acta Medica Scandinavica* 1981;**209**:121–4.

86. Watts RW, Frewin DB, Maddern JP. High renin hypertension in association with a solitary renal cyst. *Medical Journal of Australia* 1982;**1**:185–7.

87. Gordon RD, Tunny TJ, Evans EB, Fisher PM, Jackson RV. Renal venous renin ratio as a predictor of improvement in hypertension following nephrectomy for unilateral renal disease. *Clinical and Experimental Pharmacology and Physiology* 1984;**11**:403–6.

88. Gordon RD, Tunny TJ, Evans EB, Fisher PM, Jackson RV. Unstimulated renal venous renin ratio predicts improvement in hypertension following nephrectomy for unilateral renal disease. *Nephron* 1986;**44** (suppl 1):25–8.

89. Luscher TF, Vetter H, Studer A, Pouliadis G, Kuhlmann U, Glanzer K, Largiader F, Hauri D, Greminger P, Siegenthaler W, Vetter W. Renal venous renin activity in various forms of curable renal hypertension. *Clinical Nephrology* 1981;**15**:314–20.

90. Pitcock JA, Hartroft PM. The juxtaglomerular cells in man and their relationship to the level of plasma sodium and to the zona glomerulosa of the adrenal cortex. *American Journal of Pathology* 1958;**34**:863–73.

91. Dustan HP, Tarazi RC, Frohlich ED. Functional correlates of plasma renin activity in hypertensive patients. *Circulation* 1970;**41**:555–67.

92. Kaplan NM. Renin profiles. The unfulfilled promises. *JAMA* 1977;**238**,611–3.

93. Harris PE, Kendall-Taylor P. Isolated aldosterone deficiency in a patient with autoimmune adrenalitis. *American Journal of Medicine* 1991;**90**:124.

94. Oelkers W, L'age M. Control of mineralocorticoid substitution in Addison's disease by plasma renin measurement. *Klinische Wochenschrift* 1976;**54**:607–12.

95. Thompson DG, Mason AS, Goodwin FJ. Mineralocorticoid replacement in Addison's disease. *Clinical Endocrinology* 1979;**10**:499–506.

96. Smith SJ, MacGregor GA, Markandu ND, Bayliss J, Banks RA, Prentice MG, Dorrington-Ward P, Wise P. Evidence that patients with Addison's disease are undertreated with fludrocortisone. *Lancet* 1984;**i**:11–4.

97. Cutler GB, Laue L. Congenital adrenal hyperplasia due to 21-hydroxylase deficiency. *New England Journal of Medicine* 1990;**323**:1806–13.

98. Winter JSD. Marginal comment: Current approaches to the treatment of congenital adrenal hyperplasia. *Journal of Paediatrics* 1980;**97**:81–2.

99. Griffiths KD, Anderson JM, Rudd BT, Virdi NK, Holder G, Rayner PHW. Plasma renin activity in the management of congenital adrenal hyperplasia. *Archives of Disease in Childhood* 1984;**59**:360–5.

100. Lieberman J. Elevation of serum angiotensin-converting enzyme (ACE) level in sarcoidosis. *American Journal of Medicine* 1975;**59**:365–72.

101. Oparil S, Low J, Koerner TJ. Altered angiotensin I conversion in pulmonary disease. *Clinical Science and Molecular Medicine* 1976;**51**:537–43.

102. Studdy P, Bird R, James DG, Sherlock S. Serum angiotensin-converting enzyme (SACE) in sarcoidosis and other granulomatous disorders. *Lancet* 1978;**ii**:1331–4.

103. Allen R, Mendelsohn FAO, Csicsmann J, Weller RF, Hurley TH, Doyle AE. A clinical evaluation of serum angiotensin converting enzyme in sarcoidosis. *Australian and New Zealand Journal of Medicine* 1980;**10**:496–501.

104. Rohatgi PK, Ryan JW. Simple radioassay for measuring serum activity of angiotensin-converting enzyme in sarcoidosis. *Chest* 1980;**78**:69–76.

105. Romer FK, Jacobsen F. The influence of prednisone on serum angiotensin-converting enzyme activity in patients with and without sarcoidosis. *Scandinavian Journal of Clinical and Laboratory Investigation* 1982;**42**:377–82.

106. Romer FK. Angiotensin-converting enzyme in hypercalcaemic disorders. *Acta Medica Scandinavica* 1982;**211**:31–3.

107. Lufkin EG, DeRemee RA, Rohrbach MS. The predictive value of serum angiotensin-converting enzyme activity in the differential diagnosis of hypercalcaemia. *Mayo Clinic Proceedings* 1983;**58**:447–51.

108. DeRemee RA, Lufkin EG, Rohrbach MS. Serum angiotensin-converting enzyme activity. Its use in the evaluation and management of hypercalcemia associated with sarcoidosis. *Archives of Internal Medicine* 1985;**145**:677–9.

109. Lieberman J, Sastre A. Serum angiotensin-converting enzyme: Elevations in diabetes mellitus. *Annals of Internal Medicine* 1980;**93**:825–6.

110. Matsuki K, Sakata T. Angiotensin-converting enzyme in diseases of the liver. *American Journal of Medicine* 1982;**73**:549–51.

111. Johnson DA, Diehl AM, Sjogren MH, Lazar J, Cattau EL, Smallridge RC. Serum angiotensin-converting enzyme activity in evaluation of patients with liver disease. *American Journal of Medicine* 1987;**83**:256–60.

112. Nakamura Y, Takeda T, Ishii M, Nishiyama K, Yamakada M, Hirata Y, Kimura K, Murao S. Elevation of serum angiotensin-converting enzyme activity in patients with hyperthyroidism. *Journal of Clinical Endocrinology and Metabolism* 1982;**55**:931–4.

113. Falezza G, Santonastaso CL, Parisi T, Muggeo M. High serum levels of angiotensin-converting enzyme in untreated Addison's disease. *Journal of Clinical Endocrinology and Metabolism* 1985;**61**:496–8.

114. D'Onofrio GMD, Levitt S, Ilett KF. Serum angiotensin-converting enzyme in Crohn's disease, ulcerative colitis and peptic ulceration. *Australian and New Zealand Journal of Medicine* 1984;**14**:27–30.

115. Lieberman J, Rea TH. Serum angiotensin-converting enzyme in leprosy and coccidioidomycosis. *Annals of Internal Medicine* 1977;**87**:422–5.

116. Singer F, Talavera W, Zumoff B. Elevated levels of angiotensin-converting enzyme in *Pneumocystis carinii* pneumonia. *Chest* 1989;**95**:803–6.

117. Boomsma F, Michiels JJ, Prins E, Abels J, Schalekamp MADH. Angiotensin-converting enzyme: A tumour marker in malignant histiocytosis. *British Medical Journal* 1983;**286**:1106.

118. Milledge JS, Catley DM. Renin, aldosterone, and converting enzyme during exercise and acute hypoxia in humans. *American Journal of Physiology* 1982;**52**:320–3.

119. Milledge JS, Catley DM. Angiotensin converting enzyme response to hypoxia in man: Its role in altitude acclimatization. *Clinical Science* 1984;**67**:453–6.

120. Bedrossian CWM, Woo J, Miller WC, Cannon DC. Decreased angiotensin-converting enzyme in the adult respiratory distress syndrome. *American Journal of Clinical Pathology* 1978;**70**:244–7.

121. Fourrier F, Chopin C, Wallaert B, Wattre P, Mangalaboyi J, Durocher A, Dubois D, Wattel F. Angiotensin-converting enzyme in human adult respiratory distress syndrome. *Chest* 1983;**83**:593–7.

122. Metsarinne K, Fyhrquist F, Gronhagen-Riska C. Increased levels of immunoreactive plasma renin substrate during infectious peritonitis in patients on continuous ambulatory peritoneal dialysis. *Clinical Science* 1988;**75**:411–4.

123. Atkinson AB, Brown JJ, Davies DL, Leckie B, Lever AF, Morton JJ, Robertson JIS. Renal artery stenosis with normal angiotensin II values. *Hypertension* 1981;**3**:53–8.

83.10

84 BETA ADRENOCEPTOR BLOCKERS AND THE RENIN–ANGIOTENSIN SYSTEM

JAMES CONWAY AND JOHN CRUICKSHANK

INTRODUCTION

Propranolol, the first β-blocker to become generally available, was soon shown to lower plasma renin activity (PRA) [1–5]. Although β-blockers can completely suppress the renin response to renal nerve stimulation [6], in hypertensive subjects they seldom reduce PRA to very low levels, even when administered at very high doses (Fig. 84.1). At the usual clinical doses, it is rare to observe a reduction of more than 60% of the resting value [7,8]. The response is related to the initial level of PRA (Fig. 84.2).

In animal preparations, renin is released in response to a variety of homeostatic reflexes and there is a tonic inhibitory influence from the vagus [9]. Stretching the atrium decreases renin secretion [10], and stimulation of somatic afferents also leads to reflex renin release [11].

Beta-blockers reduce PRA at rest, under the stimulus of posture [12,13], during exercise [14], and in response to diuretics [15,16]. In dogs and in man, after the administration of a diuretic, β-blockers do not affect renin until significant volume depletion has occurred [17,18]. Elevation of renin by dietary sodium restriction is also affected by β-blockers but the effect is less than it is to diuretic-induced elevation of renin [19–21]. All the β-blockers reduce PRA [22], but nonselective agents are more effective than are the selective ones [23]. This is probably not due to an effect on the juxtaglomerular (JG) cells but to a prejunctional (β₂) action of the nonselective agents (see below). Plasma renin concentration does not appear to be reduced with atenolol [24] but PRA clearly is.

Since the release of renin is governed by multiple control mechanisms (see *Chapter 24*), there is a need to ensure that the changes observed after administration of β-agonists or β-blockers are directly due to the agent acting on the JG apparatus as opposed to an indirect effect which could raise renin levels; for example, changes in renal blood flow critically affect plasma renin levels [25–27].

Beta-agonists have been shown to have a direct effect on renin release from the kidney [28–32] and also from slices of renal tissue [33–35] and isolated renal cortical cells [36]. Initially, there was some difficulty in determining the receptor type responsible for the inhibition of renin release [23,36–40], but the evidence points to the β₁ adrenoceptor being the predominant, if not the only, receptor type involved [41–43] (see *Chapter 24*). Furthermore, the β₂ selective blocker, ICI 118551, failed to affect renin release due to renal nerve stimulation [44], and binding studies with this agent also point to B₁ receptors being responsible for renin release. The rabbit may be an exception since some evidence points to a β₂ receptor being involved in this species. This conclusion was reached on the basis of the effect of various

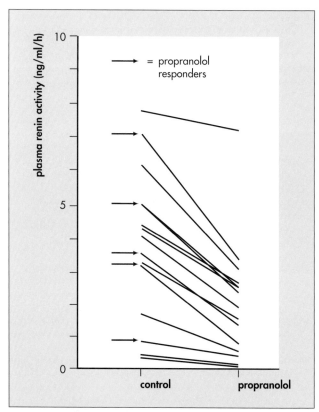

Fig. 84.1 Reduction in plasma renin levels in hypertensive patients. Propranolol responders had a fall in diastolic pressure of 12–20mmHg.

84.1

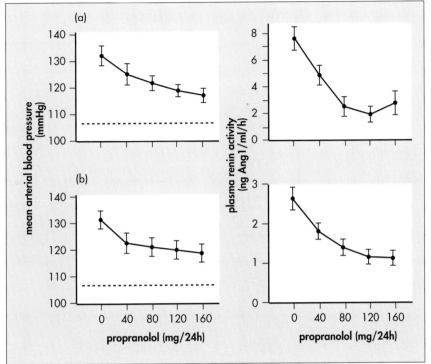

Fig. 84.2 The effect of increasing doses of propranolol on blood pressure and plasma renin activity (PRA) in hypertensive patients with high (a) and normal (b) PRA. Results are mean ± SD. Modified from Hollifield JW et al [7].

types of β-blockers on the renin response to infused isoproterenol and epinephrine [3,40]. These are, however, generalized β-stimulants and it is difficult to differentiate their direct action on the JG cells from β₂-vasodilator effects which can then induce a reflex release of renin.

Low levels of renal nerve stimulation, either directly [6,45] or by activation of the baroreflex [46,47], lead to renin release and this is prevented by β-blockers [27]. Renin release from a nonfiltering kidney after nerve stimulation is also inhibited by β-blockers [48].

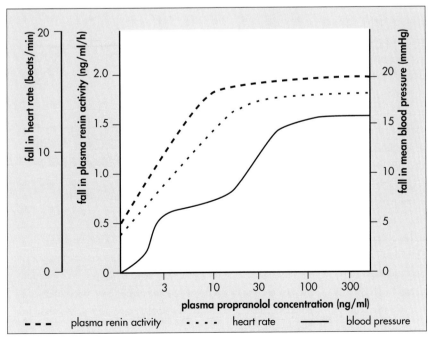

Fig. 84.3 Relationship between plasma propranolol concentration and the fall in plasma renin activity (PRA), in heart rate and in blood pressure. Note that the change in PRA and heart rate according to propranolol concentrations are approximately the same, whereas the change in blood pressure shows evidence for a two-stage process. Modified from Esler MD et al [8].

BETA-RECEPTORS ON THE JUXTAGLOMERULAR CELLS

The JG cells are richly innervated by postganglionic sympathetic nerves [49,50], and nerve stimulation releases renin [27,51], an effect which persists after concurrent changes in renal blood flow have been prevented.

Autoradiographic evidence demonstrates that the receptors on the surface of the JG cells are of the β_1-type in the guinea pig [52], dog [26,53], rat [54], and cat [6,27]; rabbit tissue has not been examined in this way. Beta$_2$ receptors are found in the kidney but these are associated with the renal tubular cells [53–55].

RENIN RELEASE IN MAN

Pharmacological evidence confirms that, as in most other mammals [56], β_1 receptors are involved in renin release in man. Beta blockers such as atenolol and metoprolol are effective in reducing renin [27,57–60] whereas the β_2 selective blocker, ICI 118551, is not [60,61].

Beta-blockers can affect renin levels by actions other than those on the JG cells. Most β-blockers reduce renal blood flow [62] and indeed the glomerular filtration rate [62–64] and hence the presentation of sodium ions to the JG cells. Thus, β-blockers may influence renin output from the kidney by an effect on blood flow and by reducing the sodium load to the tubular fluid.

Since β-agonists release renin, it is not surprising that β-blockers with intrinsic sympathomimetic activity are less effective than are nonstimulant blockers [41,64,65]. The effectiveness in reducing renin is inversely related to the level of intrinsic sympathomimetic activity [66]. For pindolol (an agent with marked intrinsic sympathomimetic activity), a biphasic response is seen in which low doses reduce PRA and high doses raise it above the control level [65]. Moreover, Waal–Manning and Simpson [67] have reported that a fall in blood pressure was observed when the dose of pindolol was reduced from an average of 48mg/d to 19mg/d. This observation is corroborated by Bjerle *et al* [68].

The dose–response relationship shows that renin reduction is achieved by modest doses of propranolol ranging between 20 and 80mg/d [7,8,69] (Fig. 84.2). The maximum effect of these doses is achieved at a plasma level of 30μg/ml [69]. The dose–response relationship for heart rate is close to that for plasma renin reduction (Fig. 84.3) [8,69]. The effect of propranolol on PRA is sustained and there is no evidence for the development of tolerance with time [2].

INDIRECT RENIN RELEASE

In addition to their direct effects on the JG cells, β-blockers can also affect renin release through their ability to block presynaptic β-receptors [70]. These are of the β_2 type and they mediate the release of norepinephrine at the sympathetic nerve terminals. Thus, β-blockade will reduce neurotransmitter release and this could contribute to the superiority of nonselective over selective agents on PRA.

The renin release in response to the Ang II antagonist, saralasin [42], and to ACE inhibitors [71,72] is reduced by propranolol.

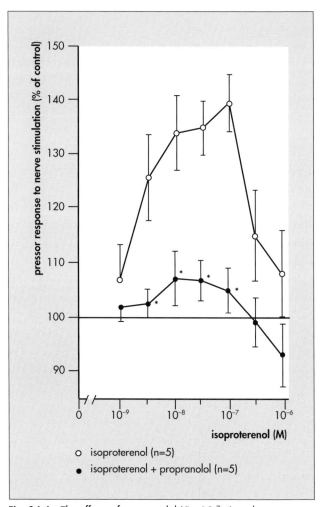

Fig. 84.4 The effects of propranolol (5×10^{-7}M) on the isoproterenol-induced pressor responses produced by sympathetic nerve stimulation in rat mesenteric arteries. Responses evoked in the presence of drugs are expressed as per cent mean of mean control ± SEM. *$P<0.05$ versus isoproterenol alone. Modified from Nakamura M *et al* [77].

RENIN RELEASE FROM VASCULAR TISSUES

The components of the RAS have been reported to be present in the walls of arteries and veins [38,73,74]. They are to be found indeed in cultured vascular smooth-muscle cells [74,75]. At this site, Ang II can not only directly affect smooth-muscle tone but it also facilitates the release of norepinephrine by a presynaptic action on sympathetic nerve terminals [76]. Isoproterenol also enhances the constrictor responses to nerve stimulation by its presynaptic action [70]. This potentiation can be blocked by propranolol, suggesting that Ang II influences the presynaptic β-receptor [77,78] (Fig. 84.4).

Angiotensin has been shown to be released by β-stimulation in rat mesenteric artery preparations and this effect is blocked by propranolol. Vascular tone then can be influenced by locally generated Ang II; its release is facilitated by β-receptors and can be blocked by propranolol. Thus, the RAS exerts a direct control of vascular tone in addition to the indirect effect through renal renin.

THE CONTRIBUTION OF CHANGES IN RENIN TO THE ANTIHYPERTENSIVE ACTION OF BETA-BLOCKERS

Beta-blockers were introduced for the treatment of ischemic heart disease [79] and it was not readily appreciated that they reduced blood pressure until Prichard and Gillam [80] and Zacharias and Cowan proved the point [81]. This activity is shared by practically all the β-blockers with a β_1 component, and an excellent account of their antihypertensive effects can be found in the review by Van Baak *et al* [82]. Their mode of action, like that of most other antihypertensive agents, has been a subject of controversy and the question has not yet been settled. As evidence has accumulated, however, the picture is becoming clearer.

When treatment with β-blockers is started, cardiac output and heart rate decline promptly [83–86]. At the same time, PRA is reduced [2,4,16]. All these changes occur within an hour of drug administration, though blood pressure does not change. There is thus an increase in peripheral resistance which is due to a reflex response to the hemodynamic changes [83,87]. The reduction of cardiac output triggers the baroreceptor reflex to maintain blood pressure by increasing sympathetic tone [88,89]. After denervation of the baroreceptors, the characteristic delay in the fall in blood pressure after the first dose of a β-blocker is greatly reduced [89,90].

In response to β-blockade, subjects with exceptionally high renin values tend to have a greater fall in blood pressure, whereas those with normal plasma renin values and those with very low values tend to have a smaller fall in pressure. It was therefore suggested that the antihypertensive action of β-blockers results from the reduction in renin [2,22,24,87]. This suggestion has been challenged on many grounds. The relationship observed between fall in blood pressure and initial renin levels depends critically upon relatively small numbers of subjects with either extremely low or very high renin levels. For the majority of patients, there is no detectable relationship between the fall in plasma renin and change in blood pressure.

Furthermore, if a β-blocker such as pindolol, with marked intrinsic sympathomimetic activity, is substituted for propranolol, blood pressure remains at its reduced level but plasma renin rises to its pretreatment value [65]. The concentrations of propranolol required to reduce renin are much lower than those required to lower blood pressure [8,91] and at high concentrations of β-blockers, the fall in blood pressure is unrelated to the change in PRA (see *Figs. 84.2* and *84.3*). This is the clearest evidence available that β-blockers lower blood pressure by at least two mechanisms.

Vasodilatation can contribute to the fall in blood pressure when β-blockers with high levels of nonselective intrinsic sympathomimetic activity are used [69,92].

It has been shown in rats that a natriuresis which is induced by β-blockers plays a part in lowering blood pressure [90]. In man, however, sodium balance is unaffected by β-blockers [63,93].

The fall in cardiac output observed after acute β-blockade tends to persist over a period of years [84,94] although stroke volume rises slightly [95].

The evidence then points to, at least, a dual action of β-blockers in lowering blood pressure [96]. At low doses, renin levels are reduced and blood pressure falls in a dose-related manner. At higher doses, blood pressure continues to fall without further change in plasma renin (see *Figs. 84.2* and *84.3*). The second mechanism probably results from the decline in cardiac output. Three β_1-selective compounds, atenolol, epanolol, and xamoterol, provide a range of drugs with graded intrinsic sympathomimetic action (β_1 selective), with which to examine this assertion. There is a profound fall in cardiac output and blood pressure with atenolol which has no sympathomimetic stimulant activity. With xamoterol, which possesses marked sympathomimetic activity, there is no change in either cardiac output or blood pressure. Epanolol, which is midway between atenolol and xamoterol in agonist activity, produces a small fall in cardiac output and also in blood pressure [85,91,96].

There have been suggestions that β-blockers may influence blood pressure through a central action or by an effect on the presynaptic β-adrenergic receptors on sympathetic nerve endings. There is no convincing evidence, however, that either of these actions plays a role in reducing blood presure [96]. There are some circumstances where circulating epinephrine levels are raised, for example, by smoking, by mental stress, or by hypoglycemia. Beta₁-selective agents may then be superior to nonselective ones in lowering arterial pressure due to preservation of β_2 vasodilatation which combats the reflex vasoconstriction [85,97]. The circulating catecholamines will have indirect effects on norepinephrine release through their presynaptic action and this will induce a release of renin. The independent part played by this action in lowering blood pressure is difficult to assess.

Renin release induced by vasodilator drugs is inhibited by β-blockers and this results in potentiation of the antihypertensive action of the former by β-blockers [98–100].

BETA-BLOCKERS AND THE RENIN–ANGIOTENSIN SYSTEM IN RELATION TO LEFT VENTRICULAR HYPERTROPHY AND REMODELING

Left ventricular wall stress can be increased by hypertension. The response of the left ventricular wall to this stress is to hypertrophy and then dilate, thereby maintaining cardiac output and restoring wall stress to normal. These compensatory mechanisms can eventually lead to a pathological state involving increased activity of pressor/growth-promoting agents such as catecholamines, serotonin, and Ang II [101]. Angiotensin II is also believed to be a stimulus for reactive perivascular fibrosis and reparative fibrosis in the heart [102,103]; in such a way, left ventricular wall compliance is decreased and coronary vessel wall hypertrophy occurs, predisposing to heart failure and impaired coronary flow reserve respectively. Hypertensive patients with left ventricular hypertrophy have, correspondingly, a poorer prognosis [110].

Angiotensin-converting enzyme inhibitors have been found to be effective in modifying the remodeling processes

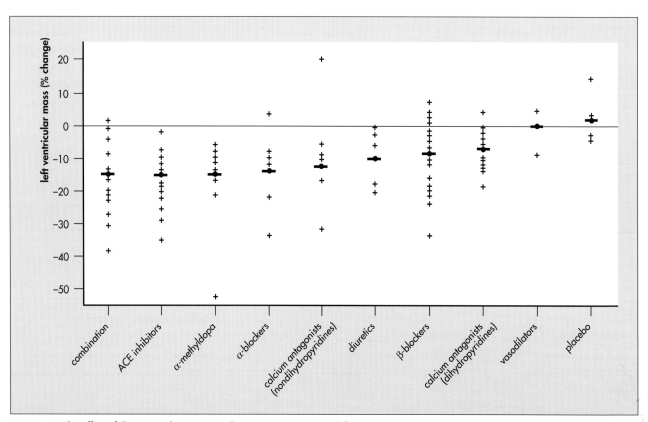

Fig. 84.5 The effect of therapy with various antihypertensive agents on left ventricular mass. For each category of treatment, results from individual trials and the overall mean are shown. Modified from Cruickshank JM *et al* [107].

leading to cardiac enlargement after myocardial infarction [104–106]. There is no experimental information concerning β-blockers in this area.

A meta-analysis of 105 published papers on the reversibility of ventricular hypertrophy with antihypertensive agents involving over 2,000 hypertensives [107] revealed that ACE inhibitors were highly effective in diminishing left ventricular mass and were superior to β-blockers in this respect (Fig. 84.5). These differences were independent of the fall in blood pressure and the duration of treatment. Beta-blockers, however, were quite effective in reducing left ventricular wall and septal thickness, and their relatively poor showing in reversing left ventricular mass could be partly due to the fact that they slightly increase ventricular volume. Another reason for the difference between the two drug classes could be the fact that β-blockers such as atenolol, unlike ACE inhibitors, do not increase arterial compliance [108] and hence decrease left ventricular afterload. Beta-blockers with vasodilating properties might prove to be effective in increasing arterial compliance and lowering afterload [109].

Angiotensin antagonists and β-blockers are associated with regression of left ventricular hypertrophy. It is not yet known whether β-receptors control the local Ang II production in the heart as they do in blood vessels.

CONCLUSION

Beta$_1$ receptors are responsible for the release of renin from the JG cells in animals and in man. The β$_1$ selective blockers reduce PRA, although the nonselective agents appear to be slightly superior in this respect probably due to their indirect effect on renal blood flow and glomerular filtration rate and/or to the antagonism of the presynaptic β$_2$-receptors on sympathetic nerve terminals.

Vascular tissue contains the components of the RAS and vascular tone has been shown to be influenced directly by locally released Ang II. This local generation of renin and hence Ang II is reduced by propranolol.

The reduction in PRA by β-blockers could play some part in the reduction of blood pressure in hypertensive patients. It is, nevertheless, clear that the antihypertensive action of β-blockers is not fully explained by suppression of renin release. Lowering of plasma renin occurs at low doses of β-blockers. The additional antihypertensive action has not been fully elucidated but it appears to be, at least in part, a consequence of a fall in cardiac output.

Angiotensin II is a growth-promoting factor that can lead to left ventricular hypertrophy involving both myocytes and fibrotic tissue [103]. Beta-blockers are only modestly capable of reversing left ventricular mass but are effective in diminishing wall thickness [107]. Beta-blockers with added vasodilating properties appear to be better than conventional β-blockers in this regard. Left ventricular remodeling postmyocardial infarction is benefited by ACE inhibitors and may be also by β-blockers, particularly when they are by coincidence already being given at the time of the infarction.

REFERENCES

1. Winer N, Chokshi DS, Walkenhorst WG. Effects of cyclic AMP, sympathomimetic amines and adrenergic receptor antagonists on renin secretion. *Circulation Research* 1971;29:239–48.

2. Buhler FR, Laragh JH, Baer L, Vaughan ED, Brunner HR. Propranolol inhibition of renin secretion. *New England Journal of Medicine* 1972;287:1209–14.

3. Michelakis AJ, Caudle J, Liddle GW. *In vitro* stimulation of renin production by epinephrine, norepinephrine, and cyclic AMP. *Proceedings of the Society for Experimental Biology and Medicine* 1969;130:748–53.

4. Michelakis AM, McAllister RG. The effect of chronic adrenergic receptor blockade on plasma renin activity in man. *Journal of Clinical Endocrinology and Metabolism* 1972;34:386–94.

5. Assaykeen TA, Ganong WF. The sympathetic nervous system and renin secretion. In: Martini E, Ganong WF, eds. *Frontiers in neuroendocrinology*. New York: Oxford University Press, 1971:67–102.

6. Ammons WS, Koyana S, Manning JW. Neural and vascular interaction in renin response to graded renal nerve stimulation. *American Journal of Physiology* 1982;242:R552–62.

7. Hollifield JW, Sherman K, Vander Zwagg R, Shand DG. Proposed mechanisms of propranolol's antihypertensive effect in essential hypertension. *New England Journal of Medicine* 1976;295:68–73.

8. Esler MD, Zweifler A, Randall O, DeQuattro V. Pathophysiologic and pharmacokinetic determinants of the antihypertensive response to propranolol. *Clinical Pharmacology and Therapeutics* 1977;22:299–308.

9. Bishop VS, Hasser EM. Arterial and cardiopulmonary reflexes in the regulation of the neurohumoral drive to the circulation. *Federation Proceedings* 1985;44:2377–81.

10. Zehr JE, Hasbargen JA, Kurz KD. Reflex suppression of renin secretion during distension of cardiopulmonary receptors in dogs. *Circulation Research* 1976;38:232–9.

11. Handa RK, Johns EJ. The role of angiotensin II in the renal responses to somatic afferent nerve stimulation in the rat. *Journal of Physiology* 1987;393:425–36.

12. DiBona GF, Johns EJ, Osborn JL. The effect of vagotomy on sodium reabsorption and renin release in anaesthetized dogs subjected to 60° head-up tilt. *Journal of Physiology* 1981;320:293–302.

13. Davies R, Slater JDH. Is the adrenergic control of renin release dominant in man? *Lancet* 1976;i:594–6.

14. Esler MD, Nestel PJ. Evaluation of practolol in hypertension. Effects on sympathetic nervous system and renin responsiveness. *British Heart Journal* 1973;**35**;469–74.

15. Attman PA, Aurell M, Johnsson G. Effects of metoprolol and propranolol on furosemide-stimulated renin release in healthy subjects. *European Journal of Clinical Pharmacology* 1975;**8**:201–4.

16. Winer N, Chokshi DS, Yoon MS, Freedman AD. Adrenergic receptor mediation of renin secretion. *Journal of Clinical Endocrinology and Metabolism* 1969;**29**:1168–75.

17. Vander AJ. Effect of catecholamines and the renal nerves on renin secretion in anesthetized dogs. *American Journal of Physiology* 1965;**209**:659–62.

18. Padfield PL, Allison MEM, Brown JJ, Lever AF, Luke RG, Robertson CC, Robertson JIS, Tree M. Effect of intravenous furosemide on plasma renin concentration: Suppression of response in hypertension. *Clinical Science and Molecular Medicine* 1975;**49**:353–8.

19. Sullivan JM, Nakano KK, Tyler HR. Plasma renin activity during levodopa therapy. Significance of long- and short-term treatment. *Journal of the American Medical Association* 1973;**224**:1726–9.

20. Vetter W, Zabuba K, Armbruster H, Beckerhoff R, Vetter H, Nussberger J, Schmied U, Reck G, Fontana A, Seigenthaler W. Effect of propranolol and pindolol on renin secretion in normal supine man. *Klinische Wochenschrift* 1975;**53**:709–11.

21. Mookerjee S, Eich RH, Obeid AI, Smulyan H. Hemodynamic and plasma renin effects of propranolol in essential hypertension. *Archives of Internal Medicine* 1977;**137**:290–5.

22. Amery A, De Plaen JF, Fagard R, Lijnen P, Reybrouck T. The relationship between beta-blockade, hyporeninaemic and hypotensive effect of two beta-blocking agents. *Postgraduate Medical Journal* 1976;**52** (suppl 4):102–8.

23. Harms HH, Gooren L, Spoelstra AJG, Hesse C, Verschoor L. Blockade of isoprenaline-induced changes in plasma free fatty acids, immunoreactive insulin levels and plasma renin activity in healthy human subjects by propranolol, pindolol, practolol, atenolol, metroprolol and acebutolol. *British Journal of Clinical Pharmacology* 1978;**5**:19–26.

24. Amery A, Billiet L, Boel A, Fagard R, Reybrouck T, Williems J. Mechanism of hypotensive effect during beta-adrenergic blockade in hypertensive patients. *American Heart Journal* 1976;**91**:634–42.

25. Blaine EH, Davis JO, Prewitt RL. Evidence for a renal vascular receptor in control of renin secretion. *American Journal of Physiology* 1971;**220**:1593–7.

26. Blair ML, Chen YH, Izzo JLJ. Influence of renal perfusion pressure on alpha- and beta-adrenergic stimulation of renin release. *American Journal of Physiology* 1985;**248**:E317–26.

27. Johns EJ. Role of the renal nerves in modulating renin release during pressure reduction at the feline kidney. *Clinical Science* 1985;**69**:185–95.

28. Haruyuki N, Nakane Y, Roux A, Corvol P, Menard J. Effects of selective and nonselective beta adrenergic agents on renin secretion in isolated perfused rat kidney. *Journal of Pharmacology and Experimental Therapeutics* 1980;**212**:34–8.

29. Holdaas H, Langaard O, Eide I, Kiil F. Conditions for enhancement of renin release by isoproterenol, dopamine, and glucagon. *American Journal of Physiology* 1982;**242**:F267–73.

30. Johns EJ, Singer B. Effect of propranolol and theophylline on renin release caused by furosemide in the cat. *European Journal of Pharmacology* 1973;**23**:67–73.

31. Nolly HL, Reid IA, Ganong WF. Effect of theophylline and adrenergic blocking drugs on the renin response to norepinephrine *in vitro*. *Circulation Research* 1974;**35**:575.

32. Ueda H, Yasuda H, Takabatake Y, Iizuka M, Iizuka T, Thori M, Sakamoto Y. Observations on the mechanism of renin release by catecholamines. *Circulation Research* 1970;**26/27** (suppl I):195–200.

33. Capponi AM, Vallotton MB. Renin release by rat kidney slices incubated *in vitro*; role of sodium and of α- and β-adrenergic receptors, and effect of vincristine. *Circulation Research* 1976;**39**:200–3.

34. Desaulles E, Miesch F, Schwartz J. Evidence for the participation of β_1-adrenoreceptors in isoprenaline-induced renin release from rat kidney slices *in vitro*. *British Journal of Pharmacology* 1978;**63**:421–5.

35. Lyons HJ, Churchill PC. Renin secretion from rat renal cortical cell suspensions. *American Journal of Physiology* 1975;**228**:1835–9.

36. Johns EJ, Richards HK, Singer B. Effects of adrenaline, noradrenaline, isoprenaline and salbutamol on the production and release of renin by isolated renal cortical cells of the cat. *British Journal of Pharmacology* 1975;**53**:67–73.

37. Capponi AM, Gourjon M, Vallotton MB. Effect of β-blocking agents and angiotensin II on isoproterenol-stimulated renin release from rat kidney slices. *Circulation Research* 1977;**40 & 41** (suppl 1):89–93.

38. Naruse M, Inagami T. Antibody-sensitive renin of adrenal and resistance vessels is markedly elevated in spontaneously hypertensive rats. *Clinical Science* 1982;**63**:187–9.

39. Salvetti A, Poli L, Arzilli F, Sassano L, Pedrinelli R, Motolese M. Effects of salbutamol and metoprolol on plasma renin activity and plasma potassium of normal subjects and of hypertensive patients. *Journal of Endocrinological Investigation* 1978;**1**:1–8.

40. Weber MA, Stokes GS, Gain Judith M. Comparison of the effects on renin release of beta adrenergic antagonists with differing properties. *Journal of Clinical Investigation* 1974;**54**:1413–9.

41. Davies R, Wiggins R, Slater JDH, Geddes D. Nature of the adrenoreceptor that mediates renin release in man. *Cardiovascular Medicine* 1978;**3**:571–5.

42. Keeton TK, Campbell WB. The pharmacologic alteration of renin release. *Pharmacological Reviews* 1980;**32**:81–227.

43. Johns EJ, Singer B. Comparison of the effects of propranolol and ICI 66082 in blocking the renin releasing effect of renal nerve stimulation in the cat. *British Journal of Pharmacology* 1974;**52**:315–8.

44. Johns EJ. An investigation into the type of β-adrenoceptor mediating sympathetically activated renin release in the cat. *British Journal of Pharmacology* 1981;**73**:749–54.

45. Holdaas H, Dibona GF, Kiil F. Effect of low-level renal nerve stimulation on renin release from nonfiltering kidneys. *American Journal of Physiology* 1981;**241**:F156–61.

46. Stella A, Zanchetti A. Effects of renal denervation on renin release in response to tilting and furosemide. *American Journal of Physiology* 1977:**232**:H500–7.

47. Zanchetti A. Neural regulation of renin release: Experimental evidence and clinical implications in arterial hypertension. *Circulation* 1977;**56**:691–8.

48. Holdaas H, Langaard O, Eide I, Kiil F. Mechanism of renin release during renal nerve stimulation in dogs. *Scandinavian Journal of Clincal and Laboratory Investigation* 1981;**41**:617–25.

49. Barajas L. Innervation of the renal cortex. *Federation Proceedings* 1978;**37**:1192–201.

50. Barajas L. Anatomy of the juxtaglomerular apparatus. *American Journal of Physiology* 1979;**237**:F333–43.

51. Dibona GF. Neural regulation of renal tubular sodium reabsorption and renin secretion. *Federation Proceedings* 1985;**44**:2816–22.

52. Lew R, Summers RJ. Autoradiographic localization of beta-adrenoceptor subtypes in guinea-pig kidney. *British Journal of Pharmacology* 1985;**85**:341–8.

53. Lew R, Summers RJ. The distribution of beta-adrenoceptors in dog kidney: An autoradiographic analysis. *European Journal of Pharmacology* 1987;**140**:1–11.

54. Healey DP, Munzel PA, Insel PA. Localization of beta-1 adrenergic and beta-2 adrenergic receptors in rat kidney by autoradiography. *Circulation Research* 1985;**57**:278–84.

55. Milavec–Krizman M, Evenou JP, Wagner H, Berthold R, Stoll A. Characterization of beta-adrenoceptor subtypes in rat kidney with new highly selective beta-1 blockers and their role in renin release. *Biochemical Pharmacology* 1985;**35**:3951–7.

56. Johns EJ. An investigation into the type of β-adrenoceptor mediating sympathetically activated renin release in the cat. *British Journal of Pharmacology* 1981;**73**:749–54.

57. Mancia C, Romero C, Shepherd JT. Inhibition of renin release by beta$_1$ receptors. *Circulation Research* 1975;**36**:529–35.

58. McLeod AA, Brown JE, Kuhn C, Mitchell BB, Sedov FA, Williams RS, Shand DG. Differentiation of hemodynamic, humoral and metabolic responses to beta-1 and beta-2-adrenergic stimulation in man using atenolol and propranolol. *Circulation* 1983;**67**:1076–84.

59. Cruickshank JM, Prichard BNC. *Beta-blockers in clinical practice.* Edinburgh: Churchill Livingstone, 1987.

60. Cruickshank JM. The clinical importance of cardioselectivity and lipophilicity in beta blockers. *American Heart Journal* 1980;**100**:160–78.

61. Vanhees L, Fagard R, Hespel P, Lijnen P, Amery A. Renin release: Beta-1 or beta-2 receptor mediated? *New England Journal of Medicine* 1985;**312**:123–4.

62. Schermeister J, Decot M, Hallauer W, Willmann H. Beta-receptoren und renal hamodynamik des Menshcen. *Arzneimittel-Forschung* 1966;**16**:847–51.

63. Wilkinson R. Beta-blockers and renal function. *Drugs* 1982;**23**:195–206.

64. Anavekar SN, Louis WJ, Morgan TO, Doyle AE, Johnston CI. The relationship of plasma levels of pindolol in hypertensive patients to effects on blood pressure, plasma renin and plasma noradrenaline levels. *Clinical Experimental Pharmacology and Physiology* 1975;**2**:203–12.

65. Stokes GS, Weber MA, Thornell IR. β-blockers and plasma renin activity in hypertension. *British Medical Journal* 1974;**1**:60–2.

66. Man in't Veld AJ, Schalekamp MADH. Hemodynamic consequences of intrinsic sympathomimetic activity and cardioselectivity in beta-blocker therapy for hypertension. *European Heart Journal* 1983;**4** (suppl D):31–41.

67. Waal–Manning HJ, Simpson FO. Paradoxical effect of pindolol. *British Medical Journal* 1975;**3**:155–6.

68. Bjerle P, Jacobsson KA, Agert G. Adrenergic beta-receptor blockade in essential hypertension: A comparison between pindolol and propranolol. *Current Therapeutic Research* 1975;**18**:387–94.

69. Leonetti G, Mayer G, Morganti A, Terzoli L, Zanchetti A, Bianchetti G, Di Salle E, Morselli PL, Chidsey CA. Hypotensive and renin suppressing activities of propranolol in hypertensive patients. *Clinical Science and Molecular Medicine* 1975;**48**:491–9.

70. Starke K. Regulation of noradrenaline release by presynaptic receptor systems. *Reviews of Physiology Biochemistry and Pharmacology* 1977;**77**:1–125.

71. Antonaccio MJ, Harris D, High JP, Rubin B. The effects of captopril, propranolol and indomethacin on blood pressure and plasma renin activity in spontaneously hypertensive and normotensive rats. *Proceedings of the Society for Experimental Biology and Medicine* 1979;**152**:429–33.

72. Harris DN, Heran CL, Goldenberg HJ, High JP, Laffan RJ, Rubin B, Antonaccio MJ, Goldberg ME. Effects of SQ 14,225 an orally active inhibitor of angiotensin converting enzyme on blood pressure, heart rate and plasma renin activity of conscious normotensive dogs. *European Journal of Pharmacology* 1978;**51**:345–9.

73. Collier JG, Robinson BF. Comparison of effects of locally infused angiotensin I and II on hand veins and forearm arteries in man: Evidence for converting enzyme activity in limb vessels. *Clinical Science and Molecular Medicine* 1974;**47**:189–92.

74. Re R, Fallon JT, Dzau V, Quay SC, Haber E. Renin synthesis by canine aortic smooth muscle cells in culture. *Life Sciences* 1982;**30**:99–106.

75. Dzau VJ. Vascular renin–angiotensin: A possible autocrine/paracrine system in control of vascular function. *Journal of Cardiovasular Pharmacology* 1984;**6**:S377–82.

76. Zimmerman BG. Actions of angiotensin on adrenergic nerve endings. *Federation Proceedings* 1978;**37**:199–202.

77. Nakamura M, Jackson EK, Inagami T. Beta adrenoreceptor mediated release of angiotensin II from mesenteric arteries. *American Journal of Physiology* 1986;**250**:H144–8.

78. Kawasaki H, Cline WH Jr, Su C. Involvement of the vascular renin–angiotensin system in beta adrenergic receptor-mediated facilitation of vascular neurotransmission in spontaneously hypertensive rats. *Journal of Pharmacology and Experimental Therapeutics* 1984;**231**:23–32.

79. Black JW, Stephenson JS. Pharmacology of a new adrenergic beta-receptor blocking compound (Nethalide). *Lancet* 1962;**ii**:311–4.

80. Prichard BNC, Gillam PMS. Use of propranolol in the treatment of hypertension. *British Medical Journal* 1964;**2**:725–7.

81. Zacharias FJ, Cowen KJ. Controlled trial of propranolol in hypertension. *British Medical Journal* 1970;**1**:471–4.

82. Van Baak MA, Struyker–Boudier HAJ, Smits JFM. Antihypertensive mechanisms of beta-adrenoceptor blockade: A review. *Clinical and Experimental Hypertension. Part A, Theory and Practice* 1985;**(A)7**:1–72.

83. Tarazi RC, Dustan HP. Beta-adrenergic blockade in hypertension. *American Journal of Cardiology* 1972;**29**:633–40.

84. Lund–Johansen P. Haemodynamic changes at rest and during exercise in long-term beta-blocker therapy of essential hypertension. *Acta Medica Scandinavica* 1974;**195**:117–21.

85. Svendsen TL, Hartling O, Trap–Jensen J. Immediate haemodynamic effects of propranolol, practolol, pindolol, atenolol and ICI 89,406 in healthy volunteers. *European Journal of Clincal Pharmacology* 1979;**15**:223–8.

86. Tsukiyama H, Otsuka K, Higuma K. Effects of beta-adrenoceptor antagonists on central haemodynamics in essential hypertension. *British Journal of Clinical Pharmacology* 1982;**13** (suppl):269–78.

87. Bühler FR, Laragh JH, Vaughan ED Jr, Brunner HR, Gavras H, Baer L. Antihypertensive action of propranolol. Specific antirenin responses in high and normal renin forms of essential, renal, renovascular and malignant hypertension. *American Journal of Cardiology* 1973;**32**:511–22.

88. Smits JFM, Struyker–Boudier HAJ. The mechanisms of antihypertensive action of the adrenergic receptor blocking drugs. *Clinical and Experimental Hypertension. Part A, Theory and Practice* 1982;**(A)4**:71–86.

89. Struyker–Boudier HAJ, Evenwel RT, Smits JFM, van Essen H. Baroreflex sensitivity during the development of spontaneous hypertension in rats. *Clinical Science* 1982;**62**:589–94.

90. Smits JFM, Coleman TG, Smith TL, Kasbergen CM, van Essen H, Struyker–Boudier HAJ. Antihypertensive effect of propranolol in conscious spontaneously hypertensive rats: Central hemodynamics, plasma volume and renal function during beta-blockade with propranolol. *Journal of Cardiovascular Pharmacology* 1982;**4**:903–14.

91. Leonetti G, Sampieri L, Caspidi C, Terzoli L, Rupoli L, Fruscio M, Gradnik R, Zanchetti A. Does β$_1$-selective agonistic activity interfere with the antihypertensive efficacy of β$_1$ selective blocking agents? *Journal of Hypertension* 1985;**3** (suppl 3):S243–5.

92. Man in't Veld AJ, Schalekamp MADH. Effects of 10 different beta-adrenoceptor antagonists on hemodynamics, plasma renin activity, and plasma norepinephrine in hypertension: The key role of vascular resistance changes in relation to partial agonist activity. *Journal of Cardiovascular Pharmacology* 1983;**5**:S30–45.

93. Weber MA, Drayer JIM. Renal effects of beta-adrenoceptor blockade. *Kidney International* 1980;**18**:686–99.

94. Lund–Johansen P. Hemodynamic consequences of long-term beta-blocker therapy: A 5-year follow-up study of atenolol. *Journal of Cardiovascular Pharmacology* 1979;**1**:487–95.

95. Wikstrand J, Trimarco B, Buzzetti G, Ricciardelli B, de Luca N, Volpe M, Condorelli M. Increased cardiac output and lowered peripheral resistance during metoprolol treatment. *Acta Medica Scandinavica* 1983;**672**:105–10.

96. Conway J, Bilski A. Beta-blockers. In: Ganten D, Mulrow P, eds. *Handbook of experimental pharmacology volume 93. Pharmacology of antihypertensive therapeutics.* Berlin: Springer–Verlag, 1990;65–104.

97. Van Herwaarden CLA, Fennis JFM, Binkhorst RA, van't Laar A. Haemodynamic effects of adrenaline during treatment of hypertensive patients with propranolol and metoprolol. *European Journal of Clinical Pharmacology* 1977;**12**:397–402.

98. Gilmore E, Weil J, Chidsey C. Treatment of essential hypertension with a new vasodilator in combination with beta-adrenergic blockade *New England Journal of Medicine* 1970;**282**:521–7.

99. Meyer DK, Peskar B, Tauchmann U, Hertting G. Potentiation and abolition of the increase in plasma renin activity seen after hypotensive drugs in rats. *European Journal of Pharmacology* 1971;**16**:278–82.

100. Pettinger WA, Keeton K. Altered renin release and propranolol potentiation of vasodilatory drug hypotension. *Journal of Clinical Investigation* 1975;**55**:236–43.

101. Morgan HE, Baker KM. Cardiac hypertrophy: Mechanical, neural and endocrine dependence. *Circulation* 1991;**83**:13–25.

102. Weber KT, Janicki JS. Angiotensin and the remodelling of the modelling. *British Journal of Clinical Pharmacology* 1989;**28**:1415–505.

103. Weber KT. Collagen matrix synthesis and degradation in the development and regression of left ventricular hypertrophy. *Cardiovascular Reviews and Reports* 1991;**12**:61–9.

104. Pfeffer MA, Lamas GA, Vaughan DE, Parisi AF, Braunwald E. Effect of captopril on progressive ventricular dilatation after anterior myocardial infarction. *New England Journal of Medicine* 1988;**319**:80–6.

105. Pfeffer MA, Braunwald E. Ventricular remodelling after myocardial infarction. *Circulation* 1990;**81**:1161–72.

106. Sharpe N, Smith H, Murphy J, Hannan S. Treatment of patients with symptomless left ventricular dysfunction after myocardial infarction. *Lancet* 1988;**i**:255–9.

107. Cruickshank JM, Lewis J, Moore V, Dodd C. Reversibility of left ventricular hypertrophy (LVH) by differing types of antihypertensive therapy. *Journal of Human Hypertension* 1992;**6**:85–90.

108. De Luca ND, Ricciardelli B, Rossillo G, Lembo G, Volpe M, Cuocolo A, Trimarco B. Stable improvement in large artery compliance after long-term anti-hypertensive treatment with enalapril. *American Journal of Hypertension* 1988;**1**:181–3.

109. Kelly R, Daley J, Avolio A, O'Rourke M. Arterial dilation and reduced wave reflection. Benefit of dilevalol in hypertension. *Hypertension* 1989;**14**:14–21.

110. Frohlich ED. Cardiac hypertrophy in hypertension. *New England Journal of Medicine* 1987;**317**:831–3.

85 RENIN INHIBITORS

KWAN Y HUI AND EDGAR HABER

INTRODUCTION

The RAS plays an important role in the regulation of blood pressure through a combination of hormonal effects on vasoconstriction, electrolyte balance, and the autonomic nervous system. The RAS has been shown to be involved in some forms of secondary hypertension and essential hypertension, as well as congestive heart failure. Nevertheless, a precise definition of its role in the etiology of essential hypertension remains elusive. This definition awaits development of clinically useful, specific antagonists of the RAS.

With the advent of captopril — an orally administered drug that inhibits an intermediate protease of the RAS, ACE — it became apparent that blocking the RAS was an effective treatment for essential hypertension, regardless of a patient's plasma renin concentration [1], and was also a means of ameliorating heart failure by reducing afterload [2]. Captopril and the other presently available ACE inhibitors, such as enalapril and lisinopril, are impressive antihypertensive drugs with low side-effect profiles. The action of ACE is, however, not specific to the RAS. In addition to its role as catalyst in the conversion of Ang I to Ang II, the very same enzyme plays a role in the inactivation of bradykinin and, probably, in the inactivation of enkephalins, as well as of other biologically active peptides. As ACE inhibitors block the degradation of bradykinin, its plasma or tissue concentration may rise, resulting both in direct effects, such as vasodilatation, and in the stimulation of the production of eicosanoids. Some of the adverse effects of ACE inhibitors, such as the development of flushing or rash, have been attributed to the elaboration of bradykinin or prostaglandins [3]. Other more serious questions about the nonspecific action of ACE inhibitors surround their intrarenal effects: is afferent renal arteriolar dilatation, with its significant effect on renal function, a consequence of the reduction of intrarenal Ang II concentration or of the production of bradykinin or prostaglandins within the kidney? Angiotensin-converting enzyme inhibitors also cause renal failure in bilateral renal artery stenosis and appear to have beneficial effects in diabetic nephropathy. Would inhibition of the RAS in a more selective manner avoid these variously adverse and beneficial results?

There is now abundant evidence that renin is synthesized in tissues other than the kidney. In these tissues, it may act locally, exerting a paracrine rather than an endocrine function [4]. In addition, several alternate enzymes capable of generating Ang II from Ang I *in vitro* are known to exist [5]. Thus, the inhibition of renin rather than ACE may be a better means of blocking Ang II formation in tissues.

Figure 85.1 lists potential targets for inhibition in the RAS. Of the presently accessible sites, the Ang II receptor and the enzyme renin itself provide opportunities for the most selective intervention. Traditionally, Ang II-receptor inhibitors have been short-lived peptides that required parenteral administration: they have had diagnostic but not therapeutic applications. Recently, there has been a major advance in the development of long-lasting and specific blockers of the Ang II receptor. Substituted imidazoles, which are nonpeptidyl and of low molecular weight, have emerged as a new class of highly specific Ang II-receptor antagonists [6,7]. There has also been considerable progress in the design of renin inhibitors. This chapter summarizes the development of specific renin inhibitors and examines their prospects.

Step in the pathway	Agent
Renin biosynthesis	Genetic-message blockers (undiscovered)
Renin secretion	β-adrenergic blockers (nonspecific)
Renin maturation	Prorenin processing-enzyme inhibitors (undiscovered)
Renin activity	Antibodies
	Peptide and peptide mimetic inhibitors of renin
ACE	Captopril, enalapril, lisinopril
Ang II receptor	Saralasin and similar peptides
	Imidazole derivatives

Fig. 85.1 Potential sites for inhibition of the RAS. Modified from Haber E and Hui KY. *Hypertension: Pathophysiology, diagnosis, and management.* New York: Raven Press, 1990:2343–50.

EARLY RENIN INHIBITORS

Although monoclonal antibodies are excellent experimental tools [8,9], the necessity of parenteral administration and potential immunogenicity prevent the use of antirenin antibodies in clinical trials. Therefore, it was necessary to search for a small organic compound that was a specific renin inhibitor. The first low molecular-weight inhibitor to block the action of renin effectively *in vivo* was reported in 1980 [10]. It was an analog of an octapeptide that Skeggs *et al* [11] had shown many years before to be the minimal substrate for renin. This substrate analog was not very potent (inhibitory constants between 1.0 and 2.3mM were reported [12,13]), and, although it was an effective hypotensive agent in the primate, at higher doses, the analog exhibited some lack of specificity [13,14].

RENIN INHIBITORS BASED ON THE SUBSTITUTION OF STATINE OR ITS VARIANTS AT THE SCISSILE BOND

More potent substrate-analog inhibitors have since been constructed by substituting various nonhydrolyzable residues for the scissile bond (the peptide bond renin cleaves in angiotensinogen). It had been noted that pepstatin, a potent inhibitor of pepsin, became a modestly potent, though nonselective, inhibitor of renin (pepsin and renin are both acid proteases) when it was modified to increase its solubility [15–17]. Investigators then learned that the selectivity of renin substrate analogs could be increased by substituting the unusual amino acid, statine (found in pepstatin and believed by some to be an analog of the transition state of the peptide bond as it undergoes enzymatic hydrolysis), for the two amino acids on either side of the scissile-bond region of the angiotensinogen sequence [18]. Several variants of statine have been reported (Fig. 85.2): these include AHPPA — (3S,4S)- 4-amino-3-hydroxy-5-phenylpentanoic acid [19], ACHPA — (3S,4S)-4-amino-3-hydroxy-5-cyclohexylpentanoic acid [19], difluorostatine [20], difluorostatone [20], 2-substituted statine [21], and 3-amino-deoxystatine [22] and its difluoro analog [23]. This class of substrate analogs has proved to be very potent, with inhibitory constants in the nanomolar range (with the exception of the difluoro-amino-deoxystatine-containing inhibitors). Among these changes, the inclusion of a cyclohexylmethyl group as the statine side chain is generally very effective in boosting potency.

Statine variant	Example of renin inhibitor *	IC_{50} (nM)†	
Statine [18,20,53]	Iva–His–Pro–Phe–His–A–Ile–Phe–NH₂	1.90	[18]
	Boc–Phe–His–A–Ile–AMP	1.70	[20]
AHPPA [19,53]	Iva–His–Pro–Phe–His–B–Leu–Phe–NH₂	2.20	[19]
ACHPA [19,42,75]	Iva–His–Pro–Phe–His–C–Leu–Phe–NH₂	0.17	[19]
Difluorostatine [20]	Boc–Phe–His–D–Ile–AMP	12.00	[20]
Difluorostatone [20,111]	Boc–Phe–His–E–Ile–AMP	0.52	[20]
2-substituted statine [21]	iBu–His–Pro–Phe–Phe–F–Leu–Phe–NH₂	1.70‡	[21]
3-amino-deoxystatine [22]	Boc–His–Pro–Phe–His–G–Ile–His–NH₂	28.00	[22]
Difluoro-amino-deoxystatine [23]	Boc–Phe–His–H–Ile–AMP	340.00	[23]

*A = statine, (3S,4S)-4-amino-3-hydroxy-6-methylheptanoic acid; B = AHPPA, (3S,4S)-4-amino-3-hydroxy-5-phenylpentanoic acid; C = ACHPA, (3S,4S)-4-amino-3-hydroxy-5-cyclohexylpentanoic acid; D = difluorostatine, (3R,4S)-4-amino-2,2-difluoro-3-hydroxy-6-methylheptanoic acid; E = difluorostatone, 4S-amino-2,2-difluoro-6-methy-3-oxoheptanoic acid; F = (2R,3S,4S)-4-amino-3-hydroxy-2-isobutyl-6-methylheptanoic acid; G = 3-amino-deoxystatine, (3R,4S)-3,4-diamino-6-methylheptanoic acid; H = difluoro-amino-deoxystatine, (3R,4S)-3,4-diamino-2,2-difluoro-6-methylheptanoic acid; Iva = isovaleryl; Boc = tertbutyloxycarbonyl; iBu = isobutyl; AMP = amino-methylpyridine. †IC_{50} values are against human plasma renin; ‡k_i value.

Fig. 85.2 Scissile-bond modifications with statine and its variants. References are given in parentheses. Modified from Haber E and Hui KY. *Hypertension: Pathophysiology, diagnosis, and management.* New York: Raven Press, 1990:2343–50.

OTHER SUBSTITUTIONS AT THE SCISSILE BOND

A number of modifications can be made to the scissile bond in order to prevent its hydrolysis by renin (Fig. 85.3). Substitutions include hydroxyethylene [24,25] and dihydroxyethylene [26] (both transition-state analogs), a reduced peptide bond (secondary amine) [27], an olefine bond [28], an aminoalcohol bond [29], an ether linkage [30] (including thioether and its oxidized derivatives [31]), a retro-inverso amide formed by diamino-hydroxyalkanes [32,33], phosphostatine [34], phosphinic isostere [35], and amino-hydroxyalkanoyl residues such as (2R,3S)-3-amino-2-hydroxy-5-methylhexanoic acid [36] (also known as norstatine [37]). In general, potency in this group of analogs relates directly to the number of amino-acid residues on either side of the substituted scissile bond. A remarkable degree of activity, however, has been reported for a dipeptide derivative, KRI-1230, which contains a scissile-bond substitution in conjunction with modifications at both termini [37].

OTHER MODIFICATIONS

Alterations to both the carboxyl and amino termini of the substrate-analog structure appear to be particularly valuable for increasing the inhibitory potency of small peptides and peptide-like molecules; Fig. 85.4 summarizes the strategies reported. Some of these alterations include substituting an

Pseudopeptide	Example of renin inhibitor*	IC_{50} (nM)†	
Secondary amine	Pro–His–Pro–Phe–His–Leu $\overset{R}{-}$ Val–Ile–His–Lys	10.0	[27]
Hydroxy isostere [24,25,112–114]	Boc–His–Pro–Phe–His–Leu $\overset{OH}{-}$ Val–Ile–His	6.9	[25]
Ether, thioether isosteres [30,31]	Pro–His–Pro–Phe–His–Leu $\overset{O}{-}$ Val–Ile–His–D–Lys	1,700	[30]
Amino-hydroxyalkanoic acid [36,37,115,116]	NMP–His–Norstatine–OCH(CH₃)₂ (KRI-1230)	7.8	[37]
Olefinic amino acid	Leu[CH=CH]Gly–Val–Phe–OCH₃	400,000‡	[28]
Amino alcohol	His–Pro–Phe–His–Leu(AA)Val–Ile–Phe–OCH₃	61§	[29]
Retro-inverso amide [32,33]	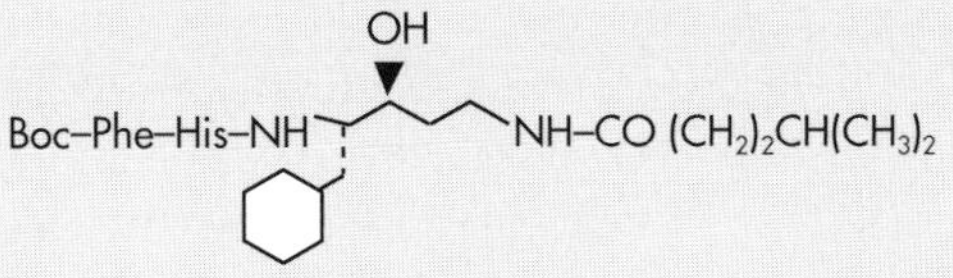 Boc–Phe–His–NH ... NH–CO (CH₂)₂CH(CH₃)₂	15§	[32]
Phosphostatine	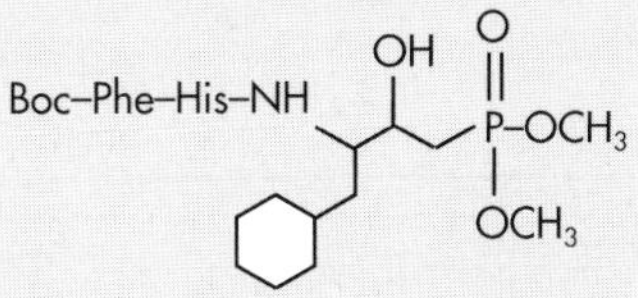 Boc–Phe–His–NH ... P–OCH₃ OCH₃	39§	[34]
Phosphinic isostere	Pro–His–Pro–Phe–His–Leu $\overset{P}{-}$ Val–Ile–His–Lys	75	[35]

*$\overset{R}{-}$, reduced peptide bond -CH₂-NH-; $\overset{OH}{-}$, hydroxyethylene -CH(OH)-CH₂-; $\overset{O}{-}$, ether linkage -CH₂-O-; $\overset{P}{-}$, phosphoric acid derivative; Norstatine, (2R,3S)-3-amino-2-hydroxy-5-methylhexanoic acid [36,37,115]; [CH=CH], trans carbon-carbon double bond; (AA), aminoalcohol -CH(OH)-CH₂-NH-; Boc, tert-butyloxycarbonyl; NMP, 2-(1-naphthylmethyl)-3-(morpholinocarbonyl)propyl; †IC_{50} values are against human plasma renin; ‡ K_i value against human amniotic renin; §IC_{50} values are against purified human kidney renin.

Fig. 85.3 Scissile-bond modifications with nonhydrolyzable pseudopeptides. References are given in parentheses. Modified from Haber E and Hui KY. *Hypertension: Pathophysiology, diagnosis, and management.* New York: Raven Press, 1990:2343–5.

Modification	Example of renin inhibitor*	IC$_{50}$(nM)†	
Internal residue substitution			
Nα–methyl and Cα-methyl amino acids [55,56]	Boc–Phe–MeHis–Statine–Ile–AMP	120	[55]
hydrophobic residues [38,40,117]	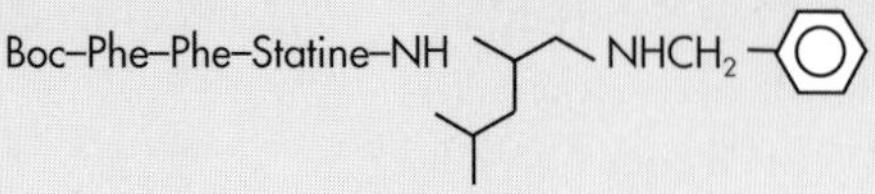 Boc–Phe–Phe–Statine–NH ... NHCH$_2$	~1,000 0.026‡	[117] [117]
amide bond isostere [57,58]	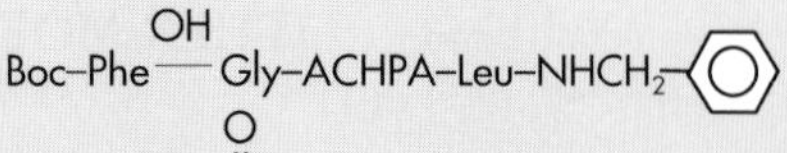 Boc–Phe OH Gly–ACHPA–Leu–NHCH$_2$	61	[58]
ionizable amino acid	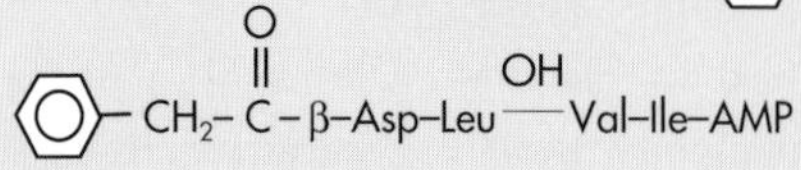 CH$_2$–C–β–Asp–Leu OH Val–Ile–AMP	3.5	[118]
Carboxy-terminal modification			
peptide aldehyde and alcohol [38–40]	Z–[3–(1-naphthyl)Ala]–His–Leucinal	80§	[38]
polar and nonpolar amides [42–46]	Boc–Phe–His–ACHPA–Leu–AMP	0.047	[43]
pseudostatine compounds [34,46–52]	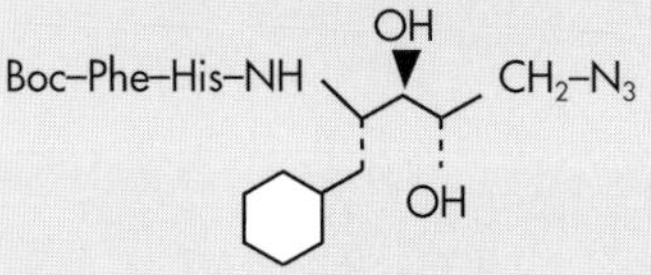 Boc–Phe–His–NH OH CH$_2$–N$_3$ OH	0.4‖	[50]
Amino-terminal modification			
Hydrophobic ring structures [37,40,42]	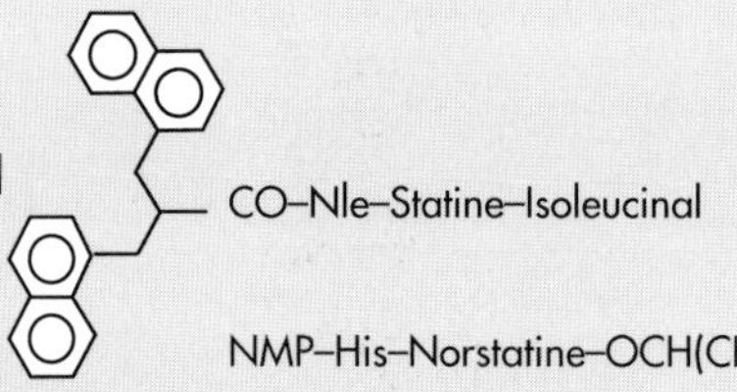 CO–Nle–Statine–Isoleucinal	3	[40]
	NMP–His–Norstatine–OCH(CH$_3$)$_2$	7.8	[37]
polar moieties [54,119,120]	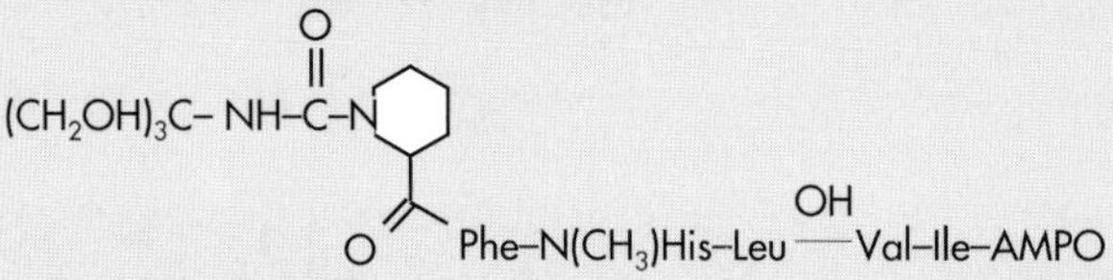 (CH$_2$OH)$_3$C–NH–C–N ... O Phe–N(CH$_3$)His–Leu OH Val–Ile–AMPO	0.58	[54]
Conformationally restricted analogs [59–65]			
	CO(CH$_2$)$_2$ CHPhCO–D–Phe–Lys–D–Trp–NH(CH$_2$)$_2$ CH(CH$_3$)$_2$	26	[65]

* Boc, tert-butyloxycarbonyl; Z, benzyloxycarbonyl; Statine, (3S,4S)-4-amino-3-hydroxy-6-methylheptanoic acid; ACHPA, (3S,4S)-4-amino-3-hydroxy-5-cyclohexylpentanoic acid; AMP, amino-methylpyridine; AMPO, 2-(aminomethyl) pyridine; Norstatine, (2R,3S)-3-amino-2-hydroxy-5-methylhexanoic acid [36,37,115]; —OH—, hydroxyethylene; Ph, phenyl. † IC$_{50}$ values are against human plasma renin; ‡ K$_i$ value against purified human kidney renin using synthetic tetradecapeptide as the substrate. § IC$_{50}$ values against purified human kidney renin using sheep angiotensinogen as the substrate; ‖ IC$_{50}$ value against purified human kidney renin.

Fig. 85.4 Other modifications to inhibitor structure. References are given in parentheses. Modified from Haber E and Hui KY. *Hypertension: Pathophysiology, diagnosis, and management.* New York: Raven Press, 1990:2343–50.

85.4

aldehyde [38,39], an alcohol [40,41], and polar or nonpolar amides [41–46] for the carboxy-terminal carboxylate, and substituting phenylalanine aminoadamantane for the entire carboxy-terminal amino acid [45]. Among the carboxy-terminal modifications reported, the incorporation of an amino-methylpyridine seems to produce the most active analog [43]. Another approach is to substitute a statine-like carboxy-terminal compound in place of the scissile-bond dipeptide [34, 46–52]. This shortens the length of the substrate-analog inhibitor and retains potency.

The amino termini of renin inhibitors are frequently protected by acetyl, isovaleryl, tert-butyloxycarbonyl, and benzyloxy-carbonyl groups. To reduce the number of amino-acid residues needed at the amino-terminal segment, and to retain potency, bis[(1-naphthyl)methyl]acetyl [40] and 2-(1-naphthyl-methyl)-3-(morpholinocarbonyl)propyl [37], which contain highly hydrophobic ring structures, have been used as the amino-terminal protecting group. Furthermore, extension of the peptide beyond the P_3 position [53] by incorporation of a bulky hydrophilic moiety also appears to enhance potency [54].

Structure	In vitro IC_{50} (nM)*	Route of administration
A-64662; enalkiren 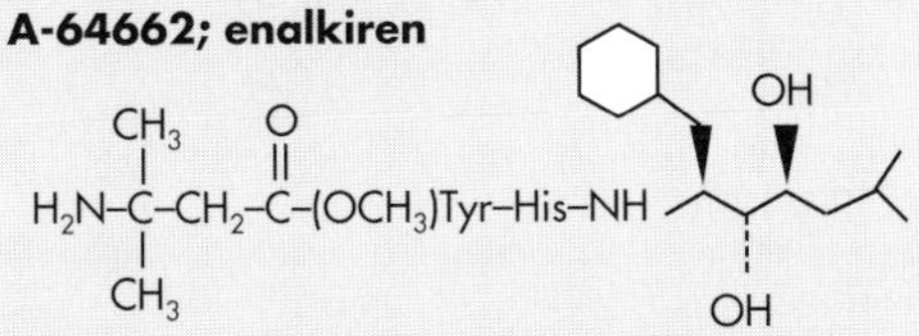	14	intravenous bolus [67]
KRI-1314 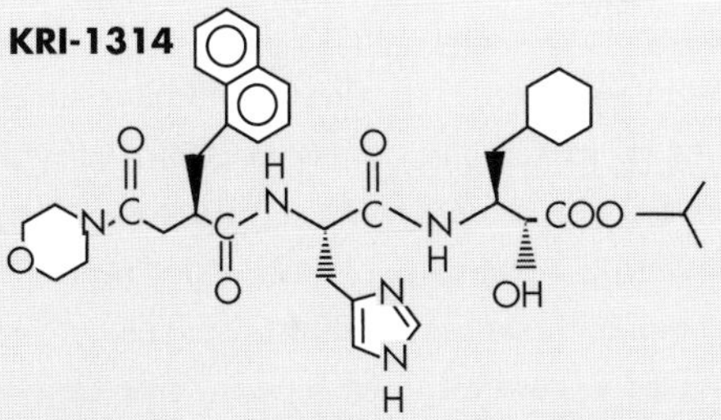	4.7	oral [68]
ES 8891 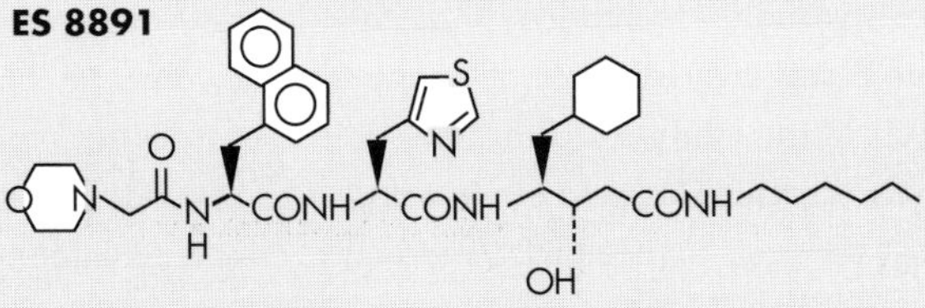	1.1	oral [69]
CGP 3856 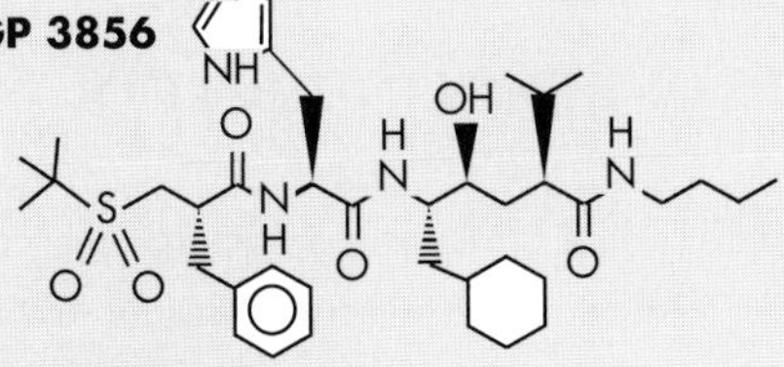	0.7	oral [70]
no compound code 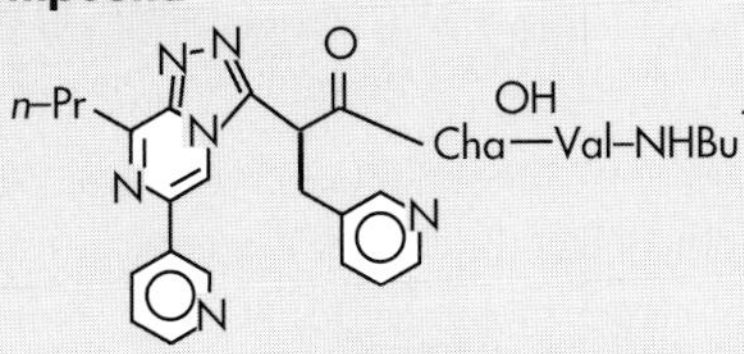	0.2‡	oral [71]

Fig. 85.5 Long-acting potent renin inhibitors. References are given in parentheses.

Unusual amino acids substituted in conjunction with modifications at the scissile bond appear to increase an analog's inhibitory constant, as well as to impart other desirable properties such as a prolonged *in vivo* half-life. Examples include substitution of N^α-methylhistidine at the P_2 position, N^α- or C^α-methylphenylalanine at the P_2 or P_3 position [55], α-methylproline at the P_4 position [56], and an amide-bond isostere at various postions within the molecule [57,58].

One of the favored approaches in the design of enzyme inhibitors has been to construct conformationally restricted polypeptides. Several such conformationally restricted renin-inhibitory substrate analogs have been described [59–65], and there has been recent progress with cyclic peptides attaining nanomolar IC_{50} values [65]. The creation of an irreversible renin inhibitor is also an attractive concept. With this in mind, investigators have incorporated into substrate-like peptides, epoxy groups that can react covalently with renin; one example is Z-Pro–Phe–Gly–NHCH(isobutyl)-CH-(epoxide)-CH-CH$_2$CO–Val–Phe–OCH$_3$, which has an IC_{50} value of 7×10^{-5}M against human amniotic renin [66]. Unfortunately, the inhibitory potency of this compound is too low for it to be of interest. This line of inquiry could, however, yield more interesting inhibitors.

By taking advantage of the sum of the past decade's experience in the design of substrate-based renin inhibitors, several groups of investigators [67–71] have synthesized relatively small molecules with high potency and long duration of activity (Fig. 85.5). A unique feature of the design of this group of compounds is the minimization or elimination of natural amino-acid components.

PRORENIN PEPTIDES

Another approach to the development of renin inhibitors would be to modify the structure of prorenin, an inactive zymogen that becomes the active enzyme after cleavage of a peptide bond and subsequent loss of an amino-terminal peptide. By reasoning that the association of this peptide with renin would render the molecule inactive, investigators believe that analogs of the prorenin peptide could act as inhibitors [72–74]. These analogs, however, have very low affinities for renin. Although the prorenin peptide analog approach is highly innovative, it does not, for the present, appear to be a promising area for development.

SPECIES SPECIFICITY

Renin inhibitors vary greatly in potency — often by over several orders of magnitude — with respect to the species of renin against which they are tested. For obvious reasons, most work has focused on the development of inhibitors selective for human renin. Yet, because of the rat's utility as an experimental animal (the availability of genetically determined models of hypertension make it particularly useful), efforts have been made to develop inhibitors selective for the renin of this species. (Renin inhibitors that are effective in man or other primates are generally quite ineffective in the rat.) Several selective rat renin inhibitors have been reported [75,76]. Since dogs are also popular animal models in which to study hemodynamic effects, renin inhibitors that are highly potent against dog renin have been designed [19,77].

ORAL ACTIVITY

All the renin inhibitors discussed thus far, although promising with respect to specificity and potency, are poorly absorbed by the gastrointestinal tract. Thus, they would be of little use in investigations of the chronic illness for which they were designed — essential hypertension. As yet, there is no general method for converting a pharmacologically active peptide into an equivalent compound that can be administered orally. Several compounds have now, however, been reported that are potent but have limited absorption [37,42,67–71,78–80]. Since absorption is still less than 20% of the administered dose, the likelihood of the inhibitors being the subjects of extensive clinical study is small. The main interest of these compounds lies in the hope they give to the search for an orally active renin inhibitor.

PRINCIPLES OF RENIN INHIBITION

As yet, our understanding of renin inhibitors has not reached a point equivalent to that of the masterful insight of Ondetti, Rubin, and Cushman [81], which generalized the principles of ACE inhibition and led to the development of the commonly used antihypertensive drugs captopril, enalapril, and lisinopril. In attempts to facilitate the design of renin inhibitors, investigators have built models of the enzyme's catalytic site on the basis of structures of related molecules [52,82–84]. Now that the human renin gene has been cloned [85] and expressed [86] and the X-ray crystallographic structure of recombinant human renin has been determined [87], it should be possible for the general principles of renin inhibition to emerge.

DO RENIN INHIBITORS HAVE A FUTURE AS CLINICALLY EFFECTIVE ANTIHYPERTENSIVE AGENTS?

Even though effective oral renin inhibitors may offer a more selective means of blocking the RAS, it is not certain whether they will provide significant clinical advantages over ACE inhibitors. One potential advantage of any new class of drugs is that it may eliminate adverse reactions associated with agents in current use. It remains to be determined, however, whether the adverse reactions common to captopril, enalapril, and lisinopril are the result of blockade of the target enzyme (ACE and kininase II are the same) or whether they are the consequence of a general inhibition of the RAS that would be a feature of any class of drugs used to block it [3]. Nonspecific effects of ACE inhibitors which could be independent of a reduction in Ang II concentration include increased bradykinin or prostaglandin concentrations, blunting of sympathetic activity, increased parasympathetic activity,

effects on the central nervous system, and redistribution of blood flow. A potential advantage of renin inhibitors may derive from enhanced cellular penetration, so that tissue as well as extracellular renins could be blocked.

Renin-specific antibodies have proved excellent models for renin inhibitors, particularly with respect to the highly selective inhibition of the enzyme in extracellular fluid. Due to their molecular size, however, antibodies are unlikely to penetrate the cell membrane and thus cannot be used to address questions about potential intracellular effects. When a monospecific antibody for renin and teprotide, an ACE inhibitor, were compared in the sodium-depleted dog, their hemodynamic effects were identical [88]. These results were confirmed later in the marmoset, in comparisons between monoclonal antibodies and enalaprilat [89,90].

As soon as peptide renin inhibitors that were effective *in vivo* became available, they were compared with ACE inhibitors under a variety of circumstances. In sodium-depleted primates, we showed that an ACE inhibitor (captopril) and a statine-containing, substrate-analog renin-inhibitory peptide (R-PEP-27) at high dose were approximately equipotent in lowering blood pressure [91] (Fig. 85.6). This lowering effect of blood pressure was associated with a parallel decrease in plasma renin

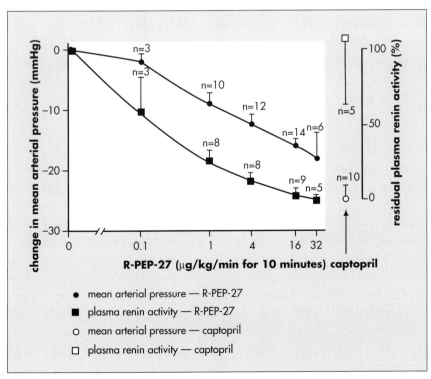

Fig. 85.6 Comparison between a renin inhibitor (R-PEP-27) and a converting-enzyme inhibitor (captopril) in a nonhuman primate model, and the biochemical events that occur as a result of renin inhibition. Modified from Hui KY *et al* [91]. (a) The change in mean arterial pressure and residual plasma renin activity of sodium-depleted primates after a 10-minute intravenous infusion of R-PEP-27 at various doses (0–32μg/kg/min), or approximately 20 minutes after an intravenous bolus injection of captopril at 400μg/k/min.

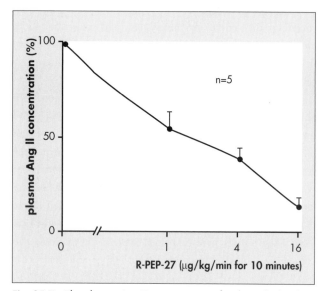

Fig. 85.7 The plasma Ang II concentration of sodium-depleted primates after a 10-minute intravenous infusion of different doses of R-PEP-27 (0, 1, 4, and 16μg/kg/min). Values are means ± SEM.

activity (PRA) and plasma Ang II concentration (Fig. 85.7). As a consequence of endogenous renin inhibition, release of both total renin and active renin was stimulated (Fig. 85.8), consistent with the theory of a negative feedback mechanism [92]. Other studies in sodium-depleted primates demonstrated similar results: ACE inhibitors and renin inhibitors lowered blood pressure equivalently [10,25,78,93]. In a very interesting model of hypertension associated with normal renin levels in the marmoset, created by ligating a branch of one renal artery, Neisius and Wood [94] showed that a renin inhibitor and an ACE inhibitor had equal effects on blood pressure. In normotensive dogs, as well as in hypertensive dogs subjected to renal artery constriction, Smith *et al* [95] also found no significant difference in hypotensive effect between enalaprilat and a potent ACHPA-containing renin inhibitor. These reports are representative of many others that fail to demonstrate a convincing difference between renin and ACE inhibitors in acute systemic or renal hemodynamic studies; other examples are known [96–98].

Although there is little difference in systemic blood-pressure effects between renin inhibitors and ACE inhibitors, there may be differences in organ-specific hemodynamic responses to these two classes of compounds: renal response is one example. In conscious dogs (uninephrectomized), intrarenal blockade of the RAS with the ACE inhibitor, teprotide, increased the glomerular filtration rate and renal plasma flow, whereas blockade with a renin inhibitor did not [99]. In another study in the dog, long-term inhibition of the RAS by a renin inhibitor and an ACE inhibitor resulted in

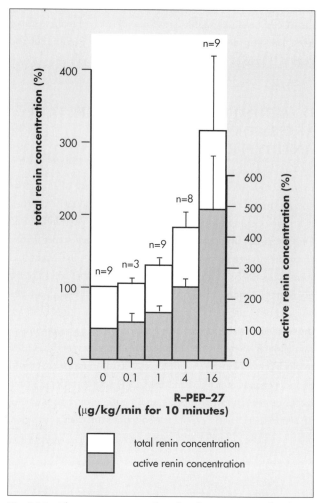

Fig. 85.8 The concentrations of total and active renins of sodium-depleted primates after a 10-minute intravenous infusion of different doses of R-PEP-27 (0, 0.1, 1, 4, and 16μg/kg/min). Bars are means ± SEM.

differences in sodium excretion and renal plasma flow [100]. In other, short-term studies, however, the renal hemodynamic profiles for the two classes of inhibitors appeared similar [95,101]. In mildly volume-depleted marmosets, Neisius *et al* [102] showed that both renin and ACE inhibitors increased renal blood flow in an equivalent manner. Since renal function is an important consideration in blood-pressure control, renal pharmacology should be an important focus in the development of renin inhibitors.

It is also possible that certain renin inhibitors possess hypotensive activity secondary to their effects on circulating renin. One such molecule is the renin inhibitor, A-64662, which caused hypotension in both normal and anephric monkeys [103]. In addition, a series of ACHPA-containing renin inhibitors exhibited more profoundly hypotensive effects than did enalaprilat [104].

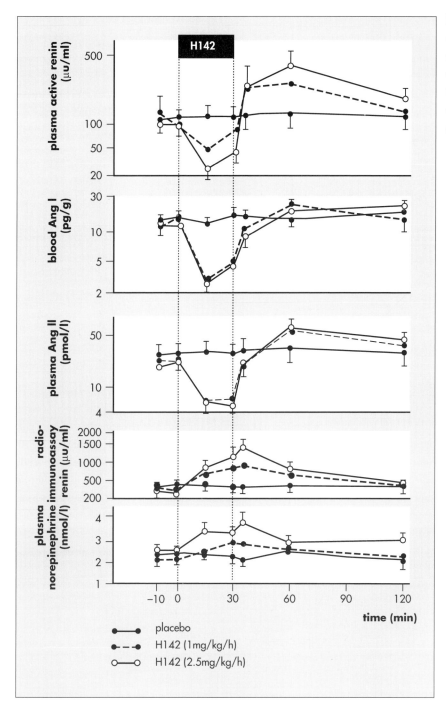

Fig. 85.9 Measurements of plasma active renin, Ang I and II, total renin, and norepinephrine before, during, and after administration of the renin inhibitor, H142, in nine human subjects. Means ± SEM derived from the original data are shown. Modified from Webb DJ *et al* [121].

At present, the notion that clear differences in effect exist between renin inhibitors and ACE inhibitors is hard to support. Since it has not been easy to differentiate systemic from local hemodynamic effects, it has been difficult to define a role for kinin inhibition or eicosanoid release in the regulation of resistance vessel tone. Differences in tissue penetration have also not been demonstrated. It must be emphasized, however, that few truly long-term animal studies have been reported [100,105,106] Studies in sodium-depleted normal human subjects began in the 1980s [14,121]. As shown in Fig. 85.9, administration of the renin inhibitor, H142, was accompanied by a fall in the concentration of circulating enzymically active renin (free active renin not bound to H142) while the concentration of immunoreactive renin rose, reflecting an increase in renin secretion. The fall in the

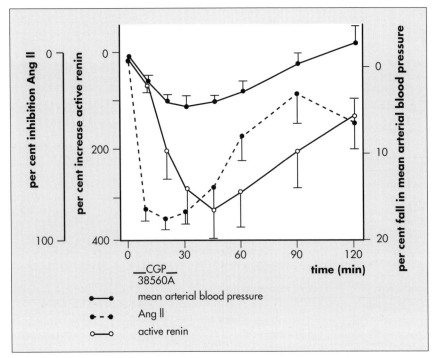

Fig. 85.10 Effects of the renin inhibitor, CGP 38560A, on mean arterial pressure, Ang II, and active renin after a 30-minute intravenous infusion into patients with hypertension. The results are expressed as a percentage of the control value. Modified from Jeunemaître X *et al* [109].

concentration of enzymically active renin was paralleled by reductions in concentrations of circulating Ang I and Ang II. At a high dose of H142, the plasma norepinephrine concentration increased [121]. Zusman *et al* [14] reported a greater hypotensive effect with 'RIP' (a moderately potent substrate analog renin inhibitor) than with captopril in subjects studied in the supine and upright positions. Other short-term studies of normal man showed moderate or no change in blood pressure associated with effective suppression of PRA and a fall in plasma Ang I and II concentrations [69,107,108,121].

In the limited number of short-term studies of patients with essential hypertension, the focus has been on the effect of renin inhibitors on blood pressure and the circulating RAS. One report [109] showed hemodynamic and biochemical profiles (Fig. 85.10) similar to those we observed in our nonhuman primate study [91]; in both studies, with increasing doses of renin inhibitor, blood pressure and plasma Ang II concentration decreased, whereas active renin concentration increased. In all the clinical studies, antihypertensive effects were transient [67,109,110,122] unless the renin inhibitor was given intravenously at high doses [67].

REFERENCES

1. Edwards CRW, Padfield PL. Angiotensin-converting enzyme inhibitors: Past, present, and bright future. *Lancet* 1985;i:30–4.

2. Sutton FJ. Vasodilator therapy. *American Journal of Medicine* 1986;**80** (suppl 2B):54–8.

3. Brunner HR, Waeber B, Nussberger J. Pharmacology of converting enzyme inhibitors. *Clinical and Experimental Hypertension. Part A, Theory and Practice* 1987;**A9**:275–88.

4. Corvol P, Waeber B, Bühler FR. Circulating and tissue renin–angiotensin system and its inhibition: Present and future. Satellite symposium of the Journées de l'Hypertension Artérielle. Paris, December 14, 1988. *Journal of Cardiovascular Pharmacology* 1989;**14** (suppl 4):S1–65.

5. Dzau VJ. Multiple pathways of angiotensin production in the blood vessel wall: Evidence, possibilities and hypotheses. *Journal of Hypertension* 1989;**7**:933–6.

6. Duncia JV, Chiu AT, Carini DJ, Gregory GB, Johnson AL, Price WA, Wells GJ, Wong PC, Calabrese JC, Timmermans PBMWM. The discovery of potent nonpeptide angiotensin II receptor antagonists: A new class of potent antihypertensives. *Journal of Medicinal Chemistry* 1990;**33**:1312–29.

7. Timmermans PBMWM, Carini DJ, Chiu AT, Duncia JV, Price WA Jr, Wells GJ, Wong PC, Wexler RR, Johnson AL. The discovery and physiological effects of a new class of highly specific angiotensin II-receptor antagonists. In: Laragh JH, Brenner BM, eds. *Hypertension: Pathophysiology, diagnosis, and management.* New York: Raven Press, 1990:2351–60.

8. Galen FX, Devaux C, Atlas S, Guyenne T, Menard J, Corvol P, Simon D, Cazaubon C, Richer P, Badouaille G, Richaud JP, Gros P, Pau B. New monoclonal antibodies directed against human renin: Powerful tools for the investigation of the renin system. *Journal of Clinical Investigation* 1984;**74**:723–35.

9. Dzau VJ, Mudgett–Hunter M, Haber E. Monoclonal antibodies as molecular probes to study structural heterogeneity between human and animal renins and other aspartyl proteinases. *Journal of Clinical Endocrinology and Metabolism* 1986;**62**:424–8.

10. Burton J, Cody RJ Jr, Herd JA, Haber E. Specific inhibition of renin by an angiotensinogen analog: Studies in sodium depletion and renin-dependent hypertension. *Proceedings of the National Academy of Sciences of the USA* 1980;**77**:5476–9.

11. Skeggs LT, Lentz KE, Kahn JR, Hochstrasser H. Kinetics of the action of renin with nine synthetic peptide substrates. *Journal of Experimental Medicine* 1968;**128**:13–34.

12. Cody RJ, Burton J, Evin G, Poulsen K, Herd JA, Haber E. A substrate analog inhibitor of renin that is effective *in vivo*. *Biochemical and Biophysical Research Communications* 1980;**97**:230–5.

13. Pals DT, DeGraaf GL, Kati WM, Lawson JA, Smith CW, Skala GF. Cardiovascular effects of a renin inhibitor in relation to posture in nonhuman primates. *Clinical and Experimental Hypertension. Part A, Theory and Practice* 1985;**A7**:105–21.

14. Zusman RM, Burton J, Christensen D, Nussberger J, Dodds A, Haber E. Hemodynamic effects of a competitive renin inhibitory peptide in humans: Evidence for multiple mechanisms of action. *Transactions of the Association of American Physicians* 1983;**96**:365–74.

15. Evin G, Castro B, Gardes J, Kreft C, Ménard J, Corvol P. Soluble derivatives of pepstatin: New, potent, *in vivo* inhibitors of renin. In: Gross E, Meienhofer J, eds. *Peptides: Structure and biological function. Proceedings of the Sixth American Peptide Symposium.* Rockford, Illinois: Pierce Chemical, 1979:165–8.

16. Eid M, Evin G, Castro B, Ménard J, Çorvol P. New renin inhibitors homologous with pepstatin. *Biochemical Journal* 1981;**197**:465–71.

17. Guégan R, Diaz J, Cazaubon C, Beaumont M, Carlet C, Clément J, Demarne H, Mellet M, Richaud J–P, Segondy D, Vedel M, Gagnol J–P, Roncucci R, Castro B, Corvol P, Evin G, Roques BP. Pepstatin analogues as novel renin inhibitors. *Journal of Medicinal Chemistry* 1986;**29**:1152–9.

18. Boger J, Lohr NS, Ulm EH, Poe M, Blaine EH, Fanelli GM, Lin T–Y, Payne LS, Schorn TW, LaMont BI, Vassil TC, Stabilito II, Veber DF, Rich DH, Bopari AS. Novel renin inhibitors containing the amino acid statine. *Nature* 1983;**303**:81–4.

19. Boger J, Payne LS, Perlow DS, Lohr NS, Poe M, Blaine EH, Ulm EH, Schorn TW, LaMont BI, Lin T–Y, Kawai M, Rich DH, Veber DF. Renin inhibitors. Syntheses of subnanomolar, competitive, transition-state analogue inhibitors containing a novel analogue of statine. *Journal of Medicinal Chemistry* 1985;**28**: 1779–90.

20. Thaisrivongs S, Pals DT, Kati WM, Turner SR, Thomasco LM, Watt W. Design and syntheses of potent and specific renin inhibitors containing difluorostatine, difluorostatone, and related analogues. *Journal of Medicinal Chemistry* 1986;**29**:2080–7.

21. Veber DF, Bock MG, Brady SF, Ulm EH, Cochran DW, Smith GM, LaMont BI, Dipardo RM, Poe M, Freidinger RM, Evans BE, Boger J. Renin inhibitors containing 2-substituted statine. *Biochemical Society Transactions* 1984;**12**:956–9.

22. Jones M, Sueiras–Diaz J, Szelke M, Leckie B, Beattie S. Renin inhibitors containing the novel amino-acid 3-amino-deoxystatine. In: Deber CM, Hruby VJ, Kopple KD, eds. *Peptides: Structure and function. Proceedings of the Ninth American Peptide Symposium.* Rockford, Illinois: Pierce Chemical, 1985:759–62.

23. Thaisrivongs S, Schostarez HJ, Pals DT, Turner SR. α, α-Difluoro-β-aminodeoxystatine-containing renin inhibitory peptides. *Journal of Medicinal Chemistry* 1987;**30**:1837–42.

24. Szelke M, Jones DM, Atrash B, Hallett A, Leckie BJ. Novel transition-state analogue inhibitors of renin. In: Hruby VJ, Rich DH, eds. *Peptides: Structure and function. Proceedings of the Eighth American Peptide Symposium.* Rockford, Illinois: Pierce Chemical, 1983:579–82.

25. Szelke M, Tree M, Leckie BJ, Jones DM, Atrash B, Beattie S, Donovan B, Hallett A, Hughes M. Lever AF, Morton JJ, Sueiras–Diaz J. A transition-state analogue inhibitor of human renin (H.261): Test *in vitro* and a comparison with captopril in the anaesthetized baboon. *Journal of Hypertension* 1985;**3**:13–8.

26. Luly JR, BaMaung N, Soderquist J, Fung AKL, Stein H, Kleinert HD, Marcotte PA, Egan DA, Bopp B, Merits I, Bolis G, Greer J, Perun TJ, Plattner JJ. Renin inhibitors. Dipeptide analogues of angiotensinogen utilizing a dihydroxyethylene transition-state mimic at the scissile bond to impart greater inhibitory potency. *Journal of Medicinal Chemistry* 1988;**31**:2264–76.

27. Szelke M, Leckie B, Hallett A, Jones DM, Sueiras J, Atrash B, Lever AF. Potent new inhibitors of human renin. *Nature* 1982;**299**:555–7.

28. Johnson RL. Inhibition of renin by substrate analogue inhibitors containing the olefinic amino acid 5(S)-amino-7-methyl-3(E)-octenoic acid. *Journal of Medicinal Chemistry* 1984;**27**:1351–4.

29. Dann JG, Stammers DK, Harris, CJ, Arrowsmith RJ, Davies DE, Hardy GW, Morton JA. Human renin: A new class of inhibitors. *Biochemical and Biophysical Research Communications* 1986;**134**:71–7.

30. TenBrink RE, Pals DT, Harris DW, Johnson GA. Renin inhibitors containing ψ[CH₂O] pseudopeptide inserts. *Journal of Medicinal Chemistry* 1988;**31**:671–7.

31. Smith CW, Saneii HH, Sawyer TK, Pals DT, Scahill TA, Kamdar BV, Lawson JA. Synthesis and renin inhibitory acitivity of angiotensinogen analogues having dehydrostatine, Leuψ[CH₂S]Val, or Leuψ[CH₂SO]Val at the P₁–P₁ cleavage site. *Journal of Medicinal Chemistry* 1988;**31**:1377–82.

32. Rosenberg SH, Plattner JJ, Woods KW, Stein HH, Marcotte PA, Cohen J, Perun TJ. Novel renin inhibitors containing analogues of statine retro-inverted at the C-termini: Specificity at the P₂ histidine site. *Journal of Medicinal Chemistry* 1987;**30**:1224–8.

33. Luly JR, Plattner JJ, Stein H, Yi N, Soderquist J, Marcotte PA, Kleinert HD, Perun TJ. Modified peptides which display potent and specific inhibition of human renin. *Biochemical and Biophysical Research Communications* 1987;**143**: 44–51.

34. Dellaria JF Jr, Maki RG, Stein HH, Cohen J, Whittern D, Marsh K, Hoffman DJ, Plattner JJ, Perun TJ. New inhibitors of renin that contain novel phosphostatine Leu–Val replacements. *Journal of Medicinal Chemistry* 1990;**33**:534–42.

35. Allen MC, Fuhrer W, Tuck B, Wade R, Wood JM. Renin inhibitors. Synthesis of transition-state analogue inhibitors containing phosphorus acid derivatives at the scissile bond. *Journal of Medicinal Chemistry* 1989;**32**:1652–61.

36. Johnson RL. Renin inhibitors. Substitution of the leucyl residues of Leu–Leu–Val–Phe–OCH₃ with 3-amino-2-hydroxy-5-methylhexanoic acid. *Journal of Medicinal Chemistry* 1982;**25**:605–10.

37. Iizuka K, Kamijo T, Kubota T, Akahane K, Umeyama H, Kiso Y. New human renin inhibitors containing an unnatural amino acid norstatine. *Journal of Medicinal Chemistry* 1988;**31**:701–4.

38. Kokubu T, Hiwada K, Murakami E, Imamura Y, Matsueda R, Yabe Y, Koike H, Iijima Y. Highly potent and specific inhibitors of human renin. *Hypertension* 1985;**7** (suppl I):I-8–11.

39. Fehrentz JA, Heitz A, Castro B, Cazaubon C, Nisato D. Aldehydic peptides inhibiting renin. *FEBS Letters* 1984;**167**:273–6.

40. Kokubu T, Hiwada K, Nagae A, Murakami E, Morisawa Y, Yabe Y, Koike H, Iijima Y. Statine-containing dipeptide and tripeptide inhibitors of human renin. *Hypertension* 1986;**8** (suppl II):II-1–5.

41. Hanson GJ, Baran JS, Lindberg T, Walsh GM, Papaioannou SE, Babler M, Bittner SE, Yang P–C, Dal Corobbo M. Dipeptide glycols: A new class of renin inhibitors. *Biochemical and Biophysical Research Communications* 1985;**132**:155–61.

42. Nisato D, Lacour C, Roccon A, Gayraud R, Cazaubon C, Carlet C, Plouzané C, Richaud J–P, Tonnerre B, Gagnol J–P, Wagnon J. Discovery and pharmacological characterization of highly potent, picomolar-range, renin inhibitors. *Journal of Hypertension* 1987;**5** (suppl 5):S23–5.

43. Bock MG, DiPardo RM, Evans BE, Freidinger RM, Whitter WL, Payne LS, Boger J, Ulm EH, Blaine EW, Veber DF. Renin inhibitors. Synthesis and biological activity of statine- and ACHPA-containing peptides having polar end groups. In: Deber CM, Hruby VJ, Kopple KD, eds. *Peptides: Structure and function. Proceedings of the Ninth American Peptide Symposium.* Rockford, Illinois: Pierce Chemical, 1985:751–4.

44. Bock MG, DiPardo RM, Evans BE, Rittle KE, Boger J, Poe M, La Mont BI, Lynch RJ, Ulm EH, Vlasuk GP, Greenlee WJ, Veber DF. Renin inhibitors. Statine-containing tetrapeptides with varied hydrophobic carboxy termini. *Journal of Medicinal Chemistry* 1987;**30**:1853–7.

45. Papaioannou S, Hansen D Jr, Babler M, Yang P–C, Bittner S, Miller A, Clare M. New class of inhibitors specific for human renin. *Clinical and Experimental Hypertension — Theory and Practice* 1985;**A7**:1243–57.

46. Natarajan S, Free CA, Sabo EF, Lin J, Spitzmiller ER, Samaniego SG, Smith S, Zanoni LM. Tripeptide aminoalcohols: A new class of human renin inhibitors. In: Marshall GR, ed. *Peptides: Chemistry and biology. Proceedings of the Tenth American Peptide Symposium.* Leiden: ESCOM, 1988:131–3.

47. Luly JR, Yi N, Soderquist J, Stein H, Cohen J, Perun TJ, Plattner JJ. New inhibitors of human renin that contain novel Leu–Val replacements. *Journal of Medicinal Chemistry* 1987;30:1609–16.

48. Bolis G, Fung AKL, Greer J, Kleinert HD, Marcotte PA, Perun TJ, Plattner JJ, Stein HH. Renin inhibitors. Dipeptide analogues of angiotensinogen incorporating transition-state, nonpeptidic replacements at the scissile bond. *Journal of Medicinal Chemistry* 1987;30:1729–37.

49. Luly JR, Bolis G, BaMaung N, Soderquist J, Dellaria JF, Stein H, Cohen J, Perun TJ, Greer J, Plattner JJ. New inhibitors of human renin that contain novel Leu–Val replacements. Examination of the P$_1$ site. *Journal of Medicinal Chemistry* 1988;31:532–9.

50. Rosenberg SH, Woods KW, Plattner JJ, Stein HH, Kleinert HD, Cohen J. Novel, subnanomolar renin inhibitors containing a postscissile site azide residue. In: Marshall GR, ed. *Peptides: Chemistry and biology. Proceedings of the Tenth American Peptide Symposium.* Leiden: ESCOM, 1988:500–2.

51. Luly JR, Fung AKL, Plattner JJ, Marcotte PA, BaMaung N, Soderquist JL, Stein HH. Transition-state analog inhibitors of human renin. In: Marshal GR, ed. *Peptides: Chemistry and biology. Proceedings of the Tenth American Peptide Symposium.* Leiden: ESCOM, 1988;487–9.

52. Rosenberg SH, Woods KW, Kleinert HD, Stein H, Nellans HN, Hoffman DJ, Spanton SG, Pyter RA, Cohen J, Egan DA, Plattner JJ, Perun TJ. Azido glycols: Potent, low molecular weight renin inhibitors containing an unusual post scissile site residue. *Journal of Medicinal Chemistry* 1989;32:1371–8.

53. Hui KY, Carlson WD, Bernatowicz MS, Haber E. Analysis of structure–activity relationships in renin substrate analogue inhibitory peptides. *Journal of Medicinal Chemistry* 1987;30:1287–95.

54. Bundy GL, Pals DT, Lawson JA, Couch SJ, Lipton MF, Mauragis MA. Potent renin inhibitory peptides containing hydrophilic end groups. *Journal of Medicinal Chemistry* 1990;33:2276–83.

55. Thaisrivongs S, Pals DT, Harris DW, Kati WM, Turner SR. Design and synthesis of a potent and specific renin inhibitor with a prolonged duration of action *in vivo. Journal of Medicinal Chemistry* 1986;29:2088–93.

56. Thaisrivongs S, Pals DT, Lawson JA, Turner SR, Harris DW. α-Methylproline-containing renin inhibitory peptides: *In vivo* evaluation in an anesthetized, ganglion-blocked, hog renin infused rat model. *Journal of Medicinal Chemistry* 1987;30:536–41.

57. Kempf DJ, de Lara E, Stein HH, Cohen J, Egan DA, Plattner JJ. Renin inhibitors based on dipeptide analogues. Incorporation of the hydroxyethylene isostere at the P$_2$/P$_3$ sites. *Journal of Medicinal Chemistry* 1990;33:371–4.

58. Kaltenbronn JS, Hudspeth JP, Junney EA, Michniewicz BM, Nicolaides ED, Repine JT, Roark WH, Stier MA, Tinney FJ, Woo PKW, Essenburg AD. Renin inhibitors containing isosteric replacements of the amide bond connecting the P$_3$ and P$_2$ sites. *Journal of Medicinal Chemistry* 1990;33:838–45.

59. Boger J. Renin inhibitors. Design of angiotensinogen transition-state analogs containing statine. In: Hruby VJ, Rich DH, eds. *Peptides: Structure and function. Proceedings of the Eighth American Peptide Symposium.* Rockford, Illinois: Pierce Chemical 1983:569–78.

60. Sham HL, Bolis G, Stein HH, Fesik SW, Marcotte PA, Plattner JJ, Rempel CA, Greer J. Renin inhibitors. Design and synthesis of a new class of conformationally restricted analogues of angiotensinogen. *Journal of Medicinal Chemistry* 1988;31:284–95.

61. Nakaie CR, Pesquero JL, Oliveira MCF, Juliano L, Pavia ACM. Renin inhibition by linear and conformationally restricted analogs of renin substrate. In: Deber CM, Hruby VJ, Kopple KD, eds. *Peptides: Structure and function. Proceedings of the Ninth American Peptide Symposium.* Rockford, Illinois: Pierce Chemical, 1985:755–8.

62. Thaisrivongs S, Pals DT, Turner SR, Kroll LT. Conformationally constrained renin inhibitory peptides: γ-lactam-bridged dipeptide isostere as conformational restriction. *Journal of Medicinal Chemistry* 1988;31:1369–76.

63. Sawyer TK, Pals DT, Smith CW, Saneii HH, Epps DE, Duchamp DJ, Hester JB, TenBrink RE, Staples DJ, DeVaux AE, Affholter JA, Skala GF, Kati WM, Lawson JA, Schuette MR, Kamdar BV, Emmert DE. 'Transition state' substituted renin inhibitory peptides: Structure–conformation–activity studies on N^{im}-formyl-Trp and Trp modified congeners. In: Deber CM, Hruby VJ, Kopple KD, eds. *Peptides: Structure and function. Proceedings of the Ninth American Peptide Symposium.* Rockford, Illinois: Pierce Chemical, 1985:729–38.

64. Dutta AS, Gormley JJ, McLachlan PF, Major JS. Novel inhibitors of human renin. Cyclic peptides based on the tetrapeptide sequence Glu-D–Phe–Lys-D–Trp. *Journal of Medicinal Chemistry* 1990;33:2552–60.

65. Dutta AS, Gormley JJ, McLachlan PF, Major JS. Inhibitors of human renin. Cyclic peptide analogues containing a D-Phe–Lys-D–Trp sequence. *Journal of Medicinal Chemistry* 1990;33:2560–8.

66. Johnson RL. Synthesis of epoxypolypeptides as inhibitors of renin. In: Hruby VJ, Rich DH, eds. *Peptides: Structure and function. Proceedings of the Eigth American Peptide Symposium.* Rockford, Illinois: Pierce Chemical, 1983:587–90.

67. Boger RS, Glassman HN, Cavanaugh JH, Schmitz PJ, Lamm J, Moyse D, Cohen A, Kleinert HD, Luther RR. Prolonged duration of blood pressure response to enalkiren, the novel dipeptide renin inhibitor, in essential hypertension. *Hypertension* 1990;15:835–40.

68. Iizuka K, Kamijo T, Harada H, Akahane K, Kubota T, Umeyama H, Ishida T, Kiso Y. Orally potent human renin inhibitors derived from angiotensinogen transition state: Design, synthesis, and mode of interaction. *Journal of Medicinal Chemistry* 1990;33:2707–14.

69. Kokubu T, Hiwada K, Murakami E, Muneta S, Kitami Y, Salmon PF. ES-8891, an orally active inhibitor of human renin. *Hypertension* 1990;15:909–13.

70. Wood JM, Criscione L, de Gasparo M, Bühlmayer P, Rüeger H, Stanton JL, Jupp RA, Kay J. CGP 38 560: Orally active, low-molecular-weight renin inhibitor with high potency and specificity. *Journal of Cardiovascular Pharmacology* 1989;14:221–6.

71. Bradbury RH, Major JS, Oldham AA, Rivett JE, Roberts DA, Slater AM, Timms D, Waterson D. 1,2,4-triazolo[4,3-a]pyrazine derivatives with human renin inhibitory activity. 2. Synthesis, biological properties and molecular modeling of hydroxyethylene isostere derivatives. *Journal of Medicinal Chemistry* 1990;33:2335–42.

72. Evin G, Devin J, Ménard J, Corvol P, Castro B. Synthesis of peptides related to the prosegment of renin precursor: A new way in the search for renin inhibitors. In: Hruby VJ, Rich, DH, eds. *Peptides: Structure and function. Proceedings of the Eighth American Peptide Symposium.* Rockford, Illinois: Pierce Chemical, 1983: 591–4.

73. Evin G, Devin J, Castro B, Ménard J, Corvol P. Synthesis of peptides related to the prosegment of mouse submaxillary gland renin precursor: An approach to renin inhibitors. *Proceedings of the National Academy of Sciences of the USA* 1984;81: 48–52.

74. Cumin F, Evin G, Fehrentz J–A, Seyer R, Castro B, Ménard J, Corvol P. Inhibition of human renin by synthetic peptides derived from its prosegment. *Journal of Biological Chemistry* 1985;260:9154–7.

75. Hui KY, Holtzman EJ, Quinones MA, Hollenberg NK, Haber E. Design of rat renin inhibitory peptides. *Journal of Medicinal Chemistry* 1988;31:1679–86.

76. Sueiras–Diaz J, Jones DM, Evans DM, Szelke M, Leckie BJ, Beattie SR, Wallace ECH, Morton JJ. Potent *in vivo* inhibitors of rat renin. In: Marshall GR, ed. *Peptides: Chemistry and biology. Proceedings of the Tenth American Peptide Symposium.* Leiden: ESCOM, 1988:510–1.

77. Hui KY, Siragy HM. Dog renin inhibitors: Structure–activity and *in vivo* studies. In: Rivier JE, Marshall GR, eds. *Peptides: Chemistry, structure and biology. Proceedings of the Ninth American Peptide Symposium.* Leiden: ESCOM, 1990: 399–401.

78. Wood JM, Gulati N, Forgiarini P, Fuhrer W, Hofbauer KG. Effects of a specific and long-acting renin inhibitor in the marmoset. *Hypertension* 1985;7:797–803.

79. Pals DT, Thaisrivongs S, Lawson JA, Kati WM, Turner SR, DeGraaf GL, Harris DW, Johnson GA. An orally active inhibitor of renin. *Hypertension* 1986;8: 1105–12.

80. Hanson GJ, Baran JS, Lowrie HS, Russell MA, Sarussi SJ, Williams K, Babler M, Bittner SE, Papaioannou SE, Yang P–C, Walsh GM. A new class of orally active glycol renin inhibitors containing phenyllactic acid at P₃. *Biochemical and Biophysical Research Communications* 1989;160:1–5.

81. Ondetti MA, Rubin B, Cushman DW. Design of specific inhibitors of angiotensin-converting enzyme: New class of orally active antihypertensive agents. *Science* 1977;196:441–4.

82. Carlson W, Karplus M, Haber E. Construction of a model for the three-dimensional structure of human renal renin. *Hypertension* 1985;7:13–26.

83. Hemmings AM, Foundling SI, Sibanda BL, Wood SP, Pearl LH, Blundell T. Energy calculations on aspartic proteinases: Human renin, endothiapepsin and its complex with an angiotensinogen fragment analogue, H-142. *Biochemical Society Transactions* 1985;13:1036–41.

84. Blundell TL, Cooper J, Foundling SI, Jones DM, Atrash B, Szelke M. On the rational design of renin inhibitors: X-ray studies of aspartic proteinases complexed with transition-state analogues. *Biochemistry* 1987;26:5585–90.

85. Hardman JA, Hort YJ, Catanzaro DF, Tellam JT, Baxter JD, Morris BJ, Shine J. Primary structure of the human renin gene. *DNA* 1984;3:457–68.

86. Fritz LC, Arfsten AE, Dzau VJ, Atlas SA, Baxter JD, Fiddes JC, Shine J, Cofer CL, Kushner P, Ponte PA. Characterization of human prorenin expressed in mammalian cells from cloned cDNA. *Proceedings of the National Academy of Sciences of the USA* 1986;83:4114–8.

87. Sielecki AR, Hayakawa K, Fujinaga M, Murphy MEP, Fraser M, Muir AK, Carilli CT, Lewicki JA, Baxter JD, James MNG. Structure of recombinant human renin, a target for cardiovascular-active drugs, at 2.5 Å resolution. *Science* 1989;243:1346–51.

88. Dzau VJ, Devine D, Mudgett–Hunter M, Kopelman RI, Barger AC, Haber E. Antibodies as specific renin inhibitors: Studies with polyclonal and monoclonal antibodies and Fab fragments. *Clinical and Experimental Hypertension. Part A, Theory and Practice* 1983;A5:1207–20.

89. Michel J–B, Wood J, Hofbauer K, Corvol P, Ménard J. Blood pressure effects of renin inhibition by human renin antiserum in normotensive marmosets. *American Journal of Physiology* 1984;246:F309–16.

90. Wood JM, Heusser C, Gulati N, Forgiarini P, Hofbauer KG. Monoclonal antibodies against human renin. Blood pressure effects in the marmoset. *Hypertension* 1986;8:600–5.

91. Hui KY, Knight DR, Nussberger J, Hartley LH, Vatner SF, Haber E. Effects of renin inhibition in the conscious primate *Macaca fascicularis*. *Hypertension* 1989;14:480–7.

92. Blair–West JR, Coghlan JP, Denton DA, Funder JW, Scoggins BA, Wright RD. Inhibition of renin secretion by systemic and intrarenal angiotensin infusion. *American Journal of Physiology* 1971;220:1309–15.

93. Miyazaki M, Etoh Y, Toda N, Kubota T, Iizuka K. Hypotension caused by inhibitors of renin and converting-enzyme in monkeys {Abstract}. *Japanese Journal of Pharmacology* 1987;43 (suppl):146P.

94. Neisius D, Wood JM, Antihypertensive effect of a renin inhibitor in marmosets with a segmental renal infarction. *Journal of Hypertension* 1987;5:721–5.

95. Smith SG III, Seymour AA, Mazack EK, Boger J, Blaine EH. Comparison of a new renin inhibitor and enalaprilat in renal hypertensive dogs. *Hypertension* 1987;9:150–6.

96. Hofbauer KG, Ménard J, Michel JB, Wood JM. Inhibition of renin in the primate *Callithrix jacchus* (common marmoset). *Clinical and Experimental Hypertension. Part A, Theory and Practice* 1983;A5:1237–47.

97. Takaori K, Hartley LH, Burton J. Hypotensive effects of the renin inhibitor (RI-78) and the converting enzyme inhibitor (teprotide) in conscious monkeys. *Clinical and Experimental Hypertension, Part A, Theory and Practice* 1987;A9:387–90.

98. Wood JM, Jobber RA, Baum H–P, Hofbauer KG. Comparison of chronic inhibition of renin and converting enzyme in the marmoset. *Clinical and Experimental Hypertension. Part A, Theory and Practice* 1987;A9:337–43.

99. Siragy HM, Howel NL, Peach MJ, Carey RM. Combined intrarenal blockade of the renin–angiotensin system in the conscious dog. *American Journal of Physiology* 1990;258:F522–9.

100. Hall JE, Mizelle HL. Control of arterial pressure and renal function during chronic renin inhibition. *Journal of Hypertension* 1990;8:351–9.

101. Pals DT, Ludens JH, DeGraaf GL. Systemic and renal haemodynamic effects of renin or angiotensin converting enzyme inhibition in non-human primates. *Journal of Hypertension* 1989;7 (suppl 2):S43–6.

102. Neisius D, Wood JM, Hofbauer KG. Renal vasodilation after inhibition of renin or converting enzyme in marmoset. *American Journal of Physiology* 1986;251:H897–902.

103. Kleinert HD, Martin D, Chekal MA, Kadam J, Luly JR, Plattner JJ, Perun TJ, Luther RR. Effects of the renin inhibitor A-64662 in monkeys and rats with varying baseline plasma renin activity. *Hypertension* 1988;11:613–9.

104. Schaffer LW, Schorn TW, Winquist RJ, Strouse JF, Payne L, Chakravarty PK, de Laszlo SE, tenBroeke J, Veber DF, Greenlee WJ, Siegl PKS. Acute hypotensive responses to peptide inhibitors of renin in conscious monkeys: An effect on blood pressure independent of plasma renin inhibition. *Journal of Hypertension* 1990;8:251–9.

105. Verburg KM, Kleinert HD, Kadam JR, Chekal MA, Mento PF, Wilkes BM. Effects of chronic infusion of renin inhibitor A-64662 in sodium-depleted monkeys. *Hypertension* 1989;13:262–72.

106. Wood JM, Jobber RA, Baum HP, de Gasparo M, Nussberger J. Biochemical effects of prolonged renin inhibition in marmosets. *Journal of Hypertension* 1989;7:615–8.

107. Nussberger J, Delabays A, De gasparo M, Cumin F, Waeber B, Brunner HR, Ménard J. Hemodynamic and biochemical consequences of renin inhibition by infusion of CGP 38560A in normal volunteers. *Hypertension* 1989;13:948–53.

108. Delabays A, Nussberger J, Porchet M, Waeber B, Hoyos P, Boger R, Glassman H, Kleinert HD, Luther R, Brunner HR. Hemodynamic and humoral effects of the new renin inhibitor enalkiren in normal humans. *Hypertension* 1989; 13:941–7.

109. Jeunemaître X, Ménard J, Nussberger J, Guyene TT, Brunner HR, Corvol P. Plasma angiotensins, renin, and blood pressure during acute renin inhibition by CGP 38 560A in hypertensive patients. *American Journal of Hypertension* 1989;2:819–27.

110. Bursztyn M, Gavras I, Tifft CP, Luther R, Boger R, Gavras H. Effects of a novel renin inhibitor in patients with essential hypertension. *Journal of Cardiovascular Pharmacology* 1990;15:493–500.

111. Fearon K, Spaltenstein A, Hopkins PB, Gelb MH. Fluoro ketone containing peptides as inhibitors of human renin. *Journal of Medicinal Chemistry* 1987;30:1617–22.

112. Kempf DJ, de Lara E, Stein HH, Cohen J, Plattner JJ. Renin inhibitors based on novel dipeptide analogues. Incorporation of the dehydrohydroxyethylene isostere at the scissile bond. *Journal of Medicinal Chemistry* 1987;30:1978–83.

113. Thaisrivongs S, Pals DT, Kroll LT, Turner SR, Han FS. Renin inhibitors. Design of angiotensinogen transition-state analogues containing novel (2R,3R,4R,5S)-5-amino-3,4-dihydroxy-2-isopropyl-7-methyloctanoic acid. *Journal of Medicinal Chemistry* 1987;30:976–82.

114. Evans BE, Rittle KE, Ulm UH, Veber DF. A stereocontrolled synthesis of hydroxyethylene dipeptide isosteres using novel, chiral aminoalkyl epoxides: New renin inhibitor analogs. In: Deber CM, Hruby VJ, Kopple KD, eds. *Peptides: Structure and function. Proceedings of the Ninth American Peptide Symposium.* Rockford, Illinois: Pierce Chemical 1985;743–6.

115. Toda N, Miyazaki M, Etoh Y, Kubota T, Iizuka K. Human renin inhibiting dipeptide. *European Journal of Pharmacology* 1986;129:393–6.

116. Johnson RL, Verschoor K. Inhibition of renin by angiotensinogen peptide fragments containing the hydroxy amino acid residue 5-amino-3-hydroxy-7-methyloctanoic acid. *Journal of Medicinal Chemistry* 1983;26:1457–62.

117. Evans BE, Rittle KE, Bock MG, Bennett CD, DiPardo RM, Boger J, Poe M, Ulm EH, LaMont BI, Blaine EH, Fanelli GM, Stabilito II, Veber DF. A uniquely potent renin inhibitor and its unanticipated plasma binding component. *Journal of Medicinal Chemistry* 1985;28:1755–6.

118. Thaisrivongs S, Mao B, Pals DT, Turner SR, Kroll LT. Renin inhibitor peptides. A beta-aspartyl residue as a replacement for the histidyl residue at the P$_2$ site. *Journal of Medicinal Chemistry* 1990;33:1337–43.

119. Bock MG, DiPardo RM, Evans BE, Freidinger RM, Rittle KE, Payne LS, Boger J, Whitter WL, LaMont BI, Ulm EH, Blaine EH, Schorn TW, Veber DF. Renin inhibitors containing hydrophilic groups. Tetrapeptides with enhanced aqueous solubility and nanomolar potency. *Journal of Medicinal Chemistry* 1988;31:1918–23.

120. Rosenberg SH, Woods KW, Sham HL, Kleinert HD, Martin DL, Stein H, Cohen J, Egan DA, Bopp B, Merits I, Garren KW, Hoffman DJ, Plattner JJ. Water-soluble renin inhibitors: Design of a subnanomolar inhibitor with a prolonged duration of action. *Journal of Medicinal Chemistry* 1990;33:1962–9.

121. Webb DJ, Manhem PJO, Ball SG, Inglis G, Leckie BJ, Lever A, Morton JJ, Robertson JIS, Murray GD, Ménard J, Hallett A, Jones DM, Szelke M. A study of the renin inhibitor H142 in man. *Journal of Hypertension* 1985;3:653–8.

122. Van den Meiracker AH, Admiraal PJJ, Man in't Veld AJ, Derkx FHM, Ritsema van Eck HJ, Mulder P, Van Brummelen P, Schalekamp MA. Prolonged blood pressure reduction by orally active renin inhibitor Ro 42-5892 in essential hypertension. *British Medical Journal* 1990;301:205–10.

86 ANGIOTENSIN ANTAGONISTS

HANS R BRUNNER, JÜRG NUSSBERGER,
AND BERNARD WAEBER

INTRODUCTION

Renin was discovered in 1898 by Tigerstedt and Bergman [1] (see *Chapter 1*). Little progress was, however, made in the next 30 years, until the classic experiments of Goldblatt *et al* [2] showed that hypertension could be caused by constricting one or both renal arteries (see *Chapter 55*). This led to reawakening of interest in the RAS [3], which was identified by a number of workers as a possible candidate as the mediator of renovascular hypertension. Surprisingly, Goldblatt himself appears to have realized the possible importance of the RAS rather late [4], his first publication referring to renin in this context appearing only in 1938 [5]. Once interest in the RAS had been revived, most attention focused on its possible involvement in renovascular hypertension, an aspect that was to prove remarkably intractable of elucidation, as is described in detail in *Chapter 55*. This early preoccupation with renovascular hypertension is indicated in the titles of books of this period which were devoted to the RAS [6,7]. Of most immediate relevance to this chapter was that, well into the 1950s and 1960s, few investigators considered that the RAS was involved either in normal cardiovascular regulation or in hypertension of etiology other than renovascular. Consequently, nearly all early attempts to develop Ang II antagonists were concerned with the investigation and/or treatment of renovascular hypertension.

IMMUNIZATION AGAINST ANGIOTENSIN II

First attempts to investigate the role of the RAS in experimental hypertension by specific blockade of Ang II were made using immunization against Ang II. In the beginning, these studies provided controversial results. Indeed, animals actively immunized against Ang II developed renovascular hypertension just the same as their nonimmunized counterparts [8–10]. In contrast, rats with 1-clip, 2-kidney renal hypertension treated with a specific Ang II antiserum obtained from immunized rabbits responded with a marked, though only transient, decrease in blood pressure [11–13]. Similarly prepared hypertensive animals treated with rabbit serum containing no Ang II antibodies exhibited no blood-pressure decrease. The explanation of this apparent contradiction came when other investigators demonstrated that following active immunization, circulating antibodies were saturated with huge amounts of Ang II, while a tiny fraction, though a considerable absolute amount, of Ang II remained unbound [14].

PEPTIDE ANALOG ANTAGONISTS OF ANGIOTENSIN II

A major advance occurred with the synthesis of Ang II analogs which exhibited clear antagonistic effects at the receptor level [15,16]. This provided the possibility to block specifically, the action of Ang II at its receptor and thus to explore in detail, the role of Ang II in the pathogenesis not only of experimental, but also of clinical, hypertension, and indeed of many other physiological and pathological conditions.

In a major review in 1974, Khosla *et al* [17] examined the structure–activity relationships of no fewer than 229 peptide analogs of Ang II. They evaluated specifically and in painstaking detail, synthetic analogs of the parent hormone Ang II and their value as its antagonists. The most widely used, but by no means the only one, of these analog antagonists was saralasin, so named because sarcosine was substituted in position 1, and alanine in position 8, of the naturally occurring bovine valine[5] Ang II [18].

The introduction of peptide analog antagonists of Ang II, following on the development of the first reliable assays for plasma renin (see *Chapter 13*) and Ang II (see *Chapter 15*), led to an explosion of knowledge and understanding of the physiological and pathophysiological role of the RAS in man and in a wide range of laboratory animals. Many of these crucial studies are quoted in the relevant chapters of this book. Two of many comprehensive surveys of the use of analog antagonists are the 1974

Volhard lecture by Davis [19], which is concerned principally with physiological issues, and the book edited by Stokes and Edwards [20], which reports on many pertinent physiological and clinical studies.

Some selected aspects of this wealth of knowledge derived from the use of analog antagonists of Ang II are illustrated by brief description of certain studies.

With this new approach, it was found that the blood pressure of rats with 1-clip, 2-kidney renal hypertension (see *Chapter 55*) could be normalized by infusing the Ang II antagonist saralasin, while this had no effect on the blood pressure of animals with one renal artery clipped and the contralateral intact kidney removed [13]. Subsequently, it could be demonstrated that these latter 1-clip, 1-kidney hypertensive animals could also be made Ang II dependent by sodium depletion [21]. Conversely, rats rendered hypertensive by the administration of desoxycorticosterone acetate (DOCA) and saline as drinking fluid ('DOCA-salt hypertension'), characterized by a very low plasma renin activity (PRA), exhibited a slight increase in blood pressure during administration of saralasin [22]. This latter phenomenon was a clear reflection of the inherent partial agonistic properties of this Ang II analog.

Later studies [23] in 1-clip, 2-kidney hypertensive rats also showed that in animals without elevated plasma renin, more prolonged infusion of saralasin, for 11 hours, could return blood pressure to normal, even though the initial blood-pressure fall was negligible. These observations were taken by Riegger *et al* [23] to indicate a saralasin-responsive slow pressor action of Ang II (see *Chapter 28*). Other workers [24], however, were unable to confirm the studies of Riegger *et al*. This difficult issue of the role of the RAS in renovascular hypertension is dealt with in detail in *Chapter 55*.

The partial agonist action of saralasin requires emphasis. As will be shown, it can cloud interpretation of experimental results. The partial agonist effect is especially relevant to the slow pressor action of Ang II. With saralasin, as also with the parent compound Ang II itself [25], prolonged administration (over several days) at doses that are not initally pressor, can eventually cause marked hypertension [26].

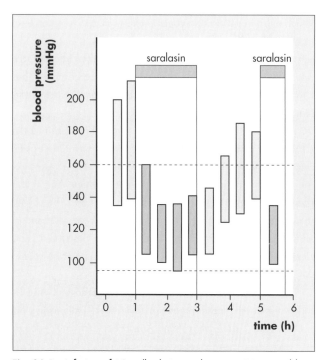

Fig. 86.1 Infusion of 10μg/kg/min saralasin in a 21-year-old patient with severe hypertension and high plasma renin activity. A marked and reproducible fall in blood pressure has been induced. Modified from Brunner HR *et al* [28].

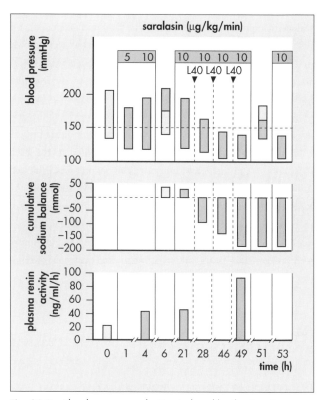

Fig. 86.2 Blood-pressure reduction induced by the Ang II inhibitor saralasin alone and after furosemide-induced sodium depletion, in a patient with hypertension due to bilateral renal artery stenosis. L40 indicates the intravenous administration of furosemide, 40mg. Modified from Brunner HR *et al* [28].

In clinical studies, infusion of the Ang II antagonist saralasin demonstratated for the first time, in a patient with severe hypertension and high PRA, that elevated blood pressure was indeed related to activation of the RAS, since it was completely normalized during the infusion (Fig. 86.1) [27,28], It rapidly became evident that in patients with a rather high PRA, blood pressure could be normalized or markedly reduced by specific blockade of the Ang II receptors [27–29], Furthermore, mimicking the previous animal experiments, it could also be shown that the efficacy of Ang II blockade was markedly enhanced by concomitant, diuretic-induced salt depletion of the hypertensive patients (Fig. 86.2) [28]. Thus, the whole concept of treating hypertension with blockade of the RAS alone or in combination with simultaneous sodium depletion, which has since become the basis for the widespread use of ACE inhibitors (*Chapters 87* and *91*), was already established using the first Ang II antagonist.

The Ang II analogs acting as receptor antagonists were also administered to explore the role of the RAS in normal blood-pressure homeostasis. It was demonstrated that normotensive volunteers became hypotensive during the infusion of the antagonist only if they were considerably salt depleted and assumed an upright posture [30]. It was further shown that the administration of the Ang II antagonist reduced aldosterone secretion, though depending on the circumstances again, an agonistic effect could prevail [31]. The same authors also pointed out the

important role of Ang II in regulating tone within the renal vascular system [32].

Last but not least, using saralasin in patients with congestive heart failure, it was demonstrated that blockade of the RAS could considerably improve pump function (Fig. 86.3) [33,34]. With the availability of converting-enzyme inhibitors, this concept was rapidly developed to become a treatment of choice for patients with congestive heart failure (see *Chapter 93*).

All early Ang II antagonists, including the most commonly used saralasin, had two main shortcomings: first, they were all analogs of Ang II and thus peptides that had to be administered parenterally; this of course excluded a priori them becoming useful therapeutic agents for chronic treatment. Second, as already mentioned, they exhibited more or less pronounced partial agonistic effects in addition to their antagonistic properties. Depending on the circumstances of administration, these agonistic effects could even become predominant [26]. Consequently, as a rule, the effects observed with these compounds probably tended to underestimate the actual extent of contribution of the RAS to the pathogenesis of the various diseases under study, being virtually confined to eliminating the acute effects of Ang II.

The fact that circulating Ang II had, for example, an immediate direct effect on both arterial pressure and plasma aldosterone, and that these effects were antagonized acutely and in proportion to the prevailing plasma Ang II concentration, by

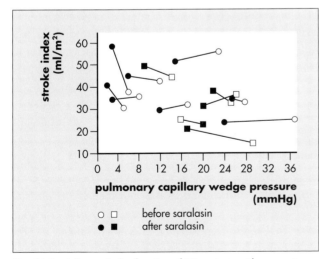

Fig. 86.3 Left ventricular function of 13 patients with congestive heart failure who underwent a saralasin infusion. All but one patient, with increased arterial pressure, experienced some degree of improvement in left ventricular function. Modified from Turini GA *et al* [33].

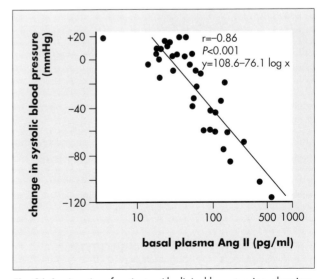

Fig. 86.4 A series of patients with clinical hypertension, showing change in systolic arterial pressure on saralasin administration in relation to the basal (presaralasin) plasma Ang II level. Modified from Brown JJ *et al* [35].

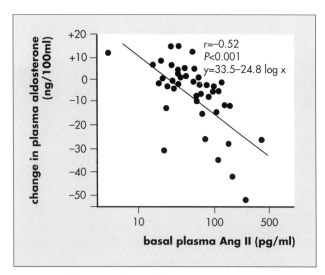

Fig. 86.5 Change in plasma aldosterone concentration on saralasin infusion in relation to the basal (presaralasin) plasma Ang II level, in a series of patients (as shown in *Fig. 86.4*) with clinical hypertension. Modified from Brown JJ *et al* [35].

infusing saralasin, is shown in Figs. 86.4 and 86.5 [35]. The longer-term effects of blockade of the RAS can, however, be very different. This was soon confirmed by the use of converting-enzyme inhibitors, which could of course be given long term, and which in general were markedly more effective than the early Ang II antagonists [36]. However, this greater efficacy of ACE inhibitors is even today still attributed by some to their possession of certain actions additional to blockade of the RAS (see *Chapter 87*).

If the Ang II antagonists were abandoned clinically in the late 1970s, it is not because the concept of specific Ang II blockade at its receptor proved to be ineffective, but rather because an orally active converting-enzyme inhibitor, captopril, became available for general clinical use. The therapeutic concept to block Ang II at its receptor was sound, but there existed at that time no orally active antagonist. The situation changed again in the late 1980s, when a new structural class of Ang II antagonists, which are active when taken orally, was developed. These newer Ang II antagonists merit detailed exposition.

DEVELOPMENT OF A NONPEPTIDE ANGIOTENSIN II-RECEPTOR ANTAGONIST

The basis for the development of nonpeptide Ang II-receptor antagonists was laid down in 1982 when Furukawa and his co-workers in Osaka obtained patents for hypotensive imidazole

derivatives with Ang II antagonistic properties [37,38]. This lead was taken up by a group of investigators led by Timmermans. These latter scientists first were able to confirm the Ang II antagonistic effect of the compounds described by the Japanese researchers [39,40] and then embarked on a program of optimizing the properties of such imidazole derivatives [41]. This led to the synthesis of losartan (DuP 753) (Fig. 86.6) which was further developed for the use in clinical pharmacology. Losartan is characterized by an IC_{50} of 1.9×10^{-8} mol/l (inhibition of Ang II binding to isolated rat adrenal cortical microsomes), by a pA_2 of 8.48 (antagonism of Ang II-induced constriction of rabbit isolated aorta) (Fig. 86.7) [42], and by antihypertensive potency in renal hypertensive rats with an ED_{30} of 0.78mg/kg. This represents an increase in receptor affinity of 2–3 orders of magnitude compared with the compounds initially described by Furukawa *et al* [37,38].

PHARMACOLOGY OF LOSARTAN

The interaction of losartan with Ang II receptors from several organ systems was evaluated *in vitro*. Losartan inhibited the specific binding of radiolabeled Ang II to receptors of rat adrenal cortical microsomes with an IC_{50} of approximately 1.9×10^{-8} mol/l [42]. This was quite close to the IC_{50} of 1×10^{-9} mol/l found for saralasin in the same preparation. Similarly, with receptors prepared from rat aortic smooth-muscle cells, the IC_{50} of losartan was again very similar to that observed with saralasin [43]. In contrast, specific Ang II binding in rat adrenal medulla and brain membranes was much more sensitive to saralasin than to losartan. This observation has led to the characterization of two different types of Ang II receptors, as will be discussed later in this chapter (for terminology see *Appendix II*). Biochemical aspects of Ang II receptors are described in detail in *Chapter 12*.

Functional antagonism of Ang II actions could be demonstrated for instance in cultured smooth-muscle cells. In these preparations, Ang II-stimulated calcium efflux could be blocked similarly by saralasin and losartan [42,44]. Since saralasin exhibits partial agonistic effects, it was important to demonstrate a lack of intrinsic agonistic properties of losartan, and this could be done at a concentration of up to 10^{-5} mol/l [42]. An equally important factor to prove for a nonpeptide antagonist was specificity. The responses of isolated aortic strips to nor-epinephrine or to potassium chloride were not inhibited by losartan [45].

In vivo, 3–10mg/kg of losartan intravenously, shifted the pressor dose–response curves to Ang II to the right by at least

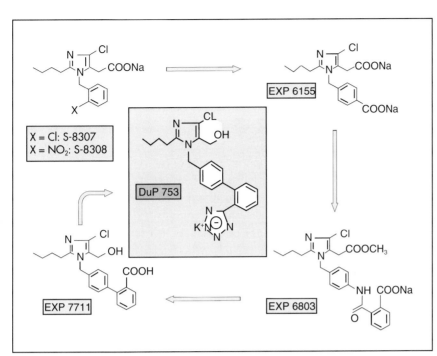

Fig. 86.6 Chemical structures of some nonpeptide Ang II-receptor antagonists, illustrating the structural modifications of the initial lead compounds, S-8307 and S-8308, into DuP 753 (losartan), a potent, orally active antagonist. Modified from Timmermans PB *et al* [41].

two orders of magnitude [46]. In normotensive rats, even doses as low as 1mg/kg reduced the pressure response to exogenous Ang II (Fig. 86.8). Similar doses of losartan were able to attenuate the increase in plasma aldosterone induced by Ang II [46]. The same doses given to furosemide-treated normotensive rats induced a mean blood-pressure drop of 20–30mmHg, while adding captopril had no additional hypotensive effect [46]. Intravenous or oral administration of losartan to rats made hypertensive by complete ligation of one renal artery six days prior to the experiment, reduced blood pressure to normotensive levels; a dose of 3mg/kg administered orally produced an antihypertensive effect that lasted for more than 24 hours [47]. Losartan given at doses of 10mg/kg intravenously, did not reduce blood pressure in DOCA-salt hypertensive rats [47]. Similarly, in conscious spontaneously hypertensive rats (SHR) with bilateral nephrectomy, losartan did not reduce blood pressure (Fig. 86.9) [48]. In SHR with intact kidneys, however, 3–10mg/kg orally of losartan markedly decreased blood pressure in a dose-dependent fashion, without accelerating heart rate (Fig 86.10) [48]. Adding captopril 60 minutes after the administration of losartan had no further effect on blood pressure [48]. In no instance, and particularly neither in the nephrectomized nor in the DOCA-salt hypertensive animals, was a losartan-induced blood-pressure rise observed; this confirms the results obtained *in vitro*, suggesting a complete lack of agonistic properties of losartan. An important observation with considerable implications for

clinical studies is the characterization of the pharmacological actions of an active metabolite of losartan termed EXP 3174 [49].

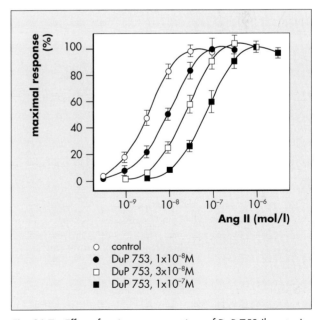

Fig. 86.7 Effect of various concentrations of DuP 753 (losartan) on the concentration–contractile response curve to Ang II in isolated rabbit aortic strips. Mean ± SEM (n=6). Modified from Chiu AT *et al* [42].

It appears that this metabolite has a markedly higher affinity for the Ang II receptor than has its mother compound losartan.

Taken together, these animal studies demonstrate that orally administered losartan, probably in part via its metabolite EXP 3174, is a potent and highly specific antagonist of Ang II at certain Ang II receptors. Losartan seems to be effective only when the renal renin system is normally operative and, unlike some of the earlier Ang II analogs, it exhibits no partial agonistic activity.

HETEROGENEITY OF ANGIOTENSIN II RECEPTORS

As already pointed out, when comparing the inhibitory effects of saralasin and losartan, it became apparent that, depending on the tissue studied, the results were not the same [43,50]. Saralasin is a much more potent inhibitor of Ang II binding than is losartan [51], particularly in receptors prepared from rat brain and adrenal medulla. When binding of Ang II was studied in microsomes from adrenal cortical cells, saralasin produced a 100% inhibition, while losartan antagonized only 75–80% of the binding, even when its concentrations were considerably increased (Fig. 86.11) [50]. After preincubation of the same microsomes from the adrenal cortex with losartan at 10μmol/l,

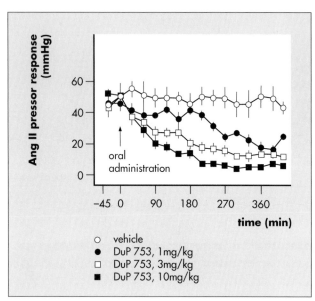

Fig. 86.8 Effects of vehicle and DuP 753 (losartan) given orally, on the pressor response to Ang II (0.1μg/kg, intravenously administered) in conscious normotensive rats. Mean ± SEM (n=4–6). Modified from Wong PC *et al* [46].

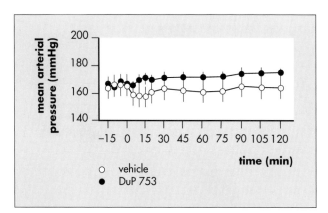

Fig. 86.9 Effects of vehicle and DuP 753 (losartan) 10mg/kg, intravenously administered, on mean arterial pressure in bilaterally nephrectomized conscious spontaneously hypertensive rats. Kidneys were removed 18–24 hours prior to the experiment. Mean ± SEM (n=5–6). Modified from Wong PC *et al* [48].

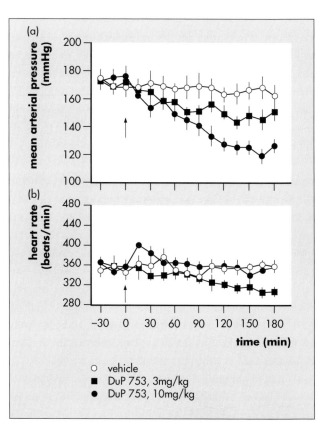

Fig. 86.10 Effects of vehicle and DuP 753 (losartan) given orally on mean arterial pressure (a) and heart rate (b) in conscious spontaneously hypertensive rats. Mean ± SEM (n=5–6). Modified from Wong PC *et al* [48].

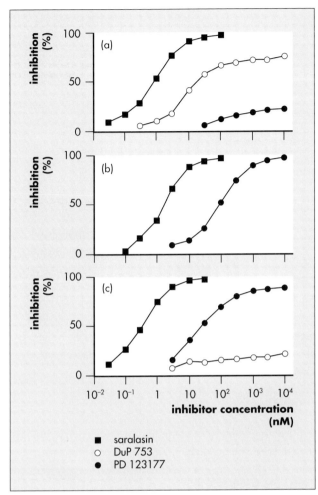

Fig. 86.11 Microsomal binding of Ang II. The inhibition of Ang II binding by saralasin, DuP 753 (losartan), and PD 123177, was determined using adrenal cortical microsomes (saralasin, IC_{50}=0.9nM; Dup 753, IC_{50}=15nM) (a), adrenal cortical microsomes with 10μM DuP 753 (saralasin, IC_{50}=1.66nM; PD 123177, IC_{50}=92nM), and adrenal medullary microsomes (saralasin, IC_{50}=0.4nM; PD 123177, IC_{50}=30nM) (c). Modified from Herblin WF *et al* [51].

the remaining Ang II binding could be completely inhibited by saralasin. Under these circumstances, similar inhibition could be obtained with a compound developed by Parke Davis, and identified as PD 123177. These studies strongly suggested that there are at least two populations of Ang II-receptor sites in the adrenal cortex. The major population was inhibited by losartan and these receptors were designated as type I (AT1). The second population of receptors, which was resistant to inhibition by losartan but blocked by PD 123177, was designated as type II (AT2) (see *Appendix I*). The different types of Ang II receptors

also appear to be coupled to different signal-transduction mechanisms [52] and may vary between species [53]. Both Ang II receptor types are blocked by saralasin. A similar picture emerged when analyzing the receptors types in microsomes from rat adrenal medulla: losartan provided only a very small degree of blockade, while PD 123177 induced potent, and nearly complete, inhibition. These results suggest that in the adrenal medulla, the receptor type AT2 is predominant.

Most of the AT2 Ang II receptors have been demonstrated in different areas of the brain [54–58], but they also seem to exist in the adrenal cortex and medulla [51,59], in the uterus [51], and in fetal rats where they can be demonstrated in many additional organs [60]. At least two antagonists are already available which selectively inhibit these AT2 receptors, the nonpeptide PD 123177 and the peptide CGP 42112 A [61]. In contrast, losartan and a subsequently developed antagonist DuP 532 seem to be quite specific for the AT1 Ang II receptors. As mentioned, saralasin blocks both receptor types [51]. Most of the well-known Ang II-related actions such as vascular constriction (see *Chapter 28*), aldosterone secretion (see *Chapter 33*), and the dipsogenic effects (see *Chapter 32*), seem to be dependent on the AT1-receptor type. This explains the considerable efficacy demonstrated with losartan in various experimental settings. Nevertheless, as shown later, it should be noted that during losartan administration, all the AT2 receptors remain exposed to rising levels of circulating Ang II, which could become a source of unsuspected and/or untoward effects. Possibly of critical importance in this connection will be the nature of the Ang II receptor responsible for the stimulation of angiotensinogen (renin substrate) secretion [62,63]. In long-term ACE inhibition, the fall in Ang II is accompanied by a reduction also in angiotensinogen [64], Ang I does not increase to the same extent as does renin [65], and thus ACE inhibition remains effective. It remains to be seen if a similar mechanism operates with, for example, long-term losartan treatment, and whether it has therapeutic relevance. A sceptical view is given in *Chapter 23*. It is likely that more types of Ang II receptors will be characterized in the future and many new antagonists with different profiles of blocking the various types (and perhaps subtypes) developed.

The heterogeneity of Ang II receptors is also discussed in *Chapter 12*.

RENAL EFFECTS OF LOSARTAN

Angiotensin II receptors have been found in the renal vasculature, in glomeruli, in the proximal convoluted tubules,

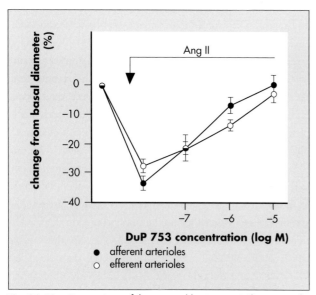

Fig. 86.12 Comparison of the reversal by DuP 753 (losartan) of Ang II-induced contractions of afferent and efferent arterioles (mean ± SEM). The two vessels responded identically to DuP 753-related receptor blockade. Modified from Loutzenhiser R et al [70].

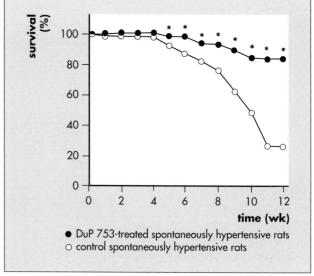

Fig. 86.13 Cumulative proportion of surviving DuP 753 (losartan)-treated and control spontaneously hypertensive stroke-prone rats, estimated on the population exposed at the beginning of each week. *P<0.01 versus control group. Modified from Camargo MJ et al [76].

and in medullary interstitial cells [66–68] (see *Chapter 25*). Angiotensin II exerts many effects in the kidney which range from inhibition of renin release to changes in renal blood flow and glomerular filtration rate (GFR), and the regulation of various tubular functions (see *Chapters 21, 26, 27,* and *40*).

In the isolated perfused kidney, losartan, as did saralasin, completely reversed the Ang II-induced increase in renal vascular resistance. Furthermore, losartan completely displaced radiolabeled Ang II bound to cultured glomerular mesangial as well as to renal medullary interstitial cells [69]. These results strongly suggest that the renal receptors studied were homogeneously of the AT1 type. In some further, very elegant studies in isolated perfused hydronephrotic kidneys, it was shown that losartan similarly reversed the Ang II-induced constriction of the afferent arterioles as well as of the efferent arterioles (Fig. 86.12) [70]. Other investigators demonstrated by *in vivo* microperfusion of the proximal convoluted tubules of Münich Wistar rats that losartan administered intravenously reduced the absorption of bicarbonate, chloride, and water in the S1 subsegment of the tubules [71]. Compared with captopril 3mg/kg intravenously, losartan 10mg/kg intravenously was significantly more effective in inhibiting sodium-chloride transport. This effect on proximal tubules was also demonstrated in normotensive Wistar–Kyoto rats and in SHR, in which losartan

induced a significant increase in fractional excretion of lithium, though urine flow and sodium excretion were not necessarily enhanced [72]. In conscious hypertensive dogs, losartan increased effective renal plasma flow, reduced renal vascular resistance, raised GFR, and lowered fractional tubular sodium reabsorption [73]. As will be seen later, in the clinical studies losartan also stimulated renin effects, confirming the strong predominance of AT1 Ang II receptors in the various renal tissues.

HEMODYNAMICS AND SURVIVAL

In a rat model of congestive heart failure induced by ligature of the proximal left coronary artery, the Ang II antagonist losartan decreased left ventricular end-diastolic pressure and mean circulatory filling pressure and also reduced end-diastolic volume index in comparison with untreated control animals [74]. These therapeutic effects of losartan were at least as great as those exerted by captopril in a third group of animals. In this same model, as well as in normal rats, it was also shown that losartan shifted the Ang II dose–response curve in a parallel fashion.

In a further evaluation of differential regional hemodynamics, losartan was administered to water-replete and water-deprived Brattleboro rats [75]. In both groups of animals, the

Ang II antagonist induced an increase in renal blood flow and a dose-dependent tachycardia. In addition, in the water-deprived animals, losartan caused dose-dependent hypotension and mesenteric artery vasodilation.

Highly suggestive are also two survival studies in different hypertensive rat models. In one of them, SH stroke-prone rats were fed a high salt diet and started, at six weeks of age when the animals were still normotensive, on losartan dissolved in drinking water, at 30mg/kg/d. Over the next 12 weeks, the treated animals developed hypertension at a much attenuated rate compared with the untreated controls, and gained significantly more weight. At 12 weeks, the survival of the animals treated with losartan was significantly and markedly better than that of the untreated controls (Fig. 86.13) [76]. Similarly, over a treatment period of 10 weeks, losartan reduced the mortality of salt-loaded Dahl-S rats even though after 10 weeks of treatment, the blood pressure of the treated animals was not different from that of the control group [77]. These data provide circumstantial evidence that Ang II may lead to an increased mortality associated with the hypertensive disease, independently of blood pressure *per se* [78,79], and that this may be reversed by specifically blocking the RAS. These matters are discussed further in *Chapters 40* and *60*.

ANGIOTENSIN II ANTAGONISTS COMPARED WITH CONVERTING-ENZYME INHIBITORS

Much that has been learned during recent years about the physiology and pathophysiology of the RAS has been based on the observation of the effect of converting-enzyme inhibitors. Though there is little doubt today that the converting-enzyme inhibitors act mostly by blocking the RAS, there nevertheless always remains some doubt as to whether some residual effect, under certain circumstances, could be due to vasodilation induced by bradykinin or prostaglandins (see *Chapters 10, 38, and 87*). Previously, attempts were made to rule out or confirm some of these effects using, for instance, bradykinin antagonists [80,81] or inhibitors of prostaglandin synthesis. A more direct approach is now possible by comparing the effect of a specific Ang II antagonist with that of converting enzyme inhibitors and/or by combining the two agents. Thus, it has been possible to demonstrate that renal hypertensive rats do not derive any further benefit from captopril after they have been treated with losartan [47]. As already mentioned, the Ang II antagonist also

had effects similar to those of captopril in the treatment of experimental congestive heart failure [74].

The contribution of kinins to the renal vasodilator effect of captopril was studied in rabbits [82]. If not all, at least most, of the renal vasodilator effect of captopril could also be produced by losartan. It is possible that the remaining effect was due to endogenous bradykinin.

Obviously, many more studies will be carried out to provide more specific answers to the question of what mechanisms are responsible for the effects of converting-enzyme inhibitors. Undoubtedly, the newer Ang II antagonists will be used predominantly to answer these questions.

CLINICAL STUDIES WITH LOSARTAN

With the nonpeptide Ang II antagonist losartan, the first clinical evaluation was carried out in normal volunteers. In principle, the aim was to assess its potency and efficacy in blocking the pressor response to exogenous Ang I or II. After a previous validation of finger photoplethysmography as a measure of the pressure response to bolus injections of Ang [83], single and repeated administration of losartan at doses up to 40mg were carried out [84]. Single administration of losartan induced a dose-dependent inhibition of the pressor response to Ang I (Fig. 86.14). The peak effect was achieved approximately three hours following the 40-mg dose, which resulted in an inhibition of the Ang I response of approximately 70%. Even 24 hours after a single dose of 40mg, the response to exogenous bolus injections of Ang I was still clearly attenuated. When the same losartan doses were administered once a day for eight days, a quantitatively similar blocking effect was observed. However, the pressor response to exogenous Ang II on the eighth day prior to losartan administration was clearly reduced, reflecting the long duration of action of the drug. As might have been expected, a dose-dependent rise in PRA and Ang II levels was observed on day one, and this was even accentuated on day eight, reflecting inhibition of the negative feedback loop exerted by Ang II on renin secretion (Fig. 86.15) (see *Chapter 24*). No effect on plasma aldosterone could be demonstrated but it has to be kept in mind that the 40-mg dose of losartan did not completely inhibit the pressor response to either Ang I or II and that in the course of the study, intermittent bolus injections of Ang I or II had been administered to these normal volunteers. During this study, following the 20- and 40-mg dose of losartan, plasma levels of losartan were measured and related to the concurrent degree of inhibition of the

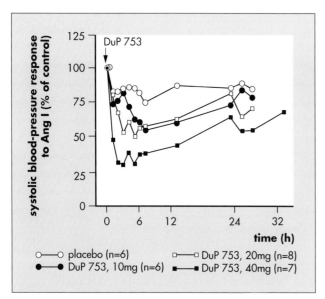

Fig. 86.14 Effects of single doses of oral DuP 753 (losartan, 10, 20, or 40mg) or placebo on systolic blood-pressure response (mean) to constant test doses of Ang I in healthy volunteers. Modified from Christen Y et al [84].

Ang-induced blood-pressure response or the plasma Ang II concentration. It became evident that there was a dissociation in time between the profile of circulating plasma drug levels and the drug effect. These results strongly suggested that in man, as shown previously in animals [49], losartan has to be metabolized, and that some active metabolite (presumably EXP 3174) is responsible for a considerable part of the drug effect.

A further investigation was carried out to assess the effects of higher doses of losartan in order to achieve as complete a blockade of Ang II as possible [85]. Equally important, in this evaluation, not only plasma losartan levels but also concentrations of the metabolite EXP 3174, were quantified. Oral doses of 40, 80, and 120mg losartan were administered. With the two higher doses, the Ang II pressor response was inhibited by more than 90% at its peak. With these higher doses of losartan, a significant fall in plasma aldosterone levels could also be demonstrated.

The plasma concentrations of both the mother compound losartan and its active metabolite EXP 3174 showed dose-dependent profiles, where the decay of the metabolite was much slower than that of losartan (Fig. 86.16). When the per cent inhibition of the Ang II response was related to circulating EXP 3174 levels, the pattern of a saturation plot emerged, and

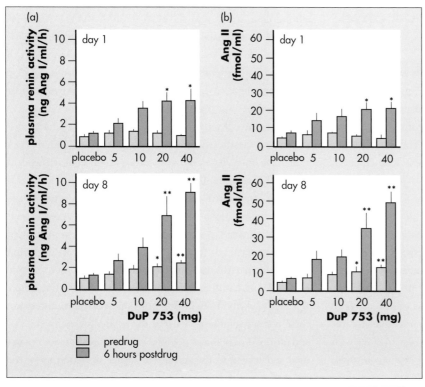

Fig. 86.15 Effects of four different doses of DuP 753 (losartan, 5, 10, 20, or 40mg, orally, once daily) or placebo (n=6) on plasma renin activity (a) and immunoreactive Ang II (b), measured before and six hours after drug intake on days one and eight of drug administration. Mean ± SEM. *$P<0.05$, **$P<0.01$ versus placebo. Modified from Christen Y et al [84].

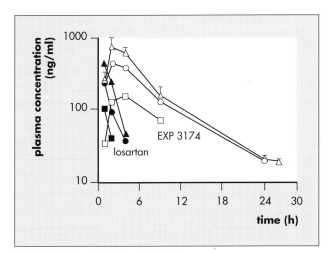

Fig. 86.16 Time profiles of the mean plasma concentrations of the parent compound losartan (closed symbols) and its active metabolite EXP 3174 (open symbols) after single oral administration of losartan (squares, 40mg; circles 80mg; triangles 120mg) in six volunteers. For clarity, standard deviations are reported only for the active metabolite following the highest dose. Modified from Munafo H *et al* [85].

accordingly, a Hill equation was fitted to these data. Based on this analysis, the 80-mg dose appeared to provide close to maximal Ang II inhibition. Moreover, circulating levels of 200–250ng/ml of EXP 3174 seemed sufficient for maximal blockade (Fig. 86.17). Indeed, virtually all of the Ang II inhibitory effect of losartan semed to be explained by circulating EXP 3174 without taking into account its mother compound. This is not to say that losartan itself is not an Ang II antagonist. It rather reflects a potentially higher affinity of EXP 3174 than of losartan for the Ang II receptor and also its much longer half-life. These studies taken together demonstrated that losartan is a potent and a highly effective Ang II antagonist in man, and that a dose of between 40 and 80mg once daily, provided close to maximal Ang II blockade for several hours.

It still remains to be seen whether losartan is able to reduce blood pressure in hypertensive patients and if so, what dose is needed to achieve this. The possibly critical issue of its effect on hepatic angiotensinogen output [64] has been mentioned earlier. Though several hundred patients have already been treated with these new Ang II antagonists, few data have been published so far. In a preliminary study of 100 hypertensive patients, the effect of losartan given once daily for five days at doses of 50, 100, and 150mg was compared with that of enalapril [86]. All three losartan doses induced significant blood-pressure reductions in relation to the placebo-treated control group. Whereas on the

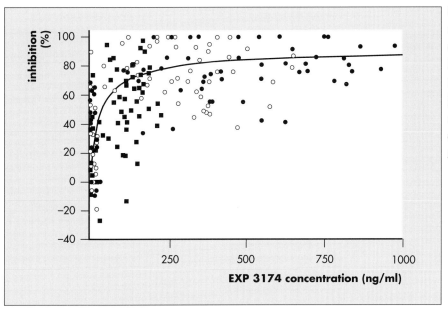

Fig. 86.17 Inhibition of the pressor response to Ang II challenge versus the concentration of the active metabolite of losartan, EXP 3174, in six volunteers. Doses of losartan were 40mg (■), 80mg (○) and 120mg (●). The solid line represents the Hill fit constructed from averaged individual parameters. Modified from Munafo H *et al* [85].

first day enalapril was clearly more effective in reducing blood pressure than was losartan, blood-pressure levels were not different on the fifth day of treatment, suggesting that long-term Ang II blockade may be as effective as converting-enzyme inhibition in reducing blood pressure of hypertensive patients. There was no difference in the effect of the three losartan doses, suggesting that 50mg daily may already provide close to maximal efficacy. This would seem to be in quite good agreement with our data obtained in normal volunteers. Obviously, these are preliminary observations and more results are awaited with great impatience.

CONCLUSIONS

Twenty years ago, the whole concept of treating hypertension and congestive heart failure by blocking the RAS was developed using Ang II peptide analogs with partial antagonistic properties. Shortly afterwards, this approach was overtaken by the use of the newly available, orally active, converting-enzyme inhibitors, which have since become a mainstay of antihypertensive therapy. Due to the further development of nonpeptide Ang II antagonists, the original and specific approach using Ang II-receptor blockade as a treatment modality can once more be pursued. With losartan and its highly effective metabolite EXP

3174, long-term blockade of the AT1 type of the Ang II receptor is now a practical possibility. This renders feasible, for the first time, testing of the real long-term contribution of the RAS to the pathogenesis of hypertension and also the evaluation of how much of the efficacy of converting-enzyme inhibitors is related to inhibition of the RAS and how much may be due to potentiation of bradykinin or to induction of vasodilating prostanoids. Thus, Ang II antagonists provide some important tools to further the understanding of the pathogenic mechanisms involved in the development of hypertension. It remains to be seen with long-term evaluation how effective these agents will be and particularly whether because of their specificity for the Ang II receptor, they may exhibit less side effects than for instance, converting-enzyme inhibitors. Last but not least, with the discovery of different types of Ang II receptors, there exists the exciting prospect of developing second- and third-generation receptor antagonists which may specifically inhibit only certain ranges of actions of Ang II.

ACKNOWLEDGMENTS

This work was supported by grants from the Swiss National Science Foundation and the Cardiovascular Research Foundation.

REFERENCES

1. Tigerstedt R, Bergman PG. Niere und Kreislauf. *Skandinavisches Archiv für Physiologie* 1898;**8**:223–71.

2. Goldblatt H, Lynch J, Hanzal RF, Summerville WW. Studies on experimental hypertension; production of persistent elevation of systolic blood pressure by means of renal ischemia. *Journal of Experimental Medicine* 1934;**59**:347–79.

3. Pickering GW, Prinzmetal M. Some observations on renin, a pressor substance contained in normal kidney, together with a method for its biological assay. *Clinical Science* 1938;**3**:211–27.

4. Goldblatt PJ. The Goldblatt experiment: A conceptual paradigm. In: Laragh JH, Brenner BM, eds. *Hypertension: Pathophysiology, diagnosis and management.* New York:Raven Press, 1990:21–32.

5. Goldblatt H. Experimental hypertension produced by renal ischemia. *Harvey Lectures* 1937–1938;**Series 33**:237–75.

6. Braun-Menendez E, Fasciolo JC, Leloir LF, Munoz JM, Taquini AC. *Renal hypertension* [transl. by Dexter L]. Springfield, Illinois: Charles C Thomas, 1946.

7. Page IH, McCubbin JW, eds. *Renal hypertension.* Chicago:Year Book Medical Publishers, 1968.

8. Eide I, Aars H. Renal hypertension in rabbits immunized with angiotensin II. *Scandinavian Journal of Clinical Investigation* 1970;**25**:119–27.

9. Johnston CI, Hutchinson JS, Mendelsohn FA. Biological significance of renin angiotensin immunization. *Circulation Research* 1970;**26** (suppl 2):215–22.

10. Macdonald GJ, Louis WJ, Renzini V, Peart WS. Renal-clip hypertension in rabbits immunized against angiotensin II. *Circulation Research* 1970;**27**:197–211.

11. Bing J, Poulsen K. Effect of anti-angiotensin II on blood pressure and sensitivity to angiotensin and renin. *Acta Physiologica Scandinavica* 1970;**78**:6–18.

12. Worcel M, Meyer P, d'Auriac GA, Papanicolaou N, Milliez P. The role of angiotensin. Indirect studies with antiangiotensin plasma. *Circulation Research* 1970;**26, 27** (suppl 2):223–34.

13. Brunner HR, Kirshman JD, Sealey JE, Laragh JH. Hypertension of renal origin: Evidence for two different mechanisms. *Science* 1971;**174**:1344–6.

14. Walker WG, Ruiz-Maza F, Horvath JS. Demonstration of free (unbound) angiotensin II in immunized rabbits. *Proceedings of the Fifth International Congress on Nephropathology.* 1972:115. Basel: Karger.

15. Marshall GR, Vine W, Needleman P. A specific competitive inhibitor of angiotensin II. *Proceedings of the National Academy of Sciences of the USA* 1970;**67**:1624–30.

16. Pals DT, Masucci FD, Sipos F, Denning GS Jr. A specific competitive antagonist of the vascular action of angiotensin II. *Circulation Research* 1971;**29**:664–72.

17. Khosla MC, Smeby RR, Bumpus FM. Structure–activity relationship in angiotensin II analogs. In: Page IH, Bumpus FM, eds. *Angiotensin.* Berlin: Springer–Verlag, 1974;126–61.

18. Türker RK, Page IH, Bumpus FM. Antagonists of angiotensin II. In: Page IH, Bumpus FM, eds. *Angiotensin.* Berlin: Springer–Verlag, 1974:162–9.

19. Davis JO. The use of blocking agents to define the functions of the renin–angiotensin system. Volhard lecture. *Clinical Science* 1975;**48** (suppl 2):3–14S.

20. Stokes GS, Edwards KDG, eds. Drugs affecting the renin–angiotensin–aldosterone system: Use of angiotensin inhibitors. *Progress in Biochemical Pharmacology* 1976;**12**:1–258.

21. Gavras H, Brunner HR, Vaughan ED Jr, Laragh JH. Angiotensin–sodium interaction in blood pressure maintenance of renal hypertensive and normotensive rats. *Science* 1973;**180**:1369–72.

22. Gavras H, Brunner HR, Laragh JH, Vaughan ED Jr, Koss M, Cote LJ, Gavras I. Malignant hypertension resulting from deoxycorticosterone acetate and salt excess; role of renin and sodium in vascular changes. *Circulation Research* 1975;**36**:300–9.

23. Riegger AJG, Lever AF, Millar JA, Morton JJ, Slack B. Correction of renal hypertension in the rat by prolonged infusion of angiotensin inhibitors. *Lancet* 1977;**ii**:1317–9.

24. Bing RF, Russell CI, Swales JD, Thurston H. Effect of 12-hour infusion of saralasin or captopril on blood pressure in conscious hypertensive rats: Relation to plasma renin, duration of hypertension, and effect of unclipping. *Journal of Laboratory and Clinical Medicine* 1981;**98**:302–10.

25. Dickinson CJ, Yu R. The progressive pressor response to angiotensin in the rabbit. *Journal of Physiology* 1967;**10**:91–9.

26. Brown AJ, Clark SA, Lever AF. Slow rise and diurnal change of blood pressure with saralasin and angiotensin II in rats. *American Journal of Physiology* 1983;**244**:F84–8.

27. Brunner HR, Gavras H, Laragh JH, Keenan R. Angiotensin II blockade in man by sar¹-ala⁸-angiotensin II for understanding and treatment of high blood pressure. *Lancet* 1973;**ii**:1045–8.

28. Brunner HR, Gavras H, Laragh JH, Keenan R. Hypertension in man. Exposure of the renin and sodium components using angiotensin II blockade. *Circulation Research* 1974;**34** (suppl 1):35–43.

29. Streeten DHP, Anderson GH, Freiberg JM, Dalakos TG. Use of an angiotensin II antagonist (saralasin) in the recognition of angiotensinogenic hypertension. *New England Journal of Medicine* 1975;**292**:657–62.

30. Posternak L, Brunner HR, Gavras H, Brunner DB. Angiotensin II blockade in normal man: Interaction of renin and sodium in maintaining blood pressure. *Kidney International* 1977;**11**:197–203.

31. Hollenberg NK, Williams GH, Burger B, Ishikawa I, Adams DF. Blockade and stimulation of renal, adrenal, and vascular angiotensin II receptors with 1-sar, 8-ala angiotensin II in man. *Journal of Clinical Investigation* 1976;**57**:39–46.

32. Ishikawa I, Hollenberg NK. Blockade of the systemic and renal vascular actions of angiotensin II with the 1-sar, 8-ala analogue in the rat. *Life Sciences* 1975;**17**:121–30.

33. Turini GA, Brunner HR, Ferguson RK, Rivier JL, Gavras H. Congestive heart failure in normotensive man: Haemodynamics, renin, and angiotensin II blockade. *British Heart Journal* 1978;**40**:1134–42.

34. Gavras H, Flessas A, Ryan TJ, Brunner HR, Faxon DP, Gavras I. Angiotensin II inhibition; treatment of congestive heart failure in a high-renin hypertension. *Journal of the American Medical Association* 1977;**238**:880–2.

35. Brown JJ, Brown WCB, Fraser R, Lever AF, Morton JJ, Robertson JIS, Agabiti-Rosei E, Trust PM. The effects of the angiotensin II antagonist saralasin on blood pressure and plasma aldosterone in man in relation to the prevailing plasma angiotensin II concentration. *Progress in Biochemical Pharmacology* 1976;**12**:230–41.

36. Case DB, Wallace JM, Keim HJ, Weber MA, Drayer JIM, White RP, Sealey JE, Laragh JH. Estimating renin participation in hypertension: Superiority of converting enzyme inhibitor over saralasin. *American Journal of Medicine* 1976;**61**:790–6.

37. Furukawa Y, Kishimoto S, Nishikawa K. Hypotensive imidazole derivatives. *US Patent 4,340,598 issued to Takeda Chemical Industries Ltd, Osaka, Japan*; 1982.

38. Furukawa Y, Kishimoto S, Nishikawa K. Hypotensive imidazole-5-acetic acid derivatives. *US Patent 4,355,040 issued to Takeda Chemical Industries Ltd, Osaka, Japan*; 1982.

39. Wong PC, Chiu AT, Price WA, Thoolen JMC, Carini DJ, Johnson AL, Taber RI, Timmermans PBMWM. Nonpeptide angiotensin II receptor antagonists. I. Pharmacological characterization of 2-n-butyl-4-chloro-1-(2-chlorobenzyl)imidazole-5-acetic acid, sodium salt (S-8307). *Journal of Pharmacology and Experimental Therapeutics* 1988;**247**:1–7.

40. Chiu AT, Carini DJ, Johnson AL, McCall DE, Price WA, Thoolen MJMC, Wong PC, Taber RI, Timmermans PBMWM. Nonpeptide angiotensin II receptor antagonists. II. Pharmacology of S-8308. *European Journal of Pharmacology* 1988;**157**:13–21.

41. Timmermans PB, Carini DJ, Chiu AT, Duncia JV, Price WA Jr, Wells GJ, Wong PC, Johnson AL, Wexler RR. The discovery of a new class of highly specific nonpeptide angiotensin II receptor antagonists. *American Journal of Hypertension* 1991;**4**:275–81S.

42. Chiu AT, McCall DE, Price WA, Wong PC, Carini DJ, Duncia JV, Wexler RR, Yoo SE, Johnson AL, Timmermans P. Nonpeptide angiotensin II receptor antagonists. VII. Cellular and biochemical pharmacology of DUP 753, an orally active antihypertensive agent. *Journal of Pharmacology and Experimental Therapeutics* 1990;**252**:711–8.

43. Chiu AT, McCall DE, Ardecky RJ, Duncia JV, Nguyen TT, Timmermans PBMWM. Angiotensin II receptor subtypes and their selective nonpeptide ligands. *Receptor* 1990;**1**:33–40.

44. Burnier M, Centeno G, Grouzmann E, Walker P, Waeber B, Brunner HR. *In vitro* effects of DuP 753, a nonpeptide angiotensin II receptor antagonist, on human platelets and rat vascular smooth muscle cells. *American Journal of Hypertension* 1991;**4**:438–43.

45. Chiu AT, McCall DE, Price WA Jr, Wong PC, Carini DJ, Duncia JV, Wexler RR, Yoo SE, Johnson AL, Timmermans PB. *In vitro* pharmacology of DuP 753. *American Journal of Hypertension* 1991;**4**:282–7S.

46. Wong PC, Price WA, Chiu AT, Duncia JV, Carini DJ, Wexler RR, Johnson AL, Timmermans PBMWM. Nonpeptide angiotensin II receptor antagonists. VIII. Characterization of functional antagonism displayed by DUP 753, an orally active antihypertensive agent. *Journal of Pharmacology and Experimental Therapeutics* 1990;**252**:719–25.

47. Wong PC, Price WA, Chiu AT, Duncia JV, Carini DJ, Wexler RR, Johnson AL, Timmermans PBMWM. Nonpeptide angiotensin II receptor antagonists. IX. Antihypertensive activity in rats of DuP 753, an orally active antihypertensive agent. *Journal of Pharmacology and Experimental Therapeutics* 1990;**252**:726–32.

48. Wong PC, Price WA, Chiu AT, Duncia JV, Carini DJ, Wexler RR, Johnson AL, Timmermans PBMWM. Hypotensive action of DuP 753, an angiotensin II antagonist in spontaneously hypertensive rats. Nonpeptide angiotensin II receptor antagonists. X. *Hypertension* 1990;**15**:459–68.

49. Wong PC, Price WA Jr, Chiu AT, Duncia JV, Carini DJ, Wexler RR, Johnson AL, Timmermans PB. Nonpeptide angiotensin II receptor antagonists. XI. Pharmacology of EXP 3174: An active metabolite of DuP 753, an orally active antihypertensive agent. *Journal of Pharmacology and Experimental Therapeutics* 1990;**255**:211–7.

50. Chiu AT, Herblin WF, McCall DE, Ardecky RJ, Carini DJ, Duncia JV, Pease LJ, Wong PC, Wexler RR, Johnson AL, Timmermans PBMWM. Identification of angiotensin II receptor subtypes. *Biochemical and Biophysical Research Communications* 1989;**165**:196–203.

51. Herblin WF, Chiu AT, McCall DE, Ardecky RJ, Carini DJ, Duncia JV, Pease LJ, Wong PC, Wexler RR, Johnson AL, Timmermans PBMWM. Angiotensin II receptor heterogeneity. *American Journal of Hypertension* 1991;**4**:299–302S.

52. Sumners C, Tang W, Zelezna B, Raizada MK. Angiotensin II receptor subtypes are coupled with distinct signal-transduction mechanisms in neurons and astrocytes from rat brain. *Proceedings of the National Academy of Sciences of the USA* 1991;**88**:7567–71.

53. Ji H, Sandberg K, Catt KJ. Novel angiotensin II antagonists distinguish amphibian from mammalian angiotensin II receptors expressed in *Xenopus laevis* oocytes. *Molecular Pharmacology* 1991;**39**:120–3.

54. Leung KH, Smith RD, Pieter B, Timmermans PB, Chiu AT. Regional distribution of the two subtypes of angiotensin II receptor in rat brain using selective nonpeptide antagonists. *Neuroscience Letters* 1991;**123**:95–8.

55. Tsutsumi K, Saavedra JM. Characterization and development of angiotensin II receptor subtypes (AT1 and AT2) in rat brain. *American Journal of Physiology* 1991;**261**:R209–16.

56. Song K, Allen AM, Paxinos G, Mendelsohn FA. Angiotensin II receptor subtypes in rat brain. *Clinical and Experimental Pharmacology and Physiology* 1991;**18**:93–6.

57. Tallant EA, Diz DI, Khosla MC, Ferrario CM. Identification and regulation of angiotensin II receptor subtypes on NG108–15 cells. *Hypertension* 1991;**17**:1135–43.

58. Grove KL, Cook VI, Speth RC. Angiotensin II receptors in the ventral portion of the bed nucleus of the stria terminalis. *Neuroendocrinology* 1991;**53**:339–43.

59. Wiest SA, Rampersaud A, Zimmerman K, Steinberg MI. Characterization of distinct angiotensin II binding sites in rat adrenal gland and bovine cerebellum using selective nonpeptide antagonists. *Journal of Cardiovascular Pharmacology* 1991;**17**:177–84.

60. Tsutsumi K, Stromberg C, Viswanathan M, Saavedra JM. Angiotensin II receptor subtypes in fetal tissue of the rat: Autoradiography, guanine nucleotide sensitivity, and association with phosphoinositide hydrolysis. *Endocrinology* 1991;**129**:1075–82.

61. Whitebread S, Mele M, Kamber B, De Gasparo M. Preliminary biochemical characterization of two angiotensin II receptor subtypes. *Biochemical and Biophysical Research Communications* 1989;**163**:284–91.

62. Khayyal M, MacGregor J, Brown JJ, Lever AF, Robertson JIS. Increase of plasma renin-substrate after infusion of angiotensin in the rat. *Clinical Science* 1973;**44**:87–90.

63. Nasjletti A, Masson GMC. Stimulation of angiotensinogen formation by renin and angiotensin. *Proceedings of the Society for Experimental Biology and Medicine* 1973;**142**:307–10.

64. Rasmussen S, Nielsen MD, Giese J. Captopril combined with thiazide lowers renin substrate concentrations: Implications for methodology in renin assays. *Clinical Science* 1981;**60**:591–3.

65. Robertson JIS, Tillman DM, Ball SG, Lever AF. Angiotensin converting enzyme inhibition in hypertension. *Journal of Hypertension* 1987;**5** (suppl 3):19–25.

66. Skorecki KL, Ballermann BJ, Rennke HJ, Brenner BM. Angiotensin receptor regulation in isolated rat glomeruli. *Federation Proceedings* 1963;**42**:3064–70.

67. Cox HM, Munday KA, Poat JA. Location of [^{125}I]-angiotensin II receptors on rat kidney epithelial cells. *British Journal of Pharmacology* 1984;**82**:891–5.

68. Douglas JG. Angiotensin receptor subtypes of the kidney cortex. *American Journal of Physiology* 1987;**253**:F1–7.

69. Fontoura BM, Nussenzveig DR, Timmermans PB, Maack T. DuP 753 is a potent nonpeptide antagonist of angiotensin II receptors in isolated perfused rat kidney and cultured renal cells. *American Journal of Hypertension* 1991;**4**: 303–8S.

70. Loutzenhiser R, Epstein M, Hayashi K, Takenaka T, Forster H. Characterization of the renal microvascular effects of angiotensin II antagonist, DuP 753: Studies in isolated perfused hydronephrotic kidneys. *American Journal of Hypertension* 1991;**4**:309–14S.

71. Xie MH, Liu FY, Wong PC, Timmermans PBMWM, Cogan MG. Proximal nephron and renal effects of DuP 753, a non-peptide angiotensin II receptor antagonist. *Kidney International* 1990;**38**:473–9.

72. Fenoy FJ, Milicic I, Smith RD, Wong PC, Timmermans PB, Roman R. Effects of DuP 753 on renal function of normotensive and spontaneously hypertensive rats. *American Journal of Hypertension* 1991;**4**:321–6S.

73. Bovee KC, Wong PC, Timmermans PB, Thoolen MJ. Effects of the nonpeptide angiotensin II receptor antagonist DuP 753 on blood pressure and renal functions in spontaneously hypertensive PH dogs. *American Journal of Hypertension* 1991;**4**:327–33S.

74. Raya TE, Fonken SJ, Lee RW, Daugherty S, Goldman S, Wong PC, Timmermans PB, Morkin E. Hemodynamic effects of direct angiotensin II blockade compared to converting enzyme inhibition in rat model of heart failure. *American Journal of Hypertension* 1991;**4**:334–40S.

75. Batin P, Gardiner SM, Compton AM, Bennett T. Differential regional haemodynamic effects of the non-peptide angiotensin II antagonist, DuP 753, in water-replete and water-deprived Brattleboro rats. *Life Sciences* 1991;**48**:733–9.

76. Camargo MJ, von Lutterotti N, Pecker MS, James GD, Timmermans PB, Laragh JH. DuP 753 increases survival in spontaneously hypertensive stroke-prone rats fed a high sodium diet. *American Journal of Hypertension* 1991;**4**:341–5S.

77. von Lutterotti N, Camargo MJ, Mueller FB, Timmermans PB, Laragh JH. Angiotensin II receptor antagonist markedly reduces mortality in salt-loaded Dahl S rats. *American Journal of Hypertension* 1991;**4**:346–9S.

78. Brunner HR, Laragh JH, Baer L, Newton MA, Goodwin FT, Krakoff LR, Bard RH, Bühler FR. Essential hypertension: Renin and aldosterone, heart attack and stroke. *New England Journal of Medicine* 1972;**286**:441–9.

79. Alderman MH, Madhavan S, Ooi WL, Cohen H, Sealey JE, Laragh JH. Association of the renin–sodium profile with the risk of myocardial infarction in patients with hypertension. *New England Journal of Medicine* 1991;**324**: 1098–104.

80. Benetos A, Gavras H, Stewart JM, Vavrek RJ, Hatinoglou S, Gavras I. Vasodepressor role of endogenous bradykinin assessed by a bradykinin antagonist. *Hypertension* 1986;**8**:971–4.

81. Waeber B, Aubert JF, Flückiger JP, Nussberger J, Vavrek R, Stewart JM, Brunner HR. Role of endogenous bradykinin in blood pressure control of conscious rats. *Kidney International* 1988;**34** (suppl 26):63–8.

82. Hajj-ali AF, Zimmerman BG. Kinin contribution to renal vasodilator effect of captopril in rabbit. *Hypertension* 1991;**17**:504–9.

83. Christen Y, Waeber B, Nussberger J, Brunner HR. Non-invasive blood pressure monitoring at the finger for studying short-lasting pressor responses in man. *Journal of Clinical Pharmacology* 1990;**30**:711–4.

84. Christen Y, Waeber B, Nussberger J, Porchet M, Borland RM, Lee RJ, Maggon K, Shum L, Timmermans PB, Brunner HR. Oral administration of DuP 753, a specific angiotensin II receptor antagonist, to normal male volunteers. Inhibition of pressor response to exogenous angiotensin I and II. *Circulation* 1991;**83**: 1333–42.

85. Munafo H, Christen Y, Nussberger J, Shum LY, Borland RM, Lee RJ, Waeber B, Biollaz J, Brunner HR. Drug concentration response relationships in normal volunteers after oral administration of losartan (DuP 753, MK 954), an angiotensin receptor antagonist. *Clinical Pharmacology and Therapeutics* 1992;in press.

86. Nelson E, Merrill D, Sweet C, Bradstreet T, Panebianco D, Byyny R, Herman T, Lasseter K, Levy B, Lewis G, McMahon FG, Reeves R, Ruff D, Shepherd A, Weidler D, Irvin J. Efficacy and safety of oral MK-954 (DuP 753), an angiotensin receptor antagonist, in essential hypertension. In Abstracts, European Society of Hypertension, Milano, 1991, No 512.

87

ANGIOTENSIN-CONVERTING ENZYME INHIBITORS

COLIN I JOHNSTON

INTRODUCTION

Angiotensin-converting enzyme inhibitors have been a significant advance in the treatment of cardiovascular diseases, particularly hypertension and cardiac failure. Since the first orally active ACE inhibitor captopril was designed in 1977 by Ondetti and Cushman, there have been rapid advances in our knowledge of the RAS and a proliferation of ACE inhibitors [1–3]. Likewise, there has been an explosion in the number of publications dealing with ACE and its inhibitors. Compared with the β-blocking agents, however, ACE inhibitors as a group are chemically quite similar. More importantly, there do not appear to be subclasses or isoenzymes of ACE as there are for adrenergic receptors.

This chapter concentrates on the general principles of ACE inhibitors and discusses their mode of action and outlines the pharmacokinetics and pharmacodynamics which are important in understanding their clinical usage. It also focuses on factors that are important in choosing between ACE inhibitors for a particular clinical circumstance and compares new drugs that are undergoing clinical trials with the index drugs captopril and enalapril.

The ACE inhibitors are most frequently prescribed for patients with essential hypertension or with cardiac failure. Details of their use in these two disorders are given in *Chapters 91* and *93*.

PHARMACEUTICAL CHEMISTRY

The design of the first orally active ACE inhibitor, captopril, was based on the action of peptides from the venom of the South American pit viper, *Bothrops jararaca*, to block ACE, together with the similarities noted by Ondetti and Cushman [4,5] between ACE and a well-studied peptidase, carboxipeptidase A. Angiotensin-converting enzyme was known to be a zinc-dependent metallopeptidase and Ondetti and Cushman realized the significance of designing an inhibitor that would bind

tightly to zinc. For this reason, they incorporated a sulfhydryl group into their original dipeptide molecule. Other important binding sites on ACE are S1, S'_1, and S'_2. Some subsequent ACE inhibitors also employed sulfhydryl zinc binders [6], but the next important development was when Patchett *et al* [7] described the substituted carboxyalkyl dipeptide, enalapril. This did not use a sulfhydryl ligand to bind to zinc, but instead used the carboxyl molecule.

Subsequent ACE inhibitors [8–10] have been developed with alternative zinc ligands [2], to increase potency [3], to prolong the duration of action [4], to produce compounds not eliminated entirely by the kidney [8–10], or to increase oral absorption. A theoretical model of the enzyme (ACE) and some of its inhibitors are depicted in Fig. 87.1.

HUMAN ANGIOTENSIN-CONVERTING ENZYME

Angiotensin-converting enzyme has now been cloned (11) and sequenced and its active site studied more accurately by expressing the enzyme *in vitro* and conducting site-directed mutagenesis [12,13]. Unlike other metallopeptidases, ACE is now known to

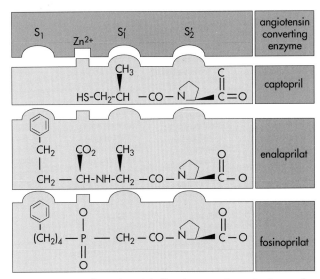

Fig. 87.1 Hypothetical model of binding sites (zinc, S_1, S'_1, and S'_2) on ACE for three different zinc ligands: a sulfhydryl (SH) group, a carboxyl (CO_2) group, and a phosphinyl (PO_2) group.

be a bilobed enzyme with two homologous arms, both of which contain an active site [12,14]. It is also known that both active sites are zinc dependent, that one zinc molecule binds per active site [15,16], and that many of the zinc-binding properties of the two active sites are identical. The catalytic activity of the two sites is very similar but the sites have different chloride requirements and display different catalytic constants [12–16] (see *Chapter 10*). Preliminary studies using different radioligands to bind to the active sites of the enzyme have suggested that the requirements for binding and inhibition at the two catalytic sites may be different [17]. This raises the interesting possibility that there may be different substrates for each site. Equally importantly, it also raises the prospect of being able to design specific inhibitors for either the carboxy-terminal active site or the amino-terminal active site of ACE (see *Chapters 10* and *16*).

Despite these advances in our knowledge, the three-dimensional structure of the enzyme and the exact conformation of the active sites, are not known. Hence, the design and construction of new ACE inhibitors continue to be made in an empiric fashion.

CLASSIFICATION

A useful classification of ACE inhibitors, based on pharmaceutical chemistry, is shown in Fig. 87.2. The compounds are classified according to their predominant method of binding to the zinc moiety of the enzyme. These include drugs binding either through a sulfhydryl group, which are derivatives of captopril, or binding (as does enalapril) with a carboxyl group of a substituted amino acid. A third major category includes compounds that use phosphorus or phosphinic acid as the predominant zinc-binding ligand [4,6]. This does not then include the ketomethylene or aminoketone tripeptides which, because of poor bioavailability, have failed to reach clinical development. It should be emphasized that the zinc ligand, although very important, is not the only significant binding site for ACE inhibitors, and subsite binding may confer additional potency and benefits.

Angiotensin-converting enzyme and its inhibitors can be measured by a variety of different methods, each with its own advantages and disadvantages. It has been reported, however, that the apparent potency and properties of the various inhibitors depend on the surrogate substrate used for measurement of enzyme activity [18]. This does not apply to radioligand-binding displacement assays which can be used both for the measurement of ACE and its inhibitors [19–22]. In this method, a radioiodinated specific inhibitor of ACE ([125]I 351A) is bound to

the active site of the enzyme in a stoichiometric, one-to-one relationship, and the ability of an inhibitor to displace this specific radioligand is a measure of its potency. Such determinations of displacement binding correlate exceedingly well with inhibition of catalytic activity. An example of the displacement of labeled 351A from ACE derived from human plasma by a panel of inhibitors, is shown in Fig. 87.3. The comparison between their ability to displace the radioligand (ID_{50}) compared with their catalytic inhibitory activity (IC_{50}) is shown in Fig. 87.4. Using such methods, it is extremely easy to measure rapidly and accurately the inhibitory potency of any compound, together with its binding characteristics. The binding characteristics, particularly the off rate of an inhibitor of ACE is an important determinant of the pharmacokinetic characteristics of the compound.

Captopril is an active ACE inhibitor but its absorption from the gastrointestinal tract is not high and is reduced if taken with food.

The next important consideration in the development of ACE inhibitors was the introduction of prodrugs. Most of the newer compounds, with the exception of lisinopril and ceranopril, are prodrugs. This has usually been achieved by adding an ester group which makes the compounds more lipophilic, improves their absorption from the gastrointestinal tract, and

Fig. 87.2
Classification of ACE inhibitors based on the chemical group that binds as the zinc ligand.

sulfhydryl ligand
  captopril
  alacepril
  pivalopril
  zofenopril
carboxyl ligand
  enalapril
  benazapril
  cilazapril
  delapril
  lisinopril
  pentopril
  perindopril
  quinapril
  ramipril
  spirapril
  trandopril
phosphinyl group
  fosinopril
  ceronapril

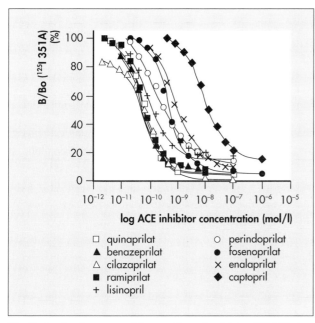

Fig. 87.3 Displacement of the specific radioinhibitor ^{125}I 351 A bound to human plasma ACE by a variety of ACE inhibitors.

increases their bioavailability. They then require deesterification, usually by the gut wall and liver, before release of the active diacid.

INHIBITION OF, AND BINDING TO, PLASMA AND TISSUE ANGIOTENSIN-CONVERTING ENZYME

Before the pharmacokinetics and mode of action of ACE inhibitors can be discussed and understood, it is important to understand the change in concept of the RAS which has occurred in recent years. It is now well recognized that the RAS is both a circulating, as well as a local tissue, system [23–27] (see *Chapters* 41–51). Accordingly, it may act as a circulating hormone, a paracrine or autocrine hormone, or even as an intracrine hormone system. Angiotensin-converting enzyme has a wide distribution, being found in high concentration not only in endothelial cells but also in epithelial transporting cells in the gastrointestinal and reproductive tracts and in neuronal cells (see *Chapters 10,41,45–47,49, and 50*). In addition to its wide distribution, converting enzyme is also a rather promiscuous enzyme, with a wide substrate susceptibility [15,28–30] (see *Chapter 10*). The enzyme will act not only as a dipeptidase on Ang I and bradykinin, but is also capable of hydrolyzing enkephalins and neurotensin. Furthermore, it functions as an endopeptidase by degrading substance P and luteinizing hormone releasing hormone *in vitro*. Whether these peptides are endogenous and physiologically important substrates has yet to be established, but it does raise the possibility that the enzyme may have different actions in different tissues. Except for the testis, however, ACE appears to be the same enzyme in all tissues studied and with the same catalytic properties [14,15,30]. In the testis, the enzyme is known

ACE inhibitor	Enzymic IC$_{50}$ (M)	ACE inhibitor	Binding displacement ID$_{50}$ (M)
quinaprilat	5.5×10^{-11}	quinaprilat	4.5×10^{-11}
cilazaprilat	8.0×10^{-10}	benazeprilat	4.8×10^{-11}
benazeprilat	1.3×10^{-9}	cilazaprilat	6.5×10^{-11}
utibaprilat	1.4×10^{-9}	ramiprilat	7.0×10^{-11}
perindoprilat	1.8×10^{-9}	lisinopril	1.7×10^{-10}
ramiprilat	1.9×10^{-9}	perindoprilat	2.5×10^{-10}
zabiciprilat	2.7×10^{-9}	utibaprilat	3.6×10^{-10}
lisinopril	4.5×10^{-9}	fosenoprilat	5.1×10^{-10}
enalaprilat	4.5×10^{-9}	enalaprilat	1.1×10^{-9}
spiraprilat	7.0×10^{-9}	captopril	1.6×10^{-9}
fosenoprilat	1.6×10^{-8}		
captopril	2.2×10^{-8}		

Fig. 87.4 Concentration of ACE inhibitors required to inhibit 50% of enzymic activities of human plasma ACE (IC$_{50}$) compared with the concentration needed to displace 50% of the radioligand ^{125}I 351 A (ID$_{50}$).

to be composed of only one unit with the carboxy-terminal catalytic site [14,16] (see *Chapter 47*).

The inhibitors of ACE block the enzyme in tissue in the same fashion and in the same rank order of potency as they do the enzyme derived from plasma [31]. This is shown for a panel of ACE inhibitors against a variety of tissues in Fig. 87.5. One can also demonstrate that following oral administration of ACE inhibitors, the enzyme is inhibited in a variety of tissues [32]. This is quantified for enalapril in Fig. 87.6 and illustrated by color-coded computerized *in vitro* autoradiograph in Plate 55. However, the degree of inhibition in the various tissues does vary and there are differences with different inhibitors [32,33,34].

The above data have given rise to the concept of variable tissue bioavailability of the various ACE inhibitors [1,30]. The degree of inhibition of the enzyme in different tissues depends on a number of factors [Fig. 87.7] including plasma concentration of the prodrug and diacid, the lipid solubility of the prodrug and the diacid, tissue penetration and whether there are active transport systems, the ability of different tissues to deesterify the compounds, and the presence of blood–tissue barriers such as the blood–brain and blood–testicular barriers. Although many of the ACE inhibitors that are esterified prodrugs are lipophilic, their active diacids generally are hydrophilic. It has been shown that many tissues besides the gut and liver contain esterases capable of converting the prodrugs to their active diacids and that the rate of deesterification does vary among the different compounds. It is theoretically possible therefore that compounds could be developed with limited access to some tissues that contain ACE. This is particularly so for the brain. It can be demonstrated that some compounds (captopril, ramipril,

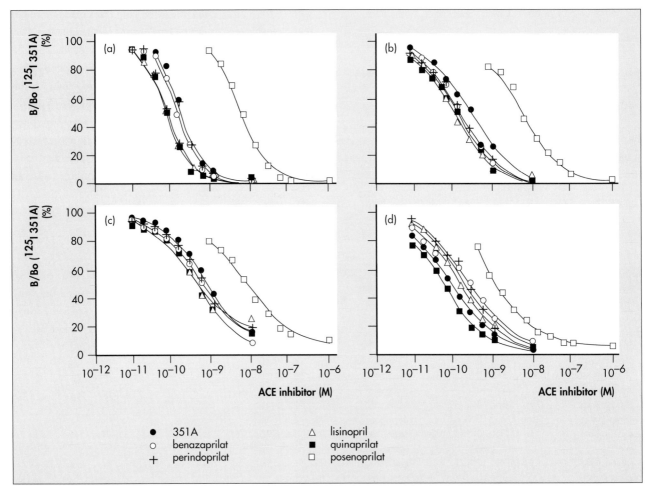

Fig. 87.5 Displacement of radioligand bound to ACE derived from rat plasma (a), lung (b), heart (c), and kidney (d) by six different ACE inhibitors.

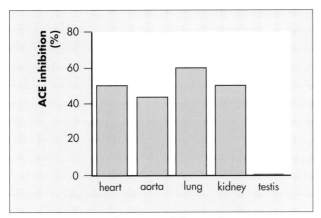

Fig. 87.6 Inhibition of tissue ACE following chronic administration of enalapril (10mg/kg/d) to rats. Tissue ACE was measured by quantitative *in vitro* autoradiography.

plasma concentration
lipid solubility
  prodrug
  diacid
tissue penetration
  lipophilicity
  specific uptake mechanism
tissue esterase activity
blood–tissue barriers
  blood–brain
  blood–testis

Fig. 87.7 Factors important in determining the bioavailability of ACE inhibitors and their prodrug form.

oral absorption/bioavailability
prodrug: biotransformation
lipophilicity
enzyme: inhibitor kinetics
  affinity (tight)
  off rate
protein binding
tissue bioavailability
metabolism
  active metabolites
  inactive metabolites
route of elimination
  hepatic excretion
  renal excretion

Fig. 87.8 Pharmacokinetic properties that distinguish between individual ACE inhibitors.

enalapril) will cross the blood–brain–barrier, whereas others (quinapril, benazapril) do not appear to do so, even after prolonged administration. This raises the question of whether the antihypertensive action of the ACE inhibitors is due to inhibition of the plasma and endothelial enzyme or whether it is dependent on also inhibiting tissue ACE in other important organs (brain, vessels, heart, kidney, adrenals). The binding of ACE inhibitors to the tissue enzyme has a very important influence on the pharmacokinetic characteristics of the individual inhibitors (see below).

PHARMACOKINETICS

It is in the field of pharmacokinetic characteristics that the ACE inhibitors vary the most [35,36]. Some of the important considerations determining the pharmacokinetics of this class of drugs are shown in Fig. 87.8. Most of the newer drugs are prodrugs that require biotransformation and are esterified to increase their gastrointestinal absorption. However, captopril, lisinopril, and ceranopril are not prodrugs and do not require deesterification. Their absorption, therefore, is influenced somewhat by meals. Most of the biotransformation in man takes place either across the gastrointestinal tract or in the liver. However, other tissues do contain esterases [37] that are capable of deesterifying these compounds. This may allow access of the prodrug to some tissues from which the active compounds would otherwise be excluded. Tissue distribution and bioavailability are dependent also on lipophilicity. This is particularly important in regard to the blood–brain barrier

Many of the ACE inhibitors are protein bound in plasma, although the significance of this in determining pharmacokinetic characteristics is doubtful, since the affinity of the inhibitors for the enzyme is far greater than that for plasma proteins.

Lisinopril does not undergo metabolism in the body and is excreted intact. Captopril, however, and other sulfhydryl-containing ACE inhibitors undergo quite complex transformation, in part because the sulfhydryl group binds to cysteine and other reducing compounds and proteins. This complicates their pharmacokinetics considerably. Captopril is converted into a series of inactive compounds in a reversible fashion which provides a depot for the drug [38]. Some of the other compounds (perindopril, spirapril, for example) are metabolized to inactive substances.

The majority of the ACE inhibitors are excreted through the kidney both by glomerular filtration and tubular secretion

[39,40]. For this reason, the dose of nearly all the ACE inhibitors should be calculated according to the level of the glomerular filtration rate (GFR). An exception is probably spirapril which is excreted in the bile. Although ramipril, quinapril, zofenopril, benazapril, and fosinopril have some hepatic inactivation, this is not sufficient to prevent drug accumulation in renal failure.

The pharmacokinetics of ACE inhibitors is complex because of varying volumes of distribution, complex metabolic pathways for some, but most importantly, because of binding of the inhibitors to tissue ACE [41,42]. In general, the detailed pharmacokinetics of the ACE inhibitors are best described by a distribution phase, followed by an initial elimination phase of between two and six hours, and then a prolonged terminal washout phase lasting many hours, often for more than 24 hours. Presumably, the long terminal washout is due to the slow dissociation of the inhibitors from tissue ACE. It is probable that the slow off rate of the inhibitor from the enzyme accounts for the long duration of action of these compounds. Apart from captopril, pivalopril, and pentopril, the other ACE inhibitors can be given once daily to patients with hypertension. A list of the important pharmacokinetic parameters for individual drugs that are in clinical use, is detailed in Fig. 87.9.

PHARMACODYNAMICS

It is likely that the pharmacodynamics of the ACE inhibitors as a group will be very similar since their effects are dependent upon inhibition of the same enzyme (however, see *Chapter 98*). The pharmacodynamic changes associated with the administration of ACE inhibitors are summarized in Fig. 87.10 and are described in detail for essential hypertension in *Chapter 91*, heart failure in *Chapter 93*, and for various other disorders as shown in the *Contents* of this book. Responses, particularly in hemodynamic indices, can differ between disorders, but a broad overview is now presented.

HEMODYNAMICS

All of the ACE inhibitors have been shown to reduce blood pressure by decreasing total peripheral resistance. This is usually associated with little or no increase in cardiac output and no change in heart rate [43,44]. This characteristic lack of reflex tachycardia is probably due to the interaction of Ang II with the sympathetic nervous system [45,46] and also the parasympathetic system (see *Chapter 37*). There is sometimes a small

fall in central venous pressure which may be particularly beneficial in patients with heart failure. Vasodilatation is greatest in the cerebral, coronary and renal vasculature. Cerebral autoregulation is reset to lower levels of arterial pressure which probably accounts for the rarity of postural symptoms and syncope when the blood pressure is reduced with these drugs. Although renal blood flow may be slightly increased, the GFR generally remains the same. There are rarely hypotensive postural effects. Although unusual, tachycardia has been reported [96] during chronic therapy. The normal hemodynamic responses to exercise are maintained during treatment with ACE inhibitors.

In patients with hypertension, it has been shown that the ACE inhibitors are associated with an increase in arterial compliance [47] and with regression of vascular and cardiac hypertrophy (see *Chapters 94–96*).

HORMONAL CHANGES

The hormonal changes include a decrease in plasma Ang II and aldosterone with reciprocal rises in plasma renin and Ang I [48–50,96]. The increase in plasma renin is due probably to both a fall in blood-pressure activating renal baroreceptors and removal of the inhibitory action of Ang II on renin release (see *Chapter 24*). Plasma renin reaches very high levels in patients treated in the long term with ACE inhibitors, and it has been shown that the reactive hyperreninemia reflects the level of plasma Ang II during chronic ACE inhibition [51]. It has been shown that plasma levels of renin substrate (angiotensinogen) are reduced during sustained treatment with ACE inhibitors.

Consistent changes in the kallikrein–kinin system have been more difficult to establish. Urinary kallikrein excretion has been shown to be reduced, but no consistent changes have been reported in plasma or urinary kinins. Studies using specific bradykinin antagonists, however, do suggest that part of the pharmacodynamic response of ACE inhibitors may be due to inhibition of bradykinin breakdown [52–55]. There are varying reports on the effects of ACE inhibitors on prostaglandins [56–58] see (*Chapter 38*) but no consistent pattern has emerged.

METABOLIC EFFECTS

Angiotensin-converting enzyme inhibitors are considered to have favorable metabolic effects. They correct the hypokalemia and other metabolic abnormalities induced by diuretics in patients with essential hypertension [59] (see *Chapter 91*). They have little effect on plasma lipid concentrations [60] and have been shown to increase insulin sensitivity [61].

Ligand	Prodrug	Bio-availability (%)	Time to maximum concentration (h)	Protein binding	Route of elimination	Daily dosage (mg)	Administration per day
sulfhydryl							
captopril	no	70	0.5–1.0		renal	25–100	twice
alacepril	yes		1.0		gastrointestinal/renal	25–100	once
fentiapril	no				renal	7.5–30	once
pivalopril	yes					10–50	twice
zofenopril	yes	80		85	renal/liver	5–10	once
carboxyl							
enalapril	yes	50	1.0		renal	5–40	once
lisinopril	no	25	5.0		renal	10–80	once
ramipril	yes	60	2.5	60	renal	25–10	once
perindopril	yes	70	2.0	20	renal	4–8	once
cilazapril	yes	55	1.0		renal/gastrointestinal	25–10	once
quinapril	yes	75	1.5	35	renal/liver	5–20	once
bunazepril	yes	80		95	renal/liver	5–20	
spirapril	yes	80	2.0		liver	12.5–50	once
delapril	yes				kidney	30–60	once
pentopril	yes					125–200	twice
trandopril	yes						
phosphinyl							
fosinopril	yes	25	3.0	95	liver/gastrointestinal/renal	5–40	once
ceronapril	no	40	10.0		renal		once

Fig. 87.9 Comparative pharmacokinetic parameters for individual ACE inhibitors in clinical use.

hemodynamic
↓ blood pressure
↓ total peripheral resistance
↑ in cerebral, renal, coronary blood flow
=↑ cardiac output
= heart rate
↓ arterial compliance
renal
↑ renal blood flow
= glomerular filtration rate
   diuresis and natriuresis
regression of vascular and cardiac hypertrophy
hormonal changes
↓ Ang II
↑ Ang I
↑ renin
↓ renin substrate
↓ aldosterone
= blood kinins
↑ urinary kinins
? prostaglandins
metabolic effects
↓ exchangeable sodium
↑ plasma potassium
↓ plasma uric acid
↑ insulin sensitivity

Fig. 87.10 Hemodynamic, hormonal, structural, renal, and metabolic effects of ACE inhibitors. ↑, increased; ↓, decreased; =, no change; ?, uncertain.

MODE OF ACTION

Despite the fact that ACE inhibitors have been in clinical use for over 10 years, it is still not clear and certainly not agreed upon, how they reduce blood pressure [62,63]. It is generally accepted that the acute hypotensive response is due to a fall in circulating levels of Ang II. The long-term effects on blood pressure, however, do not correlate closely with the fall in plasma Ang II. It is apparent that the antihypertensive effect of ACE inhibitors is complex and probably involves inhibition of tissue ACE. The difficulty in defining the factors that determine their effects on blood pressure is compounded by the fact that ACE has multiple substrates and that Ang II has multiple biological actions and also interacts with the kallikrein–kinin, sympathetic, prostaglandin, and atrial natriuretic factor (ANF) systems (see *Chapters 36–38*). There may also be induction of converting enzyme during chronic therapy. Furthermore, the pharmacokinetics of the compounds are complex due to variable

tissue binding, and their inhibition of tissue ACE, especially within the brain, varies between the individual compounds. It has been shown for example, that whereas enalapril crosses the blood–brain barrier and inhibits brain ACE, quinapril, even after two weeks of oral dosing, is unable to inhibit brain ACE. Since the two agents have similar antihypertensive effects, this suggests that inhibition of brain ACE is not essential for the hypotensive action of all ACE inhibitors. Overall, and despite the complex issues discussed above, the evidence suggests that suppression of plasma Ang II may still be an important component of the hypotensive action of ACE inhibitors during chronic therapy [41,64–67,96].

Several other mechanisms have been proposed as contributing to the long-term hypotensive effects of ACE inhibitors (Fig. 87.11). As outlined above, the development of specific bradykinin-receptor antagonists has given some indication that inhibition of bradykinin breakdown may be involved in the antihypertensive effects of ACE inhibitors [52–55].

An important component in the long-term antihypertensive effect of ACE inhibitors is likely to be their interaction with the sympathetic nervous system [45,46] (see *Chapter 37*). Angiotensin II interacts at several levels with the sympathetic nervous system. In the periphery, its most important action is probably the facilitation of norepinephrine release from

inhibition of the RAS
   plasma (endocrine)
   tissue (autocrine, paracrine)
   central versus peripheral
   interaction with sympathetic and
   parasympathetic systems
potentiation of the kallikrein–kinin system
   circulating kinins
   local kinins
   prostaglandin interactions
aldosterone–sodium homeostasis
stimulation of the prostaglandin system
suppression of the sympathetic nervous system
   peripheral
   central
effects on other peptides including neuropeptides

Fig. 87.11 Proposed mechanisms for the antihypertensive effect of ACE inhibitors.

adrenergic nerve endings. Removal of Ang II during ACE inhibition probably therefore suppresses peripheral sympathetic nerve activity and thereby contributes to the long-term antihypertensive action of these agents. The effects of ACE inhibitors on sympathetic activity have received scant attention, as have their interactions with the parasympathetic system (see *Chapter 37*).

Since the renin–angiotensin–aldosterone system is important in sodium homeostasis (see *Chapter 74*), suppression of Ang II levels and a tendency for aldosterone levels to fall during ACE inhibition often results in a state of negative sodium balance provided, of course, that arterial (and renal perfusion) pressure is not reduced excessively (see *Chapter 26*). This effect on sodium balance may contribute importantly to the long-term antihypertensive action of the ACE inhibitors [96]. Lastly, it is possible that the ACE inhibitors affect the metabolism of other neuropeptides in the brain or periphery which could influence blood-pressure control.

NEWER ANGIOTENSIN-CONVERTING ENZYME INHIBITORS

The number of new ACE inhibitors under development is impossible to determine but must approach 100. This section deals only with those agents that in 1992 were in phase III clinical trials or about to be released for clinical use. As the pharmacokinetics, pharmacodynamics, and clinical usage of captopril [68], enalapril [69], and lisinopril [70] have been covered more than adequately in review articles [1–3], and have formed the basis for most of this chapter so far, they will not be discussed here. When evaluating new ACE-inhibiting compounds, the properties shown in Fig. 87.12 need to be kept in mind [1,35]. In general, most developments have involved changes in the zinc-binding ligand, and increased bioavailability or prolongation of action. Many of the details of these can be found in the reviews by de Felice and Kortis [71] and Salvetti [36].

ALACEPRIL

Alacepril [72] is a derivative of captopril and is converted to captopril in the body. It has very similar pharmacokinetics to captopril, with oral absorption of approximately 67% and a plasma half-life of 2.6 hours. Like captopril, intestinal absorption of the drug is delayed by concomitant ingestion of food.

Compared with captopril, the onset of its effect on blood pressure is slightly delayed, but the duration of its antihypertensive action is longer.

pharmaceutical chemistry
   zinc ligand
   prodrug
biochemistry
   competitive kinetics
   noncompetitive inhibition of ACE
   affinity and potency
   lipophilicity
pharmacokinetics
   biotransformation of prodrug
   absorption and bioavailability
   distribution volume
   metabolism: active plus inactive metabolites
   route of elimination
      liver
      bile
      renal
   duration of action
tissue distribution
   ester prodrug
   tissue esterases
   active diacid
   blood–brain barrier
   blood–testicular barrier
substrate specificity
other peptide or enzymes
efficacy
adverse reactions
drug interactions
other additional actions
   prostaglandins
   free-radical scavenger

Fig. 87.12 Properties that distinguish between different ACE inhibitors.

BENAZAPRIL

Benazapril [73] is one of the most potent of the new ACE inhibitors. It is a prodrug that is rapidly and completely absorbed and is converted to the active diacid benazaprilat. Pharmacokinetics show polyphasic elimination with a very long terminal half-life. It is extensively bound to plasma protein and is eliminated predominantly by the kidney, although there is some metabolism of the drug to acylglucuronides. The dose should be reduced in patients with severe renal failure. Benazapril has been shown to be effective in treating patients with hypertension. Furthermore, it has a sustained inhibitory effect on ACE and can be used in a once-daily dosage.

CERANOPRIL

Ceranopril [4] is a phosphorus-containing ACE inhibitor. Unlike fosinopril, however, it is not a prodrug, it is well absorbed, and no biotransformation occurs. It is, like captopril and lisinopril, active in its own right. It is slightly more potent than captopril and has a much longer duration of action. Being lipophilic, it is taken up well by tissues and eliminated by the kidneys.

CILAZAPRIL

Cilazapril [74] is another nonsulfhydryl, bicyclic lactam prodrug that is converted by tissue esterases into the active dicarboxylic acid, cilazaprilat. It is almost completely absorbed and peak plasma concentrations are achieved at 1–2 hours. Inhibition of plasma ACE is rapid and prolonged, lasting more than 24 hours. Its oral absorption is slightly delayed and is reduced by food. Like most ACE inhibitors, it has fairly complex pharmacokinetics with a prolonged terminal phase. The active drug is excreted by the kidneys and plasma levels are inversely related to creatinine clearance, hence there should be an adjustment of dose in patients with reduced renal function. It is efficacious in the treatment of hypertension and congestive heart failure.

DELAPRIL

Delapril [75] was developed in Japan and is a nonsulfhydryl ester prodrug. Unlike the other ACE inhibitors, it contains an indane ring in place of proline. It is deesterified to the active diacid and also undergoes some further metabolism to both active (5-hydroxy derivative) and inactive compounds. It is approximately eight times more potent than captopril. The drug is rapidly absorbed in man, reaching a peak plasma concentration at one hour. The diacid appears a few hours later and an active 5-hydroxy metabolite has a peak plasma concentration at 2–3 hours. Despite the fact that the plasma half-life is short, inhibition of plasma ACE is prolonged. This is probably due to interconversion between the prodrug and the active metabolites. Although in animals there is some evidence for extrarenal metabolism and excretion of delapril, in man, the majority appears to be eliminated by the renal route and therefore a lower dose is necessary in patients with renal impairment. Delapril has been shown in clinical trials to be an effective antihypertensive agent.

FOSINOPRIL

Fosinopril [76] is a phosphorus zinc-binding inhibitor that has reached clinical development. It is slightly more potent than captopril but not as potent as the newer carboxylated dipeptides.

Its absorption is rapid and complete and is not influenced by food. The prodrug is converted by tissue esterases into the active compound, fosinoprilat, which reaches peak plasma concentrations within 2–3 hours. It produces prolonged inhibition of serum and tissue ACE. After a single oral dose, inhibition of serum and tissue ACE is sustained for longer than 24 hours. Fosinopril has been shown to be effective in lowering the blood pressure in hypertensive animals and man. It need be administered only once daily.

PERINDOPRIL

Perindopril [77] is a nonsulfhydryl, carboxylated dipeptide ACE inhibitor that is significantly more potent than enalapril, captopril, or lisinopril. It is a prodrug that is well absorbed, and then converted *in vivo* to the active diacid. Peak blood concentrations are achieved approximately 2–4 hours after ingestion, and inhibition of plasma and tissue ACE is prolonged. The drug has polyphasic pharmacokinetics. Excretion is mainly through the kidneys, so the dose should be reduced when given to patients with renal insufficiency. Extensive clinical trials have shown the drug to be effective in patients with hypertension or heart failure.

QUINAPRIL

Quinapril [78], another carboxylated dipeptide, is one of the most potent of the new prodrug ACE inhibitors. Oral absorption, which is approximately 60%, is not significantly altered by food. The drug is extensively converted into the active diacid quinaprilat and bound to plasma protein. Although it has a relatively short plasma half-life, the tissue half-life is probably prolonged. Quinapril produces a sustained inhibition of serum and plasma ACE, and studies in man show that its hypotensive effect lasts for at least 24 hours. Since excretion is largely by the kidneys, the dose needs to be decreased in patients with renal impairment. Quinapril is effective in the treatment of both hypertension and heart failure.

RAMIPRIL

Ramipril [79] is a another potent carboxylated dipeptide inhibitor prodrug. It is rapidly absorbed with a bioavailability of approximately 60%. It is then metabolized very rapidly and readily to the active diacid ramaprilat which is said to form an enzyme–inhibitor complex with a slow rate of dissociation, which accounts for its long antihypertensive action. Peak serum concentrations of the active drug are attained approximately two hours after ingestion and, again, pharmacokinetics are polyphasic with a very prolonged terminal half-life. It is excreted mainly by the kidneys and dosage adjustments are necessary in patients with renal failure. Ramipril is effective in hypertension and in heart failure.

SPIRAPRIL

Spirapril [80] is a monoethyl prodrug that is slightly more potent than enalapril and lisinopril. It is well absorbed from the gastrointestinal tract, has a relatively long half-life, and is transformed in the body to spiraprilat which has a short plasma half-life. Spiraprilat, unlike the other carboxylated dipeptides, undergoes metabolism in the body and is excreted mainly by the liver. Its antihypertensive action is prolonged, thus the drug can be administered once per day.

ZOFENOPRIL

Zofenopril [81], like captopril and alacepril, is a sulfhydryl-containing ACE inhibitor. The prodrug, however, is more lipophilic than captopril, which accounts for its rapid and complete absorption. It undergoes conversion to the active compound, zofenoprilat, in both the gut wall and liver. Peak blood concentrations of zofenoprilat occur approximately one hour after dosing and it is extensively bound to plasma proteins. Its volume of distribution is approximately twice that of captopril. Although zofenoprilat is eliminated by the kidneys and by the liver, its elimination is slowed in renal failure, hence drug dosage should be reduced in patients with renal insufficiency. It has a longer half-life and greater potency than captopril.

SUMMARY

The new sulfhydryl-containing ACE inhibitors (alacepril, zofenopril) are prodrugs that are converted *in vivo* to active metabolites. Compared with captopril, they have better bioavailability and a longer duration of action. Ceranopril, a phosphorus-containing ACE inhibitor, like captopril and lisinopril, is not a prodrug. The newer carboxylated dipeptides are all prodrugs, are generally very potent, and have a prolonged duration of action. All of them are eliminated by the kidneys except spirapril which is eliminated almost entirely by the liver. The phosphorus-containing ACE inhibitors are a new chemical class. Fosinopril is a prodrug but ceranopril is not. They are not much more potent than captopril but have a much longer half-life and slower onset of action. Fosinopril is partially eliminated by the liver but ceranopril appears to be eliminated by the kidneys.

ADDITIONAL CHARACTERISTICS AND DRUG INTERACTIONS

It has been postulated that some of the ACE inhibitors may have additional actions beyond inhibition of ACE. It is also claimed that some of them may have specific selectivity for tissue ACE. This is particularly true for some of the newer sulfhydryl and phosphonyl compounds which are said to inhibit cardiac ACE more than do other ACE inhibitors (37). Similarly, ramipril is reported to provide cardioprotection at doses that do not inhibit systemic plasma ACE. Other studies, however, show that the distribution of ACE inhibition is fairly uniform in various tissues and is dose and time dependent [31,32]. An additional claim is that the cardioprotection afforded by ramipril under experimental circumstances is bradykinin dependent, and that some of the cardiac actions of ACE inhibition are due to accumulation of bradykinin [82]. With the development of new methods for studying bradykinin, it should become apparent whether some of the actions and adverse reactions of the ACE inhibitors are due to bradykinin accumulation. It is to be hoped that studies with specific bradykinin-receptor antagonists will be definitive in this regard.

A number of reports indicate that the sulfhydryl-containing ACE inhibitors can act as free-oxygen scavengers [83,84]. Whereas it is true that these drugs can indeed scavenge free radicals, they are relatively weak compared with more conventional scavengers. The data on whether or not significant cardioprotection from ACE inhibition is due to free radical scavenging alone, are very controversial.

Another action that has been reported to be specific for sulfhydryl-containing ACE inhibitors is their ability to prevent nitrate intolerance [85]. This is thought by some, but not all, to be specifically dependent upon the sulfhydryl group. There are dissenting reports [86] so further studies are needed in this area (see *Chapter 98*).

Very few drug interactions have been reported for ACE inhibitors compared with other antihypertensive compounds [87]. Probably the most important is the interaction with diuretics. The ACE inhibitors have been shown to blunt or reverse the 'metabolic' effects of diuretics (see *Chapter 91*). Furthermore, diuretics potentiate the antihypertensive effect of ACE inhibitors. In patients who are treated with diuretics, the introduction of ACE inhibitors can occasionally cause symptomatic hypotension, thus it is preferable to stop, or reduce the dose of diuretics before introducing the ACE inhibitor. A more important adverse interaction is with potassium-sparing diuretics. Co-administration of an ACE inhibitor and a potassium-sparing diuretic may cause or aggravate hyperkalemia. This is particularly so in elderly patients and in those with reduced renal function. Patients treated with nonsteroidal anti-inflammatory agents may also develop hyperkalemia if an ACE inhibitor is introduced, and renal function can deteriorate (see *Chapter 99*). Nonsteroidal anti-inflammatory agents have been reported to blunt the antihypertensive effect of ACE inhibitors but this is nonspecific as they also blunt the hypotensive effect of many other classes of antihypertensive agents. Probenecid reduces the renal excretion of captopril and therefore increases its blood level. The ACE inhibitors have been reported to raise plasma lithium levels and induce lithium toxicity. There appears to be no interaction with the β-blockers, and the metabolic conversion of ACE inhibitors is little affected by β-blockade or impairment in liver function.

FUTURE DEVELOPMENTS

There are already in development, formulations that combine a conventional thiazide diuretic with an ACE inhibitor, which should prove useful in respect to compliance with therapy. More innovative is the development of a compound that is both a direct nitroso vasodilator and an ACE inhibitor [89]. The synthesis of a compound which inhibits both ACE and the enzyme neutral endopeptidase, which is responsible for the degradation

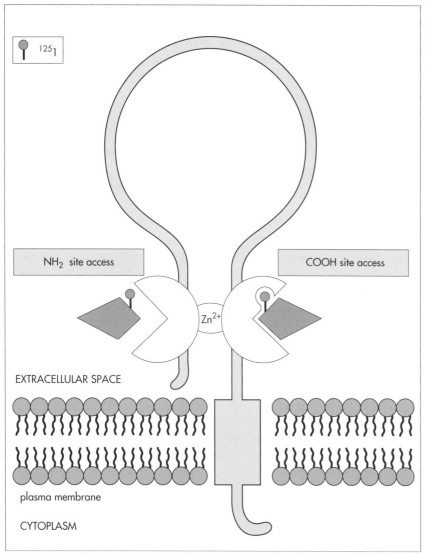

Fig. 87.13 Theoretical model of the two active sites of ACE with the different, restricted conformation requirements for each site.

of ANF is also of great potential therapeutic significance [90]. There are a large number of interactions between the RAS and ANF [91,92] (see *Chapter 36*). Atrial natriuretic factors can be regarded as endogenous inhibitors of the RAS, and an increase in circulating ANF is likely to induce a natriuresis and diuresis without activating the RAS.

Angiotensin-converting enzyme inhibitors are being evaluated further with regard to cardioprotection, renoprotection, and vasculoprotection. There are reports that captopril may be protective against experimental atherosclerosis [93]. A further exciting development is the realization that the endothelial cell is vitally important in vessel health and disease (see *Chapter 29*); contains a high concentration of ACE; and is easily damaged by high pressure, shear stress, and lipids, and that ACE inhibitors may protect against this damage [94,95].

The realization that ACE has two distinct active sites which differ in some of their characteristics (Fig. 87.13) should make possible the development of more specific inhibitors [17] that have access to and block only one catalytic site.

Such specific blockers of ACE may have more discrete effects than currently available ACE inhibitors, and their side-effect profile may prove superior.

REFERENCES

1. Johnston CI. Angiotensin-converting enzyme inhibitors. In: Doyle AE, ed. *Handbook of hypertension, volume II, second edition: Clinical pharmacology of antihypertensive drugs.* Amsterdam: Elsevier, 1988; 301–26.

2. Waeber B, Nussberger J, Brunner HR. Angiotensin-converting enzyme inhibitors in hypertension. In: Laragh JH, Brenner BM, eds. *Hypertension: Pathophysiology, diagnosis and management.* New York: Raven Press, 1990:2209–32.

3. Unger T, Gohlke P, Gruber M-G. Converting enzyme inhibitors. In: Ganten D, Mulrow PJ, eds. *Handbook of experimental pharmacology, volume 93.* Berlin: Springer-Verlag, 1990: 379–480.

4. Ondetti MA. Structural relationships of angiotensin converting enzyme inhibitors to pharmacologic activity. *Circulation* 1988;77 (suppl 1):I74–8.

5. Cushman DW, Ondetti MA. Personal and historical perspectives: History of the design of captopril and related inhibitors of angiotensin converting enzyme. *Hypertension,* 1991;17:589–92.

6. Cushman DW, Ondetti MA, Gordon EM, Natarajan S, Karanewsky DS, Krapcho J, Petrillo EW Jr. Rational design and biochemical utility of specific inhibitors of angiotensin-converting enzyme. *Journal of Cardiovascular Pharmacology.* 1987;10 (suppl 7):S17–30.

7. Patchett AA, Harris E, Tristram EW, Wyvratt MJ, Wu MT, Taub D, Peterson ER, Ikeler TJ, ten Broeke J, Payne LG, Ondeyka DL, Thorsett ED, Greenlee WJ, Lohr NS, Hoffsommer RD, Joshua H, Ruyle WV, Rothrock JW, Aster SD, Maycock AL, Robinson FM, Hirshmann R, Sweet CS, Ulm EH, Gross DM, Vassil TC, Stone CA. A new class of angiotensin-converting enzyme inhibitors. *Nature* 1980;288:280–3.

8. Cohen ML. Synthetic and fermentation-derived angiotensin-converting enzyme inhibitors. *Annual Review of Pharmacology and Toxicology* 1985;25:307–25.

9. Wyvratt MJ, Patchett AA. Recent developments in the design of angiotensin-converting enzyme inhibitors. *Medicinal Research Reviews* 1985;5:483–531.

10. Petrillo, EW Jr, Powell JR, Cushman DW, Ondetti MA. Angiotensin converting enzyme inhibitors: Accomplishments and challenges. *Clinical and Experimental Hypertension. Part A — Theory and Practice* 1987;[A] 9: 235–41.

11. Soubrier F, Alhenc-Gelas F, Hubert C, Allegrini J, John M, Tregear G, Corvol P. Two putative active centres in human angiotensin I-converting enzyme revealed by molecular cloning. *Proceedings of the National Academy of Sciences of the USA.* 1988;85:9386–90.

12. Wei L, Alhenc-Gelas F, Corvol P, Clauser E. The two homologous domains of human angiotensin I-converting enzyme are both catalytically active. *Journal of Biological Chemistry* 1991;266:9002–8.

13. Wei L, Alhenc-Gelas F, Soubrier F, Michaud A, Corvol P, Clauser E. Expression and characterization of recombinant human angiotensin I-converting enzyme. Evidence for a C-terminal transmembrane anchor and for a proteolytic processing of the secreted recombinant and plasma enzymes. *Journal of Biological Chemistry* 1991;266:5540–6.

14. Soubrier F, Hubert C, Wei L, Rigat B, Clauser E, Alhenc-Gelas F, Corvol P. Recent advances in molecular biology and biochemistry of the human angiotensin I converting enzyme. In: McGregor G, Sever P, eds. *Current advances in ACE inhibition, volume 2.* London: Churchill Livingstone, 1991;125–30.

15. Ehlers MRW, Riordan JF. Angiotensin-converting enzyme: New concepts concerning its biological role. *Biochemistry* 1989;28:5311–8.

16. Ehlers MRW, Riordan JF. Angiotensin-converting enzyme: Zinc- and inhibitor-binding stoichiometries of the somatic and testis isozymes. *Biochemistry* 1991;30:7118–26.

17. Perich RB, Jackson B, Attwood MR, Prior K, Johnsont CI. Angiotensin converting enzyme inhibitors act at two different binding sites on angiotensin converting enzyme. *Pharmaceutical and Pharmacology Letters* 1991;1:41-3.

18. Juillerat L, Nussberger J, Menard J, Mooser V, Christen, Y, Waeber B, Graf P, Brunner HR. Determinants of angiotensin II generation during converting enzyme inhibition. *Hypertension* 1990;16:564–72.

19. Johnston CI, Jackson B, Cubela R, Larmour I, Arnolda L. Evaluation of angiotensin converting enzyme (ACE) in the pharmacokinetics and pharmacodynamics of ACE inhibitors. *Journal of Cardiovascular Pharmacology* 1986;8 (suppl 1):S9–S14.

20. Jackson B, Cubela RB, Johnston CI. Inhibition of tissue angiotensin converting enzyme by perindopril: *In vivo* assessment in the rat using radioinhibitor binding displacement *Journal of Pharmacology and Experimental Therapeutics* 1988:245:950–5.

21. Strittmatter SM, Kapiloff MS, Snyder SH. [^{3}H] Captopril binding to membrane associated angiotensin converting enzyme. *Biochemistry and Biophysical Research Communications* 1983;112:1027–33.

22. Fyhrquist F, Tikkanen I, Gronhagen-Riska C, Hortling L, Hichens M. Inhibitor binding assay for angiotensin-converting enzyme. *Clinical Chemistry* 1984;30:696–700.

23. Campbell DJ. Circulating and tissue angiotensin systems. *Journal of Clinical Investigation* 1987;79:1–6.

24. Dzau VJ. Circulating versus local renin–angiotensin system in cardiovascular homeostasis. *Circulation* 1988;77 (suppl 1):I4–13.

25. Unger T, Gohlke P. Tissue renin–angiotensin systems in the heart and vasculature: Possible involvement in the cardiovascular actions of converting enzyme inhibitors. *American Journal of Cardiology* 1990;65:3–10I.

26. Swales JD, Samani NJ. Localisation and physiological effects of tissue renin–angiotensin systems. *Journal of Human Hypertension* 1989;3 (suppl 1):71–7.

27. Johnston CI. Biochemistry and pharmacology of the renin-angiotensin system. *Drugs* 1990;39 (suppl 1):21–31.

28. Erdos EG, Skidgel RA. The angiotensin I-converting enzyme. *Laboratory Investigation* 1987;56:345–8.

29. Erdos EG. Angiotensin I converting enzyme and the changes in our concepts through the years. *Hypertension* 1990;16:363–7.

30. Johnston CI, Kohzuki K. Angiotensin converting enzyme: Localization, regulation and inhibition. In: MacGregor GA, Sever PS, eds. *Current advances in ACE inhibition* London: Churchill Livingstone, 1989;3–7.

31. Johnston CI, Mendelsohn FAO, Cubela RB, Jackson B, Kohzuki M, Fabris B. Inhibition of angiotensin converting enzyme (ACE) in plasma and tissues: Studies *ex-vivo* after administration of ACE inhibitors. *Journal of Hypertension* 1988;6 (suppl 3):S17–22.

32. Johnston CI, Fabris B, Yamada H, Mendelsohn FAO, Cubela R, Sivell D, Jackson B. Comparative studies of tissue inhibition by angiotensin converting enzyme inhibitors. *Journal of Hypertension* 1989:7 (suppl 5):S11–6.

33. Cushman DW, Wang FL, Fung WC, Harvey CM, DeForrest JM. Differentiation of angiotensin-converting enzyme (ACE) inhibitors by their selective inhibition of ACE in physiologically important target organs. *American Journal of Hypertension* 1989;2:294–306.

34. Sakaguchi K, Chai SY, Jackson B, Johnston CI, Mendelsohn FAO. Inhibition of tissue angiotensin converting enzyme : Quantitation by autoradiography. *Hypertension* 1988;11:230–8.

35. Kostis JB. Angiotensin converting enzyme inhibitors. *American Journal of Hypertension* 1989;2:57–64.

36. Salvetti A. Newer ACE inhibitors. A look at the future. *Drugs* 1990;40:800–28.

37. Grover GJ, Sleph PG, Dzwonczyk, S, Wang P, Fung W, Tobias D, Cushman DW. Effects of different angiotensin-converting enzyme (ACE) inhibitors on ischemic isolated rat hearts: Relationship between cardiac ACE inhibition and cardioprotection. *Journal of Pharmacology and Experimental Therapeutics* 1991;257:919–29.

38. Drummer OH, Jarrott B, The disposition and metabolism of captopril *Medicinal Research Reviews* 1986;6:75–97.

39. Begg EJ, Bailey RR, Lynn KL, Robson RA, Frank GJ, Olson SC. The pharamacokinetics of angiotensin converting enzyme inhibitors in patients with renal impairment. *Journal of Hypertension* 1989;5 (suppl 7):S29–32.

40. Sica DA, Cutler RE, Parmer RJ, Ford NF. Comparison of the steady-state pharmacokinetics of fosinopril, lisinopril and enalapril in patients with chronic renal insufficiency. *Clinical Pharmacokinetics* 1991;20:420–7.

41. Francis RJ, Brown AN, Kler L, Fasanella d'Amore T, Nussberger J, Waeber B, Brunner HR. Pharmacokinetics of the converting enzyme inhibitor cilazapril in normal volunteers and the relationship to enzyme inhibition: Development of a mathematical model. *Journal of Cardiovascular Pharmacology* 1987;9:32–8.

42. Meredith PA, Elliott HL, Donnelly R, Reid JL. Prediction of response to antihypertensive therapy with enalapril and nifedipine. *Journal of Hypertension* 1989;7 (suppl 6):S252–3.

43. Lund-Johansen P, Omvik P. Long-term haemodynamic effects of enalapril (alone and in combination with hydrochlorothiazide) at rest and during exercise in essential hypertension. *Journal of Hypertension* 1984;2 (suppl 2):49–56.

44. Giudicelli J-F, Richer C, Richard C, Thuillez C. Angiotensin converting enzyme inhibition. Systemic and regional hemodynamics in rats and humans. *American Journal of Hypertension* 1991;4 (suppl):258S–62S.

45. Zimmerman BG. Adrenergic facilitation by angiotensin: Does it serve a physiological function? *Clinical Science* 1981;60:343–8.

46. Ajayi AA, Lees KR, Reid JL. Effects of angiotensin converting enzyme inhibitor, perindopril on autonomic reflexes. *European Journal of Clinical Pharmacology* 1986;30:177–82.

47. Simon AC, Levenson JA, Bouthier J, Maarek B, Safar ME. Effects of acute and chronic angiotensin converting enzyme inhibition on large arteries in human hypertension. *Journal of Cardiovascular Pharmacology* 1985;7 (suppl. I):S45–5.

48. Johnston CI, McGrath BP, Millar JA, Matthews PGF. Long-term effects of captopril (SQ14225) on blood pressure and hormone levels in essential hypertension. *Lancet* 1979;ii:493–6.

49. Hulthen I, Hokfelt T. The effect of the converting enzyme inhibitor SQ20.881 on kinins, renin–angiotensin–aldosterone and catecholamines in relation to blood pressure in hypertensive patients. *Acta Medica Scandinavica* 1978;204:497–502.

50. Lees KR, Reid JL. Haemodynamic and humoral effects of oral perindopril on angiotensin converting enzyme inhibitor in man. *British Journal of Clinical Pharmacology* 1987;23:159–64.

51. Mooser V, Nussberger J, Juillerat L, Burnier M, Waeber B, Bidiville J, Pauly N, Brunner HR. Reactive hyperreninemia is a major determinant of plasma angiotensin II during ACE inhibition. *Journal of Cardiovascular Pharmacology* 1990;15:276–82.

52. Clappison BH, Anderson WP, Johnston CI. Renal hemodynamic and renal kinins after angiotensin-converting enzyme inhibition. *Kidney International* 1981;20:615–20.

53. Carbonell LF, Carretero OA, Stewart JM, Scicli AG. Effect of a kinin antagonist on the acute antihypertensive activity of enalaprilat in severe hypertension. *Hypertension* 1988;11:239–42.

54. Unger T, Scholkens BA, Bonner G. Kinins and converting enzyme inhibitors. *Journal of Cardiovascular Pharmacology* 1990;15 (suppl 6):S1–109.

55. Danckwardt L, Shimizu I, Blönner G, Rettig R, Unger T. Converting enzyme inhibition in kinin-deficient brown Norway rats. *Hypertension* 1990;16:429–35.

56. Zusman RM. Effects of converting enzyme inhibitors on the renin–angiotensin–aldosterone, bradykinin and arachidonic acid-prostaglandin systems: Correlation of chemical structure and biological activity. *American Journal of Kidney Diseases* 1987;10 (suppl 1):13–23.

57. Swartz SL. The role of prostaglandins in mediating the effects of angiotensin converting enzyme inhibitors and other antihypertensive drugs. *Cardiovascular Drugs and Therapy* 1987;1:39–43.

58. Quilley J, Duchin KL, Hudes EM, McGiff JC. The antihypertensive effect of captopril in essential hypertension: Relationship to prostaglandins and the kallikrein–kinin system. *Journal of Hypertension* 1987;5:121–8.

59. Weinberger MH. Angiotensin converting enzyme inhibitors enhance the antihypertensive efficacy of diuretics and blunt or prevent adverse metabolic effects. *Journal of Cardiovascular Pharmacology* 1989;13 (suppl 3):S1–4.

60. Koskinen P. Manninen V, Eilaso A. Quinapril and blood lipids. *British Journal of Clinical Pharmacology* 1988;26:478–80.

61. Jauch KW, Hartl W, Guenther B, Wicklmayr M, Rett K. Captopril enhances insulin responsiveness of forearm muscle tissue in non-insulin-dependent diabetes mellitus. *European Journal of Clinical Investigation* 1987;17:448–54.

62. Johnston CI, Jackson B, Cubela R, Arnolda L. Mechanism for hypotensive action of angiotensin converting enzyme inhibitors. *Clinical and Experimental Hypertension* 1984;6:551–61.

63. Brunner HR, Waeber B, Nussberger J. What we would like to know about the antihypertensive mechanisms of angiotensin converting enzyme inhibition. *Journal of Hypertension* 1988;6 (suppl 3):S1–5.

64. Johnston CI, Jackson B, McGrath BP, Matthews G, Arnolda L. Relationship of antihypertensive effect of enalapril to serum MK422 levels and angiotensin converting enzyme inhibition. *Journal of Hypertension* 1983;1 (suppl I):71–5.

65. Waeber B, Nussberger J, Juillerat L, Brunner HR. Angiotensin converting enzyme inhibition: Discrepancy between antihypertensive effect and suppression of enzyme activity. *Journal of Cardiovascular Pharmacology* 1989;14 (suppl 4):S53–9.

66. Gadsbøll N, Nielsen MD, Giese J, Leth A, Lønborg-Jensen H. Diurnal monitoring of blood pressure and the renin–angiotensin system in hypertensive patients on long-term angiotensin converting enzyme inhibition. *Journal of Hypertension* 1990;8:733–40.

67. Nussberger J, Waeber B, Brunner HR. Plasma angiotensin II and the antihypertensive action of angiotensin-converting enzyme inhibition. *American Journal of Hypertension* 1989;2:286–93.

68. Romankiewicz JA, Brogden RN, Heel RC, Speight TM, Avery GS. Captopril: An update review of its pharmacological properties and therapeutic efficacy in congestive heart failure. *Drugs* 1983;25:6–40.

69. Todd PA, Heel RC. Enalapril: A review of its pharmacodynamic and pharmacokinetic properties, and therapeutic use in hypertension and congestive heart failure. *Drugs* 1986;31:198–248.

70. Lancaster SG, Todd PA. Lisinopril: A preliminary review of its pharmacodynamic and pharmacokinetic properties, and therapeutic use in hypertension and congestive heart failure. *Drugs* 1988;35:646–69.

71. DeFelice EA, Kostis JB. New ACE inhibitors. In: Kostis JB, Defelice EA, eds. *Angiotensin converting enzyme inhibitors.* New York: Alan R List, 1987:213–61.

72. Matsuno Y, Tairai I, Fujitani E, Ito S, Kadokawa I. General pharmacology of the novel angiotensin converting enzyme inhibitor, alacepril. *Arzneimittel Forschung* 1986;36:55–62.

73. Brunner HR, Salvetti A, Sever PS. Benazepril: Profile of a new ACE inhibitor. *International Congress and Symposium Series Number 166.* London: Royal Society of Medicine Services.

74. Deget F, Brogden RN. Cilazapril. A review of its pharmacodynamic and pharmacokinetic properties, and therapeutic potential in cardiovascular disease. *Drugs* 1991;41:799.

75. Oka Y, Nishikawa K, Kito G, Mayahara H, Tanayama S. et al. Delapril. *Cardiovascular Drug Reviews* 1988;6:192–205.

76. Duchin KL, Waclawski AP, Tu JI, Manning J, Frantz M, Willard DA. Pharmacokinetics, safety, and pharmacologic effects of fosinopril sodium, an angiotensin-converting enzyme inhibitor in healthy subjects. *Journal of Clinical Pharmacology* 1991;31:58.

77. Todd PA, Fitton A. Perindopril. A review of its pharmacological properties and therapeutic use in cardiovascular disorders. *Drugs* 1991;42:90–114.

78. Wadworth AN, Brogden RN. Quinapril. A review of its pharmacological properties, and therapeutic efficacy in cardiovascular disorders. *Drugs* 1991;41:378–99.

79. Todd PA, Benfield P. Ramipril. A review of its pharmacological properties and therapeutic efficacy in cardiovascular disorders. *Drugs* 1990;39:110–35.

80. Sybert EJ, Watkins RW, Ahn HS, Baum T, La Rocca P, Patrick J, Leitz F. Pharmacologic metabolic and toxicologic profile of spirapril (SCH 33844), a new angiotensin converting inhibitor. *Journal of Cardiovascular Pharmacology* 1987;10 (suppl 7):105.

81. Singhui SM, Foley IE, Willard DA, Morrison RA. Disposition of zofenopril calcium in healthy subjects. *Journal of Pharmaceutical Sciences* 1990;79:970–3.

82. Linz W, Martorana PA, Scholkens BA. Local inhibition of bradykinin degradation in ischemic hearts. *Journal of Cardiovascular Pharmacology* 1990;15 (suppl 6):S99–105.

83. Westlin W, Mullane K. Does captopril attenuate reperfusion-induced myocardial dysfunction by scavenging free radicals? *Circulation* 1988; 77 (suppl 1):I30–9

84. McMurray J, Chopra M. Influence of ACE inhibitors on free radicals and reperfusion injury; pharmacological curiosity or therapeutic hope? *British Journal of Clinical Pharmacology* 1991;31:373–9.

85. Katz RJ, Levy WS, Buff L, Wasserman AG. Prevention of nitrate tolerance with angiotensin converting enzyme inhibitors. *Circulation* 1991;83:1271–7.

86. Dupuis J, Lalonde G, Bichet D, Rouleau JL. Captopril does not prevent nitroglycerin tolerance in heart failure. *Canadian Journal of Cardiology* 1990;6:281–6.

87. Hodsman GP, Johnston CI. Angiotensin converting enzyme inhibitors: Drug interactions. *Journal of Hypertension* 1987;5:1–6.

88. Williams GH. Converting enzyme inhibitors in the treatment of hypertension. *New England Journal of Medicine* 1988;319:1517–25.

89. Shaffer JE, Lee F, Thomson S, Han B-J, Cooke JP, Loscalzo J. The hemodynamic effects of S-nitrosocaptopril in anesthetized dogs. *Journal of Pharmacology and Experimental Therapeutics* 1991;256:704–9.

90. Gros C, Noel N, Souque A, Schwartz J-C, Danvy D, Plaquevent J-C, Duhamel L, Duhamel P, Lecomte J-M, Bralet J. Mixed inhibitors of angiotensin-converting enzyme (EC 3.4.15.1) and enkephalinase (EC 3.4.24.11): Rational design, properties, and potential cardiovascular applications of glycopril and alatriopril. *Proceedings of the National Academy of Sciences of the USA* 1991;88:4210–4.

91. Johnston CI, Hodsman GP, Kohzuki M, Casley DJ, Fabris B, Phillips PA. Interaction between atrial natriuretic peptide and the renin angiotensin aldosterone system. Endogenous antagonists. *American Journal of Medicine* 1989;87:24–8S.

92. Johnston CI, Phillips PA, Arnolda I, Mooser V. Modulation of the renin–angiotensin system by atrial natriuretic peptide. *Journal of Cardiovascular Pharmacology* 1990;16 (suppl 7):S43–6.

93. Chobanian AV, Haudenschild CC, Nickerson C, Drago R. Antiatherogenic effect of captopril in the Watanabe heritable hyperlipidemic rabbit. *Hypertension* 1990;15:327–31.

94. Mark II, Freedman AM, Dickens BF, Weglicki WB. Protective effect of sulfhydryl-containing angiotensin converting enzyme inhibitors against free radical injury in endothelial cells. *Biochemical Pharmacology* 1990;40:2169–75.

95. Miller VM. Does antihypertensive therapy improve the function of vascular endothelium? *Hypertension* 1990;16:541–3.

96. Hodsman GP, Brown JJ, Cumming AMM, Davies DL, East BW, Lever AF, Morton JJ, Murray GD, Robertson JIS. Enalapril (MK421) in the treatment of hypertension with renal artery stenosis. *Journal of Hypertension* 1983; 1 (suppl 1):109–17.

88 ANGIOTENSIN-CONVERTING ENZYME INHIBITORS IN CLINICAL RENOVASCULAR HYPERTENSION

J IAN S ROBERTSON

INTRODUCTION

The participation of the RAS in the pathogenesis of renovascular hypertension is complex and crucial, as has been described in detail in *Chapter 55*. It was emphasized there that experimental renovascular hypertension has two distinct models. In so-called '1-clip, 2-kidney' renovascular hypertension (Fig. 88.1), a constriction is placed on one renal artery, the contralateral renal artery and kidney remaining untouched; this model corresponds to the more usual syndrome of unilateral renal artery stenosis encountered clinically (see Color Plate 17). In the alternative '1-clip, 1-kidney' hypertension, a constriction is placed on one renal artery, while the contralateral kidney is excised. The clinical counterpart of this latter model is less common, but not rare. Participation of the RAS in the pathogenesis of systemic hypertension is clearer in the '1-clip, 2-kidney' model, although it deserves re-emphasis that in phase II of the evolution of the raised arterial pressure in that

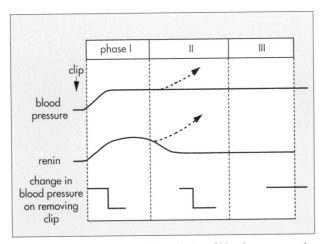

Fig. 88.1 Diagram showing the evolution of blood pressure and peripheral plasma renin in the three phases of experimental Goldblatt 1-clip, 2-kidney hypertension. The arrows and broken line in phase II indicate the course in the hyponatremic hypertensive syndrome. Modified from Robertson JIS *et al* [66].

model, plasma levels of renin and Ang II can often subside into the normal range (Fig. 88.1). This aspect is important to recognize clinically. It is also possible that the three phases in the evolution of renovascular hypertension as seen in this experimental model in the rat may be less clear in man, where the stenosis may develop gradually. Under these clinical circumstances, renal renin production may need to increase only slightly, perhaps with little detectable rise in peripheral renin or Ang II, but nevertheless sufficient to raise blood pressure via the slow pressor action of Ang II (*Chapter 28*).

In both models of renovascular hypertension, activation of the RAS in the kidney distal to the renal artery stenosis (see Color Plates 14–16) subserves important compensatory functions, partly countering the adverse consequence of the diminished renal blood flow and perfusion pressure. These comprise sustenance of glomerular filtration rate (GFR), of the capacity to excrete urea, and of renal artery pressure distal to the stenosis; they are described more fully in *Chapters 21* and *55*. The compensatory actions will be diminished or lost with the administration of ACE inhibitors. Such considerations have important implications for ACE inhibitors in the clinical counterpart of the '1-clip, 2-kidney' model; while in theory, and in the opinion of some, but by no means all, clinicians, they virtually preclude their use in the clinical syndrome corresponding to '1-clip, 1-kidney' form.

It must be recognized that the clinical conjunction of a renal artery stenosis with systemic hypertension does not necessarily imply a cause-and-effect relationship, which is required for the definition of renovascular hypertension. The establishment of the diagnosis of renovascular hypertension in man needs demonstration of relief of hypertension either by restoring patency of the narrowed renal artery, or by excision of the afflicted kidney. Alternative explanations for the association of hypertension with renal artery stenosis are the superimposition of a functionally irrelevant renal artery lesion on concurrent or pre-existent essential hypertension, or the development of a functionally significant renal artery stenosis in a patient with essential hypertension, with consequent exacerbation of the already high blood pressure [1–3]. The likely therapeutic benefit from surgical reconstruction, angioplasty, nephrectomy, or ACE inhibition will obviously differ greatly in these various circumstances.

Last, in renovascular hypertension, as in other forms of secondary hypertension, correction of the initiating lesion will return arterial pressure to the age- and sex-adjusted normal range in only some 50% of patients [1]. Accordingly, the antihypertensive effect of ACE inhibitors might be expected similarly to be limited. To complicate matters further, it is now apparent that, contrary to early predictions, ACE inhibitors often have a substantial antihypertensive effect in patients with essential hypertension, including those with low circulating levels of renin (see *Chapter 91*).

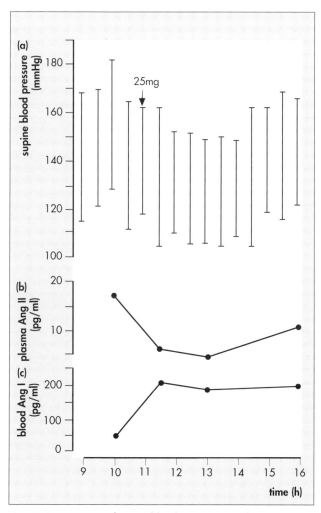

Fig. 88.2 Response of supine blood pressure (a), plasma Ang II (b), and blood Ang I (c) to initial oral dose of 25mg captopril in a young woman with unilateral renal artery stenosis, severe hypertension, and normal plasma values of renin and Ang II. Modified from Atkinson AB *et al* [5].

UNILATERAL RENAL ARTERY STENOSIS WITH SLIGHT OR MINIMAL ELEVATION OF PLASMA RENIN AND ANGIOTENSIN II

Unilateral renal artery stenosis with slight or minimal elevation of plasma renin and Ang II is the syndrome of renal artery stenosis most often encountered in man, and corresponds to the more usual evolution of phase II of experimental 1-clip, 2-kidney hypertension (see *Chapter 55*) (Fig. 88.1). Peripheral plasma levels of renin, Ang II, and aldosterone are only modestly elevated, even lying in the upper part of the normal range in many patients, there is no disturbance of the pattern of plasma electrolytes, and total body sodium and potassium content are normal. In the occasional patient, renin levels may even be in the low–normal range and a pressor (rather than depressor) response to the Ang II-receptor antagonist, saralasin, can be observed [4]. Atkinson *et al* [5] gave a detailed account of the effects of captopril in a young, severely hypertensive woman of this kind, with marked unilateral renal artery stenosis but with plasma concentrations of active renin, Ang II, and aldosterone variously only slightly elevated or in the upper part of the normal range. The initiation of captopril treatment caused an immediate fall in plasma Ang II and aldosterone, with converse increases in blood Ang I and plasma active renin concentrations; the early fall in blood pressure was modest (Fig. 88.2). With prolonged captopril treatment, plasma Ang II and aldosterone remained suppressed, while both exchangeable and total body measurements of sodium and potassium were unaltered. Blood pressure fell further, to normal values, with prolonged captopril treatment (Fig. 88.3). Subsequent surgical relief of the renal artery stenosis was curative; absolute values of arterial pressure and plasma Ang II were similar with prolonged captopril treatment to those after operation.

Hodsman *et al* [6,7] reported on a series of 10 patients with hypertension and unilateral renal artery stenosis given enalapril alone once daily for 12 weeks. These patients did not have demonstrably abnormal plasma electrolyte values. The decrease in blood pressure six hours after the initial dose of enalapril was significantly correlated with the pretreatment plasma concentrations of active renin and Ang II, and with the concurrent fall in plasma Ang II (Fig. 88.4). Blood pressure decreased further with continued treatment; the long-term blood-pressure decrease was no longer significantly correlated with the pretreatment plasma concentrations of active renin or Ang II. At three months, 24 hours after the last dose of enalapril, blood pressure, plasma Ang II, and plasma-converting enzyme activity remained low, and active renin and Ang I, high; six hours after dosing, Ang II had,

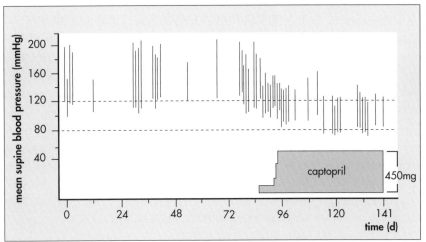

Fig. 88.3 Long-term blood-pressure response to captopril monotherapy in the patient in *Fig. 88.2*. The means of supine blood pressures taken on any particular day are shown. Modified from Atkinson AB *et al* [5].

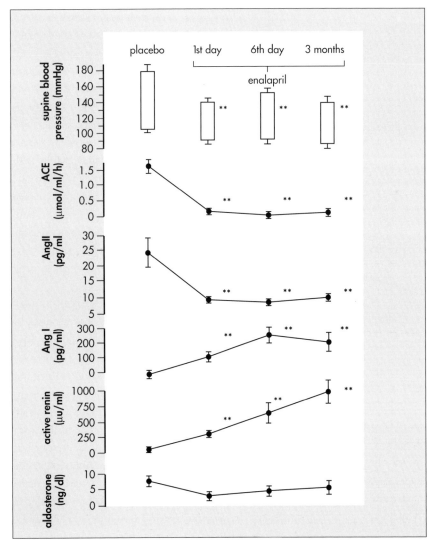

Fig. 88.4 Data from a series of 10 hypertensive patients with unilateral renal artery stenosis. Measurements were made on the final day of placebo therapy, and on the first day, sixth day, and third month of enalapril monotherapy, as a single daily dose of 10–40mg. Statistical comparisons are made with placebo values. **P<0.01. Data are means ± SEM. Note the dissociation between the continued increase of plasma active renin concentration between the sixth day and third month of treatment, while Ang I falls slightly over this period. Modified from Hodsman GP *et al* [7].

however, decreased further (Fig. 88.5). The increase in circulating active renin during long-term ACE inhibitor therapy was proportionately greater than the concurrent increase in Ang I; this was believed probably to reflect the diminution in plasma angiotensinogen concentration which occurs with prolonged ACE inhibition [8]. After three months of enalapril treatment, plasma sodium concentration was unchanged, while there was a slight average increase in plasma potassium, which was statistically, but in no instance clinically, significant. Total body potassium was unchanged. However, in contrast to the single patient reported by Atkinson et al [5] and described above, after three months of ACE

inhibitor therapy, exchangeable body sodium had fallen in nine patients, and was unchanged in the 10th (Fig. 88.6). The effect of ACE inhibition alone in causing a fall in body sodium content led the authors to caution against the indiscriminate use of diuretics in conjunction with ACE inhibitors in this disease.

While the foregoing data were gratifying in demonstrating the efficacy of ACE inhibitors in correcting systemic hypertension in this clinical syndrome of renovascular disease, they did not establish superiority of these agents over other forms of drug treatment. Evidence of such superiority was obtained by Hodsman et al [6,7] in an open study of a group of 10 patients with arteriographic evidence of unilateral or bilateral renal artery stenosis and severe hypertension which had responded poorly to a range of other antihypertensive drugs given either alone or in combination. After three months of enalapril treatment, which was combined with a diuretic in two patients, and with atenolol in two, blood pressure control was much more satisfactory than on previous therapy (Fig. 88.7).

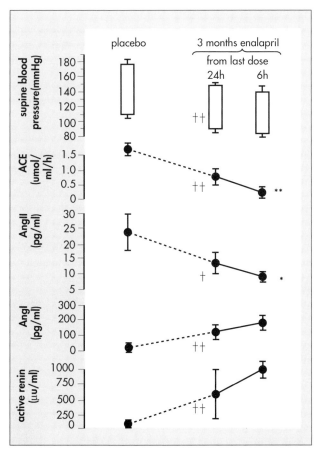

Fig. 88.5 Patients of *Fig. 88.4*. This shows a comparison of values obtained after three months of continuous once-daily oral enalapril therapy (10–40mg) with those on the final day of placebo therapy. Measurements made on enalapril were at 24 hours and 6 hours after the preceding dose. Data are means ± SEM. Comparison with values obtained on placebo is made: †*P*<0.05; ††*P*<0.01. Comparison is also made with 24-hour values: *P<0.05; **P<0.01. Modified from Hodsman GP *et al* [7].

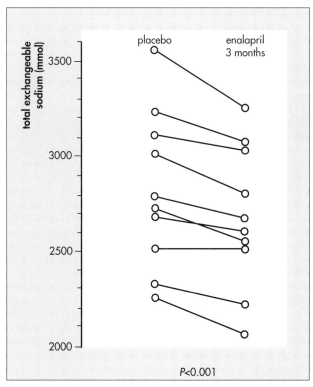

Fig. 88.6 Patients of *Figs. 88.4* and *88.5*. Total exchangeable body sodium is shown before and at the third month of enalapril treatment. Modified from Hodsman GP *et al* [7].

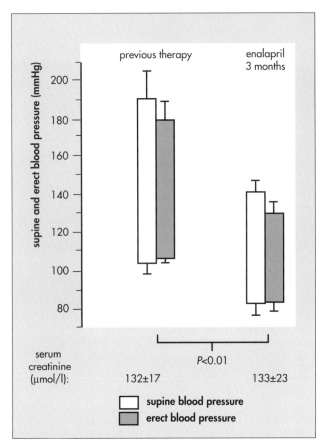

Fig. 88.7 Series of 10 patients with bilateral or unilateral renovascular disease and hypertension resistant to previous antihypertensive therapy with a variety of drugs. A comparison of supine and erect blood pressure and serum creatinine on previous therapy and at the third month of enalapril alone, 10–40mg once daily, is shown. Data are means ± SEM. Modified from Hodsman GP *et al* [7].

ANGIOTENSIN-CONVERTING ENZYME INHIBITION IN RENAL ARTERY STENOSIS WITH THE HYPONATREMIC HYPERTENSIVE SYNDROME

A rarer, but much more dramatic, mode of presentation of renovascular hypertension is as the 'hyponatremic hypertensive syndrome' [10–14] (see *Chapter 55*) (see *Fig. 88.1*). In this condition, a severe unilateral renal artery stenosis or occlusion causes very marked secretion of renin from the affected kidney, with gross elevation of peripheral plasma Ang II and consequent hypertension. However, because of the severity of the renal artery narrowing, the systemic hypertension is insufficient to moderate the signal to renin secretion, while pressure natriuresis via the contralateral kidney leads to sodium depletion and hence to yet greater renin release. Secondary aldosterone excess then causes potassium loss, with further reinforcement of the stimuli to renin release. Plasma Ang II can rise sufficiently to stimulate secretion of vasopressin. This rapidly advancing vicious cycle is usually characterized further by supervention of the malignant phase of hypertension, thirst, and polyuria.

The effect of ACE inhibitors in this syndrome contrasts strongly with that observed in the more usual form of renovascular disease described above. Atkinson *et al* [15] published an account of a woman who developed severe, malignant-phase hypertension following unilateral renal artery occlusion (Fig. 88.8). She was hyponatremic and hypokalemic, depleted of both body sodium and potassium, and had elevated peripheral blood levels of active renin, Ang I, Ang II, aldosterone,

Franklin and Smith [9] reported on a multicenter prospective double-blind comparison of enalapril plus hydrochlorothiazide with 'standard triple therapy' (hydrochlorothiazide plus hydralazine plus timolol) in a large series of patients with renal artery stenosis and hypertension. Effective control of diastolic blood pressure was achieved in 96% of 36 patients given enalapril, against 82% of 38 patients given the triple-drug regimen. These authors concluded cautiously that 'enalapril plus hydrochlorothiazide is effective in treating renovascular hypertension'.

The evidence of these three papers [6,7,9] is thus modestly suggestive of a superiority of ACE inhibition over other forms of drug therapy in controlling the most common form of clinical renovascular hypertension.

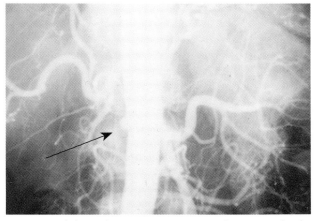

Fig. 88.8 Abdominal aortagram in a patient who presented with malignant hypertension and the hyponatremic syndrome. The right renal artery (arrowed) is occluded. Reproduced with permission from Atkinson AB *et al* [15].

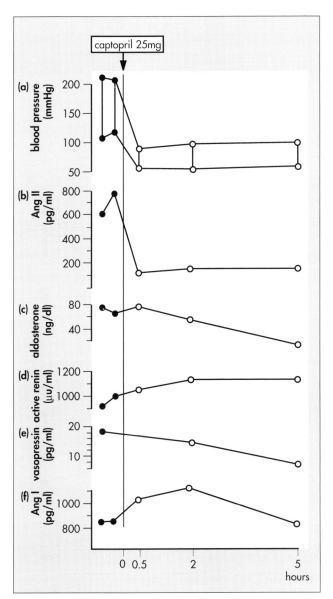

Fig. 88.9 Patient of *Fig. 88.8*. Changes in arterial pressure (a), plasma concentrations of Ang II (b), aldosterone (c), active renin (d), vasopressin (e), and blood Ang I (f) after a single oral dose of captopril 25mg are shown. Modified from Atkinson AB *et al* [15].

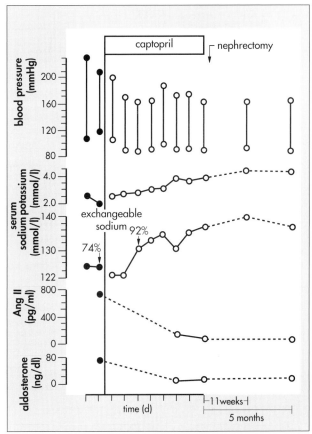

Fig. 88.10 Patient of *Figs. 88.8* and *88.9*, showing response to one week of treatment with captopril (450mg daily), followed by unilateral nephrectomy, when all treatment was stopped. Note the correction of severe hyponatremia and hypokalemia and of the deficient exchangeable body sodium with captopril. Unilateral nephrectomy is curative. Modified from Atkinson AB *et al* [15].

and vasopressin. An initial 25-mg dose of captopril led within 30 minutes, to a steep fall in plasma Ang II and in blood pressure; plasma aldosterone and vasopressin declined more slowly over the next five hours. There were converse increases in plasma active renin and in blood Ang I concentrations (Fig. 88.9). Continued captopril therapy over the subsequent seven days was accompanied by sustained suppression of plasma Ang II, restoration of the initially depleted body sodium and potassium content, correction of both hyponatremia and

hypokalemia, and less marked hypotension, although blood pressure remained controlled (Fig. 88.10). Subsequent unilateral nephrectomy was curative. The long-term postoperative blood-pressure levels resembled those during the latter days of preoperative captopril treatment, and were substantially higher than the very low values recorded immediately after the introduction of captopril (Fig. 88.10).

There can be little doubt of the specific efficacy of ACE inhibitors in this dramatic syndrome, which is notoriously unresponsive to other forms of antihypertensive drug therapy. Since the fall in blood pressure with the first dose of ACE inhibitor can be excessive, great caution is needed with initiation of treatment [14,15].

VALUE OF ANGIOTENSIN-CONVERTING ENZYME INHIBITORS IN PREDICTING SUBSEQUENT BLOOD PRESSURE RESPONSE TO SURGERY

The contrasting extent of the initial blood pressure response to ACE inhibition in the different syndromes of renovascular hypertension described above deserves emphasis. In the various forms of the disease, the fall in blood pressure following the first dose of ACE inhibitor can severally fall short of [5] or exceed [15], the long-term response. By contrast, the blood pressure values during prolonged ACE inhibitor treatment have been reported by two groups [16–18] to predict reasonably closely those achieved following reconstructive renal artery surgery, unilateral nephrectomy or transluminal angioplasty. The blood pressures obtained with long-term ACE inhibition may not only provide a useful guide to the success or otherwise of operative intervention; they can also indicate the extent of involvement of the RAS in different syndromes at various stages of the evolution of the disease, and hence insights into pathogenesis.

ADVERSE EFFECTS OF ANGIOTENSIN-CONVERTING ENZYME INHIBITION ON THE AFFECTED KIDNEY IN RENAL ARTERY STENOSIS

The compensatory intrarenal actions of the RAS in several circumstances of impaired renal blood flow, including renal artery stenosis, have previously been emphasized and their mechanisms described in detail (see *Chapter 21*). The beneficial effects include the partial preservation, despite the diminished renal circulation, of GFR, of the capacity to excrete urea, and of pressure in the main renal artery distal to the stenosis. These compensatory actions will be diminished or lost with the administration of ACE inhibitors. This aspect has been a source of concern and controversy regarding the use of these ACE inhibitors in hypertensive patients with renal artery stenosis.

Wenting *et al* [19] examined the function of the separate kidneys by isotope renography in patients with unilateral renal artery stenosis which had been demonstrated by arteriography. They observed that in 7 of 14 such patients, the renal extraction ratios of ^{131}I-sodium iodohippurate (^{131}I-hippuran) and of ^{125}I-thalamate were greatly reduced on the affected side when 50mg of captopril was given. The reduced extraction of sodium iodohippurate was considered probably to reflect a shortened plasma transit time through the kidney because of intrarenal

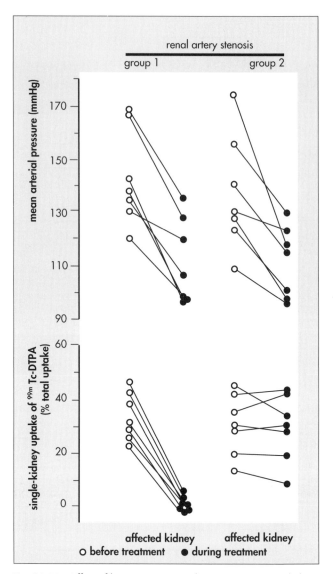

Fig. 88.11 Effect of long-term captopril treatment, 150mg daily, on mean blood pressure (diastolic plus one-third of pulse pressure) and the uptake, in the affected kidney, of ^{99m}Tc-DTPA in 14 patients with unilateral renal artery stenosis. Patients were allocated to two groups according to change in DTPA uptake. Modified from Wenting GJ *et al* [19].

vasodilatation. The reduced extraction of thalamate reflected a low filtration fraction, suggesting that the vasodilatation was, at least in part, at postglomerular arterioles. With long-term captopril treatment, the uptake of ^{99m}Tc-diethylene-triamene-penta-acetic acid (^{99m}Tc-DTPA) became almost zero in the seven patients who showed unilateral decline of renal function with captopril, indicating severe reduction in the GFR. This appeared to be an 'all-or-none' phenomenon and was not apparent in the other seven patients of the series. One week after stopping captopril, the uptake of ^{99m}Tc-DTPA had returned on the affected side. Captopril had little effect on the contralateral kidney (Fig. 88.11). Wenting *et al* [19,20] argued that these are likely to be effects specific to ACE inhibition, not simply a response to systemic blood pressure reduction.

Hodsman *et al* [7] estimated effective renal plasma flow on the two sides by ^{123}I-hippuran renography before and during long-term enalapril therapy in nine patients with hypertension and unilateral renal artery stenosis (Fig. 88.12). While effective renal

plasma flow was increased on the contralateral side, the affected kidney, already with a lower effective renal plasma flow, suffered a further decrease with enalapril therapy.

To what extent ACE inhibition may predispose to renal artery thrombosis is difficult to assess because of the frequent spontaneous progression of renal artery stenosis to occlusion. In a series of 20 hypertensive patients with renal artery stenosis given long-term enalapril, Tillman *et al* [21] noted that eight already had unilateral renal artery occlusion before starting the drug. In this series, one man suffered occlusion of a tightly stenosed renal artery by the third month of enalapril treatment (Fig. 88.13). Four further patients showed no uptake on the

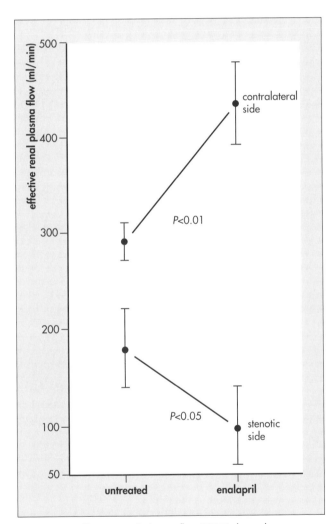

Fig. 88.12 Effective renal plasma flow (ERPF) shown by ^{123}I-hippuran renography, before and at the third month of treatment with enalapril alone, 10–40mg once daily, in a series of 10 hypertensive patients with unilateral renal artery stenosis. Data are means ± SEM. The series is the same as illustrated in *Figs. 88.4–88.6*. The already lower ERPF on the stenotic side is reduced further on enalapril, while that via the contralateral kidney is increased. Modified from Hodsman GP *et al* [7].

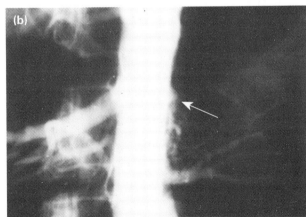

Fig. 88.13 (a) Patient with severe left renal artery stenosis, tenuous left renal artery, and small left kidney before enalapril treatment. (b) At the third month of enalapril monotherapy, left renal artery shown in (a) was occluded, while serum creatinine rose from 118 to 127µmol/l. The patient is from the series illustrated in *Figs. 88.4–88.6*. Reproduced with permission from Tillman DM *et al* [21].

affected side on ^{123}I-hippuran renography at times varying from 12–25 months from the start of therapy. Despite these findings, the decline in overall renal function either in these five patients or in the series overall was modest, indicating the capacity for the contralateral kidney to mask the adverse changes induced on the afflicted side. In the 20 patients of Tillman et al [21], serum urea rose from a basal mean (± SEM) of 5.9 ± 0.6 mmol/l to 6.6 ± 0.7 at three months (not significant) and to 7.7 ± 1.1 long term ($P<0.05$). Serum creatinine rose from 118.3 ± 10.5 mmol/l to 129.4 ± 11.5 at three months ($P<0.05$) and to 140.8 ± 14.8 long term (change from three months to long term not significant). On a more positive aspect, seven patients in the series of 20 reported by Tillman et al [21] had marked proteinuria (0.3–4.2g/24h) before starting enalapril. By the third month of treatment, this proteinuria had cleared in four patients, and was much less severe (0.13–0.9g/24h) in the remaining three. Similar clearing of proteinuria by ACE inhibitors in renovascular hypertension has been noted by other workers [22–24].

Angiotensin-converting enzyme inhibitors have been more clearly implicated in predisposing to renal artery occlusion by other workers [25]. Postma et al [26] studied retrospectively 78 patients with unilateral renal artery stenosis undergoing antihypertensive drug treatment. Renal artery thrombosis occurred in 14 patients (18%). Such occlusion could be shown to be related both to the combination of ACE inhibitor with diuretic ($P<0.05$) and to the use of an ACE inhibitor alone ($P=0.06$). Of the 14 patients who occluded the stenosed renal artery while taking an ACE inhibitor, only three showed a rise in serum creatinine.

In patients with only a single kidney supplied by a stenosed renal artery, or in many subjects with bilateral renal artery stenosis, the introduction of ACE inhibitors can often, although not invariably, provoke more serious azotemia [27,28]. There is, moreover, good evidence that the impairment of renal function induced in this way by ACE inhibition is more severe than can be explained simply by lowering systemic arterial pressure [29]. The risks are even greater if diuretics are used concurrently, because these latter agents will increase dependence on the intrarenal compensatory actions of the RAS. As was mentioned above, ACE inhibitors given alone can cause a fall in body sodium content in patients with renal artery stenosis [6,7] (see Fig. 88.6). Nevertheless, not all radiologically visible stenoses are functionally critical, and ACE inhibitors have been successfully employed in patients with bilateral renal artery lesions or with stenosis of an artery to a solitary kidney [30–32].

There can, however, be little doubt that ACE inhibitors fairly consistently, and via well-defined obvious mechanisms, further depress the function of the affected kidney in patients with renal artery stenosis. Accordingly, some authors [21] have advocated that, in patients destined for reconstructive surgery or angioplasty, ACE inhibitors should be given for no more than 2–4 weeks before operation. This should permit correction of systemic hypertension and any accompanying biochemical disturbance, while minimizing the hazard to the affected kidney. It appears clear, moreover, that these agents exacerbate the risks of progression to renal artery thrombosis. Nevertheless, in patients unsuitable for, or unwilling to undergo, corrective procedures, long-term ACE inhibitor treatment can be given usefully, albeit cautiously, with the recognition that the function of the affected, or more severely affected, kidney will almost inevitably be depressed.

These issues raise concern because of frequency of occult renovascular disease in patients with ostensible essential hypertension, especially those with evident arterial disease at other sites, and in the elderly [33–36], The use of ACE inhibitors can in these populations induce unseen renal problems. Contrasting opinions on the hazards and benefits of ACE inhibitors in patients with renovascular disease are given in Chapters 89 and 90.

ANGIOTENSIN-CONVERTING ENZYME INHIBITORS AND THE DIAGNOSIS OF RENOVASCULAR HYPERTENSION

ENHANCEMENT OF RENOGRAM FEATURES

The critically important compensatory changes mediated by the RAS within the kidney affected by renal artery stenosis, their diminution or abolition by ACE inhibition, and the consequent alterations in renographic appearances, have been discussed in some detail in the preceding paragraphs. These features [19,20] have consequently been proposed as the basis of a diagnostic procedure [37–43]. With such approaches, depression of renal function is assessed using ^{99}Tc-DPTA as an index of GFR, and/or ^{131}I-hippuran as an index of effective renal plasma flow, 45–60 minutes after the administration of a rapidly acting ACE inhibitor such as captopril. Theoretically, these tests should be useful with both unilateral and bilateral renal artery stenosis. Their merits and demerits have been argued in a number of reviews [44,45].

MAGNITUDE OF ACUTE FALL IN ARTERIAL BLOOD PRESSURE

The magnitude of acute fall in arterial blood pressure was earlier employed, using an Ang II analog antagonist such as saralasin given intravenously [46–49]. With later modification, the ACE inhibitor captopril replaced saralasin [50]. Some workers administered diuretics before the test in an attempt to enhance sensitivity and, it was hoped, specificity [51]. A particularly steep and profound fall in blood pressure was held to indicate the likelihood of renovascular hypertension.

It is now well established, however, that the magnitude of the acute fall in arterial pressure with saralasin infusion [52] (Fig. 88.14) or with an ACE inhibitor [6,7] is directly proportional to the immediately preceding plasma level of renin or Ang II. Therefore, this method is simply an indirect means of assessing the peripheral activation of the RAS. The approach thus suffers in

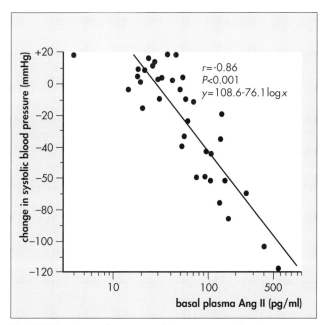

Fig. 88.14 Series of patients with hypertension, showing response of systolic blood pressure to intravenous administration of the Ang II antagonist, saralasin, in relation to the pre-saralasin peripheral plasma concentration of Ang II. The fall in blood pressure is proportional to the plasma Ang II concentration. Modified from Brown JJ *et al* [52].

this context from the same limitations as beset diagnostic procedures based on peripheral venous renin or Ang II assay, and which are discussed below.

ELEVATION OF PERIPHERAL PLASMA RENIN LEVEL

As was discussed in detail in *Chapter 55*, and more briefly earlier in this chapter, in established (phase II) renovascular hypertension, the levels of renin and Ang II in peripheral plasma are frequently only moderately elevated, and can indeed sometimes lie in the normal range. Thus, such assays are, alone, of very limited value in diagnosis [l]. However, the possibility that plasma renin might show a disproportionate increase in peripheral plasma in response to an Ang II antagonist or to an ACE inhibitor has been explored enthusiatically by several groups [53–55]. Both Imai *et al* [55] and Muller *et al* [56] have claimed that with this method, the rise in peripheral plasma renin activity (PRA) is consistently greater in patients with renovascular hypertension than in those with essential hypertension, there being virtually no overlap between the groups. Other authors have been less enthusiastic [57,58] or even dismissive [59]. More cautious reviewers [44,45,60] have, perhaps predictably, taken an intermediate position, according to this test a useful, albeit limited, diagnostic role.

ENHANCEMENT OF LATERALIZATION OF RENAL VEIN RENIN VALUES

As was described in detail in *Chapter 55*, in hypertensive patients with unilateral renal artery stenosis, plasma concentrations of active renin and Ang II, and PRA, are elevated in blood drawn from the renal vein of the affected side as compared with aortic blood. This venoarterial transrenal difference reflects both increased net secretion of renin and Ang II, and the reduction of renal blood flow. By contrast, renin secretion from the contralateral kidney is usually suppressed, with no difference in renin values between aorta and renal vein. The contralateral kidney is, more-over, a net extractor of Ang II [61]. Consequently, assay of renin in blood drawn from the two renal veins can be a useful aid to diagnosis of unilateral renal artery stenosis.

Delin *et al* [62] have emphasized further that if renin secretion is stimulated acutely, the renal vein ratio can be enhanced, with consequently greater sensitivity. Several means of stimulating renin secretion have been employed in this context, including upright tilting and the administration of drugs such as furosemide, hydralazine, or captopril [1]. Thibonnier *et al* [63] reported excellent discrimination employing captopril in this manner.

	Untreated			During enalapril		
	Arterial plasma	Renal vein plasma		Arterial plasma	Renal vein plasma	
		Affected	Contralateral		Affected	Contralateral
Active renin concentration (μu/ml)	50.5 ± 16.1	81.0 ± 25.1*	50.0 ± 14.6	1008.5 ± 163.2	1958.8 ± 419.8*	927.5 ± 156.2*
Inactive renin concentration (μu/ml)	110.2 ± 24.7	120.0 ± 26.8	116.8 ± 26.9	674.7 ± 102.2	1135.2 ± 143.1**	650.0 ± 58.1
Ang II (pmol/l)	(Venous plasma) 22.0 ± 6.4			(Venous plasma) 11.4 ± 2.9†		

Fig. 88.15 Differences of active and inactive plasma renin concentrations across the affected and unaffected kidneys in six hypertensive patients with unilateral renal artery stenosis, before and during enalapril monotherapy (10–40mg once daily). Peripheral venous plasma Ang II concentrations are also shown. Data are mean ± SEM. Comparison is made between arterial and renal vein measurements: *P<0.05; **P<0.01. Comparison of Ang II values is also made: †P<0.001. Modified from Tillman DM *et al* [64].

It must be emphasized that this enhanced lateralization is seen only transiently with acute stimulation of renin secretion. With prolonged administration of ACE inhibitors, a steady state is re-established; although renin levels in peripheral and renal venous plasma are markedly elevated during prolonged ACE inhibition, the renal vein renin ratio is unchanged [64,65] (Fig. 88.15).

A surprising finding with long-term ACE inhibition in patients with unilateral renal artery stenosis is that there is continued net inhibition of renin secretion by the contralateral kidney, which might, by contrast, have been expected to have been stimulated to secrete renin by the combined effects of systemic blood-pressure reduction and the fall in plasma Ang II [64,65]. With long-term administration of enalapril, Tillman *et al* [64] even observed net extraction of active renin across the contralateral kidney, with significantly lower values in renal vein than in aorta (Fig. 88.15). Derkx *et al* [65], employing captopril long term, found similar values of active renin in aorta and the vein of the contralateral (unaffected) kidney.

USE OF ANGIOTENSIN-CONVERTING ENZYME INHIBITORS IN THE DIAGNOSIS OF RENOVASCULAR HYPERTENSION

It will be apparent from the data presented in this section that ACE inhibitors have various effects which can assist in the diagnosis of renovascular hypertension. The sequence in which these tests should be applied is not so far agreed.

A not unreasonable approach [44,45] is to assess initially in patients considered to have possible renovascular hypertension, the response of PRA in peripheral venous blood to captopril administration. If the initial results are suggestive, this could be followed by isotope renography with captopril challenge. Then, if the diagnosis remains likely, renal vein renin assay could be undertaken, again after acute captopril challenge. These tests will of course need to be supplemented by other procedures such as arteriography, as appropriate [1].

CONCLUSIONS

The value of ACE inhibitors in lowering systemic blood pressure in patients with renovascular hypertension is most clearly seen in the rare hyponatremic syndrome. This malady is refractory to other forms of drug therapy, while the function of the affected kidney is usually already so seriously compromised that little is lost by administering an ACE inhibitor.

In the more common form of clinical renovascular hypertension, with unilateral, or predominantly unilateral, renal artery stenosis, ACE inhibitors can effectively control systemic hypertension. They are probably, but not certainly, superior to other currently available classes of orally active antihypertensive drugs in this respect.

The long-term blood-pressure response to ACE inhibition predicts that following successful surgical intervention ACE inhibitors, by eliminating intrarenal renin-mediated compensatory mechanisms, consistently depress the function of the kidney affected by renal artery stenosis. They can provoke renal failure in patients with bilateral renal artery stenosis or in those with only a single kidney supplied by a stenotic artery, especially if a diuretic is given concurrently.

Angiotensin-converting enzyme inhibitors probably predispose already narrowed renal arteries to occlusion. When given acutely, they may facilitate the diagnosis of renovascular hypertension by stimulating a rise of renin level in peripheral blood; by transiently enhancing the renal vein renin differential; and by depressing the isotopic renographic appearances on the affected side.

REFERENCES

1. Robertson JIS. Unilateral renal disease and hypertension. In: Robertson JIS, ed. *Handbook of hypertension, vol 15. Clinical aspects of hypertension.* Amsterdam: Elsevier, 1992:chapter 10.

2. Lisa JR, Eckstein D, Solomon C. Relationship between arterial sclerosis of renal artery and hypertension: Analysis of 100 necropsies. *American Journal of the Medical Sciences* 1943;**205**:701–3.

3. Eyler WR, Clark MD, Garman JE, Rian RL, Meiniger DE. Angiography of the renal areas including a comparative study of renal arterial stenoses in patients with and without hypertension. *Radiology* 1962;**78**:879–91.

4. Marks LS, Maxwell MH, Kaufman JJ. Non-renin-mediated renovascular hypertension: A new syndrome. *Lancet* 1977;**i**:615–7.

5. Atkinson AB, Brown JJ, Davies DL, Leckie B, Lever AF, Morton JJ, Robertson JIS. Renal artery stenosis with normal angiotensin II values. Relationship between angiotensin II and body sodium and potassium on correction of hypertension by captopril and subsequent surgery. *Hypertension* 1981;**3**:53–8.

6. Hodsman GP, Brown JJ, Cumming AMM, Davies DL, East BW, Lever AF, Morton JJ, Murray GD, Robertson I, Robertson JIS. Enalapril in the treatment of hypertension with renal artery stenosis. *British Medical Journal* 1983;**287**:1413–7.

7. Hodsman GP, Brown JJ, Cumming AMM, Davies DL, East BW, Lever AF, Morton JJ, Murray GD, Robertson JIS. Enalapril in the treatment of hypertension with renal artery stenosis: Changes in blood pressure, renin, angiotensin I and II, renal function, and body composition. *American Journal of Medicine* 1984;**77** (2A):52–60.

8. Rasmussen S, Nielsen MD, Giese J. Captopril combined with thiazide lowers renin substrate concentration; Implications for methodology in renin assays. *Clinical Science* 1981;**60**:591–3.

9. Franklin SS, Smith RD. Comparison of effects of enalapril plus hydrochlorothiazide versus standard triple therapy on renal function in renovascular hypertension. *American Journal of Medicine* 1985;**79** (suppl 3C):14–23.

10. Brown JJ, Davies DL, Lever AF, Robertson JIS. Plasma renin concentration in human hypertension. 1: Relationship between renin, sodium, and potassium. *British Medical Journal* 1965;**ii**:144–8.

11. Brown JJ, Davies DL, Lever AF, Robertson JIS. Renin and angiotensin: A survey of some aspects. *Postgraduate Medical Journal* 1966;**42**:153–76.

12. [Editorial]. Hyponatraemic hypertensive syndrome. *Lancet* 1986;**i**:718–9.

13. Laidlaw JC, Yendt ER, Gornall AG. Hypertension caused by renal artery occlusion simulating primary aldosteronism. *Metabolism* 1960;**9**:612–23.

14. Heslop H, Richards AM, Nicholls MG, Espiner EA, Ikram H, Maslowski AH. Hyponatraemic-hypertensive syndrome due to unilateral renal ischaemia in women who smoke heavily. *New Zealand Medical Journal* 1985;**98**:739–42.

15. Atkinson AB, Brown JJ, Davies DL, Fraser R, Leckie B, Lever AF, Morton JJ, Robertson JIS. Hyponatraemic hypertensive syndrome with renal artery occlusion corrected by captopril. *Lancet* 1979;**ii**:606–9.

16. Staessen J, Wilms G, Baert A, Fagard R, Lijnen P, Suy R, Amery A. Blood pressure during long-term converting enzyme inhibition predicts the curability of renovascular hypertension by angioplasty. *American Journal of Hypertension* 1988;**1**:208–14.

17. Atkinson AB, Brown JJ, Cumming AMM, Fraser R, Lever AF, Leckie BJ, Morton JJ, Robertson JIS, Davies DL. Captopril in the management of hypertension with renal artery stenosis: Its long-term effect as a predictor of surgical outcome. *American Journal of Cardiology* 1982;**49**:1460–6.

18. Staessen J, Bulpitt C, Fagard R, Lijnen P, Amery A. Long-term converting-enzyme inhibition as a guide to surgical curability of hypertension associated with renovascular disease. *American Journal of Cardiology* 1983;**51**:1317–22.

19. Wenting GJ, Tan–Tjiong HL, Derkx FHM, de Bruyn JHB, Man in't Veld AJ, Schalekamp MADH. Split renal function after captopril in unilateral renal artery stenosis. *British Medical Journal* 1984;**288**:886–90.

20. Wenting GJ, Derkx FHM, Tan–Tjiong HL, van Seyen AJ, Man in't Veld AJ, Schalekamp MADH. Risks of angiotensin converting enzyme inhibition in renal artery stenosis. *Kidney International* 1987;**31** (suppl 20):180–3.

21. Tillman DM, Malatino LS, Cumming AMM, Hodsman GP, Leckie BJ, Lever AF, Morton JJ, Webb DJ, Robertson JIS. Enalapril in hypertension with renal artery stenosis: Long-term follow-up and effects on renal function. *Journal of Hypertension* 1984;**2** (suppl 2):93–100.

22. Takeda R, Morimoto S, Uchida K, Kigoshi T, Sumitani T, Matsubara F. Effects of captopril on both hypertension and proteinuria. Report of case of renovascular hypertension associated with nephrotic syndrome. *Archives of Internal Medicine* 1980;**140**:1531–3.

23. Holman ND, Donker AJM, Van Der Meer J. Disappearance of renin-induced proteinuria by an ACE-inhibitor: A case report. *Clinical Nephrology* 1990;**49**: 21–30.

24. Mizuno K, Numura S, Tani M, Takahashi M, Hayashi A, Yamaguchi M, Fukuchi S. Angiotensin-converting inhibitors in the treatment of renovascular hypertension with nephrotic-range proteinuria. *Current Therapeutic Research* 1991;**49**:21–30.

25. Main J, Wilkinson R. Early renal artery occlusion after enalapril in atheromatous renal artery stenosis. *British Medical Journal* 1989;**299**:394.

26. Postma CT, Hoefnagels WHL, Barentsz JO, de Boo Th, Thien Th. Occlusion of unilateral stenosed renal arteries: Relation to medical treatment. *Journal of Human Hypertension* 1989;**3**:185–90.

27. Hricik DE, Browning PJ, Kopelman R, Goorno WE, Madias NE, Dzau VJ. Captopril-induced functional renal insufficiency in patients with bilateral renal artery stenosis or renal-artery stenosis in a solitary kidney. *New England Journal of Medicine* 1983;**308**:377–81.

28. Hricik DE. Captopril-induced renal insufficiency and the role of sodium balance. *Annals of Internal Medicine* 1985;**103**:222–3.

29. Textor SC. ACE inhibitors in renovascular hypertension. *Cardiovascular Drugs and Therapy* 1990;**4**:229–35.

30. Burris JF, Baer AM, Mroczek WJ. Successful use of captopril in a patient with renal artery stenosis of a solitary kidney. *Journal of Clinical Pharmacology* 1987;**27**:32–40.

31. Canjanello JV, Madaio MP, Madias NE. Enalapril in the management of hypertension associated with renal artery stenosis. *Journal of Clinical Pharmacology* 1987;**27**:32–40.

32. Hollenberg NK. Medical therapy of renovascular hypertension: Efficacy and safety of captopril in 269 patients. *Cardiovascular Reviews and Reports* 1983;**4**:852–79.

33. Scoble JE, Hamilton G. Atherosclerotic renovascular disease. *British Medical Journal* 1990;**300**:1670–1.

34. Choudhri AH, Cleland JGF, Rowlands PC, Tran TL, McCary M, Al-Kutoubu MAO. Unsuspected renal artery stenosis in peripheral vascular disease. *British Medical Journal* 1990;**301**:1197–8.

35. Priollet P, Lazareth I, Manière-Constantin D, Aimé F. Renal artery stenosis and peripheral vascular disease. *Lancet* 1990;**336**:879.

36. Salmon P, Brown MA. Renal artery stenosis and peripheral vascular disease: Implications for ACE inhibitor therapy. *Lancet* 1990;**336**:321.

37. Geyskes GG, Yoe Oei H, Puylaert CBAJ, Dorhout Mees EJ. Renography with captopril. *Archives of Internal Medicine* 1986;**146**:1705–8.

38. Geyskes GG, Oei HY, Puylaert C, Mees EJD. Renovascular hypertension identified by captopril-induced changes in the renogram. *Hypertension* 1987;**9**:451–8.

39. Fommei E, Ghione S, Palla L, Mosca F, Ferrari M, Palombo C, Giaconi S, Gazzetti P, Donato L. Renal scintigraphic captopril test in the diagnosis of renovascular hypertension. *Hypertension* 1987;**10**:212–20.

40. Sfakaniakis GN, Bourgoignie JJ, Jaffe D, Kyriakides G, Perez-Stable E, Duncan R. Single-dose captopril scintigraphy in the diagnosis of renovascular hypertension. *Journal of Nuclear Medicine* 1987;**28**:1383–92.

41. Dondi M, Franchi R, Levorato M, Zuccato A, Gaggi R, Mirelli M, Stella A, Marchetta F, Losinno F, Monetti N. Evaluation of hypertensive patients by means of captopril-enhanced renal scintigraphy with technetium-99mDTPA. *Journal of Nuclear Medicine* 1989;**30**:615–21.

42. Setaro JF, Saddler MC, Chen ChC, Hoffer PB, Roer DA, Markowitz DM, Meier GH, Gusberg RJ, Black HR. Simplified captopril renography in diagnosis and treatment of renal artery stenosis. *Hypertension* 1991;**18**:289–98.

43. Ritter SG, Bentley MD, Fiksen–Olsen MJ, Brown ML, Romero JC, Zachariah K. Effect of captopril on renal function in hypertensive dogs with unilateral renal artery stenosis, studied with radionuclide dynamic scintigraphy. *American Journal of Hypertension* 1990;**3**:591–8.

44. Davidson R, Wilcox CS. Diagnostic usefulness of renal scanning after angiotensin converting enzyme inhibitors. *Hypertension* 1991;**18**:299–303.

45. Kaplan NM. The captopril challenge for renovascular hypertension. *American Journal of Hypertension* 1990;**3**:588–90.

46. Marks LS, Maxwell MH, Kaufmann JJ. Saralasin bolus test. Rapid procedure for renin mediated hypertension. *Lancet* 1975;**ii**:784.

47. Streeten DH, Anderson GH, Freiberg JM, Dalakos TG. Use of angiotensin II antagonist (saralasin) in the recognition of 'angiotensinogenic' hypertension . *New England Journal of Medicine* 1975;**292**:657–62.

48. Wilson HM, Wilson JP, Slaton PE. Saralasin infusion in the recognition of renovascular hypertension. *Annals of Internal Medicine* 1977;**87**:36–42.

49. Maxwell MH, Varady P, Zawada ET, Burkhalter JF, Waks U, Marks L. Maximal discrimination of renovascular from essential hypertension by the saralasin test. *Clinical Science and Molecular Medicine* 1978;**55** (suppl 4):297–9.

50. Gavras H, Brunner HR, Turini GA. Antihypertensive effect of the oral angiotensin converting enzyme inhibitor SQ 14225 in man. *New England Journal of Medicine* 1978;**298**:991–3.

51. Streeten DHP, Anderson GH. Angiotensin-receptor blocking drugs. In: Doyle AE, ed. *Clinical pharmacology of antihypertensive drugs. Handbook of hypertension, vol. 11*. Amsterdam: Elsevier, 1988:274–300.

52. Brown JJ, Brown WCB, Fraser R, Lever AF, Morton JJ, Robertson JIS, Agabiti–Rosei E, Trust PM. The effects of the angiotensin II antagonist saralasin on blood pressure and plasma aldosterone in man in relation to the prevailing plasma angiotensin II concentration. *Progress in Biochemical Pharmacology* 1976;**12**:230–41.

53. Case DB, Atlas SA, Laragh JH. Reactive hyper-reninaemia to angiotensin blockade identifies renovascular hypertension. *Clinical Science* 1979;**57** (suppl):135–65.

54. Case DB, Laragh JH. Reactive hyper-reninaemia in renovascular hypertension after angiotensin blockade with saralasin or converting enzyme inhibitor. *Annals of Internal Medicine* 1979;**91**:153–60.

55. Imai Y, Abe K, Otsuka Y. Exaggerated response of renin secretion to captopril in renovascular hypertension. *Japanese Heart Journal* 1980;**21**:793–802.

56. Muller FB, Sealey JE, Case DB, Atlas SA, Pickering TG, Pecker MS, Preibisz JJ, Laragh JH. The captopril test for identifying renovascular disease in hypertensive patients. *American Journal of Medicine* 1986;**80**:633–44.

57. Thibonnier M, Sassano P, Joseph A, Guyenne TT, Corvol P, Raynaud A, Seurot M, Gaux JC. Diagnostic value of a single dose of captopril in renin- and aldosterone-dependent, surgically curable hypertension. *Cardiovascular Reviews and Reports* 1982;**3**:1659–68.

58. Gaul MK, Linn WD, Mulrow CD. Captopril stimulated renin secretion in the diagnosis of renovascular hypertension. *American Journal of Hypertension* 1989;**2**:335–40.

59. Salvetti A, Arzilli F, Nuccorini A, Mauro M, Giovanetti R. Does humoral and hemodynamic response to acute ACE inhibition identify true renovascular hypertension? In: Glorioso N, Laragh JH, Rapelli A, eds. *Renovascular hypertension*. New York: Raven Press, 1987:305–15.

60. Gosse P, Dupas JY, Reynaud P, Jullien E, Dallochio M. Captopril test in the detection of renovascular hypertension in a population with low prevalence of the disease; a prospective study. *American Journal of Hypertension* 1989;**2**:191–3.

61. Webb DJ, Cumming AMM, Adams FC, Hodsman GP, Leckie BJ, Lever AF, Morton JJ, Murray GD, Robertson JIS. Changes in active and inactive renin and in angiotensin II across the kidney in essential hypertension and renal artery stenosis. *Journal of Hypertension* 1984;**2**:605–14.

62. Delin K, Aurell M, Granerus G. Acute stimulation of renin release in the diagnosis of renovascular hypertension. In: Glorioso N, Laragh JH, Rapelli A, eds. *Renovascular hypertension*. New York: Raven Press, 1987:341–50.

63. Thibonnier M, Joseph A, Sassano P, Guyenne TT, Corvol P, Raynaud A, Seurot M, Gauz JC. Improved diagnosis of unilateral renal artery lesions after captopril administration. *Journal of the American Medical Association* 1984;**251**:56–60.

64. Tillman DM, Malatino LS, Lever AF, Robertson JIS. Transrenal changes in active and inactive renin and angiotensin II across the kidney in renal artery stenosis: effects of converting enzyme inhibiton. *Kidney International* 1987;**31** (suppl 20):184–90.

65. Derkx FHM, de Wind AE, Lipovsky MM, Stroes ESG, Pieterman H, van den Meiracker AH, Wenting GJ, Man in't Veld AJ, Schalekamp MADH. Renal vein renin lateralisation is not improved by captopril treatment. In: MacGregor GA, Sever PS, Caldwell ADS, eds. *Current Advances in ACE Inhibition*, Volume 2, Edinburgh: Churchill-Livingstone, 1991:213–17.

66. Robertson JIS, Morton JJ, Tillman DM, Lever AF. The pathophysiology of renovascular hypertension. *Journal of Hypertension* 1986;**4** (suppl 4) :95–103.

89

A CAUTIOUS VIEW OF THE VALUE OF ANGIOTENSIN-CONVERTING ENZYME INHIBITION IN RENOVASCULAR DISEASE

JOËL MÉNARD, JEAN BAPTISTE MICHEL, AND PIERRE-FRANÇOIS PLOUIN

Within the vast field of hypertensive diseases, renovascular hypertension has always been a matter of debate concerning the cost effectiveness of its detection, the relative importance of the RAS in its pathophysiology, and more recently, the choice of treatment between medical therapy and revascularization. A new debate has been generated by the surprising observation that a treatment that is apparently ideal for this disease, the blockade of the RAS by the inhibition of ACE, might do more harm than good, by causing functional or organic renal damage in a subgroup of patients whose characteristics still remain to be defined.

The first victims of the administration of the ACE inhibitor, captopril, to renovascular 'patients' were three rats, reported by Bengis and Coleman [1]. These three rats, extracted from a group of seven animals having malignant hypertension after clipping their single remaining kidney, responded to captopril by a fall in blood pressure, a progressive adipsia, oliguria, and uremia. One died, and the other two recovered when captopril was withdrawn, with their blood pressure rising progressively over three days; water intake, urine output, and urine sodium excretion rose to the pre-inhibition values, and renal function was normalized. Although this observation did not permit differentiation of the consequences of the fall in blood pressure from those of the intrarenal effects of ACE inhibition, it was an early pointer to the essential role of the RAS in maintaining the glomerular filtration rate (GFR) under certain circumstances such as sodium depletion, congestive heart failure, and stenosis of the renal artery [2].

Subsequently, clinical reports of renal insufficiency in patients with renovascular disease who were treated with captopril appeared in the literature [3]. These reports raised controversial views on the nature and the specificity of this adverse effect, since it was known that treatment of renovascular hypertension by drugs other than ACE inhibitors was also able to induce renal dysfunction or renal artery occlusion through a fall in blood pressure [4]. The risks of ACE inhibition in patients with bilateral lesions or solitary kidneys were studied more systematically at a later date, in consecutive series of 9 [5], 11 [6], and 4 patients [7].

The objective of this review is to make practical recommendations after a critical analysis of the experimental and clinical data and an evaluation of the benefit/risk ratio of ACE inhibition in renovascular hypertension. It should be noted that what is reported for ACE inhibition is likely to be true for inhibition of the RAS at large. Both experimental studies and carefully conducted clinical studies of renin inhibitors and Ang II antagonists are, however, needed in this situation; the effects of ACE inhibition on blood pressure and renal function could result from properties of ACE inhibitors independent of the RAS.

THE COMPLEX BILATERAL RENAL DYSFUNCTION OF RENOVASCULAR HYPERTENSION

Many experiments have examined the role of the RAS in influencing the functions of a clipped kidney and of the contralateral 'untouched' kidney (see *Chapters 21* and *55*). The two selected in this article are the experiments performed by Huang and Navar [8, 9], in the 2-kidney, 1-clip hypertensive rat model. They compared the responses of blood pressure and renal hemodynamics after removal of the clip from the clipped kidney, with the effects of ACE inhibition. Blood pressure rapidly decreased from 161 ± 4 to 118 ± 3 mmHg within 1.5 hours of clip removal. The removal of the clip also induced significant increases in GFR, renal blood flow (RBF), and urinary flow. Infusion of the ACE inhibitor SQ20881 teprotide (3mg/kg/h) also decreased mean arterial blood pressure from 157 ± 3 to 139 ± 4 mmHg after 30 minutes and then to 124 ± 3 mmHg after 2.5 hours of infusion. However, significant decreases in RBF, GFR, and urinary flow, accompanied this teprotide-induced fall in blood pressure.

The contrast between the two procedures, surgical and pharmacological, also extended to the contralateral untouched kidney. Removal of the clip decreased RBF, GFR, and urine flow of the contralateral kidney, whereas infusion of the ACE inhibitor increased these measurements.

These experiments are extremely important to our understanding of why, in renovascular hypertensive patients, two treatments that similarly control high blood pressure, the pharmacologic approach through the blockade of the RAS, or reconstruction of the renal artery by surgical revascularization or percutaneous angioplasty, will have different effects on the renal dysfunction. It is also interesting to observe that in the experiments of Navar et al [8, 9], despite a similar sodium loss, ACE inhibition was slightly less effective on blood-pressure reduction than was removal of the clip.

Another set of experiments performed in dogs with a single kidney [10,11], compared the changes with time of the responses to a fixed degree of inflation of a balloon cuff around the renal artery, with or without continuous enalapril treatment. In untreated dogs, cuff inflation increased mean aortic blood pressure by 17.1±20mmHg, while GFR and RBF returned to prestenosis levels. In enalapril-treated dogs, blood pressure increased by 23.0±2.7mmHg, but in the absence of a functional RAS, GFR remained low at 56±6% of prestenosis levels, RBF returned to normal and the renal artery pressure remained 25% lower than control values. The conclusion of these authors was that the main role of Ang II in chronic 1-kidney Goldblatt hypertension was not as a pressor hormone, but rather, through its actions within the kidney, to preserve glomerular filtration.

All the experimental evidence that has been accumulated in dogs, rats, and rabbits illustrates the complexity of the renal disease known as renovascular hypertension. The increased intrarenal generation of Ang II in the stenotic kidney preserves GFR in the face of a reduction in both RBF and perfusion pressure. The main renal arterial pressure distal to the stenosis is sustained by activation of the RAS. Intrarenal Ang II enhances mesangial-cell contraction and alters the filtering surface area of the glomerular capillary. On the other hand, it helps to maintain glomerular filtration by a predominant vasoconstrictor effect on the efferent glomerular arteriole, it exerts a tonic effect on the vasa recta by reducing the velocity of blood flow in these countercurrent systems, and it facilitates urea excretion despite the reduction in the overall RBF and GFR [12].

In the contralateral 'untouched' kidney, despite the uniform decrease in the renin content of superficial and deep glomeruli, the excess of circulating renin released from the stenotic kidney impairs sodium excretion through Ang II production [13], except when a rapid and severe rise in blood pressure induces sodium loss [14]. In renovascular hypertension, there exists, not only systemic hypertension but also dysfunction of both the stenotic kidney and its contralateral partner. This dysfunction needs its own specific therapy — correction of the renal artery stenosis. Control of blood pressure and preservation or restoration to normal of the renal functions are the dual objectives of therapy. Experimental evidence summarized above suggests that it is unlikely that the renal objective can be successfully attained through the administration of an ACE inhibitor.

EXPERIMENTAL EVIDENCE OF THE ADVERSE RENAL EFFECTS OF LONG-TERM ANGIOTENSIN-CONVERTING ENZYME INHIBITION IN RENOVASCULAR HYPERTENSION

Experimentation in rats has the advantage of a standardized procedure providing reproducible disease that is extremely sensitive to the diameter (internal gap) of the clip that is used (0.20 or 0.25mm) and to the age of the animal.

Three groups of experimental studies have been performed which have all indicated the deleterious renal effects of ACE inhibition in experimental renal hypertension in rats [Fig. 89.1].

Helmchen et al showed that in rats with bilaterally constricted renal arteries, short-term blockade of the RAS led to a significant reduction of renal excretory function [15]. Gröne and Helmchen [16] studied the effects of 14 days' treatment with enalapril once a day (mean dose 6.3±1.3mg/kg body weight/day) or with dihydralazine (13.2±1.1mg/kg bodyweight/12 hours) in 1-clip, 2-kidney hypertensive rats on a low sodium diet. These two drug treatments had similar effects on blood pressure (systolic blood pressure was between 100 and 130mmHg in treated rats, versus 200mmHg in untreated animals), and both treatments decreased heart weight (untreated: 1,299±58mg; dihydralazine: 1,067±39mg; enalapril: 1,033±30mg). There was no apparent change in plasma creatinine when both kidneys were present. However, two days after the left renal artery was unclipped and a right nephrectomy performed, plasma creatinine rose to 2.75±0.33mg/100ml in the enalapril-treated rats versus 1.12±0.18 in the dihydralazine-treated rats, compared with 1.0±0.09 in the controls. This experiment unmasked the functional alterations in the clipped kidney. Seven days later, renal function had recovered and the GFR of the remaining right kidney of enalapril- and dihydralazine-treated rats was not different. Using light microscopy, the clipped kidneys of enalapril-treated rats showed major changes in the proximal tubules after 14 days of drug therapy. The most important lesions were atrophy, with a slight degree of interstitial edema, and fibrosis. Distal tubules were almost normal. A morphological recovery was observed in the single remaining (left) kidney of rats treated by ACE inhibition seven days after the end of drug therapy, which paralleled the improvement in excretory function. This recovery may have been favored by the removal of the

Reference	Untreated hypertensive rats	ACE inhibitor-treated rats	Conventional therapy	Stenotic/contralateral kidney weight ratio
Helmchen et al (1982) [15]	2-kidney, 2-clip	low sodium captopril 4 days	low sodium dihydralazine 4 days	
Gröne and Helmchen (1986) [16]	2-kidney, 1-clip	low sodium enalapril 14 days	low sodium dihydralazine 14 days	0.63/0.45/0.62
Michel et al (1986) [17]	2-kidney, 1-clip	normal sodium perindopril 5 weeks	normal sodium* triple therapy 5 weeks	0.76/0.53/0.70
Michel et al (1987) [18]	2-kidney, 1-clip	normal sodium enalapril 5 weeks		0.66/0.34/ –
Jackson et al (1990) [20]	2-kidney, 1-clip	normal sodium enalapril 12 months	normal sodium* minoxidil 12 months	0.68/0.29/0.66

* In these groups, blood-pressure control was not achieved by treatment.

Fig. 89.1 Experimental data on the renal effects of ACE inhibition in renovascular hypertensive rats.

contralateral untouched kidney, which was performed simultaneously with unclipping of the left renal artery. In the dihydralazine-treated rats, tubular atrophy, although present, was much less marked than in the animals treated by the ACE inhibitor.

In a series of experiments, we have shown, with two different ACE inhibitors, perindopril [17] and enalapril [18,19], that the beneficial effect of the drugs on systemic blood pressure, and a reduction in heart weight, were accompanied by a decrease of the weight of the clipped kidney with an enhanced increase in size of the contralateral, untouched kidney. Triple therapy with clonidine, dihydralazine, and furosemide did not induce these renal changes; furthermore, it did not control blood pressure (173 ± 18 mmHg) of the renal hypertensive rats as effectively as perindopril (144 ± 13 mmHg) [17].

Three main morphological lesions were observed during these experiments [17,19]: nephroangiosclerosis, probably a consequence of hypertension; ischemia related either to renal artery stenosis or to nephroangiosclerosis; and glomerulosclerosis resulting from the intraglomerular effects of hypertension (Plates 56–59, see Plate Section). Ischemia is the most difficult to evaluate since it evolves with time, it is particularly heterogeneous, and it is proportional to the decrease in renal function and blood flow.

ISCHEMIA

Ischemia of the kidney involves three main morphological and progressive features: tubular lesions, glomerular lesions, and inflammation. It is uncertain if these morphological lesions are directly related to the decrease in RBF or indirectly related to loss of renal function. The primary tubular lesion in renal ischemia depends on the distal vasculature of the tubules and on the oxygen dependence of tubular function. The first histological sign is a decrease in the length of epithelial cells leading to widening of the lumen. These early tubular lesions are reversible. With time, when ischemia is more severe, the decrease in area of epithelial cells is more marked and is accompanied by a true dilatation of the cortical tubules and urine stagnation. At an advanced stage of the disease, the tubular dilatation creates pseudocysts with deformation of the kidney surface.

With renal ischemia, there is initially a shrinkage of glomerular tufts. This early lesion is grossly related to the decrease in perfusion pressure and flow within the glomerular capillary flocculus and is reversible with revascularization. At a later stage, the glomerular tuft retracts, loses its microscopic structure, and dies.

In the initial stages of ischemia, there is no inflammation in the renal interstitium. When ischemia is more severe, inflammation appears in the interstitium, probably with some cell necrosis.

Terminally, the inflammatory component becomes predominant and is associated with irreversible fibrosis.

NEPHROANGIOSCLEROSIS

Nephroangiosclerosis is the major renal lesion directly related to systemic hypertension; the clipped kidney is largely protected from this effect. In response to the increase in arteriolar wall stress and to the increase in protein and lipid deposits, arterial wall thickness increases. This increase involves smooth-muscle cell proliferation, protein deposition, and fibrosis. Later, nephroangiosclerosis leads to obstruction of the arteriolar lumen with consequent localized distal small areas of severe ischemia. The ischemic lesions related to the nephroangiosclerotic process can be compared with lacunar infarcts described in the brain. The irreversible ischemic renal lesions are associated with local small cystic formation, bordered by fibrosis.

GLOMERULOSCLEROSIS

Glomerulosclerosis is less frequent than nephroangiosclerosis in hypertension. This lesion is related to the high perfusion pressure within the glomerular capillaries. At an early stage, it appears as fibrotic scars leading to partial adherence of the glomerular tufts to the Bowman capsules. Later, the tufts are irreversibly fibrotic with complete disappearance of the normal structure.

The effects of renal revascularization on interstitial inflammation are unknown, but experimental revascularization of severely inflamed ischemic kidneys is associated with glomerulosclerosis.

In experimental renovascular hypertension, these three lesions have been observed. In the absence of treatment, the clipped kidney is usually microscopically normal or near normal, showing only some early signs of ischemia involving tubular dilatation and glomerular tuft shrinkage. During ACE inhibition, the degree of ischemia becomes more severe. Major dilatation of the tubules is observed and interstitial inflammation appears. Due to the presence of the clip on the main renal artery, ischemia is diffuse and relatively homogeneous in the clipped kidney. In contrast, in the contralateral untouched kidney, nephroangiosclerosis, and in some places, glomerulosclerosis, are prominent. The vascular lesions are distal and therefore, the secondary ischemic lesions are always focal, localized, and associated with some lesions of glomerulosclerosis in the nonischemic areas. In contrast to the worsening of lesions in the clipped kidney, ACE inhibition prevents the formation of lesions of nephroangiosclerosis in the contralateral kidney.

The physiological consequences of these anatomical lesions have been extensively investigated. After five weeks of treatment with enalapril (2mg/kg/day) or vehicle, the untouched kidney was removed, and thus renal function became exclusively dependent on the clipped kidney [18]. The treated animals were randomly divided into two groups: one in which treatment with enalapril was stopped (treated/untreated) and a second in which the treatment was continued (treated/treated). Survival rates were affected by the treatment. Three deaths occurred among 17 rats in the hypertensive untreated group, 10 among 24 rats in the treated/untreated group, and 12 among 23 rats in the treated/treated group. Moreover, in surviving animals, the concentration of plasma creatinine was correlated with the weight and the presence of lesions in the remnant kidney. As in the experiments reported by Gröne and Helmchen [16], ACE inhibition induced severe morphological alterations in the clipped kidney whose consequences were only unmasked when the contralateral untouched kidney was removed.

In other experiments performed by Jackson *et al* [20], drug treatment of 1-clip, 2-kidney hypertensive rats was continued for 12 months: enalapril was adjusted to 14mg/kg/day and minoxidil to 40mg/kg/day. At 12 months, blood pressure was 201±8mmHg (untreated control group), 181±6mmHg (minoxidil group), and 122±3mmHg (enalapril group). Of the rats, 84% survived in the enalapril group, 48% in the minoxidil group, and 15% in the untreated group, which shows the overall beneficial effect of blood pressure control. As in our experiments, the untouched kidney was protected from the histological lesions observed in the untreated group by minoxidil and enalapril. In contrast, the clipped kidney from the enalapril group was markedly reduced in size, and, on microscopic examination, had prominent cortical lesions, interstitial fibrosis, and collapse of glomerular tufts. In five animals of the enalapril group, cessation of therapy for two weeks did not lead to recovery of glomerular filtration in the clipped kidney; this was confirmed on histological examination.

These several experiments published from 1982–1990 are coherent from several viewpoints:
- Drug treatment of 1-clip, 2-kidney renovascular hypertension in rats improves survival, reduces cardiac hypertrophy, and diminishes vascular and ischemic renal lesions in the untouched kidney.
- ACE inhibition was the only really effective antihypertensive drug treatment. Minoxidil or triple therapy with clonidine, furosemide, and dihydralazine failed adequately to control blood pressure. In one experiment, however, dihydralazine was as effective as enalapril on blood pressure in rats on a sodium-free diet.

- The ACE inhibitor induced cessation of glomerular filtration in severely stenotic kidneys and generated major lesions in the glomeruli, the tubules, and the interstitium. Renal lesions were largely irreversible after treatment for five weeks or more.

The conclusion is that the functional changes induced by ACE inhibition in severely stenotic kidneys are likely to induce anatomical lesions, and the cost of blood-pressure control is the effective loss of the kidney. This can be considered as a pharmacologic nephrectomy [20].

Animal experiments, however, differ from the situation in man in several aspects [21,22]. The onset of the disease is precisely known in rats, but is frequently unknown in patients. Many cases of human atherosclerotic renovascular hypertension are secondary to essential hypertension. The experimental clip on the renal artery is a reproducible and uniform lesion, whereas in man, the size and the location of the atherosclerotic plaques are quite variable. The evolution of human atheromatous plaques is unpredictable, as is also the natural history of the different forms of fibromuscular diseases of the renal arteries. Finally, the clinical context does not exist in rats, whereas it has a predominant influence in patients. Thus, we should be cautious in transferring experimental information to clinical situations.

EVIDENCE FOR PARALLELISM BETWEEN THE RENIN-DEPENDENT FUNCTIONAL CHANGES IN THE STENOTIC KIDNEY OF MAN AND ANIMALS DURING ANGIOTENSIN-CONVERTING ENZYME INHIBITION

The obvious major question now is, are the functional consequences of activation or inhibition of the RAS in a kidney distal to a renal artery stenosis similar in rats and patients? The answer is yes, they are. A second question is, are these functional changes able to induce the same anatomical lesions in man as in rats? The answer to this second question is uncertain since the problem is more complex as a consequence of the nature and evolution of human arterial disease.

All investigations performed so far in patients with unilateral renal artery stenosis indicate similar changes in renal function after ACE inhibition to those described in animals [23]. Wenting et al [24] have shown in patients with a unilateral renal artery stenosis, that a single dose of 50mg captopril reduced the renal extraction ratios of ^{131}I-hippuran and ^{125}I-thalamate in 8 of 14 patients. The uptake of 99m Tc-diethylene triaminepenta-acetic acid, a measure

of glomerular filtration, became almost zero in the stenosed kidneys of seven patients.

Hodsman et al [25] reported a fall in effective renal plasma flow (^{123}I-hippuran renography) on the stenotic side from 162 ± 41ml/min to 102 ± 41 and a converse rise on the contralateral side from 298 ± 21ml/min to 437 ± 48ml/min after three months of enalapril treatment in a group of 10 patients with unilateral artery stenosis. Overall, creatinine clearance decreased from an initial mean ($\pm$SEM) of 105 ± 12ml/min to 88 ± 8ml/min. The concomitant increase in serum creatinine was related to the decrease in systemic arterial pressure ($r=-0.68$, $P<0.05$).

Miyamori et al [26] showed that captopril (37.5–75mg/day for one week) decreased the GFR of the stenotic kidney of five patients with unilateral renal artery stenosis from 24.3 ± 4.9 ml/min to 8.8ml/min. Effective renal plasma flow (ERPF) was unchanged. In the nonstenotic kidney, GFR did not change and the ERPF increased from 265 ± 14 to 318 ± 14ml/min. Similar changes were reported in four patients after 48 weeks of treatment.

Still more important, is the comparison of the renal effects of a fall in blood pressure induced by ACE inhibition to a similar fall in blood pressure induced by another antihypertensive treatment. Blood pressure and renal hemodynamic changes in patients with renovascular hypertension treated with captopril 25mg (n = 14) or sodium nitroprusside (n = 8) were analyzed by Textor et al [27, 28]. No significant changes in ERPF were detected. Following captopril administration, however, the GFR fell from 78 ± 8ml/min to 58 ± 6ml/min, which was below the limits observed with nitroprusside infusion (84 ± 9ml/min).

Ribstein et al [29] compared in 10 patients (six with bilateral renal artery stenosis and four with unilateral stenosis), the effects of 20mg nifedipine with the effects of 50mg captopril. The fall in blood pressure was 7.0 ± 2.9% after captopril and 19.1 ± 3.5% after nifedipine ($P<0.006$). The ERPF did not change, but creatinine clearance fell by 22.6 ± 11.7% after captopril and increased by 12.6 ± 5.5% after nifedipine ($P<0.019$). A reduction in sodium excretion induced by captopril contrasted with the nifedipine-induced natriuresis ($P=0.042$).

After four weeks of treatment with nifedipine or captopril, administered to six patients with renovascular hypertension in order to achieve the same degree of systemic blood-pressure reduction, Miyamori et al observed a decrease in GFR of the stenotic kidney from 24 ± 6ml/min to 11 ± 2ml/min ($P<0.01$) during captopril administration and a much less marked decrease (to 18.8 ± 5ml/min) during nifedipine administration [30]. The ERPF increased in the nonstenotic kidneys in response to both drugs. These results in man are at variance with the experimental observations of Huang [31] and Ploth *et al* [32], who reported a similar response of the 2-kidney, 1-clip renovascular rats to verapamil and to the blockade of the RAS. Calcium blockade, as well as ACE inhibition, increased GFR and ERPF in the contralateral unclipped kidney and decreased GFR in the clipped kidney, in parallel to the fall in blood pressure. They concluded that, during both treatments, the essential factor was an important fall of the postclip pressure, which was sufficient to explain the decrease in GFR. The conclusion from human data is at variance with these animal studies in that calcium antagonism may preferentially dilate preglomerular arterioles and reduce the renal vascular resistance with less effects on postglomerular arterioles. In contrast, ACE inhibition predominantly dilates the postglomerular arterioles in the stenotic kidney.

In conclusion, any fall in systemic blood pressure induced by a drug treatment may decrease GFR when a renal artery stenosis is present, as shown for example by the data of Textor *et al* [27]. Angiotensin-converting enzyme inhibition is certainly able to do this, but is still likely to be more dangerous than other agents because of its intrarenal effects. The reality of these effects is demonstrated when a fall in GFR occurs in the absence of a fall in systemic blood pressure, such as illustrated in a patient with stenosis of the artery to a solitary kidney [28]. Moreover, acute and chronic treatment with drugs other than ACE inhibitors, particularly calcium blockers, might be as effective as ACE inhibitors in controlling systemic blood pressure, and might preserve the GFR of the stenotic kidney.

Thus, treatment of renovascular hypertension with an ACE inhibitor will decrease perfusion pressure beyond the stenosis, and reduce efferent arteriolar resistances, therefore inducing a fall in GFR additional to that due to the stenosis itself. This adverse renal effect is the basis for a diagnostic test for renovascular hypertension by the acute administration of captopril [33]. Do we have evidence that such chronic hypofiltration has consequences on renal function and morphology, which are more serious than the transitory and apparently benign functional changes observed after a single administration of an ACE inhibitor? Furthermore, do we have evidence that a chronic state of hypofiltration induced by ACE inhibition creates lesions similar to those reported in animals, which are ischemic atrophy or 'disuse' atrophy [34]?

To the first question, we can answer that with brief ACE inhibition, interruption of treatment is accompanied by a normalization of renal function [35,36]. One of the longest instances of a captopril-induced renal insufficiency was followed for two years, monitored by an increase in plasma creatinine from 127 to 295μmol/l. Plasma creatinine came back towards its initial level on stopping ACE inhibition [36].

A wider issue is the possible facilitation of renal artery thrombosis by ACE inhibition [37]. The natural history of untreated renovascular hypertension is characterized by the occurrence of renal artery occlusion due to various mechanisms, including local thrombosis, plaque rupture, intraparietal hematoma, and dissection of the renal artery [21,22]. These complications are characteristic of the human disease, whether atherosclerotic or fibromuscular. Small series of selected patients cannot give unbiased information concerning a possibly increased incidence of renal artery occlusion specifically due to the use of ACE inhibitors [38]. The optimistic conclusions of some studies are no more valid than the occasional pessimistic observations of others [39–43]. Even in the presence of a bilateral artery stenosis, the occurrence of renal failure is not constant, probably because of the asymmetry in the severity of the occlusive disease.

Among 10 patients, Hodsman *et al* observed four occlusions of the affected artery within two years of treatment with an ACE inhibitor [25]; these were not associated with a sharp deterioration in overall renal function and were revealed only by routine renography. Moreover, these authors pointed out that the presence of this complication was already present in six of 20 patients before the start of their trial. If the fall in blood pressure induced by ACE inhibition is more rapid and more marked beyond the stenosis than it is with other antihypertensive drugs, this will certainly create the hemodynamic conditions that favor local thrombosis.

On a theoretical basis, but in the absence of firm epidemiological evidence (mainly due to the complexity of the local disease), it is justified to consider ACE inhibition as a risk factor promoting occlusion of a stenotic renal artery, particularly under two circumstances where the RAS has a critical role to support both systemic blood pressure and GFR. These circumstances are, first, in cases of severe stenosis, and second with the existence of sodium depletion, either as a consequence of progression to the hyponatremic syndrome of a malignant phase of hypertension [44], or of diuretic treatment.

Since the earlier observation of the renal effects of captopril in severe essential and renovascular hypertension, the role of sodium depletion in increasing the risk of renal deterioration has been consistently confirmed. Acute renal failure can be corrected by salt replacement, even without interrupting captopril therapy, and it may be improved by blockade of prostaglandin synthesis with aspirin [45]. In a series of 89 patients, the occurrence of occlusion of a unilateral renal artery stenosis during antihypertensive drug treatment was reviewed [37]. Complete occlusion occurred in 14 patients (18%), among whom only three showed a significant rise in serum creatinine. The combination of a diuretic and an ACE inhibitor showed an independent relationship to the development of an occlusion ($P<0.05$), and the ACE inhibitor alone also showed an almost significant relationship ($P=0.06$). However, ACE inhibition may lead to complete loss of renal function on one side without necessarily causing a rise in serum creatinine, when a functional contralateral kidney is present (see *Chapter 27*).

THE SUCCESS RATE OF DRUG TREATMENT OF RENOVASCULAR HYPERTENSION WITH AND WITHOUT ANGIOTENSIN-CONVERTING ENZYME INHIBITORS

A review of the results reported with the various drug treatments of renovascular hypertension does suggest an improvement in the quality of systemic blood-pressure control with ACE inhibitors [38]. Well adapted to the physiopathology of the disease, as well as attractive, ACE inhibitors are in several respects, an excellent treatment of renovascular hypertension.

We have reviewed the indirect and direct evidence, which suggests, unfortunately, that in a percentage of cases, ACE inhibitors may be responsible for pharmacologic 'nephrectomy' resulting from occlusion of the renal artery or a 'disuse' atrophy of the kidney. Such a risk might be justified in the absence of specific and effective radiological or surgical treatment. This, however, is not the situation. It would also be justified if the control of blood pressure were not possible by drugs other than ACE inhibitors. This again may not be correct.

An extensive prospective randomized, double-blind study was performed by Franklin and Smith [46]. They included 75 patients with renovascular disease whose diastolic blood pressure was above 95mmHg despite hydrochlorothiazide treatment (50mg daily). Both triple therapy (timolol, hydralazine, and hydrochlorothiazide) and enalapril therapy (5mg twice daily to 20mg twice daily, and hydrochlorothiazide up to 100mg daily) were effective in decreasing systolic blood pressure, respectively, by 20 and 32mmHg ($P<0.005$) and diastolic blood pressure by 18 and 20mmHg (no significant difference between groups).

A modest superiority in the control of blood pressure by ACE inhibition was thus shown. Effective control of diastolic hypertension was considered to occur in 96% of patients receiving enalapril compared with 82% in patients receiving the triple-drug regimen. However, among 49 patients participating in an extension of the study and treated with enalapril, deterioration of renal function was observed in 10 patients against only one among 39 patients treated with the triple therapy. This triple therapy included a β-blocker, timolol, which is able to decrease plasma renin activity. Unfortunately, no randomized study has yet been performed to compare the effects on systemic blood pressure and on renal function of the stenotic kidney, of the decrease in renin release induced by a β-blocker, with the blockade of the RAS induced by an ACE inhibitor.

In the study of Franklin and Smith, the main risk factor for the development of renal problems was the existence of a severe degree of unilateral or bilateral renal artery stenosis. The treatment selected in this study was probably not the most suitable. Given that enalapril alone has been shown to lower total exchangeable sodium in hypertension with renovascular disease [25], the dose of hydrochlorothiazide required (up to 100mg daily) was probably excessive. On the other hand, calcium blockers, which are also effective antihypertensive drugs with possible different intrarenal effects [29,30], were not used in the study. Thus, it remains possible that renovascular hypertension, or at any rate, hypertension with renovascular disease, can be controlled in many patients by medical treatment excluding ACE inhibitors. This medical strategy could have less risks for the affected kidney than has ACE inhibition if the fall in perfusion pressure of a stenotic kidney is better tolerated in the presence of a functional intrarenal RAS.

PRACTICAL RECOMMENDATIONS

Although opinions on the validity of surgical or percutaneous angioplastic treatment of renal artery stenosis may vary according to the success rates of surgeons or radiologists [47,48], the logical treatment of this disease is the recanalization of the abnormal renal artery. A successful procedure is the only way to obtain, simultaneously, a fall in blood pressure and the restoration and preservation of renal function.

Both atherosclerotic and fibromuscular lesions are progressive and frequently bilateral either at the time of discovery, or later [21,22]. Two kidneys are usual, not a luxury. When the diagnosis of renovascular hypertension due to unilateral or predominantly unilateral renal artery stenosis has been confirmed, the proposal to treat the condition using an ACE inhibitor for one month in the absence of diuretics, might be useful to improve cardiovascular and metabolic status and to predict the systemic blood-pressure response to the surgical or radiological intervention [49]. This, however, might also be risky if there is a severe stenosis (>80%). Diuretics should certainly be excluded from treatment.

When long-term medical treatment is selected because the experience of the radiologist or surgeon is considered insufficient, or because there is no opportunity to refer the patient to a center with the relevant expertise, ACE inhibitors should not, in our view, be considered as a first choice. Other drugs can be almost as effective in blood-pressure control with probably less renal risks. No currently available form of medical treatment, however, will protect the patient from the natural evolution of the disease towards a sudden or progressive complete occlusion of the stenotic renal artery. Moreover, compliance with drug therapy and side effects will be other limiting factors of long-term, and frequently complex, drug treatments.

When medical treatment of hypertension will include an ACE inhibitor and a diuretic, renal artery stenosis should be reasonably excluded whatever the age of the patient and even more, in elderly patients. This can be performed on the basis of a clinical strategy aiming at the recognition of a subgroup at risk (severe hypertension or hypertension of recent and rapid onset, cigarette smoking, lateralized abdominal or loin bruit, a slightly increased plasma creatinine or reduced plasma potassium, the presence of a peripheral vascular disease) [50–52]. In these patients, systematic supplementary tests should be performed (see *Chapters 55* and *88*). If the blood pressure of a compliant hypertensive patient who has previously been given an ACE inhibitor and a diuretic, becomes resistant to a previously effective treatment, or when an increase in serum creatinine is found, diuretics should be immediately stopped; renovascular hypertension previously absent or undiagnosed may exist. It should be borne in mind that severe intrarenal lesions are also able to impair renal function during ACE inhibition and to create a 'pseudo-renal artery stenosis' syndrome [53].

Angiotensin-converting enzyme inhibition has made modern medicine much more effective in patients with certain cardiac, vascular, and renal diseases. We must admit, however, that it has complicated the initial and long-term management of the hypertensive patient with renovascular disease.

REFERENCES

1. Bengis RG, Coleman TG. Antihypertensive effect of prolonged blockade of angiotensin formation in benign and malignant, one- and two-kidney Goldblatt hypertensive rats. *Clinical Science* 1979;57:53–62.

2. Hall JE. Control of sodium excretion by angiotensin II: Intrarenal mechanisms and blood pressure regulation. *American Journal of Physiology* 1986;250:R960–72.

3. Farrow PR, Wilkinson R. Reversible renal failure during treatment with captopril. *British Medical Journal* 1979;1:1680.

4. Shaw AB, Gopalka SK. Renal artery thrombosis caused by antihypertensive treatment. *British Medical Journal* 1982;285:1617.

5. Aldigier JC, Plouin PF, Guyene TT, Thibonnier M, Corvol P, Ménard J. Comparison of the hormonal and renal effects of captopril in severe essential and renovascular hypertension. *American Journal of Cardiology* 1982;49:1447–52.

6. Hricik DE, Browning PJ, Kopelman R, Goorno WE, Madias NE, Dzau V. Captopril-induced functional renal insufficiency in patients with bilateral renal-artery stenosis or renal-artery stenosis in a solitary kidney. *New England Journal of Medicine* 1983;308:373–6.

7. Curtis JJ, Luke RG, Whelchel JD, Diethelm AG, Jones P, Dustan HP. Inhibition of angiotensin converting enzyme in renal-transplant recipients with hypertension. *New England Journal of Medicine* 1983;308:377–81.

8. Huang WC, Ploth DW, Bell PD, Work J, Navar LG. Bilateral renal function responses to converting enzyme inhibitor (SQ 20,881) in two-kidney, one-clip Goldblatt hypertensive rats. *Hypertension* 1981;3:285–93.

9. Huang WC, Navar LG. Effects of unclipping and converting enzyme inhibition on bilateral renal function in Goldblatt hypertensive rats. *Kidney International* 1983;23:816–22.

10. Woods RL, Anderson PW, Korner PI. Renal and systemic effects of enalapril in chronic one-kidney hypertension. *Hypertension* 1986;8:109–16.

11. Anderson WP, Denton KM, Woods RL, Alcorn D. Angiotensin II and the maintenance of GFR and renal blood flow during renal artery narrowing. *Kidney International* 1990;38 (suppl 30):109–13.

12. Robertson JIS, Richards AM. Converting enzyme inhibitors and renal function in cardiac failure. *Kidney International* 1987;31 (suppl 20):S-216–9.

13. Ploth DW. Angiotensin-dependent renal mechanisms in two-kidney, one-clip renal vascular hypertension. *American Journal of Physiology* 1983;245:F131–41.

14. Möhring J, Möhring B, Naumann HJ, Philippi A, Homsy E, Orth H, Dauda G, Kazda S, Gross F. Salt and water balance and renin activity in renal hypertension of rats. *American Journal of Physiology* 1975;228:1847–55.

15. Helmchen U, Gröne HJ, Kirchertz EJ, Bader H, Bohle RM, Kneissler U, Khosla C. Contrasting renal effects of different antihypertensive agents in hypertensive rats with bilaterally constricted renal arteries. *Kidney International* 1982;22 (suppl 12):198–205.

16. Gröne HJ, Helmchen U. Impairment and recovery of the clipped kidney in two kidney, one clip hypertensive rats during and after antihypertensive therapy. *Laboratory Investigation* 1986;54:645–55.

17. Michel JB, Dussaule JC, Choudat L, Auzan C, Nochy D, Corvol P, Ménard J. Effects of antihypertensive treatment in one-clip, two-kidney hypertension in rats. *Kidney International* 1986;29:1011–20.

18. Michel JB, Dussaule JC, Choudat L, Nochy D, Corvol P, Ménard J. Renal damage induced in the clipped kidney of one-clip, two-kidney hypertensive rats during normalization of blood pressure by converting enzyme inhibition. *Kidney International* 1987;31 (suppl 20):168–72.

19. Michel JB, Nochy D, Choudat L, Dussaule JC, Philippe M, Chastang C, Corvol P, Ménard J. Consequences of renal morphologic damage induced by inhibition of converting enzyme in rat renovascular hypertension. *Laboratory Investigation* 1987;57:402–11.

20. Jackson B, Franze L, Sumithran E, Johnston CI. Pharmacologic nephrectomy with chronic angiotensin converting enzyme inhibitor treatment in renovascular hypertension in the rat. *Journal of Laboratory and Clinical Medicine* 1990;115:21–7.

21. Dean RH, Kieffer RW, Smith BM, Oates JA, Nadeau JHJ, Hollifield JW, Dupont WD. Renovascular hypertension. Anatomic and renal function changes during drug therapy. *Archives of Surgery* 1981;116:1408–15.

22. Schreiber MJ, Pohl MA, Novick AC. The natural history of atherosclerotic and fibromuscular renal artery disease. *Urologic Clinics of North America* 1984;II:383–92.

23. Bender W, La France N, Walker WG. Mechanism of deterioration in renal function in patients with renovascular hypertension treated with enalapril. *Hypertension* 1984;6 (suppl I):193–7.

24. Wenting GJ, Tan-Tjiong HL, Derkx FHM, de Bruyn JHB, Man in't Veld, AJ, Schalekamp MADH. Split renal function after captopril in unilateral renal artery stenosis. *British Medical Journal* 1984;288:886–90.

25. Hodsman GP, Brown JJ, Cumming AMM, Davies DL, East BW, Lever AF, Morton JJ, Murray GD, Robertson JIS. Enalapril in treatment of hypertension with renal artery stenosis. Changes in blood pressure, renin, angiotensin I and II, renal function and body composition. *American Journal of Medicine* 1984;77 (2A):52–60.

26. Miyamori I, Yasuhara S, Takeda Y, Koshida H, Ikeda M, Nagai K, Okamoto H, Morise T, Takeda R, Aburano T. Effects of converting enzyme inhibition on split renal function in renovascular hypertension. *Hypertension* 1986;**8**:415–21.

27. Textor SC, Novick AC, Tarazi RC, Klimas V, Vidt DG, Pohl M. Critical perfusion pressure for renal function in patients with bilateral atherosclerotic renal vascular disease. *Annals of Internal Medicine* 1985;**102**:308–14.

28. Textor SC, Tarazi RC, Novick AC, Bravo EL, Fouad FM. Regulation of renal hemodynamics and glomerular filtration in patients with renovascular hypertension during converting enzyme inhibition with captopril. *American Journal of Medicine* 1984;**76** (5B):29–37.

29. Ribstein J, Mourad G, Mimran A. Contrasting acute effects of captopril and nifedipine on renal function in renovascular hypertension. *American Journal of Hypertension* 1988;**1**:239–44.

30. Miyamori I, Yasuhara S, Matsubara T, Takasaki H, Takeda R. Comparative effects of captopril and nifedipine on split renal function in renovascular hypertension. *American Journal of Hypertension* 1988;**1**:359–63.

31. Huang WC. Effects of verapamil alone and with captopril on blood pressure and bilateral renal function in Goldblatt hypertensive rats. *Clinical Science* 1985;**70**:453–60.

32. Ploth DW, Kleeman K, Morrill L, Rademacher R, Jackson CA. Effects of verapamil and converting enzyme inhibition on bilateral renal function of two-kidney, one-clip hypertensive rats. *Clinical Science* 1987:**72**:657–67.

33. Geyskes GG, Oei HY, Puylaert CBAJ, Dorhout EJ. Renovascular hypertension identified by captopril-induced changes in the renogram. *Hypertension* 1987;**9**:451–8.

34. Hricik DE. Angiotensin-converting enzyme inhibition in renovascular hypertension: The narrowing gap between functional renal failure and progressive renal atrophy. *Journal of Laboratory and Clinical Medicine* 1990;**115**:8–9.

35. Dominiczak A, Isles C, Gillen G, Brown JJ. Angiotensin converting enzyme inhibition and renal insufficiency in patients with bilateral renovascular disease. *Journal of Human Hypertension* 1988;**2**:53–6.

36. Salahudeen AK, Pringle A. Reversibility of captopril-induced renal insufficiency after prolonged use in an unusual case of renovascular hypertension. *Journal of Human Hypertension* 1988;**2**:57–9.

37. Postma CT, Hoefnagels WH, Barentsz JO, de Boo T, Thien T. Occlusion of unilateral stenosed renal arteries. Relation to medical treatment. *Journal of Human Hypertension* 1989;**2**:185–90.

38. Hollenberg NK. Medical therapy of renovascular hypertension: Efficacy and safety of captopril in 269 patients. *Cardiovascular Reviews and Reports* 1983;**4**:852–78.

39. Reams GP, Bauer JH, Gaddy P. Use of the converting enzyme inhibitor enalapril in renovascular hypertension. Effect on blood pressure, renal function, and the renin–angiotensin–aldosterone system. *Hypertension* 1986;**8**:290–7.

40. Fyhrquist F, Grönhagen-Riska C, Tikkanen I, Junggren IL. Long-term monotherapy with lisinopril in renovascular hypertension. *Journal of Cardiovascular Pharmacology* 1987;**9** (suppl 3):61–5.

41. Hollenberg NK. Renal hemodynamics in essential and renovascular hypertension. Influence of captopril. *American Journal of Medicine* 1984;**76** (5B):22–8.

42. Tillman DM, Adams FG, Gillen G, Morton JJ, Robertson JIS. Ramipril for hypertension secondary to renal artery stenosis. Changes in blood pressure, the renin–angiotensin system and total and divided renal function. *American Journal of Cardiology* 1987;**59**:133–42D.

43. Canzanello VJ, Madaio MP, Madias NE. Enalapril in the management of hypertension associated with renal artery stenosis. *Journal of Clinical Pharmacology* 1987;**27**:32–40.

44. Editorial. Hyponatremic hypertensive syndrome. *Lancet* 1986;**i**:18–9.

45. Andreucci VE, Conte G, Dal Canton A, Di Minno G, Usberti M. The causal role of salt depletion in acute renal failure due to captopril in hypertensive patients with a single functioning kidney. *Renal Failure* 1987;**10**:9–20.

46. Franklin SS, Smith RD. Comparison of effects of enalapril plus hydrochlorothiazide versus standard triple therapy on renal function in renovascular hypertension. *American Journal of Medicine* 1985;**79** (3C):14–23.

47. Ramsay LE, Waller PC. Blood pressure response to percutaneous transluminal angioplasty for renovascular hypertension: An overview of published series. *British Medical Journal* 1990;**300**:569–72.

48. Jeunemaitre X, Julien J, Raynaud A, Pagny JY, Gaux JC, Plouin PF, Ménard J, Corvol P. Angioplastie endoluminale dans l'hypertension artérielle renovasculaire. Cent quatre cas. *Presse Medicale* 1990;**19**:205–9.

49. Staessen J, Wilms G, Baert A, Fagard R, Lijnen P, Suy R, Amery A. Blood pressure during long-term converting-enzyme inhibition predicts the curability of renovascular hypertension by angioplasty. *American Journal of Hypertension* 1988;**1**:208–14.

50. Salmon P, Brown MA. Renal artery stenosis and peripheral vascular disease: Implications for ACE inhibitor therapy. *Lancet* 1990;**336**:321.

51. Priollet P, Lazareth I, Manière-Constantin D, Aimé F. Renal artery stenosis and peripheral vascular disease. *Lancet* 1990;**336**:879.

52. Choudhri AH, Cleland JGF, Rowlands PC, Tran TL, McCarty M, Al-Kutoubi MAO. Unsuspected renal artery stenosis in peripheral vascular disease. *British Medical Journal* 1990;**30**:1197–8.

53. Pettinger WA, Mitchell HC, Lee HC, Redman HC. Pseudo-renal stenosis (PRAS) syndrome. *American Journal of Hypertension* 1989;**2**:349–51.

90 A BUOYANT VIEW OF THE VALUE OF ANGIOTENSIN-CONVERTING ENZYME INHIBITION IN RENOVASCULAR DISEASE

NORMAN K HOLLENBERG

A critical assessment of the role of ACE inhibitors in the treatment of renovascular hypertension must address a series of issues. What are the effectiveness and the risks of the available alternative treatment strategies, surgery, and angioplasty? If medical therapy is considered, how does the efficacy and safety of ACE inhibition compare with that of the alternative agents available? What is known of the natural history of hypertension and the renal arterial lesion? Equally important, how much of what is known has come from studies in patients with the disease, and how much from animal models? Although in some areas the available information is limited or strongly biased, a reasonable and balanced view of the data assigns, I believe, an important role for ACE inhibitors in the treatment of selected patients with renovascular hypertension. Indeed, in some patients they are, in my view, the clear treatment of choice.

SURGICAL TREATMENT OF RENOVASCULAR HYPERTENSION

Since surgical treatment is the time-honored treatment of renal arterial disease, it seems appropriate to begin with what has been learned about the effectiveness and safety of surgery for reno-vascular hypertension. There is a venerable literature. Only a few years separated the classic Goldblatt experiment in the dog in 1934 [1] and the first report of cure of hypertension by nephrectomy in 1938 [2]. By 1956, Homer Smith was able to present a sobering paper [3]: among 575 patients who underwent unilateral nephrectomy for presumed renovascular hypertension, only 26% were cured and only approximately half derived any benefit. Smith was unable to report on morbidity or mortality, but did point out that the rather discouraging results must be an under-estimate as only the best were likely to be published. By 1963, Stamey concluded that 'we are in an era of romance with renal artery stenosis. When the hue and cry is over, there will be far less enthusiasm for the surgical repair of … atherosclerotic occlusion

of the renal artery' [4]. By the mid-1970s, careful analysis supported that notion [5].

In atherosclerotic disease (Fig. 90.1), the reported cure rates for hypertension ranged from less than 25% to over 80%, with a large number of centers finding intermediate results [6–16]. The definition of improvement varied, so that at least some of the difference in reported responses could be attributable to this variation. The definition of failure, on the other hand, is unequivo-cal and the range of failure reported was 12–44%, with an average of 24%. Death occurred in 9%.

These observations can be explained. In 1962, Morris et al [6] described 200 patients with atherosclerotic renovascular disease treated by surgery. The report rapidly became a landmark and the expectation in the field. Of the patients, 80% were cured, 88% were cured or improved, and the mortality was only 6%. These results were, however, in sharp contrast to those de-scribed in other papers (Fig. 90.1). In 1965, Laragh et al assemb-led 11 publications describing 279 patients from 11 centers [7]. These described events before the report by Morris et al [6]. In the 11 centers, 42% of patients had their hypertension cured by surgery, 30% apparently showed improvement, and the failure rate was 28%, including an 8% mortality. Reports from surgical centers [12–16] generally described a low failure rate and mortality in the next two decades. Reports written by internists, on the other hand, differed substantially [8–10]. The latter described a failure rate and mortality that substantially exceeded those described in papers from surgical units. Patient selection appears to be pivotal. Surgery in the patient with advanced atherosclerosis, particularly if there is also diabetes mellitus or uremia, is associated with a very high mortality and failure rate [17,18]. The surgical teams described better results, and this, at least in part, reflected better patient selection. It seems likely that the surgeons had learned to avoid the patients at very high risk. On the other hand, such patients do require treatment.

In one report, surgical treatment of coronary and cerebral arterial disease preceded that for renovascular hypertension [16]. The Cooperative Study on Renal Vascular Hypertension enrolled 300 patients in 15 centers. The cure and failure rates and mortality were strikingly similar to those reported in the earlier analyses

Reference number	Number of patients	Number of centers	Hypertension			Dead (%)
			Cured (%)	Improved (%)	Failures (%)	
6	200	1	80	8	12	6
7	297	11	42	30	28	8
8	66	1	23	33	44	25
9	28	1	7	46	29	18
10	36	1	14	33	4	8
11	48	1	—	—	—	17
12	300	15	41	15	32	12
13	78	1	36	50	14	1
14	105	1	28	52	18	3
15	52	1	29	58	8	6
16	100	1	40	51	9	2
Total	1,310	35	45*	29*	24*	9*

*weighted means

Fig. 90.1   Results of surgery for hypertension associated with atherosclerotic renovascular disease

[17,18]. Results were substantially better for isolated unilateral renal atherosclerosis. Hypertension was cured in approximately 50% of patients, and the mortality was less than 6%, as opposed to 13.8% for those with bilateral disease. Operative deaths occurred in older individuals with advanced atherosclerosis, with evidence of vascular occlusive disease in multiple beds, and with an enlarged heart or impaired renal function.

In contrast to the results in atherosclerotic renovascular disease, surgical treatment for fibromuscular dysplasia has consistently been better (Fig. 90.2). Mortality has been rare and surgical success more frequent.

What of preservation of renal function, an often-stated indication for surgery or angioplasty? The question is particularly important in the patient with bilateral disease or with a solitary

ischemic kidney. Unfortunately, as indicated by the Cooperative Study, aggressive surgery for bilateral renal arterial disease has been associated with a higher mortality. Indeed, the suggestion has been made that surgery in such patients should be restricted to the more severely involved kidney [17,18].

PERCUTANEOUS TRANSLUMINAL ANGIOPLASTY

Despite the fact that transluminal angioplasty is a more recent technic [20], a pattern similar to that described for surgery is emerging. After initial enthusiasm, with time the reports and analyses have become much more balanced and sober. In most early

Reference number	Number of patients	Number of centers	Hypertension			Dead (%)
			Cured (%)	Improved (%)	Failures (%)	
7	62	5	61	32	7	0
8	42	1	57	19	21	2
12	179	15	64	11	25	3
19	19	1	81	5	14	5
14	159	1	63	33	4	0
15	25	1	56	40	0	4

Fig. 90.2   Results of surgery for hypertension associated with fibrous dysplasia.

Reference number	Angioplasty attempted	Excluded from analysis*	Technical failure	Response of blood pressure		
				Cured	Improved	Failed
27	31	3	5(16)	7(25)	6(21)	15(54)
28	68	0	10(15)	12(18)	38(56)	18(26)
29	70	0	2(3)	14(20)	29(41)	27(39)
25	89	0	21(24)	26(29)	22(25)	41(46)
30	98	0	7(7)	25(26)	66(67)	7(7)
31	63	8	8(13)	16(29)	17(31)	22(40)
32	94	2	12(13)	14(15)	42(46)	36(39)
33	80	0	11(14)	21(26)	29(36)	30(38)
34	65	7	5(8)	20(34)	22(38)	16(28)
35	33	1	3(9)	8(25)	15(47)	9(28)
Total	691	21	84(12)	163(24)	286(43)	221(33)
Range (%)			3–2	15–34	21–67	7–54

*excludes technical failures

Fig. 90.3 Summary of outcome after angioplasty for renal artery stenosis in 10 published series of hypertensive patients. Results are numbers (percentages) of patients. Modified from Ramsey LE and Waller PC [26].

Reference number	Atheromatous renal artery stenosis				Fibromuscular renal artery stenosis			
	Technically successful angioplasty	Response of blood-pressure			Technically successful angioplasty	Response of blood pressure		
		Cured	Improved	Failed*		Cured	Improved	Failed*
27	13	2(15)	4(31)	7(54)	8	5(63)	1(13)	2(25)
28	44	8(18)	29(66)	7(16)	9	4(44)	5(56)	0(0)
29	44	4(9)	19(43)	21(48)	21	10(48)	10(48)	1(5)
25	34	7(21)	10(29)	17(50)	27	16(59)	9(33)	2(7)
30	61	15(25)	46(75)	0(0)	27	10(37)	17(63)	0(0)
31	34	5(15)	15(44)	14(41)	13	11(85)	2(15)	0(0)
32	60	9(15)	30(50)	21(35)	20	5(25)	12(60)	3(15)
33	48	11(23)	21(44)	16(33)	21	10(48)	8(38)	3(14)
34	31	9(29)	15(48)	7(23)	22	11(50)	7(32)	4(18)
35	22	3(14)	13(59)	6(27)	7	5(71)	2(29)	0(0)
Total	391	73(19)	202(52)	116(30)	175	87(50)	73(42)	15(9)
Range (%)		9–29	29–75	0–54		25–85	13–63	0–25

*excludes technical failures

Fig. 90.4 Summary of outcome after angioplasty in 10 published series of hypertensive patients according to indication for angioplasty (atheromatous or fibromuscular renal artery stenosis). Results are numbers (percentages) of patients. Modified from Ramsey LE and Waller PC [26].

90.3

papers, the series were small and follow-up was rather short [21–23]. The two most substantial early reports were those of Schwarten et al [24] and of Sos et al [25]. During an 18-month period, Schwarten et al [24] performed transluminal angioplasty in 66 patients, including 55 with atherosclerosis. Follow-up ranged from 1 to 18 months. Technical success was high: 23 of the patients (44%) became normotensive, and an additional 25 patients (48%) improved. The success rate, at least in part, probably reflected the fact that the results for atherosclerosis and fibromuscular disease were pooled. Sos et al [25] reported similar overall results, but pointed out that the technical success rate dropped sharply in the most needy group of patients — those with bilateral atherosclerotic disease. They also emphasized the clinically important fact that an atherosclerotic lesion at the ostium, the most common location, is that least likely to do well with angioplasty.

A 'meta-analysis' carried a sobering message [26]. This paper reviewed 10 published series involving 691 patients treated by angioplasty for renovascular hypertension. There were large variations between studies in the rate of technical success and in the outcome. As was true in the case of surgery, patients with fibromuscular dysplasia had a higher cure rate than did those with atherosclerotic lesions (50% versus 19%) (Figs. 90.3 and 90.4) [27–35]. Complications occurred in 63 patients (9%) and there were three reported deaths (0.4%). These authors concluded, quite reasonably, that angioplasty in renovascular hypertension is not a panacea. The patients who have the strongest clinical need, those with advanced atherosclerosis, are those who are most likely to have a lesion that is technically difficult to correct, and to have the highest failure and complication rate. Mortality, however, seems to be substantially lower than with surgery.

MEDICAL THERAPY AND RENOVASCULAR HYPERTENSION

Until the past decade, medical therapy for renal vascular hypertension was often both poorly tolerated and ineffective (Fig. 90.5). A substantial series of patients was described by Dustan et al in 1963

Reference number	n	Follow-up	Agents*	Results (%) Controlled or much improved	Intermediate	Failure	Deaths (%)
Non-ACE inhibitor therapy							
36	32	1–6 yr	hydralazine guanethidine	41	31	28	31
37	42	0–8 yr		45	36	19	
10	72	34 mo					40
38	165	0.5–10 yr		46	30	24	30
39	83	5 yr		35	34	31	34
40	11	1–180 d	propranolol	45	27	18	
41	114	1–8 yr	methyldopa	81	16	3	
	59	7–14 yr		46	15	39	
42	44	<6 mo	propranolol	59	23	8	
	16		no propranolol	29	8	63	
ACE inhibitor therapy							
43	12	6 mo	captopril	92	8	0	
44	15	6 wk	captopril	62	23	15	
45	53	2–3 yr	captopril	68	20	17	
46	21	28±3 mo	captopril	90	10	0	
47	269	0.3–2 yr	captopril	77	18	5	
48	48		enalapril	96	0	4	

*in most patients, a thiazide diuretic was also used

Fig. 90.5 Reported responses to medical therapy in renovascular hypertension.

[36]. A combination of a thiazide, hydralazine, and guanethidine — the heroic therapy of that era, with the patients as the heroes — was used in 32 cases, with a follow-up of from 1–6 years. Hypertension was controlled in only 41%; therapy clearly failed in 28%; and 31% died during the follow-up period (Fig. 90.5). During the subsequent two decades, the experience of others was equally discouraging [10, 37–42]. Adequate control of hypertension or improvement was achieved in only 35–45%; 25% or more were failures; and during a similar follow-up period, mortality was 30–40%. The predominant lesion in these series was atherosclerosis.

Since β-adrenergic blocking agents act at least in part by blunting renin release (see *Chapter 84*), one would have expected improved experience with their use. Indeed, when the follow-up period was limited, this appeared to be the case [40]. With more prolonged observation, however, the results once again were disappointing [42].

With the advent of ACE inhibitors, a more promising pattern emerged, with much higher success and lower failure rates [43–48]. One of the largest series [47] involved 269 patients in whom captopril had been used as emergency or urgent therapy because of extreme resistance of the hypertension despite aggressive medical therapy, or because previous therapy had been intolerable. On earlier therapy, the median and mode for diastolic blood pressure exceeded 110mmHg, despite the use of three or more antihypertensive agents together in over 90% of patients. Over 40% were azotemic, and 136 of the 269 patients had either a solitary kidney or advanced bilateral renal arterial disease. The efficacy of ACE inhibition in these patients was unequivocal. Despite the severity of the disease, an ACE inhibitor employed alone or with a thiazide was ineffective in only 5% of patients. Over 80% of patients achieved striking improvement, or goal blood pressure. In 13%, adverse reactions led to discontinuation of treatment, but the captopril doses often exceeded 600mg/d in the earlier studies, and the frequency of azotemia was high [47]. Equal success rates were achieved with enalapril [48]. Thus, the efficacy of ACE inhibition in hypertension with renovascular disease is unambiguous. There are, on the other hand, legitimate sources of concern that require examination.

ANGIOTENSIN-CONVERTING ENZYME INHIBITION IN RENOVASCULAR HYPERTENSION: SOURCES OF CONCERN

One important issue is the development of acute renal failure following the initiation of ACE inhibitor therapy. The reason centers on the fact that with renal artery stenosis, the affected kidney may be dependent on locally elevated Ang II to sustain glomerular filtration and main renal artery pressure [58,71,72]. The patients with renovascular hypertension at particular risk have bilateral renal artery stenosis or a critical stenosis involving a solitary kidney. An impressive series of reports began to appear soon after the advent of ACE inhibition in renovascular hypertension [49–55]. Is acute renal failure a necessary or predictable influence of ACE inhibition, in those specifically at risk? Such case reports provide a numerator, but not a denominator. In the 269 patients described earlier [47], rapidly progressive acute renal failure, sufficient to lead to discontinuation or adjustment of treatment, occurred in eight patients (3%) during the first several weeks of study. All patients developing this syndrome had either renal artery stenosis involving a solitary kidney or advanced bilateral renal artery stenosis, and all were already azotemic when captopril therapy was started. Many also were given concomitant diuretic therapy. As ACE inhibitor therapy alone in patients with hypertension and renal artery stenosis has been shown to lead to a fall in body sodium content [71], diuretics should be employed cautiously in this context. The frequency of renal failure in the 136 specifically at risk because of bilateral arterial disease or renal arterial disease of a solitary kidney, was 6% — substantially less than might have been expected from the anecdotal reports. In some cases it was possible to adjust the captopril dose to a level providing clinically acceptable control of hypertension and a clinically acceptable level of azotemia [47].

Comparable data were found in a prospective trial of enalapril in patients with renovascular hypertension [48]. This study involved 48 patients, of whom 44% had bilateral renal artery stenosis and 32% had abnormal renal function at baseline. Goal blood pressure was achieved in 96% of the patients receiving enalapril, and oliguric acute renal failure occurred in none despite the fact that 21 had bilateral renal artery stenosis. In one patient, azotemia did develop rapidly but resolved with discontinuation of the accompanying diuretic. Such a maneuver would be considered, of course, only in the patient in whom hypertension was severe and in whom surgery or angioplasty were inappropriate, but as indicated in earlier sections, this is not a rare circumstance.

What of the long term? Three cases of renal artery occlusion were reported in patients with advanced atherosclerotic stenosis during a 13–21-week period of treatment with captopril plus hydrochlorothiazide [56]. On the other hand, no cases were observed among patients followed up for up to two years in the earlier analysis [47]. Occlusion of a stenotic renal artery, of course, can occur as a consequence of the natural course of the disease [57].

In one series of 20 patients, eight had unilateral renal artery occlusion before starting enalapril; five further patients showed evidence of unilateral renal circulatory shutdown within 3–25 months of starting enalapril. A cause-and-effect relationship is difficult to establish in these circumstances [72].

In rats, atrophy of the renal parenchyma distal to renal artery stenosis has been noted with ACE inhibition, but not with alternative agents [58, 59]. The rat, however, is particularly prone to show renal abnormalities with increasing age, and with hypertension, and may well be particularly dependent on local Ang II formation for maintaining filtration rate and overall renal function [60]. There is only limited information available at the moment to indicate that data from the rat are applicable to patients.

As an alternative treatment strategy, calcium-channel blocking agents may allow better preservation of renal function than can ACE inhibitors in patients specifically at risk [61,62]. This has been proposed, based on local intrarenal control mechanisms, in patients at risk [63]. In our experience, unfortunately, it has not been rare for patients in this category to respond inadequately to a calcium-channel blocking agent. The combination of an ACE inhibitor and a calcium-channel blocking agent, allowing the use of lower doses of the ACE inhibitor, may, however, turn out to be beneficial. Certainly, there has been substantial interest in that combination for the treatment of intractable hypertension [64–67].

CONCLUSIONS

Most physicians would prefer to identify the patients likely to do well with surgery or angioplasty in preference to long-standing medical therapy. Clearly surgery and angioplasty, when effective have an advantage preserving renal parenchyma and function. On the other hand, there are many patients with severe hypertension who are poor candidates for surgery and angioplasty and in whom the hypertension is difficult to treat. While there can be little doubt that a kidney distal to a renal artery lesion is often heavily dependent on enhanced intrarenal Ang II to preserve its function and thus is at risk with ACE inhibition [58,71,72], such treatment can be especially effective in controlling systemic hypertension. The treatment of severe hypertension is crucial. The 70 placebo-treated patients in the VA Cooperative Study in severe hypertensives experienced 28 adverse cardiovascular events in a follow-up of 11 months, versus only three events in the 73 actively treated patients [68]. Many patients with renovascular hypertension are elderly, and it is known that antihypertensive therapy in the elderly reduces risk substantially [69,70]. The widely held view that ACE inhibitors should be withheld in such patients leaves them at considerable risk of complications of their severe hypertension on an ineffective or poorly tolerated medical regimen. A balanced view would suggest that a trial of ACE inhibitor therapy is not only reasonable in such patients, it is mandatory.

REFERENCES

1. Goldblatt H, Lynch J, Hanzel R, Summerville WW. Studies on experimental hypertension. *Journal of Experimental Medicine* 1934;59:347–80.

2. Leadbetter WF, Burkland CE. Hypertension in unilateral renal disease. *Journal of Urology* 1938;39:611–26.

3. Smith HW. Unilateral nephrectomy in hypertensive disease. *Journal of Urology* 1956;76:685–701.

4. Stamey TA. *Renovascular hypertension*. Baltimore: Williams & Wilkins, 1963.

5. McNeil BJ, Adelstein SJ. Measures of clinical efficacy: The value of case finding in hypertensive renovascular disease. *New England Journal of Medicine* 1975;293:221–6.

6. Morris GC, DeBakey NE, Cooley DS. Surgical treatment of renal failure of renovascular origin. *JAMA* 1962;182:609–16.

7. Laragh JH, Cannon PJ, Meltzer JI. Recent advances in hypertension. *American Journal of Medicine* 1965;39:616–45.

8. Perloff D, Sokolow M, Wylie EH, Palubinskas AJ. Renal vascular hypertension, further experiences. *American Heart Journal* 1967;74:614–31.

9. Kirdendall WM, Fitz AE, Lawrence MS. Renal hypertension: Diagnosis and surgical treatment. *New England Journal of Medicine* 1967;276:479–86.

10. Shapiro AP, Perez-Stable E, Scheib ET. Renal artery stenosis and hypertension. *American Journal of Medicine* 1969;47:175–93.

11. Bergentz SE, Kjellbo H, Hansson LO, Hood B. Renal artery stenosis and hypertension. *Scandinavian Journal of Urology and Nephrology* 1969;3:229–34.

12. Foster JH, Maxwell MH, Franklin SS, Bleifer KH, Trippel OH, Julian OC, DeCamp PT, Varady PT. Renovascular occlusive disease: Results of operative treatment. *JAMA* 1975;231:1043–8.

13. Dean RH, Oates JA, Wilson JP, Rhamy RK, Hollifield JW, Burko H, Foster JH. Bilateral renal artery stenosis and renovascular hypertension. *Surgery* 1977;81:53–62.

14. Stanley JC, Fry WJ. Surgical treatment of renovascular hypertension. *Archives of Surgery* 1977;112:1291–7.

15. Lankford NS, Donohue JP, Grim CE, Gifford RW, Vidt D. Results of surgical treatment of renovascular hypertension. *Journal of Urology* 1979;122:439–43.

16. Novick AC, Straffon RA, Stewart BH, Gifford RW, Vidt D. Diminished operative morbidity and mortality in renal revascularization. *JAMA* 1981;246:749–53.

17. Franklin SS, Young JD, Maxwell MH, Foster JH, Palmer JM, Cerny J, Varady PT. Operative morbidity and mortality in renovascular disease. *JAMA* 1975;231:1148–53.

18. Maxwell MH. Cooperative study of renovascular hypertension: Current status. *Kidney International* 1975;8 (suppl 5):153–60.

19. Korobkin M, Perloff DL, Palubinskas AJ. Renal arteriography in the evaluation of unexplained hypertension in children and adolescents. *Journal of Pediatrics* 1976;**88**:388–93.

20. Dotter CT. Transluminal angioplasty: A long view. *Radiology* 1980;**135**: 561–4.

21. Weinberger MH, Yune HY, Grim GE, Luft FC, Klatte EC, Donohue JP. Percutaneous transluminal angioplasty for renal artery stenosis in a solitary functioning kidney. *Annals of Internal Medicine* 1979;**91**:684–8.

22. Katzen BT, Fordis M, Keiser HR. Percutaneous transluminal angioplasty: A new nonsurgical treatment for renovascular hypertension. In: Yamori Y, ed. *Prophylactic approach to hypertensive diseases.* New York: Raven Press, 1979:459.

23. Tegtmeyer CJ, Dyer R, Teates CD, Ayers CR, Carey RM, Wellons HA Jr, Stanton LW. Percutaneous transluminal dilatation of the renal arteries. *Radiology* 1980;**135**:589–99.

24. Schwarten DE, Yune HY, Klatte EC, Grim CE, Weinberger MH. Clinical experience with percutaneous transluminal angioplasty (PTA) of stenotic renal arteries. *Radiology* 1980;**135**:601–4.

25. Sos TA, Pickering TG, Sniderman K, Saddekni S, Case DB, Silane MF, Vaughan ED Jr, Laragh JH. Percutaneous transluminal angioplasty in renovascular hypertension due to atheroma or fibromuscular dysplasia. *New England Journal of Medicine* 1983;**309**:274–9.

26. Ramsay LE, Waller PC. Blood pressure response to percutaneous transluminal angioplasty for renovascular hypertension: An overview of published series. *British Medical Journal* 1990;**300**:569–72.

27. Martin EC, Mattern RF, Baer L, Pankuchen EI, Casarella WJ. Renal angioplasty for hypertension: Predictive factors for long-term success *American Journal of Roentgenology* 1981;**137**:921–4.

28. Colapinto RF, Stronell RD, Harries–Jones EP, Gildiner M, Hobbs BB, Farrow GA, Wilson DR, Morrow JD, Logan AG, Birch SJ. Percutaneous transluminal dilatation of the renal artery. Follow-up studies on renovascular hypertension. *American Journal of Roentgenology* 1982;**139**:727–32.

29. Geyskes GG, Puylaert CB, Oei HY, Dorhourt Mees EJ. Follow-up study of 70 patients with renal artery stenosis treated by percutaneous transluminal dilatation. *British Medical Journal* 1983;**287**:333–6.

30. Tegtmeyer CJ, Kellum CD, Ayers C. Percutaneous transluminal angioplasty of the renal artery. *Radiology* 1984;**153**:77–84.

31. Miller GA, Ford KK, Braun SD, Newman GE, Moore AV Jr, Malone R, Dunnick NR. Percutaneous transluminal angioplasty vs surgery for renovascular hypertension. *American Journal of Roentgenology* 1985;**144**:447–50.

32. Martin LG, Price RB, Casarella WJ, Sones PJ, Wells JO Jr, Zellmer RA, Chuang VP, Silbiger ML Jr, Berkman WA. Percutaneous angioplasty in clinical management of renovascular hypertension: Initial and long-term results. *Radiology* 1985;**155**:629–33.

33. Kaplan-Pavlobcic S, Koecli M, Obrez I, Luzar S, Licina A, Kolar B, Surlan M. Percutaneous transluminal renal angioplasty: Follow-up studies in renovascular hypertension. *Prezeglad Lekarski* 1985;**42**:342–4.

34. Kuhlmann U, Greminger P, Gruntzig A, Schneider E, Pouliadis G, Luscher T, Steurer J, Siegenthaler W, Vetter W. Long-term experience in percutaneous transluminal dilatation of renal artery stenosis. *American Journal of Medicine* 1985;**79**:692–8.

35. Bell GM, Reid J, Buist TA. Percutaneous transluminal angioplasty improves blood pressure and renal function in renovascular hypertension. *Quarterly Journal of Medicine* 1987;**63**:393–403.

36. Dustan HP, Page IH, Poutasse EF, Wilson L. An evaluation of treatment of hypertension associated with occlusive renal arterial disease. *Circulation* 1963;**27**:1018–33.

37. Peart WS. Treatment of hypertension associated with renal artery stenosis. In: Engel A, Larson T, eds. *Stroke: Thule International Symposium.* Stockholm: Nordiska Bokhandelns Forlag, 1967:

38. Kjellbo H, Lund N, Bergentz SE, Hood B. Renal artery stenosis and hypertension. *Scandinavian Journal of Urology and Nephrology* 1970;**4**:49–57.

39. Owen K. Results of surgical treatment in comparison with medical treatment of renovascular hypertension. *Clinical Science and Molecular Medicine* 1973;**45** (suppl):95–8.

40. Buhler FR, Laragh JH, Vaughan ED Jr, Brunner HR, Gavras H, Baer L. The antihypertensive action of propranolol. Specific antirenin responses in high and normal renin forms of essential, renal, renovascular and malignant hypertension. In: Laragh JH, ed. *Hypertension manual.* New York: Yorke, 1973:873–98.

41. Hunt JC, Strong CG. Renovascular hypertension: Mechanisms, natural history and treatment. In: LaraghJH, ed. *Hypertension manual*, New York: Yorke, 1976:509–36.

42. Streeten DHP, Anderson GH Jr. Outpatient experience with saralasin. *Kidney International* 1979;**15**:44–52.

43. Studer A, Luscher T, Greminger P, Siegenthaler W, Vetter W. Captopril in therapy-resistant essential and renovascular hypertension. In: H Brunner, F Gross, eds. *Recent advances in hypertensive therapy.* Amsterdam: Excerpta Medica, 1981:31–40.

44. Atkinson AB, Brown JJ, Cumming AMM, Fraser R, Lever AF, Leckie BJ, Morton JJ, Robertson JIS, Davies DL. Captopril in the management of hypertension with renal artery stenosis: Its long-term effect as a predictor of surgical outcome. *American Journal of Cardiology* 1982;**49**:1460–6.

45. Hollifield JW, Moore LC, Winn SD, Marshall MA, McCombs C, Frazer MG, Goncharenko V. Angiotensin converting enzyme inhibition in renovascular hypertension. *Cardiovascular Reviews and Reports* 1982;**3**:673–6.

46. Case DB, Atlas SA, Marion RM, Laragh JH. Long term efficacy of captopril in renovascular and essential hypertension. *American Journal of Cardiology* 1982;**49**:1440–6.

47. Hollenberg NK. Medical therapy of renovascular hypertension: Efficacy and safety of captopril in 269 patients. *Cardiovascular Reviews and Reports* 1983;**4**:852–79.

48. Franklin SS, Smith RD. Comparison of effects of enalapril plus hydrochlorothiazide versus standard triple therapy on renal function in renovascular hypertension. *American Journal of Medicine* 1985;**79** (suppl 3C): 14–23.

49. Collste P, Haglund K, Lundgren G, Magnusson G, Oatman J. Reversible renal failure during treatment with captopril. *British Medical Journal* 1979;**2**:612–3.

50. Farrow PR, Wilkinson R. Reversible renal failure during treatment with captopril. *British Medical Journal* 1979;**1**:1680.

51. Grossman A, Eckland D, Price P, Edwards CR. Captopril: Reversible renal failure with severe hyperkalemia. *Lancet* 1980;**i**:712.

52. Kawamura J, Okada Y, Nishibuchi S, Yoshida O. Transient anuria following administration of angiotensin I-converting enzyme inhibitor (SQ 14225) in a patient with renal artery stenosis of the solitary kidney successfully treated with renal autotransplantation. *Journal of Urology* 1982;**127**:111–3.

53. Silas JH, Klenka Z, Solomon SA, Bone JM. Captopril induced reversible renal failure: A marker of renal artery stenosis affecting a solitary kidney. *British Medical Journal* 1983;**286**:1702–3.

54. Hricik DE, Browning PJ, Kopelman R, Goorno WE, Madias NE, Dzau VJ. Captopril induced functional renal insufficiency in patients with bilateral renal artery stenoses or renal artery stenosis in a solitary kidney. *New England Journal of Medicine* 1983;**308**:373–6.

55. Curtis JJ, Luke RG, Whelcher JD, Diethelm AG, Jones P, Dustan HP. Inhibition of angiotensin converting enzyme in renal transplant recipients with hypertension. *New England Journal of Medicine* 1983;**308**:377–81.

56. Hoefnagels WHL, Thien T. Renal artery occlusion in patients with renovascular hypertension treated with captopril. *British Medical Journal* 1986;**292**:24–5.

57. Schreiber MJ, Pohl MA, Novick AC. The natural history of atherosclerotic and fibrous renal artery disease. *Urologic Clinics of North America* 1984;**11**:383–91.

58. Michel JB, Dussaule JC, Choudat L, Auzan C, Nochy D, Corvol P, Menard J. Effects of antihypertensive treatment in one-clip, two kidney hypertension in rats. *Kidney International* 1986;**29**:1011–20.

59. Jackson B, Franze L, Sumithran E, Johnston CI. Pharmacologic nephrectomy with chronic angiotensin-converting enzyme inhibitor treatment in renovascular hypertension in the rat. *Journal of Laboratory and Clinical Medicine* 1990;**115**: 21–7.

60. Anderson S, Rennke HG, Brenner BM. Therapeutic advantage of converting enzyme inhibitors in arresting progressive renal disease associated with systemic hypertension in the rat. *Journal of Clinical Investigation* 1986;77:1993–2000.

61. Helmchen U, Grone HJ, Kirchentz EJ, Bader H, Bohle RM, Kneissler U, Khusla MC. Contrasting renal effects of different antihypertensive agents in hypertensive rats with bilaterally constricted renal arteries. *Kidney International* 1982;22 (suppl 12):198–205.

62. Mourad G, Ribstein J, Argiles A, Mimran A, Nion C. Contrasting effects of acute angiotensin converting enzyme inhibitors and calcium antagonists in transplant renal artery stenosis. *Nephrology, Dialysis, and Transplantation* 1988;4: 66–70.

63. Loutzenhiser RD, Epstein M. Calcium antagonists and renal hemodynamics. *American Journal of Physiology* 1985;2:F619–29.

64. Mimran A, Ribstein J. Effect of chronic nifedipine in patients inadequately controlled by a converting enzyme inhibitor and a diuretic. *Journal of Cardiovascular Pharmacology* 1985;7:S92–5.

65. Brouwer RML, Bolli P, Erne P, Conen D, Kiowski W, Buhler FR. Antihypertensive treatment using calcium antagonists in combination with captopril rather than diuretics. *Journal of Cardiovascular Pharmacology* 1985;7:S88–91.

66. Singer DRJ, Markandu ND, Shore AC, MacGregor GA. Captopril and nifedipine in combination for moderate to severe essential hypertension. *Hypertension* 1987;9:629–33.

67. Pieri R, Nardecchia A, Pirrelli A. Combined nifedipine and captopril treatment in moderately severe primary hypertension. *American Journal of Nephrology* 1986;6 (suppl 1):111–4.

68. Veterans Administration Cooperative Study Group on Antihypertensive Agents. Effects of treatment on morbidity in hypertension. I. Results in patients with diastolic blood pressure averaging 115 through 129 mm Hg. *JAMA* 1967;202:1028–34.

69. European Working Party on High Blood Pressure in the Elderly. Mortality and morbidity results from the European Working Party on high blood pressure in the elderly trial. *Lancet* 1985;i:1349–55.

70. Coope J, Warrender TS. Randomized trial of treatment of hypertension in elderly patients in primary care. *British Medical Journal* 1986;293:1145–8.

71. Hodsman GP, Brown JJ, Cumming AMM, Davies DL, East BW, Lever AF, Morton JJ, Murray GD, Robertson JIS. Enalapril in the treatment of hypertension with renal artery stenosis: Changes in blood pressure, renin, angiotensin I and II, renal function, and body composition. *American Journal of Medicine* 1984;77 (2A):52–60.

72. Tillman DM, Malatino LS, Cumming AMM, Hodsman GP, Leckie BJ, Lever AF, Morton JJ, Webb DJ, Robertson JIS. Enalapril in hypertension with renal artery stenosis: Long-term follow-up and effects on renal function. *Journal of Hypertension* 1984;2 (suppl 2):93–100.

91 ANGIOTENSIN-CONVERTING ENZYME INHIBITORS IN THE TREATMENT OF ESSENTIAL HYPERTENSION

LENNART HANSSON, BJÖRN DAHLÖF, ANDERS HIMMELMANN, AND ANDERS SVENSSON

INTRODUCTION

Treatment of arterial hypertension with antihypertensive drugs became established in the 1950s. Antihypertensive therapy now constitutes one of the most common medical interventions in industrialized countries. The rapid and gratifying developments in this field over the last four decades can be attributed to a number of circumstances: the availability of effective and well-tolerated antihypertensive agents [1–4]; numerous controlled intervention trials which, albeit with various limitations and some inconsistencies, have demonstrated a reduction in morbidity and mortality when hypertension is treated [5]; and consequent increasing awareness that control of hypertension has a great potential for reducing cardiovascular morbidity and mortality [6].

Four classes of antihypertensive compounds — diuretics, β-adrenoceptor blocking agents, calcium antagonists, and ACE inhibitors — are currently accepted as suitable for initial treatment of hypertension. These classes of drug have been recommended for such use by the Joint National Committee in the USA [7], by the World Health Organization [8], and by the International Society of Hypertension [8] in their most recent guidelines for the management of hypertension. The British Hypertension Society, more cautiously [9], advocates β-blockers or diuretics as initial treatment for essential hypertension, with ACE inhibitors or calcium antagonists as ready alternatives. The diversity of mechanisms by which these four drug classes lower arterial pressure deserves emphasis. Despite increasing insight into the pathophysiology of primary ('essential') hypertension in recent years [10,11], and some hopeful but as yet still faltering attempts to treat primary hypertension by using drugs that would correct such specific causal mechanisms [12–14], current treatment remains substantially arbitrary.

It is the purpose of this chapter to review clinical aspects of the use of ACE inhibitors in the treatment of primary (essential) hypertension. When ACE inhibitors were introduced into clinical medicine, it was widely supposed that they would be effective predominantly in circumstances such as renovascular hypertension, characterized by stimulation of the systemic RAS. The value of ACE inhibitors in renovascular hypertension has indeed been established (see *Chapter 88*). The fact that ACE inhibitors should prove effective in essential hypertension, particularly in the older patient, in whom the RAS tends to be suppressed (see *Chapter 62*), was less expected, but is, nevertheless, gratifying. As discussed later in this chapter, there are now suggestions that ACE inhibitors may offer advantages over some of the earlier antihypertensive drugs, but whether such theoretical assets will eventually provide enhanced cardiovascular protection must await the outcome of prospective, randomized, large-scale intervention studies such as the Captopril Prevention Project (CAPPP) trial [15].

ANGIOTENSIN-CONVERTING ENZYME INHIBITORS: EFFICACY IN ESSENTIAL HYPERTENSION

Although individual ACE inhibitors currently available differ as regards bioavailability, metabolism, route of elimination [16], and in their onset and duration of antihypertensive effects (Fig. 91.1), they are all competitive inhibitors of ACE and they all lower blood pressure by reducing total peripheral vascular resistance [17] (see *Chapter 87*).

MONOTHERAPY

In general, ACE inhibitors can be regarded as antihypertensive drugs with similar efficacy to other blood-pressure lowering agents [18]. Their antihypertensive effect is maintained during long-term treatment [19], which is probably similar for individual ACE inhibitors, at least when assessed using conventional blood-pressure recording devices [20–22].

Twenty-one parallel-group trials comparing six different ACE inhibitors with various other antihypertensive agents in mild-to-moderate essential hypertension are summarized in Fig. 91.2.

Specifically, ACE inhibitors have been found, in comparative studies, to be similarly effective to diuretics [23], β-blockers

	Captopril	Enalapril	Lisinopril	Ramipril	Cilazapril
time to peak blood level	1	3	7	2.5	2
hypotensive response to single dose:					
onset	0.5	1–1.5	2	2	1
time to maximum effect	1	4	6	4	6
duration of effect	4–6	8–12	18	18	10

Fig. 91.1 Time–effect relationship for some ACE inhibitors, in hours. Modified from Johnston CI [16].

[24,25], calcium antagonists [26], or methyldopa [27]. In one large double-blind trial, Herrick *et al* [28] found that enalapril, 20 or 40mg daily, lowered blood pressure significantly more than did atenolol, 50 or 100mg daily. Reduction of systolic pressure was noted to be more with lisinopril than with metoprolol [25]; with enalapril than with hydrochlorothiazide (in nonblack patients) [29]; and with lisinopril than with atenolol [30]. Conversely, some studies have demonstrated a slightly greater antihypertensive effect of comparator drugs, for example of the calcium antagonist isradipine [31], and of the combined α- and β-blocker labetalol [32] when compared with enalapril. A trial by Conway *et al* demonstrated a greater fall in the mean 24-hour ambulatory blood pressure with lisinopril than with enalapril, the advantage (average 5.9/3.3mmHg) being statistically significant for systolic blood pressure [33]. Thus, there might be minor differences between ACE inhibitors, but further studies with a wide range of doses are needed before firm conclusions can be drawn.

COMBINED THERAPY

It is often estimated that only some 30–60% of hypertensive patients attain adequate blood-pressure control with a single drug [34]. This means that a substantial proportion of the treated hypertensive population requires combination therapy. Angiotensin-converting enzyme inhibitors have additive effects when used with many, but not all, classes of other antihypertensive agent. The mechanisms underlying the interactions vary [35].

Diuretics

The RAS is activated during treatment with diuretics, and the reactive rise in peripheral plasma Ang II thus limits the fall in blood pressure which would otherwise occur. Therefore, it is appropriate to combine an ACE inhibitor with a diuretic when either alone fails to normalize blood pressure. In general, an acceptable antihypertensive response with these two drug types together is greater than 80% [36], With such a combination, lower doses of hydrochlorothiazide (6.25–25mg/d) than have traditionally been used in single therapy can achieve adequate blood-pressure reduction [37,38]. An important bonus, in addition to pressure reduction, is that the ACE inhibitor tends to counter adverse effects of thiazide diuretics on plasma electrolytes, uric acid, glucose, and lipids [35]. Thus, this is a particularly attractive combination.

It is important, however, to avoid the conjoint use of an ACE inhibitor with a potassium-conserving diuretic such as spironolactone, amiloride, or triamterene [16]. Since ACE inhibitors lower plasma Ang II concentration, aldosterone secretion and plasma aldosterone levels fall (see *Chapter 33*) and plasma potassium tends to rise [39,40]. Therefore, if an ACE inhibitor and a potassium-conserving diuretic are given together, dangerous hyperkalemia can occur, especially if there is concomitant renal impairment, or occult renal artery disease (see *Chapter 88*). These problems are more likely to occur in the elderly.

Dietary salt restriction

The antihypertensive effect of ACE inhibitors is also enhanced when dietary sodium intake is reduced, and moderate restriction of dietary sodium intake can thus be an alternative to adding a diuretic in selected patients who fail to achieve normotension on ACE inhibitor monotherapy [41]. The mechanism of this reinforced action is similar to that seen with diuretics, because dietary sodium restriction also activates the RAS.

Calcium antagonists

The combination of a dihydropyridine calcium antagonist with an ACE inhibitor can be even more effective than the more traditional combination of an ACE inhibitor with a diuretic

91.2

Reference	Authors	Number of patients	Duration (wk)	Drug dosage (mg/d)	Decrease in blood pressure (systolic/diastolic) (mmHg)*	Response rate (%)[†]	Comments
captopril (C)							
19	Andren et al (1985)	50	8	C 75–300 A 50–200	31/20 24/18		HCT added in 30 cases, open study 2 years
296	Captopril Research Group of Japan (1985)	270	12	C 37.5–75 Pr 60–120	26/15 23/12		TCM added in all cases; less adverse effects with C
297	Garinin (1986)	135	16	C 50–100 E 10–20	17/14 19/16		HCT added in 26 cases
298	Rumboldt et al (1988)	69	9	C100–200 E 40–80	28/21 35/25	97 100	HCT added in 53 cases
21	Witte and Walter (1987)	222	16	C 200 R 10	20/19; 26/18[†] 22/20; 28/18[†]	83 77	HCT added in 76 cases
enalapril (E)							
299	Chrysant et al (1983)	31	18	E 5–40 P			Well tolerated, effective
300	Goodwin (1984)	367	12	E 20–40 Pr 160–240	13/13% 11/12%	77 59	
301	Helgeland et al (1986)	436[§]	16	E 20–40 A 50–100 HCT 25–50	18/12 14/13 16/9		10-week extension
302	Sassano et al (1984)	100	26	E+ T+	20/19% 17/17%		hypokalemia occurred with E
303	Thind et al (1985)	32	16	E 10–40 C 75–300	28/18 29/17	75 75	HCT 50 added to all
29	Vidt (1984)	455	8	E 20–40 HCT 50–100 E+HCT	15/11% 20/13% 33/21%	22 42 80	
lisinopril (L)							
30	Bolzano et al (1987)	490	24	L 20–80 A 50–100	89 87		
304	Gomez et al (1985)	102	6	L 1.25–80 P	16/10		
305	Merrill et al (1987)	207	8	L 20 HCT 12.5 L+HCT	9.2% 6.4% 15.7%		8.2% stopped by adverse effects
23	Pool et al (1987)	394	24	L 20–80 HCT 12.5–50 L+HCT		82 67 84	
306	Morlin et al (1987)	136	12	L 20–80 N 48–80		82 79	
25	Zachariah et al (1987)	175	8	L 40–80 M 100–200		63 65	
ramipril (R)							
307	Karlberg et al (1987)	34[‖]	4	R 5–10 P	22/9		
308	Villamil et al (1987)	86	4	R 2.5–5 P	15/18		19 patients dropped out
perindopril (Pe)							
309	Morgan et al (1987)	32	4	Pe 2–8 P	22/11 3/2		Effects of Pe were independent of sodium intake
quinapril (Q)[‖]							
310	Gavras (1984)	8	1	Q 0.625–10	27/26		

* Compared to baseline or placebo values; † responders were patients in whom diastolic blood pressure was reduced to ≤90mmHg or by ≥5–10mmHg;
‡ blood-pressure reduction with the addition of hydrochlorothiazide; § single-blind study; ‖ nonblinded study.
A = atenolol; HCT = hydrochlorothiazide; E+ = E + HCT + oxprenolol + dihydralazine; M = metoprolol; N = nifedipine; Pr = propranolol; T+ = HCT + oxprenolol + dihydralazine; TCM = trichloromethiazide; P = placebo.

Fig. 91.2 Some parallel group studies comparing ACE inhibitors with other antihypertensive agents in mild/moderate hypertension. Modified from McAreavey D and Robertson JIS [22].

91.3

[42–44] and does not adversely affect the 'metabolic profile'. It is not clear at present exactly how calcium antagonists interact with ACE inhibitors as regards sodium balance, and the possible importance of this for blood-pressure reduction has not been determined.

An increase in exchangeable sodium with nifedipine monotherapy in essential hypertension has been reported [45]. Some conflicting findings have, however, been published. Nicardipine did not cause any detectable change in total body sodium [46], while a natriuresis has been seen on withdrawal of long-term nifedipine [47].

The antiadrenergic and parasympathomimetic effects of ACE inhibitors prevent or reduce the palpitations and reflex tachycardia which can be troublesome with dihydropyridine calcium antagonists. A reduction of headache and ankle edema has been claimed after the addition of captopril to nifedipine [48].

Thus, the combination of an ACE inhibitor and a calcium antagonist is usually effective and well tolerated.

Serotonergic type 2 antagonists

Two studies have reported particularly effective blood-pressure control when the serotonergic type 2 ($5HT_2$) antagonist ketanserin has been given together with, respectively, captopril [49] or enalapril [50].

Alpha-blockers

The α_1-blocker doxazosin, in combination with captopril or enalapril, has been reported to be effective in the treatment of hypertension. In one study, 53 of 56 patients were judged as therapeutic successes, side effects were mild, and favorable lipid changes were observed [51]. Experience is still, however, limited with this potentially useful combination.

Beta-blockers

Beta-blockers and ACE inhibitors share one antihypertensive action in that they both lower circulating concentrations of Ang II (see *Chapter 84*). Thus, this combination might not seem especially promising [35 52]. Indeed, MacGregor and co-workers added hydrochlorothiazide, propranolol, or nifedipine to captopril treatment in hypertensive patients and found no further fall in blood pressure with propranolol [53]. Wing *et al* likewise found that the combination of enalapril and atenolol was relatively ineffectual [54]. In contrast, Staessen *et al* reported that propranolol induced a further significant reduction of blood pressure in patients already receiving captopril; furthermore, there was no difference in antihypertensive efficacy between propranolol and a thiazide diuretic when used as additional

treatment [55]. Belz *et al* found that whereas the ACE inhibitor cilazapril and the β-blocker propranolol each reduced diastolic blood pressure by some 10mmHg when administered alone, the combination reduced diastolic pressure by an average of 20mmHg [56].

One possible explanation for these divergent results could be differences between patient populations, amongst which, inter alia, age may be an important factor. It is well known for example that circulating levels of renin decline with advancing age (see *Chapter 74*). When 262 patients with supine diastolic blood pressure in the range 95–115mmHg, while taking atenolol 50mg once daily were given lisinopril in addition, those below the age of 50 years had a 56% greater fall in diastolic pressure than did those older than 50 [57]. However, there are several problems with presumed age-related differences of antihypertensive effects [58], and sufficiently large, randomized, prospective studies have not yet been performed to settle this question. This problem is discussed further below.

In essential hypertension, ACE inhibitors are therefore valuably effective when given alone and also when combined with a variety of other antihypertensive agents. They can be used safely and effectively in combination with thiazide diuretics or with dihydropyridine calcium antagonists. There are more limited but encouraging reports of their combination with α-blockers and serotonergic antagonists. Angiotensin-converting enzyme inhibitors are less consistently useful (indeed some workers deny their value) when given together with β-blockers. One combination to avoid is that of an ACE inhibitor and a potassium-sparing diuretic, which can cause dangerous hyperkalemia [16].

RESISTANT HYPERTENSION

Provided that adherence to the regimen can be assured, we consider that hypertension should be regarded as resistant if the blood pressure cannot be reduced to less than 150/100mmHg by a rational triple-drug regimen, including a diuretic, prescribed in nearly maximal doses and if the pretreatment blood pressure was 180/115mmHg or higher [59]. Other workers have taken slightly different definitions [34].

The most frequent reason for failure of antihypertensive treatment is probably poor patient compliance. An underlying undetected secondary form of hypertension is an alternative possibility [60].

Several classes of antihypertensive agents may cause sodium retention, and an expanded extracellular volume has been related to apparent drug resistance [61]. Accordingly, an intensified diuretic scheme can be used [62]. As discussed earlier, however, diuretics stimulate renin secretion and hence a rise in plasma Ang II which then counteracts, to a greater or lesser extent, the antihypertensive action of these drugs [63,64].

In a study of 16 patients with refractory hypertension, a low sodium diet plus diuretics reduced blood pressure, body weight, and intravascular fluid volume, and increased heart rate, peripheral vascular resistance, and plasma renin activity (PRA) [65]. There was a close negative correlation between the per cent increase in PRA and the fall in mean blood pressure per unit of weight loss, indicating that patients who had the least percentage increase in PRA achieved the greatest reduction in blood pressure. After sodium depletion, infusion of the competitive Ang II antagonist saralasin reduced total peripheral resistance and induced a further drop in blood pressure [65], These observations strongly suggest that ACE inhibitors should effectively lower blood pressure in such circumstances.

In several studies of genuinely resistant hypertension, captopril, in doses up to 450mg daily and usually in combination with a diuretic, has proved effective [39,66–71]. In 34 men with essential hypertension that was resistant to long-term therapy with metoprolol (200mg/d) plus furosemide (80mg/d), captopril or minoxidil were added in a double-blind, randomized six-month trial [69]. Blood pressure fell by 28/13mmHg with the addition of captopril and by 23/12mmHg with minoxidil (Fig. 91.3). Captopril induced a 16% decrease in left ventricular mass index, whereas minoxidil had no effect [69].

In patients with refractory hypertension, including those resistant to captopril and/or minodixil, the addition of a β-blocker and a diuretic has often proved effective [70,71],

It may be concluded that ACE inhibitors are useful as additional therapy in patients with previously resistant hypertension. Moreover, there may be further benefits such as resolution of left ventricular hypertrophy and partial reversal of diuretic-induced perturbations in biochemical indices.

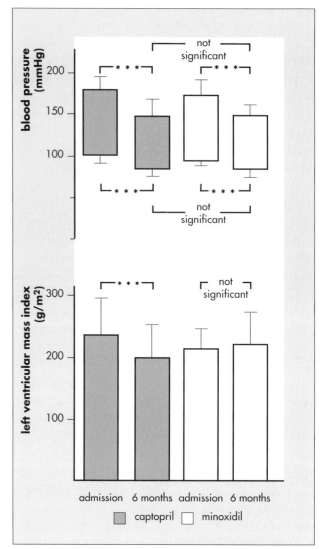

Fig. 91.3 Blood pressure and left ventricular mass index at admission in 34 male essential hypertensives with resistant hypertension after long-term treatment with 200mg/d metoprolol and 80mg/d furosemide, and after the addition of either captopril or minoxidil for six months. Data shown are mean ± SD. *** $P<0.001$. Modified from Julien J et al [69].

HYPERTENSION: URGENT TREATMENT

Circumstances in which urgent treatment of hypertension is needed are rare. Hypertensive encephalopathy, in which severe hypertension is complicated by clouding of consciousness, confusion or coma, headache, and/or convulsions does, however, require immediate therapy. Supervention of the malignant phase, recognized by the retinal appearance of hemorrhages and exudates, with or without papilledema, in a severely hypertensive patient (see *Chapter 60*), calls for hospital admission forthwith

and the institution of antihypertensive treatment within 24 hours [34]. In American parlance, 'hypertensive emergencies' are cases in which blood pressure must be lowered within one hour whereas 'hypertensive urgencies' require blood pressure to be controlled within 24 hours [72]. Great care must be exercised, however, since a rapid or excessive reduction in arterial pressure can cause cerebral hypoperfusion and ischemic brain damage [73]. The dangers of overhasty and unduly zealous blood-pressure reduction can hardly be overemphasized [74]. Moreover, sclerotic and rigid arteries, especially in the elderly, render them resistant to compression by a sphygmomanometer cuff and hence to a falsely high blood-pressure reading ('pseudohypertension'). Inappropriately aggressive therapy in such patients has led to death [75].

Hodsman et al [76] have enumerated the features likely to predict dangerously severe first-dose hypotension with an ACE inhibitor. These include old age, renal or renal artery disease, prior diuretic treatment, or other evidence of sodium depletion. (In less pressing circumstances, old patients can tolerate the introduction of ACE inhibitors with few problems, as is discussed in the following section.)

When urgent treatment is needed, orally administered captopril has been reported to give a significant and safe reduction in blood pressure, the antihypertensive effect occurring within 15 minutes [77]. Sublingual captopril [78,79] and intravenous enalaprilat [80] are also effective, their onset of action occurring within five minutes of administration. The efficacy and tolerability of sublingual captopril have been endorsed in the elderly [81,82]. Compared with ingested nifedipine, the fall in blood pressure with sublingual captopril is similar, although its antihypertensive action is more prolonged [83]. Parenthetically, it should be noted that, in these reports, although nifedipine was ostensibly 'sublingual', when given in this manner, it probably must be swallowed to work rather than being absorbed via the buccal mucosa [74,84,85]. In a randomized study in elderly hypertensives, sublingual captopril, unlike oral nifedipine, did not cause reflex tachycardia or severe hypotension [81].

In summary, ACE inhibitors appear to be relatively safe and well tolerated in hypertensive emergencies. They are probably equally as good as oral nifedipine, at least in elderly patients, although the potential hazard of causing renal impairment in the patient with bilateral renal artery stenosis must be kept in mind [22,86].

HYPERTENSION IN THE ELDERLY

Hypertension is common among the elderly, who comprise a large and progressively expanding proportion of the population [87]. Approximately 45% in the group aged 65–74 years have systolic pressures ≥160mmHg and/or diastolic pressures ≥95mmHg [88], while 64% of those in this age group have systolic pressures ≥140mmHg and/or diastolic pressures ≥90mmHg [89]. It is also clear that the absolute and relative importance of hypertension as a risk factor for cardiovascular disease and death does not decrease with age [90]. Furthermore, antihypertensive drug treatment has been shown to reduce

cardiovascular morbidity and mortality in subjects over 60 years of age [87,91]. In the Systolic Hypertension in the Elderly Program (SHEP), a double-blind placebo-controlled trial of treatment for isolated systolic hypertension in patients over 60 years of age, the total stroke incidence was reduced by 36% in the actively treated group [92]. The beneficial effects on morbidity and mortality of drug treatment in hypertensives in the age range 70–84 years have further been clearly demonstrated in the double-blind, placebo-controlled Swedish Trial in Old Patients with Hypertension (STOP-Hypertension) [93].

The pathophysiological features of essential hypertension in the elderly differ distinctly from those in younger patients [94]. In older hypertensive people, cardiac output, heart rate, and stroke volume are lower, whereas total peripheral resistance is higher, than in younger hypertensives. Angiotensin-converting enzyme inhibitors, which reduce peripheral resistance and do not impair cardiac function, would thus seem appropriate to use in the elderly. However, it was previously, and incorrectly, believed that ACE inhibitors were unsuitable for treatment of hypertension in older patients. Plasma renin falls progressively with age [94–96] and it was accordingly considered that this should make ACE inhibitors less effective in lowering blood pressure in the elderly [97]. Although some early reports seemed to support this notion [98], other studies, in healthy volunteers, revealed a greater fall in blood pressure with enalapril in the older subjects [99]. Several ACE inhibitors have now been shown to be both effective and well tolerated in elderly hypertensives [100–102].

In a multicenter surveillance study, 975 patients aged over 65 years and with severe treatment-resistant hypertension were given captopril, 50mg three times daily either as monotherapy or in combination with other antihypertensive agents [103]. In the 418 patients who were followed for one year, the systolic blood pressure fell by 18% and the diastolic pressure by 16%.

In another study, elderly patients with mild-to-moderate hypertension not responding to captopril 25mg twice daily were given either a higher dose of captopril (50mg twice daily) or the addition of hydrochlorothiazide 15mg twice daily [104]. The fall in diastolic blood pressure was greater in patients given hydrochlorothiazide than in those who received the higher dose of captopril. As in previous reports [105], the blood pressure response to an ACE inhibitor–diuretic combination was well tolerated.

Enalapril (10–20mg once daily) [106,107] and lisinopril (2.5–40mg once daily) [108–111] have also been used as monotherapy in the elderly. In a Belgian multicenter study of 3,060 patients, lisinopril was as efficacious and well tolerated in patients over 65 years as in patients younger than 65 [112]. Lisinopril treatment for one year in elderly hypertensives did not alter the glomerular filtration rate (GFR), while renal blood flow increased [113].

Newer ACE inhibitors such as cilazapril [114], delapril [115], perindopril [116], and quinapril [117,118] have also been shown to be efficacious and well tolerated in the elderly.

Compared with usual doses of diuretics [119–122,311] or of calcium antagonists [123], ACE inhibitors have similar anti-hypertensive efficacy, although formal comparisons of dose–response curves for drugs in these classes have not been reported. The metabolic disturbances associated with diuretic therapy, such as reductions in potassium and increases in urea, uric acid, glucose [119–122], and cholesterol [121], are not a feature of long-term treatment with ACE inhibitors.

Favorable effects noted with ACE inhibition in the elderly include increased exercise tolerance [124], absence of negative effects on quality of life [125] or lipid metabolism [126], and a reduction in the number and complexity of premature ventricular depolarizations [312].

Others, however, have raised caution. Atherosclerotic arterial disease is more common with aging, and the elderly subject with apparent primary (essential) hypertension may have occult renal artery stenosis [127–130]. Treatment with an ACE inhibitor could in this situation further impair the function of the affected kidney (see *Chapter 88*).

HYPERTENSION IN CHILDREN AND ADOLESCENTS

Hypertension presenting in a young person mandates a diligent search for a correctable underlying cause. Where no such form of secondary hypertension is present, initial intervention for childhood and adolescent hypertension should be non-pharmacological [11]. Antihypertensive drug therapy, however, is sometimes needed [131]. Angiotensin-converting enzyme inhibitors have proved to be both effective and well-tolerated in children and adolescents with hypertension.

In an international collaborative study, captopril was given to 73 children with severe hypertension, some with underlying secondary forms, others with essential hypertension [132]. Sixteen of these children were followed for more than one year. After three months, 62% had normalized their systolic blood pressure and 53% had normalized their diastolic blood pressure (that is, pressures were ≤95th percentile), while another 15% and 27% were considered 'responders' for either systolic or diastolic pressure, respectively (that is, there was blood-pressure reduction of at least 10%). A baseline measurement of PRA failed to predict the blood-pressure response.

Captopril has been used in hypertensive infants [133]. In an open study, all of 11 neonates, 5–84 days of age, had an antihypertensive response within 24 hours of the initial dose. Enalapril, once daily, has been used successfully in hypertensive children aged 3.5–12 months [134].

It must, nevertheless, be emphasized that because of the possible hazards of administering ACE inhibitors to pregnant women (see below), such therapy should be prescribed with caution in girls who have attained reproductive age. Due to the very limited information available regarding the use of ACE inhibitors in children, it is strongly recommended that manufacturing prescribing recommendations are followed closely and that regular patient follow-up is organized.

HYPERTENSION IN PREGNANCY

The RAS in normal and hypertensive pregnancy is discussed fully in *Chapters 50 and 52*. Angiotensin-converting enzyme inhibitors given during pregnancy in animals have been associated with high rates of fetal loss [135,136]. There are case reports of a very rare skull ossification defect in the fetus of mothers who conceived while on ACE inhibitor therapy [137,138]. Moreover, ACE inhibitor treatment in the second and third trimesters of pregnancy has been associated with oligohydramniosis and intrauterine growth retardation [138,139], as well as with hypotension and anuria in the newborn infant [140]. Although there are reports of a normal outcome of pregnancy for mothers who have been treated with captopril or enalapril [141,142], it seems that the fetus fares better if the ACE inhibitor is replaced by alternative antihypertensive agents once pregnancy is diagnosed [143].

Accordingly, ACE inhibitors are not recommended during gestation [144,145].

INITIATION AND CESSATION OF ANGIOTENSIN-CONVERTING ENZYME INHIBITOR THERAPY

Generally, a smooth reduction of blood pressure is seen upon treatment with an ACE inhibitor. Although a decrease in blood pressure can be observed within 30–120 minutes (see *Fig. 91.1*), the maximum effect may take up to four weeks [16].

In hypertensive patients who are sodium depleted, who have been given diuretics, who have treated heart failure, or who have severe or renovascular hypertension, there is a risk of 'first-dose' hypotension [76,146,147]. Patients with hyponatremia are at particular risk of this complication. Old age could be another factor, as even healthy elderly people may react with a prominent fall in blood pressure [100]. Profound falls in blood pressure have been observed in the absence of symptoms, but myocardial ischemia, transient hemiparesis, dysphasia, coma, and even death have been reported [76,146–149], It has been suggested that 5mg enalapril should be the maximum starting dose to be used in hypertensive patients already on diuretic treatment [147] at least in patients in whom the diuretic cannot be witheld for 2–3 days prior to introduction of the ACE inhibitor. Since precipitous falls in blood pressure have occurred after doses of captopril as low as 6.25mg, it is a wise precaution to withhold diuretic therapy for a few days before starting treatment with an ACE inhibitor.

The mechanisms underlying severe hypotension with the first dose of an ACE inhibitor derive from sudden and simultaneous withdrawal of several actions of Ang II. These are direct arterial constriction, sympathetic stimulation, and vagal inhibition (see *Chapter 37*). Thus, the phenomenon is likely if arterial pressure is sustained by high circulating concentrations of Ang II, if there is increased sympathetic tone, and if vagal tone is potentially high, as, for example, with concomitant cardiac glycoside therapy [146,150]. Peripheral venodilatation may also be of importance [149] when ACE inhibitors are administered. The first-dose reaction thus resembles in many respects, vasovagal syncope, with bradycardia and reduced cardiac output [151]. However, with prudence and reasonable precautions, in clinical practice, this effect is rarely a serious problem [76].

As ACE inhibitors lower blood pressure by blocking the RAS, it might seem logical to measure plasma levels of renin or Ang II in order to select those most likely to benefit from such treatment. Whereas the acute hypotensive effect of ACE inhibitors shows a correlation with pretreatment levels of plasma renin or Ang II [16,40,152], these measurements are not, however, predictive of the long-term blood-pressure response in the individual patient [153] and are not clinically useful in this context.

When most forms of antihypertensive treatment are withdrawn, blood pressure gradually returns to pretreatment levels in a majority of patients. In some cases, however, rebound or overshoot hypertension is seen and may be accompanied by hypertensive encephalopathy, by a cerebrovascular accident, or by other catastrophic cardiovascular events [154,155]. Withdrawal of centrally acting antihypertensive drugs such as methyldopa, guanfacine, and guanabenz has been reported to cause this 'withdrawal syndrome' with features of increased sympathetic activity [155]. Sudden omission of clonidine therapy, however, seems to be, by far, the most common cause of serious rebound effects, with a clinical picture resembling that of an acute pheochromocytoma crisis including hypersecretion of cathecholamines [154–156].

During treatment with ACE inhibitors, the plasma level of Ang II is reduced and there is a converse increase in circulating renin and Ang I levels [152]. It should, however, be emphasized that angiotensinogen production is heavily dependent on Ang II [157]; hence, with long-term suppression of Ang II, angiotensinogen production is depressed, and with prolonged ACE inhibition, there is a fall in plasma angiotensinogen concentration [158,159]. Thus, with such long-term ACE inhibition, the circulating concentration of Ang I is proportionately much lower than the concurrent plasma concentrations of active renin [40,152]. These complex biochemical adjustments mean that withdrawal of prolonged ACE inhibitor therapy does not result in rebound or even overshoot hypertension, because there is no steep increase in circulating Ang II [155,160–162]. Instead, there is a gradual biochemical readjustment and a slow rise in Ang II and aldosterone [160], and the increase in blood pressure is smooth and symptomless. Thus, in this respect, ACE inhibitors can be withdrawn safely in patients with hypertension or heart failure [163].

SIDE EFFECTS

Angiotensin-converting enzyme inhibitors are generally well tolerated. Their side effects are summarized in Fig. 91.4 [40,76,164–176] and are discussed in more detail in *Chapter 99*. It is worth noting that some side effects (neutropenia, agranulocytosis, proteinuria, the nephrotic syndrome, Guillain–Barré neuropathy, and taste disturbance) seem to be peculiar to captopril and are allegedly a consequence of the presence of a sulfhydryl group in that compound [4]. The more serious of the side effects earlier seen with captopril accompanied large doses (up to 450mg daily) previously in vogue. Such side effects are rarer with the more modest doses of captopril now employed, although Guillain–Barré neuropathy has been reported at a captopril dose of only 75mg daily [168].

EFFECTS OF ANTIHYPERTENSIVE TREATMENT ON MORBIDITY AND MORTALITY: ROLE OF ANGIOTENSIN-CONVERTING ENZYME INHIBITORS

A consideration of the actual and potential place of ACE inhibitors in the repertoire of antihypertensive drug therapy requires to be prefaced by a resumé of the achievements and failures of such treatment so far.

Side effects	Reference
angioneurotic edema	164
bone marrow depression	65
cholestatic jaundice	166
deterioration of asthma (not agreed by all authors)	167
first-dose hypotensive reaction	76
Guillain–Barré neuropathy	168
immune-complex glomerulopathy	169
maculopapular rash	170
nephrotic syndrome	171
nonproductive cough	172
onycholysis	173
proteinuria	174
provocation of Raynaud's phenomenon	40,67
taste disturbance	175
urticaria	176

Fig. 91.4 Side effects of ACE inhibitors.

There can be no doubt of some substantial successes. Hypertensive heart failure is now a rarity [177]. The five-year survival in malignant hypertension has improved from zero without treatment to 75% with antihypertensive drug therapy [5].

The extent of the benefit with prophylactic antihypertensive treatment is more controversial, with most of the controversy centered on the very large and expensive US Hypertension Detection and Follow-up Program (HDFP) [178]. The HDFP was not strictly a controlled trial of antihypertensive drug therapy *per se*, but rather a comparison of two systems of delivery of healthcare: Stepped Care (SC) (that is, special intervention, including a defined program of antihypertensive treatment) versus Referred Care (RC) (that is, treatment at the discretion of the patient's regular physician). Analysis of the outcome [178] showed that SC patients fared better in several respects, not only in having lower cardiovascular morbidity, including that from coronary artery disease, but also fewer deaths from causes unlikely to be related to antihypertensive treatment such as diabetes mellitus, gastrointestinal disease, and cancer. These additional benefits in the SC group have been considered by several writers [179–181], including the authors of the initial HDFP report itself [178], to have reflected possibly more ready access to diagnostic and treatment facilities than were available to the RC group of patients. The reception of the HDFP results has varied from outright dismissal ('The HDFP study … ought to be rejected because it was not a proper trial of the treatment of

hypertension' [179]), through severe criticism ('We shall never know how much of the overall benefit observed was due to antihypertensive treatment and how much to … other factors' [180]), to credulous acceptance (one of the '14 unconfounded randomized trials of antihypertensive drugs' [182]). The explanatory discursion is necessary; the inclusion or exclusion of the HDFP data substantially affects assessment of the benefits of prophylactic antihypertensive treatment.

Meta-analyses of intervention trials in hypertension which have included HDFP have found stroke morbidity to be reduced by approximately 40% and coronary heart disease morbidity by approximately 14%, the latter with very wide 95% confidence limits of from 4 to 22% [182,183]. These results are from an average period of treatment of five years and relate to a reduction in diastolic blood pressure of 5–6mmHg compared with control patients [182,183]. Not surprisingly, these meta-analyses [182,183] and their interpretation have been sharply criticized [184–186].

Setting aside the controversy, there is agreement that antihypertensive drug treatment can correct the malignant phase and hypertensive heart failure [85,177,181,187,188], can substantially prevent stroke, is effective in the elderly (aged 60–84 years) as well as in younger patients [87,93], and, moreover, can benefit those with 'isolated systolic' hypertension, where the systolic is over 159mmHg but the diastolic below 90mmHg [92]. In spite of these broadly encouraging results, it remains, nevertheless, obvious that both morbidity [189] and mortality rates [190] remain much higher in treated hypertensive patients than in matched normotensive subjects.

To some extent, discrepancies between the effects of antihypertensive treatment on stroke and coronary heart disease could be explained by differences in the underlying pathophysiology of the two conditions [85,177,191]. Antihypertensive drug treatment has hitherto, and for good reasons, focused on blood-pressure reduction as such, and has been more successful against those complications directly related to the high arterial pressure [187]. Since the protective effect against stroke, as well as coronary heart disease, is suboptimal, however, other possibilities must be considered. These various considerations are not mutually exclusive.

First, long-standing hypertension may cause irreversible cardiovascular changes and atherosclerosis, which could contribute to the increased cardiovascular risk even when the blood pressure is well controlled. This possibility was raised as long ago as 1958 when it was noted that although treatment of malignant hypertension improved survival, new problems arose as a consequence of atherosclerosis and its complications [192]. Atherosclerotic complications of hypertension have more subtle origins than high arterial pressure as such, these factors include left ventricular hypertrophy, reduced compliance in large arteries, flow turbulence, and endothelial dysfunction [85,187]. Future antihypertensive drug design needs to address these issues [193].

Second, a hitherto largely unregarded aspect of antihypertensive therapy (except in the malignant phase) is its capacity to slow the hypertension-related decline in renal function [194]. There would appear to be considerable scope for antihypertensive drugs which could usefully attack this problem.

A third possibility is that some of the excess risk could be attributable to suboptimal lowering of blood pressure [195]. The issue of whether more vigorous reduction of blood pressure would further diminish cardiovascular morbidity and mortality is being investigated in the ongoing BBB (Behandla Blodtryck Bättre: treat blood pressure better) study [196].

Fourth, even if antihypertensive drugs had sufficient efficacy to lower arterial pressure adequately, dosage may be constrained, or the patient's compliance with treatment may be overtly or covertly impaired by unwanted symptomatic side effects. Future drugs should impart a low burden of side effects; in current jargon, they should not seriously diminish the 'quality of life'.

A fifth possible explanation for the hitherto suboptimal results of antihypertensive treatment could be that some classes of drug used so far may have carried some biochemical and pathophysiological consequences which have partly offset their benefits. Amongst these are potentially adverse plasma lipid patterns resulting from the use of thiazides or β-blockers [197,198]; lowering of plasma potassium and/or magnesium, and hence the provocation of ventricular dysrhythmias by thiazides [199,200]; and adverse effects on insulin and glucose metabolism, with the consequent development or worsening of diabetes mellitus, again with either thiazides or β-blockers [201]. These are emotive issues, and both the thiazides and β-blockers have been spiritedly defended against these various charges [202–205]. Nevertheless, the advocacy of lower doses of thiazide diuretics for the treatment of hypertension [206,207], and the encouraging results of the SHEP trial [92], in which low doses of chlorthalidone (12.5 or 25mg) were given, indicate that these notions may have some foundation.

With this background, the established and potential benefits of ACE inhibitors in these respects are now considered.

ANGIOTENSIN-CONVERTING ENZYME INHIBITORS AND CARDIAC HYPERTROPHY

Left ventricular hypertrophy in hypertension implies a ventricle that empties well but fills poorly. There is a raised end-diastolic pressure, elevated circulating atrial natriuretic factor, subendocardial ischemia, and increased ventricular ectopy [85,208].

Left ventricular hypertrophy as detected by electrocardiography (EKG) or echocardiography is a very powerful risk indicator for various cardiovascular disorders in hypertensive patients [209–211]. It therefore seems potentially desirable to reverse left ventricular hypertrophy [212], even though the effects of this measure on prognosis are as yet not fully known.

RENIN–ANGIOTENSIN SYSTEM AND CARDIAC HYPERTROPHY

There is evidence the RAS plays an important role in the development of both cardiac hypertrophy and left ventricular dysfunction [213–215]. Angiotensin II may be involved either through potentiation of sympathetic nervous tone [216,217] or by direct trophic stimulation of cardiac muscle [218–221], or both (see *Chapter 31*).

Prolonged treatment with captopril in spontaneously hypertensive rats (SHR), started at an early age, has been shown to prevent completely the development of ventricular hypertrophy [222]. Several other intervention studies in animal models have shown that ACE inhibitors consistently reduce or prevent the progression of cardiac hypertrophy [223–225] while also improving left ventricular performance [226]. Whereas captopril and dihydralazine were equally effective in preventing a rise in blood pressure in SHR, captopril limited cardiovascular hypertrophy, but dihydralazine did not [223]. These observations again point to the possible importance of Ang II as a trophic factor.

Experimental evidence therefore suggests that different classes of agents, although with similar antihypertensive efficacy, affect cardiac hypertrophy differentially [214,227,228].

REVERSAL OF LEFT VENTRICULAR HYPERTROPHY WITH ANGIOTENSIN-CONVERTING ENZYME INHIBITORS IN MAN

Devereux *et al* [215] reported that the available literature in man supported the concept that antihypertensive drugs that inhibited activity of the RAS (ACE inhibitors and β-blockers), more consistently induced regression of left ventricular hypertrophy than did classes of drugs such as diuretics and vasodilators which increased activity of the RAS. Only five studies with ACE inhibitors were, however, included [229–233].

Mujais *et al* [234] evaluated the effect of captopril on ECG-voltage in hypertensive patients with evidence of left ventricular hypertrophy. They found two different response patterns: either correction of EKG abnormalities or no effect in spite of similar blood-pressure responses in the two groups [234].

Most studies in this field have used echocardiography, which is superior to the EKG both as regards sensitivity and specificity in determining left ventricular hypertrophy and in estimating ventricular mass [235,236]. Results of clinical trials that have evaluated the effect of ACE inhibitors given alone on cardiac hypertrophy in man using echocardiography, are presented in Fig. 91.5. Only four studies were controlled, that is, randomized, double-blind, and comparative [69,237–239]; the rest were open and uncontrolled [240–250]. In most of these reports (17/20, 85%), a significant reduction of left ventricular mass (range −2 to −35%) was achieved. It should be noted that most patients were included in these studies according to blood-pressure criteria rather than the presence or absence of ventricular hypertrophy.

Captopril and enalapril have also been studied in combination with other antihypertensive agents and shown to reverse cardiac hypertrophy, although any specific effect of the ACE inhibitor (as against blood-pressure reduction alone) cannot be defined under these circumstances [251,252].

The controlled studies noted above deserve further discussion. Nifedipine was compared with captopril in a small, controlled six-month study by Sheiban *et al* [237]. Both treatments induced a similar and significant reduction of left ventricular wall thickness and mass. Regression of cardiac hypertrophy was accompanied by an improvement in left ventricular function [237].

Graettinger *et al* [239] compared atenolol and lisinopril in a three-month, double-blind randomized trial. In spite of effective 24-hour blood-pressure reduction, neither drug produced significant echocardiographic changes in wall thickness or estimated muscle mass. This may be partly explained by the fact that baseline values for left ventricular mass were not in the hypertrophic range [239].

In a double-blind, parallel group study, previously untreated essential hypertensives were randomized to receive either enalapril or hydrochlorothiazide. After six months, there was a significant reduction in left ventricular mass with enalapril (15%) but a smaller insignificant reduction with hydrochlorothiazide (8%). The effect of enalapril was due mainly to regression in wall thickness; this was significantly greater than with hydrochlorothiazide [238],

Julien and co-workers [69] reported a study in patients with resistant hypertension where captopril or minoxidil were added in a double-blind fashion to patients with a diastolic pressure greater than 100mmHg while receiving metoprolol plus furosemide. The drugs were equally effective in lowering blood pressure, but only captopril reduced left ventricular mass (see *Fig. 91.3*). The increase in cardiac mass seen with minoxidil was unlikely to result from secondary fluid volume expansion, since the

---

general description
- a total of 17 studies variously with captopril (5), enalapril (8), lisinopril (2), and perindopril (2)
- average number of patients per study: 11.7 (range 7–20)
- mean follow-up: 6 months (range 3–12)

effect of treatment

change in mean arterial pressure	−15.7%	(CI: −13.9, −17.5)
change in left ventricular mass/left ventricular mass index	−15.8%	(CI: −10.8, −20.8)
change in relative wall thickness (n=13)	−9.2%	(CI: −3.7, −14.8)
change in left ventricular mass/left ventricular mass index versus change in mean arterial pressure	r=0.58	

Fig. 91.5 The effect of monotherapy with ACE inhibitors on cardiac indices, as evaluated by echocardiography in patients with essential hypertension. Data from Julien J *et al* [69], Sheiban I *et al* [237], Dahlöf B and Hansson L [238], Graettinger WF *et al* [239], Muiesan ML *et al* [240], Motz W *et al* [241], Grandi AM *et al* [242], Picca M *et al* [243], Di Bello V *et al* [244], Garavaglia G *et al* [245], Asmar RG *et al* [246,247], Shahi M *et al* [248], de Faire U *et al* [249], and Mezzetti A *et al* [250].

patients were also receiving furosemide. Reflex activation of the sympathetic nervous system is, however, a possible explanation since there was a rise in heart rate with minoxidil despite concomitant β-blocker therapy [69]. Further activation of the RAS by minoxidil may also have contributed.

In a meta-analysis of 109 studies that all used echocardiography, the effects of monotherapy were compared with ACE inhibitors, β-blockers, calcium antagonists, and diuretics on left ventricular mass. Possibly relevant confounding factors were corrected for using covariance analysis. It was evident that ACE inhibitors reduced left ventricular mass, mainly by affecting wall thickness, more effectively than did β-blockers, calcium antagonists, and in particular, diuretics. Indeed, diuretics reduced only left ventricular volume [253]. The prognostic implications of these results, although encouraging, are not yet clear. These issues are presently being investigated in the so-called CAPPP [15] (see later). The possibility that ACE inhibitors may not only reduce left ventricular mass but also suppress arrythmogenesis in essential hypertension is suggested by two reports, although one is uncontrolled [312] and the other, so far, is in abstract form only [313].

FUNCTIONAL ASPECTS

There has been some concern that any reduction of cardiac hypertrophy might adversely affect left ventricular function. Several studies [231–233,240–242,245,250] have, however, shown that there is no deterioration in left ventricular performance with ACE inhibitors, while in some cases, diastolic function has improved [69,237–242].

The effect of captopril in combination with a diuretic was evaluated in hypertensive patients with initially abnormal left ventricular diastolic function [248]. After nine months of therapy, a significant reduction in left ventricular mass was seen without change in Doppler indices of left ventricular diastolic function. This observation strengthens the premise that there is no direct relation between left ventricular mass and diastolic function.

Two prospective intervention trials in patients with asymptomatic left ventricular dysfunction following myocardial infarction have shown that various indices of cardiac function were better preserved during captopril treatment than during placebo or furosemide therapy following one year of observation [254, 255]. Moreover, ventricular dilatation was prevented by the ACE inhibitor (see Chapter 77). In one study, physical performance, assessed repeatedly during the trial, was superior in the ACE inhibitor-treated patients [255]. Bearing in mind the above-mentioned comparative failure thus far of antihypertensive treatment to diminish coronary artery disease and its consequences, such benefits, although not yet demonstrated in hypertensive patients, are of considerable potential interest.

NEW TECHNIQUES

New methods for evaluating cardiac structure and function have emerged, such as magnetic resonance imaging (MRI). With MRI, the cardiac chambers are clearly visualized without the need for contrast material. In a study of the effect of three months' treatment with the ACE inhibitor ramipril in hypertensive patients, MRI and echocardiography were used in parallel. Both techniques showed an equivalent decrease in wall thickness, but MRI provided superior images [256].

Present evidence clearly indicates that ACE inhibitors are probably the most effective antihypertensive agents in reversing cardiac hypertrophy. This effect of ACE inhibitors is not associated with impaired cardiac performance provided blood pressure is controlled, and indeed, diastolic function frequently improves. The prognostic implications of these observations remain to be elucidated and are presently under investigation [15].

MEDIAL THICKENING IN RESISTANCE ARTERIES

Folkow and his colleagues have emphasized the pathophysiological importance of medial thickening in resistance arteries in hypertension [257]. The result of such structural change is that the wall:lumen ratio is increased, and, even at full dilatation, the cross-sectional vascular luminal diameter is less. Since resistance to flow is proportional to the fourth power of the luminal radius, these changes have two important consequences: as they progress, the blood pressure is driven higher, while the efficacy of drug treatment is impaired, because even at full dilatation the arterial lumen is restricted.

Amongst the influences responsible for medial thickening in resistance arteries the RAS must be considered, whose effects here are akin to those on the left ventricle mentioned above (see Chapter 31). In experimental animals, drugs that facilitate regression of such medial thickening are generally those which also promote resolution of left ventricular hypertrophy. Angiotensin-converting enzyme inhibitors, β-blockers and methyldopa have most often been successful, while direct-acting vasodilators such as hydralazine or minoxidil, and diuretics, have not [258]. It should be emphasized, however, that the progression of left ventricular hypertrophy and of medial arteriolar thickening, and their regression with treatment, do not always proceed at the same rate implying varying dominant influences at the two tissues [258,259].

Direct biopsy studies with antihypertensive treatment in man have shown that therapy can lead to correction of medial thickening in resistance arteries, although so far these reports have not permitted comparative evaluation of different drug classes in this respect [260] (see *Chapter 96*). Indirect evaluation in hypertensive patients has indicated that, as in animals, ACE inhibitors and β-blockers are useful agents in facilitating regression of such medial thickening [258,259].

Successful correction of these structural changes would certainly be an important factor in achieving thorough blood-pressure reduction with therapy.

LARGE ARTERIAL COMPLIANCE

Physical compliance in large arteries is progressively impaired in hypertension and with aging [85,208,261] (see *Chapter 95*). Such changes lead to disproportionate elevation of systolic pressure and are associated with left ventricular hypertrophy and with increased turbulence of blood flow and hence predisposition to atherosclerosis [85,208]. For all these reasons, antihypertensive drugs are now being sought which would improve, rather than worsen, physical compliance in large arteries [193].

Comparative trials have shown that whereas propranolol is ineffective on large arterial compliance in hypertension, equipotent antihypertensive doses of enalapril improve compliance [262]. Similarly, radial artery compliance and diameter were increased 6 hours after lisinopril dosing in normotensive volunteers, whereas no definite effect was observed with either atenolol or nitrendipine [314]. While these initial results are encouraging, their prognostic import remains to be determined.

EFFECTIVE LOWERING OF SYSTOLIC BLOOD PRESSURE

Systolic blood pressure is at least as strong an indicator of cardiovascular risk as is diastolic blood pressure [263]. Control of isolated systolic hypertension has been shown to diminish cardiovascular morbidity and mortality [92]. It is interesting therefore that in a review of trials comparing the ACE inhibitor enalapril with propranolol or atenolol, it was shown that systolic blood pressures, both supine and standing, were more effectively reduced with the ACE inhibitor [264].

SCAVENGING OF FREE RADICALS

91.13

It is assumed that oxygen-derived free radicals play a pathophysiological role in many disorders, including myocardial ischemia. It is possibly relevant that ACE inhibitors may act as scavengers of free radicals [265], but it remains to be seen if this action is of any clinical relevance. So far, positive results *in vivo* have been seen in a study of patients with chronic heart failure [266]. Ceriello *et al* [267] have shown an acute antihypertensive effect of antioxidants in diabetic and hypertensive subjects.

ENDOTHELIAL FUNCTION

Endothelial lesions and disturbances of endothelial biochemical function influence the progression of arterial disease in hypertension and its response to treatment [268] (see *Chapter 29*). Antihypertensive drugs which could preserve or enhance such endothelial functions would presumably confer especial advantages in treatment [268].

In this connection, it is of interest that captopril can stimulate release of endothelium-derived relaxing factor; this action seems to be independent of ACE inhibition [269].

PRESERVATION OF RENAL FUNCTION

A potentially important, but hitherto neglected, therapeutic goal in hypertension is slowing of the gradual decline in the GFR with time [194]. Studies in patients with diabetic nephropathy have shown, even in normotensive individuals, that treatment with the ACE inhibitor captopril significantly reduces the rate of decline in the GFR [270] (see *Chapter 56*). Enalapril reduced the rate of decline in GFR to a greater extent than metoprolol in insulin-dependent diabetic patients with diabetic retinopathy, and urinary albumin excretion was 60% lower with the ACE inhibitor than during treatment with the β-blocker [315]. In nondiabetic hypertensives with chronic renal failure, treatment with an ACE inhibitor has been shown to be superior in this respect to standard antihypertensive triple therapy [271]. Aperloo *et al* [272] have found that enalapril lowers proteinuria more than atenolol does despite a similar blood-pressure reducing effect of the two drugs.

It is important to contrast these beneficial effects in hypertension and diabetes mellitus with clinical conditions such as cardiac failure, where the kidneys are underperfused and partly dependent on the RAS to sustain GFR and urea excretion (see *Chapter 76*). In these latter circumstances, by contrast, the administration of ACE inhibitors often leads to a modest decline in GFR, with a concomitant increase in serum urea and creatinine [273–276].

METABOLIC ASPECTS

Several studies have reported on the many potentially negative metabolic effects of diuretics and of those β-blockers which are devoid of intrinsic sympathomimetic activity [277]. This is in contrast to the ACE inhibitors, which can be regarded as metabolically neutral [277]. Particular interest has been directed to the benign effects of ACE inhibition on insulin and glucose metabolism [201,301]. In addition, the ACE inhibitors maintain or increase serum potassium and magnesium levels, have few or beneficial effects on the serum lipid profile and coagulation indices [278,279], and tend to increase uric acid excretion, at least in the short term [280].

ANGIOTENSIN-CONVERTING ENZYME INHIBITORS AND QUALITY OF LIFE

The ideal treatment for hypertension should reduce blood pressure without impairing the patient's quality of life [5,281]. The untreated person with mild-to-moderate essential hypertension is usually asymptomatic, and antihypertensive drugs, with their attendant symptomatic side effects, frequently impair life quality [282,283].

A growing interest in the effects of antihypertensive treatment on quality of life, and the evolution of methods for its evaluation, developed at about the same time as the introduction of ACE inhibitors. These aspects are discussed also in *Chapter 99*. The ACE inhibitors were early noted to be well tolerated and appeared to have ready patient acceptability due to minimal interference with wellbeing. It was even suspected initially that ACE inhibition could induce a euphoriant response, perhaps as a consequence of central enkephalinase inhibition [284,285].

Subsequent studies have not confirmed that ACE inhibitors cause euphoria. With some exceptions, however [286], data have been consistent in showing that wellbeing and quality of life are not markedly impaired during treatment of essential hypertension with ACE inhibitors [27,28,38,287–292,316].

Any evaluation of a patient's quality of life/wellbeing on antihypertensive therapy has to allow for observer bias related to the prior expectations of the patient and the doctor, both about the disorder itself and of its treatment. This was highlighted in a study by Jachuck *et al* [293] who found that patients, doctors, and close relatives assessed the patient's quality of life on antihypertensive therapy very differently. Such observations underscore the need to perform, wherever possible, double-blind and appropriately controlled assessments in this context. Studies with different ACE inhibitors in essential hypertension dealing with various aspects of quality of life are listed in Fig. 91.6.

In a postmarketing surveillance of 11,710 patients receiving enalapril in general practice, the drug was generally well tolerated and the most frequently reported finding was an improvement in wellbeing, which was noted in 20% of the patients [294]. Detailed evaluation of these patients revealed that most were women and/or had side effects on previous therapy. Such observations [38,294] indicate that the improvement in general wellbeing on an ACE inhibitor may in part be due to loss of side effects experienced on prior medication.

Callender *et al* [286] performed a double-blind crossover study in eight hypertensive patients using the Goldberg Health Questionnaire as well as tests for alertness and concentration. A slight but significant depression of mood was found on captopril compared with placebo.

By contrast, in a study of healthy volunteers by Olajide and Lader, enalapril and placebo were administered for two weeks and had no apparent effect on mood [287].

Lichter *et al* [288] found a slight but consistent impairment in several memory tests with atenolol monotherapy but not with enalapril.

In a trial of 36 patients with essential hypertension treated mainly with β-blockers and diuretics, wellbeing was found to increase when this therapy was substituted with placebo, and was significantly higher when patients received enalapril in place of their initial treatment [38] (Fig. 91.7).

Croog *et al* [27] performed a large study which compared captopril, propranolol, and methyldopa in 626 men with mild-to-moderate hypertension. Patients treated with captopril had a significantly better outcome with regard to general wellbeing and physical symptoms than did those given either of the other therapies. In addition, captopril affected sexual function significantly less than did propranolol, while work performance, cognition, and life satisfaction were less affected than with methyldopa. Captopril therapy was also accompanied by a lower discontinuation rate due to side effects than was either methyldopa or propranolol [27].

Such superiority of ACE inhibitors was not, however, confirmed when they were compared with more modern drugs than methyldopa or propranolol. Atenolol has been evaluated against enalapril [28,290], captopril [289,290], and delapril [291] in controlled studies of moderate size. There were no major differences between any of the ACE inhibitors and atenolol regarding the patient's assessment of quality of life.

ACE inhibitor (n)	Comparison (n)	Duration (month)	Study design	Method	Main result	Reference	
captopril (8)	placebo (8)	1.5	R, DB, CO, EH treated with bendroflumethiazide and atenolol	Goldberg Health Questionnaire	significant depression of mood	Callender et al (1983)	286
enalapril (12)	placebo (12)	0.5	R, DB, CO normal subjects	auditory evoked electrocardiography	modest effect on alertness	Olajide and Lader (1985)	287
enalapril (36)		1.5	open, EH	ASPECT scale (early version)	wellbeing significantly increased on enalapril versus previous therapy	Dahlöf et al (1985)	38
enalapril (12)	atenolol (13)	4	R, DB, PG, EH	a variety of memory tests	consistent depression of memory function on atenolol but not on enalapril	Lichter et al (1986)	288
captopril (213)	α-methyldopa (201) propranolol (212)	6	R, DB, PG, EH white men	extensive standardized evaluation on 8 main aspects of quality of life	significant positive effect on wellbeing, work performance, and life satisfaction versus α-methyldopa, less sexual dysfunction and improved wellbeing versus propranolol	Croog et al (1986)	27
enalapril (86)	atenolol (76)	3	R, DB, PG, EH	Goldberg Health Questionnaire / psychological testing	no difference enalapril versus atenolol on overall quality of life, significant improvement in attention and mental speed on enalapril	Herrick et al (1989)	28
captopril (63)	atenolol (62)	2	R, DB, PG, EH	symptom rating test	nonsignificant improvement of wellbeing for both drugs, no difference captopril versus atenolol	Fletcher et al (1990)	289
captopril (87) enalapril (84)	atenolol (88) propranolol (85)	1	R, DB, PG, EH	PGWB index and life satisfaction questionnaire	improvement of wellbeing and life satisfaction for captopril, enalapril, atenolol, but not for propranolol	Steiner et al (1990)	290
delapril (114)	atenolol (116)	4–5	R, DB, PG, EH	ASPECT scale	significant improvement of wellbeing for both drugs, no difference delapril versus atenolol	Jern et al (1991)	291
lisinopril (412)	nifedipine (416)	2.5	R, DB, PG, EH	ASPECT scale	no difference lisinopril versus nifedipine except on highest dose of nifedipine (nifedipine 80mg → detoriation)	Os et al (1991)	292

R = randomized; DB = double blind; PG = parallel group; EH = essential hypertension; CO = crossover; PGWB, psychological general wellbeing.

Fig. 91.6 The effect of ACE inhibitors on the quality of life.

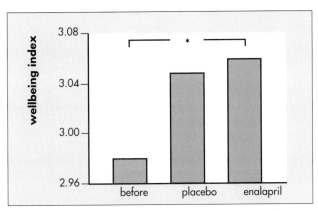

Fig. 91.7 Wellbeing indices on β-blockade/diuretics (before) and after four weeks of placebo (placebo), and six weeks of enalapril monotherapy (enalapril) in 36 patients with essential hypertension. *P<0.05. Modified from Dahlöf B *et al* [38].

In the study of essential hypertensives by Jern and co-workers which used the ASPECT scale, both atenolol and delapril improved wellbeing significantly and to a similar extent [291].

Lisinopril was compared with nifedipine in a 10-week controlled study of 828 patients with essential hypertension, approximately 50% of whom were previously untreated [292]. Quality of life was assessed using the ASPECT scale both by patients and by their spouses. No significant changes in wellbeing were observed with either drug, except for the highest dose of nifedipine (80mg) which caused a deterioration. Patients and spouses were in close agreement in their assessments [292].

In a single-dose study [295], captopril was administered to healthy subjects and compared with placebo, oxazepam, and atenolol in a double-blind manner. In contrast to the other active treatments, captopril did not affect performance, alertness, or mood. Indeed, short-term memory and ability to concentrate were improved on the ACE inhibitor [295]. It appears possible therefore that ACE inhibitors may have central actions under some circumstances.

Angiotensin-converting enzyme inhibitors do not therefore have a major negative impact on quality of life or wellbeing when used in the treatment of hypertension. They are distinctly superior to methyldopa and propranolol, and probably also to nifedipine. They have not, however, been convincingly demonstrated to be superior to β-blockers such as atenolol. There is no good evidence for a euphoriant action of ACE inhibitors, although central effects cannot be ruled out. Their high acceptability should, for obvious reasons, result in better compliance with treatment.

FUTURE DEVELOPMENTS

Most of the major intervention trials demonstrating benefit from antihypertensive drug therapy have featured thiazide diuretics and β-blockers [9]. Despite the limited (albeit distinct) advantages of such diuretic or β-blocker treatment, some workers have expressed reluctance to accept newer agents such as ACE inhibitors, which have not yet been subject to similar scrutiny [202,203].

A number of potential advantages from ACE inhibitor treatment in hypertension have been reviewed in this chapter. It remains to be demonstrated, however, whether such aspects are of theoretical interest only or whether they in fact affect cardiovascular morbidity and mortality. A Scandinavian study has been initiated to clarify this issue; it is a prospective trial in hypertensive patients, aged 25–66 years, who are randomized to either ACE inhibitor based therapy or to antihypertensive treatment that does not include an ACE inhibitor [15]. At least 7,000 patients will be studied for five years.

The STOP-II trial will randomize 6,000 elderly hypertensive patients to one of three arms: ACE inhibitor, calcium antagonist or β-blocker.

The US National Heart, Lung and Blood Institute is planning a trial to evaluate the effect of ACE inhibitors and calcium antagonists on cardiovascular morbidity and mortality in some 30,000 hypertensive patients. It is hoped that these trials will determine whether ACE inhibitor treatment in hypertension is as effective as, or superior to, currently used antihypertensive therapies in reducing cardiovascular morbidity and mortality.

REFERENCES

1. Page IH. Antihypertensive drugs: Our debt to industrial chemists. *New England Journal of Medicine* 1981;304:615–8.

2. Smith A. Image and reality: Drugs for the future. *British Medical Journal* 1982;285:761.

3. Rawlins MD. Alfred Nobel and the drug hunters: Pharmacologists have won many Nobel prizes. *British Medical Journal* 1988;297:1628.

4. Hansson L, Svensson A, Dahlöf B, Eggertsen R. Drug treatment of hypertension. In: Robertson JIS, ed. *Handbook of hypertension, vol 15, Clinical aspects of essential hypertension.* Amsterdam: Elsevier, 1992:chapter 24.

5. Hansson L, Dahlöf B. What are we really achieving with long-term antihypertensive drug therapy? In: Laragh JH, Brenner BM, eds. *Hypertension: Pathophysiology, diagnosis, and management.* New York: Raven Press, 1990:2131–41.

6. Gifford RW. Management and treatment of essential hypertension, including malignant hypertension and emergencies. In : Genest J, Kuchel O, Hamet P, Cantin M, eds. *Hypertension, 2nd edition*. New York: McGraw-Hill, 1983:1127–70.

7. 1988 Joint National Committee. The 1988 report of the Joint National Committee on Detection, Evaluation, and Treatment of High Blood Pressure. *Archives of Internal Medicine* 1988;148:1023–8.

8. WHO/ISH Fifth Mild Hypertension Conference. 1989 guidelines for the management of mild hypertension: Memorandum from a WHO/ISH meeting. *Journal of Hypertension* 1989;7:689–93.

9. Swales JD, Ramsay LE, Coope JR, Pocock S, Robertson JIS, Sever PS, Shaper AG. Treating mild hypertension: Report of the British Hypertension Society working party. *British Medical Journal* 1989;298:694–8.

10. Cusi D, Bianchi G. Genetic and molecular aspects of primary hypertension. In: Robertson JIS, ed. *Clinical aspects of hypertension*. Handbook of hypertension, vol 15. Amsterdam: Elsevier, 1992:chapter 4.

11. Beilin LJ. Environmental and dietary aspects of hypertension. In: Robertson JIS, ed. *Clinical aspects of hypertension. Handbook of hypertension, vol 15*. Amsterdam: Elsevier, 1992:chapter 5.

12. Waeber B, Burnier M, Nüssberger J, Brunner HR. Trials using crossover design and ambulatory blood pressure recordings to determine the efficacy of antihypertensive agents in individual patients. *Journal of Hypertension* 1990;8 (suppl 4):37–41.

13. Bellet M, Whalen JJ, Bodin F, Serrurier D, Tanner K, Menard J. Use of crossover trials to obtain antihypertensive dose–response curves and to study combination therapy during the development of benazepril. *Journal of Hypertension* 1990;8 (suppl 4):43–8.

14. Niutta E, Cusi D, Colombo R, Pellizoni M, Cesana B, Barlassina C, Soldat L, Bianchi G. Predicting interindividual variations in antihypertensive therapy; the role of sodium transport systems and renin. *Journal of Hypertension* 1990;8 (suppl 4):53–8.

15. The CAPPP group. The captopril prevention project: A prospective intervention trial of angiotensin converting enzyme inhibition in the treatment of hypertension. *Journal of Hypertension* 1990;8:985–90.

16. Johnston CI. Angiotensin converting enzyme inhibition. In: Doyle A, ed. *Clinical pharmacology of antihypertensive drugs: Handbook of hypertension, vol. 11*. Amsterdam: Elsevier, 1988:301–26.

17. Vanhoutte PM, Auch-Schwelk W, Biondi ML, Lorenz PR, Schini VB, Vidal MJ. Why are converting enzyme inhibitors vasodilators? *British Journal of Clinical Pharmacology* 1989;28:95–104s.

18. Waeber B, Christen Y, Perret F, Nussberger J, Brunner HR. Treatment of hypertension with angiotensin-converting enzyme inhibitors as monotherapy. In: Laragh JH, Bühler FR, eds. *The management of hypertension: Handbook of hypertension, vol 13*. Amsterdam: Elsevier, 1990:277–95.

19. Andrén L, Karlberg BE, Svensson A, Öhman P, Nilsson OR, Hansson L. Long-term effects of captopril and atenolol in essential hypertension. *Acta Medica Scandinavica* 1985;217:155–60.

20. Ayers CR, Baker KM, Weawer BA, Lehman MR. Enalapril maleate versus captopril. A comparison of the hormonal and antihypertensive effects. *Drugs* 1985;30 (suppl 1):70–3.

21. Witte PU, Walter U. The multicenter study group: Comparative double-blind study of ramipril and captopril in mild to moderate essential hypertension. *American Journal of Cardiology* 1987;59:115–20D.

22. McAreavey D, Robertson JIS. Angiotensin converting enzyme inhibitors and moderate hypertension. *Drugs* 1990;40:326–45.

23. Pool JL, Gennari J, Goldstein R, Kochar MS, Lewin AJ, Maxwell MH, McChesney JA, Mehta J, Nash DT, Nelson EB, Rastogi S, Rofman B, Weinberger M. Controlled multicenter study of the antihypertensive effects of lisinopril, hydrochlorothiazide and lisinopril plus hydrochlorothiazide in the treatment of 394 patients with mild to moderate essential hypertension. *Journal of Cardiovascular Pharmacology* 1987;9 (suppl 3):s36–42.

24. Andrén L, Karlberg B, Öhman P, Svensson A, Asplund J, Hansson L. Captopril and atenolol combined with hydrochlorothiazide in essential hypertension. *British Journal of Clinical Pharmacology* 1982;14:107–11s.

25. Zachariah PK, Bonnet G, Chrysant SG, DeBacker G, Goldstein R, Herrera J, Lindner A, Malerson BJ, Maxwell MH, McMahon FG, Merril RH, Paton RR, Rapp AD, Roginski MS, Seedat YK, Jime F, Vaicaitis JS, Weinberg MS, Zusman RM. Evaluation of antihypertensive efficacy of lisinopril compared to metoprolol in moderate to severe hypertension. *Journal of Cardiovascular Pharmacology* 1987;9 (suppl 3):s53–8.

26. Witchitz S, Serradimigni A, for the Cooperative Study Group. Lisinopril versus slow-release nifedipine in the treatment of mild to moderate hypertension: A multicentre study. *Journal of Human Hypertension* 1989;3 (suppl 1):29–33.

27. Croog SH, Levine S, Testa MA, Brown B, Bulpitt CJ, Jeakins CD, Klerman GL, Williams GH. The effects of antihypertensive therapy on the quality of life. *New England Journal of Medicine* 1986;314:1657–64.

28. Herrick AL, Waller PC, Berkin KE, Pringle SD, Callender JS, Robertson MP, Findlay JP, Murray GD, Reid JL, Lorimer AR, Weir RJ, Carmichael HA, Robertson JIS, Ball SG, McInnes GT. Comparison of enalapril and atenolol in mild to moderate hypertension. *American Journal of Medicine* 1989;86:421–6.

29. Vidt DG, for the Multiclinic Study Group. A controlled multiclinic study to compare the antihypertensive effects of MK-421, hydrochlorothiazide and MK-421 combined with hydrochlorothiazide in patients with mild to moderate essential hypertension. *Journal of Hypertension* 1984;2 (suppl 2): 81–8.

30. Bolzano K, Arriaga J, Bernal R, Bernardes H, Calderon JL, Debruyn J, Dienstl F, Drayer J, Goodfriend TL, Gross W, Guthrie GP, Holwerda N, Klein W, Krakoff L, Liebau H, Oparil S, Reams GP, Reed WG, Safar M, Schubotz R, Seedat YK, Thind GS, Veriava Y, Wollam G, Woods JW, Zusman RM. The antihypertensive effect of lisinopril compared to atenolol in patients with mild to moderate hypertension. *Journal of Cardiovascular Pharmacology* 1987;9 (suppl 3):43–7.

31. Eisner GM, Johnson BF, MacMahon P, Rudd P, Sowers JR, Vargas R, Zemel M. A multicenter comparison of the safety and efficacy of isradipine and enalapril in the treatment of hypertension. *American Journal of Hypertension* 1991;4:154–7s.

32. Applegate WB, Borhani N, DeQuattro V, Kaihlanen PM, Oishi S, Due DL, Sirgo MA. Comparison of labetalol versus enalapril as monotherapy in elderly patients with hypertension: Results of 24-hour ambulatory blood pressure monitoring. *American Journal of Medicine* 1991;90:198–205.

33. Conway J, Coats AJS, Bird R. Lisinopril and enalapril in hypertension: A comparative study using ambulatory monitoring. *Journal of Human Hypertension* 1990;4:235–9.

34. Robertson JIS, Ball SG. Hypertension. In: Julian DG, Camm AJ, Fox KM, Hall RJC, Poole-Wilson PA, eds. *Diseases of the heart*. London: Baillière-Tindall, 1989;1227–92.

35. Pickering TG. The use of angiotensin-converting enzyme inhibitors in combination with other antihypertensive agents. *American Journal of Hypertension* 1991;4:73–8s.

36. Townsend RR, Holland OB. Combination of converting-enzyme inhibitor with diuretic for the treatment of hypertension. *Archives of Internal Medicine* 1990;150:1175–83.

37. Andrén L, Weiner L, Svensson A, Hansson L. Enalapril with either a 'very low' or 'low' dose of hydrochlorothiazide is equally effective in essential hypertension. A double-blind study in 100 hypertensive patients. *Journal of Hypertension* 1983;1 (suppl 2):384–6.

38. Dahlöf B, Andrén L, Eggertsen R, Jern S, Svensson A, Hansson L. Potentiation of the antihypertensive effect of enalapril by randomized addition of different doses of hydrochlorothiazide. *Journal of Hypertension* 1985;3 (suppl 3):483–6.

39. Atkinson AB, Lever AF, Brown JJ, Robertson JIS. Combined treatment of severe intractable hypertension with captopril and diuretic. *Lancet* 1980;ii:105–8.

40. Hodsman GP, Brown JJ, Cumming AMM, Davies DL, East BW, Lever AF, Morton JJ, Murray GD, Robertson I, Robertson JIS. Enalapril in the treatment of hypertension with renal artery stenosis. *British Medical Journal* 1983;287:1413–7.

41. MacGregor GA, Markandu ND, Singer DRJ, Cappuccio FP, Shore AC, Sagnella G. Moderate sodium restriction with angiotensin converting enzyme inhibitor in essential hypertension: A double blind study. *British Medical Journal* 1987;294:531–4.

42. Eggertsen R, Svensson A, Dahlöf B, Hansson L. Additive effect of isradipine in combination with captopril in hypertensive patients. *American Journal of Medicine* 1989;86 (suppl 4A):124–6.

43. Morgan T, Anderson A, Hopper J. Enalapril and nifedipine in essential hypertension. Synergism of the hypotensive effects in combination. *Clinical and Experimental Hypertension. Part A, Theory and Practice* 1988;10:779–89.

44. Anderson A, Morgan T. Interaction of enalapril with sodium restriction, diuretics and slow-channel calcium-blocking drugs. *Nephron* 1990;55 (suppl 1):70–2.

45. Marone C, Luisolo S, Bomio F, Beretta-Piccoli C, Bianchetti MG, Weidmann P. Body sodium–blood volume state, aldosterone and cardiovascular responsiveness after calcium entry blockade with nifedipine. *Kidney International* 1985;28: 658–65.

46. Murray TS, East BW, Robertson JIS. Nicardipine versus propranolol in the treatment of essential hypertension: Effect on total body elemental composition. *British Journal of Clinical Pharmacology* 1986;22 (suppl 3):259–66.

47. Pevahouse JB, Markandu ND, Capuccio FP, Buckley MG, Sagnella GA, MacGregor GA. Long term reduction in sodium balance: Possible additional mechanism whereby nifedipine lowers blood pressure. *British Medical Journal* 1990;301:580–4.

48. Guazzi MD, DeCesare N, Galli C, Salvioni A, Tramentana C, Tamberini G, Bartorelli A. Calcium-channel blockade with nifedipine and angiotensin converting-enzyme inhibition with captopril in the therapy of patients with severe primary hypertension. *Circulation* 1984;70:279–84.

49. Lavezzaro G, Ladetto PE, Valente M, Stramignoni D, Zanna C, Assogna G, Salvetti A. Ketanserin and captopril interaction in the treatment of essential hypertensives. *Cardiovascular Drugs and Therapy* 1990;4:119–22.

50. Celentano A, Galderisi M, Mossetti G, Garofalo M, Mureddo GF, Tammaro P, Assogna G, Gravini E, de Divitiis O. Ketanserin in elderly hypertension: Comparison and combination with enalapril. In: Paoletti R, Vanhoutte PM, Brunello N, Maggi FM, eds. *Cardiovascular system, hypertension, and serotonin antagonists.* Dordrecht: Kluwer Academic Publishers, 1990:149–53.

51. Englert RG, Maursberger H. A single-blind study of doxazosin in the treatment of essential hypertension when added to nonresponders to angiotensin-converting enzyme inhibitor therapy. *American Heart Journal* 1988;116: 1826–32.

52. Hansson L. Beta-blockers with ACE-inhibitors — a logical combination? *Journal of Human Hypertension* 1989;3 (suppl 1):97–100.

53. MacGregor GA, Markandu ND, Smith SJ, Sagnella GA. Captopril: Contrasting effects of adding hydrochlorothiazide, propranolol or nifedipine. *Journal of Cardiovascular Pharmacology* 1985;7 (suppl 1):s82–7.

54. Wing LMH, Chalmers JP, West MJ, Russell AE, Morris MJ, Enalapril and atenolol in hypertension: Attenuation of hypotensive effect in combination. *Clinical and Experimental Hypertension* 1988;A10:119–33.

55. Staessen J, Fagard R, Lijnen P, Verschuren LJ, Amery A. Double-blind comparison between propranolol and bendroflumethiazide in captopril-treated resistant hypertensive patients. *American Heart Journal* 1983;106:321–8.

56. Belz GG, Breithaupt K, Erb K, Kleinbloesm CH, Wolf GK. Influence of the converting-enzyme inhibitor cilazapril and the beta-blocker propranolol and their combination on haemodynamics in hypertension. *Journal of Hypertension* 1989;7:817–24.

57. Hansson L, for the Swedish Lisinopril Study Group. Lisinopril combined with atenolol in the treatment of hypertension. *Journal of Cardiovascular Pharmacology* 1991;18:457–61.

58. Murray GD, Lesaffre E, Robertson JIS. Interpreting age-related aspects of antihypertensive treatment: Statistical defects and their remedy. *Journal of Hypertension* 1988;6 (suppl):s121–6.

59. Gifford RW. Resistant hypertension. Introduction and definitions. *Hypertension* 1988;11 (suppl II):II-65–6.

60. Kaplan NM. Argument for a minimal evaluation of the hypertensive patient. In: Bühler FR, Laragh JH, eds. *Handbook of hypertension, vol 13: The management of hypertension.* Amsterdam: Elsevier, 1990:145–53.

61. Finnerty FA. Relationship of extracellular fluid volume to the development of drug resistance in the hypertensive patient. *American Heart Journal* 1971;81: 563–5.

62. Ramsay LE, Silas JH, Freestone S. Diuretic treatment for resistant hypertension. *British Medical Journal* 1980;281:1101–3.

63. Vaughan Jr ED, Carey RM, Peach MJ, Ackerly JA, Ayers CR. The renin response to diuretic therapy: A limitation of antihypertensive potential. *Circulation Research* 1977;42:376–81.

64. Ibsen H, Leth A, Hollnagel H, Kappelgard AM, Damkjær–Nielsen M, Christensen NJ, Giese J. Renin–angiotensin system in mild essential hypertension: The functional significance of angiotensin II in untreated and thiazide-treated hypertensive patients. *Acta Medica Scandinavica* 1979;205: 547–55.

65. Gavras H, Waeber B, Kershaw GR, Liang C–S, Textor SC, Brunner HR, Tifft CP, Gavras I. Role of reactive hyperreninemia in blood pressure changes induced by sodium depletion in patients with refractory hypertension. *Hypertension* 1981;3:441–7.

66. White NJ, Rajagopalan B, Yahaya H, Ledingham JGG. Captopril and frusemide in severe drug-resistant hypertension. *Lancet* 1980;ii:108–10.

67. Havelka J, Vetter H, Studer A, Greminger P, Lücher T, Wollnik S, Siegenthaler W, Vetter W. Acute and chronic effects of the angiotensin converting enzyme inhibitor captopril in severe hypertension. *American Journal of Cardiology* 1982;49:1467–74.

68. Raine AEG, Ledingham JGG. Clinical experience with captopril in the treatment of severe drug-resistant hypertension. *American Journal of Cardiology* 1982;49:1475–9.

69. Julien J, Dufloux M–A, Prasquier R, Chatellier G, Menard D, Plouin P–F, Menard J, Corvol P. Effects of captopril and minoxidil on left ventricular hypertrophy in resistant hypertensive patients: A 6 month double-blind comparison. *Journal of the American College of Cardiology* 1990;16:137–42.

70. Traub YM, Levey BA. Combined treatment with minoxidil and captopril in refractory hypertension. *Archives of Internal Medicine* 1983;143:1142–4.

71. Seedat YK, Rawat R. Captopril combined with minoxidil, beta-blocker and furosemide in the treatment of refractory hypertension. *European Journal of Clinical Pharmacology* 1983;25:9–11.

72. Rinke CM. Hypertensive emergencies and urgencies. *Journal of the American Medical Association* 1986;255:1607–13.

73. Editorial. Dangerous antihypertensive treatment. *British Medical Journal* 1979;2:228–9.

74. Messerli FH, Kowey P, Grodzicki T. Sublingual nifedipine for hypertensive emergencies. *Lancet* 1991;338:881.

75. Littenberg B, Wolfberg C. Pseudohypertension masquerading as malignant hypertension: Case report and review of the literature. *American Journal of Medicine* 1988;84:539–42.

76. Hodsman GP, Isles CG, Murray GD, Usherwood TP, Webb DJ, Robertson JIS. Factors related to first dose hypotensive effect of captopril: Prediction and treatment. *British Medical Journal* 1983;286:832–4.

77. Biollaz J, Waeber B, Brunner HR. Hypertensive crisis treated with orally administered captopril. *European Journal of Clinical Pharmacology* 1983;25:145–9.

78. Tschollar W, Belz GG. Sublingual captopril in hypertensive crisis. *Lancet* 1985;i:34–5.

79. Hauger-Klevene JH. Captopril in hypertensive crisis. *Lancet* 1985;ii:732.

80. DiPette DJ, Ferraro JC, Evans RR, Martin M. Enalaprilat, an intravenous angiotensin-converting enzyme inhibitor, in hypertensive crisis. *Clinical Pharmacology and Therapeutics* 1985;38:199–204.

81. Marigliano V, Santilli D, Fiorani M, Ariani A, Cacciafesta M, Ferri C, Piccirillio G. Hypertensive emergencies in old age: Effects of angiotensin converting enzyme inhibition. *Journal of Hypertension* 1988;6 (suppl 1):S91–3.

82. Di Veroli C, Pastorelli R. Acute captopril treatment in elderly hypertensive patients: A controlled study. *Journal of Hypertension* 1988;6 (suppl 1):S95–6.

83. Hauger-Klevene JH. Comparison of sublingual captopril and nifedipine. *Lancet* 1986;i:219.

84. Van Harten J, Burggraaf K, Danhof M, Van Brummelen P, Breimer DD. Negligible sublingual absorption of nifedipine. *Lancet* 1987;ii:1365.

85. Spence JD, Arnold JMO, Gilbert JJ. Consequences of hypertension and effects of antihypertensive therapy. In: Robertson JIS, ed. *Clinical aspects of hypertension. Handbook of hypertension, vol 15.* Amsterdam: Elsevier, 1992:chapter 23.

86. Gifford RW. Management of hypertensive crisis. *Journal of the American Medical Association* 1991;266:829–35.

87. Robertson JIS. Hypertension and its treatment in the elderly. *Clinical and Experimental Hypertension* 1989;AII:779–805.

88. The Working Group on Hypertension in the Elderly. Statement on hypertension in the elderly. *Journal of the American Medical Association* 1986;256:70–4.

89. Subcommittee on Definition and Prevalence of the 1984 Joint National Committee. Hypertension prevalence and the status of awareness, treatment, and control in the United States. *Hypertension* 1985;7:457–68.

90. Kannel WB, Stokes J. Hypertension as a cardiovascular risk factor. In: Bulpitt CJ, ed. *Handbook of hypertension, vol 6: Epidemiology of hypertension.* Amsterdam: Elsevier, 1985:15–34.

91. Amery A, Birkenhäger WH, Brixco P, Bulpitt C, Clement D, Deruyttere M, De Schaepdryver A, Dollery C, Fagard R, Forette F, Forte J, Hamdy R, Henry JF, Joossens JV, Leonetti G, Lund-Johansen P, O'Mallery K, Petrie J, Strasser T, Tuomilehto J, Williams B. Mortality and morbidity results from the European Working Party on High Blood Pressure in the Elderly trial. *Lancet* 1985;i:1349–54.

92. SHEP Cooperative Research Group. Prevention of stroke by antihypertensive drug treatment in older persons with isolated systolic hypertension. Final results of the Systolic Hypertension in Elderly Program (SHEP). *Journal of the American Medical Association* 1991;265:3255–64.

93. Dahlöf B, Lindholm LH, Hansson L, Scherstén B, Ekbom T, Wester P-O. Morbidity and mortality in the Swedish Trial in Old Patients with Hypertension (STOP-Hypertension). *Lancet* 1991;338:1281–5.

94. Messerli FH, Sundgaard-Riise K, Ventura HO, Dunn FG, Glade LB, Frolich ED. Essential hypertension in the elderly: Haemodynamics, intravascular volume, plasma renin activity, and circulating catecholamine levels. *Lancet* 1983;ii:983–6.

95. Weidmann P, De Myttenaire-Bursztein SD, Maxwell MH, deLima J. Effects of aging on plasma renin and aldosterone in normal man. *Kidney International* 1975;8:325–33.

96. Mead TW, Imeson JD, Gordon D, Peart WS. The epidemiology of plasma renin. *Clinical Science* 1983;64:273–80.

97. Bühler FR, Bolli P, Kiowski W, Erne P, Hulthén UL, Block LH. Renin profiling to select antihypertensive baseline drugs. Renin inhibitors for high-renin and calcium entry blockers for low-renin patients. *American Journal of Medicine* 1984;77 (suppl 2A):36–42.

98. Lijnen P, Fagard R, Groeseneken D, M'Buyamba JR, Staessen J, Amery A. The hypotensive effect of captopril in hypertensive patients is age related. *Methods and Findings in Experimental and Clinical Pharmacology* 1983;5:655–60.

99. Ajayi AA, Hockings N, Reid JL. Age and pharmacodynamics of angiotensin converting enzyme inhibitor enalapril and enalaprilat. *British Journal of Clinical Pharmacology* 1986;21:349–57.

100. Reid JL. Angiotensin converting enzyme inhibitors in the elderly. *British Medical Journal* 1987;295:943-4.

101. Breckenridge A. Age-related effects of angiotensin converting enzyme inhibitors. *Journal of Cardiovascular Pharmacology* 1988;12 (suppl 8):100–4.

102. Ball SG. Age-related effects of converting enzyme inhibitors: A commentary. *Journal of cardiovascular Pharmacology* 1988;12 (suppl 8):105–7.

103. Jenkins AC, Knill JR, Dreslinski GR. Captopril in treatment of the elderly patients. *Archives of Internal Medicine* 1985;145:2029–31.

104. Tuck ML, Katz LA, Kirkendall WM, Koeppe PR, Ruoff GE, Sapir DG. Low dose captopril in mild to moderate geriatric hypertension. *Journal of the American Geriatrics Society* 1986;34:693–6.

105. Creisson C, Baulac L, Lenfant B. Captopril-hydrochlorothiazide combination in elderly patients with mild-moderate hypertension: A double blind, randomized, placebo-controlled study. *Postgraduate Medical Journal* 1986;62 (suppl I):139–41.

106. Woo J, Woo KS, Vallance-Owen J. The use of angiotensin converting enzyme (ACE) inhibitor enalapril in the treatment of mild to moderate hypertension in the elderly. *British Journal of Clinical Practice* 1987;41:845–7.

107. Mulinari R, Gavras I, Gavras H. Efficacy and tolerability of enalapril monotherapy in older patients compared to younger. *Clinical Therapeutics* 1987;9:678–89.

108. Laher MS, Natin D, Rao SK, Jones RW, Carr P. Lisinopril in elderly patients with hypertension. *Journal of Cardiovascular Pharmacology* 1987;9 (suppl 3): 569–71.

109. Thomson AH, Kelly JG, Whiting B. Lisinopril population pharmacokinetics in elderly and renal disease patients with hypertension. *British Journal of Clinical Pharmacology* 1989;27:57–65.

110. Marlier R, Vandepapeliere P, De Vriese G. Safety and efficacy of lisinopril in elderly patients with mild to moderate hypertension. *Journal of Human Hypertension* 1989;3 (suppl 1):163–7.

111. Cummings DM, Amadio P, Taylor EJ, Balaban DJ, Rocci ML, Abrams WB, Feinberg J, Vlasses PH. The antihypertensive response to lisinopril: The effect of age in a predominantly black population. *Journal of Clinical Pharmacology* 1989;29:25–32.

112. Thomson M, Droussin AM, Lame PA. The antihypertensive effect and safety of lisinopril in patients with mild to moderate essential hypertension. A Belgian multicenter study. *Acta Cardiologica* 1990;45:297–309.

113. Laher MS. Lisinopril in elderly patients with hypertension. Long term effects on renal and metabolic function. *Drugs* 1990;39 (suppl 2):55–63.

114. Kobrin I, Ben-Ishay D, Bompani R, Dixon R, Hoverman RJ, Jones RW, Kogler P, Sanchez R. Efficacy and safety of cilazapril in elderly patients with essential hypertension. A multicenter study. *American Journal of Medicine* 1989;87 (suppl 6B):33–6S.

115. Ogihara T, Kaneko Y, Ikeda M, Yamada K, Omae T, Arakawa K, Ishii M, Yoshinaga K, Kumahara Y, Kokubu T. Clinical evaluation of delapril in Japan: Report from the Japan Study Group on Delapril. *American Journal of Hypertension* 1991;4:42–5S.

116. Forette F, McClaran J, Delesalle MC, Hervy MP, Bouchacourt P, Henry-Amar M, Santoni JP. Value of angiotensin converting enzyme inhibitors in the elderly: The example of perindopril. *Clinical and Experimental Hypertension* 1989;A11 (suppl 2):587–603.

117. Canter D, Frank G. ACE inhibitors in the treatment of hypertension in the older patient. *European Heart Journal* 1990;11 (suppl D):33–43.

118. Knapp LE, Frank GJ, McLain R, Rieger MM, Posvar E, Singer R. The safety and tolerability of quinapril. *Journal of Cardiovascular Pharmacology* 1990;15 (suppl 2):S47–55.

119. Corea L, Bentivoglio M, Verdecchia P, Providenza M. Converting-enzyme inhibition versus diuretic therapy as first therapeutic approach to the elderly hypertensive patient. *Current Therapeutic Research* 1984;36:347–51.

120. Woo J, Woo KS, Kin T, Vallance-Owen J. A single blind randomized crossover study of angiotensin-converting enzyme inhibitor and triamterene and hydrochlorothiazide in the treatment of mild to moderate hypertension in the elderly. *Archives of Internal Medicine* 1987;147:1386–8.

121. Shapiro DA, Liss C, Walker JF, Lewis JL, Lengerich RA, Irvin JD. Enalapril and hydrochlorothiazide as antihypertensive agents in the elderly. *Journal of Cardiovascular Pharmacology* 1987;10 (suppl 7):160–2.

122. Grosskopf S, German R, Beilin LJ, Vandongen R, Rogers P. A randomised double blind comparison of enalapril versus hydrochlorothiazide in elderly hypertensives. *Journal of Human Hypertension* 1989;3:131–6.

123. Gilchrist NL, Nicholls MG, Ewer TC, Livesey JH, Sainsbury R. A comparison of long acting nifedipine and enalapril in elderly hypertensives: A randomized single-blind cross-over study. *Journal of Human Hypertension* 1988;2:33–9.

124. Kusaka M, Atarashi K, Matsumoto K, Sumida Y, Shingu T, Ootsuki T, Matsuura H, Kajiyama G. Effects of treatment with captopril on exercise tolerance and plasma catecholamines in elderly hypertensives. *Journal of Hypertension* 1989;7 (suppl 7):S59–61.

125. Cox JP, Duggan J, O'Boyle CA, Mee F, Walsh JB, Coakley D, O'Brien E, O'Malley K. A double-blind evaluation of captopril in elderly hypertensives. *Journal of Hypertension* 1989;7:299–303.

126. Giuntoli F, Gabbani S, Natali A, Galeone F, Saba P and the Captopril Study Group. Captopril in elderly hypertensive patients: Efficacy and tolerability in a long-term study. *Current Therapeutic Research* 1989;45:1025–30.

127. Scoble JE, Hamilton G. Atherosclerotic renovascular disease. *British Medical Journal* 1990;300:1670–1.

128. Choudhri AH, Cleland JGF, Rowlands PC, Tran TL, McCary M. Al-Kutoubi MAO. Unsuspected renal artery stenosis in peripheral vascular disease. *British Medical Journal* 1990;301:1197–8.

129. Priollet P, Lazareth I, Manière-Constantin D, Aimé F. Renal artery stenosis and peripheral vascular disease. *Lancet* 1990;336:879.

130. Salmon P, Brown MA. Renal artery stenosis and peripheral vascular disease: Implications for ACE inhibitor therapy. *Lancet* 1990;336:321.

131. Task force on blood pressure control in children. Report of the second task force on blood pressure control in children — 1987. *Pediatrics* 1989;79:1–25.

132. Mirkin BL, Newman TJ. Efficacy and safety of captopril in severe childhood hypertension. Report of the international collaborative study group. *Pediatrics* 1985;75:1091–100.

133. O'Dea RF, Mirkin BL, Alward CT, Sinaiko AR. Treatment of neonatal hypertension with captopril. *Journal of Pediatrics* 1988;113:403–6.

134. Miller K, Atkin B, Rodel Jr PV, Walker JF. Enalapril: A well tolerated and efficacious agent for the pediatric hypertensive patient. *Journal of Hypertension* 1986;4 (suppl 5):S413–6.

135. Broughton Pipkin F, Symonds EM, Turner SR. The effect of captopril (SQ 14,225) upon mother and fetus in chronically cannulated ewe and in the pregnant rabbit. *Journal of Physiology* 1982;325:415–22.

136. Keith IM, Will JA, Weir EK. Captopril: Association with fetal death and pulmonary vascular changes in the rabbit. *Proceedings of the Society for Experimental Biology and Medicine* 1982;170:378–83.

137. Duminy PC, Burger PD. Fetal abnormality associated with the use of captopril during pregnancy. *South African Medical Journal* 1981;60:805.

138. Metha N, Modi N. ACE inhibitors in pregnancy. *Lancet* 1989;ii:96.

139. Broughton Pipkin F, Baker PN, Symonds EM. ACE inhibitors in pregnancy. *Lancet* 1989;ii:96–7.

140. Rosa FW, Bosco LA, Fossum Graham C, Milstein JB, Dreis M, Creamer J. Neonatal anuria with maternal angiotensin-converting enzyme inhibition. *Obstetrics and Gynecology* 1989;74:371–4.

141. Kraft-Jais C, Plouin PF, Tchobrutsky C, Boutroy MJ. Angiotensin converting enzyme inhibitors during pregnancy: A survey of 22 patients given captopril and nine given enalapril. *British Journal of Obstetrics and Gynaecology* 1988;95:420–2.

142. Smith AM. Are ACE inhibitors safe in pregnancy? *Lancet* 1989;ii:750–1.

143. Editorial. Are ACE inhibitors safe in pregnancy? *Lancet* 1989;ii:482–3.

144. Svensson A. Hypertension in pregnancy. In: Hansson L, ed. *The International Society of Hypertension 1988 Hypertension Annual*. London: Gower Academic Journals, 1988:33–46.

145. Lubbe WF. Treatment of hypertension in pregnancy. *Journal of Cardiovascular Pharmacology* 1990;16 (suppl 7):S110–3.

146. Cleland JGF, Dargie HJ, McAlpine H, Ball SG, Morton JJ, Robertson JIS, Ford I. Severe hypotension after first dose of enalapril in heart failure. *British Medical Journal* 1985;291:1309–12.

147. Webster J. Angiotensin converting enzyme inhibitors in the clinic: First dose hypotension. *Journal of Hypertension* 1987;5 (suppl 3):27–30.

148. Packer M, Kessler PD, Gottlieb SS. Adverse effects of converting-enzyme inhibition in patients with severe congestive heart failure: Pathophysiology and management. *Postgraduate Medical Journal* 1986;62 (suppl 1):179–82.

149. Capewell S, Capewell A. 'First dose' hypotension and venodilatation. *British Journal of Clinical Pharmacology* 1991;31:213–5.

150. Ajayi AA, Campbell BC, Meredith PA, Kelman AW, Reid JL. The effect of captopril on the reflex control of heart rate: Possible mechanisms. *British Journal of Clinical Pharmacology* 1985;20:17–25.

151. Guyton AC. *Textbook of medical physiology*. London:WB Saunders, 1981.

152. Hodsman GP, Brown JJ, Cumming AMM, Davies DL, East BW, Lever AF, Morton JJ, Murray GD, Robertson JIS. Enalapril in treatment of hypertension with renal artery stenosis: Changes in blood pressure, renin, angiotensin I and II, renal function, and body composition. *American Journal of Medicine* 1984;77 (2A):52–60.

153. Waeber B, Gavras I, Brunner HR, Cook CA, Charocopos F, Gavras HP. Prediction of sustained antihypertensive efficacy of chronic captopril therapy. Relationships to immediate blood pressure response and control plasma renin activity. *American Heart Journal* 1982;103:384–90.

154. Houston MC. Abrupt cessation of treatment in hypertension: Consideration of clinical features, mechanisms, prevention and management of the discontinuance syndrome. *American Heart Journal* 1981;102:415–30.

155. Svensson A, Hansson L, Nicholls G. Rebound hypertension. In: Robertson JIS, ed. *ACE Report, vol 28*. London: Gower Medical Publishing Ltd, 1986.

156. Hansson L, Hunyor SN, Julius S, Hoobler SW. Blood pressure crisis following withdrawal of clonidine (Catapres, Catapresan) with special reference to arterial and urinary catecholamine levels and suggestions for acute management. *American Heart Journal* 1973;85:605–10.

157. Khayyal M, MacGregor J, Brown JJ, Lever AF, Robertson JIS. Increase of plasma renin-substrate concentration after infusion of angiotensin in the rat. *Clinical Science* 1973;44:87–90.

158. Rasmussen S, Nielsen MD, Giese J. Captopril combined with thiazide lowers renin substrate concentration: Implications for methodology in renin assays. *Clinical Science* 1981;60:591–3.

159. Giese J, Rasmussen S, Nielsen MD, Ibsen H. Biochemical monitoring of vasoactive peptides during angiotensin converting enzyme inhibition. *Journal of Hypertension* 1983;1 (suppl 1):31–6.

160. Boomsma F, deBruyn JHB, Derkx FHM, Schalekamp MADH. Opposite effects of captopril on angiotensin I-converting enzyme 'activity' and 'concentration'; relation between enzyme inhibition and long-term blood pressure response. *Clinical Science* 1981;60:491–8.

161. Vlasses PH, Koffer H, Ferguson RK, Green PJ, McElwain GE. Captopril withdrawal after chronic therapy. *Clinical and Experimental Hypertension* 1981;3:929–37.

162. Guthrie GP, Kotchen TA, Hammond JA. Effects of treatment with and withdrawal from enalapril in essential hypertension. *Clinical Research* 1983;31:730A.

163. Maslowski AH, Nicholls MG, Ikram H, Espiner EA, Turner JG. Haemodynamic, hormonal and electrolyte responses to withdrawal of long-term captopril treatment for heart failure. *Lancet* 1981;ii:959–61.

164. Jett GK. Captopril-induced angioedema. *Annals of Emergency Medicine* 1984;13:489–90.

165. Van Brummelen P, Willemze R, Tan WD, Thompson L. Captopril associated agranulocytosis. *Lancet* 1980;i:150.

166. Rahmat J, Gelfand RL, Gelfand MC, Winchester JF, Schreiner GF, Zimmerman HJ. Captopril associated cholestatic jaundice. *Annals of Internal Medicine* 1985;102:56–8.

167. Salena BJ. Chronic cough and the use of captopril: Unmasking of asthma. *Archives of Internal Medicine* 1986;146:202–3.

168. Chakraborty TK, Ruddell WS. Guillain–Barré neuropathy during treatment with captopril. *Postgraduate Medical Journal* 1987;63:221–2.

169. Hoorntje SJ, Kallenberg CGM, Weening JJ, Donker AMJ, The TH, Hoedemaeker PJ. Immune-complex glomerulopathy in patients treated with captopril. *Lancet* 1980;ii:1212–4.

170. Clement MI. Captopril induced eruptions. *Archives of Dermatology* 1981;117:525–6.

171. Seedat YK. Nephrotic syndrome from captopril. *South African Medical Journal* 1980;57:390.

172. Yeo WW, Ramsay LE. Persistent dry cough with enalapril: Incidence depends on method used. *Journal of Human Hypertension* 19990;4:517–20.

173. Bruggemeyer CD, Ramirez G. Onycholysis associated with captopril. *Lancet* 1984;i:1352–3.

174. Case DB, Atlas SA, Mouradian JA, Fishman RA, Sherman RL, Laragh JH. Proteinuria during long-term captopril therapy. *Journal of the American Medical Association* 1980;244:346–9.

175. Vlasses PH, Ferguson RK. Temporary ageusia related to captopril. *Lancet* 1979;**ii**:526.

176. Wood SM, Mann RD, Rawlins MD. Angio-edema and urticaria associated with angiotensin converting enzyme inhibition. *British Medical Journal* 1987;**294**: 91–2.

177. Doyle AE. Vascular complications of hypertension. In: Robertson JIS, ed. *Clinical aspects of essential hypertension. Handbook of hypertension, vol 1.* Amsterdam: Elsevier, 1983:365–77.

178. Hypertension Detection and Follow-up Program Cooperative Group. Five-year findings of the Hypertension Detection and Follow-up Program: I, reduction in mortality of persons with high blood presure, including mild hypertension. *Journal of the American Medical Association* 1979;**242**:2562–71.

179. Hampton JR. An appraisal of hypertension trials. *Medicographia* 1983;**5** (suppl 2):12–5.

180. Ramsay LE. Mild hypertension: Treat patients, not populations. *Journal of Hypertension* 1985;**3**:449–55.

181. Robertson JIS. The large studies in hypertension: What have they shown? *British Journal of Clinical Pharmacology* 1987;**24** (suppl):3–14S.

182. Collins R, Peto R, MacMahon S, Herbert P, Fierbach NH, Eberlein KA, Godwin J, Qizilbash N, Taylor JO, Hennekens CH. Blood pressure, stroke, and coronary heart disease. Part 2, short-term reductions in blood pressure: Overview of randomised trials in their epidemiological context. *Lancet* 1990;**335**:827–38.

183. MacMahon SW, Cutler JA, Furberg CD, Payne GH. The effects of drug treatment for hypertension on morbidity and mortality from cardiovascular disease: A review of randomized controlled trials. *Progress in Cardiovascular Diseases* 1986;**29** (suppl 1):99–118.

184. Alderman MH. Meta-analysis of hypertension treatment trials. *Lancet* 1990;**335**:1092–3.

185. Kaplan NM. Meta-analysis of hypertension treatment trials. *Lancet* 1990;**335**:1093.

186. Jenkinson ML. Meta-analysis of hypertension treatment trials. *Lancet* 1990;**335**:1093–4.

187. Robertson JIS. Antihypertensive therapy: Achievements, failures, and prospects. *Journal of Cardiovascular Pharmacology* 1990;**16** (suppl 7):102–4.

188. Dahlöf B, Pennert K, Hansson L. Effect of first-line antihypertensive therapy on cardiac hypertrophy: A meta-analysis in 1141 patients. *Fifth European Meeting on Hypertension, Milan 1991*, Abstract No 140.

189. Lindholm L, Ejlertsson G, Scherstén B. High risk of cerebro-cardiovascular morbidity in well treated male hypertensives. A retrospective study of 40–59-year-old hypertensives in a Swedish primary care district. *Acta Medica Scandinavica* 1984;**216**:251–9.

190. Isles CG, Walker LM, Beevers DG, Brown I, Cameron HL, Clarke J, Hawthorne V, Hole D, Lever AF, Robertson JWK, Wapshaw JA. Mortality in patients of the Glasgow Blood Pressure Clinic. *Journal of Hypertension* 1986;**4**:141–56.

191. Strandgaard S, Haunsø S. Why does antihypertensive treatment prevent stroke but not myocardial infarction? *Lancet* 1987;**ii**:658–61.

192. Dustan HP, Schneckloth RE, Corcoran AC, Page IH. The effectiveness of long-term treatment of malignant hypertension. *Circulation* 1958;**18**:644–51.

193. Robertson JIS. Should the costs of development inhibit research into new antihypertensive drugs? *Cardiovascular Drugs and Therapy* 1989;**3**:757–9.

194. Lindemann RD, Tobin JD, Schock NW. Association between blood pressure and the rate of decline in renal function with age. *Kidney International* 1984;**26**: 861–8.

195. Hansson L, Robertson JIS. Is hypertension treated adequately? *Drugs* 1987;**34** (suppl 3):1–6.

196. The BBB Study Group. The BBB Study: A prospective randomized study of intensified antihypertensive treatment. *Journal of Hypertension* 1988;**6**:693–7.

197. Ames RP. Negative effects of diuretic drugs on metabolic risk factors for coronary heart disease: Possible alternative drug therapies. *American Journal of Cardiology* 1983;**51**:632–8.

198. Fitzgerald JD. The applied pharmacology of beta-adrenoceptor antagonists (beta-blockers) in relation to clinical outcomes. *Cardiovascular Drugs and Therapy* 1991;**5**:561–76.

199. Poole-Wilson PA. Diuretics, hypokalaemia and arrhythmias in hypertensive patients: Still an unresolved problem. *Journal of Hypertension* 1987;**5** (suppl 3):S51–5.

200. Singh BN, Hollenberg NK, Poole-Wilson PA, Robertson JIS. Diuretic-induced potassium and magnesium deficiency: Relation to drug-induced QT prolongation, cardiac arrhythmias and sudden death. *Journal of Hypertension* 1992;**10**:301–16.

201. Pollare T, Lithell H, Berne C. A comparison of the effects of hydrochlorothiazide and captopril on glucose and lipid metabolism in patients with hypertension. *New England Journal of Medicine* 1989;**321**:868–73.

202. Ramsay LE, Yeo WW. First line treatment in hypertension. *British Medical Journal* 1991;**302**:352–3.

203. Moser M. In defense of traditional antihypertensive therapy. *Hypertension* 1988;**12**:324–6.

204. Freis E. The cardiotoxicity of diuretics: Review of the evidence. *Journal of Hypertension* 1990;**8** (suppl 2):23–32.

205. McInnes GT, Yeo WW, Ramsay LE, Moser M. Cardiotoxicity and diuretics: Much speculation, little substance. *Journal of Hypertension* 1992;**10**:317–35.

206. Morgan TO. Diuretics and myocardial infarction or sudden death. *Drugs* 1986;**31** (suppl 4):132–4.

207. Carlsen JE, Kober L, Torp-Pedersen C, Johansen P. Relation between dose of bendrofluazide, antihypertensive effect and adverse biochemical effects. *British Medical Journal* 1990;**300**:975–8.

208. Robertson JIS. Left ventricular, large arterial, and resistance arterial changes, the J-curve, and antiplatelet agents. *Current Opinion in Cardiology* 1989;**4**:662–7.

209. Levy D. Left ventricular hypertrophy: Epidemiological insights from the Framingham Heart Study. *Drugs* 1988;**35** (suppl 5):1–5.

210. Levy D, Garrison RJ, Savage DD, Kannel WB, Castelli WP. Prognostic implications of echocardiographically determined left ventricular mass in the Framingham Heart Study. *New England Journal of Medicine* 1990;**322**:1561–6.

211. Koren MJ, Devereux RB, Casale PN, Savage DD, Laragh JH. Relation of left ventricular mass and geometry to morbidity and mortality in uncomplicated essential hypertension. *Annals of Internal Medicine* 1991;**114**:345–52.

212. Dahlöf B. Regression of cardiovascular structural changes — a preventive strategy. *Clinical and Experimental Hypertension* 1990;**A12** (5):877–96.

213. Brunner HR, Laragh JH, Baer L, Newton MA, Goodwin FT, Krakoff LR, Bard RH, Buhler FR. Essential hypertension: Renin and aldosterone, heart attack, and stroke. *New England Journal of Medicine* 1973;**286**:441–9.

214. Dahlöf B. Factors involved in the pathogenesis of hypertensive cardiovascular hypertrophy — a review. *Drugs* 1988;**35** (suppl 5):6–26.

215. Devereux RB, Pickering TG, Cody RJ, Laragh JH. Relation of renin–angiotensin system activity to left ventricular hypertrophy and function in experimental and human hypertension. *Journal of Clinical Hypertension* 1987;**3**:87–103.

216. Zimmerman BG, Sybetz EJ, Vong PC. Editorial review. Interaction between sympathetic and renin–angiotensin system. *Journal of Hypertension* 1984;**2**:581–7.

217. Sen S, Tarazi RC, Bumpus FM. Cardiac effects of angiotensin antagonists in normotensive rats. *Clinical Science* 1979;**56**:439–43.

218. Robertson AL, Khairallah PA, Angiotensin II: Rapid localization in nuclei of smooth and cardiac muscle. *Science* 1971;**172**:1138–9.

219. Khairallah PA, Kanabus J. Angiotensin and myocardial protein synthesis. In: Tarazi RC, Dunbar, eds. *Perspectives in cardiovascular research, vol 8.* New York: Raven Press, 1983:337–47.

220. Khairallah PA, Robertson AL, Darilla D. Effect of angiotensin II on DNA, RNA and protein synthesis. In: Genest J, Koiw E, eds. *Hypertension 72.* New York: Springer-Verlag, 1972:212–20.

221. Roth RH, Hughes J. Acceleration of protein biosynthesis by angiotensin correlation with angiotensin's effect on catecholamine biosynthesis. *Biochemical Pharmacology* 1972;**21**:3182–7.

222. Sen S, Bumpus FM. Collagen synthesis in development and reversal of cardiac hypertrophy in spontaneously hypertensive rats. *American Journal of Cardiology* 1979;44:954–8.

223. Freslon JL, Giudicelli JF. Compared myocardial and vascular effects of captopril and dihydralazine during hypertension development in spontaneously hypertensive rats. *British Journal of Pharmacology* 1983;80:533–43.

224. Sen S, Tarazi RC, Bumpus FM. Effects of converting enzyme inhibitor (SQ 14.225) on myocardial hypertrophy in spontaneously hypertensive rats. *Hypertension* 1980;2:169–76.

225. Sharma JN, Fernandez PG, Kim BK, Idikio H, Triggle CR. Cardiac regression and blood pressure control in the Dahl rat treated with either enalapril maleate (MK 421, an angiotensin-converting enzyme inhibitor) or hydrochlorothiazide. *Journal of Hypertension* 1983;1:251–6.

226. Pfeffer JM, Pfeffer MA, Mirsky I, Braunwald E. Regression of left ventricular hypertrophy and prevention of left ventricular dysfunction by captopril in the spontaneously hypertensive rat. *Proceedings of the National Academy of Sciences of the USA* 1982;79:3310–4.

227. Frohlich ED, Tarazi RC. Is arterial pressure the sole factor responsible for hypertensive cardiac hypertrophy? *American Journal of Cardiology* 1979;44:959–63.

228. Rushoaho H. Regression of cardiac hypertrophy with drug treatment in spontaneously hypertensive rats. *Medical Biology* 1984;62:263–76.

229. Devereux RB, Case DB, Cody RJ, Sachs I, Laragh JH. Captopril treatment of hypertension increases low but not normal cardiac index. *Clinical Research* 1981;29:356A.

230. Lombardo M, Zaini G, Pastori F, Fusco M, Pacini S, Foppoli C. Left ventricular mass and function before and after antihypertensive treatment. *Journal of Hypertension* 1983;1:215–9.

231. Ventura HO, Frohlich ED, Messerli FH, Kobrin I, Kardon MB. Cardiovascular effects and regional blood flow distribution associated with angiotensin converting enzyme inhibition (captopril) in essential hypertension. *American Journal of Cardiology* 1985;55:1023–6.

232. Nakashima Y, Fouad FM, Tarazi RC. Regression of left ventricular hypertrophy from systemic hypertension by enalapril. *American Journal of Cardiology* 1984;53:1044–9.

233. Dunn FG, Oigman W, Ventura HO, Messerli FH, Kobrin I, Frohlich ED. Enalapril improves systemic and renal hemodynamics and allows regression of left ventricular mass in essential hypertension. *American Journal of Cardiology* 1984;53:105–8.

234. Mujais SK, Fouad FM, Tarazi RC. Reversal of left ventricular hypertrophy with captopril: Heterogeneity of response among hypertensive patients. *Clinical Cardiology* 1983;6:595–602.

235. Devereux RB, Casale PN, Wallerson DC, Kligfield P, Hammond IW, Liebson PR, Alonso DR, Laragh JH. Cost-effectiveness of echocardiography and electrocardiography for detection of left ventricular hypertrophy in patients with systemic hypertension. *Hypertension* 1987;9 (suppl II):II69–76.

236. Devereux RB, Casale PN, Hammond IW, Savage DD, Alderman MH, Campo E, Alonso DR, Laragh JH. Echocardiographic detection of pressure-overload left ventricular hypertrophy: Effect of criteria and patient population. *Journal of Clinical Hypertension* 1986;3:66–78.

237. Sheiban I, Arcaro G, Covi G, Accardi R, Zenorini C, Lechi A. Regression of cardiac hypertrophy after antihypertensive therapy with nifedipine and captopril. *Journal of Cardiovascular Pharmacology* 1987;10 (suppl 10) S187–91.

238. Dahlöf B, Hansson L. Different effects of enalapril and hydrochlorothiazide on left ventricular structure — a controlled study in untreated hypertensives. 1992.

239. Graettinger WF, Lipson JL, Klein RC, Cheung DG, Weber MA. Comparison of antihypertensive therapies by noninvasive techniques. *Chest* 1989;96:74–9.

240. Muiesan ML, Agabiti-Rosei E, Romanelli G, Castellano M, Beschi M, Muiesan G. Beneficial effects of one year's treatment with captopril on left ventricular anatomy and function in hypertensive patients with left ventricular hypertrophy. *American Journal of Medicine* 1988;84 (suppl 3A):129–32.

241. Motz W, Strauer BE. Rückbildung der hypertensiven Herzhypertrophie durch chronische Angiotensin–Konversionenzymhemmung. *Zeitschrift fur Kardiologie* 1988;77:53–60.

242. Grandi AM, Venco A, Barzizza F, Casadei B, Marchesi E, Finardi G. Effect of enalapril on left ventricular mass and performance in essential hypertension. *American Journal of Cardiology* 1989;63:1093–7.

243. Picca M, Azzollini F, Zocca A, Bisceglia I, Pelosi G. Effects of enalapril on left ventricular function in patients with essential hypertension. *Advances in Therapeutics* 1989;6 (3):149–59.

244. Di Bello V, Santoro G, Ginanni A, Caputo MT, Giusti C. Enalapril maleato nel trattamento dell'ipertensione arteriosa essenziale. Valutazione della performance ventricolare sinistra e della regressione dell'ipertrofia ventricolare: Follow-up di un anno. *Clinica Europea* 1987;6:377–90.

245. Garavaglia G, Messerli FH, Nunez BD, Schmieder RE, Frohlich ED. Immediate and short-term cardiovascular effects of a new converting enzyme inhibitor (lisinopril) in essential hypertension. *American Journal of Cardiology* 1988;62 (13):912–6.

246. Asmar RG, Juomo HJ, Lacolley PJ, Santoni JP, Billand E, Levy BI, Safar ME. Treatment for one year with perindopril: Effect on cardiac mass and arterial compliance in essential hypertension. *Journal of Hypertension* 1988;6 (suppl 3):S33–9.

247. Asmar RG, Pannier B, Santoni JPh, Laurent ST, London GM, Levy BI, Safar ME. Reversion of cardiac hypertrophy and reduced arterial compliance after converting enzyme inhibition in essential hypertension. *Circulation* 1988;78:941–50.

248. Shahi M, Thom S, Poulter N, Sever PS, Foale RA. Regression of hypertensive left ventricular hypertrophy and left ventricular diastolic function. *Lancet* 1990;336:458–61.

249. de Faire U, Lindvall K, Andersson G, Eriksson S. Regression of left ventricular hypertrophy on long-term treatment with captopril of severe hypertensives refractory to standard triple treatment. *European Journal of Clinical Pharmacology* 1989;37:291–4.

250. Mezzetti A, Guglielmi MD, Mancini M, Proietti-Franceschilli G, de Panfilis S, di Gioacchino M, Pierdomenico SD, Neri M, Marzio L, Cuccurullo F. Captopril improves blood pressure control and favours the regression of left ventricular hypertrophy in patients taking hydrochlorothiazide. *Current Therapeutic Research* 1990;47 (1):146–155.

251. Schmieder RE, Messerli FH, Sturgill D, Garavaglia GE, Nunez BD. Cardiac performance after reduction of myocardial hypertrophy. *American Journal of Medicine* 1989;87:22–7.

252. Trimarco B, de Luca N, Ricciardelli B, Rosiello G, Volpe M, Condorelli M. Cardiac function in systemic hypertension before and after reversal of left ventricular hypertrophy. *American Journal of Cardiology* 1988;62:745–50.

253. Dahlöf B, Pennert K, Hansson L. Reversal of left ventricular hypertrophy in hypertensive patients — a meta-analysis of 109 treatment studies. *American Journal of Hypertension* 1992;5:95–110.

254. Sharpe N, Murphy J, Smith H, Hannan S. Treatment of patients with symptomless left ventricular dysfunction after myocardial infarction. *Lancet* 1988;i:255–9.

255. Pfeffer MA, Lamas GA, Vaughan DE, Parisi AF, Braunwald E. Effect of captopril on progressive ventricular dilatation after anterior myocardial infarction. *New England Journal of Medicine* 1988;319:80–6.

256. Eichstaedt H, Danne O, Langer M, Cordes M, Schubert C, Felix R, Schmutzler H. Regression of left ventricular hypertrophy under ramipril treatment investigated by nuclear magnetic resonance imaging. *Journal of Cardiovascular Pharmacology* 1989;13 (suppl 3):S75–80.

257. Folkow B, Hansson L, Sivertsson R. Structural vascular factors in the pathogenesis of hypertension. In: Robertson JIS, ed. *Clinical aspects of essential hypertension. Handbook of hypertension, vol. 1.* Amsterdam: Elsevier, 1983:133–50.

258. Fouad-Tarazi FM. Structural cardiac and vascular changes in hypertension: Response to treatment. *Current Opinion in Cardiology* 1987;2:782–6.

259. Rizzoni D, Porteri E, Castellano M, Bettoni G, Agabiti-Rosei E. Time course of the development of vascular and cardiac hypertrophy in genetic hypertension. *Circulation* 1991;**84** (suppl II):562.

260. Heagerty AM, Bund SJ, Aalkjaer C. Effects of drug treatment on human resistance arteriole morphology in essential hypertension: Direct evidence for structural remodelling of resistance vessels. *Lancet* 1988;**ii**:1209–12.

261. Safar ME, Pannier BM, Soubies PL, Laurent S, Safavian A, London GM. Intrinsic alterations in the arterial wall in hypertension and the effect of antihypertensive therapy. *Current Opinion in Cardiology* 1987;**2** (suppl 1):26–32.

262. Simon AC, Levenson J, Bouthier J, Safar ME. Effects of chronic administration of enalapril and propranolol on the large arteries in arterial hypertension. *Journal of Cardiovascular Pharmacology* 1985;**7**:856–61.

263. Kannel WB. Role of blood pressure in cardiovascular morbidity and mortality. *Progress in Cardiovascular Disease* 1974;**17**:5–24.

264. Ball SG. Systolic hypertension: a comparison of the trials with enalapril and beta-antagonists. *Current Opinion in Cardiology* 1987;**2** (suppl 1):S33–8.

265. Chopra M. Captopril: A free radical scavenger. *British Journal of Clinical Pharmacology* 1989;**27**:396–9.

266. McMurray J, Chopra M, McLay J, Scott N, Bridges A, Belch J. Free radical activity in chronic heart failure and effect of captopril. *British Heart Journal* 1989;**61**:457.

267. Ceriello A, Giugliano D, Quatraro A, Lefebvre PJ. Anti-oxidants show an antihypertensive effect in diabetic and hypertensive subjects. *Clinical Science* 1991;**81**:739–42.

268. Miller VM. Does antihypertensive therapy improve the function of the vascular endothelium? *Hypertension* 1990;**16**:541–3.

269. Shultz PJ, Raij L. Effects of antihypertensive agents on endothelium-dependent and endothelium-independent relaxations. *British Journal of Clinical Pharmacology* 1989;**28** (suppl):151–7.

270. Parving HH, Hommel E, Damkjaer Nielsen M, Giese J. Effect of captopril on blood pressure and kidney function in normotensive insulin dependent diabetics with nephropathy. *British Medical Journal* 1989;**299**:533–6.

271. Rodicio JL, Praga M, Alcazar JM, Oliet A, Gutierrez-Millet V, Ruilope LM. Effects of angiotensin converting enzyme inhibitors on the progression of renal failure and proteinuria in humans. *Journal of Hypertension* 1989;**7** (suppl 7):S43–7.

272. Aperloo AJ, de Zeeuw D, Sluiter HE, de Jong PE. Differential effects of enalapril and aterolol on proteinuria and renal haemodynamics in non-diabetic renal disease. *British Medical Journal* 1991;**303**:821–4.

273. Cleland JGF, Dargie HJ, Hodsman GP, Ball SG, Robertson JIS, Morton JJ, East BW, Robertson I, Murray GD, Gillen G. Captopril in heart failure: A double blind controlled trial. *British Heart Journal* 1984;**52**:530–5.

274. Cleland JGF, Dargie HJ, Ball SG, Gillen G, Hodsman GP, Morton JJ, East BW, Robertson I, Ford I, Robertson JIS. Effects of enalapril in heart failure: A double-blind study of exercise performance, renal function, hormones, and metabolic state. *British Heart Journal* 1984;**54**:305–12.

275. The SOLVD Investigators. Effect of enalapril on survival in patients with reduced left ventricular ejection fractions and congestive heart failure. *New England Journal of Medicine* 1991;**325**:293–302.

276. Cohn JN, Johnson G, Ziesche S, Cobb F, Francis G, Tristani F, Smith R, Dunkman WB, Loeb H, Wong M, Bhat G, Goldman S, Fletcher RD, Doherty J, Hughes CV, Carson P, Cintron G, Shabetai R, Haakenson MS. A comparison of enalapril with hydralazine-isosorbide dinitrate in the treatment of chronic congestive heart failure. *New England Journal of Medicine* 1991;**325**:303–10.

277. Houston MC. New insights and new approaches for the treatment of essential hypertension: Selection of therapy based on coronary heart disease risk factor analysis, hemodynamic profiles, quality of life, and subsets of hypertension. *American Heart Journal* 1989;**117**:911–51.

278. Ernst E, Bergmann H. Influence of cilazapril on blood rheology in healthy subjects. A pilot study. *American Journal of Medicine* 1989;**87** (suppl 6B):70–1s.

279. Gupta RK, Kjeldsen SE, Motley E, Weder AB, Zweifler AJ, Julins S. Platelet function during antihypertensive treatment with quinapril, a novel angiotensin converting enzyme inhibitor. *Journal of Cardiovascular Pharmacology* 1991;**17**:13–9.

280. Leary WP, Reyes AJ, Acosta-Barrios TN, Baharaj B. Captopril once daily as monotherapy in patients with hyperuricaemia and essential hypertension. *Lancet* 1985;**i**:277.

281. Hollenberg NK. Initial therapy in hypertension: Quality-of-life considerations. *Journal of Hypertension* 1987;**5** (suppl 1):3–7.

282. Jern S. Quality of life and hypertension. In: Hansson L, ed. *1987 Hypertension Annual*. London: Gower Academic Journals, 1987:21–35.

283. Callender JS. Hypertension and quality of life. *Current Opinion in Cardiology* 1988;**3** (suppl 2):S31–6.

284. Schwartz JC, de la Baune S, Yi CC. Enkephalin metabolism in brain and its inhibition. *Progress in Neuro-psychopharmacology* 1982;**6**:665–71.

285. Zubenko GS, Nixon RA. Mood-elevating effect of captopril in depressed patients. *American Journal of Psychiatry* 1984;**141**:110–1.

286. Callender JS, Hodsman GP, Hutcheson MJ, Lever AF, Robertson JIS. Mood changes during captopril therapy for hypertension: A double blind pilot study. *Hypertension* 1983;**5** (suppl III):III-90–2.

287. Olajide D, Lader M. Psychotropic effects of enalapril maleate in normal volunteers. *Psychopharmacology* 1985;**86**:374–6.

288. Lichter I, Richardson PJ, Wyke MA. Differential effects of atenolol and enalapril on memory during treatment for essential hypertension. *British Journal of Clinical Pharmacology* 1986;**21**:641–5.

289. Fletcher AE, Bulpitt CJ, Hawkins CM, Havinga TK, ten Berge BS, May JF. Quality of life on antihypertensive therapy: A randomized double-blind controlled trial of captopril and atenolol. *Journal of Hypertension* 1990;**8**:463–6.

290. Steiner S, Friedhoff A, Wilson B, Wecker J, Santo J. Antihypertensive therapy and quality of life: A comparison of atenolol, captopril, enalapril and propranolol. *Journal of Human Hypertension* 1990;**4**:217–25.

291. Jern S for The European Delapril Study Group. Changes of quality of life during treatment with delapril and atenolol in patients with mild to moderate hypertension. *Journal of Cardiovascular Pharmacology* 1992;in press.

292. Os I, Bratland B, Dahlöf B, Gisholt K, Syvertsen JO, Tretli S. Lisinopril or nifedipine in essential hypertension? A Norwegian multicenter study on efficacy, tolerability and quality of life in 828 patients. *Journal of Hypertension* 1991;**9**:1097–104.

293. Jachuck SJ, Brierley H, Jachuck S, Willcox PM. The effect of hypotensive drugs on the quality of life. *Journal of the Royal College of General Practitioners* 1982;**32**:103–5.

294. Cooper W, Sheldon D, Brown D, Kimber G, Isitt V, Currie W. Post-marketing surveillance of enalapril: Experience in 11,710 hypertensive patients in general practice. *Journal of the Royal College of General Practitioners* 1987;**37**:346–9.

295. Currie D, Lewis RV, McDevitt DG, Nicholson AN, Wright NA. Central effects of the angiotensin-converting enzyme inhibitor, captopril. I. Performance and subjective assessments of mood. *British Journal of Clinical Pharmacology* 1990;**30**:527–36.

296. Captopril Research Group of Japan. Clinical effects of low-dose captopril plus a thiazide diuretic on mild to moderate essential hypertension: A multicenter double-blind comparison with propranolol. *Journal of Cardiovascular Pharmacology* 1985;**7** (suppl 1):S77–81.

297. Garinin G. A comparison of once-daily antihypertensive therapy with captopril and enalapril. *Current Therapeutic Research* 1986;**40**:567–75.

298. Rumboldt Z, Marinkovic M, Drinovic J. Enalapril versus captopril: A double-blind multicentre comparison in essential hypertension. *International Journal of Clinical Pharmacology Research* 1988;**8**:181–8.

299. Chrysant SG, Brown RD, Kem DC, Brown JL. Antihypertensive and metabolic effects of a new converting enzyme inhibitor, enalapril. *Clinical Pharmacology and Therapeutics* 1983;**33**:741–6.

300. Goodwin FJ. A comparative study of enalapril and propranolol in mild to moderate essential hypertension. *Symposium on the Management of Congestive Heart Failure and Hypertension* London, 1984, Abstract no L-17.

301. Helgeland A, Hagelind CH, Strommen R, Tretli S. Enalapril, atenolol and hydrochlorothiazide in mild to moderate hypertension. *Lancet* 1986;**i**:872–5.

302. Sassano P, Chatellier G, Amiot A-M, Alhenc-Gelas F, Corvol P, Ménard J. A double-blind randomized evaluation of converting enzyme inhibition as the first treatment of mild to moderate hypertension. *Journal of Hypertension* 1984;**2** (suppl 2):75–80.

303. Thind GS, Johnson A, Bhatnagar D, Herkel TW. A parallel study of enalapril and captopril and one year of experience with enalapril treatment in moderate-to-severe hypertension. *American Heart Journal* 1985;**109**:852–8.

304. Gomez HJ, Sromovsky MS, Kristianson K, Cirillo VJ, Wilhelmsson CE, Berglund G. Lisinopril dose response in mild to moderate hypertension. *Clinical Pharmacology and Therapeutics* 1985;**37**:198.

305. Merrill DD, Byyny RL, Carr A, Dauer AD, Kazilionis JE, Lester FM, Miller K, Gibson TP, Whipple J. Lisinopril/hydrochlorothiazide in essential hypertension. *Clinical Pharmacology and Therapeutics* 1987;**41**:227.

306. Morlin C, Baglivo H, Boeijinga JK, Breckinridge AM, Clement D, Johnston GD, Klein W, Kramer R, Luccioni R, Meurer KA, Richardson PJ, Rosenthal J, Six R, Witzgall H. Comparative trial of lisinopril and nifedipine in mild to severe essential hypertension. *Journal of Cardiovascular Pharmacology* 1987;**9** (suppl 3):S48–52.

307. Karlberg BE, Lindstrom T, Rosenqvist R, Ohman KP. Efficacy, tolerance and hormonal effects of a new oral angiotensin converting enzyme inhibitor, ramipril (HOE 498) in mild to moderate primary hypertension. *American Journal of Cardiology* 1987;**59**:104–9D.

308. Villamil AS, Cairns V, Witte PU, Bertolasi C. A double-blind study to compare the efficacy, tolerance and safety of two doses of the angiotensin converting enzyme inhibitor ramipril with placebo. *American Journal of Cardiology* 1987;**59**:110–4D.

309. Morgan T, Anderson A, Wilson D, Murphy J, Nowson C. The effect of perindopril on blood pressure in humans on different sodium intakes. *Journal of Cardiovascular Pharmacology* 1987;**10** (suppl 7):S119–21.

310. Gavras I. Pilot study of the effects of the angiotensin converting enzyme inhibitor CI-906 on patients with essential hypertension. *Journal of Clinical Pharmacology* 1984;**24**:343–50.

311. Schnaper HW, Stein G, Schoenberger JA, Loen AS, Tuck ML, Taylor AA, Liss C, Shapiro DA. Comparison of enalapril and thiazide diuretics in the elderly hypertensive patient. *Gerontology* 1987;**33** (suppl 1):24–35.

312. Verza M, Cacciapuoti F, Spiezia R, D'Avino M, Arpino G, D'Errico S, Sepe J, Varricchio M. Effects of the angiotensin converting enzyme inhibitor enalapril compared with diuretic therapy in elderly hypertensive patients. *Journal of Hypertension* 1988;**6** (suppl 1):S97–9.

313. Novo S, Nardi E, Abrignani MG, Adamo L, Liquori M, Longo B, Strano A. Effects of chronic treatment with enalapril and hydrochlorothiazide on blood pressure, left ventricular mass and arrhythmias in hypertensive patients. *American Journal of Hypertension* 1991;**4**:55A.

314. Perret F, Mooser V, Hayoz D, Tardy Y, Meister J-J, Etienne J-D, Farine P-A, Marazzi A, Burnier M, Nussberger J, Waeber B, Brunner H-R. Evaluation of arterial-compliance pressure curves. Effect of antihypertensive drugs. *Hypertension* 1991;**18** (suppl II):II77–83.

315. Björck S, Mulec H, Johnson SA, Nordén G, Aurell M. Renal protective effect of enalapril in diabetic nephropathy. *British Medical Journal* 1992;**304**:339–43.

316. Frimodt-Moeller J, Poulsen DL, Kiornerup HJ, Bech P. Quality of life, side effects and efficacy of lisinopril compared with metoprolol in patients with mild to moderate essential hypertension. *Journal of Human Hypertension* 1991;**5**:215–21.

92

ANGIOTENSIN-CONVERTING ENZYME INHIBITORS IN DIABETES MELLITUS

ROBERTO SN KALIL, STEPHEN A KATZ, AND
WILLIAM F KEANE

INTRODUCTION

Diabetes mellitus is a major cause of morbidity and mortality throughout the world. Death in diabetic patients commonly relates to microvascular complications, particularly diabetic nephropathy. In the United States Renal Data System Annual Report of 1990, nearly 35% of all patients with end-stage renal disease had diabetic nephropathy as the cause of renal failure [1]. These data also indicated that diabetic nephropathy as a cause of end-stage renal disease has increased progressively during the past decade [1]. Type I or insulin-dependent diabetes mellitus (IDDM) has been considered the major cause of end-stage renal disease. It has been estimated that approximately one-third of IDDM patients will develop overt diabetic nephropathy and, thereafter, end-stage renal disease [2]. Effective antihypertensive therapy can, however, postpone the development of renal failure [3,4]. Recent epidemiologic data have suggested that end-stage renal disease occurs also in patients with type II or noninsulin-dependent diabetes mellitus (NIDDM) with a frequency that equals that reported in IDDM [5]. Considering that over 80% of all diabetic patients have type II diabetes, this finding may have considerable impact on end-stage renal disease programs (*Chapter 56*).

Much of our understanding of the natural history of diabetic nephropathy has emerged from the evaluation of patients with IDDM. Relatively few reports describe the clinical course during the development of renal disease in type II diabetic patients. Recent data from the Pima Indian epidemiologic study have suggested that glycemic control, duration of diabetes, and hypertension are all important in the evolution of type II diabetic nephropathy [6]. These clinical risk factors are similar to those identified as important in IDDM patients who develop progressive renal failure.

In this chapter, evidence supporting the role of the RAS in the development and progression of diabetic nephropathy in type I and type II diabetes is reviewed, a topic touched on also in *Chapter 75*. In addition, studies which have demonstrated that ACE inhibitors slow the development of renal disease in experimental models of diabetes are evaluated. Last, the results of available studies in type I and type II diabetic patients in whom ACE inhibitors have been given, are analyzed.

RENIN–ANGIOTENSIN SYSTEM IN DIABETES

The RAS in diabetes mellitus is discussed extensively in *Chapter 75*. It is relatively clear that blockade of the RAS with ACE inhibitors in experimental models of diabetes ameliorates diabetic glomerular injury (Fig. 92.1), thus suggesting a role for the RAS in the pathogenesis of diabetic nephropathy. The exact mechanism and site of action of these agents are still somewhat problematic since ACE inhibitors could be working through direct blockade of plasma Ang II formation, or through inhibition of local renal vascular or glomerular renin systems, or both. In addition, ACE inhibitors could also mediate some of their effects through the kinin system. The finding that in the streptozotocin model of type I diabetes, ACE inhibitors, in part, reduce glomerular injury by reducing postglomerular resistance and thus, glomerular capillary pressure (Fig. 92.1), lends credence to the hypothesis that the local RAS may be important in this experimental model. Anderson *et al* have studied renal tissue renin in a rat model of type I diabetes [7]. In diabetic insulin-treated rats, they found a higher renal renin content and increased levels of renal angiotensinogen mRNA when compared with control rats. They hypothesized that the renal RAS may play an important role in the hemodynamic abnormalities of early diabetes [7] (see below).

Plasma renin activity (PRA) has been reported to be low, normal, or high in diabetic patients [8]. Variable assessments of the RAS in the diabetic state are due to a large variety of factors (see *Chapter 75*). As the diabetic state and nephropathy progress, the multiple secretory stimuli for renin (*Chapter 24*) can change; for instance, hypertension, glomerular hyperfiltration, and sodium and volume retention are all commonly associated with diabetes and each would tend to inhibit renal renin secretion via the renal baroreceptor and macula densa mechanisms. However, increased sympathetic nerve activity and alterations in Ang II responsiveness, which are sometimes associated with diabetes, could

Single agent studies

Author [reference]	Model	ACE inhibitor	SBP	MAP	UAE	GFR	SNGFR	P_{gc}	$\overline{\Delta P}$	FGS	V_g
Dunn [92]	STZ	ENA	NR	$D_{1,2}$	NR	NR	D_2	NR	D_1	NR	NR
Dunn [92]	STZ	ENA	NR	$D_{1,2}$	D_1	NR	NR	NR	NR	D_1	NR
O'Brien [93]†	STZ	RAM	NC	NR	NC	D_1	NR	NR	NR	NR	NR
Cooper [94]	STZ	ENA	NR	D_1	D_1	NR	NR	NR	NR	NR	NC
Cooper [94]	SHR–STZ	ENA	NR	D_1	D_1	NR	NR	NR	NR	NR	NC
Zatz [27]	STZ	ENA	$D_{1,2}$	NR	NR	D_2	NR	D_1	$D_{1,2}$	NR	NR
Zatz [27]	STZ	ENA	D_1	NR	D_1	NR	NR	NR	NR	D_1	NR
Rennke [95]	STZ	CAP	NR	NR	$D_{1,2}$	NR	D_2	D_1	NR	D_1	D_1
Schmitz [37]	OZ	ENA	NR	D_1	D_1	NR	NC	NC	NR	NR	NR
O'Donnell [35]	OZ	ENA	NR	D_1	D_1	NR	NR	NR	NR	D_1	NR
Cooper [96]	STZ	ENA	NR	D_2	D_2	NR	NR	NR	NR	NR	NR

Comparative studies

Author [reference]	Model	ACE inhibitor	Comparative agent	SBP	MAP	UAE	GFR	SNGFR	P_{gc}	$\overline{\Delta P}$	FGS	V_g
Anderson [29]	STZ	CAP	TRX	NR	$D_{1,2}$	NR	NC	D_2	D_1	D_1	NR	NR
Anderson [29]	STZ	CAP	NR	D_1	NR	$D_{1,2}$	NR	NR	D_3	NR	$D_{1,2,3}$	D_1
Jackson [97]	STZ+UNINEPH	ENA	VER	NR	D_2	D_1*	D_1	NR	NR	NR	NR	NR
Yoshida [98]	STZ	CAP	BEND	D_1	NR	D_1	NR	NR	NR	NR	NR	NR
Yoshida [98]	SHR–STZ	CAP	NR	D_1	NR	$D_{1,3}$	NR	NR	NR	NR	NR	NR
Cooper [31]	SHR–STZ	ENA	MET+HYD	$D_{1,2}$	$D_{1,2}$	D_1	NR	NR	NR	NR	NR	D_1
Anderson [30]	STZ+UNINEPH	FOS	NIF–HYD	NR	D_1	$D_{1,2}$‡	NR	NR	$D_{1,2}$§	NR	NR	NR
Matsushima [99]	STZ+UNINEPH	CAP	NIC	D_1	NR	I_1	NC	NR	NR	NR	NR	NR

* = protein excretion; † = rats were fed with a high protein diet; ‡ = versus both NIF and HYD; § = versus NIF.
D_1 = significant decrease (P<0.05) compared with untreated DM rats; D_2 = significant decrease (P<0.05) compared with control; D_3 = significant decrease (P<0.05) compared with other drug (monotherapy or triple therapy); I_1 = significant increase (P<0.05) compared with control.
SBP = systolic blood pressure; MAP = mean arterial pressure; UAE = urinary albumin excretion; GFR = glomerular filtration rate; SNGFR = single nephron GFR; P_{gc} = glomerular capillary pressure; $\overline{\Delta P}$ = mean glomerular transcapillary hydraulic pressure gradient; FGS = focal glomerulosclerosis index; V_g = glomerular volume.
STZ = streptozotocin; SHR = spontaneous hypertensive rats; OZ = obese zucker rats; UNINEPH = uninephrectomized rats.
ENA = enalapril; RAM = ramipril; CAP = captopril; FOS = fosinopril; TRX = HCTZ+HYD+RES; HCTZ = hydrochlorothiazide; HYD = hydralazine; RES = reserpine; VER = verapamil; BEND = benidipine; MET = metoprolol; NIF = nifedipine; NIC = nicardipine; NC = no significant changes; NR = not recorded.

Fig. 92.1 Experimental studies with ACE inhibitors in animal models of type I and type II diabetic nephropathy.

increase circulating renin by modifying β-adrenergic and Ang II receptor-mediated renin release. Thus, abnormalities in the RAS system could be the result of physiological compensations of this system to progression of the diabetic process. Alternatively, it is possible that alterations in the RAS could directly and primarily mediate pathophysiologic complications of diabetes. Finally, type I and type II diabetes do not necessarily result in the same alterations in renin secretion. Since activity of the RAS may be a function of both the type of diabetes and disease progression, as well as of blood pressure, sodium intake and retention, autonomic function, and Ang II responsiveness, it is difficult to summarize the status of the RAS in diabetes since these factors may vary from study to study. A few concepts however, appear to have emerged.

In type I diabetes, plasma levels of renin are variable but more often are normal or depressed, especially in the presence of hypertension [9–11]. Ang II pressor responsiveness is often enhanced [9,12,13]. Some data have suggested that renin and Ang II levels are increased in patients with nephropathy and hypertension [12,14]. There is agreement that plasma levels of inactive renin (or prorenin) are increased in type I diabetes. Many studies have shown elevated plasma levels of prorenin [15–20]. Prorenin is the biosynthetic precursor of active renin. Therefore, it is possible that a defect in the conversion of prorenin to renin may exist in the diabetic state. Alternatively, an unusually high synthetic rate or low degradation rate of prorenin may be responsible. Regardless of the mechanism, high prorenin levels are associated with diabetic microvascular complications [18,19] (*Chapters 6 and 7*).

In type II diabetes, PRA appears to be reduced [19–22], particularly when hypertension [21] and sodium retention [22–24] are present. An increased pressor response to vasoactive hormones can be seen in type II diabetic patients [113]. Interestingly, using a euglycemic clamp technique, physiologic increases in insulin levels were associated with an increased pressor response to norepinephrine but not to Ang II in healthy volunteers [114].

EXPERIMENTAL STUDIES IN MODELS OF DIABETES MELLITUS

The administration of streptozotocin or alloxan to rats results in marked hyperglycemia. After the development of hyperglycemia, small daily supplemental doses of insulin produce a model of diabetes with modest hyperglycemia, hypertrophy of the kidney, and increased glomerular filtration (GFR) and renal plasma flow (RPF) rates [25]. These changes are accompanied by glomerular hypertrophy, mesangial expansion, and thickening of the glomerular basement membrane. Albuminuria becomes evident after 3–4 months and ultimately segmental glomerulosclerosis develops. Although these diabetic rats are usually normotensive, if hypertension develops, renal damage is accelerated [25]. Thus, this model has many similarities to human type I diabetes and as such, has been extensively studied.

In streptozotocin diabetic rats, alterations in glomerular hemodynamic function, specifically increases in glomerular capillary pressure or glomerular hypertension, have been proposed as playing an important role in the development of renal injury [26]. This increased glomerular capillary pressure occurs even in rats in which systemic arterial pressure is normal. Experimental data suggest that increased renal tissue renin is involved in mediating these increased glomerular pressures [7]. It has also been demonstrated that ACE inhibitor therapy might provide unique benefits in preventing or slowing the development of renal disease in the normotensive, moderately hyperglycemic diabetic rat (Fig. 92.1) [27]. In these experiments, oral administration of the ACE inhibitor, enalapril, reduced systemic arterial pressure by approximately 15mmHg. Despite this modest effect on blood pressure and, in the absence of changes in glycemic control, ACE inhibitor therapy reduced glomerular capillary pressure without affecting glomerular filtration or plasma flow rates [27]. Control of glomerular hypertension was associated with limitation of albuminuria and glomerular injury to levels seen in nondiabetic rats [28]. These data suggest that changes in systemic and particularly glomerular pressures are important in reducing glomerular damage [27,28].

A subsequent study performed in moderately hyperglycemic diabetic rats demonstrated that while reduction in blood pressure with hydralazine, reserpine, and hydrochlorothiazide (so-called triple therapy) slowed the development of albuminuria (Fig. 92.2), the effect was only to delay the development of injury (Fig. 92.3), whereas comparable blood-pressure reduction (Fig. 92.4) with the ACE inhibitor, captopril, prevented the development of nephropathy in this model of type I diabetes (see *Figs. 92.1, 92.2, and 92.3*). In these experiments, the initial reduction in albuminuria was associated with a reduction in glomerular pressures; however, this effect was not sustained in the triple-therapy group [29] (Fig. 92.5). Despite continued reduction of systemic arterial pressure by approximately 10mmHg, glomerular hypertension was noted to develop late in rats treated with triple therapy and this was considered important in the development of glomerular damage [29]. Similarly, nifedipine was without effect on glomerular injury or albuminuria in this experimental model of diabetes [30] (see *Fig. 92.1*). Data comparing enalapril with hydralazine and metoprolol in

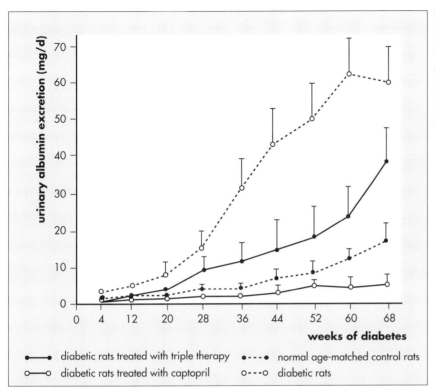

Fig. 92.2 Comparative effects of triple therapy (hydralazine, reserpine, and hydrochlorothiazide) and the ACE inhibitor, captopril, on urinary albumin excretion in long-term insulin supplemented streptozotocin-induced diabetic rats (mean ± SEM). Modified from Anderson S *et al* [29].

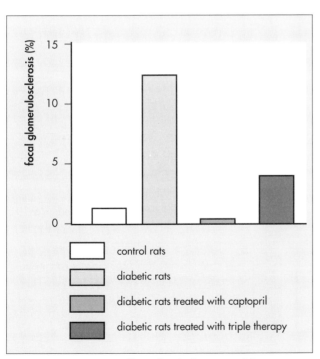

Fig. 92.3 Comparative effects of triple therapy and the ACE inhibitor, captopril, on per cent of glomerulosclerosis in long-term, insulin-supplemented, streptozotocin-induced diabetic rats. Modified from Anderson S *et al* [29].

spontaneously hypertensive diabetic rats, showed no significant difference between treatments on albumin excretion, control of blood pressure, glomerular volumes, and glomerular basement membrane thickness [31] (see *Fig. 92.1*).

The obese Zucker rat has been used to study endocrinologic and metabolic disturbances characteristic of NIDDM [32]. Obese Zucker rats spontaneously develop mild hyperglycemia, elevated plasma insulin levels, and peripheral insulin resistance. Obesity in the Zucker rat is an autosomal recessive trait. As in obese patients with NIDDM, hyperlipidemia is present. Small quantities of urinary albumin are evident in Zucker rats, at approximately 10 weeks of age, signaling the development of glomerular changes which progress to segmental glomerulosclerosis by six months of age [32]. With the development of glomerular injury, systemic hypertension develops and this appears to accentuate further glomerular damage. In contrast to the streptozotocin model of type I diabetes, neither marked glomerular hyperfiltration nor glomerular hypertension was found during the early phases of disease [33] (Figs. 92.6 and 92.7). Experimental studies suggest that the hyperlipidemia present in these rats, which is further exaggerated by the development of proteinuria, contributes to glomerular mesangial expansion as well as to the development of segmental glomerulosclerosis [34]. Studies have been conducted to evaluate whether the ACE inhibitor, enalapril, influences the

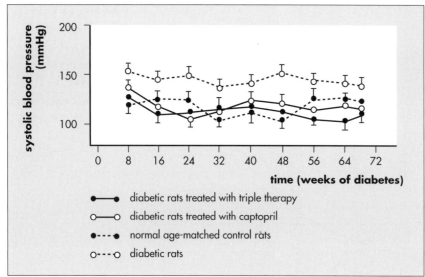

Fig. 92.4 Comparative effects of triple therapy and the ACE inhibitor, captopril, on systolic blood pressure (mean ± SEM) in long-term, insulin-supplemented, streptozotocin-induced diabetic rats. Modified from Anderson S *et al* [29].

course of renal disease in this normotensive rat model of NIDDM. These studies demonstrate that despite low plasma renin levels in obese Zucker rats, enalapril reduced systemic arterial pressure by approximately 10mmHg [35]. Albuminuria was reduced and, presumably as a consequence, serum cholesterol did not progressively increase [32–37]. Furthermore, glomerular injury was less in enalapril-treated obese Zucker rats. Kidney weights and glomerular areas were also significantly lower in the obese enalapril-treated Zucker rats. Glomerular hemodynamic function, however, particularly glomerular pressure, was not altered by enalapril therapy (see *Fig. 92.1*) [37]. These reports suggest that mechanisms other than a fall in intraglomerular pressure might protect glomeruli from damage during administration of ACE inhibitors. First, by reducing proteinuria, a favorable

effect on lipids was seen, and second, by reducing glomerular growth, amelioration of injury occurred, either because of hemodynamic effects through reduction in wall tension as described by Laplace's law, or through a mechanism involving hyperplastic/hypertrophic growth of glomerular cells presumably mediated by Ang II [38].

NATURAL HISTORY OF TYPE I DIABETIC NEPHROPATHY

Approximately 35% of patients with type I diabetes will develop end-stage renal disease. The development of renal failure in man

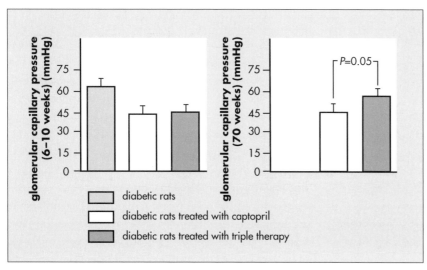

Fig. 92.5 Effect of triple therapy compared with the ACE inhibitor, captopril, on glomerular capillary pressures, early (6–10 weeks) and late (70 weeks), during the course of therapy in insulin-supplemented, streptozotocin-induced diabetic rats (mean ± SEM). Modified from Anderson S *et al* [29].

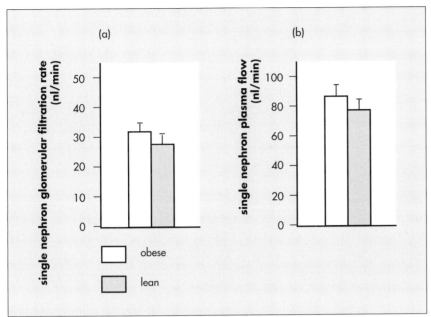

Fig. 92.6 (a) Single nephron glomerular filtration rate and (b) plasma flow in obese and lean Zucker rats in the early phase of disease, when albuminuria was minimal (mean ± SEM). Modified from O'Donnell MP *et al* [33].

is preceded by a number of identifiable stages of altered renal function (see also *Chapter 56*).

STAGES I–II

The early phases of type I diabetes are characterized by a significantly increased GFR and possibly increased RPF [39]. Temporally, these stages usually occur in the first decade after initial diagnosis of IDDM. Urinary albumin excretion rates are usually normal (<20μg/ml/min or <30mg/24h), although in some patients exercise may increase urinary albumin excretion [40].

Renal hypertrophy is also present [40]. Intensive therapy with insulin has been reported to correct the hyperfiltration, although reversal of renal hypertrophy may [115] or may not occur [41]. Morphologically, renal hypertrophy is accompanied by increased glomerular volumes [42]. During this first decade, thickening of the glomerular and tubular basement membrane evolves and a progressive expansion of the mesangial matrix is evident, signaling the transition to stage II. The increased matrix can be quantified by morphometric techniques, and an increased mesangial fractional volume has been identified as the earliest glomerular

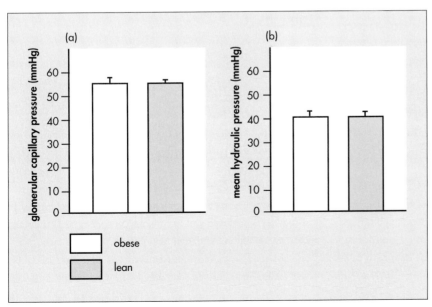

Fig. 92.7 (a) Glomerular capillary pressure and (b) mean hydraulic pressure in obese and lean Zucker rats in the early phase of disease, when albuminuria was minimal (mean ± SEM). Modified from O'Donnell MP *et al* [33].

histopathologic change in diabetic nephropathy [43]. This change may be present even in patients who do not manifest increased excretion of urinary albumin or so-called micro-albuminuria [43]. Hypertension is usually not present at these stages of disease.

STAGE III

During stage III, patients demonstrate increasing amounts of albuminuria. Usually, levels above $20\mu g/min$ or approximately $30mg/24h$ have been considered abnormal and have been termed microalbuminuria [44]. Prospective studies have demonstrated that diabetic patients with microalbuminuria have a 20-fold higher risk of developing overt nephropathy [44]. Moreover, microalbuminuria has been associated with poor glycemic control and higher levels of blood pressure even though blood pressure may be less than $130/90mmHg$ [42]. There is evidence to support the view that microalbuminuria is an indicator of early established diabetic nephropathy rather than being a true predictor of patients who will develop glomerular histologic changes [42]. Indeed, one study demonstrated that increased mesangial volume fraction was uniformly present in patients with microalbuminuria, supporting the notion that microalbuminuria is an indicator of early nephropathy rather than a predictor of those at risk of developing nephropathy [43]. Type I patients with microalbuminuria may have an elevated, normal or reduced GFR. Whether an increased GFR uniformly precedes microalbuminuria, remains to be established in man [42]. Early accounts of renal function in IDDM suggested that those patients with the greatest degree of hyperfiltration are at greatest risk of progression to overt nephropathy [45]. Not all studies, however, have confirmed this association [46]. Importantly, it is unclear if increments in GFR are related more to glycemic control [41] or to the level of protein intake [47,48], thus clouding whether the association between increased GFR and the risk of developing nephropathy is a direct or an indirect one. Nonetheless, once microalbuminuria increases above approximately $70\mu g/min$, the GFR appears to decline progressively [39]. The rate of decline in renal function appears to be accelerated by the presence of hypertension [3] and, on average, will decline at a rate of $10-12ml/year$ if blood pressure remains uncontrolled.

Blood pressure during the early phase of nephropathy is frequently in the normal range according to traditional definitions [49], although many patients with microalbuminuria have blood pressures that are above levels found in age- and disease-duration-matched diabetic patients [49]. Some data have indicated that an increase in the red blood cell Na^+/Li^+ countertransporter, considered a genetic marker for essential hypertension, is increased in type I patients with microalbuminuria [50]. Interestingly, these patients were found to have higher blood pressures as well as an atherogenic lipid profile including increased levels of low-density lipoprotein (LDL) cholesterol and decreased levels of high-density lipoprotein (HDL_2) cholesterol [51]. Whether these lipid abnormalities ultimately explain the reported three to five-fold increase in cardiovascular deaths in type I diabetics [52] remains to be established.

STAGES IV–V

In stages IV–V of the disease, renal failure, proteinuria, frequently in the nephrotic range, and severe hypertension become manifest [2]. Frequently, hypoalbuminemia develops and together with worsening renal failure, may contribute to the development of more severe lipid abnormalities. Massive proteinuria in these patients has been attributed to the development of a subpopulation of large, nonrestrictive pores in the glomerular filtration barrier [53]. Widespread microangiopathy, as well as atherosclerosis, is frequently found in patients with advanced nephropathy and reduced renal function. Indeed, the combination of hypertension and severe vascular disease accounts for the vast majority of deaths in diabetic patients with renal disease. The development of end-stage renal disease necessitating renal replacement therapy is ultimately seen in this group of IDDM patients some 25–30 years after the onset of diabetes. Indeed, some data suggest that diabetic patients with nephropathy are now living longer before requiring renal replacement therapy, than in former years [52].

NONINSULIN-DEPENDENT DIABETES MELLITUS

From an epidemiologic perspective, NIDDM appears to be more prevalent than previously reported [54]. In Minnesota, two studies performed 10 years apart indicated that in Caucasians, the prevalence of NIDDM has increased from 1.6 to 8% [55,56]. This could be the result of an aging population in general, or of longer survival of patients with NIDDM. In contrast to type I diabetic nephropathy, few data are available in NIDDM patients which detail the factors that may participate in the development of renal disease, and few studies have assessed these in a longitudinal manner. Incidence and prevalence data for type II diabetic nephropathy among different populations have, in large part, been obtained from retrospective analaysis of community- or referral-based populations. Compared with Caucasians, a higher prevalence of type II diabetes is seen in American Indians, Blacks, Hispanics, and Asians [54]. Since the glomerular histopathologic changes seen in type II diabetes are similar to those seen in type I diabetes, it is probable that many of the factors believed to contribute to renal disease in type I patients are operative also in patients with type II diabetes. Detailed epidemiologic, structural, and functional studies, however, have not been performed, and categorization of NIDDM into stages of nephropathy has not been as clearly defined as in IDDM patients.

STAGES I–II

The histologic changes seen during the early phases of NIDDM have not been reported. However, one study in Pima Indians [116] with abnormal glucose tolerance of one years' duration demonstrated that the GFR was 15% greater than in age-matched control subjects (140 ± 6 versus 122 ± 5 ml/min, respectively). Since the diabetic patients had a 16% greater body weight, only a 7% difference in the GFR was seen in the diabetic compared with control subjects (119 versus 110ml/min/1.73m^2, respectively). The urinary albumin excretion rates, although higher in the diabetic patients, were within the normal range. Evaluation of the fractional dextran-clearance profiles demonstrated that the diabetic subjects appeared to have a population of larger pores in the glomerular filtration barrier [116]. Whether these changes in renal function predict which patients progress to overt nephropathy remains to be established.

STAGE III

As in type I diabetes, the development of microalbuminuria most probably represents the earliest clinically detectable state of diabetic nephropathy. Serial epidemiologic studies, however, in which this has been monitored have not been performed. In addition, the relationship to age and the presence of essential hypertension, which may also affect urine albumin excretion, have not been evaluated in these patients. No data are available which relate microalbuminuria to structural changes in glomeruli of patients with NIDDM. Furthermore, the effect of blood-pressure control and glycemic control on microalbuminuria has not been extensively studied in NIDDM patients. Preliminary reports in small groups of Caucasian NIDDM patients matched for age, sex, and duration of diabetes demonstrated that microalbuminuria was associated with higher systolic and diastolic blood pressures, higher triglycerides, and lower HDL cholesterol levels, and with a higher incidence of cardiovascular disease [57,58]. Indeed, NIDDM patients with microalbuminuria have been reported to have a three or four-fold increase in the incidence of fatal vascular events [58].

In patients with NIDDM, hypertension appears to be more prevalent than in those with type I disease, and may antedate the clinical onset of diabetes [5]. One study in the Pima Indians showed that elevated blood pressure before the onset of NIDDM predicts albumin excretion, suggesting that hypertension associated with nephropathy is not just a consequence of the disease but may contribute to it [59]. It is not known, however, whether these patients develop hypertensive renal disease, diabetic nephropathy, other renal diseases, or a combination thereof. This is of importance in interpreting interventional studies in NIDDM patients with nephropathy, since a renal biopsy study performed on albuminuric NIDDM patients demonstrated that only 73% of patients had typical diabetic renal histologic changes [60]. The concomitant presence of retinopathy increased the likelihood that diabetic nephropathy was present [60].

The prevalence and potential importance of altered hemodynamics in NIDDM are unclear [61]. Renal function studies in Caucasian men with NIDDM have produced conflicting results [62,63]. In part, interpretation of these functional data is clouded by the fact that effects of age, body mass, and body composition have not been taken into consideration. The relationship of glomerular function to renal structure, blood pressure, glycemic control, protein intake, and microalbuminuria is not known in NIDDM. Interestingly, in one preliminary study of NIDDM patients, microalbuminuria was not associated with an increased inulin clearance or RPF [63].

STAGE IV

Proteinuria, as detected by routine techniques, progressively increases with the duration of NIDDM [62,63]. Among Caucasians, evidence for renal disease in NIDDM patients, that is, proteinuria and/or reduced renal function, has been found to occur with a frequency comparable to that described in patients with type I diabetes [5]. The ongoing epidemiological surveillance study in the Pima Indian tribe in the southwestern USA has indicated that the development of proteinuria is as high as that reported in type I diabetes [6]. In both Caucasian and American Indian populations, renal failure was present 6–8 years after proteinuria developed [6,64–66]. Hypertension and glycemic control appear to influence the development of this stage of nephropathy.

STAGE V

The progressive nature of diabetic nephropathy in NIDDM has not been as well documented as in type I patients. As indicated above, however, once proteinuria occurred in NIDDM patients, end-stage renal disease developed 6–8 years later [6,64–66]. In the Pima Indians, the prevalence of end-stage renal disease was 40.8 cases/1,000 person years at risk in those with NIDDM for >20 years, similar to that reported in patients with type I diabetes [64]. Glycemic control, duration of disease, and hypertension were significant factors that were associated with the development of end-stage renal disease [6,64–66].

TREATMENT OF DIABETIC NEPHROPATHY

Based on experimental and clinical studies addressing the pathogenesis of diabetic nephropathy, a number of therapeutic interventions have been demonstrated to benefit diabetic nephropathy. These are maintenance of euglycemia by continuous administration of insulin, treatment of hypertension, and protein restriction [4,67–70].

It is now clear that optimized insulin therapy is able to reduce hyperfiltration at least in short-term studies [68]. In addition, there are data to support the notion that the development of microalbuminuria is associated with poor metabolic control [41]. Optimized insulin therapy also reduces the degree of albuminuria [41]. The use of dietary protein restriction has been shown to reduce the rate of progression of renal disease in patients with overt diabetic nephropathy [67]. Similarly, protein restriction appears to reduce microalbuminuria in patients with incipient nephropathy [69]. Long-term studies, particularly in patients with incipient nephropathy, have not been reported. It is important to recognize that while a reduction in the amount of albuminuria is encouraging, the relationship of this effect to changes in the histopathology of diabetic nephropathy is unknown. Indeed, albuminuria may simply represent an improvement in filtration barrier characteristics, without changes of consequence in the glomerular mesangial histopathologic alterations.

Treatment of hypertension has been shown to reduce the mortality as well as the rate of loss of renal function in IDDM [3]. Based on experimental data in models of type I and type II diabetes mellitus (see *Fig. 92.1*), ACE inhibitors have been suggested as having potential benefits for IDDM and NIDDM patients with incipient and overt nephropathy, Finally, experimental studies have also supported a potential role for altered lipid metabolism, advanced glycated proteins, and the aldose-reductase

products as contributing to diabetic nephropathy. Their role in man is currently being investigated.

CLINICAL TRIALS

A variety of clinical investigations has been conducted to assess the efficacy of ACE inhibitors in the control of hypertension in diabetic patients and their impact on the progression of renal disease. While it appears clear that ACE inhibitors can effectively reduce blood pressure in diabetic patients, the influence of these agents on renal function (for example, proteinuria/albuminuria) and on the progression of renal disease has not been systematically studied. Variability in study design, end points measured, and methods of reporting results, as well as statistical techniques used, makes assessment of this body of data somewhat difficult. In some papers, patients with type I and type II diabetes are reported together. Finally, only a few studies, mostly short term, have examined properly the effectiveness of ACE inhibitors compared with other classes of antihypertensive agents, particularly with reference to potential effects of ACE inhibitors on renal function. Nonetheless, with these inherent problems in mind, we have analyzed collectively available studies in an effort to evaluate if ACE inhibitors have unique effects on albuminuria and proteinuria, and whether any such effects can be ascribed to changes in blood pressure or renal function, or both. In addition, the stage of diabetes at which therapy was initiated, the type of study performed (for example, randomized or open label), the number of subjects evaluated, and whether the study population included type I or type II diabetic patients or a mixture of both, were also evaluated. Importantly, no reported study examined the relationship between clinical improvement and histological changes with the treatment. These variables were entered into a multiple linear-regression analysis and the data were weighted depending on the number of patients studied and the strictness of the experimental design. We selected the majority of clinical trials available in the current literature and sorted them into three main groups to review. The first group consisted of diabetic patients with stages I–II nephropathy, the second group consisted of patients with incipient diabetic nephropathy (stage III), and the third group consisted of patients with overt nephropathy and chronic renal failure (stages IV and V). The duration of the studies varied from one week to 2.5 years; the number of patients per study varied from 4 to 52.

TREATMENT OF STAGES I AND II DIABETIC NEPHROPATHY WITH ANGIOTENSIN-CONVERTING ENZYME INHIBITORS

Only four trials have been performed in patients with the early stages of disease (Fig. 92.8(a)). In two of these, subjects were reported as being hypertensive. Two were short-term studies (<3 months), and two were conducted over one year [71–74]. In all four trials, blood pressure was significantly reduced not only in hypertensive but also in normotensive patients. Pedersen *et al* in a randomized double-blind, placebo-controlled trial in normotensive normoalbuminuric type I diabetic patients, demonstrated a significant reduction in albumin excretion even though urinary albumin was in the normal range [72]. This effect was seen only after three months of therapy, and the acute administration of intravenous enalapril did not have any effect on albumin excretion rates [72]. In contrast, the placebo-controlled study done by Brichard and co-workers in type I and II diabetic patients did not show significant changes in albumin excretion [74]. When renal function was examined in subjects with this stage of diabetes, no major changes in GFR or renal blood flow (RBF) were reported, particularly when assessed after prolonged therapy [73,74]. The use of ACE inhibitors during this phase of the disease is controversial and there are no reports of long-term studies examining whether this form of therapy might postpone the development of incipient nephropathy (stage III).

TREATMENT OF STAGE III DIABETIC NEPHROPATHY WITH ANGIOTENSIN-CONVERTING ENZYME INHIBITORS

Thirteen single-agent or comparative studies performed in type I and type II diabetic patients with microalbuminuria were evaluated (Figs. 92.8(b) and 92.9). The duration of these varied from two weeks to one year. The majority of trials were performed in normotensive type I patients.

Both hypertensive and normotensive type I diabetic patients with microalbuminuria showed an effect on control of blood pressure [75,76]. Patients with stage III diabetic nephropathy who were normotensive also had a significant decrease in blood pressure. In hypertensive type II diabetic patients, there was effective control of blood pressure [77].

In stage III diabetic patients, both of type I and type II, whether hypertensive or normotensive, there were no significant differences in GFR before and during the treatment with ACE

inhibitors. In two reports, however, patients with demonstrated hyperfiltration had a significant decline in GFR, while those with GFR initially in the normal range did not show any decrease [75,78]. Whether this observation is relevant to all diabetic patients with hyperfiltration remains to be established.

The majority of the trials have demonstrated that ACE inhibitors diminished urinary protein excretion. This occurred in normotensive and hypertensive patients and appeared to be sustained over many weeks. In a placebo-controlled study in type I normotensive subjects, a significant decrease in urine albumin excretion was found over a one-year interval (Fig. 92.10) [79]. A four-year trial has also been performed in normotensive, insulin-dependent patients [117]. Although renal function remained comparable in the ACE-inhibitor treated group to that in the untreated patients, urinary albumin output remained lower in the treatment group (Fig. 92.11). Moreover, 30% of the control patients progressed to overt nephropathy, as defined by albuminuria >300mg/24h, while none of the treated patients progressed to this stage of diabetic nephropathy (Fig. 92.12). Similar results have been observed in hypertensive type I diabetic patients with microalbuminuria [75]. In general, a 30–40% reduction in albuminuria was observed and was sustained. Although hypertensive patients frequently have a reduction in blood pressure greater than that in normotensive diabetic patients, the average magnitude of diminution in albuminuria was comparable (30–40%) in both groups of patients. In hypertensive type II diabetic patients, significant reductions in albumin protein/albumin excretion have also been demonstrated.

With regard to the issue of whether ACE inhibitors among antihypertensive agents have unique effects on renal function, studies comparing ACE inhibitors with calcium-channel blockers have been performed in patients with stage III diabetic nephropathy (see *Fig. 92.9*). The effect of calcium-channel blocking drugs on proteinuria or albuminuria in type I or II patients has not been as consistent as that seen with ACE inhibitors. Indeed, nifedipine has either no effect or increases urine albumin excretion, while diltiazem and nicardipine seem to decrease albumin excretion (see Fig. 92.9). Whether these differences will turn out to be clinically important remains to be determined. Many of these comparative trials are short term in duration. In 22 normotensive, type I diabetic patients, nifedipine was associated with an increase (approximately 40%), while captopril decreased (approximately 40%), in albuminuria during a six-week trial [80] (see *Fig. 92.9*). In a short-term study comparing enalapril with nicardipine in hypertensive type II diabetes mellitus patients, both agents effectively controlled blood pressure and decreased albumin excretion [77]. In a long-term trial

Author [reference]	ACE inhibitor	Type of trial	Number of patients	Duration (wks)	Type of diabetes DMI (%)	DMII (%)	HTN	Study results MAP	GFR	RBF	UAE
(a) NORMOALBUMINURIA											
Short-term studies											
Drummond [71]	ENA	DB,R,PC	18	4	100	0	N	D$_2$	NC	NC	NC
Pedersen [72]	ENA	DB,R,PC	10	13	100	0	N	NC	NC	NC	D$_2$
Long-term studies											
Passa [73]	ENA	BA	11	52	100	0	Y	D$_1$	NC	NR	NC*
Brichard [74]	PER	PC	14	52	57	43	Y	D$_2$	NC	NR	NC
(b) MICROALBUMINURIA											
Short-term studies											
Slomowitz [100]	ENA	DB,PC	6	4	100	0	N	D$_1$	NC	NC	D$_1$
Abu–Romeh [78] (HGFR)	ENA	BA	6	2	100	0	N	NC	D$_1$	NC	D$_1$
Abu–Romeh [78] (NGFR)	ENA	BA	5	2	100	0	N	NC	NC	NC	NC
Cook [76]	CAP	DB,R,PC	12	13	100	0	N	D$_1$	NC	NC	D$_1$
Casado [101]	CAP	BA	9	20	NR	NR	Y	D$_1$	NR	NR	D$_1$
Winocour [102]	CAP	BA	8	6	100	0	N	NR	NC	NC	NC
Long-term studies											
Rudberg [103]	ENA	BA	6	26	100	0	Y	NC	NC	NC	D$_2$
Rudberg [103]	ENA	BA	6	26	100	0	N	NC	NC	NC	D$_2$
Brichard [74]	PER	PC	7	52	57	43	Y	D$_2$	NC	NR	D$_2$
Marre [79]	ENA	BA	10	52	100	0	N	D$_2$	NC	I$_1$	D$_2$

*3 patients in this study were in stage III (incipient) nephropathy and all had significant reduction on albumin excretion.
I$_1$, D$_1$ = significant decrease (P<0.05) compared with baseline; D$_2$ = significant decrease (P<0.05) compared with placebo/control.
DMI = percentage of study group with type I diabetes mellitus; DMII = percentage of study group with type II diabetes mellitus; HTN = hypertension; MAP = mean arterial pressure;
GFR = glomerular filtration rate; RBF = renal blood flow; UAE = urinary albumin excretion.
ENA = enalapril; PER = perindopril; PC = placebo control; DB = double blind;
R = randomized; BA = before minus after; Y = yes; N = no; NR = not reported; NC = no significant changes.

Fig. 92.8 Results of studies of ACE inhibition in diabetic patients with (a) normoalbuminuria (stage I and II) and (b) microalbuminuria (stage III).

Author [reference]	ACE inhibitor	Type of trial	Comparative agent	Number of patients	Duration (wks)	Type of diabetes DMI (%)	DMII (%)	Stage	HTN	Study results MAP	GFR	RBF	UPE	UAE
Short-term studies														
Insua [80]	CAP	PC,R	NIF	22	6	100	0	III	N	D_1	NR	NR	NR	$D_{1,3}$
Baba [77]	ENA	DB,R,PC	NIC	7	4	0	100	III	Y	D_2	NC	NC	NR	D_2
Björck [85]	ENA	BA	MET	22	8	100	0	IV	Y	D_1	NR	NR	$D_{1,3}$	$D_{1,3}$
Bakris [87]	LIS	BA,CO	DIL	8	6	0	100	IV	Y	D_1	NC	NR	D_1	NR
Stornello [88]	CAP	BA,PC	NIC	12	4	0	100	IV	Y	D_2	NC	NC	NR	D_2
Stornello [89]	ENA	DB,R	ATE,CHL	12	6.4	0	100	IV	Y	D_2	NC	NC	NR	$D_{2,3}$†
Holdaas [104]	LIS	CO,BA,R	NIF	12	3	100	0	IV	Y	D_1	NC	I_1	NR	NC
Corcoran [105]	CAP	BA,CO	ATE,NIF,BEN	25	8	0	100	I,II,III	Y	D_3^*	NC	NR	NR	NC
Long-term studies														
Melbourne [75]	PER	DB,R	NIF	13	52	44	56	III	Y	D_1	NC‡	NR	NR	D_1
Melbourne [75]	PER	DB,R	NIF	30	52	44	56	III	N	D_1	NC	NR	NR	NC
Hollander [106]	CAP	BA	CON	10	52	81	19	IV	Y	D_1	NC	NR	$D_{1,3}$	NR

* = compared with BEN; † = compared with CHL; ‡ = patients with high GFR and significant reduction in GFR.
D_1 = significant decrease ($P<0.05$) compared with baseline; D_2 = significant decrease ($P<0.05$) compared with placebo/control; D_3 = significant decrease ($P<0.05$) compared with comparative antihypertensive agent; I_1 = significant increase ($P<0.05$) compared with baseline.
DMI = percentage of study group with type I diabetes mellitus; DMII = percentage of study group with type II diabetes mellitus; STAGE = stage of diabetic nephropathy; HTN = hypertension; MAP = mean arterial pressure; GFR = glomerular filtration rate; RBF = renal blood flow; UPE = urinary protein excretion; UAE = urinary albumin excretion; CAP = captopril; ENA = enalapril; LIS = lisinopril; PER = perindopril; PC = placebo control; R = randomized; DB = double blind; BA = before-after; CO = crossover; NIF = nifedipine; NIC = nicardipine; MET = metoprolol; DIL = diltiazem; CON = conventional therapy; ATE = atenolol; CHL = chlorthalidone; BEN = bendrofluazida.
Y = yes; N = no; NR = not reported; NC = no significant changes.

Fig. 92.9 Results of comparative studies between ACE inhibitors and other antihypertensives.

performed in Melbourne in both type I and II diabetic subjects, perindopril and nifedipine were compared [75]. It was found that in hypertensive patients, both drugs were effective in reducing blood pressure and decreasing urinary albumin excretion. By contrast, in normotensive patients with microalbuminuria, neither agent significantly changed albumin excretion, although both reduced blood pressure. Interestingly, normotensive diabetic patients who received perindopril had a 26% reduction in albumin excretion while the patients receiving nifedipine had a slight increase (4%) in urinary albumin excretion, although neither change was statistically significant. The type of diabetes did not appear to influence the response to these antihypertensive agents. Thus, the effect of nifedipine on microalbuminuria in this trial contrasts with previous reports [80].

Studies to evaluate progression of renal disease in the diabetic patient with stage III nephropathy are currently being performed. In the placebo-controlled trial of Marre and collaborators, the blood pressure rose and GFR decreased significantly in patients receiving a placebo compared with those treated with enalapril [79]. However, the rate of loss of GFR in this placebo group was 20ml/min/year, which is faster than the average (10–12ml/min/year) reported in the literature [81]. This decrease in GFR was associated with a progressive increase in albuminuria in the control group while in the enalapril-treated group, albuminuria decreased. This paper suggested a potential benefit of early

intervention in diabetic patients with incipient nephropathy. Whether alternative antihypertensive agents would exert a similar effect is presently unknown. Importantly, the implications of this effect on long-term preservation of renal structure are also uncertain. In the Melbourne trial, no significant change in renal function was observed during 12 months of therapy in either the perindopril or nifedipine groups. No placebo control group was, however, included in this study [75].

TREATMENT OF STAGES IV–V DIABETIC NEPHROPATHY WITH ANGIOTENSIN-CONVERTING ENZYME INHIBITORS

The first report using ACE inhibitors in stages IV–V diabetic patients was published in 1985 [82]. Since then, 22 papers have detailed the effects of ACE inhibitors in patients with overt diabetic nephropathy (see *Figs. 92.9* and *92.13*). Type I diabetic patients were studied in 10 trials, while patients with type II diabetes were studied in seven. Four accounts combined type I and II diabetic patients in the analyses. Hypertensive patients were evaluated in 17 reports and normotensive patients in six. In only five of these studies were ACE inhibitors compared with either a calcium-channel blocker or a β-blocker. The duration of the trials ranged from one week to 2.5 years.

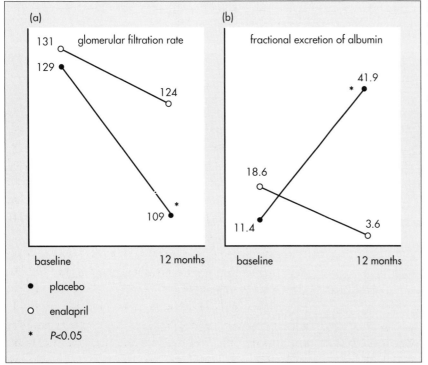

Fig. 92.10 Effects of the ACE inhibitor, enalapril, on (a) glomerular filtration rate and (b) fractional excretion of albumin, in normotensive, type I diabetic patients with incipient nephropathy. Modified from Marre M *et al* [79].

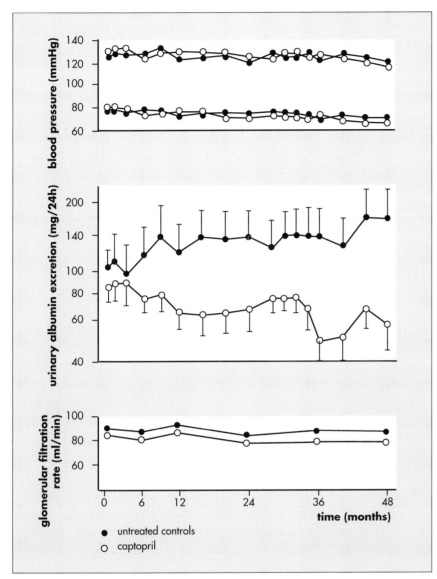

Fig. 92.11 Effect of the ACE inhibitor, captopril, versus untreated controls on blood pressure, renal function, and urinary albumin excretion in normotensive, type I diabetic patients with incipient nephropathy during a follow-up period of four years. Data are mean ± SEM. Modified from Mathiesen ER *et al* [117].

Urinary albumin excretion	Control group (n=23)	Captopril group (n=21)
decreased	8 (35%)	14 (67%)
no change/ slight increase	8 (35%)	7 (33%)
overt nephropathy (>300mg/24h)	7 (30%)	0

Fig. 92.12 Effect of the ACE inhibitor, captopril, on the progression of overt nephropathy in normotensive, type I diabetic patients, with incipient nephropathy, during a follow-up period of four years. Modified from Mathiesen ER *et al* [117].

As expected, ACE inhibitors controlled blood pressure adequately in hypertensive type I diabetic subjects. In hypertensive type II diabetic patients, adequate reduction and control of blood pressure with ACE inhibitor therapy was also achieved [83,84]. Renal hemodynamic recordings were performed in most studies and, in general, no significant differences in GFR and RBF before and during treatment were observed.

Urinary albumin and/or protein excretion decreased during ACE inhibitor therapy in most studies (see *Figs. 92.9* and *92.13*). In general, the magnitude of reduction in albuminuria was comparable with that reported in patients with stage III nephropathy, that is, a 30–40% reduction. This effect was similar in magnitude in both hypertensive and normotensive patients and appeared to be sustained over many months. In hypertensive type I diabetic patients studied for approximately two years, albumin excretion was reduced by ACE inhibitors by approximately 11%, while in control subjects, a 55% increase in albumin excretion was noted [81]. Björck demonstrated that the magnitude of reduction in urinary albumin excretion was significantly greater with ACE inhibitor therapy as compared with the β-blocker, metoprolol, despite comparable reductions in blood pressure in hypertensive type I patients with nephropathy [85]. Similar effects have been reported in a double-blind study of normotensive type II diabetic patients in whom albuminuria was significantly reduced by enalapril [86]. Not all workers have, however, demonstrated a reduction in protein excretion rate during treatment with ACE inhibitors (see *Figs. 92.9* and *92.13*).

Comparisons of ACE inhibitors with other antihypertensive agents in patients with overt nephropathy have been reported in five papers. As mentioned above, a study comparing enalapril with metoprolol in type I diabetic patients with overt nephropathy showed that both drugs effectively controlled blood pressure, but that only enalapril reduced protein excretion (by approximately 50%). There was no correlation between the decrease in albuminuria and the fall in blood pressure [85]. In type II diabetic patients with overt nephropathy, lisinopril was compared with diltiazem. Both drugs reduced blood pressure and albumin excretion and no change in GFR was observed with either agent [87]. Captopril was compared with nicardipine in type II diabetic hypertensive patients. Both drugs controlled blood pressure and decreased albumin excretion when used alone and no added effect was seen on albumin excretion rate when these agents were combined [88]. In a report by Stornello *et al* [89], in patients with overt nephropathy, hypertension, and type II diabetes mellitus, enalapril and atenolol had similar ability to reduce both blood pressure and albumin excretion. In this study, chlorthalidone was also effective in reducing blood pressure but not in reducing albumin excretion [89].

Two long-term trials addressing the issue of progression of stage IV diabetic renal disease have been reported [81,90]. The first, a case-control study in type I hypertensive patients followed for more than two years, demonstrated that the ACE inhibitor, captopril, could delay the rate of progression of renal insufficiency [81]. Patients who received active treatment had a reduction in albumin excretion of approximately 60%, with also adequate control of blood pressure, while the nontreated group had a significant increase in albuminuria [81]. Importantly, the rate of decline of GFR in patients on captopril was significantly lower than in placebo-treated control patients (10.0 versus 5.8ml/year, respectively) [81]. It is recognized, however, that other

antihypertensive agents (for example, β-blockers) have been reported to have a similar impact on the rate of loss of renal function [85]. A similar reduction in the rate of decline of renal function was reported with captopril by Björck and colleagues, although no effect on proteinuria was noted [90]. In normotensive type I patients with overt nephropathy followed for one year, patients on captopril had a rate of decline in GFR of 3.1ml/min, whereas controls had 6.5ml/min of decline in GFR [91]. At present, no long-term randomized and double-blinded study has been reported that unequivocally demonstrates that ACE inhibitor therapy preserves renal function and structure in patients with diabetic renal disease.

CONCLUSIONS: ANGIOTENSIN-CONVERTING ENZYME INHIBITOR TREATMENT IN DIABETIC NEPHROPATHY

In order to analyze the impact of ACE inhibitor therapy in diabetic nephropathy, we have combined evaluable data from 24 trials [53,71–73,75–79,81–84, 86–91,100,103,104,107,108]. To be incorporated in these analyses, studies were required to have determinations of blood pressure, GFR, and urinary albumin/protein excretion rates, both before and during treatment. These analyses also incorporated the type of diabetes and the stage of nephropathy, as well as the design and duration of the study. For purposes of these analyses, studies with a duration of greater than six months were considered 'long term'. We performed multiple linear-regression analyses to assess the relative effect of ACE inhibitor therapy on the clinical variables. The 24 trials included 328 patients who received ACE inhibitor therapy. The mean duration of the studies was 30. 7 ± 32.3 weeks. Half of these were performed in hypertensive diabetic patients of whom the majority had type I diabetes.

In both type I and II diabetic patients, blood pressure was reduced by ACE inhibitor therapy. As expected, a greater reduction in blood pressure was seen in hypertensive diabetic patients, although normotensive patients also showed a decrease. The stage of diabetic nephropathy did not seem to influence the blood-pressure fall seen with ACE inhibitor therapy. In addition, the longer the duration of therapy, the greater the fall in blood pressure.

In patients with incipient (stage III) diabetic nephropathy, ACE inhibitor therapy reduced GFR to a greater degree than was seen in patients with overt (stages IV–V) nephropathy. The

Author [reference]	ACE inhibitor	Type of trial	Number of patients	Duration (wks)	Type of diabetes DMI (%)	DMII (%)	HTN	Study results MAP	GFR	RBF	UPE	UAE
Short-term studies												
Hommel [107]	CAP	PC,R	11	12	100	0	Y	D_1	D_1	NR	NR	D_1
D'Angelo [84]	CAP	DB	10	12	100	0	Y	D_1	NC	NC	NR	NC
D'Angelo [84]	CAP	DB	10	12	0	100	Y	D_1	NC	NC	NR	NC
Taguma [82]	CAP	BA	9	8	100	0	Y	NC	NR	NR	D_1	NR
Morelli [53]	ENA	BA	16	13	100	0	N	D_1	NC	NC	NC	NR
Parving [108]	CAP	BA	14	1	100	0	Y	D_1	NC	NR	D_1	NR
Kisch [109]	CAP	BA	6	4	NR	NR	N	NC	NR	NR	D_1	NR
Casado [101]	CAP	BA	20	NR	NR	NR	Y	D_1	D_1	NR	NR	D_3
Casado [101]	CAP	BA	20	NR	NR	NR	N	NC	NC	NR	NR	D_1
Long-term studies												
Björck [90]	CAP	BA	14	107	100	0	Y	D_1	NC	NR	NC	NR
Parving [81]	CAP	BA,CC	18	134	100	0	Y	D_2	D_2	NR	NR	D_2
Brichard [74]	PER	PC	7	52	57	43	Y	D_2	NC	NC	NR	NC
Parving [91]	CAP	PC,R	17	52	100	0	N	D_2	NC	NR	NR	D_2
Valvo [83]	CAP	BA	12	26	0	100	Y	D_1	NC	NC	NC	NR
Stornello [86]	ENA	DB,R,PC	8	52	0	100	N	NC	NC	NC	NR	D_2
Romero [110]	CAP	BA	11	26	82	18	Y	D_1	NC	NR	D_1	NR
Stornello [111]	ENA	PC,R	12	26	8	92	N	NC	NC	NC	NR	D_1
Stornello [112]	CAP	BA	9	26	0	100	Y	D_2	NC	NC	NR	D_2

D_1 = significant decrease ($P<0.05$) compared with baseline; D_2 = significant decrease ($P<0.05$) compared with placebo/control; D_3 = significant decrease ($P<0.05$) compared with comparative antihypertensive agent.
DMI = percentage of study group with type I diabetes mellitus; DMII = percentage of study group with type II diabetes mellitus; HTN = hypertension; MAP = mean arterial pressure; GFR = glomerular filtration rate; RBF = renal blood flow; UPE = urinary protein excretion; UAE = urinary albumin excretion.
CAP = captopril; ENA = enalapril; PER = perindopril; PC = placebo control; DB = double blind; R = randomized; BA = before–after; CC = case control.
Y = yes; N = no; NR = not reported; NC = no significant changes.

Fig. 92.13 Results of ACE inhibition in diabetics with overt nephropathy and renal failure (stages IV and V).

reduction in GFR was most obvious in randomized, double-blinded trials. In addition, a greater reduction in GFR was seen in type I compared with type II diabetic patients.

Therapy with ACE inhibitors significantly reduced urinary albumin/protein excretion and this effect was independent of the stage of diabetic nephropathy. The greater the reduction in blood pressure, the greater was the decrease in albumin/protein excretion. Hypertensive diabetic patients (type I and II) tended to have a greater reduction in albumin/protein excretion than did normotensive patients. Interestingly, diabetic patients who were studied long term had a significantly greater reduction in protein excretion than those patients who were evaluated for a shorter interval. The long-term effect on protein/albumin excretion was also associated with a significantly greater reduction in blood pressure without any further decrease in GFR. Thus, from these analyses, it appeared that ACE inhibitor therapy reduced blood pressure, GFR, and urinary albumin/protein excretion. In addition, the duration of therapy was an important variable in the interpretation of potential benefits.

Since both blood pressure and GFR reduction could contribute to the decreased albumin/protein excretion, we examined the relative contribution of each of these factors. The blood-pressure fall could only explain 12.4% of the reduction in albumin/protein excretion, while the decrease in GFR explained only 12.6% of this effect. Thus, other mechanisms, for example intrarenal factors, may play a greater role in the decrease in albumin/protein excretion in patients with diabetic nephropathy. Whether these latter processes involve a direct influence of ACE inhibitors on glomerular hemodynamic function, or an indirect action mediated through nonhemodynamic mechanisms, for example Ang II-mediated cell proliferation and growth, or both, will require further clarification in human studies in which structure–functional correlations are performed.

REFERENCES

1. US Department of Commerce, the National Technical Information Service. Causes of ESRD. *United States National Institute of Diabetes and Kidney Diseases: US Renal Data Systems: 1990 Annual Data Report* 1990:11–6.

2. Mogensen CE, Mauer SM, Kjellstrand CM. Diabetic nephropathy. In: Schrier RW, Gottschalk CW, eds. *Diseases of the kidney: volume 3*, 4th edition. Boston: Little Brown, 1988:2395-437.

3. Parving H–H, Anderson AR, Smidt UM, Hommel E, Mathiesen ER, Svendsen PA. Effect of antihypertensive treatment on kidney function in diabetic nephropathy. *British Medical Journal* 1987;294:1443–7.

4. Mogensen CE. Long-term antihypertensive treatment inhibiting progression of diabetic nephropathy. *British Medical Journal* 1982;285:685–8.

5. Hasslacher C, Ritz E, Wake P, Michael C. Similar risks of nephropathy in patients with type I or type II diabetes mellitus. *Nephrology, Dialysis, Transplantation* 1989;4:859–63.

6. Kunzelman CL, Knowler WC, Pettit DJ, Bennett PH. Incidence of proteinuria in type 2 diabetes mellitus in the Pima indians. *Kidney International* 1989;35:681.

7. Anderson S, Bouyones B, Clarey LE, Ingelfinger JR. Intrarenal renin–angiotensin system in experimental diabetes [Abstract]. *Journal of the American Society of Nephrology* 1990;1:621.

8. Björck S. The renin angiotensin system in diabetes mellitus, a physiological and therapeutic study. *Scandinavian Journal of Urology and Nephrology* 1990; (suppl 126):1–51.

9. Tuck M. Management of hypertension in the patient with diabetes mellitus. *American Journal of Hypertension* 1988;1:384–8S.

10. Whiteside CI, Thompson J. The role of angiotensin-II in progressive diabetic glomerulopathy in the rat. *Endocrinology* 1989;125:1932–40.

11. Mann J, Ritz E. Renin–angiotensin System beim diabetischen Patienten. *Klinische Wochenschrift* 1988;66:883–91.

12. Weidmann P. Hypertension in diabetes: Pathogenesis of hypertension accompanying diabetes mellitus. In: Heidland A, Koch KM, Heidbreder E, eds. *Contributions to nephrology, volume 73*. Basel: Karger, 1989:73–90.

13. Christiansen JS, Giese J, Damkjær M, Parving H–H. The renin–angiotensin system and kidney function during initial insulin treatment in diabetic man. *Scandinavian Journal of Clinical and Laboratory Investigation* 1988;48:451–6.

14. Walker WG, Hermann J, Murphy RF, Russel RP. Prospective study of the impact of hypertension upon kidney function in diabetes mellitus. *Nephron* 1990;55 (suppl 1):21–6.

15. Björck S, Aurell M. Diabetes mellitus, the renin–angiotensin system, and angiotensin-converting enzyme inhibition. *Nephron* 1990;55 (suppl 1):10–20.

16. Amemiya S, Ishihara T, Higashida K, Kusano S, Ohyama K, Kato K. Altered synthesis of renin in patients with insulin-dependent diabetes: Plasma prorenin as a marker predicting the evolution of nephropathy. *Diabetes Research and Clinical Practice* 1990;10:115–22.

17. Bryer–Ash M, Fraze EB, Luetscher JA. Plasma renin and prorenin (inactive renin) in diabetes mellitus: Effects of intravenous furosemide. *Journal of Clinical Endocrinology and Metabolism* 1988;66:454.

18. Ubeda M. Hernandez I, Fenoy F, Quesada T. Vascular and adrenal renin like activity in chronically diabetic rats. *Hypertension* 1988;11:339-343.

19. Luetscher JA, Kraemer FB, Wilson DM. Prorenin and vascular complications of diabetes. *American Journal of Hypertension* 1989;2:382–6.

20. Luetscher JA, Kraemer FB, Wilson DM, Schwartz HC, Bryer–Ash M. Increased plasma inactive renin in diabetes mellitus. *New England Journal of Medicine* 1985;312:1412–7.

21. Misbin RI, Grant MB, Pecker MS, Atlas SA. Elevated levels of plasma prorenin (inactive renin) in diabetic and nondiabetic patients with autonomic dysfunction. *Journal of Clinical Endocrinology and Metabolism* 1987;64:964.

22. Sullivan PA, Kelleher M, Twomey M, Dineen M. Effects of converting enzyme inhibition on blood pressure plasma renin activity and plasma aldosterone in hypertensive diabetics compared to patients with essential hypertension. *Journal of Hypertension* 1985;3:359–63.

23. Trujillo A, Eggena P, Barrett J, Tuck M. Renin regulation in type II diabetes mellitus: Influence of dietary sodium. *Hypertension* 1989;13:200–5.

24. O'Hare JA, Ferriss B, Brady D, Twomey B, O'Sullivan DJ. Exchangeable sodium and renin in hypertensive diabetic patients with and without nephropathy. *Hypertension* 1985;7 (suppl II):43–8.

25. O'Donnell MP, Kasiske BL, Keane WF. Glomerular hemodynamic and structural alterations in experimental diabetes mellitus. *FASEB Journal* 1988;2:2339–47.

26. Hostetter TH, Rennke HG, Brenner BM. The case for intra-renal hypertension in the initiation and progression of diabetic and other glomerulopathies. *American Journal of Medicine* 1982;72:375–80.

27. Zatz R, Dunn BR, Meyer TW, Anderson S, Rennke HG, Brenner BM. Prevention of diabetic glomerulopathy by pharmacological amelioration of glomerular capillary hypertension. *Journal of Clinical Investigation* 1986;77:1925–30.

28. Zatz R, Anderson S, Meyer TW, Dunn BR, Rennke HG, Brenner BM. Lowering of arterial blood pressure limits glomerular sclerosis in rats with renal ablation and in experimental diabetes. *Kidney International* 1987;31 (suppl 20):S123–9.

29. Anderson S, Rennke HG, Garcia DL, Brenner BM. Short and long term effects of antihypertensive therapy in the diabetic rat. *Kidney International* 1989;36:526–36.

30. Anderson S, Rennke HG, Zayas MA, Brenner BM. Chronic calcium channel blockade fails to lower glomerular pressure and albuminuria in diabetic rats [Abstract]. *Clinical Research* 1991;39:2479.

31. Cooper ME, Allen TJ, O'Brien RC, Papazoglou D, Clarke BE, Jerums G, Doyle AE. Nephropathy in model combining genetic hypertension with experimental diabetes. *Diabetes* 1990;39:1575–9.

32. Kasiske BL, O'Donnell MP, Keane WF. The obese Zucker rat model of glomerular injury in type II diabetes. *Journal of Diabetic Complications* 1987;1:26–9.

33. O'Donnell MP, Kasiske BL, Cleary MP, Keane WF. Effects of genetic obesity on renal structure and function in the Zucker rat. II Micropuncture studies. *Journal of Laboratory and Clinical Medicine* 1985;106:605–10.

34. Kasiske BL, Cleary MP, O'Donnell MP, Keane WF. Effects of genetic obesity on renal structure and function in the Zucker rat. *Journal of Laboratory and Clinical Medicine* 1985;106:598–604.

35. O'Donnell MP, Kasiske BL, Katz SA, Schmitz PG, Keane WF. Enalapril reduces glomerular injury in obese Zucker rats. *Kidney International* 1989;35:434.

36. Kasiske BL, O'Donnell MP, Cleary MP, Keane WF. Treatment of hyperlipidemia reduces glomerular injury in obese Zucker rats. *Kidney International* 1988;33:667–72.

37. Schmitz PG, O'Donnell MP, Kasiske BL, Keane WF. Glomerular capillary pressure is increased in old obese Zucker rats and is unchanged with enalapril. *Kidney International* 1990;37:520.

38. Daniels BS, Hostetter TH. Adverse effects on dietary intake on growth in the glomerular microcirculation. *American Journal of Physiology* 1990;258:R1095–100.

39. Mogensen CE. Early glomerular hyperfiltration in insulin-dependent diabetics and late nephropathy. *Scandinavian Journal of Clinical and Laboratory Investigation* 1986;46:201–6.

40. Mogensen CE. Kidney function and glomerular permeability to macromolecules in early juvenile diabetes. *Scandinavian Journal of Clinical and Laboratory Investigation* 1971;28:79–90.

41. Wiseman MJ, Saunders AJ, Keen H, Viberti GC. Effect of blood glucose control on increased glomerular filtration rate and kidney size in insulin-dependent diabetes. *New England Journal of Medicine* 1985;312:617–27.

42. Osterby R, Parving HH, Hommel E, Jorgensen HE, Lokkegaard N. Glomerular structure and function in diabetic nephropathy; early to advanced stages. *Diabetes* 1990;39:1057–63.

43. Blous RW, Mauer SM, Sutherland DER, Steffes MW. Mean glomerular volume and rate of development of diabetic nephropathy. *Diabetes* 1989;38:1142–7.

44. Viberti GC, Hill RD, Jarret RJ, Argyropoulos A, Mahmud U, Keen H. Microalbuminuria as a predictor of clinical nephropathy in insulin-dependent diabetes mellitus. *Lancet* 1982;i:1430–2.

45. Mogensen CE, Andersen MJF. Increased kidney size and glomerular filtration rate in early juvenile diabetes. *Diabetes* 1973;22:706–12.

46. Lervang HH, Jensen S, Brochner–Mortensen J, Ditzel J. Early glomerular hyperfiltration and the development of nephropathy in the type I (insulin-dependent) diabetes mellitus. *Diabetologia* 1988;31:723–9.

47. Viberti GC, Dodds RA, Bending JJ, Bognetti E. Nonglycemic intervention in diabetic nephropathy: The role of protein intake. In: Mogensen CE, ed. *The kidney and hypertension in diabetes mellitus*. Boston: Martinus Nijhoff Publishing, 1988:205–15.

48. Kupin WL, Cortes P, Dumler F, Feldkamp CS, Kilates MC, Levin NW. Effect on renal function of a change from high to moderate protein intake in type I diabetic patients. *Diabetes* 1987;36:73–9.

49. Feldt-Rasmussen BO, Borch-Johnson K, Mathiesen ER. Hypertension in diabetes as related to nephropathy. Early blood pressure changes. *Hypertension* 1985;7 (suppl II):18–20.

50. Jones S, Trevisan R, Tariq T, Semplicini A, Mattock M, Walker JD, Nosadini R, Viberti GC. Sodium–lithium countertransport in microalbuminuric insulin-dependent diabetic patients. *Hypertension* 1990;15 (6, part 1):570–5.

51. Krowleski AS, Kosinki EJ, Warram HJ, Leland OS, Busick EJ, Asmal AC, Rand LI, Christlieb AR, Bradley RF, Kahn CR. Magnitude and determinant of coronary artery disease in juvenile-onset, insulin-dependent diabetes mellitus. *American Journal of Cardiology* 1987;59:750–5.

52. Parving HH, Hommel E. Prognosis in diabetic nephropathy. *British Medical Journal* 1989;299:230–3.

53. Morelli E, Loon N, Meyer T, Peters W, Myers BD. Effects of converting enzyme inhibition on barrier function in diabetic glomerulopathy. *Diabetes* 1990;39:76–82.

54. Harris MI, Hadden WC, Knowler WC, Bennett PH. Prevalence of diabetes and impaired glucose tolerance and plasma glucose levels in US population aged 20–74 years. *Diabetes* 1987;36:523–34.

55. French RL, Boen JR, Martinez AM, Bushhouse SA, Sprafka JM, Goetz FC. Population-based study of impaired glucose tolerance and type II diabetes in Wadena, Minnesota. *Diabetes* 1990;39:1131–7.

56. Ballard DJ, Humphrey LL, Melton III LJ, Frohnert PP, Chu CP, O'Fallon WM, Palumbo PJ. Epidemiology of persistent proteinuria in type II diabetes mellitus; population-based study in Rochester, Minnesota. *Diabetes* 1988;37:405–12.

57. Niskanem L, Usitupa M, Sarlund H, Siitonem D, Voutilainem E, Penttila I, Pyorala FK. Microalbuminuria predicts the developments of serum lipoprotein abnormalities favouring atherogenesis in newly diagnosed type 2 diabetic patients. *Diabetologia* 1990;33:237–43.

58. Jarret RJ, Viberti GC, Argyropoulos A, Hill RD, Mahmud U, Murrells TJ. Microalbuminuria predicts mortality in non-insulin-dependent diabetes. *Diabetic Medicine* 1984;1:17–9.

59. Knowler WC, Bennett PH, Nelson RG. Prediabetic blood pressure predicts albuminuria after development of NIDDM [Abstract]. *Diabetes* 1988;37:120A.

60. Owens DR, Dolben J, Uora JP, Luzio S, Williams S, Young A, Peters JR, Volund A. Retinopathy in relation to metabolic status in newly diagnosed non-insulin-dependent diabetes mellitus. In: Cameron D, Colagiuri A, Heding L, Kühl C, Mortiner R, eds. *Non insulin-dependent diabetes mellitus*. Hong Kong: Excerpta Medica, 1989:111–20.

61. Parving HH, Gall MA, Skott P, Jorgensen HE, Jorgensen F, Larsen S. Prevalence and causes of albuminuria in non insulin-dependent diabetics. *Kidney International* 1989;37:243.

62. Friedman EA, Sheih S–D, Hirsch SR, Boshell BR. No supranormal glomerular filtration in type II (non-insulin dependent) diabetes [Abstract]. *American Society of Nephrology* 1981;14:102A.

63. Vora J, Owens DR, Dolben J, Atiea J, Dean J, Peters JR. Glomerular filtration rate and effective renal plasma flow in newly presenting non-insulin dependent diabetes (NIDDM). *Diabetes Research and Clinical Practice* 1988;5 (suppl 1):57.

64. Nelson RG, Newman JM, Knowler WC, Sievers ML, Kunzelman CL, Pettit DJ, Moffett CD, Teutsch SM, Bennett PH. Incidence of end stage renal disease in type 2 diabetes mellitus in Pima indians. *Diabetologia* 1988;31:730–6.

65. Ordonez JD, Hiatt RA. Comparison of type II and type I diabetes treated for end-stage renal disease in a large prepaid health plan population. *Nephron* 1989;51:524–9.

66. Humphrey LL, Ballard DJ, Frohnert PP, Chu C–P, O'Fallon WM, Palumbo PJ. Chronic renal failure in non-insulin dependent diabetes mellitus, a population based study in Rochester, Minnesota. *Annals of Internal Medicine* 1989;111: 788–96.

67. Zeller K, Whittaker E, Sullivan L, Raskin P, Jacobson H. Effect of restricting dietary protein on the progression of renal failure in patients with insulin-dependent diabetes mellitus. *New England Journal of Medicine* 1991;324:78–84.

68. Kroc collaborative study group: Blood glucose control and the evolution of diabetic retinopathy and albuminuria. A preliminary multicenter trial. *New England Journal of Medicine* 1984;311:365–72.

69. Cohen S, Dodds R, Viberti GC. Effect of protein restriction in insulin dependent diabetics at risk of nephropathy. *British Medical Journal* 1987;294:795–8.

70. Feldt-Rasmussen BO, Mathiesen ER, Deckert T. Effect of two years of strict metabolic control on progression of incipient nephropathy in insulin-dependent diabetes. *Lancet* 1986;ii:1300–4.

71. Drummond K, Levy-Marchal C, Laborde K, Kindermans C, Wright C, Dechaux M, Czernichow P. Enalapril does not alter renal function in normotensive, normoalbuminuric, hyperfiltering type I (insulin-dependent) diabetic children. *Diabetologia* 1989;32:255–60.

72. Pedersen MM, Schmitz A, Pedersen EB, Danielson H, Christiansen JS. Acute and long-term renal effect of angiotensin converting enzyme inhibition in normotensive, normoalbuminuric insulin-dependent diabetic patients. *Diabetic Medicine* 1988;5:562-9.

73. Passa P, LeBlanc H, Marre M. Effects of enalapril in insulin-dependent diabetic subjects with mild to moderate uncomplicated hypertension. *Diabetes Care* 1987;10:200–4.

74. Brichard SM, Santoni JPh, Thomas JR, Van de Voorde K, Ketelslegers JM, Lambert AE. Long-term reduction of microalbuminuria after 1 year of angiotensin converting enzyme inhibition by perindopril in hypertensive insulin-treated diabetic patients. *Diabete et Metabolisme* 1989;16:30–6.

75. Melbourne Diabetic Nephropathy Study Group. Comparison between perindopril and nifedipine in hypertensive and normotensive diabetic patients with microalbuminuria. *British Medical Journal* 1991;302:210–6.

76. Cook J, Daneman D, Spino M, Sochett E, Perlman K, Balfe JW. Angiotensin converting enzyme inhibitor therapy to decrease microalbuminuria in normotensive children with insulin-dependent diabetes mellitus. *Journal of Pediatrics* 1990;117:39–45.

77. Baba T, Murabayashi S, Takebe K. Comparison of the renal effects of angiotensin converting enzyme inhibitor and calcium antagonist in hypertensive type 2 (non-insulin-dependent) diabetic patients with microalbuminuria: A randomized controlled trial. *Diabetologia* 1989;32:40–4.

78. Abu-Romeh SH, Nawaz MK, Ali JH, Al-Suhaili AR, Abu-Jayyab AK. Short-term effect of angiotensin-converting enzyme inhibitor enalapril in incipient diabetic nephropathy. *Clinical Nephrology* 1989;31:18–21.

79. Marre M, Chatellier G, Leblanc H, Guyene TT, Menard J, Passa P. Prevention of diabetic nephropathy with enalapril in normotensive diabetics with microalbuminuria. *British Medical Journal* 1988;297:1092–5.

80. Insua A, Ribstein J, Mimran A. Comparative effect of captopril and nifedipine in normotensive patients with incipient diabetic nephropathy. *Postgraduate Medical Journal* 1988;64 (suppl 3):59–62.

81. Parving H–H, Hommel E, Smidt UM. Protection of kidney function and decrease in albuminuria by captopril in insulin dependent diabetics with nephropathy. *British Medical Journal* 1988;297:1086–91.

82. Taguma Y, Kitamoto Y, Futaki G, Ueda H, Monama H, Ishizaki M, Takahashi H, Sekino H, Sasaki Y. Effect of captopril on heavy proteinuria in azotemic diabetics. *New England Journal of Medicine* 1985;313:1617–20.

83. Valvo E, Bedogna V, Casagrande P, Antiga L, Zamboni M, Bommartini F, Oldrizzi L, Rugiu C, Maschio G. Captopril in patients with type II diabetes and renal insufficiency: Systemic and renal hemodynamic alterations. *American Journal of Medicine* 1988;85:344–8.

84. D'Angelo A, Sartori L, Gambaro G, Giannini S, Malvasi L, Benetollo P, Lavagnini T, Crepaldi G. Captopril in the treatment of hypertension in type I and type II diabetic patients. *Postgraduate Medical Journal* 1986;62 (suppl 2): 69–72.

85. Björck S, Mulec H, Johnsen SA, Nyberg G, Aurell M. Contrasting effects of enalapril and metoprolol on proteinuria in diabetic nephropathy. *British Medical Journal* 1990;300:904–7.

86. Stornello M, Valvo EV, Scapellato L. Angiotensin converting enzyme inhibition in normotensive type II diabetics with persistent mild proteinuria. *Journal of Hypertension* 1989;7 (suppl 6):S314–5.

87. Bakris GL. Effects of diltiazem or lisinopril on massive proteinuria associated with diabetes mellitus. *Annals of Internal Medicine* 1990;112:707–8.

88. Stornello M, Valvo EV, Scapellato L. Hemodynamic, renal, and humoral effects of the calcium entry blocker nicardipine and converting enzyme inhibitor captopril in hypertensive type II diabetic patients with nephropathy. *Journal of Cardiovascular Pharmacology* 1989;14:851–5.

89. Stornello M. Valvo EV, Scapellato L. Comparative effects of enalapril, atenolol and chlorthalidone on blood pressure and kidney function of diabetic patients affected by arterial hypertension and persistent proteinuria. *Nephron* 1991;58:52–7.

90. Björck S, Nyberg G, Mulec H, Granerus G, Herlitz H, Aurell M. Beneficial effects of angiotensin converting enzyme inhibition on renal function in patients with diabetic nephropathy. *British Medical Journal* 1986;293: 471–4.

91. Parving H–H, Hommel E, Nielsen MD, Giese J. Effect of captopril on blood pressure and kidney function in normotensive insulin dependent diabetics with nephropathy. *British Medical Journal* 1989;299:533–6.

92. Dunn BR, Zatz R, Rennke HG, Meyer TW, Anderson S, Brenner BM. Prevention of glomerular capillary hypertension in experimental diabetes mellitus obviates functional and structural glomerular injury. *Journal of Hypertension* 1986;4 (suppl 5):S251–4.

93. O'Brien RG, Cooper ME, Allen TJ, Jerums G. Ramipril reduces albuminuria in diabetic rats fed a high protein diet. *Clinical and Experimental Pharmacology and Physiology* 1989;16:675–80.

94. Cooper, ME, Allen TJ, MacMillan P, Bach L, Jerums G, Doyle AE. Genetic hypertension accelerates nephropathy in the streptozotocin diabetic rat. *American Journal of Hypertension* 1988;1:5–10.

95. Rennke HG, Anderson S, Sandstrom DJ, Brenner BM. Pathogenesis of experimental diabetic microangiopathy: Differential effect of hemodynamic and metabolic factors [Abstract]. *FASEB Journal* 1989;3:A444.

96. Cooper ME, Allen TJ, MacMillan PA, Clarke BE, Jerums G, Doyle AE. Enalapril retards glomerular basement membrane thickening and albuminuria in the diabetic rat. *Diabetologia* 1989;32:326–8.

97. Jackson B, Cubela R, Debrevi L, Whitty M, Johnston CI. Disparate effects of angiotensin converting enzyme inhibitor and calcium blocker treatment on the preservation of renal structure and function following subtotal nephrectomy or streptozotocin-induced diabetes in the rat. *Journal of Cardiovascular Pharmacology* 1987;10 (suppl 10):S167–9.

98. Yoshida K, Yasujima M, Kohzuki M, Sato K, Tsunoda K, Kudo K, Kanazawa M, Yabe T, Abe K, Yoshinaga K. Calcium channel blocker (CCB) and angiotensin converting enzyme inhibitor (ACEI) in normotensive diabetic rats and hypertensive diabetic rats [Abstract]. *International Society of Nephrology, Tokyo, Japan* 1991;160A.

99. Matsushima Y, Kojima S, Kawamura M, Akabane S, Ito K. Effects of captoril and nicardipine on renal hyperfiltration and hypertrophy in uninephrectomized diabetic rats. *Japanese Journal of Nephrology* 1988;30:279–83.

100. Slomowitz LA, Bergamo R, Grosvenor M, Kopple JD. Enalapril reduces albumin excretion in diabetic patients with low levels of microalbuminuria. *American Journal of Nephrology* 1990;10:457–62.

101. Casado S, Carrasco MA, Arrieta FJ, Herrera JL. Effects of captopril in diabetic patients with different degrees of blood pressure and proteinuria [Abstract]. *Postgraduate Medical Journal* 1988;64 (suppl 3):85.

102. Winocour PH, Waldek S, Anderson DC. Converting enzyme inhibition and kidney function in normotensive diabetic patients with persistent microalbuminuria. *British Medical Journal* 1987;**295**:391.

103. Rudberg S, Aperia A, Freyschuss U. Persson B. Enalapril reduces microalbuminuria in young normotensive type 1 (insulin-dependent) diabetic patients irrespective of its hypotensive effect. *Diabetologia* 1990;**33**:470–6.

104. Holdaas H, Hartmann A, Lien MG, Nilsen L, Jervell J, Fauchald P, Endresen L, Djoseland O, Berg KJ. Contrasting effects of lisinopril and nifedipine on albuminuria and tubular transport functions in insulin dependent diabetics with nephropathy. *Journal of Internal Medicine* 1991;**229**:163–70.

105. Corcoran JS, Perkins JE, Hoffbrand BI, Yudkin JS. Treating hypertension in non-insulin-dependent diabetes: A comparison of atenolol, nifedipine, and captopril combined with bendrofluazide. *Diabetic Medicine* 1987;**4**:167–8.

106. Hollander E. Effect of antihypertensive (captopril) treatment on proteinuria in diabetic nephropathy. *Therapia Hungarica* 1988;**36**:191–5.

107. Hommel E, Parving H–H, Mathiesen E, Adsberg B, Nielsen MD, Giese J. Effect of captopril on kidney function in insulin-dependent diabetic patients with nephropathy. *British Medical Journal* 1986;**293**:467–70.

108. Parving H–H, Hommel E, Edsberg B, Mathiesen E, Nielsen MD, Giese J. The effect of captopril on glomerular filtration rate and albuminuria in insulin-dependent diabetic patients with nephropathy. *Postgraduate Medical Journal* 1986;**62** (suppl 1):65.

109. Kisch ES. Captopril and proteinuria in diabetes mellitus. *Israeli Journal of Medical Sciences* 1987;**23**:833–4.

110. Romero R, Sanmarti A, Salina I, Texidó J, Foz M, Caralps A. Utilidad de los inhibidores de la enzima conversiva de la angiotensina en el tratamiento de la nefropatía diabética. *Medicina Clinica* 1988;**90**:494–6.

111. Stornello M, Valvo EV, Puglia N, Scapellato L. Angiotensin converting enzyme inhibition with a low dose of enalapril in normotensive diabetics with persistent proteinuria. *Journal of Hypertension* 1988;**6** (suppl 4):S464–6.

112. Stornello M, Valvo EV, Vasques E, Leone S, Scapellato L. Systemic and renal effects of chronic angiotensin converting enzyme inhibition with captopril in hypertensive diabetic patients. *Journal of Hypertension* 1989;**7** (suppl 7):S65–7.

113. Weidmann P, Beretta–Piccoli C, Keusche G, Gluck Z, Mujagic M, Grimm M, Meier A, Ziegler WH. Sodium-volume factor, cardiovascular reactivity and hypotensive mechanism of diuretic therapy in mild hypertension associated with diabetes mellitus. *American Journal of Medicine* 1979;**67**:779–84.

114. Gans RO, Bilo HJG, Maarschalkerweerd WWA v, Heine RJ, Nauta JJP, Donker AJM. Exogenous insulin augments in healthy volunteers the cardiovascular reactivity of noradrenaline but not to angiotensin II. *Journal of Clinical Investigation* 1991;**88**:512–8.

115. Tuttle KR, Bruton JL, Perusek MC, Lancaster JL, Kopp DT, DeFronzo RA. Effect of strict glycemic control on renal hemodynamic response to amino acids and renal enlargement in insulin-dependent diabetes mellitus. *New England Journal of Medicine* 1991;**324**:1626–32.

116. Myers BD, Nelson RG, Williams GW, Bennett PH, Hardy SA, Berg RL, Loon N, Knowler WC, Mitch WE. Glomerular function in Pima Indians with noninsulin-dependent diabetes mellitus of recent onset. *Journal of Clinical Investigation* 1991;**88**:524–30.

117. Mathiesen ER, Hommel E, Giese J, Parving H–H. Efficacy of captopril in postponing nephropathy in normotensive insulin dependent diabetic patients with microalbuminuria. *British Medical Journal* 1991;**303**:81–7.

93 ANGIOTENSIN-CONVERTING ENZYME INHIBITORS IN THE TREATMENT OF HEART FAILURE

IAN G CROZIER, HAMID IKRAM, AND
M GARY NICHOLLS

INTRODUCTION

Heart failure is a complex pathophysiological condition resulting from impaired cardiac function that may be due either to a defect in myocardial contractility or to an excessive hemodynamic burden. Clinical features develop as a consequence of reduced cardiac output, increased filling pressures, disturbances in the balance of electrolytes and water, activation of neurohormonal systems, metabolic abnormalities within many tissues and organs, and side effects of medications. Of the neurohormonal systems, the RAS plays an important pathophysiological role which is discussed in *Chapter 76*.

Until recently, treatment for heart failure focused on augmentation of myocardial contractility and correction of fluid and electrolyte imbalance (Fig. 93.1). Digoxin, however, is the only orally effective inotrope that is so far widely available. Diuretics reduce congestive symptoms and remain a mainstay of therapy, but they do not correct the functional cardiac abnormality. Indeed, by lowering ventricular filling pressures, they can reduce cardiac output [1] (Fig. 93.1); they increase activity of the RAS [1] and the sympathetic system; and they reduce plasma and tissue potassium [2] and magnesium levels and perhaps thereby predispose to ventricular arrhythmias [193].

Attempts have been made to relieve the burden of the failing heart by the use of vasodilator drugs (Fig. 93.1). Whereas this approach is often successful under emergency conditions and in the short term, most drugs suffer from the development of 'tachyphylaxis' due, in part, to further activation of the RAS and the sympathetic system, and to fluid retention [3–7].

Following the demonstration that a competitive inhibitor of Ang II or an ACE inhibitor reduced arterial pressure, aldosterone secretion, and sodium retention in animals with heart failure [8,9], the role of these agents was examined in patients with cardiac failure. In 1977, Gavras *et al* reported that the Ang II antagonist, saralasin, increased cardiac output and decreased peripheral resistance in a patient with high plasma renin activity and severe heart failure due to renovascular hypertension [10]. One year later, it was demonstrated that an intravenous ACE inhibitor reduced systemic vascular resistance and left ventricular filling pressures while increasing cardiac output in patients with heart failure [11,12] (Fig. 93.2). Captopril, the first of the orally active ACE inhibitors, was reported to have similar effects in 1979 [13]. It soon became clear that ACE inhibitors had sustained beneficial effects [13–19], and their subsequent widespread use has revolutionized the treatment of cardiac failure.

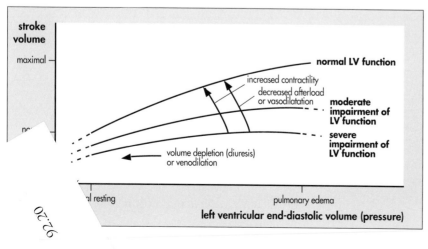

Fig. 93.1 Relationships between left ventricular (LV) end-diastolic volume (and pressure) and stroke volume, and the effects of different treatment modalities.

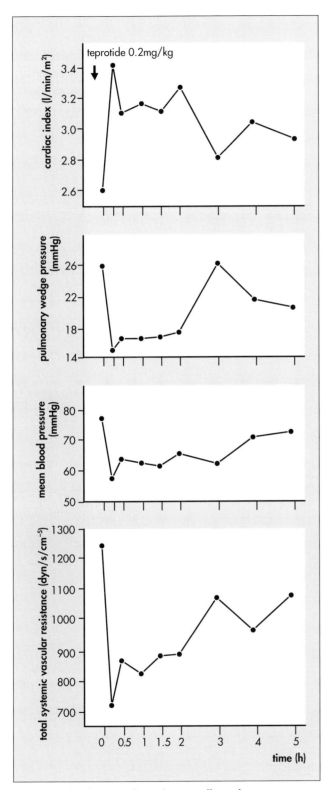

Fig. 93.2 The short-term hemodynamic effects of an intravenous injection of the ACE inhibitor, teprotide (SQ20881), in one of the first patients with cardiac failure to receive an ACE inhibitor. Modified from Gravas H *et al* [12].

EFFECTS ON HORMONES

In patients receiving diuretics and digoxin, ACE inhibitors reduce plasma ACE activity and Ang II levels, while renin levels rise. Aldosterone levels also fall and stabilize within the normal range (Fig. 93.3). These changes are prompt with the first dose of captopril [20,21] but are more gradual with other available ACE inhibitors such as enalapril [22,23], lisinopril [24], and ramipril [25]. During chronic therapy, Ang II levels remain suppressed [16,26] although measurements of Ang II are fraught with difficulties under these circumstances [27]. Following withdrawal of chronic captopril therapy, Ang II, aldosterone, and renin levels return to pretreatment values over 1–4 days without rebound hemodynamic deterioration [28].

Changes in other hormonal systems with ACE inhibition are less clearcut. The sympathetic system overall, and involving the heart and kidneys in particular, is activated in cardiac failure [29–33]. Norepinephrine levels in plasma were suppressed by ACE inhibitor therapy in many [13,30,34–39] but not all studies [7,19,22,40]. Furthermore, ACE inhibitors have been reported to suppress the plasma norepinephrine response to exercise [39,41] and also to reduce cardiac sympathetic tone [39,42]. It is not clear whether this diminution in global and cardiac sympathetic tone is due to withdrawal of a tonic stimulatory effect of Ang II on the sympathetic system [43] or to the general improvement in hemodynamic status [44]. Circulating levels of epinephrine are apparently altered little by ACE inhibitors [7,13,19,37,39], but can rise if the first dose induces symptomatic hypotension [36].

Downregulation of myocardial β-receptors and reduced myocardial responsiveness to β-adrenergic stimulation may contribute to the impairment of myocardial function in cardiac failure [45]. Angiotensin-converting enzyme inhibitors reduced downregulation of cardiac β-receptors in an animal model [46] and increased both β-adrenergic receptor density and the stimulatory guanine nucleotide regulatory protein in man [42, 47]. Furthermore, sympathetic responsiveness to volume depletion, which is impaired in heart failure, was reportedly restored with chronic ACE inhibition [29].

Whether the vasodilator actions of ACE inhibition result in part from increased bradykinin and prostaglandin levels in plasma and tissues is uncertain. Plasma bradykinin levels rose during captopril treatment according to Nishimura *et al* [48], but this needs to be confirmed. Circulating levels of prostaglandin E_2 and 6-keto-prostaglandin $F_{1\alpha}$ increased with captopril therapy [34,48], and indomethacin blunted the hemodynamic response to ACE inhibitors in patients with severe congestive failure [48].

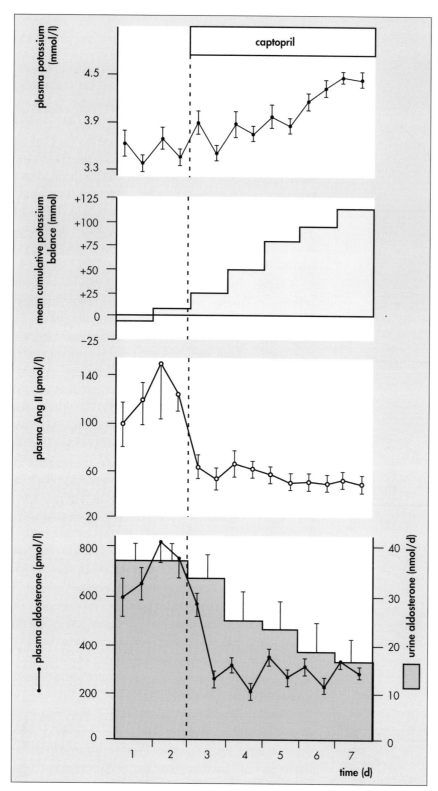

Fig. 93.3 Short-term effects of the ACE inhibitor, captopril, on plasma and cumulative potassium, Ang II, and aldosterone in patients with severe heart failure. Results are mean ± SEM. Modified from Nicholls MG *et al. Journal of Clinical Endocrinology and Metabolism* 1981;**52**:1253–6.

Angiotensin-converting enzyme inhibitors suppress cardiac secretion and circulating levels of atrial natriuretic factor (ANF) in heart failure [49]. Although the clinical relevance of this is not known, decreased ANF levels in concert with reduced renal perfusion pressure may contribute to the sodium retention that is sometimes seen following initiation of ACE inhibitor therapy.

Angiotensin-converting enzyme inhibitors have little or no effects on circulating cortisol or vasopressin levels [19,25] except in the most severe cases of heart failure where elevated levels of both hormones may fall [26,38,50].

HEMODYNAMIC EFFECTS

Angiotensin-converting enzyme inhibitors induce clear early falls in systemic vascular resistance and arterial pressure [11–20,51]. In the kidney, vascular resistance may fall by over 50% [23,25,52,53]. Lesser, but definite, vasodilation occurs in the limb, coronary, and cerebral circulations [23,25,52,54–56] (Fig. 93.4), but hepatic blood flow usually declines [52,57]. Angiotensin-converting enzyme inhibition has resulted in venodilation in most [40,58–60], but not all studies [61]. Cardiac output rises usually by 10–20% [11–19,25,36,51–53,58,62,63] although this has not been observed in all studies [22,23]. Left ventricular filling and pulmonary capillary wedge pressures fall promptly and substantially [11–20,22,25,30,51,58,62,63] (Fig. 93.5). Right atrial pressure falls to a lesser degree according to most workers [13,17,30,51,62] but in some studies, there was little or no change [18,19,25].

The beneficial effects of ACE inhibition on resting hemodynamics are also seen with exercise [63]. Furthermore, hemodynamic improvement persists during chronic treatment without evidence of 'tachyphylaxis' [23,51,62–65] (Fig. 93.5).

The magnitude of the acute hemodynamic response to ACE inhibition is only modestly related to the pretreatment plasma renin level [11,12,14,15,30,66], and the long-term response is even less closely related (Fig. 93.6). This might be explained by inhibition not only of the circulating RAS, but also of local renin systems in vessels, kidney, and the heart [67], each with its own temporal pattern of inhibition. In addition, vasodilator effects mediated by bradykinin and prostaglandins [34], sluggish changes in sodium and water balance, withdrawal of the slow pressor effect of Ang II [68] (*Chapter 28*), and reversal of Ang II-induced effects on cardiac structure and vasculature may contribute to both the magnitude and the timing of hemodynamic responses to ACE inhibition.

Although blood pressure falls in most patients and may be marked in some [36], this is not usually symptomatic. Symptomatic hypotension is more likely in patients with severe cardiac failure who are on large doses of diuretic, who have high renin levels, and who are hyponatremic [69].

Occasional patients have been reported in which the first dose of ACE inhibitor is followed by profound hypotension, severe bradycardia, and sweating [36,177]. Evidence of myocardial damage and acute reversible renal failure has been seen. The drop in blood pressure was correlated with pretreatment level of Ang II and with the fall in heart rate. The mechanisms

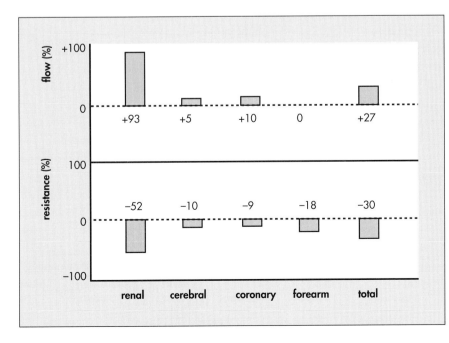

Fig. 93.4 Mean percentage changes in blood flow and resistance following two days of ACE inhibition with ramipril in 11 patients with congestive heart failure. Changes are shown for the renal, cerebral, coronary, and forearm circulations and for the total circulation. Modified from Crozier IG *et al* [25].

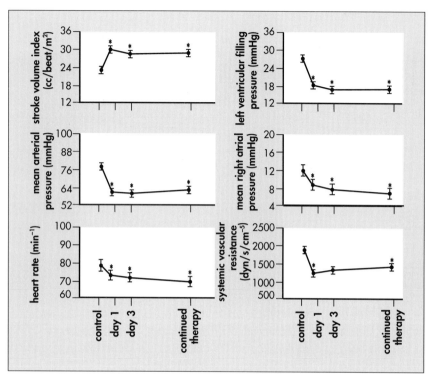

Fig. 93.5 Acute and long-term hemodynamic effects in patients with congestive heart failure who responded to an ACE inhibitor (mean ± SEM). The beneficial acute changes seen on day 1 and day 3 persist with continued therapy at 2–8 weeks. Asterisks signify statistically significant change from control; *P<0.01. Modified from Packer M et al [64].

include abrupt removal of the stimulant effect of Ang II on sympathetic tone and of its inhibitory effect on vagal tone. The latter is potentiated in heart failure by concurrent use of digoxin [177,178].

CARDIAC EFFECTS

Animal and *ex vivo* studies indicate that ACE inhibitors are coronary vasodilators as a result not only of Ang II inhibition, but also possibly via modulation of bradykinin and prostaglandin levels and perhaps by a sulfhydryl-dependent mechanism with captopril administration [70]. Studies in patients with heart failure, many of whom had normal coronary arteries, have shown coronary vasodilation and little change or an increase in coronary blood flow despite a reduction in perfusion presure [25,55,56]. In those with coronary artery disease, however, coronary blood flow tends to fall [7,71,72], presumably because diseased arteries are relatively insensitive to vasoconstricting and vasodilating influences. Nevertheless, since oxygen demand also falls, symptomatic myocardial ischemia is rarely precipitated or exacerbated.

Despite the tendency for stroke volume to increase with ACE inhibitors, cardiac work is decreased [7,55,71,72], and cardiac oxygen consumption is unaltered [55,72] or diminished [7,56, 71] as would be expected from the fall in cardiac work and improvement in myocardial efficiency [72]. The heart rate usually

falls (see *Fig. 93.5*) as a result of a decrease in cardiac sympathetic flow [39] and an increase in parasympathetic activity [73]. Extraction of oxygen across the heart is usually reduced at rest [55,71] and with few exceptions, myocardial lactate production is unaltered [71] or reduced [55]. Consequently, as noted above, symptomatic exacerbations of myocardial ischemia are rare. Indeed, a number of studies document a variable anti-anginal effect of ACE inhibitors [74,179], although exacerbation of angina was observed in one study of patients who also had cardiac failure [180].

Inhibition of the positive inotropic action of Ang II [75] by ACE inhibitors might be expected to result in a reduction in myocardial contractility. Although this is difficult to measure in intact man, an intracoronary infusion study of enalaprilat in patients with dilated cardiomyopathy did result in an acute impairment of left ventricular function [56]. This effect was small, however, perhaps because the failing myocardium is less sensitive to Ang II [76], and because high levels of Ang I may have a positive inotropic action [77].

Most studies show an overall improvement in left ventricular systolic function with ACE inhibitors [16,18,20,25,58,63, 65,78], presumably because the reduction in afterflood outweighs any negative inotropic effect. Impaired left ventricular relaxation, which is a common and important myocardial abnormality [79, 80], is also improved by ACE inhibitors [81–83], presumably through inhibition of some of the adverse actions of the RAS on left ventricular distensibility (Fig. 93.7) and cardiac structure

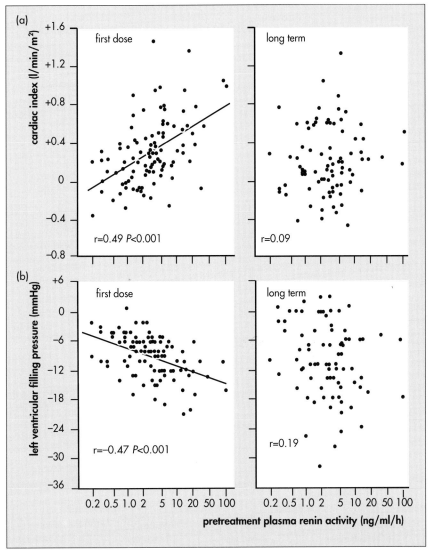

Fig. 93.6 Relations between pretreatment plasma renin activity and changes in (a) cardiac index and (b) left ventricular filling pressure after the first dose of the ACE inhibitor, captopril, and with long-term treatment in patients with congestive heart failure. A weak relationship was noted initially but not with long-term ACE inhibition. Modified from Packer M *et al* [66].

(*Chapter 94*). The latter must contribute to the marked effect of ACE inhibitors on left ventricular filling pressures, which is greater than can be explained by changes of preload and afterload alone [84]. The beneficial effects of ACE inhibition on left ventricular relaxation are not seen with direct vasodilators [85].

Finally, ACE inhibitors reduce the frequency and complexity of ventricular arrhythmias according to most [35,37,86,87] but not all authors [88], although the underlying mechanisms remain to be defined.

RENAL EFFECTS

Angiotensin II has many effects, direct and indirect, on renal function (see *Chapters 26* and *27*), some of which are especially important in heart failure [89] (see *Chapter 76*). It is not surprising

therefore, that the renal response to ACE inhibitors is complex and variable [90,91]. The severity of cardiac failure, the presence or absence of edema, the dose of maintenance diuretic, the dose of ACE inhibitor, and the magnitude of fall in arterial pressure, are major determinants of the renal response. There is usually a fall in glomerular filtration rate (GFR) in edema-free patients with the most severe grades of heart failure in whom high-dose loop or combinations of diuretics are maintained and who exhibit a fall in arterial pressure toward the lower limit of autoregulation for GFR [90–93]. On the other hand, GFR is maintained or improves during ACE inhibition in less-severe cardiac failure, if the dose of diuretics is reduced, and where the fall in arterial pressure is small.

The policy regarding diuretic therapy is important. Studies where maintenance diuretic doses were reduced during treatment with an ACE inhibitor, report no change or an improvement in GFR [16, 94]. By contrast, GFR tends to fall and plasma urea and

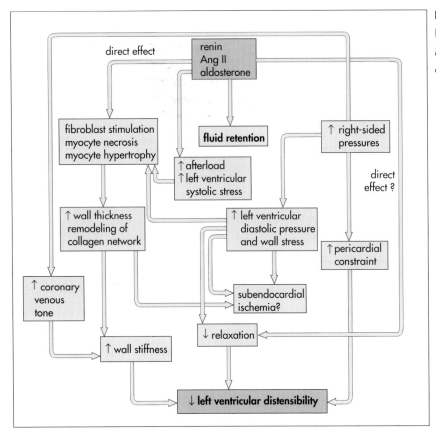

Fig. 93.7 Interrelationships between the RAS and left ventricular diastolic function. Modified from Pouleur H (unpublished data).

creatinine levels to rise, at least in the short term, when diuretic doses are unchanged [35,37,95–97]. Under these circumstances, the fall in GFR is most obvious in those with the highest baseline levels of renin and the lowest levels of achieved arterial pressure [93,98]. In the longer term, however, the GFR may return to baseline levels despite unchanged diuretic therapy [93].

Packer and his colleagues have proposed that certain patients, namely those with diabetes, with hyponatremia, or with azotemia, are at particular risk from a sustained decline in GFR during ACE inhibition [92,99]. The possibility of underlying bilateral renal artery stenosis must be considered when a major decline in GFR occurs.

The comparative effect of various ACE inhibitors has received limited attention. When high doses of captopril and enalapril were compared in patients with severe heart failure in whom furosemide doses were held constant, endogenous creatinine clearance declined over 1–3 months with enalapril but remained steady with captopril [96]. Giles and colleagues reported that blood urea nitrogen levels rose more commonly with a long-acting ACE inhibitor (lisinopril) than with the shorter-acting captopril during a three-month study in which diuretic doses 'were continued uninterrupted' [100]. Although these studies are

of interest, the outcome cannot be extrapolated to clinical practice which favors lower doses of ACE inhibitors and a reduction in the maintenance diuretic dose. Finally, Fitzpatrick and colleagues reported that intermittent ACE inhibition had similar effects on endogenous creatinine clearance to continuous ACE inhibition in pacing-induced cardiac failure in sheep [101].

Renal blood flow may change little or fall acutely after a high first dose of an ACE inhibitor [93,102]. Contrary findings have been reported, however [52,53], and with more prolonged treatment, renal blood flow increases by 10–60% [23,93,103,104].

The possibility that renal hemodynamic and GFR responses during ACE inhibition depend upon changes in kinins or prostaglandins, has been considered. Since the kallikrein inhibitor, aprotonin, did not affect the captopril-induced rise in renal plasma flow and decline in filtration fraction in patients with severe congestive heart failure, Kubo and colleagues concluded that the kallikrein–kinin system played little role in the acute renal response [105]. Although there is a dearth of objective information, the GFR deteriorates, sometimes alarmingly, when prostaglandin-synthetase inhibitors are combined with ACE inhibitors in cardiac failure. Since prostaglandin inhibitors alone can reduce the GFR in cardiac failure, it remains to be shown whether ACE inhibitor-related changes in renal function involve changes in renal prostaglandins.

ELECTROLYTE EFFECTS

Complex and variable changes in sodium balance can occur with ACE inhibition [90,91]. The urinary sodium response depends on the degree of hemodynamic improvement, alterations in renal blood flow and renal perfusion pressure, withdrawal of the direct and indirect actions of Ang II on the kidney, and changes in ANF and aldosterone levels and perhaps in sympathetic stimulation of the kidney. Furthermore, ACE inhibitors enhance the natriuretic action of loop diuretics [106].

The addition of ACE inhibitors to loop diuretics in edematous patients with heart failure often results in a natriuresis [16,52]. In contrast, net sodium and water retention occurs over the first few days in edema-free patients on high-dose diuretic therapy in whom major falls in arterial pressure occur [22,25,93,98]. With long-term therapy in the latter group of patients, there is usually little effect on sodium balance [35] or a modest natriuresis [21,93], allowing for a reduction of diuretic dosage [25,65]. Angiotensin-converting enzyme inhibitors, however, do not substitute for diuretic therapy in severe heart failure and cannot alone be relied upon to prevent the recurrence of pulmonary edema [107].

With ACE inhibition, plasma sodium changes little, or may fall initially in patients with previously normal plasma sodium concentrations [19,98,108,109]. In patients with hyponatremia, however, the effects are very different. The intrarenal mechanisms by which marked elevation of Ang II causes hyponatremia and azotemia in severe heart failure have been described in detail elsewhere [91,181]. With severe hyponatremia, the earlier compensatory intrarenal effects of modest elevation of Ang II have been lost, and a gross excess of Ang II now is causing renal circulatory shutdown. Angiotensin-converting enzyme inhibition in these latter circumstances is beneficial, and can correct both hyponatremia and azotemia [16,108,181] (Fig. 93.8). Potassium excretion is decreased and plasma potassium and magnesium levels rise [16,19,21,35,37] (see *Fig. 93.3*). Total body potassium, which may well be deficient, has been found to increase significantly with ACE inhibition, in proportion to pretreatment plasma renin levels, while total-body sodium and chloride, and weight, remained unchanged [183]. Hyperkalemia may occur in patients taking potassium supplements [16], potassium-conserving diuretics, or nonsteroidal anti-inflammatory drugs.

EFFECTS ON THE CEREBRAL CIRCULATION

In patients with congestive heart failure, cerebral blood flow is reduced [54,110] but tends to rise, without alteration in regional distribution, during ACE inhibition [25,54,110]. Some studies suggest that, as in experimental animals [111], ACE inhibitors reduce the lower limit of cerebral autoregulation in heart failure [54], possibly through inhibition of locally generated Ang II in larger cerebral vessels [112]. These favorable effects ensure that ACE inhibitors rarely cause symptoms of cerebral ischemia unless the fall in pressure, especially with the first dose, is extreme.

EFFECTS ON THE PERIPHERAL CIRCULATION

Short-term ACE inhibition induces little change in vascular resistance and blood flow in the resting limb [25,40]. Likewise, maximum global oxygen consumption, total exercise capacity, maximal leg blood flow at peak exercise, and maximal leg oxygen

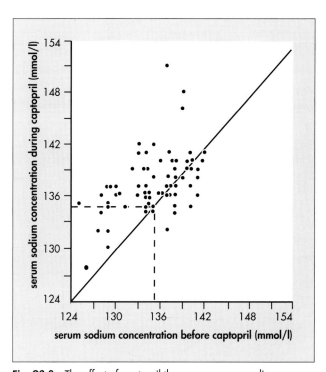

Fig. 93.8 The effect of captopril therapy on serum sodium concentration in 70 patients with severe congestive heart failure. Hyponatremia was corrected completely in 26 of 32 patients and partially so in the remainder. The diagonal line represents the line of identity. Modified from Packer M *et al* [108].

consumption are not usually altered in the short term [113,114]. Long-term therapy, however, results in a rise in resting limb blood flow [115] and total exercise capacity, peak exertional global oxygen consumption, and leg blood flow and leg oxygen consumption [116,117]. Furthermore, there is greater extraction of oxygen by the limb during exercise [117]. The mechanisms underlying these effects are unknown but may include alterations in kinin and prostaglandin levels, inhibition of local renin systems in vessel walls, changes in the water and electrolyte content of vessels, alterations in structure of myocardium and vessel walls, and gradual improvements in myocardial performance as well as a fall in circulating Ang II.

CLINICAL EFFECTS

In severe heart failure, addition of ACE inhibitors to diuretics results in resolution of pulmonary edema, a reduction in systemic venous congestion, less exertional dyspnea and lethargy, and improved exercise capacity and general wellbeing [6,16,17,19,22,25,35,37,51,58,62,63,65,78]. In many cases, the clinical improvement is substantial and may result in previously bed-bound patients being able to resume normal daily activities [16]. In contrast to direct vasodilators or postsynaptic α-blockers whose initial hemodynamic effects [59,60] are not usually sustained [3,5,6], ACE inhibitors produce a gradual symptomatic improvement that tends to increase over the first three months of therapy [78] (Fig. 93.9) and is sustained for at least 18 months [51]. The acute hemodynamic response, however, is a poor predictor of the subsequent clinical outcome [64]. A small number of patients who initially respond to an ACE

inhibitor later show hemodynamic deterioration [64,118]. This is almost certainly due to progression of the underlying disease rather than to the development of tolerance to ACE inhibition.

The mechanisms underlying these beneficial clinical effects are complex and multiple. The reduction in left ventricular filling pressure results in clearing of pulmonary edema and lessening of dyspnea. Falls in heart rate, in chamber diameter, and in arterial pressure reduce myocardial work and contribute to the increase in cardiac output, which in turn, contributes to the improvement in exercise capacity, reduction in exertional dyspnea, and general wellbeing. A decline in arterial pressure and left ventricular filling pressure alters the conditions under which the left ventricle operates and decreases left ventricular systolic and diastolic volumes [35], thereby reducing functional mitral regurgitation [119]. These effects contribute to the overall improvement in myocardial efficiency [72] and in left ventricular systolic and diastolic function. Changes in regional blood flow and especially the increase in cerebral blood flow, no doubt contribute to the notable improvement in general wellbeing.

EFFECTS ON MORTALITY

Congestive heart failure carries a grave prognosis. The five-year mortality was 62% in men and 42% in women in the Framingham study [120], and is higher in patients with severe heart failure [121] and with marked activation of the RAS [122]. Approximately half of the patients die of progressive heart failure and the other half die suddenly [121], presumably from ventricular arrhythmias. A trend towards a decrease in mortality was noted in the captopril multicenter research trial [78], with vasodilators in

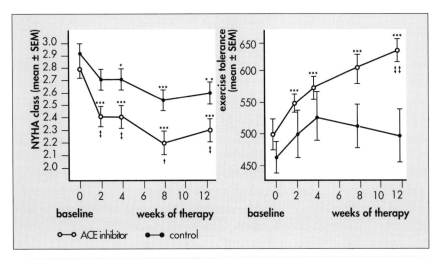

Fig 93.9 Progressive improvements in New York Heart Association (NYHA) functional class ratings and exercise tolerance (in seconds) in patients with heart failure treated with an ACE inhibitor for 12 weeks as compared with controls (mean ± SEM). *P<0.05, **P<0.01, ***P<0.001. Modified from Captopril Multicenter Research Group [78].

general [123], and with the combination of hydralazine and isosorbide dinitrate [124]. A retrospective analysis showed that survival was prolonged by ACE inhibition in the subgroup of patients with severe heart failure and hyponatremia [125].

The first clear evidence of improved survival with ACE inhibitors was provided by the CONSENSUS study which examined the effects of enalapril in severe heart failure. After an average follow-up period of six months, the mortality was 44% in the placebo group and 26% in the enalapril group (Fig. 93.10). The effect was confined to a reduction in deaths due to progressive heart failure (44 versus 22), whereas there were a similar number of sudden deaths in both groups (14 versus 14) [126]. Benefit continued in terms of decreased mortality following completion of the trial, and with addition of an ACE inhibitor in the placebo group [122]. Enalapril abolished the relationship between activity of the RAS and mortality, which suggests that activation of the RAS may itself contribute to the demise of patients with severe heart failure [122]. Although no formal survival study has been reported with ACE inhibitors other than enalapril, the tendency towards beneficial effects with captopril [78,123,127]

suggests that ACE inhibitors as a group decrease mortality in moderate and severe grades of heart failure. On the other hand, a retrospective analysis of patients randomized to xamoterol or placebo revealed a higher mortality in patients receiving captopril than in those receiving enalapril or lisinopril [128]. The significance of this finding is unclear at present, but may reflect less-sustained ACE inhibition with captopril, or specific interactions between xamoterol and individual ACE inhibitors.

A meta-analysis of 11 randomized studies reported that the reduction in mortality with ACE inhibitors was greatest in patients with heart failure due to myocardial ischemia [129]. This may relate to effects of ACE inhibitors on progressive left ventricular dilation and dysfunction, which occurs with established heart failure and in asymptomatic patients following acute myocardial infarction [130,131] (Fig. 93.11).

The CONSENSUS Study was made in patients with the most severe grades (NYHA Functional Class IV) of cardiac failure. The Studies of Left Ventricular Dysfunction (SOLVD) were designed to assess the effect on mortality of enalapril in patients with reduced left ventricular ejection fractions (≤ 0.35).

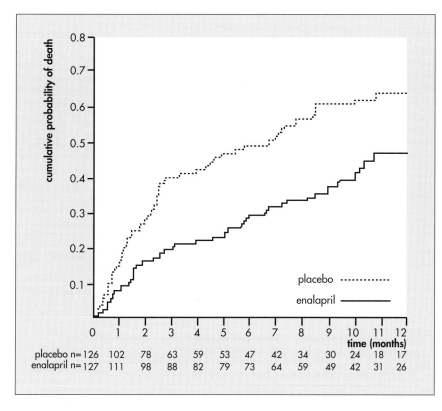

Fig. 93.10 Kaplan Meier curves for patients in the CONSENSUS study of patients with severe heart failure. After six months of therapy, the mortality was lower in the enalapril group, entirely as a result of a reduction in deaths from progressive cardiac failure. n = number of patients. Modified from The CONSENSUS Trial Study Group [126].

In the latter study, patients with overt heart failure, mostly in NYHA Functional Class II or III, were entered in the 'treatment trial' where they were randomized double-blind to receive placebo (n=1284) or enalapril (n=1285) at doses of 2.5–20mg/day for an average period of 41.4 months. The majority of patients were also receiving a diuretic and a digitalis preparation. There were fewer deaths in those receiving enalapril (452) than in the placebo group (510), which represents a 16% reduction in risk of death [184]. The chief difference in mortality was in deaths due to progressive heart failure (209 in the enalapril group, 251 in the placebo group), but of note also were the fewer fatal myocardial infarctions in enalapril-treated, versus placebo-treated patients (40 versus 53). Furthermore, the group receiving placebo required 971 hospitalizations for heart failure, compared with 683 in the enalapril group.

This study and the CONSENSUS trial indicate that enalapril prolongs survival in mild, moderate and severe symptomatic cardiac failure. The question, of course, arises as to whether ACE inhibitors also prolong life in those with left ventricular dysfunction but without overt symptomatic heart failure.

In the 'prevention arm' of SOLVD, presented at the 64th Annual Scientific Section of the American Heart Association (11–14 November 1991, Anaheim, California), patients with a left ventricular ejection fraction of ≤0.35, not receiving digitalis or diuretics, and mostly in NYHA Functional Class I or II, received enalapril or placebo for an average follow-up period of 48 months. Mortality curves for the two groups remained together for 18 months then began to diverge in favor of enalapril, but differences failed to reach pre-set levels of statistical significance ($P<0.025$). Of note is the fact that approximately half of the patients in the

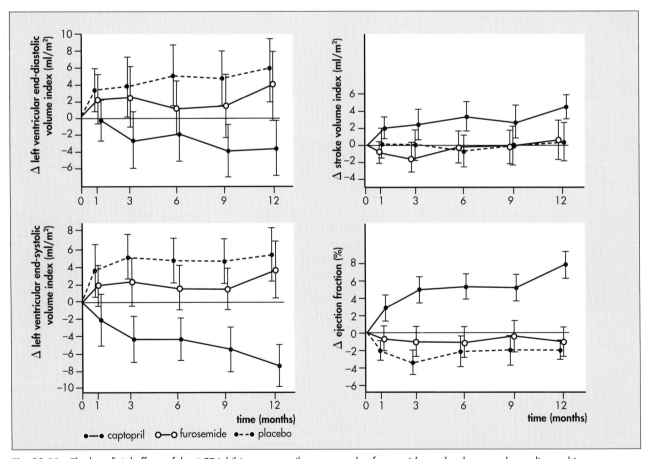

Fig. 93.11 The beneficial effects of the ACE inhibitor, captopril, as opposed to furosemide or placebo, on echocardiographic measurements of left ventricular size and function after acute myocardial infarction. The figure shows changes in left ventricular end-diastolic volume index, end-systolic volume index, stroke volume index, and ejection fraction. Values are least squares means with upper and lower least significant difference intervals ($P<0.05$). Modified from Sharpe N et al [130].

placebo group were receiving open-label ACE inhibitors by the end of the study, thus any beneficial effect from enalapril may have been partly obscured. Interpretation of the data awaits its publication in full.

The question of whether the ACE inhibitor enalapril, or the combination of hydralazine–isosorbide dinitrate is more effective in prolonging life in chronic congestive heart failure, was assessed in the Multicentre Veterans Administration Co-operative Vasodilator–Heart Failure Trial (V-HeFT II). In this Study of 804 men, mostly in NYHA Functional Class II or III, the mortality at 2 years was lower in the enalapril group (18%) than in the combined vasodilator group (25%) although the overall mortality difference was not statistically significant ($P<0.08$). Of note were the fewer sudden deaths in patients receiving enalapril (57 compared with 92 in those on the combination of vasodilators) and the between-group difference was statistically significant and most evident in patients with less severe grades of heart failure [185].

A somewhat similar study compared captopril with the hydralazine–isosorbide dinitrate combination, but in only 106 patients who were being considered for cardiac transplantation [186]. Again the ACE inhibitor increased survival over a 12-month period compared with the combined vasodilator regimen. Full details of this study are awaited.

As already mentioned, the frequency of ventricular arrhythmias is reduced by ACE inhibition according to most [35,37,86,87], but not all authors [88], possibly by effects on potassium or other electrolytes, changes in left ventricular dimensions, or a reduction in sympathetic activity. So far, however, there is little evidence [188] that the incidence of sudden death is reduced by ACE inhibition [126].

Provisional data from a small study suggest that captopril may reduce progression and mortality in mild grades of heart failure [132], but full results from this study are awaited.

DRUG ADMINISTRATION

The first dose of an ACE inhibitor should be low (for example, captopril 6.25mg, enalapril 2.5mg, or lisinopril 2.5mg) and taken with the patient supine after reduction or cessation of maintenance diuretic therapy for some days. Some workers have proposed, in order to minimize the duration of problems should severe first-dose hypotension occur, that treatment be initiated with a short-acting agent such as captopril; however, this has not found general acceptance [187]. Medical supervision, preferably in hospital, is advisable for patients with severe heart failure and especially if there is hyponatremia, hypotension, azotemia, or requirement for high-dose loop diuretics (for example, furosemide 80mg daily or more) or diuretic combinations. In less-severe heart failure, ACE inhibitors have been started by the patient at home.

Although the pharmacokinetics of some ACE inhibitors are altered in cardiac failure, perhaps due to delays in absorption or hydrolysis [133], maintenance doses should depend upon the level of renal function, except in the case of newer agents that are excreted by the liver. Whether high-dose treatment, to obtain maximal suppression of circulating Ang II and perhaps of tissue renin systems, is advisable, remains to be determined.

The intravenous route may be required for patients who are unable to take or absorb oral medication, or if a rapid response is required. Intravenous captopril results in a 30% fall in systemic vascular resistance and a 20% increase in cardiac output with maximal effects five minutes after injection, while left and right atrial pressures fall more slowly to a nadir at 60–75 minutes [134] (Fig. 93.12). Intravenous enalaprilat has a

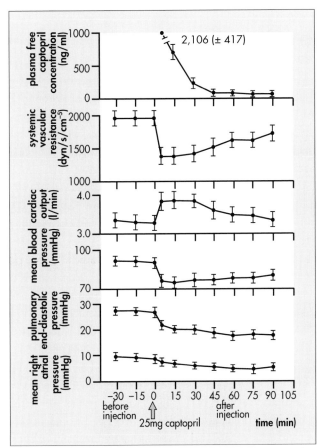

Fig. 93.12 The hemodynamic response to a 25-mg injection of the ACE inhibitor, captopril, given intravenously over five minutes in 14 patients with severe congestive heart failure (mean ± SEM). Modified from Rademaker M *et al* [134].

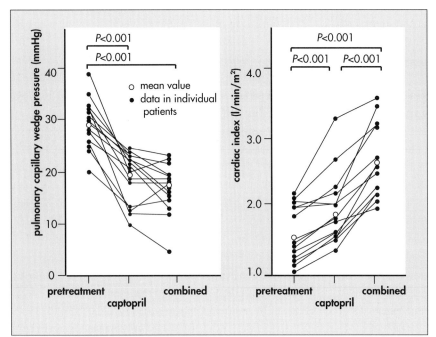

Fig. 93.13 Additive acute hemodynamic effects of hydralazine when combined with the ACE inhibitor, captopril, in patients with congestive heart failure. Modified from Massie BM *et al* [141].

prompt onset of action, with peak hemodynamic effects at 30–60 minutes [53].

Finally, the sublingual route has been used for captopril with apparent success in severe congestive heart failure [135].

COMBINATION THERAPY

Early studies utilized ACE inhibitors as third-line therapy for patients in whom digoxin and high-dose diuretics had proved insufficient. With the demonstration of beneficial effects in mild heart failure [87], ACE inhibitors are now indicated in all grades of heart failure. Given alone, however, they do not necessarily correct fluid overload [106], and although effective in some patients with mild heart failure [136], they do not always prevent fluid accumulation in patients with prior pulmonary edema [107].

We believe that initial therapy for most patients with heart failure should be the combination of an ACE inhibitor and a low-dose loop diuretic. Digoxin is also of value in the treatment of heart failure due to impaired left ventricular systolic function even in patients with sinus rhythm [87,137] and has additive hemodynamic effects with ACE inhibitors at least when given acutely [138]. Despite its not infrequent side effects and its adverse effects on mortality under some circumstances [139], results from

carefully controlled studies have demonstrated that withdrawal of digoxin therapy in the absence [191] or presence of concomitant ACE inhibitor therapy [192], results in hemodynamic, symptomatic and function deterioration in patients with mild-to-moderate chronic heart failure who are in sinus rhythm. Attention to the dose of digoxin may be necessary when used with an ACE inhibitor since digoxin clearance is decreased by captopril in severe cardiac failure independent of change in renal function [97], although there is apparently no such effect in mild heart failure [188].

In patients who continue to have fluid overload and systemic or pulmonary congestion despite the combination of an ACE inhibitor and high-dose loop diuretic, addition of a thiazide diuretic or low-dose spironolactone may initiate a diuresis [140]. Fluid and electrolyte status and renal function must be monitored closely, however, because of the risks of volume depletion, hyperkalemia, and renal impairment [140]. Beneficial acute hemodynamic responses have been reported by adding prazosin or hydralazine [118,141] (Fig. 93.13), but the long-term effectiveness of these combinations has not been evaluated. Finally, positive inotropic drugs, including dobutamine, elicit useful short-term hemodynamic effects in patients already on an ACE inhibitor/diuretic combination [142]. Such an approach may 'turn-the-tide' when all else has failed in severe cardiac failure.

COMPARISONS BETWEEN INDIVIDUAL ANGIOTENSIN-CONVERTING ENZYME INHIBITORS

Few studies have compared the clinical efficacy and adverse effects of different ACE inhibitors in heart failure. Interpretation is hampered by the fact that the drugs have individual pharmacokinetic profiles and differing potencies, yet only single-dose studies have been performed. Furthermore, as noted earlier, maintenance doses of diuretics were not altered in these studies, and the consequences regarding the renal and electrolyte responses may be quite different between long- and short-acting ACE inhibitors under the circumstances.

In one study, enalapril induced more episodes of symptomatic hypotension and greater renal functional impairment than did captopril [96], while in the study of Giles et al [100] symptomatic improvement was more obvious with lisinopril than with captopril but at the expense of a higher blood–urea–nitrogen level. In our view, and in the experience of others [143], there is no clear evidence at this stage that any one ACE inhibitor is superior to another with regard to efficacy or side-effect profile in the treatment of heart failure.

MILD HEART FAILURE

Angiotensin-converting enzyme inhibitors improve exercise time and functional capacity in patients with mild impairment of left ventricular function, the magnitude of improvement being similar to, or greater than, with digoxin [87,144]. Furthermore, patients with left ventricular dysfunction following acute myocardial infarction improve their functional capacity with ACE inhibition [131].

Captopril treatment decreased left ventricular mass and the amount of myocardial necrosis and calcification in a murine myocarditis (Coxsackievirus B3) model [145]. In dogs with cardiac failure, ACE inhibitor pretreatment reduced sodium retention and attenuated the hemodynamic deterioration [146, 147]. As already noted, for patients with left ventricular dysfunction following acute myocardial infarction, ACE inhibitors prevented the progressive increase in left ventricular size and the decline in ventricular function that otherwise occurred with either placebo or diuretic therapy [130,131] (see Fig. 93.11). The distinct possibility that ACE inhibition may slow or prevent the progression of left ventricular dysfunction and improve the prognosis for all grades of cardiac functional impairment, is

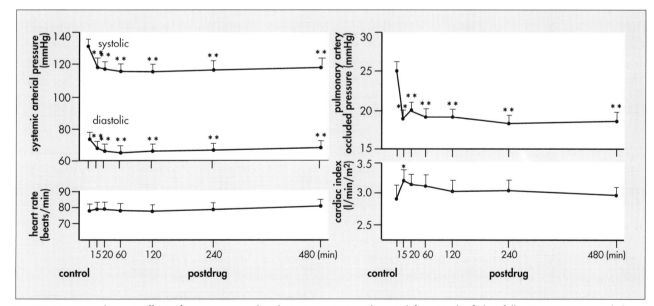

Fig. 93.14 Hemodynamic effects of intravenous enalaprilat in 15 patients with acute left ventricular failure following acute myocardial infarction (mean ± SEM). **P<0.01 versus control. Modified from Taylor SH [150].

currently being examined in multicenter placebo-controlled trials.

HYPERTENSIVE HEART FAILURE

In human hypertension, ACE inhibitors induce regression of left ventricular hypertrophy and improve diastolic dysfunction. In theory, these drugs may more effectively prevent the development of cardiac failure than alternative antihypertensive drugs which less regularly reverse left ventricular hypertrophy or stimulate activity of the RAS and the sympathetic system. Evidence, however, is lacking. The presence of hypertension in a patient with heart failure should not alter the approach to treatment with an ACE inhibitor.

HEART FAILURE IN ISCHEMIC HEART DISEASE

Angiotensin-converting enzyme inhibition is generally well tolerated in patients with ischemic heart disease and cardiac failure, probably because of the favorable effects on the balance of myocardial oxygen demand and supply. Furthermore, a preliminary report suggests that the ACE inhibitor-induced reduction in mortality of patients with heart failure is most obvious in those with underlying ischemic heart disease [129], perhaps due to their anti-ischemic effects.

In the situation of acute left ventricular failure following acute myocardial infarction, pilot studies suggest that ACE inhibitors are useful. As discussed more fully by Waeber (see *Chapter 77*), the RAS is activated after acute myocardial infarction, especially so in those who develop left ventricular failure [148]. Small, uncontrolled studies in such patients have shown that both oral captopril and intravenous enalaprilat decrease right heart and systemic arterial pressures and increase cardiac output [149,150] (Fig. 93.14). Administration of ACE inhibitors either before or after experimental myocardial infarction, limits infarct size [151]. These drugs also reduce acute ischemic and reperfusion arrhythmias [152,153]. Following experimental myocardial infarction in animals, ACE inhibitors can prevent the development of left ventricular hypertrophy and the increase in connective tissue [154]. Furthermore, they can limit progressive postinfarction dilatation and decreased diastolic compliance in the left ventricle [81,155] while also reducing mortality [156]. Data from studies in man are less comprehensive but as noted above, it is clear that ACE inhibitors reduce or prevent progressive left ventricular dysfunction over the first 12 months following acute myocardial infarction [130,131] (see *Fig. 93.11*).

VALVAR HEART FAILURE

Valvar heart disease remains an important cause of cardiac failure. Vasodilators reduce regurgitant volume acutely, increase forward cardiac output [157], and improve symptomatic status and functional capacity [158]. Long-term treatment with vasodilators results in favorable effects on left ventricular size and function [159] and might reasonably be expected to improve the natural history of regurgitant valvar heart disease.

Captopril has been shown to reduce the regurgitant volume in aortic incompetence [160], and patients with mitral regurgitation respond favorably [161]. In rats with aortic incompetence, chronic treatment with captopril reduced left ventricular hypertrophy and dilatation [155]. Our experience is that patients with either aortic or mitral incompetence respond well to ACE inhibition, but there is no information as to whether such treatment is more or less effective than with other vasodilators.

Surgical relief is the treatment of choice for patients with symptomatic aortic stenosis, but many require medical therapy where surgery is unavailable or is contraindicated. Traditional teaching is that vasodilators are contraindicated because of the risks of hypotension and decreased coronary perfusion. Nevertheless, patients with moderate aortic stenosis, impaired left ventricular systolic function, and congestive heart failure, have shown an increase in cardiac output acutely without symptomatic hypotension following vasodilation [162]. Angiotensin-converting enzyme inhibition may possibly be of value in this group of patients, but in the absence of objective data, extreme caution is required. Likewise, vasodilators are said to be contraindicated in mitral stenosis, and severe hypotension has been noted with captopril [163]. Angiotensin-converting enzyme inhibition may be of value in patients with combined mitral stenosis and incompetence, or mitral stenosis together with left ventricular functional impairment, but as yet, this has not been formally assessed.

HEART FAILURE IN CHILDREN

In children with cardiac failure due to dilated cardiomyopathy or regurgitant valvar disease, ACE inhibitors improve symptoms and hemodynamics [164,189]. Their use in children with restrictive cardiomyopathy is less secure [189]. For congenital heart disease with a systemic-to-pulmonary shunt, ACE inhibitors decrease pulmonary flow [165,166], are clinically useful, and have infrequent adverse effects [167,168]. In more complex congenital lesions and in those with pulmonary-to-systemic shunts, arterial vasodilators can increase both the shunting and the systemic hypoxia with deleterious results. Reports of ACE inhibition under these circumstances are sparse, but one documents severe hypotension following captopril administration in patients with complicated lesions such as a single ventricle and tetralogy of Fallot [163].

HEART FAILURE IN THE ELDERLY

Age-related changes in the healthy heart mimic those seen with cardiac diseases; for example, the left ventricle becomes hypertrophied, diastolic compliance is reduced [169], and inotropic reserve is reduced [170]. The maximum achievable heart rate is reduced [171], and aortic impedance is increased [172], which further compromises cardiac performance and reserve. Deposition of amyloid [173] may contribute to both left ventricular hypertrophy and reduced diastolic compliance. Due to these structural and functional changes, elderly subjects are at greater risk of developing cardiac failure in the face of a cardiac insult. While the immediate causes of heart failure in the elderly are the same as in all adults, aortic stenosis is particularly common and may be difficult to diagnose on clinical grounds.

Provided aortic stenosis and other obstructive cardiac lesions are excluded, ACE inhibitors are effective therapy for cardiac failure in the elderly [174]. Certain precautions, however, should be taken. The elderly have diminished baroreceptor sensitivity [175] and are prone to postural hypotension. Angiotensin-converting enzyme inhibitors should therefore be introduced cautiously, in low dose, and after reduction in the maintenance dose of diuretics. Renal function, which is usually impaired, must be monitored regularly, and the dosage of renally excreted ACE inhibitors modified accordingly.

It has been suggested that the responsiveness of the RAS may diminish with age. However, in a comparison of patients with heart failure over and under the age of 65, resting plasma renin and Ang II were similar and rose on standing with a further increase with exercise; there were no significant differences between the age groups. This implied that the efficacy of ACE inhibitors is likely to be maintained in the elderly patient [190].

CONCLUSION

Angiotensin-converting enzyme inhibitors are the most important advance in the medical treatment of heart failure in the last 20 years. They are distinct from, and superior to, other vasodilator drug groups [6,84,176]. Not only do they have a sustained effect to relieve symptoms and improve exercise capacity, but they also retard the progression of left ventricular dysfunction and reduce mortality in moderate-to-severe heart failure. Results of ongoing studies are awaited to determine their effects on cardiac function and mortality in milder grades of heart failure and asymptomatic left ventricular dysfunction [147].

Angiotensin-converting enzyme inhibitors are effective in all classes of heart failure and should be introduced when diuretics are first administered. They are effective whether heart failure is due to dilated cardiomyopathy, ischemic heart disease, or hypertension. Efficacy has also been shown in valvar heart disease and in pediatric patients with left-to-right shunts, but they are currently contraindicated in severe stenotic valvar disease and probably also in certain types of congenital heart disease.

The role of ACE inhibitors immediately following acute myocardial infarction is currently being evaluated (see *Chapter 77*). Further research is required to evaluate their use in combination with other vasodilators and positive inotropic agents in resistant heart failure, and as intravenous therapy for acute heart failure.

REFERENCES

1. Ikram H, Chan W, Espiner EA, Nicholls MG. Haemodynamic and hormone responses to acute and chronic frusemide therapy in congestive heart failure. *Clinical Science* 1980;59:443–9.

2. Nicholls MG. Interaction of diuretics and electrolytes in congestive heart failure. *American Journal of Cardiology* 1990;65:17–21E.

3. Packer M, Meller J, Gorlin R, Herman MV. Hemodynamic and clinical tachyphylaxis to prazosin-mediated afterload reduction in severe chronic congestive heart failure. *Circulation* 1979;59:531–9.

4. Colucci WS, Williams GH, Alexander RW, Braunwald E. Mechanisms and implications of vasodilator tolerance in the treatment of congestive heart failure. *American Journal of Medicine* 1981;71:89–96.

5. Braunwald E, Colucci WS. Vasodilator therapy of heart failure: Has the promissory note been paid? *New England Journal of Medicine* 1984;310:459–61.

6. Bayliss J, Norell MS, Canepa–Anson R, Reid C, Poole–Wilson P, Sutton G. Clinical importance of the renin–angiotensin system in chronic heart failure: Double blind comparison of captopril and prazosin. *British Medical Journal* 1985;290:1861–5.

7. Daly P, Rouleau J–L, Cousineau D, Burgess JH, Chatterjee K. Effects of captopril and a combination of hydralazine and isosorbide dinitrate on myocardial sympathetic tone in patients with severe congestive heart failure. *British Heart Journal* 1986;56:152–7.

8. Johnson JA, Davis JO. Angiotensin II: Important role in the maintenance of arterial blood pressure. *Science* 1973;179:906–7.

9. Watkins L, Burton JA, Haber E, Cant JR, Smith FW, Barger AC. The renin–angiotensin–aldosterone system in congestive failure in conscious dogs. *Journal of Clincial Investigation* 1976;57:1606–17.

10. Gavras H, Flessas A, Ryan TJ, Brunner HR, Faxon DP, Gavras I. Angiotensin II inhibition. Treatment of congestive cardiac failure in a high-renin hypertension. *Journal of the American Medical Association* 1977;238:880–2.

11. Curtis C, Cohn JN, Vrobel T, Franciosa JA. Role of the renin–angiotensin system in the systemic vasoconstriction of chronic congestive heart failure. *Circulation* 1978;58:763–9.

12. Gavras H, Faxon DP, Berkoben J, Brunner HR, Ryan TJ. Angiotensin converting enzyme inhibition in patients with congestive heart failure. *Circulation* 1978;58:770–6.

13. Turini GA, Gribic M, Brunner HR, Waeber B, Gavras H. Improvement of chronic congestive heart-failure by oral captopril. *Lancet* 1979;i:1213–5.

14. Davis R, Ribner HS, Keung E, Sonnenblick EH, LeJemtel TH. Treatment of chronic congestive heart failure with captopril, an oral inhibitor of angiotensin-converting enzyme. *New England Journal of Medicine* 1979;301:117–21.

15. Tarazi RC, Fouad FM, Ceimo JK, Bravo EL. Renin, aldosterone and cardiac decompensation: Studies with an oral converting enzyme inhibitor in heart failure. *American Journal of Cardiology* 1979;44:1013–9.

16. Dzau VJ, Colucci WS, Williams GH, Curfman G, Meggs L, Hollenberg NK. Sustained effectiveness of converting-enzyme inhibition in patients with severe congestive heart failure. *New England Journal of Medicine* 1980;302:1373–9.

17. Levine TB, Franciosa JA, Cohn JN. Acute and long-term response to an oral converting-enzyme inhibitor, captopril, in congestive heart failure. *Circulation* 1980;62:35–41.

18. Sharpe DN, Coxon RJ, Douglas JE, Long B. Low-dose captopril in chronic heart failure: Acute haemodynamic effects and long-term treatment. *Lancet* 1980;ii:1154–7.

19. Maslowski AH, Nicholls MG, Ikram H, Espiner EA. Haemodynamic, hormonal, and electrolyte responses to captopril in resistant heart failure. *Lancet* 1981;i:71–4.

20. Cody RJ, Covit A, Schaer G, Williams G. Captopril pharmacokinetics and the acute hemodynamic and hormonal response in patients with severe chronic congestive heart failure. *American Heart Journal* 1982;104:1180–3.

21. Atlas SA, Case DB, Yu ZY, Laragh JH. Hormonal and metabolic effects of angiotensin converting enzyme inhibitors. Possible differences between enalapril and captopril. *American Journal of Medicine* 1984;77 (2A):13–7.

22. Fitzpatrick D, Nicholls MG, Ikram H, Espiner EA. Haemodynamic, hormonal, and electrolyte effects of enalapril in heart failure. *British Heart Journal* 1983;50:163–9.

23. Levine TB, Olivari MT, Garberg V, Sharkey SW, Cohn JN. Hemodynamic and clinical response to enalapril, a long-acting converting-enzyme inhibitor, in patients with congestive heart failure. *Circulation* 1984;69:548–53.

24. Dickstein K. Hemodynamic, hormonal, and pharmacokinetic aspects of treatment with lisinopril in congestive heart failure. *Journal of Cardiovascular Pharmacology* 1987;9 (suppl 3):S73–81.

25. Crozier IG, Ikram H, Nicholls MG, Jans S. Global and regional hemodynamic effects of ramipril in congestive heart failure. *Journal of Cardiovascular Pharmacology* 1989;14:688–93.

26. Nicholls MG, Ikram H, Espiner EA, Maslowski AH, Scandrett MS, Penman T. Hemodynamic and hormonal responses during captopril therapy for heart failure: Acute, chronic and withdrawal studies. *American Journal of Cardiology* 1982;49:1497–501.

27. Brunner HR, Waeber B, Nussberger J. Angiotensin-converting enzyme inhibition versus blockade of the renin–angiotensin system. *American Journal of Medicine* 1989;87 (6B):15–20S.

28. Maslowski AH, Ikram H, Nicholls MG, Espiner EA, Turner JG. Haemodynamic, hormonal, and electrolyte responses to withdrawal of long-term captopril treatment for heart failure. *Lancet* 1981;ii:959–61.

29. Cody RJ, Franklin KW, Kluger J, Laragh JH. Sympathetic responsiveness and plasma norepinephrine during therapy of chronic congestive heart failure with captopril. *American Journal of Medicine* 1982;72:791–6.

30. Wenting GJ, Man In'T Veld AJ, Woittiez AJ, Boomsma F, Laird–Meeter K, Simoons ML, Hugenholtz PG, Schalekamp MADH. Effects of captopril in acute and chronic heart failure. Correlations with plasma levels of noradrenaline, renin, and aldosterone. *British Heart Journal* 1983;49:65–76.

31. Creager MA, Faxon DP, Cutler SS, Kohlmann O, Ryan TJ, Gavras H. Contribution of vasopressin to vasoconstriction in patients with congestive heart failure: Comparison with the renin–angiotensin system and the sympathetic nervous system. *Journal of the American College of Cardiology* 1986;7:758–65.

32. Hasking GJ, Esler MD, Jennings GL, Burton D, Johns JA, Korner PI. Norepinephrine spillover to plasma in patients with congestive heart failure: Evidence of increased overall and cardiorenal sympathetic nervous activity. *Circulation* 1986;73:615–21.

33. Leimbach WN, Wallin BG, Victor RG, Aylward PE, Sundlof G, Mark AL. Direct evidence from intraneural recordings for increased central sympathetic outflow in patients with heart failure. *Circulation* 1986;73:913–9.

34. Silberbauer K, Punzengruber C, Sinzinger H. Endogenous prostaglandin E2 metabolite levels, renin–angiotensin system and catecholamines versus acute hemodynamic response to captopril in chronic congestive heart failure. *Cardiology* 1983;70:297–307.

35. Cleland JGF, Dargie HJ, Hodsman GP, Ball SG, Robertson JIS, Morton JJ, East BW, Robertson I, Murray GD, Gillen G. Captopril in heart failure. A double blind controlled trial. *British Heart Journal* 1984;52:530–5.

36. Cleland J, Semple P, Hodsman P, Ball S, Ford I, Dargie H. Angiotensin II levels, hemodynamics, and sympathoadrenal function after low-dose captopril in heart failure. *American Journal of Medicine* 1984;77:880–5.

37. Cleland JGF, Dargie HJ, Ball SG, Gillen G, Hodsman GP, Morton JJ, East BW, Robertson I, Ford I, Robertson JIS. Effects of enalapril in heart failure: A double blind study of effects on exercise performance, renal function, hormones, and metabolic state. *British Heart Journal* 1985;54:305–12.

38. Riegger GAJ, Kochsiek K. Vasopressin, renin and norepinephrine levels before and after captopril administration in patients with congestive heart failure due to idiopathic dilated cardiomyopathy. *American Journal of Cardiology* 1986;58:300–3.

39. Mulligan IP, Fraser AG, Lewis MJ, Henderson AH. Effects of enalapril on myocardial noradrenaline outflow during exercise in patients with chronic heart failure. *British Heart Journal* 1989;61:23–8.

40. Faxon DP, Halperin JL, Creager MA, Gavras H, Schick EC, Ryan TJ. Angiotensin inhibition in severe heart failure: Acute central and limb hemodynamic effects of captopril with observations on sustained oral therapy. *American Heart Journal* 1981;101:548–54.

41. McGrath BP, Arnolda LF. Enalapril reduces the catecholamine response to exercise in patients with heart failure. *European Journal of Clinical Pharmacology* 1986;30:485–7.

42. Bristow MR, Gilbert EM. Anti-adrenergic actions of angiotensin converting enzyme inhibitors. *Current Opinion in Cardiology* 1989;4 (suppl 2):S45–50.

43. Zimmerman BG, Sybertz EJ, Wong PC. Interactions between sympathetic and renin–angiotensin system. *Journal of Hypertension* 1984;2:581–7.

44. Crozier IG, Teoh R, Kay R, Nicholls MG. Sympathetic nervous system during converting enzyme inhibition. *American Journal of Medicine* 1989;87 (suppl B): 29–32S.

45. Bristow MR, Ginsburg R, Minobe W, Cubicciotti RS, Sageman WS, Lurie K, Billingham ME, Harrison DC, Stinson EB. Decreased catecholamine sensitivity and β-adrenergic receptor density in failing human hearts. *New England Journal of Medicine* 1982;307:205–11.

46. Maisel AS, Phillips C, Michel MC, Ziegler MG, Carter SM. Regulation of cardiac β-adrenergic receptors by captopril: Implications for congestive heart failure. *Circulation* 1989;80:669–75.

47. Horn EM, Corwin SJ, Steinberg SF, Chow YK, Neuberg GW, Cannon PJ, Powers ER, Bilezikian JP. Reduced lymphocyte stimulatory guanine nucleotide regulatory protein and β-adrenergic receptors in congestive heart failure and reversal with angiotensin converting enzyme inhibitor therapy. *Circulation* 1988;78:1373–9.

48. Nishimura H, Kubo S, Ueyama M, Kubota J, Kawamura K. Peripheral hemodynamic effects of captopril in patients with congestive heart failure. *American Heart Journal* 1989;117:100–5.

49. Crozier IG, Nicholls MG, Ikram H, Espiner EA, Yandle TG. Atrial natriuretic peptide levels in congestive heart failure in man before and during converting enzyme inhibition. *Clinical and Experimental Pharmacology and Physiology* 1989;16:417–24.

50. Fitzpatrick D, Nicholls MG, Ikram H, Espiner EA. Acute haemodynamic, hormonal and electrolyte effects and short-term clinical response to enalapril in heart failure. *Journal of Hypertension* 1983;1 (suppl 1):147–53.

51. Captopril Multicentre Research Group. A cooperative multicentre study of captopril in congestive heart failure: Hemodynamic effects and long term response. *American Heart Journal* 1985;110:439–47.

52. Creager MA, Halperin JL, Bernard DB, Faxon DP, Melidossian CD, Gavras H, Ryan TJ. Acute regional circulatory and renal hemodynamic effects of converting-enzyme inhibition in patients with congestive heart failure. *Circulation* 1981;64:483–8.

53. Maskin CS, Ocken S, Chadwick B, LeJemtel TH. Comparative systemic and renal effects of dopamine and angiotensin-converting enzyme inhibition with enalaprilat in patients with heart failure. *Circulation* 1985;72:846–52.

54. Paulson OB, Jarden JO, Godtfredsen J, Vorstrup S. Cerebral blood flow in patients with congestive heart failure treated with captopril. *American Journal of Medicine* 1984;76 (5B):91–5.

55. DeMarco T, Daly PA, Liu M, Kayser S, Parmley WW, Chatterjee K. Enalaprilat, a new parenteral angiotensin-converting enzyme inhibitor: Rapid changes in systemic and coronary hemodynamic and humoral profile in chronic heart failure. *Journal of the American College of Cardiology* 1987;9:1131–8.

56. Foult J–M, Tavolaro O, Antony I, Nitenberg A. Direct myocardial and coronary effects of enalaprilat in patients with dilated cardiomyopathy: Assessment by a bilateral intracoronary infusion technique. *Circulation* 1988;77:337–44.

57. Crossley IR, Bihari D, Gimson AES, Westaby D, Richardson PJ, Williams R. Effects of converting enzyme inhibition on hepatic blood flow in man. *American Journal of Medicine* 1984;76:62–5.

58. Awan NA, Evenson MK, Needham KE, Win A, Mason DT. Efficacy of oral angiotensin-converting enzyme inhibition with captopril therapy in severe chronic normotensive congestive heart failure. *American Heart Journal* 1981;101:22–31.

59. Hermanovich J, Awan NA, Lui H, Mason DT. Comparative analysis of the hemodynamic actions of captopril and sodium nitroprusside in severe congestive heart failure. *American Heart Journal* 1982;104:1211–9.

60. Packer M, Medina N, Yushak M. Contrasting hemodynamic responses in severe heart failure: Comparison of captopril and other vasodilating drugs. *American Heart Journal* 1982;104:1215–20.

61. Olivari MT, Levine TB, Cox T, Cohn JN. Contrasting capacitance effects of captopril and nitroglycerin in congestive heart failure [Abstract]. *Circulation* 1982;66 (suppl II):209.

62. Ader R, Chatterjee K, Ports T, Brundage B, Hiramatsu B, Parmley W. Immediate and sustained hemodynamic and clinical improvement in chronic heart failure by an oral angiotensin-converting enzyme inhibitor. *Circulation* 1980;61:931–6.

63. Kramer BL, Massie BM, Topic N. Controlled trial of captopril in chronic heart failure: A rest and exercise hemodynamic study. *Circulation* 1983;67:807–15.

64. Packer M, Medina N, Yushak M, Meller J. Hemodynamic patterns of response during long-term captopril therapy for severe chronic heart failure. *Circulation* 1983;68:803–12.

65. Sharpe DN, Murphy J, Coxon R, Hannan SF. Enalapril in patients with chronic heart failure: A placebo-controlled, randomized, double-blind study. *Circulation* 1984;70:271–8.

66. Packer M, Medina N. Yushak M, Lee WH. Usefulness of plasma renin activity in predicting haemodynamic and clinical responses and survival during long term converting enzyme inhibition in severe chronic heart failure. Experience in 100 consecutive patients. *British Heart Journal* 1985;54:298–304.

67. Dzau VJ. Circulating versus local renin–angiotensin system in cardiovascular homeostasis. *Circulation* 1988;77 (suppl I):4–9.

68. Lever AF. Slow pressor mechanisms in hypertension: A role for hypertrophy of resistance vessels? *Journal of Hypertension* 1986;4:515–24.

69. Packer M, Medina N, Yushak M. Relation between the serum sodium concentration and the hemodynamic and clinical responses to converting enzyme inhibition with captopril in severe heart failure. *Journal of the American College of Cardiology* 1984;3:1035–43.

70. van Gilst WH, Scholtens E, de Graeff PA, de Langen CDJ, Wesseling H. Differential influences of angiotensin converting-enzyme inhibitors on the coronary circulation. *Circulation* 1988;77 (suppl I):I24–9.

71. Chatterjee K, Rouleau J–L, Parmley WW. Haemodynamic and myocardial metabolic effects of captopril in chronic heart failure. *British Heart Journal* 1982;47:233–8.

72. Halperin JL, Faxon DP, Creager MA, Bass TA, Melidossian CD, Gavras H, Ryan TJ. Coronary hemodynamic effects of angiotensin inhibition by captopril and teprotide in patients with congestive heart failure. *American Journal of Cardiology* 1982;50:967–72.

73. Osterziel KJ, Dietz R, Schmid W, Mikulaschek K, Manthey J, Kübler W. ACE inhibition improves vagal reactivity in patients with heart failure. *American Heart Journal* 1990;120:1120–9.

74. Ikram H, Low CJS, Shirlaw T, Webb CM, Richards AM, Crozier IG. Antianginal, hemodynamic and coronary vascular effects of captopril in stable angina pectoris. *American Journal of Cardiology* 1990;66:164–7.

75. Fowler NO, Holmes JC. Coronary and myocardial actions of angiotensin. *Circulation Research* 1964;14:191–201.

76. Moravec CS, Schluchter MD, Paranandi L, Czerska B, Stewart RW, Rosenkranz E, Bond M. Ionotropic effects of angiotensin II on human cardiac muscle *in vitro. Circulation* 1990;82:1973–84.

77. Hirakata H, Fouad–Tarazi FM, Bumpus M, Khosla M, Healy B, Husain A, Urata H, Kumagai H. Angiotensins and the failing heart: Enhanced positive inotropic response to angiotensin I in cardiomyopathic hamster heart in the presence of captopril. *Circulation Research* 1990;66:891–9.

78. Captopril Multicenter Research Group. A placebo controlled trial of captopril in refractory chronic congestive heart failure. *Journal of the American College of Cardiology* 1983;2:755–63.

79. Grossman W, McLaurin LP, Rolett EL. Alterations in left ventricular relaxation and diastolic compliance in congestive cardiomyopathy. *Cardiovascular Research* 1979;13:514–22.

80. Pouleur H. Diastolic dysfunction and myocardial energetics. *European Heart Journal* 1990;11 (suppl C):30–4.

81. Pfeffer JM, Pfeffer MA, Braunwald E. Influence of chronic captopril therapy on the infarcted left ventricle of the rat. *Circulation Research* 1985;57:84–95.

82. Konstam MA, Kronenberg MW, Udelson JE, Metherall J, Dolan N, Edens TR, Howe DM, Yusuf S, Youngblood M, Toltsis H, SOLVD Investigators. Effects of acute angiotensin converting enzyme inhibition of left ventricular filling in patients with congestive heart failure. Relation to right ventricular volumes. *Circulation* 1990;**81** (suppl III):115–22.

83. Rousseau MF, Gurné O, van Eyll C, Benedict CR, Pouleur H. Effects of benazeprilat on left ventricular systolic and diastolic function and neurohumoral status in patients with ischemic heart disease. *Circulation* 1990;**81** (suppl III):123–9.

84. Packer M, Meller J, Medina N, Yushak M. Quantitative differences in the hemodynamic effects of captopril and nitroprusside in severe chronic heart failure. *American Journal of Cardiology* 1983;**51**:183–7.

85. Carroll JD, Lang RM, Neumann AL, Borow KM, Rajfer SI. The differential effects of positive ionotropic and vasodilator therapy on diastolic properties in patients with congestive cardiomyopathy. *Circulation* 1986;**74**:815–25.

86. Webster MWI, Fitzpatrick MA, Nicholls MG, Ikram H, Wells JE. Effect of enalapril on ventricular arrhythmias in congestive heart failure. *American Journal of Cardiology* 1985;**56**:566–9.

87. The Captopril–Digoxin Multicentre Research Group. Comparative effects of therapy with captopril and digoxin in patients with mild to moderate heart failure. *Journal of the American Medical Association* 1988;**259**:539–44.

88. de Graeff PA, Kingma JH, Viersma JW, Wesseling H, Lie KI. Acute and chronic effects of ramipril and captopril in congestive heart failure. *International Journal of Cardiology* 1989;**23**:59–67.

89. Ichikawa I, Pfeffer JM, Pfeffer MA, Hostetter TH, Brenner BM. Role of angiotensin II in the altered renal function of congestive heart failure. *Circulation Research* 1984;**55**:669–75.

90. Nicholls MG. Overview: Angiotensin, angiotensin converting enzyme inhibition, and the kidney — congestive heart failure. *Kidney International* 1987;**31** (suppl 20):S200–2.

91. Robertson JIS, Richards AM. Converting enzyme inhibitors and renal function in cardiac failure. *Kidney International* 1987;**31** (suppl 20):S216–9.

92. Packer M, Lee WH, Medina N, Yushak M, Kessler PD. Functional renal insufficiency during long-term therapy with captopril and enalapril in severe chronic heart failure. *Annals of Internal Medicine* 1987;**106**:346–54.

93. Mujais SK, Fouad FM, Textor SC, Tarazi RC, Bravo EL, Hart N. Gifford RW. Transient renal dysfunction during initial inhibition of converting enzyme in congestive heart failure. *British Heart Journal* 1984;**52**:63–71.

94. Uretsky BF, Shaver JA, Liang C–S, Amin D, Shah PK, Levine TB, Walinsky P, LeJemtel T, Linnemeier T, Rush JE, Langendorfer A, Snapinn S. Modulation of hemodynamic effects with a converting enzyme inhibitor: Acute hemodynamic dose–response relationship of a new angiotensin converting enzyme inhibitor, lisinopril, with observations on long-term clinical, functional, and biochemical responses, *American Heart Journal* 1988;**116**:480–8.

95. Cleland JGF, Dargie HJ. Heart failure, renal function, and angiotensin converting enzyme inhibitors. *Kidney International* 1987;**31** (suppl 20): S220–8.

96. Packer M, Lee WH, Yushak M, Medina N. Comparison of captopril and enalapril in patients with severe chronic heart failure. *New England Journal of Medicine* 1986;**315**:847–53.

97. Cleland JGF, Dargie HJ, Pettigrew A, Gillen G, Robertson JIS. The effects of captopril on serum digoxin and urinary urea and digoxin clearances in patients with congestive heart failure. *American Heart Journal* 1986;**112**:130–5.

98. Pierpont GL, Francis GS, Cohn JN. Effect of captopril on renal function in patients with congestive heart failure. *British Heart Journal* 1981;**46**:522–7.

99. Packer M, Lee WH, Medina N, Yushak M, Kessler PD, Gottlieb SS. Influence of diabetes mellitus on changes in left ventricular performance and renal function produced by converting enzyme inhibition in patients with severe chronic heart failure. *American Journal of Medicine* 1987;**82**:1119–26.

100. Giles TD, Katz R, Sullivan JM, Wolfson P, Haugland M, Kirlin P, Powers E, Rich S, Hackshaw B, Chiaramida A, Rouleau JL, Fisher MB, Pigeon J, Rush JE. Short- and long-acting angiotensin-converting enzyme inhibitors: A randomised trial of lisinopril versus captopril in the treatment of congestive heart failure. *Journal of the American College of Cardiology* 1989;**13**:1240–7.

101. Fitzpatrick MA, Rademaker MT, Frampton CM, Espiner EA, Yandle TG, A'Court G, Ikram H. Renal effects of ACE inhibition in ovine heart failure: A comparison of intermittent and continuous ACE inhibition. *Journal of Cardiovascular Pharmacology* 1990;**16**:629–35.

102. Powers ER, Bannerman KS, Stone J, Reison DS, Escala EL, Kalischer A, Weiss MB, Sciacca RR, Cannon PJ. The effect of captopril on renal, coronary and systemic hemodynamics in patients with severe congestive heart failure. *American Heart Journal* 1982;**104**:1203–10.

103. Faxon DP, Creager MA, Halperin JL, Bernard DB, Ryan TJ. Redistribution of regional blood flow following angiotensin-converting enzyme inhibition. *American Journal of Medicine* 1984;**76** (suppl 5B):104–10.

104. Bayliss J, Canepa–Anson R, Norell M, Poole-Wilson P, Sutton G. The renal response to neuroendocrine inhibition in chronic heart failure: Double-blind comparison of captopril and prazosin. *European Heart Journal* 1986;**7**:877–84.

105. Kubo S, Nishioka A, Nishimura H, Kawamura K, Takatsu T. Effects of converting-enzyme inhibition on cardiorenal hemodynamics in patients with chronic congestive heart failure. *Journal of Cardiovascular Pharmacology* 1985;**7**:753–9.

106. Dzau VJ, Hollenberg NK. Renal response to captopril in severe heart failure: Role of furosemide in natriuresis and reversal of hyponatremia. *Annals of Internal Medicine* 1984;**100**:777–82.

107. Richardson A, Scriven AJ, Poole–Wilson PA, Bayliss J, Parameshwar J, Sutton GC. Double-blind comparison of captopril alone against frusemide plus amiloride in mild heart failure. *Lancet* 1987;**ii**:709–11.

108. Packer M, Medina N, Yushak M. Correction of dilutional hyponatremia in severe heart failure by converting-enzyme inhibition. *Annals of Internal Medicine* 1984;**100**:782–9.

109. Jungmann E, Storger H, Althoff PH, Hadler D, Fasbinder W, Bussmann WD, Kaltenbach M, Schoffling K. Aldosterone and prolactin responsiveness after prolonged treatment of congestive heart failure with captopril. *European Journal of Clinical Pharmacology* 1985;**28**:1–4.

110. Rajagopalan B, Raine AEG, Cooper R, Ledingham JGG. Changes in cerebral blood flow in patients with severe congestive cardiac failure before and after captopril treatment. *American Journal of Medicine* 1984;**76** (suppl 5B):86–9.

111. Barry DI, Paulson OB, Jarden JO, Juhler M, Graham DI, Strandgaard S. Effects of captopril on cerebral blood flow in normotensive and hypertensive rats. *American Journal of Medicine* 1984;**76** (suppl 5B):79–85.

112. Paulson OB, Waldemar G, Andersen AR, Barry DI, Pedersen EV, Schmidt JF, Vorstrup S. Role of angiotensin in autoregulation of cerebral blood flow. *Circulation* 1988;**77** (suppl I):I55–8.

113. Wilson JR, Ferraro N. Effect of the renin–angiotensin system on limb circulation and metabolism during exercise in patients with heart failure. *Journal of the American College of Cardiology* 1985;**6**:556–63.

114. Kugler J, Maskin C, Frishman WH, Sonnenblick EH, LeJemtel TH. Regional and systemic metabolic effects of angiotensin-converting enzyme inhibition in patients with severe heart failure. *Circulation* 1982;**66**:1256–61.

115. Mancini DM, Davis L, Wexler JP, Chadwick B, LeJemtel TH. Dependence of enhanced maximal exercise performance on increased peak skeletal muscle perfusion during long-term captopril therapy in heart failure. *Journal of the American College of Cardiology* 1987;**10**:845–50.

116. Cowley AJ, Stainer K, Rowley JM, Hampton JR. Effects of captopril on abnormalities of the peripheral circulation and respiratory function in patients with severe heart failure. *Lancet* 1984;**ii**:1120–4.

117. Drexler H, Banhardt U, Meinertz T, Wollschlager H, Lehmann M, Just H. Contrasting peripheral short-term and long-term effects of converting enzyme inhibition in patients with congestive heart failure. *Circulation* 1989;**79**:491–502.

118. Kugler J, Maskin CS, Frishman W, Sonnenblick EH, LeJemtel TH. Variable clinical response to long-term angiotensin inhibition in severe heart failure: Demonstration of additive benefits of alpha-receptor blockade. *American Heart Journal* 1982;**104**:1154–9.

119. Stevenson LW, Brunken RC, Belil D, Grover–McKay M, Schwaiger M, Schelbert HR, Tillisch JH. Afterload reduction with vasodilators and diuretics decreases mitral regurgitation during upright exercise in advanced heart failure. *Journal of the American College of Cardiology* 1990;15:174–80.

120. McKee PA, Castelli WP, NcNamara PM, Kannel WB. The natural history of congestive heart failure: The Framingham study. *New England Journal of Medicine* 1971;285:1441–6.

121. Franciosa JA, Wilen M, Ziesche S, Cohn JN. Survival in men with severe chronic left ventricular failure due to either coronary heart disease or idiopathic dilated cardiomyopathy. *American Journal of Cardiology* 1983;51:831–6.

122. Swedberg K, Eneroth P, Kjekshus J, Snapinn S. Effects of enalapril and neuroendocrine activation on prognosis in severe congestive heart failure (follow-up of the CONSENSUS trial). *American Journal of Cardiology* 1990;66 (suppl D):40–5D.

123. Furberg CD, Yusuf S. Effect of vasodilators on survival in chronic congestive heart failure. *American Journal of Cardiology* 1985;55:1110–3.

124. Cohn JN, Archibald DG, Ziesche S, Franciosa JA, Harston WE, Tristani FE, Dunkman WB, Jacobs W, Francis GS, Flohr KH, Goldman S, Cobb FR, Shah PM, Saunders R, Fletcher RD, Loeb HS, Hughes VC, Baker B. Effect of vasodilator therapy on mortality in chronic congestive heart failure. *New England Journal of Medicine* 1986;314:1547–55.

125. Lee WH, Packer M. Prognostic importance of serum sodium concentration and its modification by converting-enzyme inhibition in patients with severe chronic heart failure. *Circulation* 1986;73:257–67.

126. The CONSENSUS Trial Study Group. Effects of enalapril on mortality in severe congestive heart failure. *New England Journal of Medicine* 1987;316:1429–35.

127. Newman TJ, Maskin CS, Dennick LG, Meyer JH, Hallows BG, Cooper WH. Effects of captopril on survival in patients with heart failure. *American Journal of Medicine* 1988;84 (3A):140–4.

128. Pouleaur H, Rousseau MF, Oakley C, Ryden L. Difference in mortality between patients treated with captopril or enalapril in the xamoterol in severe heart failure study. *American Journal of Cardiology* 1991;68:71–4.

129. Nony P, Boissel JP, Chifflet R. Evaluating the effect of angiotensin converting enzyme inhibitors on mortality: Role of the etiology (ischemic or non-ischemic) of heart insufficiency [Abstract]. *European Heart Journal* 1990;11 (suppl):56.

130. Sharpe N, Smith H, Murphy J, Hannan S. Treatment of patients with symptomless left ventricular dysfunction after myocardial infarction. *Lancet* 1988;i:255–9.

131. Pfeffer MA, Lamas GA, Vaughan DE, Parisi AF, Braunwald E. Effect of captopril on progressive left ventricular dilatation after anterior myocardial infarction. *New England Journal of Medicine* 1988;319:80–6.

132. Kleber FX, Laube A, Osterkorn K, Konig E. Captopril in mild to moderate heart failure over 18 months: Effects on morbidity and mortality [Abstract]. *Journal of the American College of Cardiology* 1987;9:42A.

133. Dickstein K, Till AE, Aarsland T, Tjelta K, Abrahamsen AM, Kristianson K, Gomex HJ, Gregg H, Hichens M. The pharmacokinetics of enalapril in hospitalized patients with congestive heart failure. *British Journal of Clinical Pharmacology* 1987;23:403–10.

134. Rademaker M, Shaw TRD, Williams BC, Duncan FM, Corrie J, Eglen A, Edwards CRW. Intravenous captopril treatment in patients with severe cardiac failure. *British Heart Journal* 1986;55:187–90.

135. Hauda M, Steffen W, Erbel R, Meyer J. Sublingual administration of captopril versus nitroglycerin in patients with severe congestive heart failure. *International Journal of Cardiology* 1990;27:351–9.

136. Riegger GAJ. The effects of ACE inhibitors on exercise capacity in the treatment of congestive heart failure. *Journal of Cardiovascular Pharmacology* 1990;15 (suppl 1):S41–6.

137. Guyatt GH, Sullivan MJJ, Fallen EL, Tihal H, Rideout E, Halcrow S, Nogradi S. Townsend M, Taylor DW. A controlled trial of digoxin in congestive heart failure. *American Journal of Cardiology* 1988;61:371–5.

138. Gheorghiade M, Hall V, Lakier JB, Goldstein S. Comparative hemodynamic and neurohormonal effects of intravenous captopril and digoxin and their combinations in patients with severe heart failure. *Journal of the American College of Cardiology* 1989;13:134–42.

139. Bigger JT, Fleiss JL, Rolnitzky LM, Merab JP, Ferrick KJ. Effect of digitalis treatment on survival after acute myocardial infarction. *American Journal of Cardiology* 1985;55:623–30.

140. Ikram H, Webster MWI, Nicholls MG, Lewis GRJ, Richards AM, Crozier IG. Combined spironolactone and converting-enzyme inhibitor therapy for refractory heart failure. *Australian and New Zealand Journal of Medicine* 1986;16:61–3.

141. Massie BM, Packer M, Hanlon JT, Combs DT. Hemodynamic responses to combined therapy with captopril and hydralazine in patients with severe heart failure. *Journal of the American College of Cardiology* 1983;2:338–44.

142. Ikram H, Maslowski AH, Nicholls MG. Haemodynamic effects of dobutamine in patients with congestive heart failure receiving captopril. *British Heart Journal* 1981;46:428–530.

143. Manthey J, Osterziel KJ, Röhrig N, Dietz R, Hackenthal E, Schmidt–Gayk H, Kübler W. Ramipril and captopril in patients with heart failure: Effects on hemodynamics and vasoconstrictor systems. *American Journal of Cardiology* 1987;59:171–5D.

144. Alicandri C, Fariello R, Boni E, Zaninelli A, Muiesan G. Comparison of captopril and digoxin in mild to moderate heart failure. *Postgraduate Medical Journal* 1986;62 (suppl 1):170–5.

145. Rezkalla S, Kloner RA, Khatib G, Khatib R. Effects of delayed captopril therapy on left ventricular mass and myonecrosis during acute coxsackievirus murine myocarditis. *American Heart Journal* 1990;120:1377–81.

146. Freeman RH, Davis JO, Williams GM, DeForrest JM, Seymour AA, Rowe BP. Effects of the oral converting enzyme inhibitor, SQ 14225, in a model of low cardiac output in dogs. *Circulation Research* 1979;45:540–5.

147. Riegger GAJ, Liebau G, Holzchuh M, Witkowski D, Steilner H, Kochsiek K. Role of the renin–angiotensin system in the development of congestive heart failure in the dog as assessed by chronic converting-enzyme blockade. *American Journal of Cardiology* 1984;53:614–8.

148. McAlpine HM, Morton JJ, Leckie B, Rumley A, Gillen G, Dargie HJ. Neuroendocrine activation after acute myocardial infarction. *British Heart Journal* 1988;60:117–24.

149. McAlpine HM, Morton JJ, Leckie B, Dargie HJ. Haeemodynamic effects of captopril in acute left ventricular failure complicating myocardial infarction. *Journal of Cardiovascular Pharmacology* 1987;9 (suppl 2):S25–30.

150. Taylor SH, Verma SP, Silke B. Enalaprilat in heart failure complicating acute myocardial infarction. *Current Opinion in Cardiology* 1989;4 (suppl 2):S37–43.

151. Ertl G, Kloner RA, Alexander RW, Braunwald E. Limitation of experimental infarct size by an angiotensin-converting enzyme inhibitor. *Circulation* 1982;65:40–7.

152. Elfellah MS, Ogilvie RI. Effect of vasodilator drugs on coronary occlusion and reperfusion arrhythmias in anesthetized dogs. *Journal of Cardiovascular Pharmacology* 1985;7:826–32.

153. Linz W, Scholkens BA, Han Y–F. Beneficial effects of the converting enzyme inhibitor, ramipril, in ischemic rat hearts. *Journal of Cardiovascular Pharmacology* 1986;8 (suppl 10):S91–9.

154. Michel JB. Relationship between decrease in afterload and beneficial effects of ACE inhibitors in experimental cardiac hypertrophy and in congestive heart failure. *European Heart Journal* 1990;11 (suppl D):17–26.

155. Gay RG. Early and late effects of captopril treatment after large myocardial infarction in rats. *Journal of the American College of Cardiology* 1990;16:967–77.

156. Pfeffer MA, Pfeffer JM, Steinberg C, Finn P. Survival after an experimental myocardial infarction: Beneficial effects of long-term therapy with captopril. *Circulation* 1985;72:406–12.

157. Miller RR, Vismara LA, DeMaria AN, Salel AF, Mason DT. Afterload reduction therapy with nitroprusside in severe aortic regurgitation: Improved cardiac performance and reduced regurgitant volume. *American Journal of Cardiology* 1976;38:564–6.

158. Greenberg BH, Rahimtoola SH. Long-term vasodilator therapy in aortic insufficiency. *Annals of Internal Medicine* 1980;93:440–2.

159. Greenberg B, Massie B, Bristow JD, Cheitlin M, Siemienczuk D, Topic N, Wilson RA, Szlachcic J, Thomas D. Long term vasodilator therapy of chronic aortic insufficiency. *Circulation* 1988;78:92–103.

160. Reske SN, Heck I, Kropp J, Mattern H, Ledda R, Knopp R, Winkler C. Captopril mediated decrease of aortic regurgitation. *British Heart Journal* 1985;54:415–9.

161. Evangelista A, Bruguera J, Serrat R, Robles A, Galve E, Soler–Soler J. Influence of mitral regurgitation in the response to captopril therapy for heart failure [Abstract]. *European Heart Journal* 1990;11 (suppl):289.

162. Greenberg BH, Massie BM. Beneficial effects of afterload reduction therapy in patients with congestive heart failure and moderate aortic stenosis. *Circulation* 1980;61:1212–6.

163. Liebau G, Riegger AJG, Schanzenbacher P, Steilner H, Oehrlein S. Captopril in congestive heart failure. *British Journal of Clinical Pharmacology* 1982;14 (suppl 2):193–9S.

164. Artman M, Graham TP. Guidelines for vasodilator therapy of congestive heart failure in infants and children. *American Heart Journal* 1987;113:994–1005.

165. Schneeweiss A. Cardiovascular drugs in children: Angiotensin-converting enzyme inhibitors. *Paediatric Cardiology* 1988;9:109–15.

166. Montigny M, Davignon A, Fouron J-C, Biron P, Fournier A, Elie R. Captopril in infants for congestive heart failure secondary to a large ventricular left-to-right shunt. *American Journal of Cardiology* 1989;63:631–3.

167. Scammell AM, Arnold R, Wilkinson JL. Captopril in treatment of infant heart failure: A preliminary report. *International Journal of Cardiology* 1987;16:295–301.

168. Shaw NJ, Wilson N, Dickinson DF. Captopril in heart failure secondary to a left to right shunt. *Archives of Diseases of Children* 1988;63:360–3.

169. Gerstenblith G, Frederiksen J, Yin FCP, Fortuin NJ, Lakatta EG, Weisfeldt ML. Echocardiac assessment of a normal adult aging population. *Circulation* 1977;56:273–8.

170. Rodeheffer RJ, Gerstenblith G, Becker LC, Fleg JL, Weisfeldt ML, Lakatta EG. Exercise cardiac output is maintained with advancing age in healthy human subjects: Cardiac dilatation and increased stroke volume compensate for a diminished heart rate. *Circulation* 1984;69:203–13.

171. Gerstenblith G, Lakatta EG, Weisfeldt ML. Age changes in myocardial function and exercise response. *Progress in Cardiovascular Disease* 1976;19:1–21.

172. Yin FCP, Weisfeldt ML, Milnor WR. Role of aortic input impedance in the decreased cardiovascular response to exercise with aging in dogs. *Journal of Clinical Investigation* 1981;68:28–38.

173. Pomerance A. Senile cardiac amyloid. *British Heart Journal* 1965;27:711–6.

174. Impallomeni MG, Maruthappu J. Can captopril replace diuretics in the treatment of chronic heart failure in the elderly? *Geriatric Cardiovascular Medicine* 1988;1:215–9.

175. McGarry K, Laher M, Fitzgerald D, Horgan J, O'Brian E, O'Malley K. Baroreflex function in elderly hypertensives. *Hypertension* 1983;5:763–6.

176. Schofield PM, Brooks NH, Lawrence GP, Testa HJ, Ward C. Which vasodilator drug in patients with chronic heart failure? A randomised comparison of captopril and hydralazine. *British Journal of Clinical Pharmacology* 1991;31:25–32.

177. Cleland JGF, Dargie HJ, McAlpine H, Ball SG, Morton JJ, Robertson JIS, Ford I. Severe hypotension after first dose of enalapril in heart failure. *British Medical Journal* 1985;291:1309–12.

178. Osterziel KJ, Röhrig N, Dietz R, Manthey J, Hecht J, Kübler W. Influence of captopril on the arterial baroreceptor reflex in patients with heart failure. *European Heart Journal* 1988;9:1137–45.

179. Gibbs JSR, Crean PA, Mockus L, Wright C, Sutton GC, Fox KM. The variable effects of angiotensin converting enzyme inhibition on myocardial ischaemia in chronic stable angina. *British Heart Journal* 1989;62:112–7.

180. Cleland JGF, Henderson E, McLenachan J, Findlay IN, Dargie HJ. Effect of captopril, an angiotensin-converting enzyme inhibitor, in patients with angina pectoris and heart failure. *Journal of American College of Cardiology* 1991;17:733–9.

181. Brown JJ, Davies DL, Johnson VW, Lever AF, Robertson JIS. Renin relationships in congestive cardiac failure, treated and untreated. *American Heart Journal* 1970;80:329–42.

182. Montgomery AJ, Shepherd AN, Elmslie–Smith B. Severe hyponatraemia and cardiac failure successfully treated with captopril. *British Medical Journal* 1982;284:1085–6.

183. Cleland JGF, Dargie HJ, East BW, Robertson I, Hodsman GP, Ball SG, Gillen G, Robertson JIS, Morton JJ. Total body and serum electrolyte composition in heart failure: The effects of captopril. *European Heart Journal* 1985;6:681–8.

184. The SOLVD Investigators. Effect of enalapril on survival in patients with reduced left ventricular ejection fractions and congestive heart failure. *New England Journal of Medicine* 1991;325:293–302.

185. Cohn JN, Johnson G, Ziesche S, Cobb F, Francis G, Tristani F, Smith R, Dunkman WB, Loeb H, Wong M, Bhat G, Goldman S, Fletcher RD, Doherty J, Hughes CV, Carson P, Cintron G, Shabetai R, Haakenson C. A comparison of enalapril with hydralazine–isosorbide dinitrate in the treatment of chronic congestive heart failure. *New England Journal of Medicine* 1991;325:303–10.

186. Fonarow G, Chelimsky-Fallick C, Stevenson LW, Luu M, Hamilton M, Moriguchi J, Walden J, Albanese E, Tillisch J. Survival with angiotensin-converting-enzyme inhibition vs. direct vasodilation for the same hemodynamic goals in advanced heart failure [Abstract]. *Journal of the American College of Cardiology* 1991;17:274.

187. Robertson JIS. Ramipril — a new converting enzyme inhibitor: Concluding remarks. *American Journal of Cardiology* 1987;59:176–7D.

188. Miyakawa T, Shionoiri H, Takasaki I, Kobayashi K, Ishii M. The effect of captopril on pharmacokinetics of digoxin in patients with mild congestive heart failure. *Journal of Cardiovascular Pharmacology* 1991;17:576–80.

189. Bengur AR, Beckman RH, Rocchini AP, Crowley DC, Schork MA, Rosenthal A. Acute hemodynamic effects of captopril in children with a congestive or restrictive cardiomyopathy. *Circulation* 1991;83:523–7.

190. Cleland JGF, Dargie HJ, Robertson JIS, Ball SG, Hodsman GP. Renin and angiotensin responses to posture and exercise in elderly patients with heart failure. *European Heart Journal* 1984;5 (suppl E):9–11.

191. Young JB, Uretsky BF, Shahidi FE, Yellen LG, Harrison MC, Jolly MK and the PROVED Study Investigators. Multicenter, double-blind, placebo-controlled randomized withdrawal trial of the efficacy and safety of digoxin in patients with mild to moderate chronic heart failure not treated with converting enzyme inhibitors [Abstract]. *Journal of the American College of Cardiology* 1992;19:259.

192. Packer M, Gheorghiade M, Young JB, Smith LK, Costantini PJ, Adams KF, Cody RJ, Butman SM, Gourley LA, Jolly MK and the RADIANCE Study Investigators. Randomized, double-blind, placebo-controlled, withdrawal study of digoxin in patients with chronic heart failure treated with converting-enzyme inhibitors [Abstract]. *Journal of the American College of Cardiology* 1992;19:260.

193. Singh BN, Hollenberg NK, Poole-Wilson PA, Robertson JIS. Diuretic-induced potassium and magnesium deficiency: Relation to drug-induced QT prolongation, cardiac arrhythmias and sudden death. *Journal of Hypertension* 1992;10:301–6.

94 THE RENIN–ANGIOTENSIN SYSTEM, ACE INHIBITORS, AND CARDIAC STRUCTURE

IAN G CROZIER, A MARK RICHARDS, HAMID IKRAM, AND M GARY NICHOLLS

INTRODUCTION

Cardiac structure is influenced not only by the hemodynamic load, but also by diverse neurohumoral factors, including the RAS, α- and β-adrenergic stimulation, and thyroxine. Increased left ventricular afterload, acute or chronic ventricular injury, and stimulation of neurohormonal systems promote the development of left ventricular hypertrophy and augment left ventricular systolic function in the short and medium term. In the long term, however, diastolic dysfunction and myocyte necrosis, fibrosis, and myocellular energy depletion develop and contribute ultimately to left ventricular dilatation and failure.

Abnormalities of structure which commonly occur in cardiac disease include left ventricular hypertrophy and dilatation. Left ventricular hypertrophy may be 'primary' (as in hypertrophic cardiomyopathy) or can be a secondary response to increased wall stress caused by hypertension, cardiac valvar disease, or cardiac injury, most commonly myocardial infarction.

Cardiac myocytes hypertrophy in response to increased wall stress (tension). This hypertrophy of individual myocytes in turn results in left ventricular wall hypertrophy which tends to normalize wall tension as predicted by the Laplace relation ($T = P.r/2L$, where T = ventricular wall tension, P = left ventricular pressure, r = ventricular radius, and L = ventricular wall thickness). Increased tension is a direct stimulus to myocyte hypertrophy both in isolated tissue preparations [1] and in the intact heart [2]. These effects of tension on myocytes may be mediated by mechanotransducer ion channels, possibly by modifying intracellular pH or the concentration of intracellular messengers such as cAMP which, in turn, increase mRNA and protein production. Myocardial stretch may also increase mRNA directly via deformation of the nucleus [3]. In addition, Ang II has been shown, at least under experimental circumstances, to have a direct trophic effect on myocardial cells (see *Chapter 31*), perhaps by interaction with the sympathetic nervous system [3]. The hypertrophic response to cardiac stress or injury may be mediated or modulated by neurohumoral factors, including activity of the RAS and the sympathetic nervous system.

Despite the fact that unit wall tension declines as hypertrophy develops, left ventricular hypertrophy is of major prognostic significance in essential hypertension and in the population at large [4–9]. In the report by Koren *et al* [8], the prognostic significance of left ventricular mass, as measured by echocardiography, was assessed in 280 patients with essential hypertension. Follow-up at 10 years revealed a 28-fold increase in cardiovascular deaths (14% versus 0.5%) and an eight-fold increase in death from all causes, in patients with increased left ventricular mass (greater than $125g/m^2$) compared with those without left ventricular hypertrophy. It is apparent also that left ventricular hypertrophy is an independent risk factor for cardiovascular death and sudden cardiac death in the population at large [9]. This heightened cardiovascular risk is likely to be multifactorial involving, in the heart, decreased coronary vascular reserve and subendocardial ischemia [10], an increased frequency of ventricular arrhythmias [11], and myocardial fibrosis [12], as well as hypertension *per se*. James and Jones [121] have suggested that left ventricular hypertrophy predisposes to arrhythmias provoked by diuretic-induced hypokalemia.

Left ventricular dilatation generally occurs as a later change after direct myocardial damage or long-sustained left ventricular hypertrophy. This compensatory response permits maintenance of stroke volume in association with reduced cardiac systolic wall stress, but at the expense of an increase in unit wall stress. Ventricular dilatation often heralds a progressive deterioration in cardiac function and the onset of frank heart failure. Indeed, White *et al* [13] reported that left ventricular systolic volume was the major determinant of survival after myocardial infarction, with a left ventricular systolic volume in excess of 100ml being associated with a particularly steep decline in survival.

In this chapter, the effects of the RAS on cardiac structure, a topic covered in more detail in *Chapters 31* and *40*, are discussed briefly. Changes in cardiac structure during treatment with ACE inhibitors are subsequently outlined: definitive data from studies in man are not available, thus, much of the discussion is centered on experimental information from animal studies.

THE RENIN–ANGIOTENSIN SYSTEM AND CARDIAC STRUCTURE

The RAS appears to be intimately involved in the structural response of the left ventricle to diverse stimuli (see *Chapter 31*). First, Ang II may contribute to left ventricular hypertrophy via its direct and widespread arterial and arteriolar vasoconstrictor action and subsequent effects on left ventricular afterload. Second, Ang II can indirectly stimulate myocyte hypertrophy via its interaction with sympathetic tone [3]. Third, Ang II has a direct trophic effect on mammalian myocytes, both as a circulating hormone and probably also via the local cardiac RAS (see *Chapter 31*). Fourth, at high plasma levels, Ang II can be shown to have a myocardial toxic effect (see *Chapter 40*). Fifth, Ang II can, directly or indirectly, stimulate fibroblast proliferation [14,15] and hence the formation of collagen. Sixth, Ang II is a potent constrictor of coronary arteries [16] and may thereby contribute to myocardial ischemia in patients with coronary artery disease. Selected aspects of these effects are now discussed in brief.

Under experimental circumstances, Ang II has direct trophic effects on the myocardium (see *Chapter 31*). Angiotensin II stimulates DNA and RNA turnover in isolated myocytes [17], and protein synthesis is augmented within hours of exposure to Ang II [17-19]. These effects appear to be modulated via protein kinase C, cytosolic calcium, and activation of growth-modulating protooncogenes [20,21] (see *Chapter 31*) following localization of Ang II in the nuclear zone of the myocyte [22]. In addition, Ang II induces expression of the early growth-response gene I in rabbit myocytes [23].

The relative roles of the RAS, other trophic hormones, and hemodynamic influences on the development of ventricular hypertrophy in animals and man, have not been defined with certainty. The prevalence of an increased left ventricular mass index or wall thickness index is high in human essential hypertension [24], and despite the fact that relationships between blood-pressure levels and indices of left ventricular mass are often statistically weak [25], there seems little doubt that cardiac afterload *per se* is the major determinant of left ventricular mass. Nevertheless, it is likely that other factors are codeterminants. Positive statistical associations, which may or may not reflect cause and effect, have been noted between left ventricular mass (or wall thickness) and numerous indices including dietary intake (or urinary output) of sodium [26,27]; body weight [28,29] or body build [30]; blood viscosity [31]; plasma catecholamines [32]; and increasing age [33].

A number of authors have reported on statistical associations between activity of the RAS and indices of left ventricular mass in man. In essential hypertension, some workers report that the degree of activation of the circulating RAS is related in a positive, if statistically weak, fashion, to left ventricular hypertrophy [34–36], left ventricular systolic function [37], or cardiac index [38]. Others, however, have not found this to be so; for example, Russell and colleagues reported that electrocardiogram (EKG) voltages and the incidence of left ventricular hypertrophy (on EKG) were less in high-renin, than in normal-renin essential hypertensives [39]. Hammond *et al* [40] observed that in patients with sustained hypertension, low levels of plasma renin were associated with left ventricular hypertrophy as assessed by M-mode echocardiography. Suzuki and colleagues reported that the left ventricular mass index and relative wall thickness were similar in patients with unilateral renovascular (high-renin) hypertension and in age-, sex-, and blood-pressure-matched patients with primary (low-renin) hyperaldosteronism [41]. Furthermore, treatment of primary hyperaldosteronism results in regression of left ventricular hypertrophy [42], despite rising levels of renin and Ang II. These observations indicate that activation of the circulating RAS is not essential for the development of left ventricular hypertrophy in man. Unfortunately, the data do not clarify the role of the cardiac RAS in patients with left ventricular hypertrophy.

As discussed in *Chapter 40*, Ang II has toxic effects on the myocardium, at least under experimental circumstances. Early studies showed that cardiac myocyte injury occurred in the setting of renal ischemia [43–45]. Infusion of ischemic renal extracts or renin in nephrectomized dogs resulted in myocyte injury, while in separate experiments, myocyte necrosis could be avoided by removal of ischemic kidneys [44]. Exogenous infusion of high doses of Ang II results in focal myocardial necrosis [46,47] (see *Chapter 40*) which appears to be due, in part, to ischemia, secondary to the vascular effects of Ang II [48]. Myocyte injury is seen in association with pathophysiological levels of Ang II in such states as renovascular hypertension and heart failure. Tan and colleagues [49] showed that even low doses of exogenous Ang II administered to rats resulted in membrane changes and myocytolysis within two days and before the development of any significant rise in arterial pressure. These effects were seen with exogenous Ang II and also with increased endogenous Ang II secondary to renal ischemia. In addition to myocytolysis, fibroblast proliferation was seen within two days, and microscopic scarring at two weeks [49].

The possibility that the level of circulating Ang II in patients with mild or moderate essential hypertension modulates the risk of acute myocardial infarction is raised by the study of Alderman et al [50]. Whether this could result from an action of Ang II on the coronary vasculature, the myocardium, or both, is not known. Additional studies are needed to confirm the results of Alderman et al. These matters are reviewed in more detail in Chapter 40.

The trophic and cardiotoxic effects of Ang II may play a role in the initial cardiac response to hemodynamic overload and subsequent decompensation as described by Meerson [51] and as reviewed by Weber and Janicki [14] and Katz [52]. The initial response to hemodynamic overload as occurs with hypertension and acute myocardial infarction, is myocyte hypertrophy. While systolic function is initially preserved, progressive diastolic dysfunction, myocellular energy depletion, and myocyte necrosis and fibrosis leads to progressive left ventricular dysfunction and heart failure [52]. It seems likely that the RAS, by its known positive inotropic, trophic, and cardiotoxic effects, contributes to cardiac compensation in the short term and cardiac decompensation in the long term.

THE EFFECT OF ANGIOTENSIN-CONVERTING ENZYME INHIBITORS ON CARDIAC STRUCTURE

HYPERTENSION

Studies in man confirm that ACE inhibitors, more consistently perhaps than any other group of antihypertensive agents, reduce left ventricular mass in patients with essential hypertension [53–66,120]. The study by Shahi et al [67], however, showed no change in either left ventricular mass index or diastolic function in 20 patients with essential hypertension and diastolic dysfunction during treatment with captopril for six months. These discrepant observations are difficult to explain unless, as mentioned below, there are differential effects of individual ACE inhibitors on cardiac structure and function.

Despite concerns from animal studies that regression of left ventricular mass may have adverse consequences regarding coronary flow reserve or ventricular systolic function [68], the consensus is that systolic functioning of the left ventricle (as assessed by echocardiographic techniques) is well preserved during treatment with ACE inhibitors, and diastolic function frequently improves [53–57,59–64,66,67].

The possibility that individual ACE inhibitors have different effects on cardiac structure depending upon their varying

actions to inhibit the cardiac RAS, is raised by the study of Garavaglia [58] which reported a two-fold greater reduction in left ventricular mass with enalapril administration than with captopril or lisinopril in patients with essential hypertension, despite similar antihypertensive effects. This study requires confirmation, however, since patient numbers were small (n=8–12 per group), dose–response relationships may differ between drugs, and racial characteristics of patients in the different treatment groups were not reported.

There are, of course, limitations on the information available from echocardiography, and the results give little clue as to the structural changes in the left ventricle which result from ACE inhibitor therapy. Some insight can be gained from studies in experimental animals.

In spontaneously hypertensive rats (SHR), ACE inhibitors prevent the development, and induce regression, of established left ventricular hypertrophy to normal or near normal [67–73]. Whereas captopril and dihydralazine were equally effective in

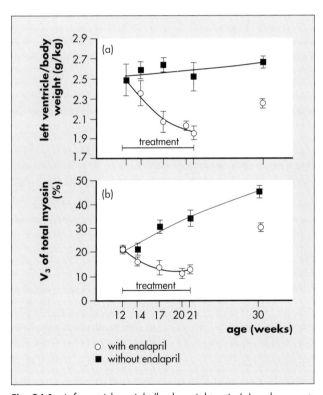

Fig. 94.1 Left ventricle weight/body weight ratio (a) and per cent myosin isoform V_3 (b) (mean ± SEM) in spontaneously hypertensive rats (SHR) with or without enalapril treatment. Twelve-week-old SHR were treated with enalapril for 0–9 weeks after which time, treatment was withdrawn. Modified from Childs TJ et al [71].

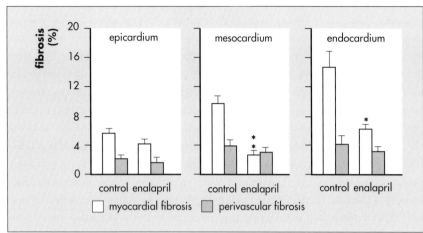

Fig. 94.2 Replacement fibrosis in the left ventricular myocardium (open bars) and around intramural vessels (tinted bars) in spontaneously hypertensive rats receiving no treatment (controls) or enalapril. Results are mean ± SEM. *P<0.02, **P<0.001 versus the control group. Modified from Pahor M et al [74].

preventing a rise in blood pressure in SHR, only the former limited cardiac hypertrophy [70]. The fact that inhibition of Ang II formation is central to the reversal of hypertrophy in these experiments in SHR is suggested by the observation that Ang II infusion during perindopril administration not only prevented the antihypertensive effect of the ACE inhibitor, but also resulted in the development of greater heart weights than in animals receiving no ACE inhibitor at all [72]. Additional effects of ACE inhibitors in SHR are normalization of the myosin isoform proportion [71] (Fig. 94.1), reduction of excess fibrosis and collagen content [69,73,74] (Fig. 94.2), improvement in cardiac performance [73,75], and a reduction in the frequency of cardiac arrhythmias [74]. Clozel and colleagues [10] reported that chronic ACE inhibition with cilazapril in SHR improved coronary vascular reserve in left and right ventricles by more than 50%, more prominently in the subendocardium than in the subepicardium. Cilazapril also increased the density and cross-sectional surface area of myocardial capillaries (Fig. 94.3) and decreased the wall/lumen ratio of arterioles in the left ventricle [10].

Similarly, in rats with 2-kidney, 1-clip renovascular hypertension, treatment with ACE inhibitors prevents the development of left ventricular hypertrophy [76] or results in regression of established left ventricular hypertrophy [73,77–79], whereas alternative antihypertensive agents fail to do so [80] and minoxidil may actually induce ventricular hypertrophy in this model [78]. Angiotensin-converting enzyme inhibition results also in normalization of the myosin isoform pattern [73,77,79,80], reduces fibrosis [76], and preserves left ventricular diastolic compliance [76]. By contrast, the increase in creatine kinase MB and BB isoforms in the myocardium of 2-kidney,

1-clip hypertensive rats was not reversed by captopril administration which might permit more efficient use of energy-rich phosphates [79].

The ACE inhibitor quinapril prevented left ventricular hypertrophy in dogs associated with intermittent hindquarter compression, whereas minoxidil failed to do so despite its antihypertensive action [81].

In rats with experimental constriction of the abdominal aorta, the circulating RAS is stimulated temporarily [82], both ACE activity [83] and angiotensinogen mRNA are increased in cardiac tissue [82], and left ventricular hypertrophy is a regular

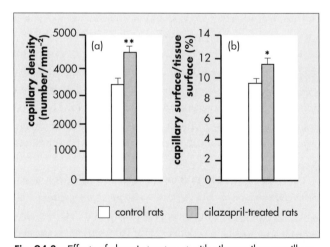

Fig. 94.3 Effects of chronic treatment with cilazapril on capillary density (a) and capillary cross-sectional surface area (b) in spontaneously hypertensive rats. *P<0.05, **P<0.001 compared to controls. Results are mean ± SEM. Modified from Clozel J-P et al [10].

occurrence [82,83]. The results from Baker *et al* [82] are of particular interest in that rats given enalapril did not develop left ventricular hypertrophy despite the fact that their cardiac afterload was similar to that in animals not receiving enalapril. These data point to Ang II having a direct trophic effect on the left ventricle in this rat model, although alternative explanations (such as a role for bradykinin or prostaglandins) are also possible. The fact that the cardiac RAS may be of importance in this regard is suggested by Linz *et al* [84] who reported that low doses of ramipril (10µg/kg) which were insufficient to reduce arterial pressure and had little effect on plasma levels of Ang II, nevertheless induced regression of left ventricular hypertrophy. These authors, using the same aortic-banded model, showed subsequently that whereas ramipril prevented the development of left ventricular hypertrophy when given from the time of surgery and induced regression when administered six weeks after surgery, the nonpeptide Ang II antagonist, losartan (DuP 753), failed to prevent hypertrophy although like ramipril, it induced regression [85]. This discrepancy could relate to involvement of different Ang II receptors in the development of ventricular hypertrophy, but it again raises the question of whether some effects of ACE inhibition on the heart might be explained by effects other than inhibition of Ang II formation.

Kromer and colleagues [86] showed that whereas quinapril failed to alter the increase in left ventricular mass in rats with supravalvular aortic stenosis if given immediately after surgery, it induced an 80% regression of established hypertrophy of the left ventricle when administered six weeks postoperation. These data differ from those of Linz [85], and suggest the possibility that individual ACE inhibitors have different effects on cardiac structure, although experimental details differ between the two studies. Zierhut *et al* [87] administered ramipril to rats with stenosis of the aortic arch, but failed to observe any effects on the development of left ventricular hypertrophy (or hypertrophy of myocytes). The explanation for this discrepant report is not obvious but could relate to the strain, age, or sex of the rats used, the site of the stenotic lesion, or the ACE inhibitor (and dose) chosen.

In rats with deoxycorticosterone (DOC)-salt hypertension, ACE inhibition failed to reduce blood pressure, reverse left ventricular hypertrophy, or alter the isomyosin pattern [88]. By contrast, in rats made hypertensive by 5/6 renal ablation and a high sodium intake, perindopril (3mg/kg) prevented the usual increase in left ventricular weight in spite of the fact that circulating renin and Ang II levels are low in this model and the ACE inhibitor did not affect the rise in arterial pressure [89]. Many

possible explanations could be invoked to explain these discrepant observations, thus more data are needed.

MYOCARDIAL ISCHEMIA, MYOCARDIAL INFARCTION, AND HEART FAILURE

The RAS appears to be important in the development and progression of left ventricular dysfunction and heart failure in ischemic heart disease. As already mentioned, Ang II is a potent constrictor of coronary arteries and, in concert with its positive inotropic action [16,90], may have adverse effects on coronary vascular reserve. The ACE inhibitors are coronary vasodilators which, in the case of very high doses of captopril and under experimental circumstances, may be augmented by a sulfhydryl-dependent vasodilating action [91]. Inhibition of ACE has been shown to limit the size of experimental myocardial infarction and to increase collateral blood flow [92]. Furthermore, ACE inhibition reduces ischemic and reperfusion arrhythmias [93–95] in association with decreased indices of myocardial ischemia [94] while also diminishing the inducibility of left ventricular arrhythmias [95]. The antifibrillatory effect of enalapril was greater than captopril, nifedipine, felodipine, or ketanserin during postischemic reperfusion in anesthetized dogs [93]. Captopril has been shown to improve postischemic contractile function [96] and while similar observations have been made with enalapril [97], conflicting data have also been reported [96], which raises the possibility that this effect may be mediated, at least in part, by the capacity of the sulfhydryl group to scavenge oxygen-free radicals.

After myocardial infarction, surviving myocytes undergo compensatory hypertrophy [98], the left ventricle dilates, remodeling occurs, [99,100], fibroblasts proliferate, and connective tissue is laid down [101]. These changes are associated with increased cardiac ACE activity [102]. Following experimental myocardial infarction in rats, ACE inhibition reduced left ventricular dilation [100,103], decreased both left ventricular mass [73,100,103,104] and fibrosis [73], and limited the decline in norepinephrine content of the noninfarcted left ventricular free wall [104]. Furthermore, left ventricular function was improved with decreased left ventricular filling pressures [100,103], normalization of the peak stroke-volume index [100], and an increased left ventricular ejection fraction [103]. These salutory effects on left ventricular structure and function persisted during captopril treatment for four months and were of similar magnitude whether the ACE inhibitor was started immediately or was delayed for 21 days after myocardial infarction [103]. Long-term follow-up of rats subjected to experimental infarction has shown that mortality is reduced, especially in animals with moderate-sized infarctions (105).

Similar beneficial effects of ACE inhibition on cardiac structure have been observed in nonischemic animal models of heart failure. In mice with Coxsackie virus B3 murine myocarditis, captopril decreased the amount of necrosis and dystrophic calcification and reduced left ventricular mass [106]. In the cardiomyopathic hamster, quinapril reduced left ventricular volumes and tended to decrease left ventricular mass in association with improved left ventricular function and increased long-term survival [107]. In rats with left ventricular volume overload secondary to aortic incompetence, captopril decreased left ventricular volume and mass [108].

Human studies following myocardial infarction have shown that captopril reduces [109,110] or prevents [111] the progressive left ventricular dilatation and decrease in left ventricular ejection fraction observed in untreated patients or in those treated with a loop diuretic. Furthermore, the SAVE trial showed that captopril reduced mortality in patients with a reduced left ventricular ejection fraction after acute myocardial infarction (*Chapter 77*). Intervention with the ACE inhibitor enalapril in human heart failure has also been shown to exert important beneficial effects on morbidity and mortality [112,113] (see *Chapter 93*). Details of the effects of ACE inhibitors on cardiac structure in man after myocardial infarction and in heart failure, however, are not available.

The mechanisms by which ACE inhibitors exert beneficial effects on cardiac structure in myocardial ischemia and in heart failure may result from a nonspecific decline in cardiac workload, the fall in circulating levels of Ang II, inhibition of the cardiac RAS, and changes in bradykinin or prostaglandin concentrations. Although hemodynamic factors are no doubt important, subhypotensive doses of ramipril prevented *ex vivo* postischemic arrhythmias and improved cardiodynamic variables after ischemia-reperfusion injuries in rats [114]. Furthermore, captopril (but not reserpine, propranolol, or phenoxybenzamine) prevented myocyte injury and fibroplasia induced by high-dose Ang II infusion in rats [49], while in cell culture studies, a specific Ang II-receptor antagonist prevented the increase in protein synthesis induced by Ang II (18). The fact that inhibition of cardiac ACE may have salutory structural effects [115] is suggested by studies showing that ramipril in doses that inhibited cardiac ACE but not the circulating enzyme, reduced myocardial infarct size and reperfusion arrhythmias in dogs [114]. Some of the responses may be accounted for by accumulation of bradykinin since the cardioprotective effect of ACE inhibitors after myocardial ischemia in dogs was mimicked by bradykinin and abolished by a bradykinin antagonist [114,116].

SYSTEMIC SCLEROSIS

The ACE inhibitors are indicated for patients with scleroderma renal crisis (see *Chapter 79*), but benefits additional to those relating to kidney function and control of arterial pressure have been reported. Kazzam and colleagues [117] documented by echocardiography, improvements in both systolic and diastolic functioning of the left ventricle in 22 patients who received captopril for 11–15 months. It is noteworthy that these patients were normotensive prior to treatment, and captopril had little or no effect on arterial pressure. The authors speculated that the effects of captopril might have been due to dilatation of coronary arterioles or inhibition of the cardiac RAS. Cardiac structural changes associated with treatment were not, of course, reported.

A report from Kahan *et al* [118] demonstrated improvements in thallium 201 myocardial perfusion in patients with systemic sclerosis who received captopril, most likely as a result of reversal in coronary microvascular dysfunction. It is possible, but unproven, that ACE inhibitors might thereby preserve cardiac structure and function in systemic sclerosis.

AGEING

In that ACE inhibitors, as discussed above, can prevent and reverse left ventricular hypertrophy and alter collagen content and myosin isoforms under some circumstances, it is relevant to enquire whether they also modify ageing-related changes in cardiac structure and function in normal, healthy individuals. Whereas no information from studies in man is known to the authors, data from experiments in rats have been reported.

Michel *et al* [88] demonstrated that ACE inhibition prevented the age-related increase in absolute and relative left ventricular weights in normotensive Wistar and Wistar–Kyoto rats. The isomyosin profile was altered by captopril toward a predominantly V_1 form in normotensive Wistar–Kyoto rats whereas ageing is usually associated with a shift toward the V_3 form [88]. In the same rats, ACE inhibition significantly decreased the collagen content of the left ventricle, but failed to alter the relative amount of collagen in the heart in adult Wistar rats [88].

Normotensive Dahl salt-resistant rats taking either a high or low salt diet exhibited a reduction in the heart weight/body weight ratio with enalapril administration [119].

While these results are of considerable interest, design of comparable studies in healthy man might present formidable problems.

SUMMARY

Angiotensin II appears to contribute to left ventricular hypertrophy and myocyte necrosis and fibrosis, and cardiac dilatation under some circumstances. It may exert its effects through hemodynamic (vasoconstrictor) actions which increase cardiac load, and also through direct or indirect trophic and/or toxic effects on the myocardium. Converting-enzyme inhibitors reverse or prevent left ventricular hypertrophy in most forms of experimental and clinical hypertension. These agents also confer important hemodynamic and prognostic benefit in cardiac failure and can prevent cardiac remodeling and progression to heart failure after experimental and clinical myocardial infarction. It appears likely that much of the benefit of ACE inhibitors is the direct result of suppression of Ang II formation. Unanswered questions include the relative importance of circulating versus tissue (cardiac) renin systems and the contribution of non-Ang II-related effects of ACE inhibition in preventing or reversing adverse changes in cardiac structure.

REFERENCES

1. Kent RL, Hoober JK, Cooper G. Load responsiveness of protein synthesis in adult mammalian myocardium: Role of cardiac deformation linked to sodium influx. *Circulation Research* 1989;64:74–85.

2. Kira Y, Kochel PJ, Gordon EE, Morgan HE. Aortic perfusion pressure as a determinant of cardiac protein synthesis. *American Journal of Physiology* 1984;246:C247–58.

3. Morgan HE, Baker KM. Cardiac hypertrophy. Mechanical, neural and endocrine dependence. *Circulation* l991;83:13–25.

4. Devereux RB. Importance of left ventricular mass as a predictor of cardiovascular morbidity in hypertension. *American Journal of Hypertension* 1989;2:650–4.

5. MacMahon S, Collins G, Rautaharju P, Cutler J, Neaton J, Prineas R, Crow R, Stamler J. Electrocardiographic left ventricular hypertrophy and effects of antihypertensive drug therapy in hypertensive participants in the multiple risk factor intervention trial. *American Journal of Cardiology* 1989;63:202–10.

6. Cooper RS, Simmons BE, Castaner A, Santhanam V, Ghali J, Mar M. Left ventricular hypertrophy is associated with worse survival independent of ventricular function and number of coronary arteries severely narrowed. *American Journal of Cardiology* 1990;65:441–5.

7. Dunn FG, McLenachan J, Isles CG, Brown I, Dargie HJ, Lever AF, Lorimer AR, Murray GD, Pringle SD, Robertson JWK. Left ventricular hypertrophy and mortality in hypertension: An analysis of data from the Glasgow Blood Pressure Clinic. *Journal of Hypertension* 1990;8:775–82.

8. Koren MJ, Devereux RB, Casale PN, Savage DD, Laragh JH. Relation of left ventricular mass and geometry to morbidity and mortality in uncomplicated essential hypertension. *Annals of Internal Medicine* 1991;114:345–52.

9. Levy D, Garrison RJ, Savage DD, Kannel WB, Castelli WP. Prognostic implications of echocardiographically determined left ventricular mass in the Framingham heart study. *New England Journal of Medicine* 1990;322:1561–6.

10. Clozel J-P, Kuhn H, Hefti F. Effect of chronic ACE inhibition on cardiac hypertrophy and coronary vascular reserve in spontaneously hypertensive rats with developed hypertension. *Journal of Hypertension* 1989;7:267–75.

11. Messerli FH, Ventura HO, Elizardi DJ, Dunn FG, Frohlich ED. Hypertension and sudden death. Increased ventricular ectopic activity in left ventricular hypertrophy. *American Journal of Medicine* 1984;77:18–22.

12. Weber KT, Janicki JS, Shroff SG, Pick R, Chen RM, Bashey RI. Collagen remodeling of the pressure-overloaded, hypertrophied nonhuman primate myocardium. *Circulation Research* 1988;62:757–65.

13. White HD, Norris RM, Brown MA, Brandt PWT, Whitlock RML, Wild CJ. Left ventricular end-systolic volume as the major determinant of survival after recovery from myocardial infarction. *Circulation* 1987;76:44–51.

14. Weber KT, Janicki JS. Angiotensin and the remodelling of the myocardium. *British Journal of Clinical Pharmacology* 1989;28 (suppl):141–50S.

15. Ganten D, Schelling P, Flugel RM, Ganten U. Effect of angiotensin and an angiotensin antagonist on iso-renin and cell growth in 3T3 mouse cells. *International Research Communications* 1975;3:327–32.

16. Fowler NO, Holmes JC. Coronary and myocardial actions of angiotensin. *Circulation Research* 1964;14:191–201.

17. Khairallah PA, Robertson AL, Davila D. Effects of angiotensin II on DNA, RNA and protein synthesis. In: Genest J, Koiw E, eds. *Hypertension 1972*. New York:Springer–Verlag, 1972:212–8.

18. Aceto JF, Baker KM. [Sar¹]angiotensin II receptor-mediated stimulation of protein synthesis in chick heart cells. *American Journal of Physiology* 1990;258:H806–13.

19. Baker KM, Aceto JF. Angiotensin II stimulation of protein synthesis and cell growth in chick heart cells. *American Journal of Physiology* 1990;259:H610–8.

20. Hoh E, Komuro I, Kurabayashi M, Katoh Y, Shibazaki Y, Yazaki Y. The molecular mechanism of angiotensin II-induced c-*fos* gene expression on rat cardiomyocytes [Abstract]. *Circulation* 1990;82 (suppl III):351.

21. Izumo S, Nadal-Ginard B, Mahdavi V. Proto-oncogene induction and reprogramming of cardiac gene expression produced by pressure overload. *Proceedings of the National Academy of Sciences of the USA* 1988;85:339–43.

22. Robertson AL, Khairallah PA. Angiotensin II: Rapid localization in nuclei of smooth and cardiac muscle. *Science* 1971;172:1138–9.

23. Neyses L, Vetter H, Sukhatme VP, Williams RS. Angiotensin II induces expression of the early growth response gene 1 in isolated adult cardiomyocytes [Abstract]. *Circulation* 1989;80 (suppl II):450.

24. Laufer E, Jennings GL, Korner PI, Dewar E. Prevalence of cardiac structural and functional abnormalities in untreated primary hypertension. *Hypertension* 1989;13:151–62.

25. Frohlich ED. Left ventricular hypertrophy, cardiac diseases and hypertension: Recent experiences. *Journal of the American College of Cardiology* 1989;14:1587–94.

26. du Cailar G, Ribstein J, Grolleau R, Mimran A. Influence of sodium intake on left ventricular structure in untreated essential hypertensives. *Journal of Hypertension* 1989;7:S258–9.

27. Schmieder RE, Messerli FH, Garavaglia GE, Nunez BD. Dietary salt intake. A determinant of cardiac involvement in essential hypertension. *Circulation* 1988;78:951–6.

28. Egan B, Fitzpatrick MA, Juni J, Buda AJ, Zweifler A. Importance of overweight in studies of left ventricular hypertrophy and diastolic function in mild systemic hypertension. *American Journal of Cardiology* 1989;64:752–5.

29. Suurkula MB, Wikstrand J, Berglund G, Sivertsson R. Body weight is more important than family history of hypertension for left ventricular function. *Hypertension* 1991;17:661–8.

30. McLenachan JM, Henderson E, Morris KI, Dargie HJ. Electrocardiographic diagnosis of left ventricular hypertrophy: Influence of body build. *Clinical Science* 1988;75:589–92.

31. Devereux RB, Drayer JIM, Chien S, Pickering TG, Letcher RL, DeYoung JL, Sealey JE, Laragh JH. Whole blood viscosity as a determinant of cardiac hypertrophy in systemic hypertension. *American Journal of Cardiology* 1984;54:592–5.

32. Trimarco B, Ricciardelli B, De Luca N, De Simone A, Cuocolo A, Galva MD, Picotti GB, Condorelli M. Participation of endogenous catecholamines in the regulation of left ventricular mass in progeny of hypertensive patients. *Circulation* 1985;72:38–46.

33. Tuzcu EM, Golz SJ, Lever HM, Salcedo EE. Left ventricular hypertrophy in persons aged 90 years and older. *American Journal of Cardiology* 1989;63:237–40.

34. Jorgensen H, Sundsfjord JA. The relation of plasma renin activity to left ventricular hypertrophy and retinopathy in patients with arterial hypertension. *Acta Medica Scandinavica* 1974;196:307–13.

35. Schmieder RE, Messerli FH, Garavaglia GE, Nunez B, MacPhee AA, Re RN. Does the renin–angiotensin–aldosterone system modify cardiac structure and function in essential hypertension? *American Journal of Medicine* 1988;84 (suppl 3A):136–41.

36. Bauwens FR, Duprez DA, De Buyzere ML, De Backer TL, Kaufman JM, Van Hoecke J, Vermeulen A, Clement DL. Influence of the arterial blood pressure and nonhemodynamic factors on left ventricular hypertrophy in moderate essential hypertension. *American Journal of Cardiology* 1991;68:925–9.

37. Dustan HP, Tarazi RC, Frohlich ED. Functional correlates of plasma renin activity in hypertensive patients. *Circulation* 1970;41:555–67.

38. London GM, Safar ME, Weiss YA, Corvol PL, Menard JE, Simon AC, Milliez PL. Relationship of plasma renin activity and aldosterone levels with hemodynamic functions in essential hypertension. *Archives of Internal Medicine* 1977;137:1042–7.

39. Russell GI, Bing RF, Thurston H, Swales JD. Plasma renin in hypertensive patients: Significance in relation to clinical and other biochemical features. *Quarterly Journal of Medicine* 1980;49:385–94.

40. Hammond IW, Devereux RB, Alderman MH, Lutas EM, Spitzer MC, Crowley JS, Laragh JH. The prevalence and correlates of echocardiographic left ventricular hypertrophy among employed patients with uncomplicated hypertension. *Journal of the American College of Cardiology* 1986;7:639–50.

41. Suzuki T, Abe H, Nagata S, Saitoh F, Iwata S, Ashizawa A, Kuramochi M, Omae T. Left ventricular structural characteristics in unilateral renovascular hypertension and primary aldosteronism. *American Journal of Cardiology* 1988;62:1224–7.

42. Pringle SD, Macfarlane PW, Isles CG, Cameron HL, Brown IA, Lorimer AR, Dunn FG. Regression of electrocardiographic left ventricular hypertrophy following treatment of primary hyperaldosteronism. *Journal of Human Hypertension* 1988;2:157–9.

43. Winternitz MC, Mylan E, Waters LL, Katzenstein R. Studies on the relation of the kidney to cardiovascular disease. *Yale Journal of Biology and Medicine* 1940;12:623–74.

44. Muirhead EE. Renal tissue and extracts vs cardiovascular injury. *Archives of Pathology* 1963;76:613–9.

45. Bhan RD, Giacomelli F, Wiener J. Ultrastructure of coronary arteries and myocardium in experimental hypertension. *Experimental and Molecular Pathology* 1978;29:66–81.

46. Gavras H, Brown JJ, Lever AF, Macadam RF, Robertson JIS. Acute renal failure, tubular necrosis, and myocardial infarction induced in the rabbit by intravenous angiotensin II. *Lancet* 1971;ii:19–22.

47. Gavras H, Kremer D, Brown JJ, Gray B, Lever AF, MacAdam RF, Medina A, Morton JJ, Robertson JIS. Angiotensin- and norepinephrine-induced myocardial lesions: Experimental and clinical studies in rabbits and man. *American Heart Journal* 1975;89:321–32.

48. Bhan RD, Giacomelli F, Wiener J. Adrenoreceptor blockade in angiotensin-induced hypertension. Effect on rat coronary artery and myocardium. *American Journal of Pathology* 1982;108:60–71.

49. Tan L-B, Jalil JE, Pick R, Janicki JS, Weber KT. Cardiac myocyte necrosis induced by angiotensin II. *Circulation Research* 1991;69:1185–95.

50. Alderman MH, Madhavan S, Ooi WL, Cohen H, Sealey JE, Laragh JH. Association of the renin–sodium profile with the risk of myocardial infarction in patients with hypertension. *New England Journal of Medicine* 1991;324:1098–104.

51. Meerson FZ. On the mechanism of compensatory hypertension and insufficiency of the heart. *Cor Vasa* 1961;3:161–77.

52. Katz AM. Cardiomyopathy of overload. A major determinant of prognosis in congestive heart failure. *New England Journal of Medicine* 1990;322:100–10.

53. Fouad FM, Tarazi RC, Bravo EL. Cardiac and haemodynamic effects of enalapril. *Journal of Hypertension* 1983;1 (suppl 1):135–42.

54. Dunn FG, Oigman W, Ventura HO, Messerli FH, Kobrin I, Frohlich ED. Enalapril improves systemic and renal hemodynamics and allows regression of left ventricular mass in essential hypertension. *American Journal of Cardiology* 1984;53:105–8.

55. Nakashima Y, Fouad FM, Tarazi RC. Regression of left ventricular hypertrophy from systemic hypertension by enalapril. *American Journal of Cardiology* 1984;53:1044–9.

56. Ventura HO, Frohlich ED, Messerli FH, Kobrin I, Kardon MB. Cardiovascular effects and regional blood flow distribution associated with angiotensin converting enzyme inhibition (captopril) in essential hypertension. *American Journal of Cardiology* 1985;55:1023–6.

57. Sheiban I, Arcaro G, Covi G, Accardi R. Zenorini C, Lechi A. Regression of cardiac hypertrophy after antihypertensive therapy with nifedipine and captopril. *Journal of Cardiovascular Pharmacology* 1987;10 (suppl 10):S187–91.

58. Garavaglia GE, Messerli FH, Nunez BD, Schmieder RE, Frohlich ED. Angiotensin converting enzyme inhibitors. Disparities in the mechanism of their antihypertensive effect. *American Journal of Hypertension* 1988;1:214–6S.

59. Muiesan ML, Agabiti-Rosei E, Romanelli G, Castellano M, Beschi M, Muiesan G. Beneficial effects of one year's treatment with captopril on left ventricular anatomy and function in hypertensive patients with left ventricular hypertrophy. *American Journal of Medicine* 1988;84 (suppl 3A):129–32.

60. Trimarco B, De Luca N, Ricciardelli B, Rosiello G, Volpe M, Condorelli G, Lembo G, Condorelli M. Cardiac function in systemic hypertension before and after reversal of left ventricular hypertrophy. *American Journal of Cardiology* 1988;62:745–50.

61. Grandi AM, Venco A, Barzizza F, Casadei B, Marchesi E, Finardi G. Effect of enalapril on left ventricular mass and performance in essential hypertension. *American Journal of Cardiology* 1989;63:1093–7.

62. Sanchez RA, Traballi CA, Marco EJ, Cianciulli T, Giannone CA, Ramirez AJ. Long-term evaluation of cilazapril in severe hypertension. Assessment of left ventricular and renal function. *American Journal of Medicine* 1989;87 (suppl 6B) 56–60S.

63. Julien J, Dufloux M-A, Prasquier R, Chatellier G, Menard D, Plouin P-F, Menard J, Corvol P. Effects of captopril and minoxidil on left ventricular hypertrophy in resistant hypertensive patients: A 6 month double-blind comparison. *Journal of the American College of Cardiology* 1990;16:137–42.

64. Schneeweiss A, Rosenthal J, Marmor A. Comparative evaluation of the acute and chronic effects of cilazapril and hydrochlorothiazide on diastolic cardiac function in hypertensive patients. *Journal of Human Hypertension* 1990;4:535–9.

65. Angermann CE, Spes CH, Willems S, Dominiak P, Kemkes BM, Theisen K. Regression of left ventricular hypertrophy in hypertensive heart transplant recipients treated with enalapril, furosemide, and verapamil. *Circulation* 1991;84:583–93.

66. Grandi AM, Venco A, Barzizza F, Petrucci E, Scalise F, Perani G, Marchesi E, Folino P, Finardi G. Double-blind comparison of perindopril and captopril in hypertension. *American Journal of Hypertension* 1991;4:516–20.

67. Shahi M, Thom S, Poulter N, Sever PS, Foale RA. The effects of blood pressure reduction on abnormal left ventricular diastolic function in hypertensive patients. *European Heart Journal* 1991;12:974–9.

68. Liebson PR. Clinical studies of drug reversal of hypertensive left ventricular hypertrophy. *American Journal of Hypertension* 1990;3:512–7.

69. Sen S, Tarazi RC, Bumpus FM. Effect of converting enzyme inhibitor (SQ14,225) on myocardial hypertrophy in spontaneously hypertensive rats. *Hypertension* 1980;2:169–76.

70. Freslon JL, Giudicelli JF. Compared myocardial and vascular effects of captopril and dihydralazine during hypertension development in spontaneously hypertensive rats. *British Journal of Clinical Pharmacology* 1983;80:533–43.

71. Childs TJ, Adams MA, Mak AS. Regression of cardiac hypertrophy in spontaneously hypertensive rats by enalapril and the expression of contractile proteins. *Hypertension* 1990;16:662–8.

72. Harrap SB, Van der Merwe WM, Griffin SA, Macpherson F, Lever AF. Brief angiotensin converting enzyme inhibitor treatment in young spontaneously hypertensive rats reduces blood pressure long-term. *Hypertension* 1990;16:603–14.

73. Michel J-B. Relationship between decrease in afterload and beneficial effects of ACE inhibitors in experimental cardiac hypertrophy and congestive heart failure. *European Heart Journal* 1990;11 (suppl D):17–26.

74. Pahor M, Bernabei R, Sgadari A, Gambassi G, Giudice PL, Pacifici L, Ramacci MT, Lagrasta C, Olivetti G, Carbonin P. Enalapril prevents cardiac fibrosis and arrhythmias in hypertensive rats. *Hypertension* 1991;18:148–57.

75. Pfeffer JM, Pfeffer MA, Mirsky I, Braunwald E. Regression of left ventricular hypertrophy and prevention of left ventricular dysfunction by captopril in the spontaneously hypertensive rat. *Proceedings of the National Academy of Sciences of the USA* 1982;79:3310–4.

76. Jalil JE, Janicki JS, Pick R, Weber KT. Coronary vascular remodeling and myocardial fibrosis in the rat with renovascular hypertension. Response to captopril. *American Journal of Hypertension* 1991;4:51–5.

77. Sen S, Young DR. Role of sodium in modulation of myocardial hypertrophy in renal hypertensive rats. *Hypertension* 1986;8:918–24.

78. Leenen FHH, Prowse S. Time-course of changes in cardiac hypertrophy and pressor mechanisms in two-kidney, one clip hypertensive rats during treatment with minoxidil, enalapril or after uninephrectomy. *Journal of Hypertension* 1987;5:73–83.

79. Pauletto P, Nascimben L, Piccolo D, Secchiero S, Vescovo G, Scannapieco G, Libera LD, Carraro U, Pessina AC, Palu CD. Ventricular myosin and creatine-kinase isoenzymes in hypertensive rats treated with captopril. *Hypertension* 1989;14:556–62.

80. Dussaule J-C, Michel J-B, Auzan C, Schwartz K, Corvol P, Menard J. Effect of antihypertensive treatment on the left ventricular isomyosin profile in one-clip, two kidney hypertensive rats. *Journal of Pharmacology and Experimental Therapeutics* 1986;236:512–8.

81. Julius S, Li Y, Brandt D, Krause L, Taylor D. Quinapril, an angiotensin converting enzyme inhibitor, prevents cardiac hypertrophy during episodic hypertension. *Hypertension* 1991;17:1161–6.

82. Baker KM, Chernin MI, Wixson SK, Aceto JF. Renin–angiotensin system involvement in pressure-overload cardiac hypertrophy in rats. *American Journal of Physiology* 1990;259:H324–32.

83. Lorrell BH, Schunkert H, Grice WN, Tang SS, Apstein CS, Dzau VJ. Alteration in cardiac angiotensin converting enzyme activity in pressure overload hypertrophy. [Abstract]. *Circulation* 1989;80 (suppl II):297.

84. Linz W, Scholkens BA, Ganten D. Converting enzyme inhibition specifically prevents the development and induces regression of cardiac hypertrophy in rats. *Clinical and Experimental Hypertension. Part A, Theory and Practice* 1989;A11:1325–50.

85. Linz W, Henning R, Scholkens BA. Role of angiotensin II receptor antagonism and converting enzyme inhibition in the progression and regression of cardiac hypertrophy in rats. *Journal of Hypertension* 1991;9 (suppl 6):S400–1.

86. Kromer EP, Elsner D, Riegger GAJ. Role of neurohumoral systems for pressure induced left ventricular hypertrophy in experimental supravalvular aortic stenosis in rats. *American Journal of Hypertension* 1991;4:521–4.

87. Zierhut W, Zimmer H-G, Gerdes AM. Effect of angiotensin converting enzyme inhibition on pressure-induced left ventricular hypertrophy in rats. *Circulation Research* 1991;69:609–17.

88. Michel J-B, Salzmann J-L, Cerol M de L, Dussaule J-C, Azizi M, Corman B, Camilleri J-P, Corvol P. Myocardial effect of converting enzyme inhibition in hypertensive and normotensive rats. *American Journal of Medicine* 1988;84 (suppl 3A):12–21.

89. Nakamura F, Nagano M, Higaki J, Higashimori K, Katahira K, Morishita R, Mikami H, Ogihara T. Regression of left ventricular hypertrophy by angiotensin converting enzyme inhibitor in reduced renal mass hypertensive rats. *Journal of Hypertension* 1991;9 (suppl 6):S398–9.

90. Moravec CS, Schluchter MD, Paranandi L, Czerska B, Stewart RW, Rosenkranz E, Bond M. Inotropic effects of angiotensin II on human cardiac muscle *in vitro*. *Circulation* 1990;82:1973–84.

91. van Gilst WH, van Wijngaarden J, Scholtens E, de Graeff PA, de Langen CDJ, Wesseling H. Captopril-induced increase in coronary flow: An SH-dependent effect on arachidonic acid metabolism? *Journal of Cardiovascular Pharmacology* 1987;9 (suppl 2):S31–6.

92. Ertl G, Kloner RA, Alexander RW, Braunwald E. Limitation of experimental infarct size by an angiotensin-converting enzyme inhibitor. *Circulation* 1982;65:40–8.

93. Elfellah MS, Ogilvie RI. Effect of vasodilator drugs on coronary occlusion and reperfusion arrhythmias in anesthetized dogs. *Journal of Cardiovascular Pharmacology* 1985;7:826–32.

94. Linz W, Scholkens BA, Han Y-F. Beneficial effects of the converting enzyme inhibitor, ramipril, in ischemic rat hearts. *Journal of Cardiovascular Pharmacology* 1986;8 (suppl 10):S91–9.

95. de Langen CDJ, de Graeff PA, van Gilst WH, Bel KJ, Kingma JH, Wesseling H. Effects of angiotensin II and captopril on inducible sustained ventricular tachycardia two weeks after myocardial infarction in the pig. *Journal of Cardiovascular Pharmacology* 1989;13:186–91.

96. Westlin W, Mullane K. Does captopril attenuate reperfusion-induced myocardial dysfunction by scavenging free radicals? *Circulation* 1988;77 (suppl I):I30–9.

97. Przyklenk K, Kloner RA. Acute effects of hydralazine and enalapril on contractile function of postischemic 'stunned' myocardium. *American Journal of Cardiology* 1987;60:934–6.

98. Anversa P, Loud AV, Levicky V, Guideri G. Left ventricular failure induced by myocardial infarction. I. Myocyte hypertrophy. *American Journal of Physiology* 1985;248:H876–82.

99. Hutchins GM, Bulkley BH. Infarct expansion versus extension: Two different complications of acute myocardial infarction. *American Journal of Cardiology* 1978;41:1127–32.

100. Pfeffer JM, Pfeffer MA, Braunwald E. Influence of chronic captopril therapy on the infarcted left ventricle of the rat. *Circulation Research* 1985;57:84–95.

101. Vracko R, Thorning D, Frederickson RG. Connective tissue cells in healing rat myocardium. *American Journal of Pathology* 1989;134:993–1006.

102. Hirsch AT, Talsness CE, Schunkert H, Paul M, Dzau VJ. Tissue-specific activation of cardiac angiotensin converting enzyme in experimental heart failure. *Circulation Research* 1991;69:475–82.

103. Gay RG. Early and late effects of captopril treatment after large myocardial infarction in rats. *Journal of the American College of Cardiology* 1990;16:967–77.

104. Ribout C, Mossiat C, Devissaguet M, Rochette L. Beneficial effect of perindopril, an angiotensin-converting enzyme inhibitor, on left ventricular performance and noradrenaline myocardial content during cardiac failure development in the rat. *Canadian Journal of Physiology and Pharmacology* 1990;68:1548–51.

105. Pfeffer MA, Pfeffer JM, Steinberg C, Finn P. Survival after an experimental myocardial infarction: Beneficial effects of long-term therapy with captopril. *Circulation* 1985;72:406–12.

106. Rezkalla S, Kloner RA, Khatib G, Khatib R. Effect of delayed captopril therapy on left ventricular mass and myonecrosis during acute Coxsackie virus murine myocarditis. *American Heart Journal* 1990;120:1377–81.

107. Haleen SJ, Weishaar RE, Overhiser RW, Bousley RF, Keiser JA, Rapundalo SR, Taylor DG. Effects of quinapril, a new angiotensin converting enzyme inhibitor, on left ventricular failure and survival in the cardiomyopathic hamster. *Circulation Research* 1991;68:1302–12.

108. Gay R. Captopril reduces left ventricular enlargement induced by chronic volume overload. *American Journal of Physiology* 1990;259:H796–803.

109. Pfeffer MA, Lamas GA, Vaughan DE, Parisi AF, Braunwald E. Effect of captopril on progressive ventricular dilatation after anterior myocardial infarction. *New England Journal of Medicine* 1988;319:80–6.

110. Oldroyd KG, Pye MP, Ray SG, Christie J, Ford I, Cobbe SM, Dargie HJ. Effects of early captopril administration on infarct expansion, left ventricular remodeling and exercise capacity after acute myocardial infarction. *American Journal of Cardiology* 1991;68:713–8.

111. Sharpe N, Murphy J, Smith H, Hannan S. Treatment of patients with symptomless left ventricular dysfunction after myocardial infarction. *Lancet* 1988;i:255–9.

112. Consensus Trial Study Group. Effects of enalapril on mortality in severe congestive heart failure. *New England Journal of Medicine* 1987;316:1429–35.

113. The SOLVD Investigators. Effect of enalapril on survival in patients with reduced left ventricular ejection fractions and congestive heart failure. *New England Journal of Medicine* 1991;325:293–302.

114. Scholkens BA, Linz W, Martorana PA. Experimental cardiovascular benefits of angiotensin-converting enzyme inhibitors: Beyond blood pressure reduction. *Journal of Cardiovascular Pharmacology* 1991;18 (suppl 2):S26–30.

115. Unger T, Ganten D, Lang RE. Effect of converting enzyme inhibitors on tissue converting enzyme and angiotensin II: Therapeutic implications. *American Journal of Cardiology* 1987;59:18–22D.

116. Martorana PA, Linz W, Scholkens BA. Does bradykinin play a role in the cardiac antiischemic effect of the ACE-inhibitors? *Basic Research in Cardiology* 1991;86: 293–926.

117. Kazzam E, Caidahl K, Hallgren R, Gustafsson R, Waldenstrom A. Non-invasive evaluation of long-term cardiac effects of captopril in systemic sclerosis. *Journal of Internal Medicine* 1991;230:203–12.

118. Kahan A, Devaux JY, Amor B, Menkes CJ, Weber S, Venot A, Strauch G. The effect of captopril on thallium 201 myocardial perfusion in systemic sclerosis. *Clinical Pharmacology and Therapeutics* 1990;47:483–9.

119. Sharma JN, Fernandez PG, Kim BK, Idikio H, Triggle CR. Cardiac regression and blood pressure control in the Dahl rat treated with either enalapril maleate (MK 421, an angiotensin converting enzyme inhibitor) or hydrochlorothiazide. *Journal of Hypertension* 1983;1:251–6.

120. Dahlöf B, Pennert K, Hansson L. Reversal of left ventricular hypertrophy in hypertensive patients. A metaanalysis of 109 treatment studies. *American Journal of Hypertension* 1992;5:95–110.

121. James MA, Jones JV. An interaction between LVH and potassium in human hypertension. *Journal of Human Hypertension* 1991;5:475–8.

95 ANGIOTENSIN-CONVERTING ENZYME INHIBITORS AND LARGE ARTERIAL STRUCTURE AND FUNCTION

MICHEL E SAFAR AND BERNARD I LEVY

Angiotensin II receptors are widely distributed throughout the vascular tree from resistance arterioles to the aorta [1]. Administration of Ang II causes a rise in blood pressure due to an increase in systemic vascular resistance, that is, a reduction in the caliber of small arteries. Angiotensin II also produces contractions in aortic strips or rings [2] as well as in isolated femoral, carotid, and coronary arteries [3–5], suggesting that the RAS acts in addition on large arteries and consequently modifies their function.

In different types of experimental hypertension, significant interactions between the RAS and large vessels have been observed. Aortic renin concentrations were found to be increased in hypertensive rats compared with normotensive controls [6,7]. In the spontaneously hypertensive rat (SHR), Asaad and Antonaccio [7] reported that the concentration of arterial wall renin correlated well with blood-pressure levels. Okamura et al [8] observed that aortic, mesenteric, and renal arterial ACE activities were increased during chronic 1-clip, 2-kidney renovascular hypertension in the rat, despite normal plasma renin activity (PRA) (see *Chapter 55*). These findings suggest that Ang II generation was increased in the arterial wall under these experimental circumstances [9–11]. Functional activity of the aortic RAS was suggested by the finding that the vascular response to ACE inhibitors was more closely correlated with vascular wall renin and ACE levels than with circulating plasma levels of renin or ACE [9–11]. Finally, there is a large body of evidence from experimental studies suggesting that the RAS and ACE inhibitors act specifically on large arterial vessels, in particular through actions on the local tissue RAS, as described in detail elsewhere in this book (see *Chapters 41–48*). It was concluded from these studies that changes in the aortic RAS were principally related to concurrent changes in blood pressure, with a cause and effect relationship being subsequently proposed. This is rather surprising since large vessels such as the aorta have no resistance function and have therefore no direct effect on the control of the level of blood pressure. The aorta has only capacitance functions which relate to the visco-elastic properties of its arterial wall [12,13].

In recent years, both experimental and clinical studies have shown that the RAS acts on the capacitance properties of the arterial system and thus *per se* influences the status of large arteries. Before considering the principal features of the RAS, ACE inhibition, and arterial vessels, it is important to consider some basic aspects of the structure and function of large arteries in animals and man.

BASIC CONCEPTS IN THE STUDY OF LARGE ARTERIES

The arterial system has two distinct but interrelated functions: to deliver an adequate supply of blood to body tissues (conduit function) and to smooth out pulsations resulting from intermittent ventricular ejection (cushioning function). These two functions may be considered independently by studying both steady and oscillatory phenomena [12–14] as shown in Fig. 95.1.

The function of arteries as conduits depends on steady components, that is, mean arterial pressure (MAP) and flow (Q), and their relationship in determining peripheral vascular resistance (VR): VR = MAP/Q. The efficiency of the conduit function depends on the caliber of small arteries and the constancy of the steady component of the pressure wave, with an almost imperceptible MAP gradient from the ascending aorta to peripheral arteries. In this respect, it has long been known that activation of the RAS increases vascular resistance, whereas ACE inhibition has the opposite effect. These findings indicate that the RAS can alter the caliber of small arteries. There is, however, much less information on interrelationships between the RAS and large arteries.

In contrast with the conduit function, the cushioning function of arteries (Windkessel effect) depends on oscillatory components of flow and pressure and their frequency-dependent relationship, that is, vascular impedance. The oscillatory component of blood pressure, which is clinically represented by pulse pressure (Fig. 95.1), varies in amplitude between central and peripheral arteries and is determined by the geometrical and visco-elastic properties of the vessels. The efficiency of the cushioning function is altered for example, with increasing age, by

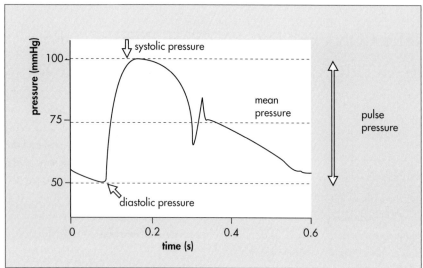

Fig. 95.1 Steady and pulsatile components of blood pressure. Any cyclic phenomenon such as blood pressure has two components: a steady component (mean arterial pressure) and a pulsatile component, which represents the cyclic variations of blood pressure around the mean and is expressed clinically by the pulse pressure. Whereas mean arterial pressure is principally influenced by vascular resistance, pulse pressure is determined largely by arterial compliance and distensibility (see text and references 12–14).

stiffening of the vessel walls, and by a reduction of the visco-elastic properties of arteries which results in a selective increase in pulse pressure without change in mean arterial pressure.

Normally, large arteries offer little resistance to flow but are distensible and consequently are able to dampen the pulsatile systolic output of the left ventricle. During ejection, the aorta and its large branches become distended, because of their storage capacity. At aortic valve closure, the elastic aorta and its branches recoil, thus sustaining the pressure head and rendering the blood flow to the periphery steadier than it would otherwise be. This characteristic buffering function is related to the visco-elastic properties of the aortic and large artery walls. Since the arteries are tube shaped, their physical properties are usually described in terms of compliance, which is measured by increasing the distending pressure (P) within the tube and recording the concomitant change in radius (or in volume, V). The volume change (dV) divided by the pressure change (dP) is arterial compliance and is represented by the slope (dV/dP) of the pressure–volume relationship (Fig. 95.2). This can be used as a quantitative index to describe the storage capacity of the arterial system. The arterial wall, which is composed of a mixture of smooth-muscle cells and connective tissue containing collagen and elastin fibers, becomes stiffer (less compliant) as it is distended [12,13]. The pressure–volume relation is thus curvilinear, and arterial compliance varies with the level of pressure. At any particular pressure level, however, compliance is also influenced by the structure of the arterial wall and by arterial smooth-muscle tone. The RAS and ACE inhibition may act on both of these aspects, as described more fully below.

In most studies described in the literature, stiffness of the arterial wall in hypertensive animals has been evaluated in strips or rings of arterial tissue [12,13,15]. Such information is limited since endothelial integrity was often not assessed, and little was done to evaluate arterial stiffness *in situ*. More recently, investigations have been carried out in living anesthetized rats with renovascular hypertension and in spontaneously hypertensive rats (SH rats). Wistar–Kyoto (WKY) (normotensive) rats served as controls [16–18]. A novel preparation utilizing 18–20mm of nonexposed common carotid large artery *in situ* has been developed in order to establish pressure–volume relationships over a wide range of transmural pressures [16–18]. As summarized in Fig. 95.3, different values of carotid compliance were obtained with increasing levels of transmural pressure in SHR and WKY rats. The relationship was parabolic in both groups. Mean carotid

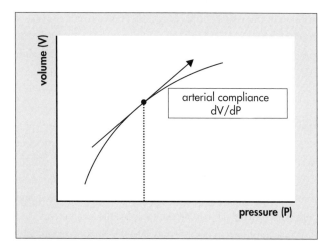

Fig. 95.2 Schematic representation of the pressure–volume relationship in a given large artery.

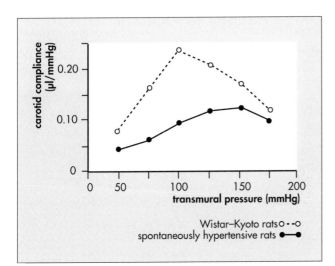

Fig. 95.3 Carotid preparation: relationships between carotid compliance and transmural pressure in normotensive (WKY) and hypertensive (SHR) rats under baseline conditions. Modified from Levy BI *et al* [16,18].

compliance varied from 0.07μl/mmHg to 0.22μl/mmHg in WKY rats and from 0.05μl/mmHg to 0.13μl/mmHg in SHR. For pressures varying from 75 to 150mmHg, the carotid compliance values in SH and WKY rats were significantly different, that is, the carotid arterial wall was stiffer in the SHR group.

In order to evaluate the influence of smooth-muscle tone on the increased arterial stiffness of hypertensive animals, the artery of the carotid preparation was washed and filled with a solution of potassium cyanide (KCN) in saline. Abolition of vascular smooth-muscle tone with the KCN solution resulted in a significant increase in carotid compliance for each level of transmural pressure (Fig. 95.4). Even after treatment with KCN, however, carotid compliance remained less in SHR than in WKY rats, suggesting that structural changes were central to the reduction in compliance in the hypertensive animals. Nevertheless, the KCN experiment indicates that smooth-muscle tone also contributed to the change in compliance.

Compliance reserve related to smooth-muscle tone (Fig. 95.4) is dependent on neurohumoral factors such as the sympathetic and the renin–angiotensin systems [12,13]. The vascular endothelium, through release of vasoactive substances [19], may also be a determinant of compliance reserve. In the carotid preparation, removal of the endothelium produced a significant increase in carotid compliance [18], which raises the possibility that altered endothelial function may contribute to compliance changes in hypertensive rats.

In conclusion, these experiments clearly show that numerous factors act on arterial compliance independent of changes in

pressure. Modifications in compliance may be mediated primarily by arterial smooth-muscle tone, with or without involvement of the endothelium. It seems likely that the RAS and ACE inhibition may modify compliance via these mechanisms. However, reduced arterial compliance is also related to structural alterations of the arterial wall, an aspect which may involve an increase in arterial smooth-muscle mass and modifications in the extra-cellular matrix. Since the RAS is capable of altering vascular structure [9–11], this mechanism is a key factor in understanding the effects of the RAS and ACE inhibition on the arterial wall.

EXPERIMENTAL STUDIES IN ANIMALS WITH HYPERTENSION

The pressure–volume relation was recorded in the carotid artery of normotensive and hypertensive rats before and after acute local administration of the ACE inhibitor, lisinopril [18]. In the presence of intact endothelium, lisinopril increased carotid compliance by 23% in WKY rats and by 14% in SHR, indicating that ACE inhibition increased arterial compliance through a reduction in arterial smooth-muscle tone. After removal of endothelium,

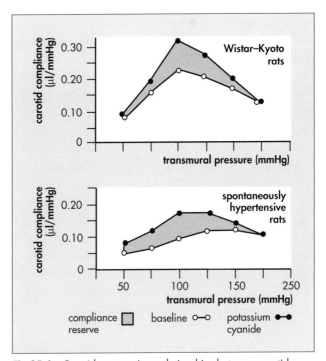

Fig.95.4 Carotid preparation: relationships between carotid compliance and transmural pressure before and after abolition of smooth-muscle tone by potassium cyanide. Modified from Levy BI *et al* [16,18].

lisinopril did not significantly increase carotid compliance in either strain, which suggests that an intact endothelium is necessary for this effect of ACE inhibition.

Carotid compliance was also evaluated during long-term treatment with the ACE inhibitor, perindopril [16, 17]. The study was performed in1-clip, 2-kidney Goldblatt hypertensive rats and in SHR. Both groups were compared to normotensive WKY rats. Treatment with perindopril for four weeks induced a significant increase in carotid compliance in both hypertensive and normotensive rats. In particular, treatment normalized carotid compliance in the renovascular hypertensive rats as compared with normotensive rats. Potassium cyanide did not produce any additional effect in the hypertensive rats, whereas it caused an increase in carotid compliance in the normotensive animals. Thus, ACE inhibition increased arterial compliance in normotensive and hypertensive rats independent of the blood-pressure level. Based on KCN experiments, these effects resulted from changes in both structural and vasomotor components of arterial compliance.

In addition to these local studies of carotid compliance, systemic hemodynamic variables were recorded at the beginning and end of the treatment period with perindopril [16,17]. The indices measured included instantaneous aortic pressure and flow velocity as recorded by the ultrasonic Doppler method. Morphological measures of the aortic media, including medial thickness, smooth muscle cells, nuclear density and size, and relative density of interstitial matrix proteins, were studied using an automated morphometrical system. In untreated animals, hypertension was associated with an increase in the characteristic impedance of the aorta and a decrease in aortic compliance. Treatment with perindopril completely reversed these *in vivo* hemodynamic markers of arterial stiffness. Morphometric analysis of the aortic wall revealed histopathological improvement in rats with renovascular hypertension (Fig. 95.5) and to a lesser extent in SHR. Treatment with perindopril reversed the increase in thickness of aortic media, with a less obvious regression of the increased absolute collagen content, and a significant decrease in the mass of arterial smooth muscle (*Fig. 95.5*). These experiments show clearly that ACE inhibition can reverse, at least in part, both the structural and the functional components of the reduced arterial compliance of hypertensive rats.

CLINICAL STUDIES

Clinical studies carried out over many years have shown that the hemodynamic abnormalities in hypertension are not limited to arterioles but also involve large arteries and result in a decrease in arterial compliance [20,21]. More recent echographic and Doppler

	Normotensive		Hypertensive	
Medial thickness (µm)		**		
Untreated	97.5 ± 4.4	***	122.3 ± 3.7	
	***	***	**	*
Treated	90.7 ± 2.7		103 ± 4.8	
Elastin density (%)		**		
Untreated	38.6 ± 12.8		31.9 ± 8.3	
		*		NS
Treated	42.5 ± 9.2		34.9 ± 5.7	
Elastin fiber thickness (µm)		NS		
Untreated	3.21 ± 0.40		3.25 ± 0.26	
				NS
Treated	3.38 ± 0.42		3.15 ± 0.16	
Collagen density (%)		**		
Untreated	7.3 ± 2.4		8.6 ± 3.6	
		**		NS
Treated	7.0 ± 2.14	**	10.6 ± 2.8	
Collagen fiber thickness (µm)		**		
Untreated	1.29 ± 0.04	**	1.38 ± 0.12	
		**		NS
Treated	1.30 ± 0.04	**	1.37 ± 0.07	
Nucleus density (numbers/field)		NS		
Untreated	38.4 ± 4.2		35.4 ± 5.5	
		**		*
Treated	40.7 ± 5.2		39.3 ± 5.3	
Nucleus cross-sectional area (µm²)		*		
Untreated	7.38 ± 0.78	**	8.58 ± 1.54	
				NS
Treated	7.55 ± 0.74		7.47 ± 0.94	

* = P<0.05 *** = P<0.001

** = P<0.01 NS = not significant.

Fig. 95.5 Histopathological changes of the aortic wall before and after converting-enzyme inhibition in 1-clip, 2-kidney hypertensive rats and in normotensive (Wistar–Kyoto) rats. Data are means ± 1 SEM. Modified from Levy BI *et al* [16].

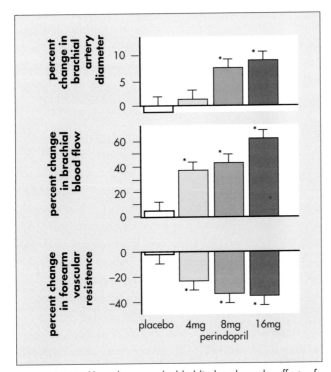

Fig. 95.6 Healthy volunteers: double-blind study on the effects of placebo and various doses of perindopril on brachial artery diameter and blood flow, and forearm vascular resistance (mean ± 1SEM). Significant changes are indicated by asterisks. Modified from Richer C *et al* [24].

methods have permitted noninvasive investigation of large arteries *in situ* [22,23]; for example it has been possible to study the

inner diameter and cross-sectional area of straight superficial arteries, and the brachial and the common carotid arteries. Since it is not possible to evaluate the overall pressure–volume relationship of a given large artery in man, it has been necessary to develop and validate satisfactory models for the determination of forearm and systemic compliance [20, 21]. When evaluating the effect of ACE inhibitors on large arteries, it must be remembered that a decrease in the distending blood pressure *per se* modifies the geometry of the arterial vessel, resulting in a passive decrease in arterial diameter (D) and volume (V) and hence a change in arterial compliance (dV/dP) (see *Figs. 95.1* and *3*). If an antihypertensive agent acts specifically on the arterial wall, independent of transmural pressure, one or both of the following characteristics may be observed: an increase in arterial diameter despite blood-pressure reduction or a change in compliance unrelated to the level of blood pressure.

In healthy volunteers given an unrestricted sodium diet, increasing doses of the ACE inhibitor perindopril were administered orally [24]. At low doses the drug induced preferential dilation of arterioles and had little effect on systemic blood pressure. In contrast, increases in brachial and carotid arterial diameter required doses that were two or three times higher (Fig. 95.6). Since ACE activity disappeared from the plasma even at the lower doses, diameter enlargment of the larger arteries might relate to inhibition of tissue ACE with higher doses of perindopril.

In patients with sustained essential hypertension, the oral administration of captopril caused a significant acute increase in the diameter of the brachial and, to a much lesser extent, the carotid arteries [23]. With intravenous perindoprilat, the

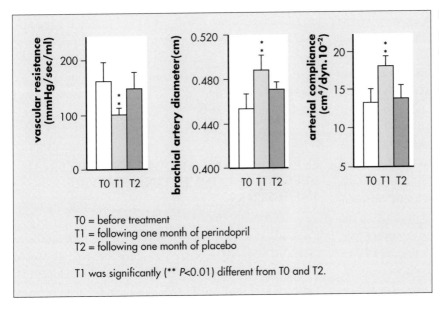

TO = before treatment
T1 = following one month of perindopril
T2 = following one month of placebo

T1 was significantly (** *P*<0.01) different from T0 and T2.

Fig. 95.7 Effects of long-term treatment by perindopril on brachial artery diameter and compliance and forearm vascular resistance in comparison with placebo (mean ± SEM). Modified from Asmar RG *et al* [29].

increase in brachial artery diameter of hypertensives was obtained with higher doses than was needed for forearm arteriolar dilatation [25], as had been observed earlier in normotensive subjects [24]. With ramipril, the response was shown to be long lasting with a somewhat greater increase in diameter in hypertensive compared with normotensive subjects for the same dosage [26,27]. With chronic oral administration of enalapril or perindopril, the increase in diameter was maintained during treatment periods of 1–12 months in hypertensive subjects [28–30] (Fig. 95.7).

Since the above findings were obtained in the presence of a significant fall in blood pressure, it seems clear that the dilating effect of ACE inhibition overcomes any pressure-related tendency for arterial diameter to decrease. Indeed it has been shown for the brachial artery that the greater the blood-pressure reduction during captopril administration the less was the associated increase in arterial diameter [31]. Thus clinical studies strongly suggest that in normotensive and hypertensive subjects, ACE inhibition has a special effect on the geometry of the walls of large arteries, independent of blood-pressure changes.

In man, the pharmacological effects of ACE inhibition on the vessel wall have been related principally to blockade of the RAS. Injections of Ang I and Ang II, with and without various ACE inhibitors, into the brachial artery indicate involvement of the RAS in regulating forearm vascular tone [32]. Additional factors may also be involved, including local increases in bradykinin and prostaglandins, and autonomic nervous system blockade [32–34]. In man, it is probable that each of these contributes to large artery dilatation during ACE inhibition. However, the intravenous administration of subpressor doses of Ang II in normotensive and hypertensive subjects induced no change in brachial artery diameter [35]. One possible explanation for this apparent discrepancy is that ACE inhibition acts not only on the systems noted above but also through a change in endothelial function, as suggested by animal experiments [18]. Indeed, vascular endothelial cells are one of the specific sites of action for bradykinin and ACE, and might be involved in producing an increase in brachial diameter with ACE inhibition [9,10].

In hypertensive subjects, the increase in brachial artery diameter following ACE inhibition was found to be associated with an increase in blood-flow velocity [29,30]. This raised the question of whether the velocity change (due to forearm arteriolar dilation) contributed to the increase in arterial diameter via the mechanism of high flow dilation, which in turn is dependent upon the status of the endothelium [36–38]. Studies in dogs have shown that both epicardial coronary and femoral arteries dilate in response to an increase in blood flow. Any factor that increases flow, such as

release of a transient arterial occlusion, causes dilatation of large arteries. If the increase in flow is prevented by a limiting stenosis, however, no dilatation of the large vessels occurs. Removal of the endothelium in isolated perfused canine coronary or femoral arteries *in situ* also abolishes flow-dependent dilatation [39].

In a study with perindopril in hypertensive subjects, the role of flow-dependent dilatation in the brachial artery was evaluated by studying the hemodynamic effects of wrist occlusion at a supra-systolic blood-pressure level [29,30]. This maneuver caused a consistent reduction in brachial artery diameter and blood-flow velocity during administration of either placebo or perindopril. Although brachial arterial diameter decreased with wrist occlusion during perindopril treatment, it remained greater than during placebo administration. These findings support the hypothesis that high flow dilatation accounts in part for the increase in brachial artery diameter, but also suggest that direct smooth-muscle relaxation occurs following inhibition of ACE.

Acute and long-term administration of captopril, enalapril, perindopril, or ramipril [26–31] in patients with essential hypertension resulted in a significant increase in arterial compliance, which was observed both in the systemic and in the brachial circulations, and in an increase in arterial diameter (Fig. 95.7). Several mechanisms may contribute to the increase in compliance [26,29,30,40,41]. A reduction in blood pressure *per se* lessens stretch of the arterial wall thereby favoring a compliance increase. With ACE inhibition however, the increase in diameter would tend to maintain stretch despite the reduction in blood pressure. Indeed stretch is related to tangential tension, which is the product of blood pressure and arterial radius. The effects of ACE inhibition on smooth muscle would favor arterial relaxation with a resulting increase in compliance, as has been observed in studies of animal hypertension. Finally, in clinical studies, it is probable that ACE inhibition improves the functional component of arterial compliance. Since it is not as yet possible to measure arterial wall thickness in man, however, it is difficult to evaluate the effects of ACE inhibition on the structural component of arterial compliance, as described above in animal experiments.

CONTRASTING CARDIAC AND ARTERIAL EFFECTS OF CONVERTING-ENZYME INHIBITION

There is a close interrelationship between the heart and large vessels in the regulation of blood flow. In this respect, the load on the heart comprises not only vascular resistance (resulting from constriction of small arteries) but also a number of other factors including capacitance of the arterial system [12,13]. Thus, changes in aortic compliance may influence the structure and function of the heart.

Studies in our laboratory [42–44] have shown that the degree of cardiac hypertrophy in man is influenced not only by levels of blood pressure and vascular resistance, but also by aortic distensibility and compliance. For a given value of mean blood pressure, there is an inverse relationship between aortic distensibility and the degree of left ventricular hypertrophy. Since cardiac hypertrophy in clinical hypertension is more closely correlated with systolic than with diastolic pressure, it seems possible that a reduction in aortic distensibility and compliance favors a disproportionate increase in systolic pressure, thus causing a more pronounced elevation of end-systolic stress and ultimately in cardiac mass. Here, it should be noted that dihydralazine-like drugs, which do not modify arterial compliance, have minimal effects on cardiac hypertrophy [45,46]. In contrast, antihypertensive drugs which increase arterial distensibility and compliance, such as ACE inhibitors, are able to reverse cardiac

hypertrophy substantially [29,30,45]; for example, perindopril therapy for three months caused a significant decrease in left ventricular mass in patients with essential hypertension, principally because of a decrease in septal and posterior-wall thickness [29,30]. Four weeks after treatment was stopped, cardiac mass remained low, whereas blood pressure and brachial artery compliance had returned toward baseline values. Re-introduction of perindopril for one year resulted in a further decrease in cardiac mass while brachial artery compliance increased again to values obtained after three months of treatment. Such findings strongly suggest that the time constants for reversal of cardiac and arterial changes are different in treated hypertensive subjects. One possible explanation is that reversion of structural changes in large arteries is limited because of their relatively high content of collagen [47,48].

The dissociation between cardiac and arterial effects during long-term treatment by perindopril was also studied in normotensive (WKY) and hypertensive (SHR) rats [49] (Fig. 95.8). The blood-pressure reduction was associated with a

| | Normotensive rats (WKY) | | Hypertensive rats (SHR) | | ANOVA Difference between: | |
	Placebo	Perindopril	Placebo	Perindopril	Strains	Treatments
mean arterial pressure (mmHg)	96 ± 3	* 81 ± 5	132 ± 6	*** 102 ± 7	***	***
heart rate (beats/min)	308 ± 7	NS 320 ± 12	372 ± 10	NS 349 ± 10	***	NS
cardiac output (ml/min)	58 ± 2	* 68 ± 5	39 ± 2	* 49 ± 6	***	**
total peripheral resistance (mmHg/ml/sec)	100 ± 5	NS 75 ± 6	212 ± 16	** 157 ± 27	***	**
systemic arterial compliance (μl/mmHg)	5.9 ± 0.3	** 8.2 ± 1.1	3.1 ± 0.2	* 5.0 ± 0.7	***	**
body weight (g)	416 ± 9	NS 439 ± 7	388 ± 3	NS 379 ± 9	***	NS
left ventricular weight (mg)	741 ± 11	NS 842 ± 29	1019 ± 30	* 940 ± 29	***	NS
left ventricular weight/body weight (mg/g)	1.79 ± 0.02	NS 1.92 ± 0.05	2.64 ± 0.06	* 2.48 ± 0.06	***	NS
medial thickness (μm)	99.8 ± 1.3	NS 98.3 ± 1.9	129.3 ± 4.1	*** 108.3 ± 3.1	***	***

* = $P < 0.05$; ** = $P < 0.01$; *** = $P < 0.001$; NS = Not significant.

Fig. 95.8 Hemodynamic and morphological changes in the heart and aorta following long-term treatment by perindopril. Data are means ± 1 SEM. Modified from Levy BI et al [49].

decrease in vascular resistance and an increase in systemic arterial compliance. The latter change was substantially more pronounced in normotensive than in hypertensive rats. In normotensive rats, there was no change in cardiac mass or aortic medial thickness. In hypertensive rats, while aortic medial thickness returned toward normotensive values, left ventricular mass decreased significantly but was not normalized.

Here again, there was a dissociation between effects on arterial and cardiac structure. In this respect, it is important to note that before treatment with the ACE inhibitor, a negative relationship was observed between cardiac hypertrophy and systemic arterial compliance in both the SHR and WKY rats. This relationship disappeared with treatment, once more confirming the dissociation between cardiac and arterial changes.

In conclusion, both clinical and experimental data clearly indicate that cardiac and arterial effects may be dissociated following long-term treatment with ACE inhibitors. Whether this is related to different time constants for remodeling of separate components of the cardiovascular system, to sluggish reversal of collagen changes or to other factors, remains to be determined.

Investigation of this dissociation may be important in clinical medicine for understanding the effects of long-term antihypertensive therapy. Indeed, the complications of hypertension can be separated into those that are pressure related such as stroke, aneurysm, left ventricular hypertrophy, and congestive heart failure, and those which relate to microvascular changes and atherosclerosis and predispose to cerebral, coronary, renal, and limb ischemia or infarction. The disturbing failure of antihypertensive drugs to reduce the incidence of myocardial infarction [50] has focused attention on structural and functional alterations within the arterial system and has stimulated a search for a better understanding of the effects of specific antihypertensive drugs on the arterial wall. It appears that with some forms of drug treatment, blood pressure is significantly decreased whereas arterial and cardiac lesions are little affected. Whether the specific arterial effects of ACE inhibitors have implications for the prevention of some complications in patients with hypertension has not been demonstrated and requires further investigation.

REFERENCES

1. Lin SY, Goodfriend TL. Angiotension receptors. *American Journal of Physiology* 1970;218:1319–28.

2. Penit J, Faure M, Jard S. Vasopressin and angiotensin II receptors in rat aortic smooth muscle cells in culture. *American Journal of Physiology* 1983;244:E72–82.

3. Toda N. Endothelium dependent relaxation induced by angiotensin II and histamine in isolated arteries of dog. *British Journal of Pharmacology* 1984;81:301–7.

4. Bolton TB. Mechanisms of action of transmitters and other substances on smooth muscle. *Physiological Reviews* 1979;68:606–24.

5. Ichikawa I, Brenner BM. Glomerular action of angiotensin II. *American Journal of Medicine* 1984;76:43–9.

6. Aguilera G, Catt K. Regulation of vascular angiotensin II receptors in the rat during altered sodium intake. *Circulation Research* 1981;49:751–8.

7. Asaad MM, Antonaccio MJ. Vascular wall renin in spontaneously hypertensive rats; potential relevance to hypertension maintenance and antihypertensive effect of captopril. *Hypertension* 1982;4:487–93.

8. Okamura T, Myazaki M, Inagami T, Toda N. Vascular renin–angiotensin system in two kidney, one clip hypertensive rats. *Hypertension* 1986;8:560–71.

9. Dzau VJ. Significance of vascular renin–angiotensin pathways. *Hypertension* 1986;8:553–9.

10. Dzau VJ, Safar ME. Large conduit arteries in hypertension: Role of the vascular renin–angiotension system. *Circulation* 1988;77:947–53.

11. Dzau VJ. Vascular renin–angiotensin: A possible autocrine or paracrine system in control of vascular function. *Journal of Cardiovascular Pharmacology* 1984;6 (suppl):377–82.

12. Milnor WR. *Hemodynamics.* Baltimore: Williams and Wilkins, 1972.

13. O'Rourke MF. *Arterial function in health and disease.* Edinburgh: Churchill-Livingstone Publishers, 1982.

14. Safar ME. Pulse pressure in essential hypertension: Clinical and therapeutical implications: Editorial review. *Journal of Hypertension* 1989;7:769–76.

15. Dobrin PB. Vascular mechanics. In: Shepherd JT, Abboud FM, eds. *Handbook of Physiology, sect. 2, The cardiovascular system, vol III, Peripheral circulation and organ blood flow, pt 1.* Bethesda, Maryland: American Physiological Society 1983:65–102.

16. Levy BI, Michel JB, Salzmann JL, Azizi M, Poitevin P, Safar ME, Camilleri JP. Effects of chronic inhibition of converting enzyme on mechanical and structural properties of arteries in rat renovascular hypertension. *Circulation Research* 1988;63:227–9.

17. Levy BI, Michel JB, Salzmann JL, Azizi M, Poitevin P, Camilleri JP, Safar ME. Arterial effects of converting enzyme inhibition in renovascular and spontaneously hypertensive rats. *Journal of Hypertension* 1988;6 (suppl 3): 23–5.

18. Levy BI, Benessiano J, Poitevin P, Safar ME. Endothelium-dependent mechanical properties of the carotid artery in WKY and SHR; role of angiotensin converting enzyme inhibition. *Circulation Research* 1990;66:321–8.

19. Furchgott RF. Role of the endothelium in responses of vascular smooth muscle. *Circulation Research* 1983;53:557–69.

20. Safar ME, Simon ACh. Hemodynamics in systolic hypertension. In: Zanchetti A, Tarazi RC, eds. *Handbook of Hypertension, vol 7, Pathophysiology of Hypertension, Cardiovascular Aspects.* Amsterdam: Elsevier Science Publishers, 1986:255–61.

21. Safar ME, London GM. Arterial and venous compliance in sustained essential hypertension. *Hypertension* 1987;10:133–9.

22. Safar ME, Peronneau PP, Levenson JA, Simon ACh. Pulsed Doppler: Diameter, velocity and flow of the brachial artery in sustained essential hypertension. *Circulation* 1981;63:393–400.

23. Bouthier JD, Safar ME, Benetos A, Simon ACh, Levenson JA, Hugue ChM. Haemodynamic effects of vasodilating drugs on the common carotid and brachial circulations of patients with essential hypertension. *British Journal of Clinical Pharmacology* 1986;21:136–42.

24. Richer C, Thuillez C, Giudicelli JP. Perindopril, converting enzyme blockade, and peripheral arterial hemodynamics in the healthy volunteer. *Journal of Cardiovascular Pharmacology* 1987;9:94–102.

25. Benetos A, Santoni JP, Safar ME. Vascular effects of intravenous infusion of the ACE inhibitor perindoprilat. *Journal of Hypertension* 1990;8:819–26.

26. Safar ME, Laurent SL, Bouthier JD, London GM, Mimran AR. Effects of converting enzyme inhibitors on hypertensive large arteries in humans. *Journal of Hypertension* 1986;4 (suppl 5):285–9.

27. Benetos A, Vasmant D, Drouhin K, Safar M. Arterial effects of acute and chronic ACE inhibition [Abstract]. *American Journal of Hypertension* 1990;3:124.

28. Simon ACh, Levenson JA, Bouthier JE, Benetos A, Achimastos A, Fouchard M, Maarek Safar M. Comparison of oral MK 421 and propranolol in mild to moderate essential hypertension and their effects on arterial and venous vessels of the forearm. *American Journal of Cardiology* 1984;53:781–5.

29. Asmar RG, Pannier B, Santoni JPh, Laurent St, London GM, Levy BI, Safar ME. Reversion of cardiac hypertrophy and reduced arterial compliance following converting enzyme inhibition in essential hypertension. *Circulation* 1988;78:941–50.

30. Asmar RG, Journo HJ, Lacolley PJ, Santoni JP, Billaud E, Safar ME. One year treatment with perindopril: Effect on cardiac mass and arterial compliance in essential hypertension. *Journal of Hypertension* 1988;6 (suppl 3):33–9.

31. Simon ACh, Levenson JA, Bouthier JL, Safar ME. Captopril-induced changes of large arteries in essential hypertension. *American Journal of Medicine* 1984;76 (5B):71–6.

32. Webb DJ, Collier JG, Seidelin PH, Struthers AD. Regulation of regional vascular tone: The role of angiotensin conversion in human forearm resistance vessels. *Journal of Hypertension* 1988;6 (suppl 3):57–9.

33. Webb DJ, Collier JG. Vascular angiotensin conversion in humans. *Journal of Cardiovascular Pharmacology* 1986;9 (suppl 10):40–4.

34. Webb DJ, Seidelin PH, Benjamin N, Collier JG, Struthers AD. Sympathetically mediated vasoconstriction is augmented by angiotensin II in man. *Journal of Hypertension* 1988;6 (suppl 4):542–3.

35. Laurent S, Lacolley P, Billaud E, Arcaro G, Safar M. Large and small forearm arteries of essential hypertensives are less reactive to angiotensin II than to noradrenaline. *Journal of Hypertension* 1989;7 (suppl 6):76–7.

36. Hantze TH, Vatner SF. Reactive dilation of large coronary arteries in conscious dogs. *Circulation Research* 1984;54:50–7.

37. Jaffe MD. High flow dilation. *Lancet* 1981;i:1237–8.

38. Hilton SM. A peripheral arterial conducting mechanism underlying dilation of the femoral artery and concerned in functional vasodilatation in skeletal muscle. *Journal of Physiology* 1959;149:93–111.

39. Pohl U, Holtz J, Busse R, Bassenge E. Crucial role of endothelium in the vasodilator response to increased flow *in vivo*. *Hypertension* 1986;8:37–44.

40. Simon AC, Levenson J, Bouthier JD, Safar ME. Effects of chronic administration of enalapril and propranolol on the large arteries in essential hypertension. *Journal of Cardiovascular Pharmacology* 1985;7:856–61.

41. Safar ME, Laurent S, Bouthier JA, London GM. Comparative effects of captopril and isosorbide dinitrate on the arterial wall of hypertensive human brachial arteries. *Journal of Cardiovascular Pharmacology* 1986;8:1257–61.

42. Bouthier JD, De Luca N, Safar ME, Simon ACh. Cardiac hypertrophy and arterial distensibility in essential hypertension. *American Heart Journal* 1985;109:1345–52.

43. Safar ME, Totomoukouo JJ, Bouthier JA, Asmar RE, Levenson JA, Simon ACh, London GM. Arterial dynamics, cardiac hypertrophy and anti-hypertensive treatment. *Circulation* 1987;75 (suppl 1):156–61.

44. Isnard RN, Pannier BM, Laurent ST, London GM, Diebold, Safar ME. Pulsatile diameter and elastic modulus of the aortic arch in essential hypertension: A noninvasive study. *Journal of the American College of Cardiology* 1989;13:399–405.

45. Tarazi RC. Regression of left ventricular hypertrophy: Partial answers for persistent questions. *Journal of the American College of Cardiology* 1984;3:1349–54.

46. Bouthier JA, Safar ME, Curien ND, London GM, Levenson JA, Simon AC. Effects of cadralazine on brachial artery hemodynamics and forearm venous tone in essential hypertension. *Clinical Pharmacology and Therapeutics* 1986;39:82–8.

47. Rorive GL, Carlier PG, Foidart JM. The structural responses of the vascular wall in experimental hypertension. In: Zanchetti A, Tarazi RC, eds. *Handbook of hypertension, vol 7. Pathophysiology of hypertension. Cardiovascular aspects.* Amsterdam: Elsevier 1986:427–53.

48. Ooshima A, Fuller GC, Cardinate GJ, Spector S, Udenfriend S. Increased collagen synthesis in blood vessels of hypertensive rats and its reversal by antihypertensive agents. *Proceedings of the National Academy of Sciences of the USA* 1974;71:3019–23.

49. Levy BI, Michel JB, Salzmann JL, Devissaguet M, Safar ME. Remodeling of heart and arteries by chronic converting enzyme inhibition in spontaneously hypertensive rats. *American Journal of Hypertension* 1991;4:2405–55.

50. Thompson SG. An appraisal of the large scale trials of antihypertensive treatment. In: Bulpitt CJ, ed. *Handbook of hypertension, vol 6, epidemiology of hypertension.* Amsterdam: Elsevier, 1985:331–3.

96 ANGIOTENSIN-CONVERTING ENZYME INHIBITORS AND RESISTANCE ARTERIAL STRUCTURE

ANTHONY M HEAGERTY, ALEX A OLDHAM, AND SARAH J BARNES

INTRODUCTION

In established human essential hypertension, it has been demonstrated that there is an increase in peripheral vascular resistance and that cardiac output is normal [1]. Furthermore, this increase in resistance to blood flow appears to be maintained by a pressure-induced rise in the wall thickness-to-lumen diameter ratio in resistance vessels. During reactive hyperemia, there is good evidence to indicate that vascular resistance in the forearm and hand remains high even under resting conditions [2,3]. Direct examination of subcutaneous resistance vessels in human essential hypertension has confirmed that there is an adaptive structural alteration proportional to the degree of hypertension, and that there is no evidence of increased sensitivity to vasoconstrictor stimuli such as norepinephrine [4]. Indirect measurements of the coronary circulation suggest that such changes are also present in the myocardial resistance vessels and serve to reduce coronary reserve in hypertension [5].

In the light of these findings and due to the disappointing impact that antihypertensive treatment has had on death from coronary heart disease, attention has turned towards the possibility of not only lowering blood pressure but also reversing the structural changes in the circulation. While the exact nature of the histological change that human hypertension brings about in resistance vessels still remains controversial [6,7], this field has been given added impetus by the findings from cultured smooth-muscle cells that pressor stimuli such as Ang II can induce pressure-independent growth responses [8]. Thus, there is the intriguing possibility that agents that not only lower blood pressure but also interfere with the generation of Ang II may be superior to other drugs in achieving the goal of reversing vascular structural changes.

The purpose of this chapter is to examine the effects of ACE inhibitors in this context. To date, most of the work in this area has employed the spontaneously hypertensive rat (SHR) as a model of human hypertension. Thus, reports on the effects of ACE inhibitors on resistance vessel structure in the SHR will be cited together with their possible drawbacks. The effects of ACE inhibitors on other components of the circulation such as the heart and large arteries, are discussed in *Chapters 77, 94*, and *95*.

BACKGROUND

In the SHR, the histological change that underlies the adaptive structural alterations of the resistance vasculature is still a contentious issue, but a large body of evidence suggests that there is hyperplasia of the medial muscle layers that encroach upon the lumen by inward growth. Some workers maintain that this hyperplasia is present, to a certain degree, in the prehypertensive state and that the adaptive change induced by the rise in pressure is then one of hypertrophy superimposed upon early exaggerated growth [9]. Therefore, when treating the genetically hypertensive rat at least, there is the opportunity to reverse a structural change in resistance vessels which can be ascribed to growth of the media.

Folkow and colleagues demonstrated that if part of a vascular bed in the young SHR is protected from the rise in blood pressure, or if neurogenic excitatory influences are interrupted by immunosympathectomy in neonatal SHR, the structural adjustments largely fail to develop [10,11]. Prolonged treatment of young SHR with β-adrenoreceptor antagonists will produce similar results [12]. These studies are mentioned because of the probable importance of autonomic overactivity in initiating genetic hypertension and the subsequent structural changes seen in the circulation; this may be of considerable significance when examining the effects of ACE inhibitors in treating SHR. In determining the implications of cardiovascular structural alterations induced by hypertension, it is interesting that treatment of SHR with hydralazine and guanethidine from the age of 10 weeks until eight months, prevented the development of vascular growth and also prolonged survival [13]. It is also important to note that such regression was not seen when rats with established structural changes were treated [13].

STUDIES WITH ANGIOTENSIN-CONVERTING ENZYME INHIBITORS

In accord with the above findings, when ACE inhibitors were used to treat young SHR, it soon became clear that the subsequent development of hypertension could be substantially attenuated [14]. The first observations on vascular structure appeared in 1980 when Giudicelli and colleagues administered captopril (100mg/kg), atenolol (200mg/kg), or hydralazine (25mg/kg) daily to SHR from 6 until 20 weeks of age [15]. They reported that captopril almost completely inhibited the development of hypertension but so also did atenolol and hydralazine. A derived estimate of peripheral vascular resistance was reported for control and captopril-treated SHR only, which indicated that the increased vascular resistance seen in the control SHR did not occur to the same extent in the treated rats, although it did rise significantly with time. The interesting observation was that when treatment was withdrawn at 20 weeks of age, the blood pressure of the rats that had received atenolol or hydralazine promptly rose to levels seen in comparably aged SHR that had never received therapy, whereas only a small, slow rise in pressure was seen in the animals that had been given captopril (Fig. 96.1) [15].

The same group of workers subsequently examined resistance vessel structure directly [16]. Spontaneously hypertensive rats were treated as before with dihydralazine or captopril from the age of six weeks until the experiment ended at 20 weeks [16], and vascular morphology was examined at 20 and 27 weeks. Both drugs attenuated the rise in blood pressure to a similar extent during the treatment period, but pressures rose more rapidly after withdrawal of dihydralazine. Resistance artery structure was examined in the first-order branches of the mesenteric arcade and the results were expressed in terms of medial wall thickness to lumen diameter ratio (M:L ratio). At 20 weeks of age, both drugs had produced a reduction in the M:L ratio, the effect being greater in the captopril-treated group. Seven weeks after withdrawal of therapy, the dihydralazine-treated animals had M:L ratios only slightly less than those recorded in untreated SHR, but in captopril-treated animals, the ratios remained significantly lower. It is interesting that the rise in the M:L ratio in hydralazine-treated rats after drug withdrawal was 18%, whereas in the captopril-treated animals it was 30.2% despite the greater rise in pressure in the former group of animals. This suggests that factors other than changes in vascular structure may contribute to the subsequent rise in pressure. This is further discussed later.

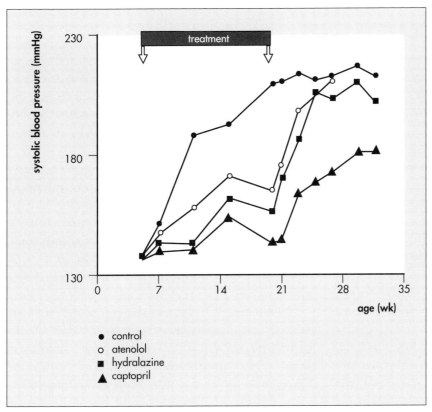

Fig. 96.1 Treatment of spontaneously hypertensive rats (SHR) with atenolol, hydralazine, or captopril for 14 weeks. After cessation of therapy, there is an abrupt rise in pressure to untreated SHR blood-pressure levels in the atenolol and hydralazine groups but only a slow rise in the captopril group. Modified from Giudicelli JF et al [15].

In an attempt to study what happens to established vascular structure, Limas *et al* treated 21 one-week-old SHR with hydralazine (20–22mg/kg) and hydrochlorothiazide (12mg/kg), captopril (50–60mg/kg) and hydrochlorothiazide (12mg/kg), or hydrochlorothiazide alone (12mg/kg) [17]. Animals were sacrificed at week 27 or 28. Each regimen lowered blood pressure although the effect was less in the diuretic-treated group. Quantitative study of the intrarenal arterial vessels demonstrated that untreated SHR had greater M:L ratios compared with normotensive Wistar–Kyoto (WKY) rats. The captopril–hydrochlorothiazide combination almost completely restored the M:L ratio to normotensive values. Hydralazine combined with hydrochlorothiazide also reduced the M:L ratio but not as effectively as captopril plus diuretic. Hydrochlorothiazide alone had no impact on the M:L ratio, and the overall impression was that the degree of regression was dependent on the efficacy of treatment in lowering pressure [17].

More recently, studies of the chronic effects of ACE inhibitors have been carried out. Harrap *et al* treated SHR with perindopril (3mg/kg daily) or vehicle from 4–16 weeks of age and reported that the blood pressure failed to rise to untreated levels after cessation of therapy [18]. It should be pointed out, however, that no other drugs were used for comparison. These findings were confirmed and extended by Cadilhac and Giudicelli [19], who also reported that perindopril (16mg/kg daily) normalized the internal luminal diameter of the first-order branches of the mesenteric arcade, although this had returned to untreated values seven weeks after therapy was stopped. In contrast to a previous study where norepinephrine vasoconstrictor responses in the mesenteric bed were reportedly abolished by captopril and reduced by enalapril [20], perindopril did not affect reactivity to norepinephrine [19].

The overall impression of the data reviewed thus far is that ACE inhibitors might be superior to other agents in their effects on vascular structure in SHR. To address this issue further, Christensen *et al* reported a large complex study where the effects of treating SHR with two ACE inhibitors were compared with those seen when other antihypertensive drugs were used. Young SHR were treated from 4–24 weeks with perindopril (1.5mg/kg per day), captopril (60mg/kg per day), hydralazine (25mg/kg per day), isradipine (42mg/kg per day) or metoprolol (130mg/kg per day) [21]. At 24 weeks, 24-hour mean blood pressures, invasively measured, were 121mmHg (perindopril), 137mmHg (captopril), 140mmHg (hydralazine), 149mmHg (isradipine) and 146mmHg (metoprolol) compared with 177mmHg (untreated SHR) and 132mmHg (WKY rats). Two weeks after discontinuation of therapy, the blood pressure had returned to untreated SHR levels in the isradipine-, metoprolol-, and hydralazine-treated animals. The characteristic slow rise in pressure after discontinuation of ACE inhibitors was observed [21]. The M:L ratio from mesenteric vessels was completely normal in the perindopril-treated group of rats but was not influenced by metoprolol, and was only partially affected by isradipine and hydralazine. In the captopril-treated group, only partial normalization of the M:L ratio was observed, although it should be pointed out that blood-pressure control with captopril was less satisfactory than in the perindopril group. If there were a close association between the ability of a drug to prevent the development of structural changes and the subsequent recrudescence of hypertension when therapy was withdrawn, then the perindopril-treated group should have shown the slowest increase in pressure, then captopril, and so on. While this held true for perindopril (slowest) and metoprolol (fastest), there was no correlation between vascular structure and the rate of rise of pressure for the other drugs tested (including captopril) [22]. Thus, although captopril, isradipine, and hydralazine produced similar effects on resistance vessel M:L ratios at 24 weeks, blood pressure remained low post-treatment in the captopril group while rising rapidly in the other groups.

The impression is that the prolonged post-treatment effects of ACE inhibitors on blood pressure cannot be ascribed solely to modifications in resistance vessel structure. This is supported by the results of a subsequent study using perindopril in doses of 0.4 and 0.8mg/kg daily to treat SHR from 4–24 weeks [23]. Again, withdrawal of the ACE inhibitor resulted in very little change in blood pressure. Combining results from two reports, the preventive effects of perindopril on the M:L ratio were dose dependent, yet the effects on blood pressure were more striking than those on vascular structure, and the blood pressure 12 weeks after withdrawal of treatment was essentially the same for all doses of perindopril [21,23].

Thus, ACE inhibitors act via some mechanism other than just a direct effect on the structure of resistance vessels. This view is reinforced by the work of Hefti *et al* which demonstrated attenuation of the expected blood-pressure rise in young SHR by chronic treatment with the ACE inhibitor cilazepril and prevention of the increase in peripheral vascular resistance, yet the blood pressure returned to untreated levels within four days of drug withdrawal [24].

Nevertheless, ACE inhibitors can have a sustained effect upon resistance vessel morphology, and evidence to support this has appeared. Harrap *et al* treated SHR with perindopril (3mg/kg/day) for just four weeks from the ages of 6–10 weeks and found that the M:L ratio remained low at the age of 32 weeks [25]. These workers believe that the early treatment of SHR with ACE inhibitors brings about long-term antihypertensive effects by preventing the full expression of genetic hypertension.

The ultimate test of the hypothesis of Harrap *et al* [25] would be to treat SHR from *in utero* until long into adulthood, and a study with this design has been published. Lee and co-workers treated female SH and WKY rats by the addition of captopril (100mg/kg/day) to the drinking water throughout pregnancy and lactation [26]. After weaning, the pups were maintained on 50mg/kg/day of captopril until 28–30 weeks of age. Once again blood pressure was reduced by the ACE inhibitor to levels seen in the normotensive rat strain. In the mesenteric resistance vessels, treatment significantly reduced the ratios of thickness of various vessel-wall components to that of the lumen in both SH and WKY rats, but more so in the SHR to the extent that after treatment, differences between SH and WKY rats in the intima-to-lumen and media-to-lumen ratios were eliminated. There was a significant correlation of the blood pressure with cross-sectional area of the media and the number of medial smooth-muscle cell layers. A perfusion study of the mesenteric vascular bed showed that sensitivity to norepinephrine was increased in SHR by captopril therapy. The authors concluded that long-term treatment with captopril before and after birth prevented the development of hypertension and the accompanying structural and functional changes in resistance vessels [26].

SUMMARY

A review of reports involving animals with genetic hypertension reveals a strikingly small number of studies where ACE inhibitors have been given after hypertension was established. In the one study of note, the ACE inhibitor controlled the blood pressure and reversed structural changes in the vasculature [17]. All other studies have concentrated upon preventing the development of hypertension and the resulting structural changes in SHR. The results uniformly suggest that ACE inhibitors are extremely efficient in this context and are perhaps superior to other available antihypertensive drugs. The number of direct comparisons with other agents, however, is small. There is good evidence that ACE inhibitors have long-term antihypertensive effects because all reports suggest that blood pressure remains low after therapy is withdrawn, the exception perhaps being with cilazepril. Prevention of the development of structural morphologic changes in arteries is likely to be only one mechanism, and this is discussed below. The effects described above are not unique to ACE inhibitors since they have been reported in rats treated from a young age with hydralazine, reserpine, or guanethidine [13,27,28] or

following immunosympathectomy. In some of these latter studies, however, hypertension was rapidly re-established after cessation of treatment, and survival was improved in one study [13]. No such reports have been made thus far with ACE inhibitors.

DOSE OF ANGIOTENSIN-CONVERTING ENZYME INHIBITORS

Compared with the maximum recommended doses of ACE inhibitors in man, the amounts used in all animal studies cited earlier are very high. The most often quoted reason for this is that the rat metabolizes drugs much faster than does man. Nevertheless, it is possible to lower blood pressure in SHR with lisinopril in daily oral doses of 0.312–5mg/kg [29]. In order to produce normotensive levels of blood pressure for prolonged periods, however, with the studies above, far higher doses are needed [29]. This raises the possibility that inhibition of tissue ACE is required for such effects. What is clear is that to obtain similar plasma levels of an ACE inhibitor, the dose required in rats per unit body weight is much higher [29] than in man at least for longer-acting ACE inhibitors such as lisinopril [30,31]. For other ACE inhibitors, the situation may be somewhat different: high concentrations may be achieved initially in response to oral dosing in the rat, for example with enalapril [32] and perindopril [30], but these are not maintained in contrast to plasma concentrations in man. This can be explained by differences in pharmacokinetics of the drugs between rat and man [33,34]. With prodrug ACE inhibitors, studies *in vitro* suggest that in the dog and man, in contrast to other species, the liver might play a greater role than plasma in hydrolysis [32]. Furthermore, the rat has a much greater number of nephrons per kilogram of body weight than has man; thus, renal clearance of ACE inhibitors is much more rapid [35]. Ideally therefore, ACE inhibitors such as captopril which are short acting in man should be given more frequently in the rat to achieve a similar therapeutic effect. Otherwise, if once-daily gavage routines are used, or the drug is administered in drinking water, overdosing will be required to obtain a sustained antihypertensive effect thereby producing extremely high peak levels. This is illustrated by the study of Richer *et al* [36] in which captopril (100mg/kg), enalapril (25mg/kg), perindopril (5mg/kg), trandolapril (5mg/kg), and ramipril (5mg/kg) were given by gavage to SHR. The drugs produced identical decreases in blood pressure but this was achieved using captopril at the equivalent of 48 times the maximum daily recommended dose in man compared with perindopril at 45 times and ramipril at 36 times the maximum recommended human dose.

A number of points should be emphasized. Firstly, as indicated above, blood pressure can be reduced to some extent with much smaller doses of these drugs than were used in the studies described, but to obtain normal blood pressure larger doses are needed. Secondly, the shorter-acting agents at least could be administered more frequently at lower doses to achieve the same effect. Thirdly, in terms of vascular structure, blood-pressure control over 24 hours is probably all-important. To illustrate this point, a study compared captopril (100mg/kg per day) with the Ang II receptor antagonist, DuP753 [37] (15mg/kg/day) in young SHR. After four weeks, the blood pressure was lower in both the captopril and DuP753 groups compared with controls, although the fall was greater in the captopril group. Only captopril prevented morphological vascular changes in mesenteric resistance vessels, and, whereas captopril in the dose used produces good 24-hour blood-pressure control [21], DuP753 may not.

SITE OF ACTION

The apparent dissociation between prevention of structural changes in resistance vessels and the prolonged lowering of blood pressure after withdrawal of ACE inhibitors [21,23], as well as the need to use large doses of drugs to keep pressure normal, raise a number of further issues. Perhaps the most important of these is the question of the underlying mechanisms of action of the ACE inhibitors. It is tempting to speculate that their effects on vascular structure when given in high doses reflect prolonged inhibition of ACE in tissues. Angiotensin-converting enzyme is present in virtually all mammalian organs and body fluids [38], and in the vascular beds of virtually all organs where it is bound to the plasma membrane of endothelial cells [39–41]. Studies with ACE inhibitors suggest that high doses can penetrate tissues and inhibit ACE *in situ*; for example, 5mg/kg perindopril reduced ACE activity in the rat aorta to 65% [42] although lower doses were much less effective (Fig. 96.2). However, it is difficult to assess whether *ex vivo* determinations of ACE inhibitory activity accurately reflect the situation *in vivo*. In addition, as yet, there are no reported studies of the effects of ACE inhibitors on tissue ACE in resistance vessels.

The possibility that mechanisms other than those discussed above explain the failure of blood pressure to rise to untreated levels after withdrawal of ACE inhibitors in chronically treated SHR should be considered. In this regard, some [16–19,23,25] but not all reports [15,20,26] show that SHR treated with ACE inhibitors failed to gain weight as they aged. Whereas most

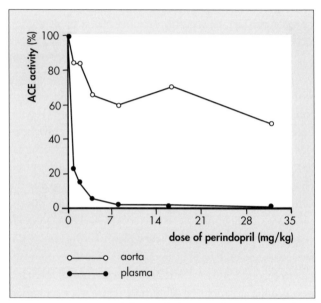

Fig. 96.2 Increasing inhibition of plasma and aortic ACE with increasing doses of perindopril in rats. Note that large doses of drug are required to reduce tissue ACE. Modified from Jackson B *et al* [42].

studies using captopril, and the trial with cilazepril [24], found no impairment in weight gain, the longer-acting ACE inhibitor, perindopril had a dose-dependent effect on body weight (Fig. 96.3) [23]. Indeed, in the study of Harrap *et al* [25] in three perindopril-treated groups of SHR, the growth rate appeared to slow during treatment compared with controls; thus, body weights were significantly lower than in controls at the end of treatment. In rats that received only four weeks' treatment, the growth rate seemed to recover when therapy was stopped, and by the end of the experiment, much of the deficit had been regained. In animals treated for eight weeks, however, the effect on growth was more pronounced and there was little tendency for these rats to catch up lost growth after treatment was stopped.

In the above studies, SHR received perindopril 3mg/kg/day. Christensen *et al* used the same drug in doses up to 1.5mg/kg/day [23]. There was a dose-dependent failure to gain weight during therapy which, however, had normalized 12 weeks after stopping the drug (Fig. 96.3). Other studies with perindopril confirm this pattern [19]. While captopril is less prone to inhibit growth, it is also less effective in preventing structural vascular abnormalities [21].

Perhaps the most attractive explanation for the prolonged effect of these drugs after withdrawal is an action on the central nervous system which could be due to inhibition of brain ACE.

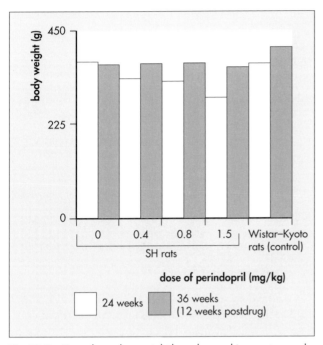

Fig. 96.3 Dose-dependent weight loss observed in spontaneously hypertensive rats treated with perindopril (0–1.5mg/kg/day) from 6 until 24 weeks of age. The weight reduction had been corrected 12 weeks after withdrawal of treatment (36 weeks). Modified from Christensen KL *et al* [21] and Christensen HRL *et al* [23].

The acute administration of Ang II into the brain of experimental animals produces transient pressor effects, a marked increase in drinking, release of vasopressin, an increase in total peripheral resistance, and an increase in sympathetic outflow [43]. The ability of ACE inhibitors to penetrate the central nervous system parallels their lipid solubility. Captopril penetrates rapidly into the brain and produces modest, short-lasting inhibition. Perindopril in high doses also crosses the blood–brain barrier and at the doses used in the vascular structure studies cited can produce marked ACE inhibition within the central nervous system [44]. It should be noted that in the experiments of Christensen *et al*, the daily water intake increased 26% in rats receiving captopril and 52% in those on perindopril [21]. It has been demonstrated that the chronic intracerebroventricular administration of captopril in doses that were ineffective (or less effective) when given

intravenously, attenuates the development of hypertension in SHR, probably due to a blunting of vascular reactivity to vasoconstriction and potentiation of the baroreflex [45]. In addition, there is evidence that orally administered captopril alters Ang II receptor binding in various areas of the brain [46] and that intracerebroventricular captopril alters the hormonal response of SHR to stress [47].

It seems most likely, therefore, that the administration of ACE inhibitors to young SHR prevents the development of hypertension by effects on the central nervous system. Angiotensin-converting enzyme has been found on the endothelial surface of moderate-sized cerebral arteries, the choroid plexus, and on the forebrain circumventricular organs; in the magnocellular division of the hypothalamic paraventricular and supraoptic nuclei; and around the basal ganglia, hippocampus, and cerebellum [48,49]. Differential effects of ACE inhibitors could be explained in terms of lipid solubility and their subsequent ability to cross the blood–brain barrier as well as their binding affinity for ACE.

CONCLUSIONS

A review of the literature provides good evidence that ACE inhibitors can prevent both the development of hypertension in SHR and the subsequent adaptive structural changes in resistance vessels. The blood pressure rises sluggishly after withdrawal of treatment, but this effect cannot be ascribed solely to the prevention of structural changes in the vasculature. The doses of ACE inhibitors required to keep the blood pressure near normal are, per unit body weight, far in excess of those used in man. This seems to reflect differences between SHR and man in the pharmacokinetic handling of such drugs and the frequency with which they are administered. There is evidence that a number of the effects of ACE inhibitors result from binding to tissue ACE in the central nervous system and perhaps also in blood vessels. Prolonged survival in SHR treated with ACE inhibitors from a young age has yet to be clearly demonstrated. Treatment of established hypertension in SHR with these drugs also reduces the blood pressure and ameliorates changes in resistance vessels. Studies to determine whether these effects will also occur in hypertensive man, and thereby result in a reduction in mortality from coronary and cardiac disease, are eagerly awaited.

REFERENCES

1. Lund–Johansen P. Haemodynamics in essential hypertension. State of the art review. *Clinical Science* 1980:59 (suppl):343–54s.

2. Folkow B, Grimby G, Thulesius O. Adaptive structural changes of the vascular walls in hypertension and their relation to the control of the peripheral resistance. *Acta Physiologica Scandinavica* 1958;44:255–72.

3. Sivertsson R. The haemodynamic importance of structural vascular changes in essential hypertension. *Acta Physiologica Scandinavica* 1970;(suppl 343):1–56.

4. Aalkjaer C, Heagerty AM, Petersen KK, Swales JD, Mulvany MJ. Evidence for increased media thickness, increased neuronal amine uptake and depressed excitation – coupling in isolated resistance vessels from essential hypertensives. *Circulation Research* 1987;61:181–6.

5. Strauer BE. The coronary circulation in hypertensive heart disease. *Hypertension* 1984;6 (suppl III):74–80.

6. Mulvany MJ, Aalkjaer C. Structure and function of small arteries. *Physiological Reviews* 1990;70:921–61.

7. Heagerty AM, Bund SJ, Izzard AS. Long-term structural changes in human hypertensive vessels. *Basic Research in Cardiology* 1991;86:19–23.

8. Heagerty AM. Angiotensin II: Vasoconstrictor or growth factor? *Journal of Cardiovascular Pharmacology* 1991;in press.

9. Lee RMKW. Structural and functional consequence of antihypertensive treatments on blood vessels. In: Lee RMKW, ed. *Blood vessel changes in hypertension: Structure and function.* Boca Raton: CRC Press Inc, 1989:163–90.

10. Folkow B, Gurevich M, Hallback M, LundgrenY, Weiss L. Haemodynamic consequences of regional hypotension in spontaneously hypertensive and normotensive rats. *Acta Physiologica Scandinavica* 1971;83:532–41.

11. Folkow B, Hallback M, LundgrenY, Weiss L. Effects of 'immunosympathectomy' on blood pressure and vascular 'reactivity' in normal and spontaneously hypertensive rats. *Acta Physiologica Scandinavica* 1972;84:512–3.

12. Weiss L, Lundgren Y, Folkow B. Effects of prolonged treatment with adrenergic beta-receptor antagonists on blood pressure, cardiovascular design and reactivity in spontaneously hypertensive rats (SHR). *Acta Physiologica Scandinavica* 1974;91:447–57.

13. Weiss L. Long-term treatment with antihypertensive drugs in spontaneously hypertensive rats (SHR). Effects on blood pressure, survival rate and cardiovascular design. *Acta Physiologica Scandinavica* 1974;91:393–408.

14. Ferrone RA, Antonaccio MJ. Prevention of the development of spontaneous hypertension in rats by captopril (SQ 14,225). *European Journal of Pharmacology* 1979;60:131–7.

15. Giudicelli JF, Freslon JL, Glasson S. Richer C. Captopril and hypertension development in the SHR. *Clinical and Experimental Hypertension. Part A. Theory and Practice* 1980;A2:1083–96.

16. Freslon JL, Giudicelli JF. Compared myocardial and vascular effects of captopril and dihydralazine during hypertension development in spontaneously hypertensive rats. *British Journal of Pharmacology* 1983;80:533–43.

17. Limas CV, Westrum B, Limas CJ. Comparative effects of hydralazine and captopril on the cardiovascular changes in spontaneously hypertensive rats. *American Journal of Pathology* 1984;117:360–71.

18. Harrap SB, Nicolacci JA, Doyle AE. Persistent effects on blood pressure and renal haemodynamics following chronic angiotensin converting enzyme inhibition with perindopril. *Clinical and Experimental Pharmacology and Physiology* 1986;13:753–65.

19. Cadilhac M, Giudicelli JF. Myocardial and vascular effects of perindopril, a new converting enzyme inhibitor during hypertension development in spontaneously hypertensive rats. *Archives Internationales de Pharmacodynamie et de Therapie* 1986;284:114–26.

20. Richer C, Doussau MP, Giudicelli JF. Effects of captopril and enalapril on regional vascular resistance and reactivity in spontaneously hypertensive rats. *Hypertension* 1983;5:312–20.

21. Christensen KL, Jespersen LT, Mulvany MJ. Development of blood pressure in spontaneously hypertensive rats after withdrawal of long-term treatment related to vascular structure. *Journal of Hypertension* 1989;7:83–90.

22. Mulvany MJ. Vascular structure and blood pressure during and after treatment with ACE inhibitors and other drugs. *American Journal of Hypertension* 1991;in press.

23. Christensen HRL, Nielsen H, Christensen KL, Baandrup U, Jespersen LT, Mulvany MJ. Long-term hypotensive effects of an angiotensin converting enzyme inhibitor in spontaneously hypertensive rats: Is there a role for vascular structure? *Journal of Hypertension* 1988;6 (suppl 3):s27–31.

24. Hefti F, Fischli W, Gerold M. Cilazepril prevents hypertension in spontaneously hypertensive rats. *Journal of Cardiovascular Pharmacology* 1986;8:641–8.

25. Harrap SB, Van der Merwe WM, Griffin SA, Macpherson F, Lever AF. Brief angiotensin converting enzyme inhibitor treatment in young spontaneously hypertensive rats reduces blood pressure long-term. *Hypertension* 1990;16:603–14.

26. Lee RMKW, Berecek KH, Tsoporis J, McKenzie R, Triggle CR. Prevention of hypertension and vascular changes by captopril treatment. *Hypertension* 1991;17:141–50.

27. Freis ED, Ragan D, Pillsbury H, Mathews M. Alteration of the course of hypertension in the spontaneously hypertensive rat. *Circulation Research* 1972;s31:1–7.

28. Limas C, Westrum B, Limas CJ. Effect of antihypertensive therapy on the vascular changes of spontaneously hypertensive rats. *American Journal of Pathology* 1983;111:380–93.

29. Sweet CS, Ulm EH. Lisinopril. *Cardiovascular Drug Reviews* 1988;6:181–91.

30. Johnston CI, Cubela R, Jackson B. Relative inhibitory potency and plasma drug levels of angiotensin converting enzyme inhibitors in the rat. *Clinical and Experimental Pharmacology and Physiology* 1988;15:123–9.

31. Case DE. The clinical pharmacology of lisinopril. *Journal of Human Hypertension* 1989;3 (suppl 1):127–31.

32. Tocco DJ, de luna FA, Duncan AEW, Vassil TC, Ulm EH. The physiological disposition and metabolism of enalapril maleate in laboratory animals. *Drug Metabolism and Disposition. The Biological Fate of Chemicals* 1982;10:15–9.

33. Lees KR, Reid JL. Age and the pharmacokinetics and pharmacodynamics of chronic enalapril treatment. *Clinical Pharmacology and Therapeutics* 1987;41:597–602.

34. Doucet L, De Veyrac B, Delaage M, Cailla H, Bernheim C, Devissaguet M. Radioimmunoassay of a new angiotensin-converting enzyme inhibitor (perindopril) in human plasma and urine: Advantages of coupling anion-exchange column chromatography with radioimmunoassay. *Journal of Pharmaceutical Sciences* 1990;79:741–5.

35. Lin JH, Chen I-Wu, Ulm EH, Duggen DE. Differential renal handling of angiotensin-converting enzyme inhibitors enalaprilat and lisinopril in rats. *Drug Metabolism and Disposition. The Biological Fate of Chemicals* 1988;16:392–6.

36. Richer C, Doussau M-P, Giudicelli JF. Systemic and regional haemodynamic profile of five angiotensin I converting enzyme inhibitors in the spontaneously hypertensive rat. *American Journal of Cardiology* 1987;59:12D–7D.

37. Morton JJ, Beattie EC, MacPherson F. Differential effects of captopril and the angiotensin receptor antagonist DuP753 on cardiovascular remodelling in the SHR [Abstract]. *Blood Vessels* 1991;28:319–20.

38. Soffer RL. Angiotensin-converting enzyme. In: Soffer RL, ed. *Biochemical regulation of blood pressure.* New York: John Wiley and Sons, 1981:123–64.

39. Ryan JE, Ryan US, Schultz DR, Whitaker C, Chung A, Dover FE. Subcellular localization of pulmonary angiotensin converting enzyme (Kininase II). *Biochemical Journal* 1975;146:497–9.

40. Caldwell PRB, Seegal BC, Hsu KC, Das M, Soffer RL. Angiotensin-converting enzyme: Vascular endothelial localization. *Science* 1976;191:1050–1.

41. Wigger HJ, Stalcup SA. Distribution and development of angiotensin converting enzyme in the foetal and newborn rabbit. An immunofluorescence study. *Laboratory Investigation* 1978;**38**:581–5.

42. Jackson B, Cubela RB, Johnston CI. Effects of perindopril on angiotensin converting enzyme in tissues of the rat. *Journal of Hypertension* 1988;**6** (suppl 3): 51–4.

43. Buckley JP. The central effects of the renin–angiotensin system. *Clinical and Experimental Hypertension. Part A. Theory and Practice* 1988;**A10**:1–16.

44. Johnston CI, Mendelsohn FAO, Cubela RB, Jackson B, Kohzuki M, Fabris B, Inhibition of angiotensin converting enzyme (ACE) in plasma and tissues: Studies *ex-vivo* after administration of ACE inhibitors. *Journal of Hypertension* 1988;**6** (suppl 3):s17–22.

45. Berecek KH, Okuno T, Nagahama S, Oparil S. Altered vascular reactivity and baroreflex sensitivity induced by chronic central administration of captopril in the spontaneously hypertensive rat. *Hypertension* 1983;**5**:689–700.

46. Wilson KM, Magargal W, Berecek KH. Long-term captopril treatment. Angiotensin II receptors and responses. *Hypertension* 1988;**11** (suppl 1):148–52.

47. Berecek KH, Coshatt G, Narkates AJ, Oparil S, Wilson KM, Robertson J. Captopril and the response to stress in the spontaneously hypertensive rat. *Hypertension* 1988;**11** (suppl 1):144–7.

48. Oldfield BJ, Ganten D, McKinley MJ. An ultrastructural analysis of the distribution of angiotensin II in the rat brain. *Journal of Neuroendocrinology* 1991;in press.

49. Pickel VM, Chan J, Ganten D. Dual peroxidase and colloidal gold-labelling study of angiotensin converting enzyme and angiotensin-like immunoreactivity in the rat subfornical organ. *Journal of Neuroscience* 1986;**6**:2457–69.

97 ANGIOTENSIN-CONVERTING ENZYME INHIBITORS AND RAYNAUD'S PHENOMENON

J IAN S ROBERTSON

Raynaud's phenomenon was described in the 19th century [1–3]. It is characterized by strictly demarcated digital ischemia affecting mainly the fingers, with the toes less often involved. The thumb is rarely afflicted, but one or more of the other digits can be attacked. The classic sequence is of pallor, cyanosis, and then lastly, redness as the digital arteries reopen, with reactive hyperemia. In some patients, the attack comprises only pallor or cyanosis.

Primary Raynaud's phenomenon affects mainly young women. Various trophic lesions can occur, although necrosis of the finger tips is rare. The pathophysiology remains obscure [2–4].

Secondary forms of Raynaud's phenomenon can result from a wide range of causes, including connective tissue disorders and several drugs [3]. Gangrenous digital lesions are more likely to supervene in many forms of secondary Raynaud's phenomenon (see Chapter 79). Pathogenesis is often, but not in all syndromes, less obscure in secondary than in primary Raynaud's phenomenon. Although in many diseases, high circulating concentrations of renin and Ang II are not evidently accompanied by Raynaud's phenomenon, with connective tissue disorders, and particularly scleroderma, high plasma Ang II levels have been invoked in this connection, and may lead to worsening of digital necrosis (see Chapter 79).

ANGIOTENSIN-CONVERTING ENZYME INHIBITORS IN THE TREATMENT OF PRIMARY RAYNAUD'S PHENOMENON

Uncontrolled studies have indicated both subjective and objective benefit from the use of captopril in primary Raynaud's phenomenon [5,6]. A placebo-controlled study, however, did not show a decrease in either the frequency or the severity of the attacks, although various measures of finger blood flow increased [7].

Miyazaki et al [8] provided evidence in one case that the acute vasodilator effect of captopril was blocked by serine proteinase inhibitors, while a competitive Ang II antagonist had no effect on digital blood flow. Since captopril was beneficial long term in this patient, they concluded that any efficacy was the result of accumulation of kinins rather than inhibition of Ang II formation.

The data have been received with varied enthusiasm. Some reviewers have accepted that captopril has been shown to be beneficial in patients with primary Raynaud's phenomenon [2]. Others have been more critical, and have emphasized the need for further controlled trials [3,9].

ANGIOTENSIN-CONVERTING ENZYME INHIBITORS IN THE TREATMENT OF SECONDARY RAYNAUD'S PHENOMENON

The use of ACE inhibitors in the treatment of Raynaud's phenomenon secondary to connective tissue disorders is considered in detail in Chapter 79.

An early open study indicated the capacity of captopril to heal digital ulcers of scleroderma [10]. In contrast, Tosi et al [6] found that captopril administration was of benefit only in primary Raynaud's phenomenon and not in that secondary to scleroderma.

Zimran et al [11] reported striking benefit with captopril administration in a patient with cyanotic, pulseless hands and feet due to ergotamine ingestion.

The need for definitive studies in secondary, as in primary Raynaud's phenomenon, has been emphasized [3].

ANGIOTENSIN-CONVERTING ENZYME INHIBITORS AS A CAUSE OF RAYNAUD'S PHENOMENON

An apparently rare, and unexpected, finding is of Raynaud's phenomenon either provoked de novo, or worsened, by ACE inhibitors. This has been reported as a minor but distinct side effect of both captopril [12] and enalapril [13] therapy. In one double-blind comparison of enalapril with atenolol in hypertension, the problem was sufficiently severe to lead to withdrawal of one of 86 patients allocated to enalapril. None of the 76 comparative patients given atenolol suffered this side effect [14]. It is possible that because of the supposed improbability of Raynaud's phenomenon as a consequence of ACE inhibition, the side effect has been misattributed, and hence underreported.

While the problem is a minor one, the fact that ACE inhibitors can sometimes provoke Raynaud's phenomenon emphasizes our present inadequate comprehension of the pathophysiology of this fascinating malady.

REFERENCES

1. Raynaud M, Barlow T. On local asphyxia and symmetrical gangrene of the extremities. *The Sydenham Society, London,* 1888:99–150.

2. Cooke ED, Nicolaides AN. Raynaud's syndrome. *British Medical Journal* 1990;**300**:553–5.

3. Coffman JD. Raynaud's phenomenon: An update. *Hypertension* 1991;**17**:593–602.

4. Brouwer RML, Wenting GJ, Schalekamp MA. Acute effect and mechanism of action of ketanserin in patients with Raynaud's phenomenon. *Journal of Cardiovascular Pharmacology* 1990;**15**:868–76.

5. Trubestein G, Wigger E, Trubestein R, Ludwig M, Wilgalis M, Stumpe KO. Behandling des Raynaud-Syndrom mit captopril. *Deutsche Medizinische Wochenschrift* 1984;**109**:857–60.

6. Tosi S, Marchesoni A, Messina K, Bellintani C, Sironi G, Faravelli C. Treatment of Raynaud's phenomenon with captopril. *Drugs under Experimental and Clinical Research* 1987;**13**:37–42.

7. Rustin MHA, Almond NE, Beacham JA, Brooks RJ, Jones DP, Cooke ED, Dowd PM. The effect of captopril on cutaneous blood flow in patients with primary Raynaud's phenomenon. *British Journal of Dermatology* 1987;**117**:751–8.

8. Miyazaki S, Miura K, Kasai Y, Abe K, Yoshinaga K. Relief from digital vasospasm by treatment with captopril and its complete inhibition by serine proteinase inhibitors in Raynaud's phenomenon. *British Medical Journal* 1982;**284**:310–1.

9. Challenor VF, Donaldson K, Waller DG. Raynaud's syndrome. *British Medical Journal* 1990;**300**:1015–6.

10. Lopez–Ovejero JA, Soal SD, d'Angelo WA, Cheigh JS, Stenzal KH, Laragh JH. Reversal of vascular and renal crisis of scleroderma by oral angiotensin-converting enzyme blockade. *New England Journal of Medicine* 1979;**300**:1417–9

11. Zimran A, Ofek B, Hershko C. Treatment with captopril for peripheral ischaemia induced by ergotamine. *British Medical Journal* 1984;**288**:364.

12. Havelka J, Vetter H, Studer A, Greminger P, Lüscher T, Wollnik S, Siegenthaler W, Vetter W. Acute and chronic effects of the angiotensin-converting enzyme inhibitor captopril in severe hypertension. *American Journal of Cardiology* 1982;**49**:1467–74.

13. Hodsman GP, Brown JJ, Cumming AMM, Davies DL, East BW, Lever AF, Morton JJ, Murray GD, Robertson JIS. Enalapril in the treatment of hypertension with renal artery stenosis. *British Medical Journal* 1983;**287**:1413–7.

14. Herrick AL, Waller PC, Berkin KE, Pringle SD, Callender JS, Robertson MP, Findlay JG, Murray GD, Reid JL, Lorimer AL, Weir RJ, Carmichael HA, Robertson JIS, Ball SG, McInnes GT. Comparison of enalapril and atenolol in mild to moderate hypertension. *American Journal of Medicine* 1989;**86**:421–6.

98 DIFFERENTIAL EFFECTS OF VARIOUS ANGIOTENSIN-CONVERTING ENZYME INHIBITORS

TERENCE BENNETT AND SHEILA M GARDINER

GENERAL INTRODUCTION

The brief history of ACE inhibitors provides a fascinating view of the interplay between basic and clinical research, and the influence of market forces (*Chapter 87*). Thus, the initial development of captopril was founded on the assumption that the systemic effects of Ang II might be involved in the etiology of some forms of renin-dependent hypertension. The remarkable and unexpected actions of captopril, however, then paved the way for the elucidation of local renin—angiotensin systems and the putative involvement of these in cardiovascular pathophysiology in low renin states.

The initial adverse effects seen with high doses of captopril were attributed, originally, to the presence of 'undesirable' sulfhydryl groups, and thus followed a second generation of nonsulfhydryl-containing ACE inhibitors. We have now, however, come the full circle and, for reasons that were totally unknown to the designers of captopril, it transpires that sulfhydryl groups in ACE inhibitors may offer additional advantages.

The potential profitability of this general therapeutic area has led to the development of many different ACE inhibitors, and some of these are being touted on the basis of unique profiles of effect. In the majority of cases, however, any novel effects have been described only in experimental animals, and, even in these cases, comparative studies of different ACE inhibitors have been extremely rare. Furthermore, *in vivo* animal studies on the effects of ACE inhibitors are often of dubious clinical significance because the doses of the drugs used are far in excess of those necessary to inhibit plasma ACE. Of course, this raises the question of the basis of the action of ACE inhibitors. If their effects are not to do with inhibition of plasma ACE, then how does one choose a clinically relevant dose? In theory, the choice could be made by reference to the degree of inhibition of ACE in an appropriate effector tissue (for example, heart, brain, kidney, and so on), but this assumes that the activity of a particular local ACE is relevant to the pharmacological effects of the ACE inhibitor in question. Furthermore, the measurement of tissue ACE inhibition *ex vivo* is not entirely

straightforward (see *Chapters 10* and *16*). If one assumes nothing about the mode of action of the ACE inhibitor under study, doses could be selected on the basis of functional effects. Then, however, one has to decide which variables are relevant; if hemodynamics are being monitored and the ACE inhibitor changes the pattern of regional and cardiac hemodynamics, how does one decide clinically relevant doses from these? One approach is to consider a range of doses, from subthreshold to supramaximal, with respect to all the variables measured [1]. Such a functional approach also allows comparative studies on different ACE inhibitors without the need to consider differing degrees of ACE inhibition in different tissues, at least with acute dosing [1]. The latter protocol, however, does not simulate the clinical condition in which chronic treatment with different ACE inhibitors could give rise to differential effects that were not apparent with acute dosing, or conversely, could obliterate differential effects that were observed with acute dosing.

Another major problem rarely acknowledged is the profound influence that anesthesia can have to activate the renal RAS sufficiently to cause systemic effects. This, in our view, renders measurements made in the presence of anesthesia of dubious significance, particularly when ACE inhibitors are used which tend to cause marked hypotension under such circumstances.

At some stage in the future, if the multitude of different ACE inhibitors becoming available [2] (*Chapter 87*) are to survive in the market on the basis of each having its own therapeutic niche due to some particular attribute, then appropriate comparative clinical trials will have to be carried out. In the interim, it is clear that comparative assessments of different ACE inhibitors in experimental animals are essential if all the theoretical possibilities for their differential effects are to be tested. Furthermore, this basic research needs to take into account the doses of the different ACE inhibitors to be studied, and the rationale behind the choice of doses; possible differences between acute and chronic effects of different ACE inhibitors, and the confounding effects of anesthesia on the interpretation of experimental data.

Evidently, such studies would be costly and, even if they were not, they would not be of interest to pharmaceutical companies unless the companies could be assured that the outcome would be favorable to their product. Hence, it is difficult to believe that such comparative studies will be forthcoming, unless the scientific community perceives them to be of importance. Assuming the latter is the case, we consider below a series of questions that seem to us relevant to any future investigations into possible differential effects of different ACE inhibitors.

IS ANGIOTENSIN-CONVERTING ENZYME THE SAME IN ALL TISSUES?

There is good evidence for the existence of ACE in many tissues (Fig. 98.1) (see *Chapter 10*). Although there is an indication that ACE in the heart and lung shows some difference with regard to association constants for ligand binding [3], the biological significance of this observation is not clear. Fabris *et al* [3], however, pointed out that, if there were differences in amino-acid sequence or tertiary structure of ACE in different tissues, then it was feasible that new ACE inhibitors could be designed to interact specifically with the structure of the active site.

In addition to such subtle differences, it is clear that the mRNA transcribed for endothelial ACE possesses an amino-terminal domain that is absent in the transcript for the testicular enzyme [4], but the implications of this for the enzymic properties of ACE are unknown. Furthermore, it remains to be determined if different ACE inhibitors show different profiles of effect against endothelial and testicular ACE (apart from the differences attributable to the presence of a blood–testicular barrier).

There is some evidence that the ACE from lung and brain are functionally different since Rogerson *et al* [5] found that substance P (1–3) was more active than substance P itself in inhibiting brain ACE, whereas substance P (1–3) was inactive against the lung enzyme. This interaction is notable because, at least *in vitro* ACE can cleave substance P, and brain ACE is also capable of cleaving neurokinin A, whereas lung ACE is not. The putative involvement of these additional effects of ACE in the responses to ACE inhibitors [6–11] (Fig. 98.2), are considered in the relevant sections below. Thus, in theoretical terms, there is the possibility

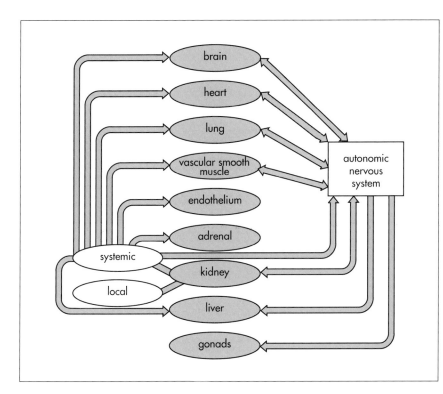

Fig. 98.1 Schematic representation of tissues containing local renin–angiotensin systems and their functional interrelations. The systemic effects of the renal RAS are far-reaching and amplified through the positive, prejunctional actions of Ang II on noradrenergic neuroeffector transmission (although this may be regionally differentiated). Likewise, locally generated Ang II may influence neuroeffector transmission selectively. Access of circulating Ang II to brain areas outside the blood–brain barrier (for example, circumventricular organs and area postrema) allows the modulation of functions such as thirst, vasopressin release, and cardiovascular control, although these variables are also influenced by local brain renin–angiotensin systems. Although it is not yet demonstrated that all the tissues listed normally synthesize and utilize all the components of the RAS, it is likely this is the case. Furthermore, such systems are probably involved in normal and pathophysiological functions including tissue growth and remodeling.

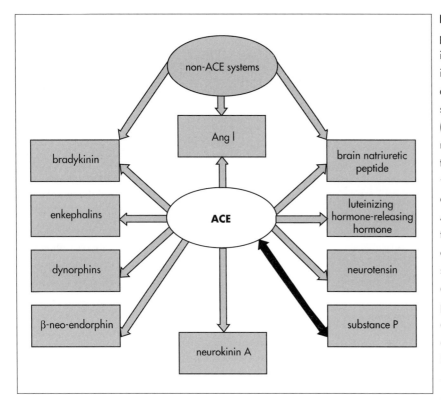

Fig. 98.2 Schematic representation of the putative enzymic activities of ACE. As indicated in the text, it is possible that ACE in different tissues has different functional attributes, so the details of the relations shown here may vary from tissue to tissue (for example, lung ACE does not cleave neurokinin A). Although it is not clear if all these properties of ACE are expressed *in vivo*, they should be borne in mind when considering the functional consequences of ACE inhibition. Particular points of note are that enzyme systems other than ACE are capable of generating Ang II, and may do so by acting on angiotensinogen. In addition, enzymes other than ACE may produce Ang II from Ang I; alternatively, enzymes other than ACE may act on Ang I and cleave the C-terminal tripeptide. Neutral endopeptidase (NEP) (E.C. 3.4.24.11) falls into this category and is notable because it also acts on bradykinin, brain natriuretic peptide, and enkephalins. In the latter case, the action of ACE on metenkephalin heptapeptide produces a dipeptide (L-arginyl-L-phenylalanine) with potent cardiovascular effects (see text). The two-way arrow between ACE and substance P indicates the latter inhibits the former. It is not known if different ACE inhibitors influence non-ACE systems differentially.

that there may be differences between ACE in different tissues, and that different ACE inhibitors might interact with tissue angiotensin-converting enzymes differentially. In addition, in disease states there might be induction of tissue ACE that might be of a normal or novel form. Obviously, such postulated disease-related changes could have consequences for the effects of ACE inhibitors.

Another point to note is that enzymes other than ACE may be involved in the production of Ang II [12] (Fig. 98.2) and these systems may be differentially affected by different ACE inhibitors. As with ACE, there is the possibility that non-ACE systems for the production of Ang II could be induced in disease states and/or with chronic ACE therapy, and thereby make

important contributions to the generation of Ang II under these circumstances (see *Chapters 5* and *23*).

There is some evidence for the existence of a non-ACE, Ang II-generating enzyme system in the human heart [13,14], although the functional significance of this system and its putative role during chronic ACE inhibition have yet to be assessed, as has the possibility that such a system might be differentially influenced by different ACE inhibitors (Fig. 98.3). In this context, it is notable that Lindpaintner *et al* [15] found no evidence for a captopril-resistant generation of Ang II from Ang I in the isolated rat heart, so it may be that species differences exist, although the human heart tissue studied by Urata *et al* [13,14] was not from normal subjects. This

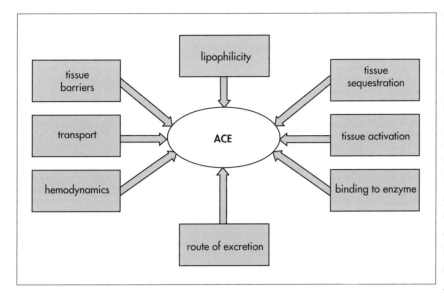

Fig. 98.3 Schematic representation of the factors that could influence the ability of any particular ACE inhibitor to suppress ACE activity in any particular tissue. The lipophilicity of the compound could influence tissue sequestration, and, if it were a prodrug, then tissue activation (through the influence of esterases, for example) could be an important variable. Clearly, the chemical interaction between the ACE inhibitor and ACE could influence the duration of action of the compound, and its route of excretion could affect its interaction with the renal RAS; for example, if it were cleared through renal filtration and tubular secretion, the ACE inhibitor might exert particularly potent renal effects. Tissue delivery of the ACE inhibitor could be influenced by its own hemodynamic effects. In the case of brain structures within the blood–brain barrier, lipophilicity could influence access, but there is a theoretical possibility that ACE inhibitors might gain entry to the brain via transport mechanisms (associated with neuronal processes). Furthermore, in disease states, the blood–brain barrier might be breached, allowing freer movement of the ACE inhibitors into the central nervous system.

emphasizes the need to know whether or not tissue ACE and other Ang II-generating systems are induced in pathophysiological states.

DO DIFFERENT ANGIOTENSIN-CONVERTING ENZYME INHIBITORS HAVE DIFFERENT EFFECTS ON TISSUE ANGIOTENSIN-CONVERTING ENZYME?

Various factors could influence the ease with which different ACE inhibitors interact with ACE in different tissues (Fig. 98.3), but until recently, hard data on which to base an answer to this question were not available. Studies by Cushman *et al* [16], however, have been designed to provide comparative quantification of the effects of seven different ACE inhibitors on ACE in a series of different tissues. Acknowledging the problem with

regard to choice of dose, Cushman *et al* [16] calculated doses to achieve equivalent inhibition of plasma ACE with the different compounds. This they managed, although it should be noted that their study involved only single oral doses in spontaneously hypertensive rats, and the *ex vivo* assessment of ACE inhibition was prone to the problems produced by sample dilution. Nonetheless, against the background of similar degrees of inhibition of plasma ACE, Cushman *et al* [16] observed that ramipril, lisinopril, and zofenopril had particularly marked effects on lung and aortic ACE, and these effects lasted 3–4 days. In contrast, the effects of captopril on aortic ACE lasted no more than one day, while the effects of fosinopril and enalapril were even more transient. Interestingly, these profiles of effect on aortic ACE did not mirror those on renal ACE in all cases. Dissociation between aortic ACE inhibition and brain ACE inhibition was even more striking, with ramipril causing no inhibition, fosinopril causing sustained inhibition, and the phosphonic acid, SQ 29,852, causing delayed inhibition, of brain ACE. These measurements, however, were made on whole brain samples and hence would not have detected regional differences. This proposition is consistent with the finding that the same dose of lisinopril as that used by Cushman *et al* [16], in the hands of Sakaguchi *et al* [17], caused significant inhibition of ACE in the subfornical organ and the organum vasculosum lamina terminalis four hours postdosing, whereas ACE activity in structures inside the blood–brain barrier (for example, caudate putamen and globus pallidus) was unchanged. It should be remembered, however, that the integrity of the blood–brain barrier may be compromised in disease states such as hypertension, and hence the influence of ACE inhibitors on brain ACE under these conditions may be more extensive than normal. In addition, since there are possibilities for molecules to gain access to the brain via transport within neuronal processes and other structures, it is perfectly feasible that ACE inhibitors that appear not to influence brain ACE following acute administration would do so following chronic dosing. Furthermore brain access seems, for some ACE inhibitors, to be dose dependent, since following administration of high doses, perindopril gains access to structures inside the blood–brain barrier, whereas following low doses, it does not [18]. On balance, however, it is probable that highly lipophilic ACE inhibitors could exert more extensive effects on brain ACE than compounds that less easily gained access to the central nervous system.

The data from Cushman *et al* [16] are notable also because all the compounds tested had relatively less effect on cardiac ACE than on ACE in other peripheral tissues, so it is not likely that differences in tissue perfusion account simply for the differences in effects seen. Clearly, tissue access and uptake, and (where relevant), activation, binding to ACE, hemodynamic effects, and the route of excretion, could all differentially affect the pharmacological profiles of different ACE inhibitors (Fig. 98.3). Moreover, additional features are probably involved, since Grover and his colleagues [19] have shown recently that differences in the degree of cardiac ACE inhibition are not sufficient to explain differences in the ability of different ACE inhibitors to provide cardioprotection following ischemia (see later).

While the doses of the ACE inhibitors used by Cushman *et al* [16] were matched for their effects on plasma ACE, they were, in functional terms, well above the levels achieving maximal effects, at least as regards acute changes in regional hemodynamics [1]. Observations such as these indicate that actions, in addition to inhibition of ACE, may be involved in many of the novel effects of ACE inhibitors seen in experimental investigations. There clearly is, however, a need for acute and chronic studies utilizing a range of doses of different ACE inhibitors to determine if the profiles of effect described by Cushman *et al* [16] are seen under all conditions.

DO DIFFERENT ANGIOTENSIN-CONVERTING ENZYME INHIBITORS HAVE DIFFERENT EFFECTS ON BRADYKININ DEGRADATION?

A corollary of this question is, does bradykinin contribute differentially to the effects of different ACE inhibitors? Since ACE is kinase II [9] (see *Chapter 10*), then variations in the extent of ACE inhibition in different tissues in the presence of different ACE inhibitors should be reflected in parallel variations in tissue accumulation of bradykinin (see *Figs. 98.1* and *98.2*). Tissue bradykinin levels, however, have not been measured under these conditions, and it is unlikely that circulating bradykinin levels could represent changes in the tissues. In addition, it should be remembered that the degradation of bradykinin can occur through various pathways not involving kinase II [9]. Hence, it does not follow that ACE inhibition would necessarily lead to accumulation of endogenous bradykinin, particularly since, under these conditions, other pathways for bradykinin degradation may take over [6].

At present, it would be fair to say there is little evidence for bradykinin involvement in the cardiovascular responses to ACE inhibition in animals or man [20, 21]. Certainly, observations such as those indicating that captopril, in the presence of the Ang II-receptor antagonist, DuP 753 (losartan), has no additional hemodynamic effects in conscious Brattleboro rats [22,23] argue against bradykinin involvement, at least when captopril is administered acutely. The studies of Danckwardt *et al* [24], however, showed that the hypotensive response to ramipril in kinin-deficient, Brown Norway rats with renal hypertension was attenuated, indicating that the involvement of bradykinin in the effects of acute ACE inhibition may be strain dependent. It is also feasible that different subgroups of human subjects would show different degrees of involvement of bradykinin-mediated mechanisms following administration of ACE inhibitors, but an important point to bear in mind in this connection is that bradykinin is a very potent peptide that, *in vivo*, does not cause vasodilatation only. Thus, even if ACE inhibition brought about local (or even systemic) accumulation of bradykinin, it does not follow this would contribute straightforwardly to the hemodynamic effects seen; for example, bradykinin can cause stimulation of afferent neuronal systems and adrenal medullary catecholamine release. *In vivo* administration of exogenous bradykinin does not cause uniform vasodilatation in all vascular beds, and in the vascular beds that do vasodilate, the response seems to involve both nitric oxide-dependent and nitric oxide-independent mechanisms, modified by baroreflex input [25]. A further complication is that low doses of exogenous bradykinin cause increases, rather than decreases, in mean systemic arterial blood pressure in conscious rats (Gardiner SM *et al*, unpublished observations), and this effect is probably due to myocardial stimulation.

There have been no comparative studies concerned with the possibility that different ACE inhibitors might exert differential effects on the regional hemodynamic actions of circulating Ang I or bradykinin.

DO DIFFERENT ANGIOTENSIN-CONVERTING ENZYME INHIBITORS HAVE DIFFERENT EFFECTS ON PROSTAGLANDIN SYNTHESIS?

Although Ang II itself increases tissue prostanoid synthesis, it has been claimed that the hemodynamic effects of ACE inhibitors are associated with increased production of prostaglandin E_2 and prostacyclin [20]. One explanation proposed for this effect is the suppression of bradykinin degradation by ACE inhibitors, since bradykinin has been shown to stimulate prostanoid release [26]. If this were the case, however, then all ACE inhibitors would be expected to enhance prostanoid synthesis since, as pointed out in the previous section, there is no evidence that these substances have differential effects on bradykinin accumulation. At least *in vitro*, nonetheless, it has been found that captopril and epicaptopril (both sulfhydryl-containing compounds, although the latter has only weak ACE inhibiting activity) increased prostaglandin E_2 production, whereas an analog of captopril without a sulfhydryl moiety was devoid of such activity [20]. These findings indicate that sulfhydryl groups, rather than ACE inhibition, are responsible for activation of prostanoid-mediated mechanisms, and this proposition is consistent with the finding that enalaprilat did not stimulate prostanoid production *in vitro* [27]. These data are, however, at variance with *in vivo* findings [2,20,28]. Furthermore, although it has been reported that the cyclo-oxygenase inhibitor, indomethacin, attenuates the hypotensive action of captopril, this has not been shown to be a specific or straightforward effect [29]. Similar doubt surrounds the involvement of prostanoids in the hemodynamic responses to enalapril, cilazapril, and lisinopril [28,30]. Moreover, if prostanoid-mediated mechanisms are involved in the effects of captopril, but not in those of nonsulfhydryl-containing ACE inhibitors, this does not result in obvious

differences in their acute hemodynamic effects [1]. Considering the putative interactions between ACE inhibitors, bradykinin and prostanoids, however, there is clearly a need for acute and chronic comparative studies on different ACE inhibitors under conditions in which bradykinin and/or prostanoid-mediated processes are selectively ablated. These topics are also discussed in *Chapter 38*.

DO DIFFERENT ANGIOTENSIN-CONVERTING ENZYME INHIBITORS HAVE DIFFERENT EFFECTS ON THE HEART?

As in other areas, it is important to consider acute and chronic effects. Furthermore, in the case of the myocardium, the direct trophic role of Ang II is particularly relevant (Fig. 98.4) (see *Chapters 31* and *42*), but not easily distinguished from the secondary consequences of changes in afterload *in vivo*. Thus, for example, although chronic treatment with perindopril has been shown to reduce cardiac mass in essential hypertension [31] it is not known if this is a direct cardiac effect; whatever the explanation, it does not seem to be specific to perindopril [31].

Grover *et al* [19] studied the ability of structurally different ACE inhibitors to inhibit cardiac ACE *in vitro*, and to improve postischemic cardiac function and suppress cell death. They found that the active sulfhydryl forms of zofenopril and fosinoprilic acid were the most potent of the free inhibitors, but zofenopril and 5-benzoylcaptopril were even more effective because they were rapidly hydrolyzed by cardiac esterases. Fosinopril, ramipril, and enalapril, however, were only poorly active. Captopril and the sulfhydryl form of zofenopril were found to improve postischemic myocardial function and also to suppress cell death, although neither zofenopril nor captopril had any effect on coronary blood flow, before or after ischemia. However, even when fosinoprilic acid, ramiprilat, or enalaprilat were perfused at a concentration sufficient to cause complete inhibition of cardiac ACE, they had no cardioprotective effects. Grover *et al* [19] concluded that ACE inhibition alone was insufficient to provide cardioprotection in their model, and that the sulfhydryl group seemed to be important in this regard.

It is necessary to be aware that the outcome of any assessment of the myocardial effects of acute or chronic ACE inhibition may depend on the variables measured. Thus, the data of Grover *et al* [19] were generated on the basis of assessing acute myocardial function following ischemia, whereas those of others have dealt with prevention of reperfusion arrhythmias and reduction of infarct size [32–40].

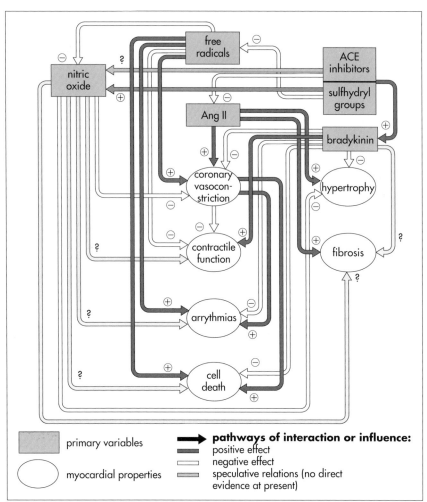

Fig. 98.4 Schematic representation of the interacting factors that could influence acute and chronic myocardial structure and function, and the effect of ACE inhibitors on them. Many other relevant variables (catecholamines, purines, prostanoids, etc), are not shown.

The earlier study of van Gilst *et al* [32] showed that captopril reduced fibrillation and purine overflow and improved myocardial function following coronary ligation of the isolated rat heart, but these effects were not compared with those of other ACE inhibitors. Subsequently, van Gilst *et al* [33] examined the effects of captopril, enalapril, ramipril, and ramiprilat in the same model; it is not clear why they did not include enalaprilat in this protocol. Captopril and ramiprilat, but not enalapril or ramipril, caused significant reduction in ventricular fibrillation and increase in cardiac function. The effect of captopril on the latter was abolished by indomethacin, but van Gilst *et al* [33] did not examine the effect of indomethacin on the response to ramiprilat. The cardioprotective effects of captopril and ramiprilat were associated with inhibition of norepinephrine overflow during reperfusion, and this effect of captopril was also abolished by indomethacin. van Gilst *et al* [33] found that enalapril was without the above-mentioned beneficial effects seen with captopril and

ramiprilat, although it did inhibit purine overflow during reperfusion. They [33] omitted, however, to emphasize that the effects seen with ramiprilat were not obtained with ramipril, and hence the failure of enalapril to exert any influence is not too surprising; obviously, a more meaningful comparison would have included enalaprilat. Nonetheless, these earlier studies have given rise to additional investigations showing that inhibition of Ang II production and bradykinin degradation probably contribute to the cardioprotective effect of ramiprilat (and of ramipril, if administered *in vivo*) following ischemia in the isolated rat heart, and in anesthetized dogs [34,36–39] (Fig. 98.4).

In other experimental models, captopril, enalapril, ramipril, and perindopril have been shown to exert cardioprotective effects independent of prostanoids [35,41]. Furthermore, in the isolated rat heart, enalaprilat, DuP 753 (a nonpeptide antagonist at the AT-1 receptors for Ang II), and CGP 44099A (an inhibitor of rat renin), given before ischemia, reduced the duration of ventricular fibrillation on reperfusion to similar extents [42]. None of the compounds, however, influenced creatine phosphokinase release or the recovery of left ventricular developed pressure on reperfusion. Thus, Fleetwood *et al* [42] concluded that Ang II, generated from angiotensinogen through the mediation of renin and ACE, was involved in the genesis of postischemic ventricular fibrillation, but did not contribute to the associated depression of myocardial function in the isolated rat heart.

In the context of cardioprotection, captopril appears the most effective of the ACE inhibitors tested [43], although the point about therapeutically relevant dose (see earlier) and dose-matching for different ACE inhibitors needs to be considered in these, as in all, experiments. In some studies, however, it has been found that sulfhydryl-containing compounds such as N-acetylcysteine, which do not inhibit ACE, counteract hypoxia-induced coronary vasoconstriction to the same extent as does captopril [41]. Hence, it appears that inhibition of cardiac ACE may provide protective effects, depending on the model of myocardial injury studied, whereas there is a consensus that sulfhydryl groups exert beneficial effects. There are at least two interrelated ways in which sulfhydryl groups could act to protect the myocardium: by scavenging oxygen-derived free radicals, and by complexing with endogenous nitric oxide, thereby enhancing its effects (Fig. 98.4).

There is considerable evidence that free radicals are involved in myocardial injury following reperfusion [44], and that sulfhydryl-containing compounds such as captopril, epicaptopril, zofenopril, and N-acetylcysteine afford cardioprotection under these conditions [43, 45–49]. Furthermore, there is evidence that captopril, epicaptopril, zofenopril, and N-acetylcysteine scavenge free radicals *in vitro* [43,49–51]. It has been claimed, however, that at therapeutic concentrations, captopril, epicaptopril, SQ 26,703, and N-acetylcysteine do not act as free radical scavengers [52,53], and that the earlier results were due to technical problems. The finding that sulfhydryl-containing ACE inhibitors offer greatest protection to the myocardium following ischemia, then, still requires an explanation.

As mentioned above, complexation between sulfhydryl groups and endogenous nitric oxide could account for some of the beneficial effects of sulfhydryl-containing ACE inhibitors. Although only recently identified as the major endothelium-derived relaxing factor [54], nitric oxide (generated from L-arginine) is now known to play a pivotal role in myocardial function and in the control of coronary vascular tone, as well as acting as a potent anti-aggregatory and antiproliferative agent generally [54]. It is particularly notable that oxygen-derived free radicals interact with and destroy the bioactivity of nitric oxide, whereas drugs such as

captopril can interact with nitric oxide to form S-nitrosocaptopril, a compound with potent vasodilator properties [55]. Hence, it is quite feasible that many of the positive features of sulfhydryl-containing ACE inhibitors are due to preservation, or enhancement, of nitric oxide-mediated mechanisms (Fig. 98.4). While these possibilities are based on experimental, rather than clinical, observations, Schneider *et al* [56] have provided some indirect evidence for such interactions in hypertensive man.

Although inhibiting the generation of Ang II might be beneficial in offsetting any putative coronary vasoconstrictor effects of this peptide, there is the theoretical possibility that loss of the positive myocardial effects of Ang II would be detrimental (Fig. 98.4). While in animals, however, ACE inhibitors can abolish the cardiac generation of Ang II from Ang I, the human myocardium has been shown to possess what Urata *et al* [13,14] have called angiotensin convertase. Thus, it may be that the beneficial effects of Ang II on the heart are maintained in the presence of ACE inhibition due to the action of alternative enzyme systems.

Even in the acute setting, little is known of the comparative cardiac effects of different ACE inhibitors. Thus, it clearly would be useful to utilize a series of experimental paradigms (for example, postischemic myocardial function, incidence of arrhythmias, cell death, infarct size, intracardiac generation of Ang II, indices of nitric oxide-mediated processes, and so on), and to compare different classes of ACE inhibitors in them.

A great deal of interest centers around the use of ACE inhibitors following myocardial infarction and in congestive heart failure (see *Chapters 76, 77,* and *93*). In the latter case, there is evidence that enalapril prolongs survival, but it is not clear that this attribute is unique, or that it is due to cardiac actions rather than effects on hemodynamics. In the context of chronic disorders, it is worth reiterating that there may be changes in tissue ACE systems and also in other systems for generating Ang II, so it is possible that even the acute actions of ACE inhibitors in such circumstances would be different from those under normal conditions.

Studies by Johnston *et al* [57] have shown that four weeks after myocardial infarction, caused by coronary artery ligation, in Wistar rats, there was marked cardiac hypertrophy and increased concentrations of ACE in all chambers of the heart, particularly in the scar tissue of the infarcted area. However, rats treated chronically with enalapril following coronary ligation showed no increase in cardiac weight or ACE concentration. It is not clear from this study [57] whether or not the prevention of myocardial hypertrophy by enalapril was due to direct effects on the heart. Furthermore, Johnston *et al* [57] did not comment on the extent to which the reduction in apparent ACE activity with chronic enalapril treatment was due to inhibition of *de novo* synthesis of enzyme, rather than occupancy of binding sites by enalaprilat. Moreover, they did not investigate the possibility that, following myocardial infarction, there might be induction of non-ACE systems for generating Ang II.

The extent to which various ACE inhibitors differ in their ability to influence postinfarction left ventricular dilatation and/or hypertrophy, myocardial fibrosis, and structural remodeling [11, 58] (Fig. 98.4) with chronic administration has yet to be assessed fully, but there are preliminary experimental data showing that captopril treatment, beginning three weeks after myocardial infarction (induced by ligation of the left anterior descending coronary artery) and continuing for two weeks, restored resting cardiac output and cardiac output during volume loading [59]. Neither benazepril nor the nonpeptide Ang II-receptor antagonist, DuP 753, showed these effects, indicating that the action of captopril was due to an effect other than, or in addition to, ACE inhibition.

Subsequent studies showed that captopril treatment, instituted immediately after experimental myocardial infarction, attenuated the hypertrophic response of the noninfarcted ventricular myocardium and blocked the increase in DNA synthesis seen in the ventricular myocardium in untreated rats following coronary ligation. Such effects were not seen with DuP 753 and were not mimicked by giving hydralazine to achieve the same hemodynamic profile as that with captopril administration [60]. It must be acknowledged, however, that administration of hydralazine may not give an identical hemodynamic profile to that of captopril in a chronic setting; for example, cardiac sympathetic effects may differ in the two circumstances. Obviously, it will be important to establish if the chronic effects seen with captopril pertain to other sulfhydryl-containing ACE inhibitors. If this is the case, then the possibility of interactions between sulfhydryl groups and free radicals, as this impinges on the L-arginine/nitric oxide system, could be relevant since nitric oxide is a potent antimitogenic agent. It would be interesting to know if in infarcted myocardial tissue there is induction of nitric oxide

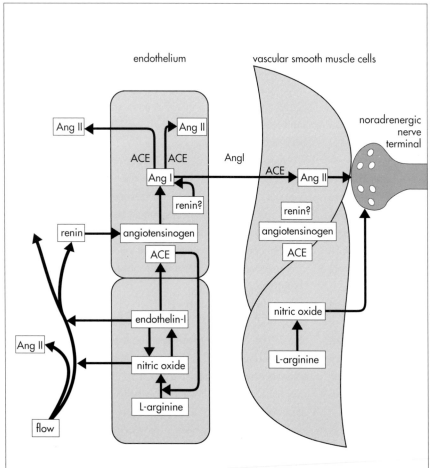

Fig. 98.5 Schematic representation of the functional relations between endothelial cells, vascular smooth muscle, and noradrenergic nerve terminals with respect to local renin–angiotensin systems. The local blood flow can deliver Ang II and renin to specific tissues and also prompt nitric oxide and endothelin-1 release. The latter can enhance ACE activity, but it is not known if ACE or ACE inhibitors affect nitric oxide synthase. Endothelin-1, nitric oxide, and Ang II generated by endothelial cells can affect vascular smooth muscle, both acutely and chronically, as could Ang II generated by the vascular smooth muscle itself. It seems, however, that nitric oxide synthase is only expressed in vascular smooth muscle under pathological conditions. There is evidence that Ang II exerts positive prejunctional effects on efferent noradrenergic vasomotor function that may be attributable to local and systemic Ang II. The question marks relate to unresolved questions regarding *de novo* synthesis of renin in the endothelial and vascular smooth-muscle cells.

synthase as is seen in other tissues during inflammation [61]. If this does occur, then it might have an important bearing on the chronic therapeutic effectiveness of different classes of ACE inhibitor following myocardial infarction, and in congestive heart failure, amongst other conditions. We also need to know whether or not ACE inhibitors have any effects on nitric oxide synthase in different systems. A summary of factors that could be influenced by ACE inhibitors is given in Fig. 98.4.

DO DIFFERENT ANGIOTENSIN-CONVERTING ENZYME INHIBITORS HAVE DIFFERENT EFFECTS ON THE VASCULAR SYSTEM?

There is some evidence that different ACE inhibitors exert somewhat different regional hemodynamic effects when administered acutely; for example, when comparing a range of doses of captopril, enalaprilat, and lisinopril, all three ACE inhibitors caused particularly marked renal and mesenteric vasodilatation under conditions of activation of the RAS in conscious rats [1]. Although there were no differences in the hypotensive effects of captopril, enalaprilat, and lisinopril, the rank order of maximal effect on renal vascular conductance was enalaprilat > captopril > lisinopril, whereas on mesenteric vascular conductance, it was captopril > enalaprilat > lisinopril. Similar differences were apparent in the blood flows to these regions, and hence it is feasible that other ACE inhibitors might have more marked differential effects on regional hemodynamics (Fig. 98.5). Moreover, since epicaptopril (the isomer of captopril with 100-fold less ACE-inhibiting activity) at a dose of 2mg/kg, caused an additional mesenteric vasodilatation similar to that seen with captopril at the same dose, it is feasible that the sulfhydryl groups of these compounds were acting to protect endothelium-derived nitric oxide and hence augment its vasodilator actions [1] (Fig. 98.5). Once again, it must be borne in mind that these results were obtained with acute doses of a limited number of ACE inhibitors and it does not follow that similar effects would be seen with chronic dosing, or in pathophysiological states. No clinical data comparing the detailed, regional hemodynamic effect of different ACE inhibitors are available.

A question that is attracting much attention currently is whether or not different ACE inhibitors have differential effects on the development of tolerance to nitrovasodilators. This question relates to the etiology of nitrate tolerance; if it is due to reduced availability of tissue sulfhydryl groups, then sulfhydryl supplementation should suppress tolerance, whereas if it is due to

activation of the RAS, then ACE inhibitors should diminish tolerance. Furthermore, if both sulfhydryl depletion and activation of the RAS underlie the development of nitrate tolerance, then sulfhydryl-containing ACE inhibitors should be particularly effective in suppressing it.

Publications in this area, however, are no less contradictory than in any other; for example, there is evidence both for [62–64] and against [65–67] increased availability of sulfhydryl groups preventing the development of nitrate tolerance. In addition, there is evidence both for [68–70] and against [71,72] captopril suppressing nitrate tolerance, although it should be noted that there are marked differences between the experimental procedures used in the different studies. The only comparative investigations of the effects of different ACE inhibitors on the development of nitrate tolerance are those of van Gilst et al [69] and Katz et al [73], and their approaches were dissimilar. van Gilst et al [69] studied the isolated rat heart and showed that the coronary vasodilator effects of isosorbide dinitrate were enhanced by cysteine or captopril, but not by ramiprilat. In contrast, Katz et al [73] carried out a randomized, placebo-controlled trial in normal volunteers of the effects of enalapril and captopril on the venodilator effects of glyceryl trinitrate. Both ACE inhibitors suppressed the development of nitrate tolerance and this effect was associated with an inhibition of the increase in body weight seen in the placebo-treated subjects. Hence, these results indicate that effects on fluid and electrolyte balance associated with ACE inhibition, rather than availability of sulfhydryl groups, might be the more important factor in suppressing nitrate tolerance in the clinical setting. It is feasible, however, that patients with depleted tissue sulfhydryl levels might show a more positive response than normal subjects to the use of sulfhydryl-containing ACE inhibitors in conjunction with nitrovasodilators, but such studies remain to be done.

Apart from differential hemodynamic effects of different ACE inhibitors, it is feasible that chronic treatment might influence vascular structure through inhibition of a local RAS and/or through additional mechanisms (Fig. 98.5). There is some evidence that chronic treatment with perindopril caused a normalization of the passive pressure–volume relationship in the carotid artery of rats with renal hypertension, but not in rats with spontaneous hypertension. The medial hypertrophy seen in rats with renal hypertension was reversed by perindopril whereas that in spontaneously hypertensive rats was not [74]. This study, however, did not consider other ACE inhibitors, and although the measurement of carotid compliance was carried out in vivo, it was performed under static, that is, no-flow conditions.

The same technique was used by Levy et al [75] who showed that removal of the endothelium, or treatment with lisinopril in the presence of the endothelium, increased carotid compliance (see also *Chapter 95*). It is difficult, nevertheless, to concede that this measurement relates straightforwardly to the *in vivo* circumstance, where flow in the carotid artery must modulate endothelial cell nitric oxide and endothelin-1 release, particularly since the effects of ACE inhibitors would likely cause changes in carotid flow patterns and hence changes in release of such vasoactive factors from endothelial cells. This is an important point, not the least because changes in endothelin release could influence endothelial ACE activity [76], and ACE inhibitors may augment endothelium-dependent vasodilator responses [77–79]. Whether or not this latter effect is due to changes in nitric oxide-mediated mechanisms is unknown, but if it is, then the antiproliferative effects of nitric oxide and its ability to inhibit endothelin release may be germane to the chronic effects of ACE inhibitors. It seems likely, however, that the hemodynamic and structural changes following chronic ACE inhibition can be dissociated [80], but it is not known if these effects differ with different ACE inhibitors. Clearly, if they do, then such differences might relate to variation in tissue ACE inhibition and/or to unique additional effects of particular ACE inhibitors.

Although we have emphasized the possibility that ACE inhibitors might have effects due to factors other than, or in addition to, suppression of Ang II formation, it is important to acknowledge that this peptide has potent effects on cardiovascular structure [81,82] (Fig. 98.5). Although there are indications, however, that the 'slow pressor' effects seen with chronic infusions of Ang II may be associated with hypertrophy of resistance vessels (see *Chapter 28*), it is notable that following cessation of Ang II infusion, systemic arterial blood pressure returns to normal within two hours [83]. Hence, even though Ang II may be capable of causing substantial changes in cardiovascular structure *in vivo*, these effects are not sufficient to cause irreversible hypertension.

DO DIFFERENT ANGIOTENSIN-CONVERTING ENZYME INHIBITORS HAVE DIFFERENT EFFECTS ON THE KIDNEY?

ACE inhibitors that undergo renal tubular secretion as well as filtration could theoretically reach higher tubular concentrations than others, particularly those metabolized in the liver, and such differences in handling could contribute to differential effects on renal tubular function (see *Chapter 26*) as could differences in their renal hemodynamic effects. However, whether or not different ACE inhibitors have such differential renal effects, either acutely

or chronically, has yet to be determined in experimental animals, or in the clinical setting, although the adverse effects of ACE inhibition in patients with renal artery stenosis and in some with congestive heart failure are well known (see *Chapters 76, 88–90, and 93*).

One aspect of the renal effects of ACE inhibitors that has received much attention is their ability to suppress the rate of progression of nephropathy (as judged by albuminuria), particularly in patients with diabetes mellitus (see *Chapter 92*). At present, it is unclear if this is a unique renoprotective effect of ACE inhibitors, separate from their ability to lower systemic arterial blood pressure [84,85]. Needless to say, there is no comparative information about different ACE inhibitors in this context.

DO DIFFERENT ANGIOTENSIN-CONVERTING ENZYME INHIBITORS HAVE DIFFERENT EFFECTS ON THE BRAIN?

Mention has been made already of the observation that access of different ACE inhibitors to the brain may vary according to factors such as lipophilicity, dose, and duration of treatment, and hence there are theoretical reasons [86] for postulating that they may exert differential effects due to these factors (see *Fig. 98.3*). In addition, it is possible there are differences in the influence of various ACE inhibitors on cerebral blood flow [87], although there are no comparative data bearing on this latter point.

Early experimental studies indicated that administration of captopril into the cerebroventricular system caused a greater fall in mean arterial blood pressure than did the same dose given peripherally [88]. This was attributed to inhibition of the cerebral production of Ang II, rather than accumulation of bradykinin, since central administration of exogenous bradykinin caused a rise rather than a fall in mean arterial blood pressure [88]. It must not be forgotten, however, that ACE cleaves several peptides besides Ang II and bradykinin; these occur in abundance in the brain [7] and hence could be involved in any central effects of ACE inhibitors (see *Fig 98.2* and Fig. 98.6). An example that is particularly interesting in this respect relates to the metabolism of metenkephalin heptapeptide. Angiotension-converting enzyme acts on this molecule and liberates the C-terminal dipeptide, L-arginyl-L-phenylalanine (Arg-Phe) [7]. Thiemermann *et al* [89] showed that Arg-Phe is a potent pressor agent in the anesthetized rat and suggested that it might be responsible for the previously described actions of the peptide, Phe-Met-Arg-Phe amide. We have found that Arg-Phe causes substantial rises in

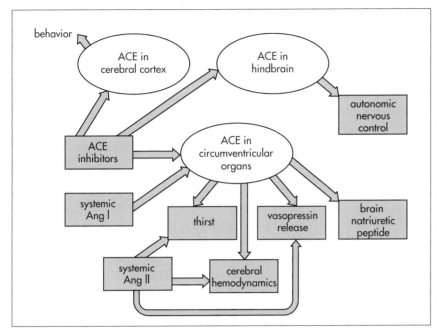

Fig. 98.6 Schematic representation of brain renin–angiotensin systems. Angiotensin-converting enzyme exists in different areas in the brain and may be associated with modulation of fluid and electrolyte balance (through actions of Ang II on thirst, vasopressin, and brain natriuretic peptide release), cardiovascular function (through influences on the medullary control of autonomic neuronal outflow to heart, blood vessels, and adrenal medulla), and behavior. These functions may also be influenced by systemic Ang I and Ang II. All of these processes may be susceptible to the influence of ACE inhibitors, particularly where ACE is located outside the blood–brain barrier (for example, circumventricular organs and area postrema).

mean arterial blood pressure in conscious rats, associated with tachycardia and regional vasoconstrictions (Gardiner SM *et al*, unpublished observations). These effects are abolished by ganglion blockade, consistent with the suggestion of Thiemermann *et al* [89] that Arg-Phe may exert its effects centrally. If this is the case, then it raises the intriguing possibility that central actions of ACE inhibitors to lower blood pressure could be due to suppression of the production of Arg-Phe from metenkephalin heptapeptide. It is noteworthy that the dipeptide, Phe-Arg, exerts no obvious cardiovascular effects in anesthetized rats [89], since this is the dipeptide cleaved from bradykinin by ACE [7].

It is not known if different ACE inhibitors interact with metenkephalin systems differentially, or to what extent such interactions could be involved in the putative effects of ACE inhibitors on mood and behavior. Observations, however, showing that peripheral administration of DuP 753 has an anxiolytic profile similar to captopril in various animal models [90,91], indicate this effect might be more specific for central Ang II-mediated processes (acting through AT-1 receptors) (Fig. 98.6). The finding that both captopril and perindopril [92] have behavioral effects, albeit in different paradigms, suggests that this is not an exclusive attribute of sulfhydryl-containing ACE inhibitors. Furthermore, analogs of captopril and perindopril with little ACE-inhibiting activity seem to be devoid of behavioral effects [90,92]. Thus, although there is good evidence for L-arginine/nitric oxide systems in the brain concerned with processes of nociception and long-term modulation [93, 94], there

is currently no evidence for a specific interaction between nitric oxide and sulfhydryl-containing ACE inhibitors as a basis for any central effects of the latter. At present, there are few [86] comparative studies on the chronic central effects of different ACE inhibitors, and no studies have been carried out with clinically relevant ranges of doses of the different compounds.

DO DIFFERENT ANGIOTENSIN-CONVERTING ENZYME INHIBITORS HAVE DIFFERENT EFFECTS ON THE AUTONOMIC NERVOUS SYSTEM?

Evidently, differential effects of different ACE inhibitors on brain function could produce differential effects on autonomic nervous activity (see *Chapters 37* and *41*) (Fig. 98.6), but we have found no data bearing directly on this point.

It is generally asserted that ACE inhibitors lower blood pressure without causing tachycardia, but it depends on the circumstances. Although unusual, tachycardia is a well-recognized, occasional accompaniment of clinical antihypertensive therapy with ACE inhibitors [95]. Furthermore, acute intravenous administration of captopril, enalaprilat, or lisinopril in conscious, water-deprived, Brattleboro rats causes hypotension associated with tachycardia [1], as does administration of DuP 753 [22,23]. The tachycardia, however, may not be as great as would be expected if mean arterial blood pressure were lowered by a similar amount with other agents. One explanation of this difference is the loss of the sympathoexcitatory and vagolytic actions of Ang II [96,97] following ACE inhibition (see *Figs. 98.5* and *98.6*), although changes in baroreflex sensitivity under these conditions have not been demonstrated convincingly in man [98–101], and there is no evidence of differential effects of various ACE inhibitors in this context. Finally, in conscious dogs, captopril may cause selective inhibition of renal nerve activity through an indomethacin-sensitive mechanism [102], but it is not known if other ACE inhibitors share this property.

DO DIFFERENT ANGIOTENSIN-CONVERTING ENZYME INHIBITORS HAVE DIFFERENT EFFECTS ON INSULIN SENSITIVITY?

There are studies (usually involving captopril, but some concerned with enalapril, ramipril, and perindopril) showing either increased insulin sensitivity [103–110] or no change in insulin sensitivity [84,111–114] during therapy. In the study of Retti

et al [103], the positive effect of captopril on insulin sensitivity was mimicked by exogenous bradykinin and these workers suggested inhibition of degradation of endogenous bradykinin by captopril was responsible for the change in insulin sensitivity. This does not, however, apply to the stimulation by captopril of glucose oxidation in human thrombocytes and mononuclear leucocytes [115]. Thus, although there have been no direct comparisons of the effect of different ACE inhibitors on insulin sensitivity, there are reasons for believing that such an effect, if real, would be an attribute of all ACE inhibitors. These matters are also discussed in *Chapter 92*.

CONCLUSIONS

As indicated at the outset, this chapter has been a parade of unanswered questions. As posed here, however, many of them are capable of being addressed, and evidently, the answers may be of clinical relevance. Hopefully, in the future, those who have read this review will examine critically the claims that any specific ACE inhibitor has unique effects on any particular function.

REFERENCES

1. Muller AF, Gardiner SM, Compton AM, Bennett T. Regional haemodynamic effects of captopril, enalaprilat and lisinopril in conscious water-replete and water-deprived Brattleboro rats. *Clinical Science* 1990;**79**:393–401.

2. Salvetti A. Newer ACE inhibitors. A look at the future. *Drugs* 1990;**40**:800–28.

3. Fabris B, Yamada H, Cubela R, Jackson B, Mendelsohn FAO, Johnston CI. Characterization of cardiac angiotensin converting enzyme (ACE) and *in vivo* inhibition following oral quinapril to rats. *British Journal of Pharmacology* 1990;**100**:651–5.

4. Alhenc-Gelas F, Soubrier F, Hubert C, Allegrini J, Lattion AL, Corvol P. The angiotensin I-converting enzyme (Kininase II): Progress in molecular and genetic structure. *Journal of Cardiovascular Pharmacology* 1990;**15** (suppl 6); S25–9.

5. Rogerson FM, Livett BG, Scanlon D, Mendelsohn FAO. Inhibition of angiotensin converting enzyme by N-terminal fragments of substance P. *Neuropeptides* 1989;**14**;213–7.

6. Skidgel RA, Schulz WW, Tam L-T, Erdös EG. Human renal angiotensin I converting enzyme and neutral endopeptidase. *Kidney International* 1987;**31** (suppl 20):S45–8.

7. Skidgel RA, Defendini R, Erdös EG. Angiotensin I converting enzyme and its role in neuropeptide metabolism. In: Turner AJ, ed. *Neuropeptides and their peptidases*. London: Ellis Horwood, 1987:165–82.

8. Erdös EG. Angiotensin I converting enzyme and the changes in our concepts through the years. *Hypertension* 1990;**16**:363–70.

9. Erdös EG. Some old and some new ideas on kinin metabolism. *Journal of Cardiovascular Pharmacology* 1990;**15** (suppl 6):S20–4.

10. Ehlers MRW, Riordan JF. Angiotensin-converting enzyme. Biochemistry and molecular biology. In: Laragh JH, Brenner BM, eds. *Hypertension: Pathophysiology, diagnosis and management*. New York: Raven Press, 1990: 1217–31.

11. MacFadyen RJ, Lees KR, Reid JL. Tissue and plasma angiotensin converting enzyme and the response to ACE inhibitor drugs. *British Journal of Clinical Pharmacology* 1991;**31**:1–13.

12. Dzau VJ. Multiple pathways of angiotensin production in the blood vessel wall: Evidence, possibilities and hypotheses. *Journal of Hypertension* 1989;**7**:933–6.

13. Urata H, Healy B, Stewart RW, Bumpus FM, Husain A. Angiotensin II-forming pathways in normal and failing human hearts. *Circulation Research* 1990;**66**:883–90.

14. Urata H, Kinoshita A, Misono KS, Bumpus FM, Husain A. Identification of a highly specific chymase as the major angiotensin II-forming enzyme in the human heart. *Journal of Biological Chemistry* 1990;**265**:22348–57.

15. Lindpaintner K, Jin M, Niedermaier N, Wilhelm MJ, Ganten D. Cardiac angiotensinogen and its local activation in the isolated perfused beating heart. *Circulation Research* 1990;**67**:564–73.

16. Cushman DW, Wang FL, Fung WC, Harvey CM, DeForrest JM. Differentiation of angiotensin-converting enzyme (ACE) inhibitors by their selective inhibition of ACE in physiologically important target organs. *American Journal of Hypertension* 1989;**2**:294–306.

17. Sakaguchi K, Chai SY, Jackson B, Johnston CI, Mendelsohn FAO. Inhibition of tissue angiotensin converting enzyme, quantitation by autoradiography. *Hypertension* 1988;**11**:230–8.

18. Johnston CI. Angiotensin converting enzyme inhibitors: Differences and advantages for first line therapy in hypertension. *Clinical and Experimental Hypertension* 1989;**A11**:1097–115.

19. Grover GJ, Sleph PG, Dzwonczyk S, Wang P, Fung W, Tobias D, Cushman DW. Effects of different angiotensin-converting enzyme (ACE) inhibitors on ischemic rat hearts: Relationship between cardiac ACE inhibition and cardioprotection. *Second International Symposium on ACE inhibition* 1991; Abstract O-5B.5.

20. Ujhelyi MR, Ferguson RK, Vlasses PH. Angiotensin-converting enzyme inhibitors: Mechanistic controversies. *Pharmacotherapy* 1989;9:351–62.

21. Waeber B, Juillerat-Jeanneret L, Aubert J-F, Schapira M, Nussberger J, Brunner HR. Involvement of the kallikrein–kinin system in the antihypertensive effect of the angiotensin converting enzyme inhibitors. *British Journal of Clinical Pharmacology* 1989;27:175–80S.

22. Batin P, Gardiner SM, Compton AM, Bennett T. Differential regional haemodynamic effects of the non-peptide angiotensin II antagonist, DuP 753, in water-replete and water-deprived Brattleboro rats. *Life Sciences* 1991;48:733–9.

23. Batin P, Gardiner SM, Compton AM, Kemp PA, Bennett T. Cardiac haemodynamic effects of the non-peptide, angiotensin II-receptor antagonist, DuP 753, in conscious Long Evans and Brattleboro rats. *British Journal of Pharmacology* 1991;103:1585–91.

24. Danckwardt L, Shimizu I, Bönner G, Rettig R, Unger T. Converting enzyme inhibition in kinin-deficient brown Norway rats. *Hypertension* 1990;16:429–35.

25. Gardiner SM, Compton AM, Kemp PA, Bennett T. Regional and cardiac haemodynamic responses to glyceryl trinitrate, acetylcholine, bradykinin and endothelin-l in conscious rats: Effects of N^G-nitro-L-arginine methyl ester. *British Journal of Pharmacology* 1990;101:632–9.

26. Schrör K. Converting enzyme inhibitors and the interaction between kinins and eicosanoids. *Journal of Cardiovascular Pharmacology* 1990;15 (suppl 6):S60–8.

27. Zusman MR. Renin- and non-renin-mediated antihypertensive actions of converting enzyme inhibitors. *Kidney International* 1984;25:969–83.

28. Oparil S, Horton R, Wilkins LH, Irvin J, Hammett DK. Antihypertensive effect of enalapril in essential hypertension: Role of prostacyclin. *American Journal of the Medical Sciences* 1987;294:395–402.

29. Quilley J, Duchin KL, Hudes EM, McGiff JC. The antihypertensive effect of captopril in essential hypertension: Relationship to prostaglandins and the kallikrein–kinin system. *Journal of Hypertension* 1987;5:121–8.

30. Kirch W, Stroemer K, Hoogkamer JFW, Kleinbloesem CH. The influence of prostaglandin inhibition by indomethacin on blood pressure and renal function in hypertensive patients treated with cilazapril. *British Journal of Clinical Pharmacology* 1989;27:297–301S.

31. Asmar RG, Journo HJ, Lacolley PJ, Santoni JP, Billaud E, Levy BI, Safar ME. Treatment for one year with perindopril: Effect on cardiac mass and arterial compliance in essential hypertension. *Journal of Hypertension* 1988;6 (suppl 3):S33–9.

32. van Gilst WH, de Graeff PA, Kingma JH, Wesseling H, de Langen CDJ. Captopril reduces purine loss and reperfusion arrhythmias in the rat heart after coronary artery occlusion. *European Journal of Pharmacology* 1984;100:113–7.

33. van Gilst WH, de Graeff PA, Wesseling H, de Langen CDJ. Reduction of reperfusion arrhythmias in the ischemic isolated rat heart by angiotensin converting enzyme inhibitors: A comparison of captopril, enalapril, and HOE 498. *Journal of Cardiovascular Pharmacology* 1986;8:722–8.

34. Linz W, Schölkens BA, Han Y-F. Beneficial effects of the converting enzyme inhibitor, ramipril, in ischemic rat hearts. *Journal of Cardiovascular Pharmacology* 1986;8 (suppl 10):S91–9.

35. Ribuot C, Rochette L. Converting enzyme inhibitors (captopril, enalapril, perindopril) prevent early post-infarction ventricular fibrillation in the anaesthetized rat. *Cardiovascular Drugs and Therapy* 1987;1:51–5.

36. Schölkens BA, Linz W, Lindpaintner K, Ganten D. Angiotensin deteriorates but bradykinin improves cardiac function following ischaemia in isolated rat hearts. *Journal of Hypertension* 1987;5 (suppl 5):S7–9.

37. Schölkens BA, Linz W, König W. Effects of the angiotensin converting enzyme inhibitor, ramipril, in isolated ischaemic rat heart are abolished by a bradykinin antagonist. *Journal of Hypertension* 1988;6 (suppl 4):S25–8.

38. Linz W, Martorana PA, Grötsch H, Bei-Yin Q, Schölkens BA. Antagonizing bradykinin (BK) obliterates the cardioprotective effects of bradykinin and angiotensin-converting enzyme (ACE) inhibitors in ischemic hearts. *Drug Development Research* 1989;19:393–408.

39. Linz W, Martorana PA, Schölkens BA. Local inhibition of bradykinin degradation in ischemic hearts. *Journal of Cardiovascular Pharmacology* 1990;15 (suppl 6):S99–109.

40. Martorana PA, Kettenbach B, Breipohl G, Linz W, Schölkens BA. Reduction of infarct size by local angiotensin-converting enzyme inhibition is abolished by a bradykinin antagonist. *European Journal of Pharmacology* 1990;182:395–6.

41. Mezzetti A, Scarinci A, Parlangeli C, Proietti-Franceschilli G, Guglielmi MD, Mancini M, Lapenna D, Porreca E, Cuccurullo F. Angiotensin-converting enzyme inhibitors counteract hypoxia-induced coronary constriction in the isolated rat heart. *Current Therapeutic Research* 1990;48:1075–85.

42. Fleetwood G, Boutinet S, Meier M, Wood JM. Involvement of the renin–angiotensin system in ischemic damage and reperfusion arrhythmias in the isolated perfused rat heart. *Journal of Cardiovascular Pharmacology* 1991;17:351–6.

43. Westlin W, Mullane K. Does captopril attenuate reperfusion-induced myocardial dysfunction by scavenging free radicals? *Circulation* 1988;77 (suppl 1):I-30–9.

44. Lucchesi BR. Myocardial ischemia, reperfusion and free radical injury. *American Journal of Cardiology* 1990;65:14–23I.

45. Sonnenblick EH, Zhao M, Eng C, LeJemtel TH, Factor SM, Capasso J, Anversa P. ACE inhibitors in acute and chronic ischaemia: Current status and future promise. *British Journal of Clinical Pharmacology* 1989;28:159–65S.

46. Przyklenk K, Kloner RA. Relationships between structure and effects of ACE inhibitors: Comparative effects in myocardial ischaemic/reperfusion injury. *British Journal of Clinical Pharmacology* 1989;28:167–75S.

47. Mak IT, Freedman AM, Dickens BF, Weglicki WB. Protective effects of sulfhydryl-containing angiotensin converting enzyme inhibitors against free radical injury in endothelial cells. *Biochemical Pharmacology* 1990;40:2169–75.

48. Koerner JE, Anderson BA, Dage RC. Protection against postischemic myocardial dysfunction in anesthetized rabbits with scavengers of oxygen-derived free radicals: Superoxide dismutase plus catalase, N-2-mercaptopropionyl glycine and captopril. *Journal of Cardiovascular Pharmacology* 1991;17:185–91.

49. Tang L-D, Sun J-Z, Wu Kl, Sun C-P, Tang Z-M. Beneficial effects of N-acetylcysteine and cysteine in stunned myocardium in perfused rat heart. *British Journal of Pharmacology* 1991;102:601–6.

50. Chopra M, Scott N, McMurray J, McLay J, Bridges A, Smith WE, Belch JJF, Captopril: A free radical scavenger. *British Journal of Clinical Pharmacology* 1989;27:396–9.

51. Chopra M, McMurray J, Stewart J, Dargie HJ, Smith WE. Free radical scavenging: A potentially beneficial action of thiol-containing angiotensin converting enzyme inhibitors. *Biochemical Society Transactions* 1990;18:1184–5.

52. Kukreja RC, Kontos HA, Hess ML. Captopril and enalaprilat do not scavenge the superoxide anion. *American Journal of Cardiology* 1990;65:24–72I.

53. Mehta JL, Nicolini FA, Lawson DL. Sulfhydryl group in angiotensin converting enzyme inhibitors and superoxide radical formation. *Journal of Cardiovascular Pharmacology* 1990;16:847–9.

54. Moncada S, Higgs EA. *Nitric oxide from L-arginine: A bioregulatory system.* Amsterdam: Excerpta Medica, 1990.

55. Shaffer JE, Lee F, Thomson S, Han BJ, Cooke JP, Loscalzo J. The hemodynamic effects of S-nitrosocaptopril in anesthetized dogs. *Journal of Pharmacology and Therapeutics* 1991;256:704–9.

56. Schneider R, Iscovitz H, Ilan Z, Bernstein K, Gros M, Iaina A. Oxygen free radical scavenger system intermediates in essential hypertensive patients before and immediately after sublingual captopril administration. *Israel Journal of Medical Science* 1990;26:491–5.

57. Johnston CI, Mooser V, Sun Y, Fabris B. Changes in cardiac angiotensin converting enzyme after myocardial infarction and hypertrophy in rats. *Clinical and Experimental Pharmacology and Physiology* 1991;18:107–10.

58. Dzau VJ. Mechanism of action of angiotensin-converting enzyme (ACE) inhibitors in hypertension and heart failure. Role of plasma versus tissue ACE. *Drugs* 1990;39 (suppl 2):11–16.

59. Smits JFM, Schoemaker RG, Daemen MJAP, Debets JJM. Haemodynamic consequences of interference with the renin–angiotensin system following myocardial infarction in rats. *British Journal of Pharmacology* 1991;102:99.

60. Van Krimpen C, Celeutjens JPM, Schoemaker RG, Smits JFM, Daemen MJAP. Effects of early angiotensin II receptor blockade on structural alterations of the rat heart after infarction. *Second International Symposium on ACE inhibition*, 1991;Abstract 0-9B.9.

61. Rees DD, Cellek S, Palmer RMJ, Moncada S. Dexamethasone prevents the induction by endotoxin of a nitric oxide synthase and the associated effects on vascular tone: An insight into endotoxin shock. *Biochemical and Biophysical Research Communications* 1990;173:541–7.

62. Horowitz JD, Antman EM, Lorell BH, Barry WH, Smith TW. Potentiation of the cardiovascular effects of nitroglycerin by N-acetylcysteine. *Circulation* 1983;68:1247–53.

63. Bertel O, Noll G. Effects of N-acetylcysteine on nitroglycerin responsiveness before and during nitrate therapy of congestive heart failure. *European Heart Journal* 1987;8 (suppl 1):44.

64. Levy WS, Katz RJ, Ruffolo RL, Leiboff RH, Wasserman AG. Potentiation of the hemodynamic effects of acutely administered nitroglycerin by methionine. *Circulation* 1988;78:640–5.

65. Gruetter CA, Lemke SM. Dissociation of cysteine and glutathione levels from nitroglycerin-induced relaxation. *European Journal of Pharmacology* 1985;111:85–95.

66. Hogan JC, Lewis MJ, Henderson AH. N-acetylcysteine fails to attenuate haemodynamic tolerance to glyceryl trinitrate in healthy volunteers. *British Journal of Clinical Pharmacology* 1989;28:421–6.

67. Stewart DJ, Münzel T, Holtz J, Bassenge E. Discrepancy between initial and steady-state resistance vessel responsiveness to short-term nitroglycerin exposure in the hindlimb of conscious dogs. *Journal of Cardiovascular Pharmacology* 1988;12:144–51.

68. Fahmy NR, Gavras HP. Impact of captopril on hemodynamic and hormonal effects of nitroprusside. *Journal of Cardiovascular Pharmacology* 1985;7:869–74.

69. van Gilst WH, de Graeff PA, Scholtens E, de Langen CDJ, Wesseling H. Potentiation of isosorbide dinitrate-induced coronary dilatation by captopril. *Journal of Cardiovascular Pharmacology* 1987;9:254–5.

70. Lawson DL, Nichols WW, Mehta P, Mehta JL. Captopril-induced reversal of nitroglycerin tolerance: Role of sulfhydryl group vs ACE-inhibitory activity. *Journal of Cardiovascular Pharmacology* 1991;17:411–8.

71. Clementi WA, Durst NL, McNay JL, Keeton TK. Captopril modifies the hemodynamic and neuroendocrine responses to sodium nitroprusside in hypertensive patients. *Hypertension* 1986;8:229–37.

72. Dakak N, Makhoul N, Flugelman MY, Merdler A, Shehadeh H, Schneeweiss A, Halon DA, Lewis BS. Failure of captopril to prevent nitrate tolerance in congestive heart failure secondary to coronary artery disease. *American Journal of Cardiology* 1990;66:608–13.

73. Katz RJ, Levy WS, Buff L, Wasserman AG. Prevention of nitrate tolerance with angiotensin converting enzyme inhibitors. *Circulation* 1991;83:1271–7.

74. Levy BI, Michel J-B, Salzmann JL, Azizi M, Poitevin P, Camilleri JP, Safar ME. Arterial effects of angiotensin converting enzyme inhibition in renovascular and spontaneously hypertensive rats. *Journal of Hypertension* 1988;6 (suppl 3):S23–5.

75. Levy BI, Benessiano J, Poitevin P, Safar ME. Endothelium-dependent mechanical properties of the carotid artery in WKY and SHR. *Circulation Research* 1990;66:321–8.

76. Kawaguchi H, Sawa H, Yasuda H. Effect of endothelin on angiotensin converting enzyme activity in cultured pulmonary artery endothelial cells. *Journal of Hypertension* 1991;9:171–4.

77. Vanhoutte PM, Auch-Schwelk W, Biondi ML, Lorenz RR, Schini VB, Vidal MJ. Why are converting enzyme inhibitors vasodilators? *British Journal of Clinical Pharmacology* 1989;28:95–104S.

78. Shultz PM, Raij L. Effects of antihypertensive agents on endothelium-dependent and endothelium-independent relaxations. *British Journal of Clinical Pharmacology* 1989;28:151–7S.

79. Clozel M, Kuhn H, Hefti F. Effects of angiotensin converting enzyme inhibitors and of hydralazine on endothelial function in hypertensive rats. *Hypertension* 1990;16:532–40.

80. Christensen HRL, Nielsen H, Christensen KL, Baandrup U, Jespersen LT, Mulvany MJ. Long-term hypotensive effects of an angiotensin converting enzyme inhibitor in spontaneously hypertensive rats: Is there a role for vascular structure? *Journal of Hypertension* 1988;6 (suppl 3):S27–31.

81. Scott-Burden T, Hahn AWA, Resink TJ, Bühler FR. Modulation of extracellular matrix by angiotensin II: Stimulated glycoconjugate synthesis and growth in vascular smooth muscle cells. *Journal of Cardiovascular Pharmacology* 1990;16 (suppl 4):S36–41.

82. Schelling P, Fischer H, Ganten D. Angiotensin and cell growth: A link to cardiovascular hypertrophy? *Journal of Hypertension* 1991;9:3–15.

83. Brown AJ, Casals-Stenzel J, Gofford S, Lever AF, Morton JJ. Comparison of fast and slow pressor effects of angiotensin II in the conscious rat. *American Journal of Physiology* 1981;241:H381–8.

84. Melbourne Diabetic Nephropathy Study Group. Comparison between perindopril and nifedipine in hypertensive and normotensive diabetic patients with microalbuminuria. *British Medical Journal* 1991;302:210–6.

85. Johnston CI, Mooser V, Jackson B, Fabris B. Renoprotective effects of angiotensin converting enzyme (ACE) inhibitor. *Second International Symposium of ACE inhibition* 1991; Abstract 0-2.4.

86. Unger T, Ganten D, Lang RE, Schölkens BA. Is tissue converting enzyme inhibition a determinant of the antihypertensive efficacy of converting enzyme inhibitors? Studies with the two different compounds, Hoe 498 and MK 421, in spontaneously hypertensive rats. *Journal of Cardiovascular Pharmacology* 1984;6:872–80.

87. Waldemar G, Paulson OB. Angiotensin converting enzyme inhibition and cerebral circulation — a review. *British Journal of Clinical Pharmacology* 1989;28:177–82S.

88. Unger T, Ganten D, Lang RE. Tissue converting enzyme and cardiovascular actions of converting enzyme inhibitors. *Journal of Cardiovascular Pharmacology* 1986;8 (suppl 10):S75–81.

89. Thiemermann C, Al-Damluji S, Hecker M, Vane JR. FMRF-amide and L-ARG-L-PHE increase blood pressure and heart rate in the anaesthetised rat by central stimulation of the sympathetic nervous system. *Biochemical and Biophysical Research Communications* 1991;175:318–24.

90. Costall B, Domeney AM, Gerrard PA, Horovitz ZP, Kelly ME, Naylor RJ, Tomkins DM. Effects of captopril and SQ 29,852 on anxiety-related behaviours in rodent and marmoset. *Pharmacology, Biochemistry & Behaviour* 1990;36:13–20.

91. Barnes NM, Costall B, Kelly ME, Murphy DA, Naylor RJ. Anxiolytic-like action of DuP 753, a non-peptide angiotensin II receptor antagonist. *Second International Symposium on ACE inhibition* 1991; Abstract P-39.

92. Martin P, Massol J, Scalbert E, Puech AJ. Involvement of angiotensin-converting enzyme inhibition in reversal of helpless behaviour evoked by perindopril in rats. *European Journal of Pharmacology* 1990;187:165–70.

93. Moore PK, Oluyomi AO, Babbedge RC, Wallace P, Hart SL. L-N^G-nitro arginine methyl ester exhibits antinociceptive activity in the mouse. *British Journal of Pharmacology* 1991;102:198–202.

94. Shibuki K, Okada D. Endogenous nitric oxide release required for long-term synaptic depression in the cerebellum. *Nature* 1991;349:326–8.

95. Hodsman GP, Brown JJ, Cumming AMM, Davies DL, East BW, Lever AF, Morton JJ, Murray GD, Robertson JIS. Enalapril (MK421) in the treatment of hypertension with renal artery stenosis. *Journal of Hypertension* 1983;1 (suppl 1);109–17.

96. Scroop GC, Lowe RD. Efferent pathways of the cardiovascular response to vertebral artery infusions of angiotensin in the dog. *Clinical Science* 1969;37:605–19.

97. Joy MD. The vasomotor centre and its afferent pathways. *Clinical Science and Molecular Medicine* 1975;48:253–6s.

98. Morganti A, Grassi G, Sala C, Capozi A, Turolo L, Sabadini E, Bolla G, Mancia G, Zanchetti A. Acute and chronic converting enzyme inhibition reduces the vasomotor response to reflex sympathetic activation in man. *Journal of Hypertension* 1985;3 (suppl 3):259–62.

99. Ajayi AA, Reid JL. The effect of enalapril on baroreceptor mediated reflex function in normotensive subjects. *British Journal of Clinical Pharmacology* 1986;21:338–9.

100. Ajayi AA, Lees KR, Reid JL. Effects of angiotensin converting enzyme inhibitor, perindopril, on autonomic reflexes. *European Journal of Clinical Pharmacology* 1986;30:177–82.

101. Elliott HL, Ajayi AA, Reid JL. The influence of cilazapril on indices of autonomic function in normotensives and hypertensives. *British Journal of Clinical Pharmacology* 1989;27:303–7S.

102. Zucker IH, Chen J-S, Wang W. Renal sympathetic nerve and hemodynamic responses to captopril in conscious dogs: Role of prostaglandins. *American Journal of Physiology* 1991;260:H260–5.

103. Rett K, Jauch KW, Wicklmayr M, Dietze G, Fink E, Mehnert H. Angiotensin converting enzyme inhibitors in diabetes: Experimental and human experience. *Postgraduate Medical Journal* 1986;62 (suppl 1):59–64.

104. Pollare T, Lithell H, Berne C. A comparison of the effects of hydrochlorothiazide and captopril on glucose and lipid metabolism in patients with hypertension. *New England Journal of Medicine* 1989;321:868–73.

105. Arauz-Pacheco C, Ramirez LC, Rios JM, Raskin P. Hypoglycemia induced by angiotensin-converting enzyme inhibitors in patients with non-insulin-dependent diabetes receiving sulfonylurea therapy. *American Journal of Medicine* 1990;89:811–3.

106. Ueda Y, Aoi W, Yamachika S, Shikaya T. Beneficial effects of angiotensin-converting enzyme inhibitor on renal function and glucose homeostasis in diabetics with hypertension. *Nephron* 1990;55 (suppl 1):85–9.

107. Janka HU, Nuber A, Mehnert H. Metabolic effects of ramipril treatment in hypertensive subjects with non-insulin-dependent diabetes mellitus. *Arzneimittel Forschung* 1990;40:432–5.

108. Kodama J, Katayama S, Tanaka K, Itabashi A, Kawazu S, Ishii J. Effect of captopril on glucose concentration. Possible role of augmented postprandial forearm blood flow. *Diabetes Care* 1990;13:1109–11.

109. Lithell HO, Pollare T, Berne C. Insulin sensitivity in newly detected hypertensive patients: Influence of captopril and other antihypertensive agents on insulin sensitivity and related biological parameters. *Journal of Cardiovascular Pharmacology* 1990;15 (suppl 5):S46–52.

110. Torlone E, Rambotti AM, Perriello G, Botta G, Samteusanio F, Bruetti P, Bolli GB. ACE-inhibition increases hepatic and extrahepatic sensitivity to insulin in patients with Type 2 (non-insulin-dependent) diabetes mellitus and arterial hypertension. *Diabetologia* 1991;34:119–25.

111. Mathews DM, Wathen CG, Bell D, Collier A, Muir AL, Clarke BF. The effect of captopril on blood pressure and glucose tolerance in hypertensive non-insulin dependent diabetics. *Postgraduate Medical Journal* 1986;62 (suppl 1):73–5.

112. Shionoiri H, Iino S, Inoue S. Glucose metabolism during captopril mono- and combination therapy in diabetic hypertensive patients: A multiclinic trial. *Clinical and Experimental Hypertension — Theory and Practice* 1987;A9:671–4.

113. Prince MJ, Stuart CA, Padia M, Bandi Z, Hollan OB. Metabolic effects of hydrochlorothiazide and enalapril during treatment of the hypertensive diabetic patient. *Archives of Internal Medicine* 1988;148:2363–8.

114. Seefeldt T, Ørskov L, Mengel A, Rasmussen O, Pedersen MM, Møller N, Christiansen JS, Schmitz O. Lack of effects of angiotensin-converting enzyme (ACE)-inhibitors on glucose metabolism in type 1 diabetes. *Diabetic Medicine* 1990;7:700–4.

115. Haeckel R, Colic D. Influence of captopril on glucose and fatty acid oxidation in human thrombocytes and mononuclear leucocytes. *Arzneimittel Forschung* 1991;41:37–9.

99

SIDE EFFECTS ASSOCIATED WITH INHIBITORS OF ANGIOTENSIN-CONVERTING ENZYME

ASTRID E FLETCHER AND COLIN T DOLLERY

INTRODUCTION

It is easier to understand, and thereby minimize adverse reactions to drugs if they are considered within a conceptual framework.

EFFECTS RELATED TO THE MAIN PHARMACOLOGICAL ACTION

Many adverse effects are directly related to a drug's main pharmacological action. They are largely predictable and exhibit a dose–response relationship. With ACE inhibitors, effects of this kind include hypotension and renal impairment in patients whose blood pressure is Ang II dependent. Such effects may be more prominent in patients with severe heart failure on fixed and high doses of loop diuretics and usually also a cardiac glycoside, who are given moderate to high doses of ACE inhibitors as initiation therapy.

EFFECTS RELATED TO SUBSIDIARY PHARMACOLOGICAL ACTIONS

Many drugs have more than one action. With ACE inhibitors, there has been interest in the possibility that other peptidase functions (for example, enkephalinase actions) might be inhibited and thereby affect mood or memory. The evidence in man for such actions is slight.

IDIOSYNCRATIC CLASS EFFECTS

Patients may be more susceptible to a drug because of their genetic make-up. Two sporadic effects of ACE inhibitors — cough and angioneurotic edema — appear to be of this susceptible type, although a genetic component has not been demonstrated. These side effects have been described, sporadically, with all widely used ACE inhibitors and are therefore most probably due to inhibition of peptidyl dipeptidase in patients who have some, as yet unknown reason, for enhanced susceptibility.

COMPOUND-SPECIFIC EFFECTS

Some adverse effects depend upon a feature of the chemical structure which is unique to that compound. When captopril was first introduced, it was frequently used in high doses in severely hypertensive patients who often had renal impairment. A group of effects was described which included proteinuria, nephrotic syndrome, granulocytopenia, taste disturbance, morbilliform rash, Guillain–Barré neuropathy, and so on. These effects, reminiscent of penicillamine toxicity, appear to exhibit a steep dose–response curve because, following reductions in the recommended dose of captopril, they are now only rarely reported.

THE BURDEN OF ADVERSE EFFECTS

Etiological classification of adverse effects is satisfying in a scientific sense, but to a patient who is taking a drug, the total burden of unwanted effects is of greater significance. Attention must be paid to the discomfort, disability, and reduction in the quality of life from such effects. Measurement of side effects has moved from the description of the occurrence of symptoms to an evaluation of the effects of these on the patients' everyday lives, that is, 'quality of life'. This includes assessment of psychological and general wellbeing, cognitive functioning, work performance, and other areas such as sleep quantity and quality and sexual function.

The severity of the disease under treatment, and the degree of benefit expected, form the other side of the equation. A moderate symptom burden may be poorly tolerated by a patient with mild essential hypertension while much more severe effects might be readily accepted by a patient with advanced heart failure. In heart failure, ACE inhibitors have been shown to improve survival [1] while in hypertension, their popularity is based on a belief that they are associated with fewer and less-severe side effects than are other forms of antihypertensive treatment.

This chapter reviews the side effects of ACE inhibitors in terms of quality of life and specific symptons, and also considers changes in biochemical and hematological variables that occur with ACE inhibitors. Data are available from a variety of sources. Randomized controlled trials provide an estimate of the comparative effects of ACE inhibitors on quality of life against other antihypertensive drugs. Data on absolute effects are not available since no large trial has included a comparison against a placebo group. Consideration of the effects of ACE inhibitors on cognitive function will include studies in animals and in normotensive subjects. The review of specific symptoms includes spontaneous reports from postmarketing surveillance studies and other longitudinal data bases such as prescription-event monitoring as well as randomized controlled trials. Spontaneous reporting may be biased by physicians' preconceptions of 'legitimate' side effects, particularly when the complaint, such as cough, occurs frequently in the background population. The advantage of this method is that it can be used in large studies and provides some indication of the occurrence of less-frequent side effects. Data on side effects from randomized controlled trials reduce reporting bias but may provide an incomplete picture: the trials are often small, and questionnaires will not include unknown side effects. These problems are encountered when the major symptomatic side effects of ACE inhibitors are discussed: cough, angioneurotic edema and rash.

QUALITY OF LIFE AND ANGIOTENSIN-CONVERTING ENZYME INHIBITORS IN HYPERTENSION

In 1986, Croog and colleagues published the results of a major trial using quality of life evaluation methods [2]. This was a double-blind trial of six months' duration in 626 men with mild to moderate hypertension, randomized to treatment with captopril, methyldopa, or propranolol. Hydrochlorothiazide was added as needed to control the blood pressure. The trial employed interviewers and used a large number of measures of quality of life. After six months of treatment, a significant benefit for captopril compared with methyldopa was shown in measures of overall wellbeing, of physical symptoms, in self-rated work performance, in a measure of cognitive function, and in overall quality of life satisfaction. There were fewer differences between captopril and propranolol, with significant differences being found in favor of captopril in general wellbeing, sexual function, and physical symptoms. Patients taking propranolol did better than did those on methyldopa in work performance. These results were obtained from patients who completed the 24 weeks of the trial and may thus have minimized differences between treatment modalities due to the exclusion of the withdrawals. Of patients on methyldopa, 20% withdrew compared with 8% on captopril and 13% on propranolol. Most withdrawals from all three drugs were because of fatigue [2].

Since this publication [2], several trials have examined

whether these benefits for ACE inhibitors are also found when compared with newer antihypertensive drugs [3–8]. Figure 99.1 summarizes the features of these trials, including patient characteristics and numbers, treatment groups, and duration of therapy. The trials were conducted in hypertensive patients in both Europe and the USA. Only one trial [5] excluded women. A further study by Croog and colleagues [6] was of a black hypertensive population. None of the trials was conducted in a specifically elderly population; the average age of subjects was 50–56 years. All trials were double blind. The duration of treatment ranged from six weeks in a crossover trial, to six months. In the report by Steiner and colleagues [5], there were two randomized ACE-inhibitor groups (captopril and enalapril), and two β-blocker groups (atenolol and propranolol). The ACE inhibitor used in the other trials was captopril (three studies), enalapril (one study), and cilazapril (one study). In all studies, atenolol was one of the comparator drugs, and in two trials, the third treatment group was administered a calcium-channel blocker, either verapamil or nifedipine.

Study [reference]	Male: Female	Average age (years)	Treatment groups	Duration (months)
Herrick et al [3]	93:69	51	enalapril atenolol	3
Fletcher et al [4]	58:67	51	captopril atenolol	2
Steiner et al [5]	360:0	not given	captopril propranolol enalapril atenolol	2
Croog et al [6]	195:199	50	captopril atenolol verapamil	2
Palmer et al [7]	163:133	56	captopril atenolol (crossover)	1.5
Fletcher et al [8]	308:232	54	cilazapril atenolol nifedipine	6

Fig. 99.1 Randomized double-blind trials assessing the comparative effects of ACE inhibitors in hypertension on quality of life.

Similar dimensions of quality of life were assessed in all trials and included those aspects that might potentially be affected by antihypertensive treatment. The questionnaires used to measure quality of life included validated standard instruments with reasonable reassurance about their reliability and ability to show changes. All trials included a measure of psychological wellbeing, and the authors usually also reported on the subscales of depression, anxiety, confusion, and irritability. Not all the trials used the same methods, but there was overlap in some, allowing direct comparisons to be made. Symptomatic complaints were measured in all but one study. Not all trials measured the same complaints or in the same way. Additional aspects of quality of life were covered by several of the reports; these included evaluation of work performance, of sexual dysfunction, of sleep dysfunction, and of overall life satisfaction. Other assessments made in some studies included objective tests of cognitive performance, and two trials included an independent assessment by a partner or relative.

The results of the trials have been reviewed elsewhere [9] and are described below.

GLOBAL MEASURES

The trials found no differences between ACE inhibitors, atenolol, and the calcium-channel blockers (verapamil or nifedipine) in global measures of psychological and general wellbeing and life satisfaction. The adverse effect of propranolol that was suggested in the 1986 study [2], was confirmed in the trial by Steiner and

Study [reference]	Differences		
Croog et al 1986 [2]	captopril — methyldopa	3.8	P<0.01
	captopril — propranolol	2.5	
Steiner et al 1990 [5]	captopril — propranolol	1.7	
	captopril — atenolol	0.3	
	enalapril — atenolol	0.7	
	enalapril — propranolol	2.1	
Croog et al 1990 [6]	captopril — atenolol		
	men	1.0	
	women	−0.8	
Fletcher et al 1991 [8]	cilazapril — atenolol	0.7	
	95% confidence interval	(−1.9, 3.4)	
	cilazapril — nifedipine	0.5	
	95% confidence interval	(−2.2, 3.1)	

Fig. 99.2 Between drug differences in general wellbeing: observations in four trials using the Psychological General Well Being Index.

colleagues [5]. Both atenolol and enalapril were associated with positive changes on the life-satisfaction scale compared with negative changes on propranolol.

Figure 99.2 gives the changes in a measure of overall wellbeing, the Psychological Well Being Index, which was used in four of the trials. In the original Croog study [2], significant differences of 3.8 units were observed between captopril and methyldopa, and of 2.5 units between captopril and propranolol [2]. In general, the differences observed between ACE inhibitors and atenolol were of a smaller order than those seen for ACE inhibitors versus propranolol or methyldopa. In the trial comparing cilazapril with atenolol and nifedipine, the largest of the recent trials and of the same duration as the 1986 study [2], the 95% confidence intervals exclude an effect between cilazapril and atenolol, and between cilazapril and nifedipine of the size seen earlier for methyldopa [2] but do not exclude the difference of 2.5 units between captopril and propranolol [8]. The average result shows only a very small difference between the ACE inhibitor and both atenolol (0.7 units) and nifedipine (0.5 units) when administered to patients with hypertension. These results suggest that the initial enthusiasm for ACE inhibitors based on the results of the study of Croog and colleagues in 1986 needs to be tempered. Angiotensin-converting enzyme inhibitors appear to have similar effects on overall wellbeing to atenolol and nifedipine.

MOOD

Measures of overall wellbeing may conceal specific effects on mood. In Steiner's study, both captopril and enalapril were significantly different from atenolol and propranolol in the depressed mood subscale although the effect for atenolol was less, the differences favoring the ACE inhibitors [5]. None of the other trials reviewed found significant differences in measures of depression. The percentage increase in score on measures of depressed mood ranged from 3% in favor of atenolol to an increase of 19% by atenolol, with 95% confidence limits from the two largest trials of −22% to +22%. Differences between ACE inhibitors and β-blockers may also reflect improvements in mood as a result of ACE inhibition.

In the early days of ACE-inhibitor therapy, there were suggestions from uncontrolled observations of an antidepressant [10] or indeed a potentially euphoric effect [11]. This possibility was investigated in a small double-blind crossover trial of eight patients with mild hypertension receiving fixed dozes of atenolol plus bendrofluazide, and further randomized to six weeks of additional treatment with captopril or placebo. This trial found no evidence for a euphoriant effect of captopril; indeed the converse was found with captopril significantly being associated with a small lowering of mood [12]. Steiner found similar improvements in vitality and positive wellbeing with ACE inhibitors and atenolol but not with propranolol [5]. Little change was observed with ACE inhibitors compared with either atenolol or with nifedipine in measures of vigor [7,8]. Overall, these results do not support an association of ACE inhibitors with mood elevation, but the instruments used may not have been sensitive to more subtle effects.

COGNITIVE FUNCTION

The literature on ACE inhibitors and cognitive function includes trials in hypertensives and studies on normotensive volunteers and laboratory animals.

Early animal studies suggested that captopril did not cross the blood–brain barrier [13,14]. Inhibition of ACE activity in the brain was subsequently shown in rats given captopril by a variety of routes including subcutaneously [15]. Johnston suggested that esterified ACE inhibitors such as enalapril are more lipophilic and more likely to cross the blood–brain barrier [16]. At therapeutic doses, however, enalapril was found to inhibit brain ACE only in the circumventricular organs that are outside the blood–brain barrier. At higher doses, esterified ACE inhibitors blocked converting enzyme within the blood–brain barrier, but only small amounts of esterified drug reach systemic plasma after oral doses in man.

In animal studies, ACE inhibitors have been shown to aid learning in mice, and to prevent the disruptive effects of scopolamine [17,18]. Captopril prevented blood-pressure elevation in mice reared in 'stressful' housing conditions which otherwise induced elevations in pressure of approximately 20mmHg [19]. The function of angiotensin-converting enzymes in the brain is not well understood. Both Ang II and its peptide analog antagonist, saralasin, improve memory and learning in rats, suggesting that cognitive effects are mediated indirectly (possibly through stimulation of central dopaminergic activity) rather than directly through Ang II receptors [20,21] (see *Chapter 41*).

In man, there are reports on the effects of ACE inhibitors on a variety of tests which broadly assess performance in terms of psychomotor speed and concentration, verbal memory, and visual memory.

PSYCHOMOTOR SPEED AND CONCENTRATION

The Trail Making B test measures the time taken to join letters and numbers in sequence, and was used in several of the randomized trials in hypertensive patients [2,6,8] (Fig. 99.3). Significant

Study [reference]	Trail making B — differences (s)	
Croog *et al* 1986 [2]		
captopril — methyldopa	8	P<0.05
captopril — propranolol	2	
Croog *et al* 1990 [6]		
captopril — atenolol	−12	men
captopril — atenolol	+ 4	women
Fletcher *et al* 1991 [8]		95% confidence interval
cilazapril — atenolol	−2	(−6, +3)
cilazapril — nifedipine	−3	(−7, +2)
+ = improved performance between drugs		

Fig. 99.3 Results of a test of cognitive function.

differences were found between captopril and methyldopa (eight seconds in favour of captopril) but not between captopril and propranolol (two seconds). In the study of black hypertensives, there were differences in favor of atenolol for men (12 seconds) and in favor of captopril for women (four seconds) [6]. The sample sizes were, however, small and these differences were not statistically significant. Very small differences were observed between cilazapril, atenolol, and nifedipine with atenolol- and nifedipine-treated patients being 2–3 seconds faster in performing the test than were cilazapril-treated patients [8]. The 95% confidence intervals for the differences ranged from −7 to +2, thus excluding the size of difference earlier found between captopril and methyldopa [2]. This suggests that the differences previously observed [2] reflected adverse effects of methyldopa rather than improvements with captopril.

Several workers have found differences between ACE inhibitors and β-blockers in other measures of psychomotor speed and alertness (Fig. 99.4). Herrick and co-workers reported that, in the Digit Symbol Substitution Test (DSST) and Paced Auditory Serial Addition Task, hypertensive patients treated with enalapril showed greater improvement from baseline than did atenolol-treated patients [3]. In young healthy male volunteers, neither atenolol nor captopril produced changes in DSST that were significantly different from placebo [22]. In the same study, both captopril and atenolol significantly increased the number of letters cancelled compared with placebo, with no apparent difference between the two drugs. The effect for captopril was found only at doses of 25mg and not at 12.5 or 50mg. No significant differences from placebo were found for either drug in tests of choice reaction time, or in critical flicker-fusion tests. Atenolol was associated with a significant reduction in the rate of finger tapping compared with placebo, but no improvement in tapping rate was observed with captopril over placebo.

An earlier study in healthy volunteers had found some evidence of increased alertness with enalapril shown by improvement in finger tapping over placebo, but no changes in other measures (DSST and Auditory Reaction time) of alertness [23] (Fig. 99.4). A further study found that finger tapping and symbol copying improved with enalapril compared with propranolol and atenolol [24]. It is possible that inconsistencies in the results of these studies are due to the use of different ACE inhibitors. The evidence that enalapril improves alertness is stronger than for captopril.

VERBAL AND VISUAL MEMORY

In three trials (Fig. 99.4) verbal memory was assessed using Digit Span tests (repetition of digits both forwards and backwards). No differences were found between ACE inhibitors, propranolol, atenolol, and verapamil [3,5,6]. Steiner's trial [5] also showed no differences between drug groups on a range of other tests of verbal memory. No differences were reported [2,3] between ACE inhibitors, β-blockers, and methyldopa in tests of visual memory.

In a small (n=25) single-blind randomized trial in hypertensive patients, verbal and visual memory-performance scores were significantly lower on atenolol compared with placebo, while no change was observed on enalapril [25]. Differences between drugs were not tested. The authors suggested that

	Drugs compared	Alertness		Memory	
		Digit symbol substitution	Finger tapping	Verbal digit span	Visual (various tests)
Hypertensives					
Herrick et al [3]	enalapril atenolol	↑ enalapril	not included	↔	↔
Steiner et al [5]	captopril verapamil atenolol propranolol	not included	not included	↔	↔
Croog et al [6]	captopril verapamil atenolol	not included	not included	↔	↔
Lichter et al [25]	atenolol enalapril	not included	not included	↓ atenolol ↔ enalapril	specially devised tests of verbal and visual memory
Normotensives Currie et al [22]	captopril atenolol	*compared to placebo* ↔ ↔	↔ captopril ↓ atenolol	*compared to placebo* ↔ ↔	
Olajide & Lader [23]	enalapril	↔	↑ enalapril		
Frcka & Lader [24]	enalapril atenolol propranolol	↔ ↔ ↔	↑ enalapril ↓ atenolol ↓ propranolol	↓ enalapril ↓ atenolol ↓ propranolol	↓ enalapril ↓ propranolol ↓ atenolol

↑   Improved
↔   No difference
↓   Reduction
Only differences significant at 5% level or more are given.

Fig. 99.4 Effects of ACE inhibitors on cognitive function tests.

99.5

atenolol interfered with memory while enalapril produced no change.

Studies on young healthy volunteers have also not shown consistent results in the effects of ACE inhibitors on memory (Fig. 99.4). In one study, immediate recall was not affected by either captopril or atenolol [22], but another found that enalapril, propranolol, and atenolol significantly impaired immediate recall as compared with placebo, while delayed recall was significantly worse on enalapril and propranolol compared with atenolol and placebo [24].

No differences in a scale of self-reports of problems with memory or concentration were found between ACE inhibitors and atenolol in two large trials [7,8]. A benefit for both captopril and propranolol in comparison with methyldopa in self-reported work performance was found by Croog and colleagues [2], but it is not clear to what extent this reflected poor performance on methyldopa. Patients taking propranolol showed little change. In summary, it is possible that some ACE inhibitors may bring about minor improvements in the performance of tests of alertness. It is unlikely that they produce either deleterious or beneficial effects on memory.

SEXUAL SYMPTOMS

Angiotensin-converting enzyme inhibitors do not appear to affect sexual function adversely. In one study, men treated with captopril showed little change in various aspects of sexual performance, while men treated with propranolol had a higher frequency of problems, particularly impotence [26]. This finding for propranolol was not confirmed in the study by Steiner who found no differences between captopril, enalapril, atenolol, and propranolol other than an increased frequency of morning erections on propranolol [5]. Other studies have found no differences in sexual function between captopril or cilazapril and atenolol [7,8].

Study [reference]	ACE inhibitor	Average daily dose (mg)	Population	Patient number	Years of follow-up (maximum)	Type of study
Groel et al [47]	captopril	160	mild to severe hypertension	6,737	1	manufacturer's data base
Chalmers et al [29]	captopril	66–72	mild to moderate hypertension	13,295	1.5	manufacturer's data base
Schoenberger et al [30]	captopril	58	mild to moderate hypertension	30,515	(7 weeks)	manufacturer's open follow-up
Inman et al [31] Speirs et al [70]	enalapril	?	any prescription of enalapril	12,543	1	prescription-event monitoring
Cooper et al [48]	enalapril	?	mild to moderate hypertension	11,710	(6 weeks)	manufacturer's data base
Coulter & Edwards [28], Coulter [56]	captopril enalapril	66 17	hypertension and heart failure	4,774 captopril 974 enalapril	5 3	prescription-event monitoring
Cameron & Higgins [34]	lisinopril	?	mild to severe hypertension and heart failure	3,270	3.5	manufacturer's data base
Knapp et al [35]	quinapril	20–40	mild to severe hypertension and heart failure	2,697	3	manufacturer's data base

Fig. 99.5 Postmarketing studies of ACE inhibitors. Information from the drug manufacturer's data base usually includes uncontrolled open follow-up studies, but may also include double-blind comparative studies.

99.6

Study [reference]	Design	Method of reporting	ACE inhibitor	Cough (%)	Rash (%)	Taste disturbance (%)
Groel et al [47]	PMS	SR	captopril	—	5–10	3–6
Chalmers et al [29]	PMS	SR+	captopril	0.2	0.8	0.3
Schoenberger et al [30]	PMS	SR	captopril	0.8	1.1	0.9
Fletcher et al [4]	DB RCT	Q	captopril	22	—	3.5
Palmer et al [7]	DB RCT	Q	captopril	17	—	—
Inman et al [31]	PEM	GP	enalapril	2.9	3	0.2
Cooper et al [48]	PMS	SR	enalapril	1	0.5	0.2
Coulter & Edwards [28], Coulter [56]	PEM	SR+	captopril / enalapril	1.1 / 2.8	— / —	6 (Q)
Yeo & Ramsay [32]	DB RCT	Q	enalapril	22	—	—
Fletcher et al [8]	DB RCT	Q	cilazapril	14	—	—
Cameron & Higgins [34]	PMS	SR	lisinopril	3	4 CHF NK HYP	—
Knapp et al [35]	PMS	SR	quinapril	2.1	0.2	—

PEM = Prescription-event monitoring; PMS = Postmarketing surveillance;
DB RCT = Double-blind randomized controlled trial; + = Leading to withdrawal;
SR = Spontaneous reporting; Q = Questionnaire;
GP = Information from general practitioner's notes; NK = Not known;
CHF = Treated for congestive heart failure; HYP = Treated for hypertension;

Fig. 99.6   Incidence of three side effects of ACE inhibitors according to the method of data collection.

SYMPTOMATIC SIDE EFFECTS

COUGH

An association of ACE inhibitors with cough has been known since 1982, when Havelka *et al* [27] reported unproductive cough developing in 4 of 67 patients (6%) treated with captopril. Estimates from postmarketing survey studies (Figs. 99.5 and 99.6) give prevalence figures of 0.2%, 0.8%, and 1.1% based on spontaneous reports of suspected adverse reactions with captopril and enalapril [28–30]. Inman reported dry cough in 2.9% of patients over a 12-month period in a large prescription-event monitoring survey of enalapril [31]. Yeo and Ramsay also found similar figures for enalapril based on spontaneous reporting [32].

Much higher figures have been reported in double-blind, randomized controlled trials using a standard questionnaire on side effects (Fig. 99.6). The percentage increase in cough over baseline was between 14 and 22%, and was much higher than the 2% or less reported for the comparator drug [4,7,8,32]. The ACE inhibitors were captopril [3,7], cilazapril [8], and enalapril [32]. The proportions of patients with cough were similar after six weeks of treatment compared with six months, which suggests that the symptom does not diminish with time. Angiotensin-converting enzyme inhibitor cough disappears on average 3–6 days after drug withdrawal [28]. Three randomized trials did not include this complaint in the symptom questionnaire and cough was not reported by the physicians [1,5,6]. At the time, these trials were initiated, cough was probably not generally recognized as an ACE inhibitor-related side effect, so the findings emphasize the poor reliability of reporting of side effects by physicians.

Several studies have reported that cough is more common in women than in men [28,32,33], but results showing a higher prevalence in nonsmokers compared with smokers are not consistent [32,33]. Angiotensin-converting enzyme inhibitor cough was shown to be a troublesome side effect in Yeo and Ramsay's study [32]. A high proportion of patients reported the cough as moderate to severe (71%), being present day and night (81%) and disturbing sleep (71%). In 21%, the cough caused vomiting. Sore throat (10% excess) and voice changes (14% excess) were also reported more frequently in patients on enalapril.

One measure of the severity of cough is the number of patients who are withdrawn from treatment because of it. In the controlled studies, this ranged from 1% or less over a period from six weeks to six months [7,8], and up to 6% in an observational study over a three-year period [32]. This latter figure represented 47% of the patients with a cough. Withdrawal rates in trials may not reflect everyday practice since in trials there is more pressure for patients to stay on randomized treatment.

It has been suggested that cough may be more common with enalapril [28]. In the New Zealand intensive-medicines monitoring programme, cough was reported in 1.1% of patients treated with captopril and 2.8% with enalapril [28]. Furthermore, the cough appeared more rapidly with enalapril and took longer to disappear after treatment withdrawal [28]. At present, there is inadequate evidence to confirm these suggestions. The reported incidence of cough has been similar in studies with enalapril [32] and captopril [7,8] but direct comparisons are unreliable due to different methods and treatment durations. Similarly, the higher prevalence figures of cough from postmarketing studies of new ACE inhibitors such as lisinopril (3%) [34] and quinapril (2%), [35] compared with captopril or enalapril (1%) probably reflect increased awareness of this symptom with time rather than real differences in pharmacological effects.

Crossover studies are a useful way to determine whether such differences between ACE inhibitors do exist. McEwen and colleagues tested the possibility of idiosyncratic responses in a small double-blind crossover trial of 20 patients receiving enalapril, ramipril, and placebo in a random order for one week with a one week between-treatment washout period [36]. Three patients who complained of cough did so on both enalapril and ramipril but not on placebo.

The mechanisms responsible for ACE inhibitor cough are not fully understood. Increased sensitivity of the cough reflex has been shown in ACE patients who develop a cough [37,38]. Morice and colleagues found that administration of captopril caused a significant shift in the capsaicin dose–response curve in normal subjects [39], but this result has been questioned. Asthmatics appear to be particularly susceptible to ACE inhibitor-induced cough, but not all asthmatics develop cough on these drugs [37,38]. Increased bronchial reactivity has been reported both in asthmatics [39] and nonasthmatics who developed an ACE inhibitor cough [40]. Lipworth described a case of asthma developing *de novo* during captopril treatment, with persistent bronchial hyperreactivity five months after treatment was stopped [41].

One postulated mechanism for ACE inhibitor cough is an increase in tissue bradykinin [42] because this mediator is degraded by ACE. Fuller and colleagues showed that enalapril enhanced cutaneous responses to bradykinin [43,44] but the response to inhaled bradykinin was not potentiated by ramipril [45]. Tachykinin (substance P) has also been suggested as a candidate peptide for increasing the sensitivity of the cough reflex due to interference with its breakdown by ACE inhibitors. There is also the possibility that both bradykinin and substance P mediate their action through other messengers such as prostaglandins. Sulindac, a cyclo-oxygenase inhibitor, has been shown to reduce the sensitivity of the cough reflex in subjects with ACE inhibitor cough but not in cases of unrelated cough [43]. The difficulty with all these theories is to explain why the ACE inhibitor cough is both sporadic and very variable in its severity.

Yeo and colleagues have suggested that genetic polymorphism may explain the incidence of ACE inhibitor-related cough [46]. The proportion (16%) of the population homozygous for ACE is similar to the incidence of cough. Homozygous individuals appear to have low serum ACE levels and in these, ACE treatment may reduce ACE levels to a critical threshold for activation of the cough reflex.

RASH

Cutaneous rash was one of the most frequently reported side effects in early studies with captopril. The rash was usually a maculopapular eruption on the arms and upper body, often accompanied by pruritus. The highest incidence of rash was in the earliest report where the average daily dose of captopril was 317 mg [47]. Later studies that used lower average daily doses of 46 and 60mg [29,30] reported the incidence of rash to be 1% or less. Moreover, the initial experience with captopril was in patients with severe hypertension who often had renal impairment. There was some indication from these studies that side effects tended to be more common in subjects taking the highest doses (over 150mg daily) and who had the highest serum creatinine levels (more than 136μm/l).

Rashes have also been described with ACE inhibitors other than captopril. Postmarketing surveillance studies in hypertensive patients reported rash (sometimes leading to drug withdrawal) in 0.8% [29], 1% [30], and 6% [47] of patients taking captopril, and in 0.5% [48] and 1.5% [49] taking enalapril. Inman *et al* [31] reported skin events in 3% of patients receiving enalapril, including angioedema (0.2%) and urticaria (0.3%). Jackson and colleagues described 11 patients who developed various side effects on captopril, principally taste disturbance and rash, which resolved in 10 patients when enalapril was substituted [50]. This led the authors to conclude that these side effects were specific to captopril rather than being a class effect.

None of the randomized trials reported a significant excess of rash with ACE inhibitors compared with alternative antihypertensive agents, although an increase with captopril was observed in one study [2]. This suggests that, unlike cough, the incidence of rash is not greater when assessed by patient questionnaire in double-blind randomized trials than by spontaneous reports.

ANGIOEDEMA

Angioedema is the most serious cutaneous response to ACE inhibitors, and has been reported in 0.2% of patients taking enalapril [31], and 0.2% of patients receiving captopril [49]. When angioedema involves the lips, tongue, glottis, larynx or mouth, it may cause obstruction of the upper airway, and deaths have been reported. In a study pooling data from the three very large postmarketing studies on enalapril [51], 39 cases of angioedema were identified out of some 36,000 patients (0.1%). In two-thirds of cases, angioedema developed within the first week of therapy.

Details on a further 138 case reports from the drug manufacturer's worldwide data base showed that the incidence of angioedema was similar in men and women, and could occur whether the ACE inhibitor was prescribed for hypertension or heart failure. Of the cases, 22%, most of which occurred in the first week of therapy, were considered life-threatening. Cases occurring later in treatment were milder and resolved spontaneously on discontinuation of therapy. Fourteen patients who developed angioedema on enalapril had also taken captopril, either before or after enalapril; seven of these experienced urticaria or angioedema while taking each drug, and the other seven while on enalapril but not on captopril. Complementary data on patients who reacted to captopril but not enalapril were not available. These observations led the authors to conclude that angioedema is a reaction to ACE

inhibitors as a group, but it is possible that some individuals may react to a specific agent only. No criteria have been defined for identifying patients who are at particular risk, although there are several case reports of life-threatening angioedema developing with ACE inhibitor treatment in patients with a history of idiopathic angioedema [52].

In cases of angioneurotic edema, the ACE inhibitor should be discontinued. Angioneurotic edema of the face, extremities, lips, tongue, glottis and/or larynx has been reported rarely in patients treated with ACE inhibitors. In such cases, the ACE inhibitor should be discontinued promptly and appropriate monitoring should be instituted to ensure complete resolution of symptoms prior to dismissing the patient. In those instances where swelling has been confined to the face and lips the condition generally resolved without treatment, although antihistamines have been useful in relieving symptoms.

Angioneurotic edema associated with laryngeal edema may be fatal. Where there is involvement of the tongue, glottis or larynx, likely to cause airway obstruction, appropriate therapy such as subcutaneous epinephrine solution 1:1000 (0.3–0.5 ml) should be administered promptly.

Suggested mechanisms of angioedema involve potentiation of the actions of bradykinin which may activate the kallikrein–kinin system in susceptible individuals with a hereditary deficiency of kallikrein inhibitor. This hypothesis, however, is unproven.

More recently, anaphylactoid responses to ACE inhibitors in patients on hemodialysis have been reported [53,54]. These reactions occurred only in ACE-treated patients on high-flux polyacrylonitrile (AN69) dialysis membranes. The proportion of patients affected was high; in one study, 9 out of 14 patients on AN69 dialysis and receiving ACE inhibitors were affected [54]. No similar reactions were observed in patients not on ACE inhibitor treatment.

RAYNAUD'S PHENOMENON

This is an unusual, but apparently genuine, side effect of ACE-inhibitor therapy, and has been reported with both captopril [27] and enalapril [3,55].

TASTE DISTURBANCE

Disturbance or loss of taste sensation was, like rash, commonly reported in the early days of captopril therapy. In more recent postmarketing studies, taste disturbances (sometimes leading to withdrawal of therapy) have been reported in 0.3% and 0.9% of patients on captopril [29,30], and 0.2% on enalapril [31,48]. Using a postal questionnaire sent to patients, Coulter reported no differences in sweet or salty taste on captopril compared with nifedipine, with a trend for more patients on captopril to report metallic taste [56]. Loss of taste was significantly associated with captopril, there being an excess incidence of 6% compared with nifedipine. In 25% of these patients, the symptom disappeared during continued treatment with captopril. In another study, abnormal recognition thresholds for salty, sweet, bitter, and sour tastes were found in patients on captopril compared with hypertensive controls, with the abnormality being most marked in the group treated for over six months [57]. Only one patient, however, complained of taste disturbance.

In one study, women were four times more likely than men to be withdrawn from captopril because of taste disturbance [29]. This gender difference has not been reported by others.

Disturbances of smell have also been reported and may be a factor influencing reports of taste disturbances, since taste is closely linked to smell [58]. Taste disturbance has been postulated to relate to the zinc-binding properties of the sulfhydryl group of captopril, leading to an increased excretion of zinc. The association between zinc and taste disturbances has been shown in other groups of patients with decreased zinc levels such as those on dialysis or after renal transplantation [57].

HYPOTENSION

The early use of captopril in high doses produced hypotensive symptoms (faintness, dizziness) in 5% of patients [47]. Symptoms appeared rapidly, usually with the first dose, and were most frequently observed in patients with volume depletion resulting from diuretic treatment in heart failure and particularly in those with hyponatremia [59,60]. Bradycardia accompanied hypotension in some patients, particularly those in heart failure and receiving cardiac glycosides [60]. The physiological basis was sudden loss of the direct vasoconstrictor effect of high levels of Ang II, with, in particular in cardiac failure, concomitant removal of the octapeptide's sympathotonic and vagal inhibitory actions.

Hypotension was the principal reason for patient withdrawal in the CONSENSUS heart failure trial; seven patients (5.5%) on enalapril withdrew for this reason compared with none taking placebo [1]. Manufacturers now recommend much lower starting doses in patients with heart failure than in those with hypertension, and withdrawal or reduction of diuretic dosage before starting the ACE inhibitor is an important preventive measure.

In a prescription-event monitoring study of patients treated with enalapril (for hypertension or heart failure), hypotension was reported in 1.8% of patients, and syncope and dizziness in 1.2% and 3.9%, respectively [31].

Postmarketing surveillance studies in hypertensive patients reported hypotensive symptoms (sometimes leading to withdrawal of captopril) in 0.8% [29] and 1.6% [30] of patients. Hypotension was reported in 0.3% of patients with enalapril but this increased to 2% when other orthostatic symptoms were included [48]. Hypotension tends to develop 0.5–1.5 hours after the oral administration of captopril and 4–6 hours after the prodrug enalapril, that is, at the time when plasma Ang II values are at their nadir [60].

EFFECTS ON BLOOD AND BIOCHEMICAL VARIABLES

NEUTROPENIA

Initially, neutropenia was considered to be a serious side effect of captopril. Cooper described 63 cases with a white-cell count of $<1,000mm^{-3}$ (1.1%) which were considered to be drug related in a review of 5,632 patients treated with captopril up to mid-1983 [61]. As noted already, very high doses of captopril were used in early studies. Furthermore, most cases of neutropenia occurred in patients with high serum creatinine levels and often with collagen vascular disorders. There was only one case of neutropenia in 4,554 patients with no history of collagen disease and normal serum creatinine levels [61]. Neutropenia was observed within the first three months of therapy, and there were no lasting effects after therapy was discontinued. Thrombocytopenia also occurred in 11 cases.

In postmarketing studies of patients with uncomplicated essential hypertension, reports of neutropenia or low white-cell counts have been infrequent. No cases were reported in 11,710 patients treated with enalapril [48], and only one unconfirmed case was noted in another group of 1,600 patients receiving enalapril [49]. In 3 out of 13,295 patients treated with captopril, total white-cell counts of between 2,000 and $3,500mm^{-3}$ were reported but none was of sufficient severity to warrant classification as neutropenia [30]. Two cases of leukopenia were recorded in prescription-event monitoring of enalapril but were not considered to be drug related [31]. An average fall of 5% in white-cell count from baseline was reported in one trial of hypertensive patients receiving captopril [7]. In another study of captopril in heart failure, there was a tendency for the drug to reduce white-cell count, although the lowest individual count was $4,000 \times 10^{6}/1$ [62].

It has been suggested that the sulfhydryl group in the captopril molecule predisposes to neutropenia. DiBianco concluded, however, that the risk of neutropenia with low doses of captopril in uncomplicated hypertension was low and there was insufficient evidence that, in these patients, the frequency was any different with captopril compared with either enalapril or other nonsulfhydryl-containing ACE inhibitors [59].

NEUROPATHY

A rare, but possibly important association with captopril therapy is neuropathy, which can be associated with high protein values in cerebrospinal fluid (Guillain–Barré syndrome) [63,64]. This has occurred with captopril doses of only 75 mg/day [64].

RENAL ADVERSE EFFECTS

Proteinuria (>1g/day, sometimes with the nephrotic syndrome) has been reported in 0.6–1.7% of patients on captopril, but this reflects initial use of the drug at high-dose levels and in hypertensive patients with vasculitis or renal disease [47,49,59,65]. The frequency varied from 0.2% in patients with no history of renal disease and receiving less than 150mg captopril daily, to 3.5% in patients with renal disease and taking more than 150mg per day of captopril [47]. Since the recommended maximum dose was reduced, reports of heavy proteinuria have been rare. Early reports suggested that the sulfhydryl group in the captopril molecule induced a glomerulonephropathy, but this was not supported in subsequent biopsy studies [59,66]. The Captopril Collaborative Study Group reported that many of the immunological and histological findings previously attributed to captopril occurred also in hypertensive patients who had not received the drug [66].

Enalapril has been reported to induce proteinuria although this has been contested [49]. In fact, for patients with pre-existing glomerular protein loss, the ACE inhibitors as a group may reduce proteinuria [67]. Numerous studies have now demonstrated that albuminuria in diabetes mellitus is reduced by ACE inhibition. The postulated mechanisms include removal of Ang II-mediated constriction of efferent arterioles with a resulting fall in intraglomerular pressure (see *Chapters 75* and *92*).

Acute renal failure has been reported in patients with bilateral renal artery stenosis treated with ACE inhibitors [68,69] and raises concern about the possible risks of ACE inhibitors in patients with occult renovascular disease particularly where measurements of renal function are not performed soon after the introduction of these drugs. Fears that treatment with ACE inhibitors might lead, through various mechanisms, to thrombosis of narrowed renal arteries, appear to have been exaggerated, although opinions are divided on this issue (see *Chapters 88–90*).

Evidence from postmarketing studies regarding the effects of ACE inhibitors on kidneys is confounded by the independent association between the conditions being treated (hypertension and heart failure) and deteriorating renal function. Reports on the incidence of ACE inhibitor-induced renal disease range from none in a manufacturer's study of hypertensive patients over a six-week period [48] to 0.13% in an 18-month study of captopril [29]. Eighty-two cases of renal failure were reported (0.7%) in a prescription-event monitoring study of enalapril [31]. In a detailed examination of 913 deaths in this study, enalapril was considered to have contributed to a decline in renal function and subsequent death in 10 cases [70]. Possible contributory factors were high doses of loop diuretics, fluid loss due to diarrhea or vomiting, concomitant administration of a nonsteroidal anti-inflammatory drug, and hyperkalemia resulting from the use of the ACE inhibitor in combination with a potassium-conserving diuretic or with potassium supplements. Most patients were being treated for heart failure; one was discovered to have bilateral renal artery stenoses at postmortem examination, and four had pre-existing renal disease. The survey suggested that enalapril should be used with great caution in patients whose blood pressure was likely to be highly Ang II dependent. The combination of an ACE inhibitor with amiloride or triamterene is particularly hazardous because a reduction in glomerular filtration, as a result of hypotension, potentiates the action of these drugs that are excreted unchanged in the urine.

The renal function of patients with uncomplicated hypertension appears to be at little risk, since none out of 12,543 such patients who were surveyed died of renal failure while taking enalapril. General advice is that serum creatinine should be measured before starting ACE inhibitors and again after the first few weeks of treatment, but more frequent monitoring is required in patients with severe heart failure.

In advanced renal disease, ACE inhibitors may have beneficial effects although extreme care is needed. These drugs appear to reduce the rate of deterioration in renal function in diabetic patients with proteinuria or other evidence of renal impairment [71] (see *Chapters 75* and *92*).

HYPERKALEMIA

Angiotensin-converting enzyme inhibitors increase serum potassium levels by an average of 0.1–0.2mmol/l in patients with uncomplicated essential hypertension [7,59,65], but severe hyperkalemia is rare in such patients [59]. A major mechanism is the reduction in Ang II-dependent aldosterone secretion. Problems are most likely to occur in azotemic patients and in those receiving concomitant potassium supplements or potassium-sparing diuretics.

EFFECTS ON LIPIDS

Recent interest in the management of risk factors in hypertensive patients has focused attention on lipid profiles of antihypertensive treatments. It has usually been considered that ACE inhibitors have neutral or minor effects on total plasma cholesterol and triglyceride levels [72,73]. Beneficial effects of ACE inhibitors on various lipoprotein fractions have been shown. Captopril was associated with a rise in the apolipoproteins A1 and A2 [74] and HDL-cholesterol [75]. Stronger evidence of the effects on a variety of lipid fractions will be provided by the Treatment of Mild Hypertension Study (TOMHS) [76].

MISCELLANEOUS SIDE EFFECTS

Some studies have reported headache, diarrhea, and lassitude as minor side effects associated with ACE inhibitors as a class [3,31,48,85,86]. Other studies have found no increase from baseline in the reporting of headache [4,6–8] or diarrhea [6–8]. Tiredness or fatigue was significantly reduced with captopril compared with methyldopa or propranolol [2] in one study, while others have reported either no effect [5–7] or a possible adverse effect on fatigue when compared with nifedipine [8]. On balance, we conclude that the evidence for attributing these side effects to ACE inhibitors is not substantial.

DRUG INTERACTIONS

Adverse effects of ACE inhibitors may occur due to potentiation of ACE inhibitor-related effects by other drugs. The most likely of these is hyperkalemia when potassium supplements or potassium-conserving diuretics are given with ACE inhibitors, particularly in patients with renal impairment.

Adverse effects of ACE inhibitors with concomitant use of nonsteroidal anti-inflammatory agents have also been reported. These include attenuation of the hypotensive effect [77] and nephrotoxicity [78]. Seelig et al described three cases of reversible renal failure in 162 patients treated with a combination of nonsteroidal anti-inflammatory drugs and ACE inhibitors and none with either drug used as monotherapy (2,278 on nonsteroidal anti-inflammatory agents and 328 with ACE inhibitors) [78].

Some interactions have so far been reported only for specific ACE inhibitors. Decreased clearance of digoxin has been shown in patients also receiving captopril [79] but this was not found for enalapril [80], possibly as a result in differences in renal metabolism. The mode of elimination of captopril may also be affected by other drugs; probenecid reduced the clearance of captopril probably at the renal tubular level [81]. Beneficial effects of ACE inhibitors may also be attenuated by concomitant administration of other antihypertensive drugs. A significant rise in blood pressure occurred when propranolol was given to captopril-treated patients [82]. This effect did not occur with cardioselective β-blockers such as atenolol which augmented the blood-pressure lowering effect of captopril and enalapril [83,84]. The use of ACE inhibitors in combination with other antihypertensive agents is discussed in detail in *Chapter 91*.

CONCLUSIONS

A historical review of the literature on adverse effects of ACE inhibitors shows an initial period, when captopril was first introduced, associated with a high frequency of side effects such as proteinuria, neutropenia, skin rash, and taste disturbance. Following a reduction in the dosage of captopril, the incidence of these side effects has been much reduced. At the same time, considerable enthusiasm developed for the apparent benefits of ACE inhibitors on quality of life. When enalapril was introduced, there were grounds for believing that it would be free of some of the specific toxic effects associated with high doses of captopril. Enthusiasm for the apparent safety of enalapril was probably a factor in the incautious use of this drug in patients with severe heart failure, which led to considerable anxiety about induction of hypotension and renal failure. Following a sharp lowering of the recommended starting dose, greater experience of enalapril use, and awareness that maintenance doses of diuretics need to be reduced in many cases, these problems too have become much less frequent. Thus, the first two available ACE inhibitors suffered because the initial recommended doses were too high.

The early history of the clinical use of ACE inhibitors reflects the apparently unavoidable pattern of medical experience and opinion concerning the benefits and risks of new drugs. Patients included in clinical trials (and in organized postmarketing surveillance) are often very carefully chosen to exclude those with contra-indications or a high risk of complications. Once the drug is in general use, these precautions are frequently overlooked and clinical situations and drug combinations are tested which had not been foreseen. Manufacturers, for commercial reasons, prefer drugs that can be given once a day in a fixed dose or in a very limited dose range. A dose chosen to suit the average patient is thus likely to prove excessive in a minority.

Detection and reporting of adverse drug reactions have improved but still have many deficiencies, particularly for hitherto unrecognized effects. A persistent, irritant dry cough is now regarded as the most common side effect of treatment with ACE inhibitors, but was not mentioned in some early review articles. The high frequencies of cough were seen in double-blind randomized controlled trials where bias in reporting side effects is reduced (Fig. 99.6).

Our understanding of the nature and importance of the side effects of ACE inhibitors is still incomplete, and in particular there is uncertainty whether or not there are significant differences between ACE inhibitors (see *Chapter 98*). The present state of knowledge indicates that ACE inhibitors do not adversely affect mood or cognition and have few unwanted metabolic effects.

Claims of enhanced mood and memory remain unproven. The most serious adverse effects are hypotension and renal failure, but greater experience, use of lower doses of the ACE inhibitors, and reduction of diuretic doses have minimized serious problems. As many as 15–20% of patients may develop a cough, and less than 1–2% a rash or some alteration of taste. Serious toxic effects such as neutropenia and angioedema probably occur in less than 1 in 10,000 and 1 in 1,000, respectively. Neuropathy is even rarer.

REFERENCES

1. The Consensus Trial Study Group. Effects of enalapril on mortality in severe congestive heart failure. Results of the Cooperative North Scandinavian Enalapril Survival Study (CONSENSUS). *New England Journal of Medicine* 1987;316: 1429–35.

2. Croog SH, Levine S, Testa MA, Brown B, Bulpitt CJ, Jenkins CD, Klerman GL, Williams GH. The effects of antihypertensive therapy on the quality of life. *New England Journal of Medicine* 1986;314:1657–64.

3. Herrick AL, Waller PC, Berkin KE, Pringle SD, Callender JS, Robertson MP, Findlay JG, Murray GD, Reid JL, Lorimer AR, Weir RJ, Carmichael HJ, Robertson JIS, Ball SG, McInnes GT. Comparison of enalapril and atenolol in mild to moderate hypertension. *American Journal of Medicine* 1989;86: 421–6.

4. Fletcher AE, Bulpitt CJ, Hawkins CM, Havinga TK, ten Berge BS, May JF, Schuurman FH, van der Veur E, Wesseling H. Quality of life on antihypertensive therapy: A randomised double blind controlled trial of captopril and atenolol. *Journal of Hypertension* 1990;8:463–6.

5. Steiner SS, Friedhoff AJ, Wilson BL, Wecker JR, Santo JP. Antihypertensive therapy and quality of life: A comparison of atenolol, captopril, enalapril and propranolol. *Journal of Human Hypertension* 1990;4:217–25.

6. Croog SH, Kong W, Levine S, Weir MR, Baume RM, Saunders E. Hypertensive black men and women. Quality of life and effects of antihypertensive medications. *Archives of Internal Medicine* 1990;150:1733–41.

7. Palmer AJ, Fletcher AE, Rudge P, Andrews C, Callaghan TS, Bulpitt CJ. Quality of life in hypertensives treated with atenolol or captopril: A double blind cross over trial. *Hypertension* in press.

8. Fletcher AE, Bulpitt CJ, Chase D, Collins WCJ, Furberg CD, Goggin TK, Hewett AJ, Neiss AM. Quality of life on three antihypertensive treatments: Cilazapril, atenolol, nifedipine. *Hypertension*.

9. Fletcher AE, Bulpitt CJ. Quality of life on ACE inhibitors. A review of recent trials in hypertension. In: Sever P, McGregor G, eds. *Current advances in ACE inhibition*. Edinburgh: Churchill Livingstone, 1991:286–8.

10. Zubenko GS, Nixon RA. Mood-elevating effect of captopril in depressed patients. *American Journal of Psychiatry* 1984;141:110–1.

11. Steine SM, Yang HYT, Costa E. Inhibition of *in situ* metabolism of [^{3}H] (met^5)-enkephalin and potential of (met^5)-enkephalin analgesia by captopril. *Brain Research* 1980;188:110–1.

12. Callender JS, Hodsman GP, Hutcheson MJ, Lever AF, Robertson JIS. Mood changes during captopril therapy for hypertension. A double blind pilot study. *Hypertension* 1983;5 (suppl III):90–3.

13. Vollmer RR, Boccagno JA. Central cardiovascular effects of SQ 14,225, an angiotensin converting enzyme inhibitor in chloralose-anaesthetized cats. *European Journal of Pharmacology* 1977;45:117–25.

14. Mann JFE, Rascher W, Dietz R, Schomig A, Ganten D. Effects of an orally active converting-enzyme inhibitor, SQ 14,225, on pressor responses to angiotensin administered into the brain ventricles of spontaneously hypertensive rats. *Clinical Science* 1979;56:585–9.

15. Evered MD, Robinson MM, Richardson MA. Captopril given intracerebroventricularly, subcutaneously or by gavage inhibits angiotensin converting enzyme inhibition in the brain. *European Journal of Pharmacology* 1980;68:443–9.

16. Johnston CI. Angiotensin coverting enzyme inhibitors: Differences and advantages for first line therapy in hypertension. *Clinical and Experimental Hypertension* 1989;A11 (5&6):1097–115.

17. Costall B, Horovitz ZP, Kelly ME, Naylor RJ, Tomkins DM. Ability of ACE inhibitors to improve basic performance and to antagonise scopolamine impairment in a mouse habituation test. *Psychopharmacology* 1988;96:S11.

18. Nicholson AN, Wright NA, Zetlein MB, Currie D, McDevitt DG. Central effects of the angiotensin converting enzyme inhibitor, captopril. II. Electroencephalogram and body sway. *British Journal of Clinical Pharmacology* 1990;30:537–46.

19. Webb RC, Hamlin MN, Henry JP, Stephens PM, Vander AJ. Captopril, blood pressure and vascular reactivity in psychosocial hypertensive mice. *Hypertension* 1986;8 (suppl I):119–22.

20. Baranowska D, Braszko JJ, Wisniewski K. Effect of angiotensin II and vasopressin on acquisition and extinction of conditioned avoidance in rats. *Psychopharmacology* 1983;81:247–51.

21. Braszko JJ, Wisniewski K. Effect of angiotensin II and saralasin on motor activity and the passive avoidance behaviour of rats. *Peptides* 1988;9:475–9.

22. Currie D, Lewis RV, McDevitt DG, Nicholson AN, Wright NA. Central effects of the angiotensin-converting enzyme inhibitor, captopril. I. Performance and subjective assessments of mood. *British Journal of Clinical Pharmacology* 1990;30:527–36.

23. Olajide O, Lader M. Psychotropic effects of enalapril maleate in normal volunteers. *Psychopharmacology* 1985;86:374–6.

24. Frcka G, Lader M. Psychotropic effects of repeated doses of enalapril, propranolol and atenolol in normal subjects. *British Journal of Clinical Pharmacology* 1988;25:67–73.

25. Lichter I, Richardson PJ, Wyke MA. Differential effects of atenolol and enalapril on memory during treatment for essential hypertension. *British Journal of Clinical Pharmacology* 1986;21:641–5.

26. Croog SH, Levine S, Sudilovsky A, Baume RM, Clive J. Sexual symptoms in hypertensive patients. A clinical trial of antihypertensive medications. *Archives of Internal Medicine* 1988;148:788–94.

27. Havelka J, Vetter H, Studer A, Greminger P, Luschner T, Wollnik S, Siegenthaler W, Vetter W. Acute and chronic effects of the angiotensin-converting enzyme inhibitor captopril in severe hypertension. *American Journal of Cardiology* 1982;49:1467–73.

28. Coulter DM, Edwards IR. Cough associated with captopril and enalapril. *British Medical Journal* 1987;294:1521–3.

29. Chalmers D, Dombey SL, Lawson DH. Post marketing surveillance of captopril (for hypertension): A preliminary report. *British Journal of Clinical Pharmacology* 1987;24:343–9.

30. Schoenberger JA, Testa M, Ross AD, Brennan WK, Bannon JA. Efficacy, safety, and quality of life assessment of captopril antihypertensive therapy in clinical practice. *Archives of Internal Medicine* 1990;**150**:301–6.

31. Inman WHW, Rawson NSB, Wilton LV, Pearce GL, Speirs CJ. Post-marketing surveillance of enalapril I. Results of prescription-event monitoring. *British Medical Journal* 1988;**297**:826–9.

32. Yeo WW, Ramsay LE. Epidemiology of cough with enalapril. *Hypertension* in press.

33. Berkin KE, Ball SG. Cough and angiotensin converting enzyme inhibition. *British Medical Journal* 1988;**296**:1279–80.

34. Cameron HA, Higgins TJC. Clinical experience with lisinopril. Observations on safety and tolerability. *Journal of Human Hypertension* 1989;**3**:177–86.

35. Knapp LE, Frank GJ, McLain R, Rieger MM, Posvar E, Singer R. The safety and tolerability of quinapril. *Journal of Cardiovascular Pharmacology* 1990;**15**:S47–55.

36. McEwen JR, Choudry N, Street R, Fuller RW. Change in cough reflex after treatment with enalapril and ramipril. *British Medical Journal* 1989;**299**:13–16.

37. Fuller RW, Choudry NB. Increased cough reflex associated with angiotensin converting enzyme inhibitor cough. *British Medical Journal* 1987;**295**:1025–6.

38. Bucknall CE, Neilly JB, Carter R, Stevenson RD, Semple PF. Bronchial hyperreactivity in patients who cough after receiving angiotensin converting enzyme inhibitors. *British Medical Journal* 1988;**296**:880–8.

39. Morice AH, Brown MJ, Higenbottam T. Cough associated with angiotensin converting enzyme inhibition. *Journal of Cardiovascular Pharmacology* 1989;**13** (suppl 3):S59–62.

40. Town GI, Hallwright GP, Maling TJB, O'Donnell TV. Angiotensin converting enzyme inhibitors and cough. *New Zealand Medical Journal* 1987;**100**:161–3.

41. Lipworth BJ, McMurray JJ, Clark RA, Struthers AD. Development of persistent late onset asthma following treatment with captopril. *European Respiratory Journal* 1989;**2**:586–8.

42. Semple PF. Bronchial hyperreactivity in patients who cough after receiving angiotensin converting enzyme inhibitors. *British Medical Journal* 1988;**296**: 86–8.

43. Fuller R. Cough associated with angiotensin converting enzyme inhibitors. *Journal of Human Hypertension* 1989;**3**:159–61.

44. Fuller RW, Warren JB, McCusker M, Dollery CT. Effect of enalapril on the skin response to bradykinin in man. *British Journal of Clinical Pharmacology* 1987;**23**:88–90.

45. Dixon CMS, Fuller RW, Barnes PJ. The effect of angiotensin converting enzyme inhibition, ramipril on bronchial responses to inhaled histamine and bradykinin in asthmatic subjects. *British Journal of Pharmacology* 1987;**23**:91–3.

46. Yeo WW, Ramsay LE, Morice AH. ACE inhibitor cough: A genetic link? *Lancet* 1991;**337**:187.

47. Groel JT, Tadros SS, Dreslinski GR, Jenkins AC. Long term antihypertensive therapy with captopril. *Hypertension* 1983;**5** (suppl III):141–51.

48. Cooper WD, Sheldon D, Brown D, Kimber GR, Isitt VL, Currie WJC. Post marketing surveillance of enalapril: Experience in 11,710 patients in general practice. *Journal of the Royal College of General Practitioners* 1987;**37**:346–9.

49. Edwards CRW, Padfield PL. Angiotensin converting enzyme inhibitors: Past, present and bright future. *Lancet* 1985;**i**:30–4.

50. Jackson B, Maher D, Matthews PG, McGrath BP, Johnston CI. Lack of cross sensitivity between captopril and enalapril. *Australian and New Zealand Journal of Medicine* 1988;**18**:21–7.

51. Slater EE, Merrill DD, Guess HA, Roylance PJ, Cooper WD, Inman WHW, Ewan PW. Clinical profile of angioedema associated with angiotensin converting enzyme inhibition. *JAMA* 1988;**260**:967–70.

52. Orfan N, Patterson R, Dykewicz MS. Severe angioedema related to ACE inhibitors in patients with a history of idiopathic angioedema. *JAMA* 1990;**264**:1287–9.

53. Tielemans C, Madhoun P, Lenaers M, Schandene L, Goldman M, Vanherweghem J–L. Anaphyloid reactions during haemodialysis on AN69 membranes in patients receiving ACE inhibitors. *Kidney International* 1990;**38**:982–4.

54. Verresen L, Waer M, Vanrenterghem Y, Michielsen P. Angiotensin-converting enzyme inhibitors and anaphylactoid reactions to high-flux membrane dialysis. *Lancet* 1990;**336**:1360–2.

55. Tillman DM, Malatino LS, Cumming AMM, Hodsman GP, Leckie BJ, Lever AF, Morton JJ, Webb DJ, Robertson JIS. Enalapril in hypertension with renal artery stenosis: Long term follow-up and effects on renal function. *Journal of Hypertension* 1984;**2** (suppl 2):93–100.

56. Coulter DM. Eye pain with nifedipine and disturbance of taste with captopril: A mutually controlled study showing a method of postmarketing surveillance. *British Medical Journal* 1988;**296**:1086–7.

57. Abu-Hamadan DK, Desai H, Sonheimer J, Felicetta J, Mahajan S, McDonald F. Taste acuity and zinc metabolism in captopril treated hypertensive male patients. *American Journal of Hypertension* 1988;**1** (suppl):303–8S.

58. Neil-Dwyer G, Marus A. ACE inhibitors in hypertension: Assessment of taste and smell function in clinical trials. *Journal of Human Hypertension* 1989;**3**: 169–76.

59. DiBianco RD. Adverse reactions with angiotensin converting enzyme inhibitors. *Medical Toxicology* 1986;**1**:122–41.

60. Cleland JGF, Dargie HJ, McAlpine H, Ball SG, Morton JJ, Robertson JIS, Ford I. Severe hypotension after first dose of enalapril in heart failure. *British Medical Journal* 1985;**291**:1309–12.

61. Cooper RA. Captopril associated neutropenia. Who is at risk? *Archives of Internal Medicine* 1983;**143**:659–60.

62. Cleland JGF, Dargie HJ, Hodsman GP, Ball SG, Robertson JIS, Morton JJ, East BW, Robertson I, Murray GD, Gillen G. Captopril in heart failure. A double blind controlled trial. *British Heart Journal* 1984;**52**:530–5.

63. Atkinson AB, Brown JJ, Lever AF, McAreavey D, Robertson JIS, Behan PO, Melville ID, Weir AI. Neurological dysfunction in two patients receiving captopril and cimetidine. *Lancet* 1980;**ii**:36–7.

64. Chakrabarty TK, Ruddell WSJ. Guillain-Barré neuropathy during treatment with captopril. *Postgraduate Medical Journal* 1987;**63**:221–2.

65. Frohlich ED, Cooper RA, Lewis EJ. Review of the overall experience of captopril in hypertension. *Archives of Internal Medicine* 1984;**144**:1441–4.

66. Captopril Collaborative Study Group. Does captopril cause renal damage in hypertensive patients? *Lancet* 1982;**i**:988–90.

67. Raine AEG. ACE inhibition and the kidney: Diagnostic and therapeutic implications. *Journal of Human Hypertension* 1990;**4**:57–62.

68. Hrick DE, Browning PJ, Kopelman R, Goorno WE, Madias NE, Dzau VJ. Captopril induced functional renal insufficiency in patients with bilateral renal artery stenosis or renal artery stenosis in a solitary kidney. *New England Journal of Medicine* 1983;**308**:373–6.

69. Watson MI, Bell GM, Muir AL, Buist TAS, Kellet RJ, Padfield PL. Captopril/diuretic combination in severe renovascular disease: A cautionary note. *Lancet* 1983;**ii**:404.

70. Speirs CJ, Dollery CT, Inman WHW, Rawson NSB, Wilton LV. Postmarketing surveillance of enalapril. II: Investigation of the potential role of enalapril in deaths with renal failure. *British Medical Journal* 1988;**297**:830–2.

71. Williams GH. Converting enzyme inhibitors in the treatment of hypertension. *New England Journal of Medicine* 1988;**319**:1517–25.

72. Edelson JT, Weinstein MC, Tosteson ANA, Williams L, Lee TH, Goldman L. Long term cost effectiveness of various initial monotherapies for mild to moderate hypertension. *JAMA* 1990;**263**:408–13.

73. Agner E. Antihypertensive therapy and blood lipids: Ace inhibitors. *Scandinavian Journal of Clinical and Laboratory Investigation* 1990;**50** (suppl 19): 55–9.

74. Sasaki J, Arakawa K. Effect of captopril on serum lipids, lipoproteins, and apolipoproteins in patients with mild essential hypertension. *Current Therapeutic Research* 1986;**40**:898–902.

75. Salvedt E, Andreassen P, Dahl K, Dyb S. Flogstad R, Hallan H, Moum B, Sandersen S, Sandvei P, Torvik D, Wessel-Aas T, Wideroe TE. An improved serum lipid profile in hypertensives during captopril treatment. *Postgraduate Medical Journal* 1986;**62** (suppl 1):78.

76. Stamler J, Prineas RJ, Neaton JD, Grimm RH, McDonald RH, Schnaper HW, Schoenberger JA, Elmer PJ, Cutler JA. Background and design of the new US trial on diet and drug treatment of 'mild' hypertension (TOMHS). *American Journal of Cardiology* 1987;59:51–60G.

77. Moore JT, Crantz FR, Hollenberg NK, Koletsky RJ, Leboff MS, Swartz SL, Levine L, Podolsky S, Dluhy RG, Williams GH. Contribution of prostaglandins to the antihypertensive action of captopril in essential hypertension. *Hypertension* 1981;3:168–73.

78. Seelig CB, Maloley PA, Campbell JR. Nephrotoxicity associated with concomitant ACE inhibitor and NSAID therapy. *Southern Medical Journal* 1990;83:1144–8.

79. Cleland JFG, Dargie HJ, Pettigrew A, Gillen G, Robertson JIS. The effects of captopril on serum digoxin and urinary urea and digoxin clearances in patients with congestive heart failure. *American Heart Journal* 1986;112:130–5.

80. Douze-Blazy P, Blanc M, Monastruc JL, Conte D, Cotonat J, Galinier F. Is there any interaction between digoxin and enalapril. *British Journal of Clinical Pharmacology* 1986;22:752–3.

81. Singhvi SM, Duchin KL, Willard DA, McKinstry DN, Migdalof BH. Renal handling of captopril: Effect of probenecid. *Clinical Pharmacology and Therapeutics* 1982;32:182–9.

82. MacGregor GA, Markandu N, Banks RA, Bayliss J, Roulston JE, Jones JC. Captopril in essential hypertension; contrasting effects of adding hydrochlorothiazide or propranolol. *British Medical Journal* 1982;284:693–6.

83. Potter JF, Beevers DG. Atenolol improved blood pressure control in patients taking captopril and frusemide. *Journal of Human Hypertension* 1987;1:127–30.

84. Franz IW, Behr V, Ketelhur R. Resting and exercise blood pressure with atenolol, enalapril and a low dose combination. *Journal of Hypertension* 1987;5:537–41.

85. McAreavey D, Robertson JIS. Angiotensin converting enzyme inhibitors and moderate hypertension. *Drugs* 1990;40:326–45.

86. Edwards IR, Coulter DM, Macintosh D. Intestinal effects of captopril. *British Medical Journal* 1992;304:359–60.

100 CONCLUSIONS: THE FUTURE

J IAN S ROBERTSON AND M GARY NICHOLLS

The ambivalent title, be it solecism or otherwise, of this final chapter, is chosen deliberately. We intend herein, Janus-like, to survey briefly how knowledge of the RAS has accumulated, and perceptions have clarified, over the past 100 years, while indulging selfishly in the luxury of speculations on likely, or at least possible, prospective revelations and developments. Such indulgence recognizes nevertheless the uncertainty in making predictions.

Our readers are reminded that we enjoined contributors to take a broad view, indeed wherever appropriate to include an historical perspective, of their various topics. Thus they were not to be limited solely to the most recent developments in their several fields, exciting and important as these often were, but also to place these newer insights in the context of the continuing explication of the subject. There is no doubt that some of our authors found this burdensome; yet others, probably more numerous, found it educational. We hope that our readers will not see it as tiresome.

Misguided or otherwise, such an approach should have revealed and emphasized that the RAS is not an atrophic evolutionary remnant, devoid of physiological function (a view which has nevertheless been propounded in the recent past). This system is not a biologically irrelevant curiosity, capable at most of providing diversion for world-weary pharmacologists. In constrast, the evidence suggests to us that the RAS has undergone repeated diversification, being adapted time and again throughout evolution to mediate different physiological and pathophysiological requirements in a wide range of tissues, organs, and syndromes.

Thus we can rationalize the biochemical complexity of the RAS, to range no more widely than the circulation. We observe, in peripheral plasma, the active enzyme renin, the concentration of which is elaborately regulated. The concentration of its substrate, angiotensinogen, is controlled largely but not completely by independent mechanisms. Concurrently, substantial quantities of inactive prorenin, of still imperfectly defined function, also

circulate. The principal initial product of the reaction of renin with angiotensinogen, the decapeptide Ang I, is inactive; two amino acid residues require to be removed by the action of angiotensin-converting enzyme (ACE) before the active octapeptide, Ang II, is formed. Further truncation forms the heptapeptide Ang III, with generally more muted, but still discernible, physiological actions. There is, moreover, substantial evidence of alternative pathways to those described above for the generation of Ang II and Ang III. Such elegant biochemical complexity speaks for the need, adequately fulfilled, to deliver appropriate but often very different concentrations of the active peptides at several tissues, thus achieving regulated physiological function while minimizing the risks of forming toxic quantities at any given site.

A beautiful example of purposeful physiological evolution in relation to the RAS is seen in cardiac failure. In normal man, the RAS and the atrial natriuretic factor (ANF) system subserve opposing functions: the former to protect, *inter alia*, against saline and volume depletion, the effects of hemorrhage, and hypotension; the latter to prevent or limit salt and fluid overload. Thus in normal physiology there is a consistent inverse correlation between circulating renin (and Ang II) and ANF. This inverse relation is not merely a result of passive responses to opposing forces; increases in circulating ANF within the physiological range reinforce the inverse correlation by inhibiting renin secretion. The supervention of congestive heart failure requires, however, that ANF and renin be recruited together; ANF to limit the tendency to abnormal retention of salt and water, renin to sustain renal function despite the reduction in renal blood flow. The concomitant increase of both ANF and renin is contrived because the inhibitory action of ANF on renin secretion is lost or markedly diminished when renal perfusion is impaired, as it is in cardiac failure. Thus in heart failure, ANF and renin are both secreted in enhanced amounts, and their respective concentrations in peripheral blood are, quite abnormally, positively correlated. Moreover, in these circumstances, their usually antagonistic actions are modified so that the two systems become mutually reinforcing. ANF minimizes, in this disease, some of the unwanted peripheral actions of the RAS, such as stimulation of aldosterone secretion, while enhancing its beneficial renal effects.

Similar evolutionary drives probably account for the existence of the numerous local extracirculatory renin–angiotensin systems, subserving autocrine and paracrine functions which are as yet often ill-defined.

Yet another biological stratagem for enabling one hormone to perform distinct and different functions in different tissues, the possession of various types of receptor with differential affinities and purposes, is clearly available to the RAS. Hitherto, the extent to which these several Ang II receptors have been exploited phylogenetically has been little studied. This is an area in which we can confidently foresee intensive study in the immediate future .

The therapeutic success of agents designed to antagonize the RAS, and especially that of the orally-active ACE inhibitors, has, gratifyingly, greatly exceeded the expectations and forecasts of even a decade ago. Even so, ACE inhibitors, as has been repeatedly emphasized, are not specific for the RAS, and it is possible that some at least of their benefits derive from additional actions, such as the extension of survival of kinins. The more specific inhibitors of renin have been disappointingly slow to achieve satisfactory oral availability and hence have so far made less therapeutic impact than had been predicted. The orally active Ang II antagonists offer great promise, and are very likely to aid illumination of many presently obscure therapeutic aspects in the near future.

Finally requiring comment is that, despite much study and numerous speculations often supported by persistent and spirited advocacy, the role, if any, of renin in human primary (essential) hypertension remains uncertain. The insertion of renin and angiotensinogen genes into the germlines of rats and mice, with the resulting hypertensive transgenic animals, is providing data of compelling interest, despite the relationship of the findings to human essential hypertension being unknown at present. So far, polymorphism of the renin gene in man has not been established as being related to, much less causally connected with, hypertension. These avenues can confidently be expected to be extensively explored in the immediate future.

We shall conclude with a final prediction, that the second century of study of the RAS will be at least as exciting and fruitful as the first. However, unless the advances in the second hundred years are sensationally spectacular and rapid, it is not likely that either of us will be available to learn of the outcome of this forecast.

APPENDIX I: NOMENCLATURE

M GARY NICHOLLS AND J IAN S ROBERTSON

Tigerstedt and Bergman [1] gave the name 'renin' to the pressor material they obtained from the rabbit renal cortex. This name was ready to hand when interest in renin revived in the 1930s, and was subsequently employed when renin was shown to be an enzyme. The peptide product of the enzymic reaction was initially given different names by two of the groups working in the field; they, with a commendable amity unfortunately not always seen in other quarters, agreed on the hybrid term 'angiotensin' [2] (Appendix Ia).

There has subsequently been gratifying consistency in nomenclature despite the increasingly evident complexity of the renin–angiotensin system (RAS). The International Society of Hypertension reported on nomenclature of the RAS in 1979 [3]. That nomenclature was revised and updated by a Joint Nomenclature and Standardization Committee of the International Society of Hypertension, The American Heart Association and the World Health Organization in 1987 [4] (Appendix Ib).

Nomenclature for angiotensin receptors was proposed by a Nomenclature Committee of the Council for High Blood Pressure Research of the American Heart Association in 1991 [5] (Appendix Ic).

The numerous important interrelationships between the RAS and the biologically active atrial peptides (ANF) required that the atrial peptide system also be given standard nomenclature. This was done by the Joint Nomenclature and Standardization Committee of the International Society of Hypertension, the American Heart Association, and the World Health Organization in 1987 [4] (Appendix Id).

In these evidently increasingly complex areas it is to be hoped that this so far excellent harmony in communication and legislation will be maintained.

APPENDIX Ia

'Concurrent discovery has become commonplace, almost as though a mental sputnik regularly circled the earth, distributing with abandon our most exciting thoughts. The vasoactive peptide resulting from the action of renin on an alpha-globulin was thus discovered by two groups of investigators with the result that the peptide received two trivial names, angiotonin and hypertensin. Synthesis of the octapeptide has now brought a degree of certainty about the identity of this peptide and justifies dropping the double nomenclature. We propose the simplified name, *angiotensin*, and its derivatives *angiotensinase* and *angiotensinogen*. *Angiotensin* is a hybrid word but does, we think, have the advantage of being easy to pronounce even with a variety of accents, and it is euphonious and is understandable despite the most recalcitrant microphone.

There will be many who from habit will want no change, but we hope usage will make the heart grow fonder.' [2]

APPENDIX Ib[1]

NOMENCLATURE OF THE RENIN–ANGIOTENSIN SYSTEM

'The committee agreed that the nomenclature will conform with the rules laid down by the Commission on Biochemical Nomenclature of the International Union of Pure and Applied Chemistry (IUPAC) and the International Union of Biochemistry (IUB).

1. Most of the established trivial names, with a few exceptions, have been retained (Table 1).
2. The amino acid sequence of the components of the human renin–angiotensin system is used as reference, and the numbering of peptides follows that of angiotensin I-(1–10) decapeptide.
3. All synthetic angiotensin peptides should be named in conformity with the IUPAC and IUB rules.

---

[1] From a report of the Joint Nomenclature and Standardization Committee of the American Heart Association, and the World Health Organization [4], with permission.

Trivial name	Abbreviations	Systematic name	Comments
Angiotensinogen	Ang-N (pro-Ang I)		Naturally occurring protein renin substrate from which angiotensin I-(1–10) decapeptide is cleaved by hydrolytic action of renin.
	TDP renin substrate	tetradecapeptide renin substrate-(1–14)	1 2 3 4 5 6 7 8 9 10 Asp-Arg-Val-Tyr-Ile-His-Pro-Phe-His-Leu- 11 12 13 14 Leu-Val-Tyr- Ser
	TriDP renin substrate (human)	tridecapeptide renin substrate-(1–13) (human)	1 2 3 4 5 6 7 8 9 10 Asp-Arg-Val-Tyr-Ile-His-Pro-Phe-His-Leu- 11 12 13 Val-Ile- His
			The above sequences serve as references. Substrates of other animal species and other synthetic substrates, substituted analogues or fragments follow the same rules as outlined for angiotensin numbering.
Preangiotensinogen			Primary translational product of Ang-N mRNA, i.e., biosynthetic precursor of Ang-N that contains an N-terminal signal polypeptide (presegment).
N-terminal-extended angiotensinogen	$(aa)_n$–Ang-N		Ang-N with an N-terminal polypeptide extension that may be part of the native presegment.
des-Ang I angiotensinogen			The polypeptide generated from Ang-N after cleavage of Ang I.
Angiotensin I	Ang I Ang-(1–10)	angiotensin-(1–10) decapeptide	The term angiotensin (Ang) is reserved for a group of peptides with amino acid sequence and biological function similar to angiotensin-(1–8) octapeptide. The amino acid sequence of human [Ile⁵]angiotensin-(1–10) decapeptide: 1 2 3 4 5 6 7 8 9 10 Asp-Arg-Val-Tyr-Ile-His-Pro-Phe-His-Leu serves as reference for all angiotensin peptides. If not defined differently, numbers indicate the amino acid of human angiotensin I.
	[Val⁵]Ang I [Val⁵]Ang-(1–10)	[Val⁵]angiotensin-(1–10) decapeptide	e.g., ox ("beef") angiotensin I
Angiotensin II	Ang II Ang-(1–8)	angiotensin-(1–8) octapeptide	e.g., human, rat angiotensin II
	[Val⁵]Ang II [Val⁵]Ang-(1–8)	[Val⁵]angiotensin-(1–8) octapeptide	e.g., ox ("beef"), sheep angiotensin II
Angiotensin III (des-Asp Ang II)	Ang III Ang-(2–8)	angiotensin-(2–8) heptapeptide	e.g., human, rat angiotensin III
	[Val⁵]Ang-(2–8)	[Val⁵]angiotensin-(2–8) heptapeptide	e.g., ox ("beef"), sheep angiotensin III

Table 1 Nomenclature of the renin–angiotensin system.

Trivial name	Abbreviations	Systematic name	Comments
Fragments of angiotensin and analogues	Ang-(4–8)	angiotensin-(4–8) pentapeptide	Sequence defined from human Ang I as: 4 5 6 7 8 Tyr-Ile-His-Pro-Phe
	[Phe^4]Ang-(4–8)	[Phe^4]angiotensin-(4–8) pentapeptide	4 5 6 7 8 Tyr-Ile-His-Pro-Phe
Saralasin	[Sar^1,Val^5,Ala^6]Ang II [Sar^1,Val^5,Ala^5]Ang-(1–8)	[Sar^1,Val^5,Ala^6] angiotensin-(1–8) octapeptide	Angiotensin antagonist; analogous nomenclature for other angiotensin-receptor antagonists.
	[Tyr^{4a}]Ang II [Tyr^{4a}]Ang-(1–8) [endo-Tyr^{4a}]Ang II	[Tyr^{4a}]angiotensin-(1–8) nonapeptide	Insertion of a residue. Amino acid sequence: 1 2 3 4 4a 5 6 7 8 Asp-Arg-Val-Tyr-Tyr-Ile-His-Pro-Phe
Renin–angiotensin system	RAS		
Renin (EC 3.4.23.15)		Ang-N–Ang I hydrolase	An enzyme that cleaves angiotensin-(1–10) decapeptide from angiotensinogen and that has no angiotensinase activity. Renin occurs in the kidney and in extrarenal organs. The major component of the human kidney enzyme serves as renin reference.
Reninlike enzyme	RLE	Ang-N–Ang I hydrolase	An operational term that should be used temporarily for an enzyme that has not been clearly identified. Information concerning the physicochemical characterization and the source of the enzyme are to be indicated.
Prorenin			Primary gene product and biosynthetic precursor (zymogen) of renin.
Preprorenin			Primary translational product of renin mRNA. Precursor of prorenin (pre-zymogen), which contains an N-terminal signal polypeptide.
Inactive renin			Operational term for inactive forms of renin that have not been clearly identified and that can be activated in vitro. This term excludes denatured enzyme. Inactive renin is to be defined by the method of activation, source of material, and physicochemical properties.
Angiotensin converting enzyme (EC 3.4.15.1)	ACE	peptidyl-dipeptide carboxyhydrolase	Converts Ang I into Ang II by cleaving His-Leu from Ang I. The enzyme is not specific for Ang I (e.g., it also cleaves bradykinin and other related peptides). The enzyme should have physiological function.
Angiotensin II forming enzyme		Ang-N–Ang II hydrolase	A group of enzymes capable of cleaving Ang II directly from Ang-N.
Angiotensinase			A group of enzymes capable of degrading Ang I, Ang II, Ang III, and other peptides; the enzymes may be amino-, carboxy-, endo-, or exo-peptidases of various specificities.

Table 1 *Continued.*

4. The source (species, tissue) and the physicochemical characteristics (e.g., isoelectric point, molecular weight) must be specified in the initial description of each component. In the case of measurements of inactive forms of renin, the method of activation (e.g., acid activation) and molecular weight should be indicated (e.g., inactive renin; molecular weight 60,000).

5. Several terms have been deleted from the nomenclature. These include the trivial name *isorenin*.

6. Guidelines for renin and related gene nomenclature will follow that recommended by the international committees concerned with mouse and human genetic analysis. The nomenclature for rat is patterned on guidelines prevailing for mouse.

'For the renin gene, there is general agreement that the structural gene locus be abbreviated *Ren*. In mouse, the genotype designation is *Ren* (in italics) and in human *REN* (in italics). Since in some mice there are two closely linked loci both encoding a protein with the properties of renin, the loci are distinguished as members of a series as follows: *Ren-1, Ren-2*. This situation does not appear to pertain to humans.

'Analysis of renin structural gene sequences in the mouse has indicated that alleles at these loci are evident. The accepted format for designating alleles in the mouse nomenclature is a superscript letter (e.g., *Ren-1*^{a} versus *Ren-1*^{b}). In computer-generated symbols the superscript may be denoted by prefixing an asterisk, as in *Ren-1*a*. In the human system, alleles are designated on the same line as the locus and are set off by an asterisk (e.g. *REN*A*). Conventions for expressing phenotypes also differ between these systems, for example:

	Genotype	Phenotype	Gene product
mouse	*Ren-1*^{a}/*Ren-1*^{b}	REN-1AB	renin-1
	Ren-2^a/*Ren-2*^{b}	REN-2AB	renin-2
human	*REN*A*/*REN*B*	REN A-B	renin

'Nomenclature systems for pseudogenes (artificial insertions — e.g., *Ren* gene transgenics in mice) and restriction fragment length polymorphisms (RFLPs) are also covered in the cited references. Investigators are urged to acquaint themselves with the relevant guidelines and, if at all feasible, to keep their designations in line with the general guidelines already published by these groups. In both mouse and human genetics, locus and allele designations are expected to be supported by genetic tests.'

APPENDIX Ic[2]

NOMENCLATURE FOR ANGIOTENSIN RECEPTORS

'In choosing an abbreviation for the angiotensin receptor, we decided AT (angiotensin) would be more appropriate than Ang (the standard abbreviation for angiotensin peptides) because using the former would avoid confusion with angiotensin II and its fragments, which have varying degrees of biological activity. The subclassification of AT receptors were denoted as subscript 1, 2, 3, and so on [Table 2]. Selective antagonists displaying differences in potency of at least two orders of magnitude were used to subclassify AT receptors as AT_1 and AT_2. The prototypical antagonist of the AT_1 receptor is DuP 753 [losartan]. The prototypical antagonists of the AT_2 receptor are CGP 42112A, PD 123177, and PD 123319. At present we realize that the classification of the AT_2 as a receptor must be tentative until a function or a physiological response can be attributed to this angiotensin II binding site. Additionally, the designation of the ligands CGP 42112A, PD 123177, and PD 123319 as antagonists is tentative since a physiological response has not as yet been attributed to this angiotensin II binding site. If, on the basis of results with selective agonists or antagonists, convincing evidence can be presented for the further subdivision of the AT_1 or AT_2 receptor, we recommend that the subscripts A, B, C, and so on be used (e.g., AT_{1A}). Finally, we recommend that 1) the AT_1 notation replace the previous terminology (e.g., the type 1 angiotensin II receptor, the type B angiotensin II receptor, and the angiotensin II$_\alpha$ receptor), and that 2) the AT_2 notation replace the previous terminology (e.g., the type 2 angiotensin II receptor, the type A angiotensin II receptor, and the angiotensin II$_\beta$ receptor).'

APPENDIX Id[3]

NOMENCLATURE FOR BIOLOGICALLY ACTIVE ATRIAL PEPTIDES

'The committee favored the terms *atrial natriuretic factor* as the trivial name and the abbreviation *ANF*. The committee was unanimous in agreeing that the human form of material be designated *human*, not *h* or *Met*, and that the rat form be designated *rat*, not *r* or *Ile*. It was also agreed that the amino acid position

[2] From a report of the Nomenclature Committee of the Council for High Blood Pressure Research [5].

[3] From a report of the Joint Nomenclature and Standardization Committee of the American Heart Association, and the World Health Organization [4], with permission.

Proposed nomenclature*	AT₁	AT₂
Previous names	AII-1; AII-B; AII$_\alpha$	AII-2; AII-A; AII$_\beta$
Potency order	Angiotensin II > angiotensin III	Angiotensin II = angiotensin III
Selective antagonists†	DuP 753 [losartan]	PD 123177; PD 123319; CGP 42112A
Effector pathways	IP₃/DG	—
	cAMP ↓	

Endogenous ligands: Angiotensin II, angiotensin III. Other fragments of angiotensin II may show selectivity among receptor subtypes.

Other receptor/binding sites: A soluble angiotensin binding protein, isolated from the liver and other tissues, displays a high affinity for CGP 42112A but not PD 123319 or DuP 753; this binding protein may represent a subtype of the AT₂ receptor.

* If angiotensin receptor subtypes can be further subdivided based on selective agonists or antagonists, we propose that AT₁ and AT₂ be subdivided as follows: AT$_{1A}$, AT$_{1B}$, AT$_{2A}$, AT$_{2B}$, and so on.

† Chemical names: DuP 753: 2-n-butyl-4-chloro-5-(hydroxymethyl)-1-[[2'-(1H-tetrazol-5-yl)biphenyl-4-yl]methyl]imidazole;

PD 123177: 1-[[(4-amino-3-methylphenyl) methyl]-5-diphenylacetyl)-4,5,6,7-tetrahydro-1H-imidazol[4,5-c]pyridine-6-carboxylic acid;

PD 123319: (S)-1-[[4-(di-methylamino)-3-methylphenyl]methyl]-5-(diphenylacetyl)-4,5,6,7-tetrahydro-1H-imidazo[4,5-c]pyridine-6-carboxylic acid;

CGP 42112A: nicotinyl-Tyr-(N$^\alpha$-benzyloxycarbonyl-Arg)Lys-His-Pro-Ile-OH.

Table 2 Angiotensin Receptors.

should be numbered from the N-terminus (not the C-terminus) after having excluded the signal peptide or leader sequence. In accordance with the view of the committee, material previously known as αhANF will now be referred to as *human atrial natriuretic factor-(99–126)* and abbreviated *human ANF-(99–126)*.

'Any synthetic peptides will be named according to the above designation and in conformity with the IUB and IUPAC rules. For example, the substitution of tyrosine at position 126 by phenylalanine will be designated *human [Phe^{126}] ANF-(99–126)*. Human pre-ANF-(1–126) represents the primary translational product from messenger RNA and is the biosynthetic precursor of human ANF-(1–126) with an N-terminal signal polypeptide. The trivial name for human pre-ANF-(1–126) is *human prepro-ANF*. Human ANF-(1–126) has been shown to be the major storage form in the atrial granules and is the precursor of the circulating form. The trivial name for human ANF-(1–126) is *human pro-ANF*.

'Evidence suggests that the predominant circulating form of rat ANF and human ANF is the 28 amino acid peptide derived from the C-terminus (i.e., 99–126). However, the committee feels that it would be inappropriate to report plasma ANF when measured by radioimmunoassay after extraction as human ANF-(99–126). The committee recommends that ANF so reported be designated as *immunoreactive human* ANF and that the method of extraction or separation be specified. When a direct radioimmunoassay is performed on plasma without prior extraction, the result should be reported as *immunoreactive ANF* and the absence of plasma extraction should be clearly stated.'

REFERENCES

1. Tigerstedt R, Bergman PG. Niere und Kreislauf. *Skandinavisches Archiv für Physiologie* 1898;8:223–71.
2. Braun-Menendez E, Page IH. Suggested revision of nomenclature: Angiotensin. *Science* 1958;127:242.
3. Nomenclature Committee of the International Society of Hypertension. Nomenclature of the renin–angiotensin system: Report. *Hypertension* 1979;1:654–6.
4. Joint Nomenclature and Standardization Committee of the International Society of Hypertension, the American Heart Association, and the World Health Organization: Special report. *Hypertension* 1987;10:461–4.
5. Nomenclature Committee of the Council for High Blood Pressure Research, American Heart Association: A report. Nomenclature for angiotensin receptors. *Hypertension* 1991;17:720–1.

APPENDIX II. STANDARDIZATION AND STANDARDS

J IAN S ROBERTSON AND M GARY NICHOLLS

Standardization has been over the years, and remains, one of the less commendable aspects of the RAS. Such will be apparent from a careful reading of Dr Stephen Poole's restrained, but slightly sad, *Chapter 17*.

The deficiencies, the reasons for them, and the then urgent requirements, were set out with grim clarity by Sir George Pickering at a major international meeting in 1963 [1] (Appendix IIa). This was when the first reliable and quantitative assays for renin and Ang II in plasma were appearing. Pickering accepted that much of the blame for deficiencies in renin standardization up to that time attached to him. Nearly all the leading authorities on the RAS attended that meeting, and there can be no doubt that the issues were presented with lucidity and force.

The problems were further exposed by the results of an international collaborative study of renin assay in 1975 [2]. An International Reference Preparation of human renin, together with Research Standard preparations for Ang I and Ang II, was then made available [2] (Appendices IIb, IIc, IId). The proposed adoption of a new International Renin Standard, and new Research Preparations of Ang I and Ang II, are described in *Chapter 17*.

Nevertheless, many working in this field still pursue what Pickering castigated three decades ago as the 'hillbilly' method of assay standardization [1]. It is impossible for the two of us, who have spent the last few months editing chapters for this book, not to have been vividly reminded that, as Pickering complained so long ago, 'Many workers do not even use a standard. You cannot compare results from day to day, from one laboratory to another, from country to country' [1] (see Appendix IIa). These same strictures still apply, although we have gathered here contributions from the world's leading authorities. Whether the deficiencies stem from ignorance, fear, laziness, simple cussedness, or all four, is uncertain. One or more must apply, however unlikely and however improbable it would have seemed if predicted in 1963 [1]. What is certain is that study of the RAS has been immensely retarded by these failings, that our knowledge consequently lags behind that in otherwise comparable disciplines, and that a vast quantity of hard work has been squandered and potential knowledge lost.

The question of standardization of an atrial natriuretic factor (ANF) assay was recognized and acted upon much earlier in the history of that hormonal system. An international collaborative assay study was conducted and reported upon in 1988 [3], and an International Standard Preparation of Human ANF was established and made available to all (Appendix IIe). It is to be hoped that the sorry story of the inadequacies of renin standardization will not be repeated for ANF.

APPENDIX IIa[1]

'In the last 25 years, we have made rather heavy weather, I think, of the renin–angiotensin problem. I think we have made heavy weather for some reasons which are inherent. These are difficult substances to deal with chemically, particularly renin. But two of the difficulties are of our own making and I would like to go into them further.

'The first is the insufficient characterization of vasoactive substances. It is not right to assume that because you have a substance that raises blood pressure it is renin or angiotensin.

'The second difficulty is biological assay. I would thus like to remind you that assay is measurement. All measurements are comparisons, and in the modern scientific world the standard with which an unknown is measured is something which is quite well defined and which is constant. You will remember that in the English-speaking world the unit of measurement is the yard — the length of a man's arm. As we became more civilized, this was replaced by the standard yard, which was kept at Winchester, because the length of man's arm differed. In biological assay the standard is as pure as possible a preparation of the substance to be assayed. The standard preparation must be stable. The first step in assay is to find the dose of the unknown that gives the same response as a given dose of standard, and secondly, this dose is then given between smaller and larger doses of standard simply to confirm that it lies between those two.

[1] From Pickering GW [1], with permission.

A.7

'This is the standard method of biological assay. Another method is the hillbilly method. You take the unknown in one hand and put stones in a bucket in the other hand until the bucket feels the same weight as the unknown. Then you guess the weight of the stones. Sometimes the methods used to assay renin and angiotensin seem to me to be very much like the hillbilly method. Even today we have no agreed unit for the assay of renin. Many workers do not even use a standard. You cannot compare results from day to day, from one laboratory to another, from country to country.

'Whether or not we shall get some sort of international standard for renin we do not know. On looking back, I am clear as to who is to blame for the failure to get an international standard for renin, and that is myself. In 1938, Prinzmetal and I described a method of assay for renin, [and] compared responses of the unknown with standard alcohol-dried rabbit kidney. This standard was stable over a period of at least six years. This standard should have been made available to other workers in the field. It was not, because rabbit kidneys were difficult to get hold of, and I thought that the answer would come quickly; then the war happened. But the real reason was a personality defect in Pickering.' [1]

APPENDIX IIb[2]

THE INTERNATIONAL REFERENCE PREPARATION OF HUMAN RENIN
(established 1974)
'A batch of 2000 ampoules coded 68/356.

Content
'Each ampoule contains: freeze-dried residue of extract of human kidneys (exact quantity unknown but not more than 0.272mg); lactose, 5mg; dried residue from 1ml of 0.1mol/l phosphate buffer; nitrogen gas at slightly less than atmospheric pressure.'

Use
'For practical purposes each ampoule contains the same quantity (±1%) of the above materials.

'The solid contents of each ampoule should be completely dissolved in a known volume of distilled water; no attempt should be made to weigh out portions of the freeze-dried plug in which the renin may not be homogeneously distributed.

'All subsequent dilutions should be made with a solution of buffer containing not less than 0.5mg/ml of a suitable inert carrier protein (such as albumin free from peptidase activity) to prevent loss due to adsorption to surfaces. For economy of use the solution may be subdivided into small containers, frozen rapidly to a low temperature (e.g. –80°C) and stored preferably at below –30°C.

'Although this material was sterilized by membrane filtration, it contains no bacteriostat and should not be assumed to be sterile.'

Biological activity
'By definition each ampoule contains 0.1 international unit. No angiotensinase could be detected on incubation with angiotensin I or II *in vitro*.'

Stability
'Results of accelerated degradation studies show that the biological activity in the unopened ampoule is stable under the conditions recommended for storage (below –20°C in the dark). The Renin Standard showed no evidence of acid activation after dialysis at pH 3.0 for 24h at 4°C in human plasma.'

Distribution into ampoules
'The bulk material consisted of 1.3115g of an extract of human kidneys (batch 181) made by the eight-step procedure of Haas, Goldblatt & Gipson (1965) [7], and generously provided by Dr E. Haas and Dr H. Goldblatt.

'In June 1968 1.155g of the material (moisture content unstated) was dissolved without further drying in 4.25 l of solvent at 4°C. The solvent consisted of 0.5% lactose in 0.1mol/l sodium phosphate buffer, pH 7.0 (a mixture of Na_2HPO_4 and NaH_2PO_4 dissolved in double glass-distilled water). The solution of renin was filtered at 4°C through a Millipore membrane (HA grade; average pore size 0.45μm), and then equal amounts of the solution were distributed as one batch into some 4050 neutral glass ampoules. (The mean content of seventy-one individually weighed ampoules was 1.014g±0.99%.)

'The solution was kept at +4°C until completion of the fill, and was then freeze-dried.

'The ampoules were then fitted with plastic capillary plugs and dried to constant weight by secondary desiccation over P_2O_5 at 0.02 Torr, when they were filled with pure dry nitrogen and sealed by glass fusion. After testing for leaks the ampoules have been stored at –20°C in the dark.'

'The Draft Final Report of the International Collaborative study of Renin Assay was considered by the 26th meeting of the

[2] From Bangham *et al* [2], with permission.

Laboratory no.	No. of house units found to be equivalent to one unit of Standard Renin 68/356	To convert approximately from house units/litre into micro-units of Standard Renin/ml multiply by	Reference
2 ("Skinner" unit)	10^5	0.010	4
3 ("Glasgow" unit)	200	5.26	5
4	180		
6 ("Goldblatt" unit)	1.0	1000	6–8
8	0.98		

Table 1 Relation of various house units of renin to the unit defined by the Renin Standard.

Expert Committee on Biological Standardization, World Health Organization, Geneva, in December 1974 (W.H.O. Technical Report Series no. 565: 26th Report of Expert Committee on Biological Standardization, 1975). The Renin Standard 68/356 employed in this study was established as the International Reference Preparation of Human Renin. The Committee defined the International Unit for Human Renin as the activity contained in 188.7mg of the International Reference Preparation; this value is equivalent to the 0.1 unit per ampoule agreed upon by the participants, thus ensuring continuity of the unit defined by the Renin Standard 68/356.'

APPENDIX IIc[3]

RESEARCH STANDARD A FOR ANGIOTENSIN I (ASP[1], ILEU[5]) (CODED 71/328)

'A batch of ampoules containing synthetic angiotensin I for use as a research standard for the bioassay or radioimmunoassay of angiotensin I (Asp[1], Ileu[5]).'

Content

'Each ampoule contains: angiotensin I (Asp[1], Ileu[5]; synthetic), nominal 9µg; mannitol, 2mg; trace of acetic acid; nitrogen gas at slightly less than atmospheric pressure.'

Use

'For practical purposes each ampoule contains the same quantity ± 1% of the above materials.

'The solid contents of each ampoule should be completely dissolved in a known volume of distilled water, saline or buffer of pH 4 or below, and no attempt should be made to weigh out portions of the freeze-dried plug, which may not be homogeneous.'

'For economy of use the contents of the ampoule may be dissolved in 0.5ml of solvent or less (to maintain an acceptable peptide concentration and thus minimize loss by surface adsorption), subdivided into small aliquots and stored at −20°C or below the eutectic of the solvent used. It is advised that further dilutions should be made in a diluent containing suitable protein such as heat-inactivated albumin to avoid surface-adsorption losses.'

'Although the material was sterilized by membrane filtration it contains no bacteriostat and should not be assumed to be sterile.'

Bulk material

'Source: synthetic angiotensin I (Asp[1], Ileu[5]) free acid was prepared by solid-phase synthesis (Oparil, Tregear, Koerner, Barnes & Haber, 1971 [9]) and provided by Professor E. Haber, Boston. A ninhydrin-positive peptide impurity (about 5%) was detected after: (a) thin-layer chromatography on cellulose with butanol–acetic acid–water (60:15:25), R_F main component 0.75, impurity 0.82; (b) two-dimensional separation on thin layer cellulose, employing electrophoresis at pH 1.9 in the first dimension and chromatography with the solvent system described in (a) in the second dimension; (c) column chromatography of the mono-iodinated peptide on DEAE-Sephadex, when a "shoulder" was observed in the elution profile of the peptide. No other iodinated peak was observed. This impurity has not been identified.'

Distribution into ampoules

'In 1972, 23.45mg of the material (peptide content 85 ± 5%) was dissolved without further drying in 268ml of 1.0% mannitol in double glass-distilled water, pH 4.

[3] From Bangham *et al* [2], with permission.

'The solution was passed through a Millipore filter membrane (mean pore size 0.45μm) and distributed at 4°C in 0.2ml aliquots into 1220 ampoules. These were frozen in liquid nitrogen and freeze-dried. The ampoules were then fitted with plastic capillary plugs and dried to constant weight by secondary desiccation over P_2O_5 at 0.02 Torr; they were then filled with pure dry nitrogen and sealed by glass fusion. After testing for leaks the ampoules have been stored at $-20°C$ in the dark.

'The peptide content of each ampoule was estimated to be 9.0μg, based on the recovery of valine as determined by amino acid analysis after hydrolysis of the contents of six ampoules. Data obtained so far indicate that biological activity did not change on storage at $-20°C$.

APPENDIX IId[4]

RESEARCH STANDARD A FOR ANGIOTENSIN II (ASP[1], ILEU[5]) (CODED 70/302)

'A batch of ampoules containing synthetic angiotensin II for use as a research standard for the bioassay or radioimmunoassay of angiotensin II (Asp[1], Ileu[5]).

Content

'Each ampoule contains: angiotensin II (Asp[1], Ileu[5]; synthetic), nominal 25.0μg: mannitol, 2mg; trace of acetic acid; nitrogen gas at slightly less than atmospheric pressure.'

Use

'Details for use are the same as those given in the preceding section for angiotensin I.'

Bulk material

'Source: synthetic angiotensin II (Asp[1], Ileu[5]) free acid was supplied by Miles Laboratories, Indiana, as 25mg of batch no. 69620. Amino acid analysis was consistent with a homogeneous peptide and it gave a single spot on paper electrophoresis when stained with ninhydrin, Pauli and Sakaguchi reagents. Under conditions which would separate the β-isomer, only one spot reacting with ninhydrin was observed after paper electrophoresis at pH 2.4.'

Distribution into ampoules

'In 1971, 24.5mg of the material was dissolved in 398ml of 0.5% mannitol in double glass-distilled water, pH 4.2.

'The solution was filtered through a Millipore HA filter membrane (mean pore size 0.45μm) and distributed at 4°C in 0.4ml aliquots into 946 ampoules. These were frozen in liquid nitrogen and freeze-dried. The ampoules were then fitted with plastic capillary plugs and dried to constant weight by secondary desiccation over P_2O_5 at 0.02 Torr; they were then filled with pure dry nitrogen and sealed by glass fusion. After testing for leaks the ampoules have been stored at $-20°C$ in the dark.

'The peptide content of each ampoule was found to be 24.3μg based on isoleucine determination by amino acid analysis after hydrolysis of the contents of two groups of six ampoules'.

APPENDIX IIe

INTERNATIONAL REFERENCE PREPARATION OF HUMAN ANF (ESTABLISHED 1987)

'At its 37th meeting in Geneva in December 1987, the Expert Committee on Biological Standardization of the World Health Organization established preparation 85/669 as the international standard for human ANF-(99–126) with a unitage of 2.5 international units per ampoule. The standard may be obtained by writing to the Director, National Institute for Biological Standards and Control, Blanche Lane, South Mimms, Potters Bar, Hertfordshire, EN6 3QG, UK. A small handling fee will be charged.' [3].

REFERENCES

1. Pickering GW. Concluding remarks, International Symposium on Angiotensin, Sodium and Hypertension, Quebec, Canada, October 11–14, 1963. *Canadian Medical Association Journal* 1964;90:340–1.

2. Bangham DR, Robertson I, Robertson JIS, Robinson CJ, Tree M. An international collaborative study of renin assay: Establishment of the international reference preparation of human renin. *Clinical Science and Molecular Medicine* 1975;48 (suppl):135–59.

3. Poole S, Gaines Das R, Dzau VJ, Richards AM, Robertson JIS. The international standard for atrial natriuretic factor: Calibration by an international collaborative study. *Hypertension* 1988;12:629–34.

4. Skinner SL. Improved assay methods for renin concentration and activity in human plasma. *Circulation Research* 1967;20:391–402.

5. Brown JJ, Davies DL, Lever AF, Robertson JIS, Tree M. Estimation of renin in human plasma. *Biochemical Journal* 1964;93:594–600.

6. Haas E, Goldblatt H. Indirect assay of plasma-renin. *Lancet* 1972;i:1330–2.

7. Haas E, Goldblatt H, Gipson EC. Extraction, purification and acetylation of human renin. *Archives of Biochemistry and Biophysics* 1965;110:534–43.

8. Haas E, Gould AB, Goldblatt H. Estimation of endogenous renin in human blood. *Lancet* 1968;i:657–60.

9. Oparil S, Tregear GW, Koerner T, Barnes BA, Haber E. Mechanism of pulmonary conversion of angiotensin I to angiotensin II in the dog. *Circulation Research* 1971;29:682–90.

---

[4] From Bangham *et al* [2], with permission.

INDEX

INDEX

102. Winocour PH, Waldek S, Anderson DC. Converting enzyme inhibition and kidney function in normotensive diabetic patients with persistent microalbuminuria. *British Medical Journal* 1987;**295**:391.

103. Rudberg S, Aperia A, Freyschuss U. Persson B. Enalapril reduces microalbuminuria in young normotensive type 1 (insulin-dependent) diabetic patients irrespective of its hypotensive effect. *Diabetologia* 1990;**33**:470–6.

104. Holdaas H, Hartmann A, Lien MG, Nilsen L, Jervell J, Fauchald P, Endresen L, Djoseland O, Berg KJ. Contrasting effects of lisinopril and nifedipine on albuminuria and tubular transport functions in insulin dependent diabetics with nephropathy. *Journal of Internal Medicine* 1991;**229**:163–70.

105. Corcoran JS, Perkins JE, Hoffbrand BI, Yudkin JS. Treating hypertension in non-insulin-dependent diabetes: A comparison of atenolol, nifedipine, and captopril combined with bendrofluazide. *Diabetic Medicine* 1987;**4**:167–8.

106. Hollander E. Effect of antihypertensive (captopril) treatment on proteinuria in diabetic nephropathy. *Therapia Hungarica* 1988;**36**:191–5.

107. Hommel E, Parving H–H, Mathiesen E, Adsberg B, Nielsen MD, Giese J. Effect of captopril on kidney function in insulin-dependent diabetic patients with nephropathy. *British Medical Journal* 1986;**293**:467–70.

108. Parving H–H, Hommel E, Edsberg B, Mathiesen E, Nielsen MD, Giese J. The effect of captopril on glomerular filtration rate and albuminuria in insulin-dependent diabetic patients with nephropathy. *Postgraduate Medical Journal* 1986;**62** (suppl 1):65.

109. Kisch ES. Captopril and proteinuria in diabetes mellitus. *Israeli Journal of Medical Sciences* 1987;**23**:833–4.

110. Romero R, Sanmarti A, Salina I, Texidó J, Foz M, Caralps A. Utilidad de los inhibidores de la enzima conversiva de la angiotensina en el tratamiento de la nefropatía diabética. *Medicina Clinica* 1988;**90**:494–6.

111. Stornello M, Valvo EV, Puglia N, Scapellato L. Angiotensin converting enzyme inhibition with a low dose of enalapril in normotensive diabetics with persistent proteinuria. *Journal of Hypertension* 1988;**6** (suppl 4):S464–6.

112. Stornello M, Valvo EV, Vasques E, Leone S, Scapellato L. Systemic and renal effects of chronic angiotensin converting enzyme inhibition with captopril in hypertensive diabetic patients. *Journal of Hypertension* 1989;**7** (suppl 7):S65–7.

113. Weidmann P, Beretta–Piccoli C, Keusche G, Gluck Z, Mujagic M, Grimm M, Meier A, Ziegler WH. Sodium-volume factor, cardiovascular reactivity and hypotensive mechanism of diuretic therapy in mild hypertension associated with diabetes mellitus. *American Journal of Medicine* 1979;**67**:779–84.

114. Gans RO, Bilo HJG, Maarschalkerweerd WWA v, Heine RJ, Nauta JJP, Donker AJM. Exogenous insulin augments in healthy volunteers the cardiovascular reactivity of noradrenaline but not to angiotensin II. *Journal of Clinical Investigation* 1991;**88**:512–8.

115. Tuttle KR, Bruton JL, Perusek MC, Lancaster JL, Kopp DT, DeFronzo RA. Effect of strict glycemic control on renal hemodynamic response to amino acids and renal enlargement in insulin-dependent diabetes mellitus. *New England Journal of Medicine* 1991;**324**:1626–32.

116. Myers BD, Nelson RG, Williams GW, Bennett PH, Hardy SA, Berg RL, Loon N, Knowler WC, Mitch WE. Glomerular function in Pima Indians with noninsulin-dependent diabetes mellitus of recent onset. *Journal of Clinical Investigation* 1991;**88**:524–30.

117. Mathiesen ER, Hommel E, Giese J, Parving H–H. Efficacy of captopril in postponing nephropathy in normotensive insulin dependent diabetic patients with microalbuminuria. *British Medical Journal* 1991;**303**:81–7.

93
ANGIOTENSIN-CONVERTING ENZYME INHIBITORS IN THE TREATMENT OF HEART FAILURE

IAN G CROZIER, HAMID IKRAM, AND
M GARY NICHOLLS

INTRODUCTION

Heart failure is a complex pathophysiological condition resulting from impaired cardiac function that may be due either to a defect in myocardial contractility or to an excessive hemodynamic burden. Clinical features develop as a consequence of reduced cardiac output, increased filling pressures, disturbances in the balance of electrolytes and water, activation of neurohormonal systems, metabolic abnormalities within many tissues and organs, and side effects of medications. Of the neurohormonal systems, the RAS plays an important pathophysiological role which is discussed in *Chapter 76*.

Until recently, treatment for heart failure focused on augmentation of myocardial contractility and correction of fluid and electrolyte imbalance (Fig. 93.1). Digoxin, however, is the only orally effective inotrope that is so far widely available. Diuretics reduce congestive symptoms and remain a mainstay of therapy, but they do not correct the functional cardiac abnormality. Indeed, by lowering ventricular filling pressures, they can reduce cardiac output [1] (Fig. 93.1); they increase activity of the RAS [1] and the sympathetic system; and they reduce plasma and tissue

potassium [2] and magnesium levels and perhaps thereby predispose to ventricular arrhythmias [193].

Attempts have been made to relieve the burden of the failing heart by the use of vasodilator drugs (Fig. 93.1). Whereas this approach is often successful under emergency conditions and in the short term, most drugs suffer from the development of 'tachyphylaxis' due, in part, to further activation of the RAS and the sympathetic system, and to fluid retention [3–7].

Following the demonstration that a competitive inhibitor of Ang II or an ACE inhibitor reduced arterial pressure, aldosterone secretion, and sodium retention in animals with heart failure [8,9], the role of these agents was examined in patients with cardiac failure. In 1977, Gavras *et al* reported that the Ang II antagonist, saralasin, increased cardiac output and decreased peripheral resistance in a patient with high plasma renin activity and severe heart failure due to renovascular hypertension [10]. One year later, it was demonstrated that an intravenous ACE inhibitor reduced systemic vascular resistance and left ventricular filling pressures while increasing cardiac output in patients with heart failure [11,12] (Fig. 93.2). Captopril, the first of the orally active ACE inhibitors, was reported to have similar effects in 1979 [13]. It soon became clear that ACE inhibitors had sustained beneficial effects [13–19], and their subsequent widespread use has revolutionized the treatment of cardiac failure.

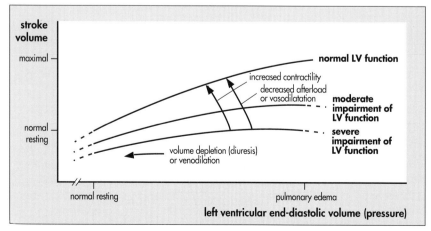

Fig. 93.1 Relationships between left ventricular (LV) end-diastolic volume (and pressure) and stroke volume, and the effects of different treatment modalities.